ANABOLICS 2005

by William Llewellyn

DISCLAIMER: This information was gathered from sources including textbooks, medical journals, and pharmaceutical reports, as well as interviews with athletes, steroid dealers, and medical experts. Neither the author nor publisher assumes any liability for the information presented in this text. This book is not intended to provide medical advice. The purpose of this reference book is only to provide a compendium of information for the reader, for entertainment purposes only. None of the information in this book is meant to be applied. Readers are advised that many of the substances described in this reference book may be prohibited or used only under a physician's care in many jurisdictions. Readers should consult with appropriate medical authorities before using any drug, and the proper legal authorities if unsure of the status of substances described herein. The author does not advocate readers engage in any illegal activities.

Published by:
Body of Science
5500 Military Trail, Ste. 22-318
Jupiter, FL 33458
888-655-5536
www.anabolicsbook.com

Contributing Researchers/Photographers
Ronny Tober
Marko Lalic
Patrik Iden
Dr. Alberto Gomez
Flanker
J. Berthelette
Steven Thomas (whitewolve41)
Big Bear 25
And a special thanks you to my many readers who sent in empty packaging samples

TABLE OF CONTENTS

Forward	6		

PART I: ANABOLIC OVERVIEW

An Introduction To Testosterone	10		
Direct and Indirect Anabolic Effects	12		
Free vs. Bound Testosterone	14		
Estrogen Aromatization	15		
DHT Conversion	17		
A Brief History of Anabolic/Androgenic Steroids	19		
Synthetic AAS Development	20		
Synthetic AAS Chemistry	25		
Steroid Nomenclature	30		
Side Effects	31		
Steroid Safety: Studies with Real-World Dosages	40		

PART II: PRACTICAL APPLICATION

Steroid Cycles	44		
Sample Steroid Stacks	47		UPDATED
Giving the Injection	56		
Steroid Lab Test Results	58		UPDATED
Paper Steroids	65		
Underground Manufacturers	66		UPDATED
Counterfeit Steroids	67		
Country Specifics	70		UPDATED
Security Stickers	73		**NEW
Designer Steroids	75		UPDATED
Anabolic Steroids and the Law	77		**NEW

PART III: DRUG PROFILES

ANABOLIC/ANDROGENIC STEROIDS

1-Testosterone (dihydroboldenone)	84		UPDATED
Anabolic DN® (nandrolone cypionate)	86	E1	
Anabolic NA® (nandrolone/methandriol blend)	88		
Anabolicum Vister® (quinbolone)	89		
Anadrol® (oxymetholone)	90	E1	UPDATED
Anadur® (nandrolone hexyloxyphenylpropionate)	94		
Anatrofin (stenbolone acetate)	95		**NEW
Anavar (oxandrolone)	96	E6	UPDATED
Andractim® (dihydrotestosterone)	99		
Andriol® (testosterone undecanoate)	100	E9	UPDATED
Androderm® (testosterone)	103	E10	
Androgel® (testosterone)	104	E10	
Cheque Drops® (mibolerone)	106		
Danocrine® (danazol)	108		

Deca-Durabolin® (nandrolone decanoate)	109	E11	UPDATED
Deposterona® (testosterone blend)	113	E21	
Dianabol® (methandrostenolone)	114	E21	UPDATED
Dinandrol (nandrolone blend)	119	E29	
Drive® (boldenone undecylenate/methylandrostenediol dipropionate)	120	E30	
Durabolin® (nandrolone phenylpropionate)	121	E30	UPDATED
Dynabolon® (nandrolone undecanoate)	123	E31	
Equilon 100 (boldenone blend)	125		
Equipoise® (boldenone undecylenate)	126	E31	UPDATED
Equitest 200 (testosterone blend)	129		
Esiclene® (formebolone)	130		
Genabol (norbolethone)	131		**NEW
Halotestin® (fluoxymesterone)	132	E36	
Hydroxytestosterone (4-hydroxy-testosterone)	134		UPDATED
Laurabolin® (nandrolone laurate)	135	E37	
Libriol (nandrolone/methandriol blend)	137	E37	
Masteron® (drostanolone propionate)	138	E37	UPDATED
Megagrisevit-Mono® (clostebol acetate)	140		
Mestanolone (methyldihydrotestosterone)	141		**NEW
Methandriol (methylandrostenediol)	142	E38	
Methyl-1-testosterone	144	E38	**NEW
Methyldienolone	146		**NEW
Methylhydroxynandrolone	148		**NEW
Methyltestosterone	149	E38	
Metribolone (methyltrienolone)	151		**NEW
Miotolan® (furazabol)	153		
Myagen (bolasterone)	154		
Neotest 250 (testosterone decanoate)	155		
Nilevar® (norethandrolone)	156	E39	
Omnadren® (testosterone blend)	158	E39	
Orabolin® (ethylestrenol)	160	E40	
Oral Turinabol (4-chlorodehydromethyltestosterone)	162	E40	UPDATED
Oranabol (oxymesterone)	164		**NEW
Parabolan® (trenbolone hexahydrobenzylcarbonate)	166	E41	UPDATED
Primobolan® (methenolone acetate)	168	E41	UPDATED
Primobolan® Depot (methenolone enanthate)	170	E42	UPDATED
Protabol (thiomesterone)	173		**NEW
Proviron® (mesterolone)	175	E46	
Sanabolicum (nandrolone cyclohexylpropionate)	177		
Spectriol (testosterone/nandrolone/methandriol blend)	178	E48	
Sten (testosterone blend)	179	E48	
Steranabol Ritardo (oxabolone cypionate)	180		UPDATED
Sustanon® (testosterone blend)	181	E48	UPDATED
Synovex® (testosterone propionate & estradiol)	184	E54	
Test 400®	185	E54	
Testolent (testosterone phenylpropionate)	186	E55	
Testosterone bucciclate	187		**NEW
Testosterone butyrate	189	E55	**NEW
Testosterone cyclohexylpropionate	190		
Testosterone cypionate	191	E55	UPDATED
Testosterone enanthate	195	E60	UPDATED
Testosterone propionate	198	E67	UPDATED
Testosterone suspension	201	E73	UPDATED
Testoviron® (testosterone blend)	204	E75	UPDATED
THG (tetrahydrogestrinone)	206		**NEW

Trenbolone acetate	208	E76	UPDATED
Trenbolone enanthate	211	E79	**NEW
Tribolin (nandrolone/methandriol blend)	213		
Trinabol 150 (trenbolone blend)	214	E79	**NEW
Triolandren (testosterone blend)	215		
Winstrol® (stanozolol)	216	E79	UPDATED

ANABOLIC AGENTS (NON-STEROID)

Arachidonic acid	221		UPDATED
Kynoselen®	223	D7	
Lutalyse® (diniprost)	224	D7	

ANALGESICS

NSAIDs (Non-Steroidal Anti-Inflammatory Drugs)	226		
Nubain® (nalbuphine HCL)	227		
Opiate Analgesics	228		

ANTI-ESTROGENS

Arimidex® (anastrozole)	232	D4	
Aromasin® (exemestane)	233		
Clomid® (clomiphene citrate)	234	D4	
Cyclofenil	236	D5	
Cytadren® (aminoglutethimide)	237	D5	
Evista (raloxifene)	239		**NEW
Fareston® (toremifene citrate)	241		
Faslodex® (fulvestrant)	242		
Femara® (letrozole)	243		
Lentaron® (formestane)	244	D7	
Nolvadex® (tamoxifen citrate)	245	D7	
Teslac® (testolactone)	247		

APPETITE STIMULANTS

Periactin	249		**NEW

DIURETICS

Aldactazide® (spironolactone/hydrochlorthiazide)	252	D3	
Aldactone® (spironolactone)	253	D4	
Dyazide® (triamterene and hydrochlorothiazide)	254		
Hydrodiuril® (hydrochlorthiazide)	255		
Lasix® (furosemide)	256	D7	
Lasilactone® (spironolactone/furosemide)	258		

ENDURANCE/ERYTHROPOIETIC DRUGS

Aranesp® (darbepoetin alfa)	260		
Epogen® (epoietin alfa)	261	D6	
Provigil (modafinil)	262		**NEW

FAT LOSS AGENTS – SYMPATHOMIMETICS

Albuterol	266		
Clenbuterol	267	D4	
Ephedrine (ephedrine hydrochloride)	269	D6	
HELIOS (clenbuterol/yohimbine hcl blend)	271	D7	
Meridia (sibutramine)	272		****NEW**
Yohimbine hydrochloride	273		
Zaditen® (ketotifen)	274	D8	

FAT LOSS AGENTS – THYROID

Cytomel® (liothyronine sodium)	276	D5	
Synthroid® (levothyroxine sodium)	277	D8	
Triacana® (tiratricol)	278		

FAT LOSS AGENTS – OTHER

Adipex-P® (phentermine hydrochloride)	280	D3	
DNP (2,4-Dinitrophenol)	281		
Capoten® (captopril)	282	D4	
Parlodel® (bromocriptine mesylate)	283	D8	
Thiomucase® (mucopolysaccharidase)	284	D8	

GROWTH HORMONES & RELATED

Catapres® (clonidine hydrochloride)	286	D4	
GH-RH (sermorelin acetate)	287		
Human Growth Hormone (somatropin)	288	D1	UPDATED
IGF-1 (Insulin-like Growth Factor-1)	291	D3	****NEW**
Nutropin AQ® (somatropin aqueous suspension)	294		
Nutropin Depot® (somatropin)	293		
Protropin® (somatrem)	297	D1	UPDATED

HYPOGLYCEMICS

Glucophage® (metformin Hcl)	300		
Insulin	301	D7	
Rezulin® (troglitazone)	304		

LIVER DETOXIFICATION

LIV-52®	308		
Silymarin (Milk Thistle Extract)	309		
Tationil® (reduced glutathione)	310	D9	

MASKING AGENTS

Epitestosterone	312		
Probenecid	313		

REDUCTASE INHIBITORS

Avodart® (dutasteride)	316	D4	UPDATED
Proscar® (finasteride)	318	D8	

SITE ENHANCEMENT

Caverject® (alprostadil)	322	
Nolotil® (metamizol)	323	
Synthol	324	D8

TANNING AGENTS

Trisoralen® (trioxsalen)	326	
Oxsoralen (methoxsalen)	327	

TESTOSTERONE STIMULATING DRUGS

HCG (Human chorionic gonadotropin)	330	D6

BIBLIOGRAPHY

APPENDIX

Drug Availability Tables: Listings by Generic Name	A	UPDATED
Drug Availability Tables: Listings by Brand Name	B	UPDATED
Drug Availability Tables: Listings by Country	C	UPDATED
Pharmaceuticals Photo Library (Ancillary Drugs)	D	UPDATED
Pharmaceuticals Photo Library (Anabolic/Androgenic Steroids)	E	UPDATED
Drug Security Stickers	F	****NEW**

Sections updated or new since the release of Anabolics 2004 are indicated in the right column.

FOREWORD

By Rick Collins, J.D.

In my extensive legal work involving anabolic steroid cases, I've corresponded with countless self-professed steroid authorities from the medical, scientific and academic fields. These are individuals with impressive credentials and doctoral degrees. You'd think they'd be fountains of knowledge. But they are mostly armchair experts or professional alarmists far more interested in pushing their own agenda than in engaging in any objective discussion. Bill Llewellyn is different.

Bill and I were both raised on Long Island, where a robust gym culture has flourished since the 1980s. Bill was part of that culture, and his experiences in the trenches and as a purely self-taught scientist have shaped his perspectives and influenced his writings as an author and columnist. By his own straightforward admission, Bill has taken a great deal of steroids. "I couldn't imagine writing so much about something I had little firsthand experience with," he said in a 2003 *Muscular Development* interview. What he has learned through the years he now passes down, in the belief that lack of reliable information presents far greater dangers than open discussion. He has little patience for trendy terms like "guru," instead describing himself as "a researcher with a reverence for the truth."

Bill's approach neither demonizes nor glamorizes anabolic steroids. From his monthly columns in *Muscular Development* to his original ANABOLICS 2000, Bill has striven to tell the truth as he sees it about a topic he knows a great deal about. Of course, his choice for frankness rather than dogmatic condemnation has made him a controversial figure. The cover of *ESPN The Magazine* once pictured him as a mysterious robed renegade, with a story that portrayed him as the representative of all those who would undermine the movement to eradicate performance-enhancing substances from sports. In actuality, Bill has little interest in the ethics issue concerning steroids in competitive athletics. His motivation has always been to study the "cosmetic" application of steroids for bodybuilding – the same application that attracts the great majority of steroid users.

When I was researching my book on steroids and the law, Bill was one of my invaluable resources on complex issues of steroid chemistry, real-world pharmacology, and product history/contents/counterfeiting. In my day-to-day practice, I have often found the previous editions of his book to be an indispensable reference. I can't imagine anyone involved with steroids in almost any capacity not having the latest edition of Bill's book.

Rick Collins, J.D.
Author, LEGAL MUSCLE: ANABOLICS IN AMERICA

Part I

Anabolic Overview

An Introduction to Testosterone

Anabolic steroids are a class of medications that contain a synthetically manufactured form of the hormone testosterone, or a related compound that is derived from (or similar in structure and action to) this hormone. In order to fully grasp how anabolic steroids work, it is, therefore, important to understand the basic functioning of testosterone.

Testosterone is the primary male sex hormone. It is manufactured by the Leydig's cells in the testes at varying amounts throughout a person's life span. The effects of this hormone become most evident during the time of puberty, when an increased output of testosterone will elicit dramatic physiological changes in the male body. This includes the onset of secondary male characteristics such as a deepened voice, body and facial hair growth, increased oil output by the sebaceous glands, development of sexual organs, maturation of sperm, and an increased libido. Indeed the male reproductive system will not function properly if testosterone levels are not significant. All such effects are considered the masculinizing or "androgenic" properties of this hormone.

Increased testosterone production will also cause growth promoting or "anabolic" changes in the body, including an enhanced rate of protein synthesis (leading to muscle accumulation). Testosterone is the reason males carry more muscle mass than women, as the two sexes have vastly contrasting amounts of this hormone. More specifically, the adult male body will manufacture between 2.5 and 11mg per day[1] while females only produce about ¼ mg. The dominant sex hormone for women is estrogen, which has a significantly different effect on the body. Among other things, a lower androgen and high estrogen level will cause women to store more body fat, accumulate less muscle tissue, have a shorter stature, and become more apt to bone weakening with age (osteoporosis).

The actual mechanism in which testosterone elicits these changes is somewhat complex. When free in the blood stream, the testosterone molecule is available to interact with various cells in the body. This includes skeletal muscle cells, as well as skin, scalp, kidney, bone, central nervous system, and prostate tissues. Testosterone binds with a cellular target in order to exert its activity, and will, therefore, effect only those body cells that posses the proper hormone receptor site (specifically the androgen receptor). This process can be likened to a lock and key system, with each receptor (lock) only being activated by a particular type of hormone (key). During this interaction, the testosterone molecule will become bound to the intracellular receptor site (located in the cytosol, not on the membrane surface), forming a new "receptor complex". This complex (hormone + receptor site) will then migrate to the cell's nucleus where it will attach to a specific section of the cell's DNA, referred to as the hormone response element. This will activate the transcription of specific genes, which in the case of a skeletal muscle cell will ultimately cause (among other things) an increase in the synthesis of the two primary contractile proteins, actin and myosin (muscular growth). Carbohydrate storage in muscle tissue may be increased due to androgen action as well.

Once this messaging process is completed, the complex will be released, and the receptor and hormone will disassociate. Both are then free to migrate back into the cytosol for further activity. The testosterone molecule is also free to diffuse back into circulation to interact with other cells. The entire receptor cycle, including hormone binding, receptor-hormone complex migration, gene transcription and subsequent return to cytosol is a slow process, taking hours, not minutes, to complete. For example, in studies using a single injection of nandrolone, it is measured to be 4 to 6 hours before free androgen receptors migrate back to the cytosol after activation. It is also suggested that this cycle includes the splitting and formation of new androgen receptors once returned to cytosol, a possible explanation for the many observations that androgens are integral in the formation of their own receptor sites[2].

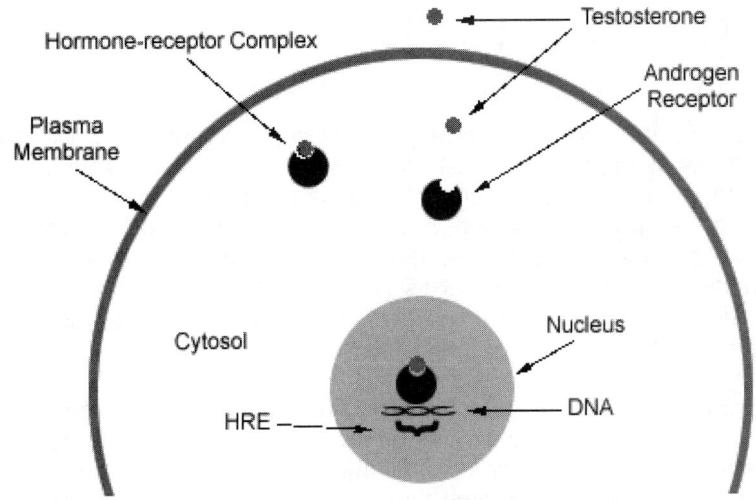

Cellular Diagram: Testosterone freely diffuses through the plasma membrane and binds with an intracellular androgen receptor. The hormone-receptor complex then enters the cell nucleus to bind with a specific segment of DNA (the Hormone Response Element), activating the transcription of specific genes.

In the kidneys, this same process works to allow androgens to augment erythropoiesis (red blood cell production)[3]. It is this effect that leads to an increase in red blood cell concentrations, and possibly increased oxygen transport capacity, during anabolic/androgenic steroid therapy. Many athletes mistakenly assume that oxymetholone and boldenone are unique in this ability, due to specific uses or mentions of this effect in drug literature. In fact, stimulation of erythropoiesis occurs with nearly all anabolic/androgenic steroids, as this effect is simply tied with activation of the androgen receptor in kidney cells. The only real exceptions might be compounds such as dihydrotestosterone and some of its derivatives[4], which are rapidly broken down upon interaction with the 3alpha-hydroxysteroid dehydrogenase enzymes (kidney tissue has a similar enzyme distribution to muscle tissue, see "anabolic/androgenic dissociation" section), and therefore display low activity in these tissues.

Adipose (fat) tissues are also androgen responsive, and here these hormones support the lipolytic (fat mobilizing) capacity of cells[5]. This may be accomplished by an androgen-tied regulation of beta-adrenergenic receptor concentrations or general cellular activity (through adenylate cyclase)[6]. We also note that the level of androgens in the body will closely correlate (inversely) with the level of stored body fat. As the level of androgenic hormones drops, typically the deposition of body fat will increase[7]. Likewise as we enhance the androgen level, body fat may be depleted at a more active rate. The ratio of androgen to estrogen action is in fact most important, as estrogen plays a counter role by acting to increase the storage of body fat in many sites of action[8]. Likewise, if one wished to lose fat during steroid use, estrogen levels should be kept low. This is clearly evidenced by the fact that non-aromatizing steroids have always been favored by bodybuilders looking to increase the look of definition and muscularity while aromatizing compounds are typically relegated to bulking phases of training due to their tendency to increase body fat storage. Aromatization is discussed in more detail in a following section (see: Estrogen Aromatization).

As mentioned, testosterone also elicits androgenic activity, which occurs by its activating receptors in what are considered to be androgen responsive tissues (often through prior conversion to dihydrotestosterone See: DHT Conversion). This includes the sebaceous glands, which are responsible for the secretion of oils in the skin. As the androgen level rises, so does the release of oils. As oil output increases, so does the chance for pores becoming clogged (we can see why acne is such a common side effect of steroid use). The production of body, and facial hair is also linked to androgen receptor activation in skin and scalp tissues. This becomes most noticeable as boys mature into puberty, a period when testosterone levels rise rapidly, and androgen activity begins to stimulate the growth of hair on the body and face. Some time later in life, and with the contribution of a genetic predisposition, androgen activity in the scalp may also help to initiate male-pattern hair loss. It is a misconception that dihydrotestosterone is an isolated culprit in the promotion of hair loss, however; as in actuality it is the general activation of the androgen receptor that is to blame (see: DHT Conversion). The functioning of sex glands and libido are also tied to the activity of androgens, as are numerous other regions of the central nervous/neuromuscular system.

Direct and Indirect Anabolic Effects

Although testosterone had been isolated, synthesized, and actively experimented with for many decades now, there is still some debate today as to exactly how steroids effect muscle mass. At this point in time, the primary mode of anabolic action with all anabolic/androgenic steroids is understood to be direct activation of the cellular androgen receptor and increases in protein synthesis. As follows, if we are able to increase our androgen level from an external source by supplementing testosterone or a similar anabolic steroid, we can greatly enhance the rate in which protein is retained by the muscles. This is clearly the primary cause for muscle growth with all anabolic/androgenic steroids. As our hormone levels increase, so does androgen receptor activation, and ultimately the rate of protein synthesis.

But other indirect mechanisms could possibly affect muscle growth outside of the normally understood androgen action on protein synthesis. An indirect mechanism is one that is not brought about by activation of the androgen receptor, but the affect androgens might have on other hormones, or even the release of locally acting hormones or growth promoters inside cells (perhaps mediated by other membrane bound receptors). We must remember also that muscle mass disposition involves not only protein synthesis, but also other factors such as tissue nutrient transport and protein breakdown. We need to look at androgenic interaction with these factors as well to get a compete picture. Concerning the first possibility, we note that studies with testosterone suggest that this hormone does not increase tissue amino acid transport[9]. This fact probably explains the profound synergy bodybuilders have noted in recent years with insulin, a hormone that strongly increases transport of nutrients into muscle cells. But regarding protein breakdown, we do see a second important pathway in which androgens might affect muscle growth.

Anti-Glucocorticoid Effect of Testosterone

Testosterone (and synthetic anabolic/androgenic steroids) may help to increase mass and strength by having an anti-catabolic effect on muscle cells. Considered one of the most important indirect mechanisms of androgen action, these hormones are shown to effect the actions of another type of steroid hormone in the body, glucocorticoids (cortisol is the primary representative of this group)[10]. Glucocorticoid hormones actually have the exact opposite effect on the muscle cell than androgens, namely sending an order to release stored protein. This process is referred to as catabolism, and represents a breaking down of muscle tissue. Muscle growth is achieved when the anabolic effects of testosterone are more pronounced overall than the degenerative effects of cortisol. With intense training and a proper diet, the body will typically store more protein than it removes, but this underlying battle is always constant.

When administering anabolic steroids however, a much higher androgen level can place glucocorticoids at a notable disadvantage. With their effect reduced, fewer cells will be given a message to release protein, and more will be accumulated in the long run. The primarily mechanism believed to bring this effect out is androgen displacement of glucocorticoids bound to the glucocorticoid receptor. In fact, in-vitro studies have supported this notion by demonstrating that testosterone has a very high affinity for this receptor[11], and further suggesting that some of its anabolic activity is directly mediated through this action[12]. It is also suggested that androgens may indirectly interfere with DNA binding to the glucocorticoid response element[13]. Although the exact underlying mechanism is still in debate, what is clear is that steroid administration inhibits protein breakdown, even in the fasted state, which seems clearly indicative of an anti-catabolic effect.

Testosterone and Creatine

In addition to protein synthesis, a rise in androgen levels should also enhance the synthesis of creatine in skeletal muscle tissues[14]. Creatine, as creatine phosphate (CP), plays a crucial role in the manufacture of ATP (adenosine triphosphate), which is a main store of energy for the muscles. As the muscle cells are stimulated to contract, ATP molecules are broken down into ADP (adenosine diphosphate), which releases energy. The cells will then undergo a process using creatine phosphate to rapidly restore ADP to its original structure, in order to replenish ATP concentrations. During periods of intense activity however, this process will not be fast enough to compensate and ATP levels will become lowered. This will cause the muscles to become fatigued and less able to effort a strenuous contraction. With increased levels of CP available to the cells, ATP is replenished at an enhanced rate and the muscle is both stronger and more enduring. This effect will account for some portion of the early strength increases seen during steroid therapy. Although perhaps not technically considered an anabolic effect as tissue hypertrophy is not a direct result, androgen support of creatine synthesis is certainly still looked at as a positive and growth supporting result in the mind of the bodybuilder.

Testosterone and IGF-1

It has also been suggested that there is an indirect mechanism of testosterone action on muscle mass mediated by Insulin-Like Growth Factor. To be more specific, studies note a clear link between androgens and tissue release of[15], and responsiveness to, this anabolic hormone. For example, it has been demonstrated that increases in IGF-1 receptor concentrations in skeletal muscle are noted when elderly men are given replacement doses of testosterone[16]. In essence, the cells are becoming primed for the actions of IGF-1, by testosterone. Alternately we see marked decreases in IGF-1 receptor protein levels with androgen deficiency in young men. It also appears that androgens are necessary for the local production and function of IGF-1 in skeletal muscle cells, independent of circulating growth hormone, and IGF-1 levels[17]. Since we do know for certain that IGF-1 is at least a minor anabolic hormone in muscle tissue, it seems reasonable to conclude that this factor, at least at some level, is involved in the muscle growth noted with steroid therapy.

Direct and Indirect Steroids?

In looking over the proposed indirect effects of testosterone, and pondering the effectiveness of the synthetic anabolic/androgenic steroids, we must resist the temptation to believe we can categorize steroids as those which directly, and those which indirectly, promote muscle growth. The belief that there are two dichotomous groups or classes of steroids ignores the fact that all commercial steroids promote not only muscle growth but also androgenic effects. There is no complete separation of these traits at this time, making clear that all activate the cellular androgen receptor. I believe the theory behind direct and indirect steroid classifications originated when some noted the low receptor binding affinity of seemingly strong anabolic steroids like oxymetholone and methandrostenolone[18]. If they bind poorly, yet work well, something else must be at work. This type of thinking fails to recognize other factors in the potency of these compounds, such as their long half-lives, estrogenic activity and weak interaction with restrictive binding proteins (see: Free vs. Bound Testosterone). While there may possibly be differences in the way various compounds could foster growth indirectly, such that advantages might even be found with certain synergistic drug combinations, the primary mode of action with all of these compounds is the androgen receptor. The notion that steroid X and Y must never be stacked together because they both compete for the same receptor when stimulating growth, while X and Z should be combined because they work via different mechanisms, should likewise not be taken too seriously. Such classifications are based on speculation only, and upon reasonable investigation are clearly invalid.

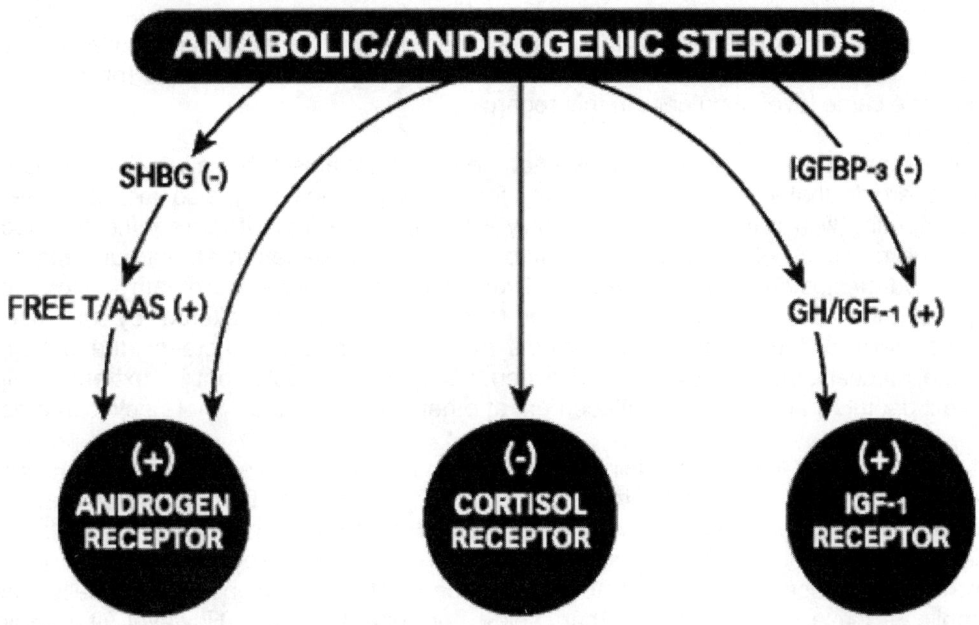

MECHANISM OF ACTION DIAGRAM: The mechanism of anabolic action due to the administation of anabolic/androgenic steroids. AAS causes not only direct stimulation of the androgen receptor, but also supports muscle growth by increasing the levels of free androgens, increasing androgen receptor density, inhibiting corticosteroid action, increasing GH/IGF-1, and suppressing IGF-1 binding proteins.

Free vs. Bound Testosterone

A very small amount of testosterone actually exists in a free state, where interaction with cellular receptors is possible. The majority will be bound to the proteins SHBG (sex hormone binding globulin, also referred to as sex steroid binding globulin and testosterone-estradiol binding globulin) and albumin, which temporarily prevent the hormone from exerting activity. Steroid hormones actually bind much more avidly to SHBG than albumin (with approximately 1,000 times greater affinity), however albumin is present in a level 1,000 times greater than SHBG. Therefore, the activity of both binding proteins in the body is relatively equal. The distribution of testosterone in men is typically 45% of testosterone bound to SHBG, and about 53% bound to albumin. The remaining 2% of the average blood concentration exists in a free, unbound state. In women, the percentage of free testosterone is lower, measured to be approximately 1%. A binding protein called ABP (androgen binding protein) also helps to mediate androgen activity in the reproductive system, although since it is found exclusively in these tissues, it is not relevant to muscle growth.

The level of free testosterone available in the blood is likewise an important factor mediating its activity, as only a small percentage is really active at any given time. It must also be noted that as we alter testosterone to form new anabolic/androgenic steroids, we also typically alter the affinity in which the steroid will bind to plasma proteins. This is an important consideration, as the higher percentage we have of free hormone, the more active the compound should be on a milligram for milligram basis. And the variance can be substantial between different compounds. For example, Proviron® (1-methyl dihydrotestosterone) binds with SHBG many times more avidly than testosterone[19], while mibolerone (7,17 dimethyl-nandrolone) and bolasterone (7,17 dimethyl-testosterone) show virtually no affinity for this protein at all (clearly the reason these steroids are such potent androgens).

The level of SHBG present in the body is also variable, and can be altered by a number of factors. The most prominent seems to be the concentration of estrogen and thyroid hormones present in the blood. We generally see a reduction in the amount of this plasma binding protein as estrogen and thyroid content decreases, and a rise in SHBG as they increase. A heightened androgen level due to the administration of anabolic/androgenic steroids has also been shown to lower levels of this protein considerably. This is clearly supported by a 1989 German study, which noted a strong tendency for SHBG reduction with the oral anabolic steroid stanozolol (Winstrol®)[20]. After only 3 days of administering a daily dose of .2mg/kg body-weight (about 18mg for a 200lb man), SHBG was lowered nearly 50% in normal subjects. Similar results have been obtained with the use of injectable testosterone enanthate; however, milligram for milligram, the effect of stanozolol was much greater in comparison. The form of administration may have been important in reaching this level of response. Although the injectable was not tried in the German study, we can refer to others comparing the effect of oral vs. transdermal estrogen[21]. These show a much greater response in SHBG levels when the drug is given orally. This is perhaps explained by the fact that SHBG is produced in the liver. Therefore, we cannot assume that injectable Winstrol® (or injectable steroids in general) will display the same level of potency in this regard.

Lowering the level of plasma binding proteins is also not the only mechanism that allows for an increased level of free testosterone. Steroids that display a high affinity for these proteins may also increase the level of free testosterone by competing with it for binding. Obviously if testosterone finds it more difficult to locate available plasma proteins in the presence of the additional compound, more will be left in an unbound state. A number of steroids including dihydrotestosterone, Proviron®, and Oral-Turinabol (chlorodehydromethyltestosterone) display a strong tendency for this effect. If the level of free-testosterone can be altered by the use of different anabolic/androgenic steroids, the possibility also exists that one steroid can increase the potency of another through these same mechanisms. For example, Proviron® is a poor anabolic, but its extremely high affinity for SHBG might make it useful by allowing the displacement of other steroids that are more active in these tissues.

We must not let this discussion lead us into thinking that binding proteins serve no valuable function. In fact they play a vital role in the transport and functioning of endogenous androgens. Binding proteins act to protect the steroid against rapid metabolism, ensure a more stable blood hormone concentration, and facilitate an even distribution of hormone to various body organs. The recent discovery of a specific receptor for Sex Hormone-Binding Globulin (SHBG-R) located on the membrane surface of steroid responsive body cells also suggests a much more complicated role for this protein than soley hormone transport. However, it remains clear that manipulating the tendency of a hormone to exist in an unbound state is an effective way to alter drug potency.

Estrogen Aromatization

Testosterone is the primary substrate used in the male body for the synthesis of estrogen (estradiol), the principal female sex hormone. Although the presence of estrogen may seem quite unusual in men, it is structurally very similar to testosterone. With a slight alteration by the enzyme aromatase, estrogen is produced in the male body. Aromatase activity occurs in various regions of the male body, including adipose[22], liver[23], gonadal[24], central nervous system[25], and skeletal muscle[26] tissues. In the context of the average healthy male, the amount of estrogen produced is generally not very significant to one's body disposition, and may even be beneficial in terms of cholesterol values (See Side Effects: Cardiovascular Disease). However, in larger amounts it does have potential to cause many unwanted effects including water retention, female breast tissue development (gynecomastia), and body fat accumulation. For these reasons, many focus on minimizing the build-up or activity of estrogen in the body with aromatase inhibitors such as Arimidex and Cytadren, or anti-estrogens such as Clomid or Nolvadex, particularly at times when gynecomastia is a worry or the athlete is attempting to increase muscle definition.

We must, however, not be led into thinking that estrogen serves no benefit. It is actually a desirable hormone in many regards. Athletes have known for years that estrogenic steroids are the best mass builders, but it is only recently that are we finally coming to understand the underlying mechanisms why. It appears that reasons go beyond the simple size, weight, and strength increases that one would attribute to estrogen-related water retention, with this hormone actually having a direct effect on the process of anabolism. This is manifest through increases in glucose utilization, growth hormone secretion, and androgen receptor proliferation.

Glucose Utilization and Estrogen

Estrogen may play a very important role in the promotion of an anabolic state by affecting glucose utilization in muscle tissue. This occurs via an altering of the level of available glucose 6-phosphate dehydrogenase, an enzyme directly tied to the use of glucose for muscle tissue growth and recuperation[27 28]. More specifically, G6PD is a vital part of the pentose phosphate pathway, which is integral in determining the rate nucleic acids and lipids are to be synthesized in cells for tissue repair. During the period of regeneration after skeletal muscle damage levels of G6PD are shown to rise dramatically, which is believed to represent a mechanism for the body to enhance recovery when needed. Surprisingly, we find that estrogen is directly tied to the level of G6PD that is to be made available to cells in this recovery window.

The link between estrogen and G6PD was established in a study demonstrating levels of this dehydrogenase enzyme to rise after administration of testosterone propionate. The investigation further showed that the aromatization of testosterone to estradiol was directly responsible for this increase, and not the androgenic action of this steroid[29]. The non-aromatizable steroids dihydrotestosterone and fluoxymesterone were tested alongside testosterone propionate, but failed to duplicate the effect of testosterone. Furthermore, the positive effect of testosterone propionate was blocked when the aromatase inhibitor 4-hydroxyandrostenedione (formestane) was added, while 17-beta estradiol administration alone caused a similar increase in G6PD to testosterone propionate. The inactive estrogen isomer 17-alpha estradiol, which is unable to bind the estrogen receptor, failed to do anything. Further tests using testosterone propionate and the anti-androgen flutamide showed that this drug also did nothing to block the positive action of testosterone, establishing it as an effect independent of the androgen receptor.

Estrogen and GH/IGF-1

Estrogen may also play an important role in the production of growth hormone and IGF-1. IGF-1 (insulin-like growth factor) is an anabolic hormone released in the liver and various peripheral tissues via the stimulus of growth hormone (See Drug Profiles: Growth Hormone). IGF-1 is responsible for the anabolic activity of growth hormone such as increased nitrogen retention/protein synthesis and cell hyperplasia (proliferation). One of the first studies to bring this issue to our attention looked at the effects of the anti-estrogen tamoxifen on IGF-1 levels, demonstrating it to have a suppressive effect[30]. A second, perhaps more noteworthy, study took place in 1993, which looked at the effects of testosterone replacement therapy on GH and IGF-1 levels alone, and compared them to the effects of testosterone combined again with tamoxifen[31]. When tamoxifen was given, GH and IGF-1 levels were notably suppressed, while both values were elevated with the administration of testosterone enanthate alone. Another study has shown 300mg of testosterone enanthate weekly to cause a slight IGF-1 increase in normal men. Here the 300mg of testosterone ester caused an elevation of estradiol levels, which would be expected at such a dose. This was compared to the effect of the same dosage of nandrolone decanoate; however, this steroid failed to produce the same increase. This result is quite interesting, especially when we note that estrogen levels were actually lowered[32] when this steroid was given. Yet another demonstrated that GH and IGF-1 secretion is increased with testosterone administration on males with delayed puberty, while dihydrotestosterone (non-aromatizable) seems to suppress GH and IGF-1 secretion[33].

Estrogen and the Androgen Receptor

It has also been demonstrated that estrogen can increase the concentration of androgen receptors in certain tissues. This was shown in studies with rats, which looked at the effects of estrogen on cellular androgen receptors in animals that underwent orchiectomy (removal of testes, often done to diminish endogenous androgen production). According to the study, administration of estrogen resulted in a striking 480% increase in methyltrienolone (a potent oral androgen often used to reference receptor binding in studies) binding in the levator ani muscle[34]. The suggested explanation is that estrogen must either be directly stimulating androgen receptor production, or perhaps diminishing the rate of receptor breakdown. Although the growth of the levator ani muscle is commonly used as a reference for the anabolic activity of steroid compounds, it is admittedly a sex organ muscle, and different from skeletal muscle tissue in that it possesses a much higher concentration of androgen receptors. However, this study did look at the effect of estrogen in fast-twitch skeletal muscle tissues (tibialis anterior and extensor digitorum longus) as well, but did not note the same dramatic increase as the levator ani. Although discouraging at first glance, the fact the estrogen can increase androgen receptor binding in any tissue remains an extremely significant finding, especially in light of the fact that we now know androgens to have some positive effects outside of muscle tissue.

Anti-Estrogens and the Athlete

So what does this all mean to the bodybuilder looking to gain optimal size? Basically I think it calls for a cautious approach to the use of estrogen maintenance drugs if mass is the objective. Obviously, anti-estrogens should be used if there is a clear need for them due to the onset of estrogenic side effects, or at the very least, the drugs being administered should be substituted for non-estrogenic compounds. Gynecomastia is certainly an unwanted problem for the steroid user, as are noticeable fat mass gains. But if these problems have not presented themselves, the added estrogen due to a cycle of testosterone or Dianabol, for example, might indeed be aiding in the buildup of muscle mass. An individual confident they will notice, or are not prone to getting, these side effects, may therefore want to hold off using estrogen maintenance drugs so as to achieve the maximum gains in tissue mass as possible.

DHT Conversion

As we see from our discussion with estrogen, in considering the physiological effects of any steroid, we must look at all of its active metabolites, and not just the initial compound. This includes not only estrogenic products, but androgenic metabolites as well. With this in mind, it is important to note that the potency of testosterone is considerably increased in many androgen responsive tissues when it converts to dihydrotestosterone. More commonly referred to by the three-letter abbreviation DHT, this hormone is, in fact, measured to be approximately three to four times stronger than testosterone. It is the most potent steroid found naturally in the human body, and important to discuss if we are to understand the full activity of testosterone, as well as other anabolic/androgenic steroids that undergo a similar conversion.

Testosterone is converted to dihydrotestosterone upon interaction with the 5-alpha reductase enzyme. More specifically, this enzyme removes the C4-5 double-bond of testosterone by the addition of two hydrogen atoms to its structure (hence the name di-hydro testosterone). The removal of this bond is important, as in this case it creates a steroid that binds to the androgen receptor much more avidly than its parent steroid. 5-alpha reductase is present in high amounts in tissues of the prostate, skin, scalp, liver and various regions of the central nervous system, and as such represents a mechanism for the body to increase the potency of testosterone specifically where strong androgenic action is needed. In these areas of the body little testosterone will actually make its way to the receptor without being converted to dihydrotestosterone, making DHT by far the active form of androgen here.

DHT and Androgenic Side Effects

In some regards this local potentiation of testosterone's activity may be unwelcome, as higher androgenic activity in certain tissues may produce a number of undesireable side effects. Acne, for example, is often triggered by dihydrotestosterone activity in the sebaceous glands, and the local formation of dihydrotestosterone in the scalp is typically blamed for triggering male pattern hair loss. You should know that it is a terrible misconception among bodybuilders that dihydrotestosterone is an isolated culprit when it comes to these side effects. All anabolic/androgenic steroids exert their activities, both anabolic and androgenic, through the same cellular androgen receptor. Dihydrotestosterone is no different than any other steroid except that it is a more potent activator of this receptor than most, and can be formed locally in certain androgen-sensitive tissues. All steroids can cause androgenic side effects in direct relation to their affinity for this receptor, and DHT has no known unique ability in this regard.

Benefits of DHT

While a lot of attention is being paid to the negative side effects of the androgen dihydrotestosterone, you should know that there are some known benefits to the strong androgenic activity brought about by this hormone as well. For example, DHT plays an important role in the organization and functioning of the central nervous system. Many neural cells contain active androgen receptors, and it is thought that there may even be a specific importance of dihydrotestosterone in this area of the body. Studies have shown DHT to have a profoundly greater impact in these cells compared to testosterone. More specifically, animal models demonstrated that both testosterone and DHT would result in increased androgen receptor proliferation in neural cells three and seven hours after being administered, however only DHT was able to sustain this increase at the twenty-one hour mark[35]. Although some might contend that this difference is simply due to DHT forming a more stable and lasting complex with the androgen receptor, others suggest that DHT and testosterone might even be affecting neural cells differently, such that the dihydrotestosterone-receptor complex and testosterone-receptor complex might be activating the transcription of different target genes.

The strong interaction between the central nervous system and skeletal muscles, collectively referred to as the neuromuscular system, is of key importance to the athlete. There appears to be little doubt that the ability of the body to adapt to training, and to activate nerve endings in muscle tissue, is reliant on the interactions of the neuromuscular system. Inhibiting the formation of DHT during a testosterone cycle may therefore inadvertently interfere with strength and muscle mass gains. This would explain why bodybuilders commonly report a drop in steroid potency when they add the 5-alpha reductase inhibitor finasteride to a testosterone cycle. Many complain strength and even muscle mass gains slow significantly when this medication is added, which would not make sense if testosterone and androgen receptor activation in muscle tissue were solely responsible for growth. Clearly more is involved, and we cannot look at dihydrotestosterone simply as a side-effect hormone.

A Brief History of Anabolic/Androgenic Steroids

While it had been clear for many centuries that the testicles were crucial for the male body to properly develop, it was not until modern times that an understanding of testosterone began to form. The first solid scientific experiments in this area, which eventually led to the discovery and replication of testosterone (and related androgens), were undertaken in the 1800's. During this century a number of animal experiments were published, most of which involved the removal and/or implantation of testicular material from/in a subject. Although very crude in design by today's standards, these studies certainly laid the foundation for the modern field of endocrinology (the study of hormones). By the turn of the century, scientists were able to produce the first experimental androgen injections. These were actualized either through the filtering of large quantities of urine (for active hormones), or by extracting testosterone from animal testicles. Again, the methods were rough but the final results proved to be very enlightening.

Chemists finally synthesized the structure of testosterone in the mid 1930's, sparking a new wave of interest in this hormone. With the medical community paying a tremendous amount of attention to this achievement, the possible therapeutic uses for a readily available synthetic testosterone quickly became an extremely popular focus. Many believed the applications for this type of a medication would be extremely far reaching, with uses ranging from the maintenance of an androgen deficiency, to that of a good health and well being treatment for the sickly or elderly. During the infancy of such experimentation, many believed they had crossed paths with a true "fountain of youth".

Dihydrotestosterone and nandrolone, two other naturally occurring steroids, were also isolated and synthesized in the early years of steroid development. To make things even more interesting, scientists soon realized that the androgenic, estrogenic and anabolic activity of steroid hormones could be adjusted by altering their molecular structure. The goal of many researchers thereafter became to manufacture a steroid with extremely strong anabolic activity, but will display little or no androgenic/estrogenic properties. This could be very beneficial, because side effects will often become pronounced when steroid hormones are administered in supraphysiological amounts. A "pure" anabolic would theoretically allow the patient to receive only the beneficial effects of androgens (lean muscle mass gain, increased energy and recuperation etc.), regardless of the dosage. Some early success with the creation of new structures convinced many scientists that they were on the right track. Unfortunately none of this progress led researchers the their ultimate goal. By the mid 1950's, well over one thousand testosterone, nandrolone, and dihydrotestosterone analogues had been produced, but none proved to be purely anabolic compounds.

The failure to reach this goal was primarily due to an initial flawed understanding of testosterone's action. Scientists had noticed high levels of DHT in certain tissues, and believed this indicated an unusual receptor affinity for this hormone. This led to the belief that the human body had two different androgen receptors. According to this theory, one receptor site would respond only to testosterone (eliciting the beneficial anabolic effects), while the other is activated specifically by the metabolite, dihydrotestosterone. With this understanding, eliminating the conversion of testosterone to DHT was thought capable of solving the problem of androgenic side effects, as these receptors would have little or none of this hormone available for binding. More recently however, scientists have come to understand that only one type of androgen receptor exists in the human body. It is also accepted that no anabolic/androgenic steroid can possibly be synthesized that would participate only with receptors in tissues related to anabolism. DHT, which was once thought not to bind to the same receptor as testosterone, is now known to do so at approximately three to four times the affinity of its parent, and the unusual recovery of DHT from androgen responsive tissues is now attributed to the distribution characteristics of the 5a-reductase enzyme.

Synthetic AAS Development

In order to develop products that would be effective therapeutically, chemists needed to solve a number of problems with using natural steroid hormones for treatment. For example, oral dosing was a problem, as our basic steroids testosterone, nandrolone and dihydrotestosterone are ineffective when administered this way. The liver would efficiently break down their structure before reaching circulation, so some form of alteration was required in order for a tablet or capsule to be produced. Our natural steroid hormones also have very short half-lives in the body, so when administered by injection, an extremely frequent and uncomfortable dosing schedule is required if a steady blood level is to be achieved. Therefore, extending steroid activity was a major goal for many chemists during the early years of synthetic AAS development. Scientists also focused on the nagging problems of possible excess estrogenic buildup in the blood, particularly with testosterone, which can become very uncomfortable for patients undergoing therapy.

Methylated Compounds and Oral Dosing

Chemists realized that by replacing the hydrogen atom at the steroid's 17th alpha position with a carbon atom (a process referred to as *alkylation*), its structure would be notably resistant to breakdown by the liver. The carbon atom is typically added in the form of a methyl group (CH3), although we see oral steroids with an added ethyl (C2H5) grouping as well. A steroid with this alteration is commonly described as a C-17 alpha alkylated oral, although the terms methylated or ethylated oral steroid are also used. The alkyl group cannot be removed metabolically, and therefore inhibits reduction of the steroid to its inactive 17-ketosteroid form by occupying one of the necessary carbon bonds. Before long, pharmaceutical companies had utilized this advance (and others) to manufacture an array of effective oral steroids including methyltestosterone, Dianabol, Winstrol®, Anadrol 50®, Halotestin®, Nilevar, Orabolin and Anavar. The principle drawback to these compounds is that they place a notable amount of stress on the liver, which in some instances can lead to actual damage to this organ.

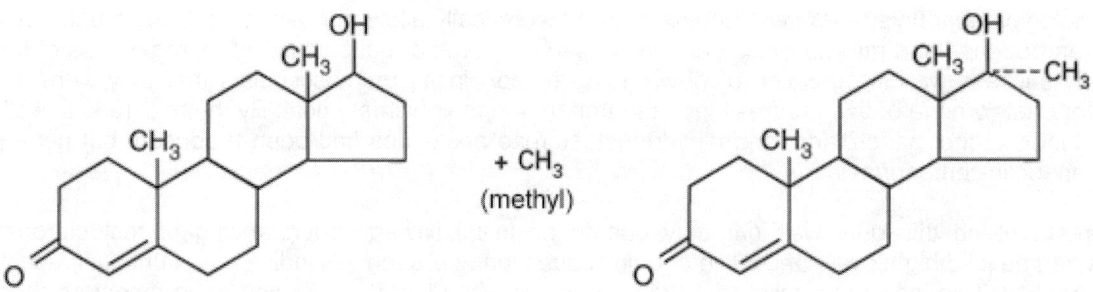

Testosterone Methyltestosterone

Because the alkyl group cannot be removed, it mediates the action of the steroid in the body. Methyltestosterone, for example, is not simply an oral equivalent of testosterone, as the added alkylation changes the activity of this steroid considerably. One major change we see is an increased tendency for the steroid to produce estrogenic side effects, to spite the fact that it actually lowers the ability of the hormone to interact with aromatase[36]. Apparently with 17-alkylation present on a steroid, aromatization (when possible) produces a more active form of estrogen (typically 17alpha-methyl or 17alpha-ethyl estradiol). These estrogens are more biologically active than estradiol due to their longer half-life and weaker tendency to bind with serum proteins. In some instances, 17alpha-alkylation will also enhance the ability of the initial steroid compound to bind with and activate the estrogen or progesterone receptor[37]. An enhancement of estrogenic properties is also obvious when we look at methandrostenolone, which is an alkylated form of boldenone (Equipoise®), and Nilevar, which is an alkylated form of the mild anabolic nandrolone. Dianabol is clearly more estrogenic than Equipoise®, a drug not noted for producing strong side effects of this nature. The same holds true for the comparison of Nilevar to Deca, a compound that we also know to be extremely mild in this regard.

C17 alpha alkylation also typically lowers the affinity in which the steroid binds to the androgen receptor, as is noted with the weak relative binding affinity of such popular agents as Dianabol and Winstrol (stanozolol). However, since this alteration also greatly prolongs the half-life of a steroid, as well as increases the tendency for it to exist in an unbound state, it creates a more potent anabolic/androgenic agent in both cases. This explains why Dianabol and stanozolol are notably effective in relatively lower weekly doses (often 140mg weekly will produce notable growth) compared to injectables such as testosterone and nandrolone, which often need to reach doses of 300-400mg weekly for a similar level of effect.

Non-Alkylated Orals

In an attempt to solve the mentioned problems with liver toxicity we see with c17-alpha alkylated compounds, a number of other orals with different chemical alterations (such as Primobolan®, Proviron®, Andriol® and Anabolicum Vister) were created. Primobolan® and Proviron® are alkylated at the one position (methyl), a trait which also slows ketosteroid reduction. Andriol® uses a 17beta carboxylic acid ester (used with injectable compounds, discussed below), however, here the oil-dissolved steroid is sealed in a capsule and is intended for oral administration. This is supposed to promote steroid absorption through intestinal lymphatic ducts, bypassing the first pass through the liver. In addition to 1 methylation, Primobolan® also utilizes a 17 beta ester (acetate) to further protect against reduction to inactive form (here there is no lymphatic system absorption). Anabolicum Vister uses 17beta enol ether linkage to protect the steroid, which is very similar to esterification as the ether breaks off to release a steroid base (boldenone in this case). While all of these types of compounds do not place the same stress on the liver, they are also much less resistant to breakdown than 17 alkylated orals, and are ultimately less active milligram for milligram.

Esters and Injectable Compounds

You may notice that many injectable steroids will list long chemical names like testosterone cypionate and testosterone enanthate, instead of just testosterone. In these cases, the cypionate and enanthate are esters (carboxylic acids) that have been attached to the 17-beta hydroxyl group of the testosterone molecule, which increase the active life span of the steroid preparation. Such alterations will reduce the steroid's level of water solubility, and increase its oil solubility. Once an esterified compound has been injected, it will form a deposit in the muscle tissue (depot) from which it will slowly enter circulation. Generally the larger the ester chain, the more oil soluble the steroid compound will be, and the longer it will take for the full dosage to be released. Once free in circulation, enzymes will quickly remove the ester chain and the parent hormone will be free to exert its activity (while the ester is present the steroid is inert).

There are a wide number of esters, which can provide varying release times, used in medicine today. To compare, an ester like decanoate can extend the release of active parent drug into the blood stream for three to four weeks, while it may only be a extended for a few days with an acetate or propionate ester. The use of an ester allows for a much less frequent injection schedule than if using a water based (straight) testosterone, which is much more comfortable for the patient. We must remember when calculating dosages, that the ester is figured into the steroids measured weight. 100mg of testosterone enanthate, therefore, contains much less base hormone than 100mg of a straight testosterone suspension (in this case it equals 72mg of testosterone). In some instances, an ester may account for roughly 40% or more of the total steroid weight, but the typical measure is somewhere around 15% to 35%. Below are the free base equivalents for several popular steroid compounds.

100 mg of steroid as:	Approximate Free Equivalent:
Trenbolone acetate	87mg
Testosterone propionate	83mg
Testosterone enanthate	72mg
Testosterone cypionate	70mg
Testosterone undecanoate	63mg
Nandrolone phenylpropionate	67mg
Nandrolone decanoate	64mg

It is also important to stress the fact that esters do not alter the activity of the parent steroid in any way. They work only to slow its release. It is quite common to hear people speak about the properties of different esters, almost as if they can magically alter a steroid's effectiveness. This is really nonsense. Enanthate is not more powerful than cypionate (perhaps a few extra milligrams of testosterone released per injection, but nothing to note), nor is Sustanon some type of incredible testosterone blend. Personally, I have always considered Sustanon a very poor buy in the face of cheaper 250mg enanthate ampules. Your muscle cells see only testosterone; ultimately there is no difference. Reports of varying levels of muscle gain, androgenic side effects, water retention etc. are only issues of timing. Faster releasing testosterone esters will produce estrogen buildup faster simply because there is more testosterone free in the blood from the start of the cycle. The same is true when we state that Durabolin® is a milder nandrolone for women compared to Deca. It is simply easier to control the blood level with a faster acting drug. Were virilization symptoms to become apparent, hormone levels will drop much faster once we stop administeration. This should not be confused with the notion that the nandrolone in Durabolin® acts differently in the body than that released from a shot of Deca-Durabolin®.

It is also worth noting that while the ester is typically hydrolyzed in general circulation, some will be hydrolyzed at the injection site where the steroid depot first contacts blood. This will cause a slightly higher concentration of both free steroid and ester in the muscle where the drug had been administered. On the plus side, this may equate to slightly better growth in this muscle, as more hormone is made available to nearby cells. Many bodybuilders have come to swear by the use of injection sites such as the deltoids, biceps and triceps, truly believing better growth can be achieved if the steroid is injected directly into these muscles. The negative to this is that the ester itself may be irritating to the tissues at the site of injection once it is broken free. In some instances it can be so caustic that the muscle itself will become swollen and sore due to the presence of the ester, and the user may even suffer a low-grade fever as the body fights off the irritant (the onset of such symptoms typically occurs 24-72 hours after injection). This effect is more common with small chain esters such as propionate and acetate, and can actually make a popular steroid such as Sustanon (which contains testosterone propionate) off-limits for some users who experience too much discomfort to justify using the drug. Longer chain esters such as decanoate and cypionate are typically much less irritating at the site of injection, and therefore are preferred by sensitive individuals.

Anabolic/Androgenic Dissociation

Although never complete, scientists had some success in their quest to separate the androgenic and anabolic properties of testosterone. A number of synthetic anabolic steroids had been developed as a result, with many being notably weaker and stronger than our base androgen. In order to first assess the anabolic and androgenic potential of each newly developed steroid, scientists had generally used rats as a model. To judge androgenic potency the typical procedure involved the post-administration measure (% growth) of the seminal vesicles and ventral prostate. These two tissues will often respond unequally to a given steroid, however, so an average of the two figures is used. Anabolic activity was most commonly determined by measuring the growth of the levator ani, a sex organ (not skeletal) muscle. This tissue may not be the most ideal one to use though, as it contains more androgen receptor than most skeletal muscles (the AR is still less abundant here than in target tissues such as the ventral prostate)[38 39]. In integrating both measures, the anabolic index is used, which relates the ratio of anabolic to androgenic response for a given steroid. An anabolic index greater than one indicates a higher tendency for anabolic effect, and therefore classifies the drug as an anabolic steroid. A measure lower than one in turn assesses the steroid as androgenic. There is some variance between experimental results and the actual real world experiences with humans, but (with a few exceptions) designations based on the anabolic index are generally accepted. Below are discussed a few factors that greatly effect anabolic/androgenic dissociation.

Nandrolone and 19-norandrogens

The section of this book dealing with DHT conversion is important, because it helps us understand the anabolic steroid nandrolone and many of its derivatives. Nandrolone is identical to testosterone except it lacks a carbon atom in the 19th position, hence its other given name 19-nortestosterone. Nandrolone is very interesting because it offers the greatest ratio of anabolic to androgenic effect of the three natural steroids (see: Synthetic AAS Chemistry). This is because it is metabolized into a less potent structure (dihydronandrolone) in androgen target tissues with high concentrations of the 5-alpha reductase enzyme, which is the exact opposite of what happens with testosterone. Apparently the removal of the c4-5 double bond, which normally increases the androgen receptor binding capability of testosterone, causes an unusual lowering of this ability with nandrolone. Instead of becoming three to four times more potent, it becomes several times weaker. This is a very desirable trait if you want to target anabolic effects over androgenic. This characteristic also carries over to most synthetic steroids derived from nandrolone, making this an attractive base steroid to use in the synthesis of new, primarily anabolic, steroids.

5-alpha Irreducible Steroids

When we look at the other mild anabolic steroids Primobolan®, Winstrol® and Anavar, none of which are derived from nandrolone, we see another interesting commonality. These steroids are DHT derivatives that are unaffected by 5alpha-reductase, and therefore neither become weaker or stronger in androgen responsive target tissues with high concentrations of this enzyme. In essence, they have a very balanced effect between muscle and androgen tissues, making them outwardly less androgenic than testosterone.

This is why these steroids are technically classified as anabolics, and are undeniably less troublesome than many other steroids in terms of promoting androgenic side effects. However, if we wanted to look for the absolute least androgenic steroid, the title would still go to nandrolone (or perhaps one of its derivatives). Female bodybuilders should likewise take note that to spite the recommendations of others, steroids like Anavar, Winstrol and Primo are not the least risky steroids to use. This is of great importance, as male sex hormones can produce many undesirable and permanent side effects when incorrectly taken by females (See: Side Effects, Virilization).

3-alpha Hydroxysteroid Dehydrogenase

The 3-alpha hydroxysteroid dehydrogenase enzyme is also important, because it can work to reduce the anabolic potency of certain steroids considerably. As follows, not all potent binders of the androgen receptor are, as a rule, great muscle-building drugs, and this enzyme is an important factor. Dihydrotestosterone is a clear example. Just as the body converts testosterone to DHT as a way to potentiate its action in certain tissues (skin, scalp, prostate etc.), it also has ways of countering the strong activity of DHT, in other tissues where it is unneeded. This is accomplished by the rapid reduction of DHT to its inactive active metabolites, namely androstanediol, before it reaches the androgen receptor. This activity occurs via interaction with the 3-alpha hydroxysteroid dehydrogenase enzyme. This enzyme is present in high concentrations in certain tissues, including skeletal muscle, and DHT is much more open to alteration by it than other steroids that possess a c4-5 double-bond (like testosterone)[40]. This causes dihydrotestosterone to be an extremely poor anabolic, to spite the fact that it actually exhibits a much higher affinity for the cellular androgen receptor than most other steroids. Were it able to reach the cellular androgen receptor without first being metabolized by 3a-HSD, it certainly would be a formidable muscle-building steroid. Unfortunately this is not the case, explaining why injectable dihydrotestosterone preparations (no longer commercially produced) were never favorite drugs among athletes looking to build mass. This trait is also shared by the currently popular oral androgen Proviron®, which is, in essence, just an oral form of DHT (1-methyl dihydrotestosterone to be specific) and known to be an extremely poor tissue builder.

Anabolics and Potency

One must remember that being classified as an anabolic just means that the steroid is more inclined to produce muscle growth than androgenic side effects. Since both effects are mediated through the same receptor, and growth is not produced by androgen receptor activation in muscle tissue alone (other CNS tissues, for example, are integral to this process as well), we find that a reduction in the androgenic activity of a compound will often coincide with a similar lowering of its muscle-building effectiveness. If we are just looking at overall muscle growth, androgenic steroids (usually potent due to their displaying a high affinity to bind with the androgen receptor in all tissues) are typically much more productive muscle-builders than anabolics, which usually bind with lower affinity in many tissues. In fact, with all of the analogues produced throughout the years, the base androgen testosterone is still considered to be one of the most effective bulking agents. The user must simply endure more side effects when acquiring his or her new muscle with this type of drug. Individuals wishing to avoid the stronger steroids will, therefore, make a trade-off, accepting less overall muscle gain in order to run a more comfortable cycle.

RBA Assay:

Another way of evaluating the potential ratio of anabolic to androgenic activity is the more recent practice of simply comparing the relative binding affinity (RBA) of various steroids for the androgen receptor in rat skeletal muscle versus prostate. When we look at the detailed study published in 1984, we see a clear trend of uniformity. Aside from dihydrotestosterone and Proviron® (mesterolone) which undergo rapid enzymatic reduction in muscle tissue, the remaining anabolic/androgenic steroids seem to bind with near equal affinity to receptors in both tissues. This study also discusses the unique activity of testosterone and nandrolone compounds, which are good substrates for the 5a-reductase enzyme found in androgen target tissues (such as the prostate), and seem to provide the most notable variance between anabolic and androgenic effect in humans. When it comes to real-world use, these particular substrates tend to behave differently (somewhat more so that other steroids) in regards to their anabolic and androgenic profiles than the animal models would suggest.

Compound	Human SHBG	Rabbit Muscle	Rat Muscle	Rat Prostate	Ratio M vs. P
methyltrienolone	<.01	1	1	1	1
dihydrotestosterone	1	.07	<.01	.46	.03
mesterolone	4.4	.21	.08	.25	.32
testosterone	.19	.07	.23	.15	1.53
nandrolone	.01	.20	.24	.60	.4
methyltestosterone	.05	.1	.11	.13	.85
methenolone	.03	.09	.24	.14	1.67
stanozolol	.01	.03	.02	.03	.6
methandrostenolone	.02	.02	.02	.03	.75
fluoxymesterone	<.01	.02	.01	.02	.77
oxymetholone	<.01	<.01	<.01	<.01	1.54
ethylestrenol	<.01	.01	<.01	<.01	2

RBA of various anabolic/androgenic steroids as competitors for human SHBG binding of DHT, and for receptor binding of methyltrienolone in cytosol from rabbit, rat skeletal muscle and prostate. Source: Endocrinology 114(6):2100-06 1984 June, "Relative Binding Affinity of Anabolic-Androgenic Steroids...", Saartok T; Dahlberg E; Gustafsson JA.

Synthetic AAS Chemistry

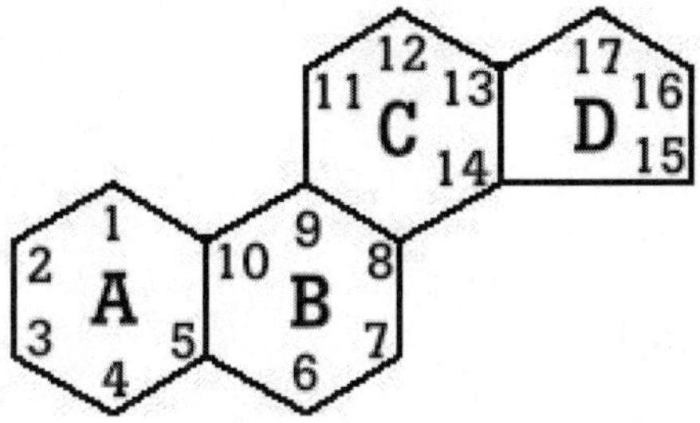

Steran Nucleus
(All natural and synthetic AAS hormones share this base structure)

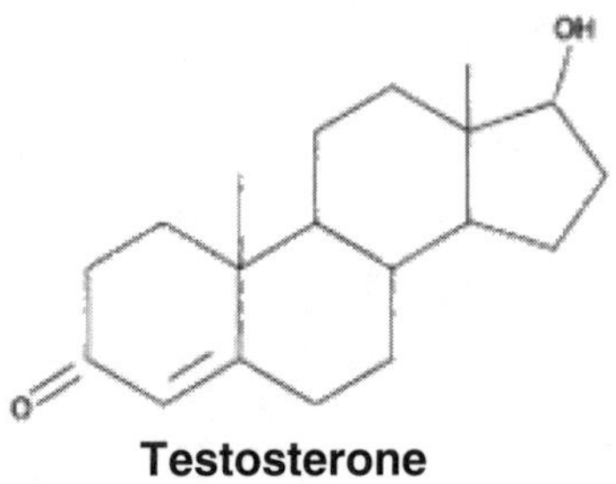

Testosterone

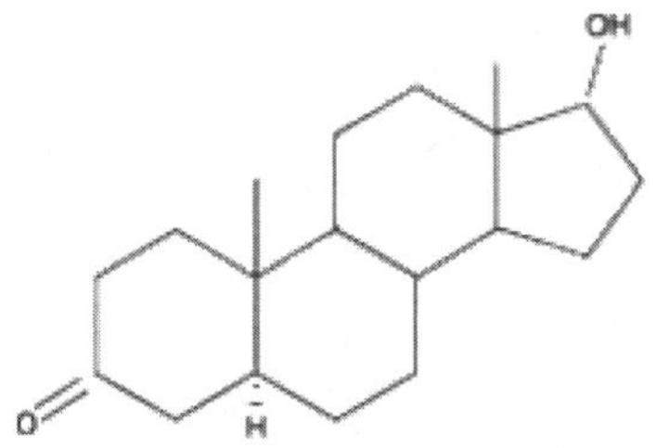

Dihydrotestosterone

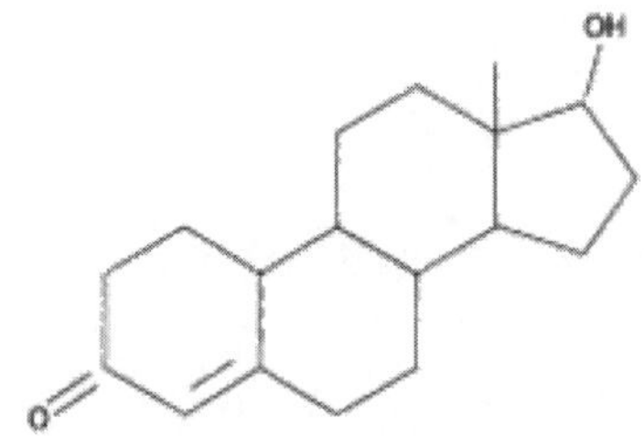

Nandrolone

All anabolic/androgenic steroids are preparations containing one of the above three natural steroid hormones, or chemically altered derivatives thereof. In creating new synthetic compounds, one of the three natural hormones is selected as a starting point, typically due to the possession of particular traits that may be beneficial for the new compound. For instance, of the three natural steroids above, dihydrotestosterone is the only steroid devoid of the possibility of aromatization and 5-alpha reduction. It was likewise a very popular choice in the creation of synthetics that lack estrogenic activity and/or exhibit a more balanced androgenic to anabolic activity ratio. Nandrolone was typically used when even lower androgenic action is desired, due to its weakening upon interaction with the 5-alpha reductase enzyme. Nandrolone also aromatizes much more slowly than testosterone. Testosterone is our most powerful muscle-building hormone, and also exhibits strong androgenic activity due to its conversion to a more potent steroid (dihydrotestosterone) via 5-alpha reductase.

Testosterone derivatives

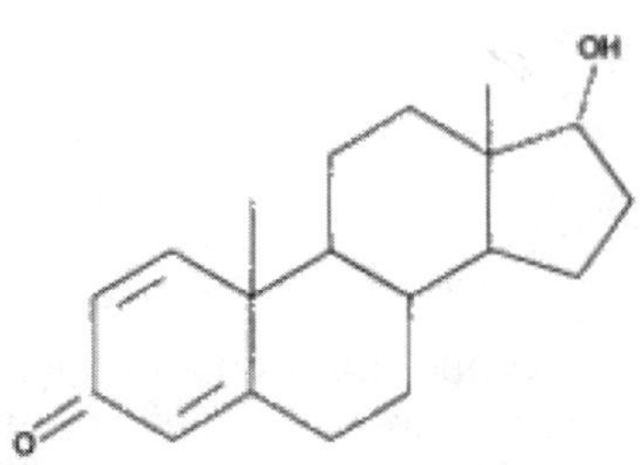

Boldenone (+c1-2 double bond)

Boldenone is testosterone with an added double-bond between carbon atoms one and two. However, this bond changes the activity of the steroid considerably. First, it dramatically slows aromatization, such that boldenone converts to estradiol at about half the rate of testosterone. Secondly, this bond causes the steroid to be a very poor substrate for the 5-alpha reductase enzyme. The more active 5-alpha reduced metabolite 5alpha-dihydroboldenone is produced only in very small amounts in humans. The hormone instead tends to convert via 5-

beta reductase to 5beta-dihydroboldenone (a virtually inactive androgen). This makes it lean towards being an anabolic instead of an androgen, although both traits are still notably apparent with this steroid. The c1-2 double bond also slows the hepatic breakdown of the structure, increasing its resistance to 17-ketosteroid deactivation and its functional half-life and oral bioavailability.

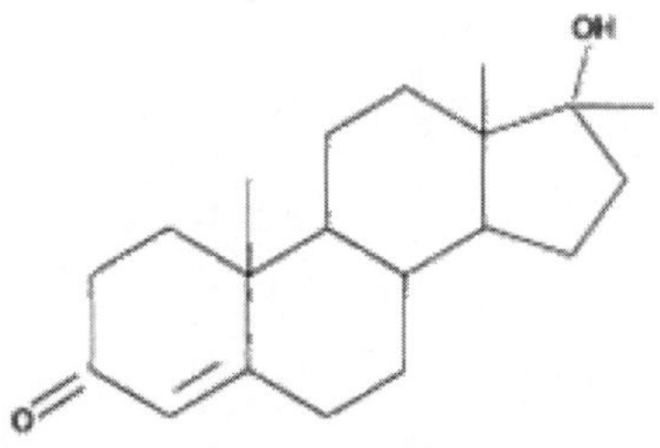

Methyltestosterone (+ 17alpha methyl)

This is the most basic derivative of testosterone, differing only by the added 17-alpha methylation that makes the steroid orally active. Conversion to 17-alpha methylestradiol makes this steroid extremely estrogenic, to spite the fact that this alteration actually reduces interaction with the aromatase enzyme.

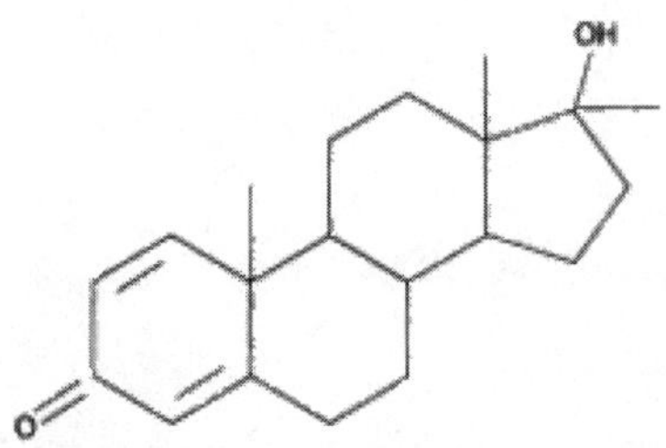

Methandrostenolone (+c 1-2 double bond; 17-alpha methyl)

In many regards, methandrostenolone is very similar to boldenone, as it too exhibits reduced estrogenic and androgenic activity due to the c1-2 double-bond. However, this steroid does have a reputation of being somewhat estrogenic though, owing to the fact that it converts to a highly active form of estrogen (17alpha-methylestradiol See: Methylated Compounds and Oral Dosing). Methandrostenolone is also much more active milligram for milligram, as the 17-alpha methyl group also gives it a longer half-life and allows it to exist in a more free state than its cousin boldenone.

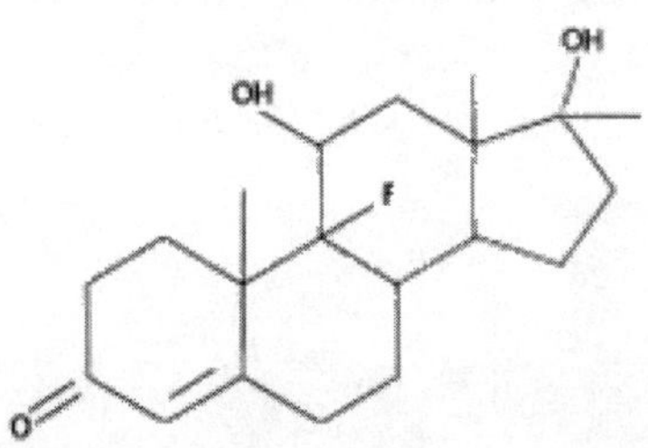

Fluoxymesterone (+11-beta hydroxyl; 9-fluoro; 17-alpha methyl)

Halotestin is a c-17alpha alkylated oral derivative of testosterone. The 11-beta group functions to inhibit aromatization, so there is no estrogen conversion at all with this steroid. It also works to lower the affinity of this steroid toward restrictive serum binding proteins. I have no explanation for the function of the 9-fluoro group at this time, however, can say that it neither blocks aromatization nor 5-alpha reduction. This is supported by the fact that other 9-fluoro steroids have been shown to aromatize, as well as studies showing fluoxymesterone to be an active substrate for the 5-alpha reductase enzyme.

Nandrolone derivatives

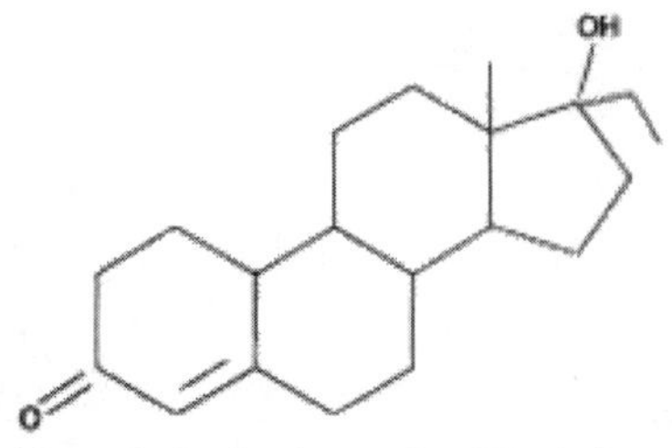

Norethandrolone (+ 17-alpha ethyl)

Norethandrolone is simply nandrolone with an added 17-alpha ethyl group. This alteration is rarely used with anabolic/androgenic steroids, and is much more commonly found with synthetic estrogens and progestins. Although 17-ethylation inhibits 17-ketosteroid reduction just as well as 17-methylation, and therefore allows this steroid to exhibit a similarly high level of oral activity, this group also tends to increase progesterone receptor binding. Norethandrolone is clearly a "troublesome" hormone in terms of water retention, fat gain and gynecomastia, which may in part be due to its heightened binding to this receptor.

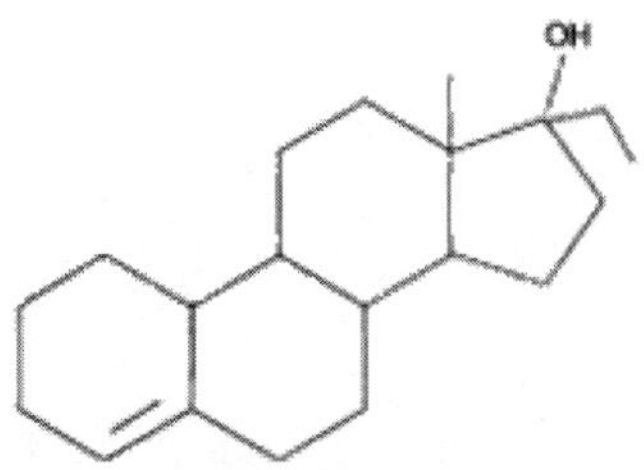

Ethylestrenol (+17-alpha ethyl; - 3 Keto)

Ethylestrenol is an oral derivative of nandrolone, very similar in structure to norethandrolone. In fact, it differs from this steroid only by the removal of the 3-keto group, which is vital to androgen receptor binding. As such, ethylestrenol is possibly the weakest steroids milligram for milligram ever sold commercially. Any activity this steroid does exhibit is likely from its conversion to norethandrolone, which does seem to occur with some affinity (apparently the 3 oxygen group is metabolically added to this compound without much trouble). This is probably the most interesting trait of ethylestrenol, which is an undistinguished compound otherwise.

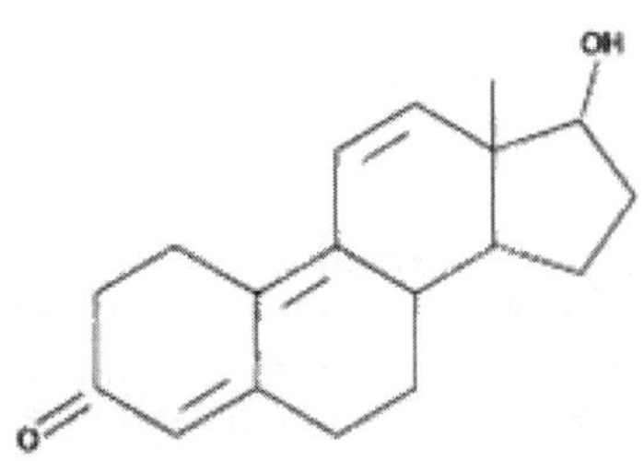

Trenbolone (+ c9-10 double bond; c11-12 double bond)

Although a derivative of nandrolone, the two additional double-bonds present on trenbolone make any similarities to its parent hormone extremely difficult to see. First, the 9-10 bond inhibits aromatization. Nandrolone is very slowly aromatized, however, some estrogen is still produced from this steroid. Not so with trenbolone. The 11-12 bond additionally increases androgen receptor binding. This steroid also does not undergo 5-alpha reduction like nandrolone, and as such does not share the same dissociation between anabolic and androgenic effects (trenbolone is much more androgenic in comparison).

Dihydrotestosterone derivatives

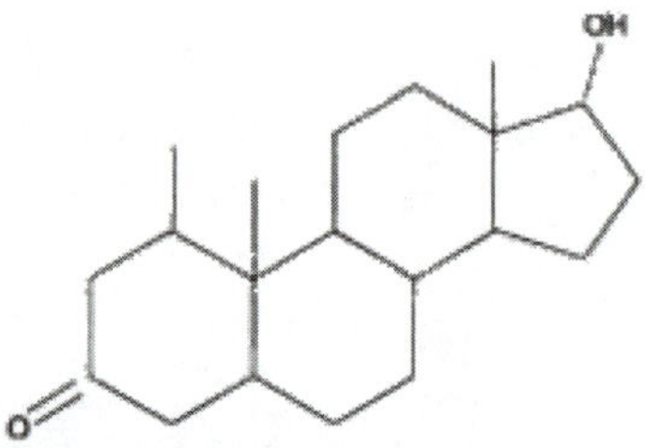

Mesterolone (+ 1-methyl)

Mesterolone is a potent orally active derivative of dihydrotestosterone. Similar to methenolone, it possesses a non-toxic 1-methyl group, which increases its resistance to hepatic breakdown. This alteration does not increase the stability of the 3-keto group however, and as such, this steroid is a poor anabolic like its parent.

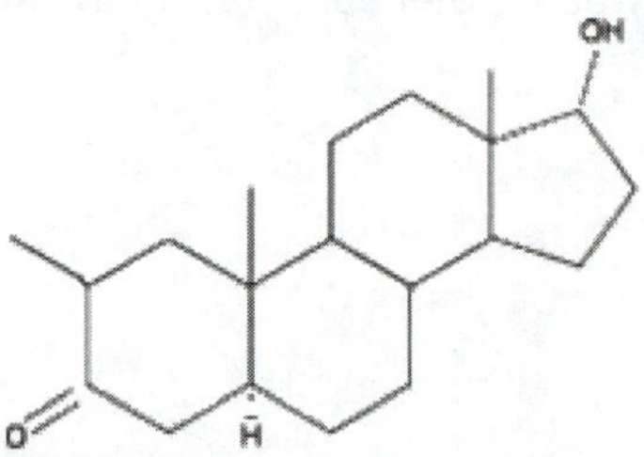

Drostanolone (+ 2-methyl)

Drostanolone is simply dihydrotestosterone with an added 2-methyl group. This addition greatly increases the stability of the 3-keto group, vital to androgen binding. As such, the activity of this steroid in muscle tissue is greatly enhanced (see: Anabolic/Androgenic Dissociation).

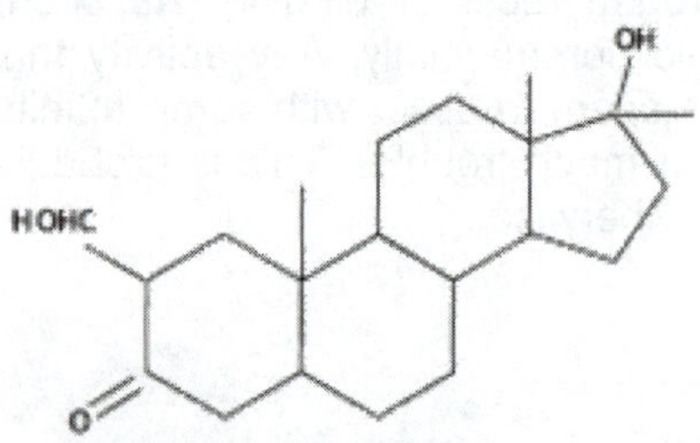

Oxymetholone (+2 hydroxymethylene; 17alpha-methyl)

Oxymetholone is an orally active derivative of dihydrotestosterone. The 17-methyl group is well understood at this point as we have discussed it with many steroids, however, the 2-hydroxymethylene group is not seen on any other commercial steroid. We do know that this group greatly enhances anabolic potency by increasing the stability of the 3-keto group, and that the configuration of this substituent also appears to allow this steroid to bind and activate the estrogen receptor.

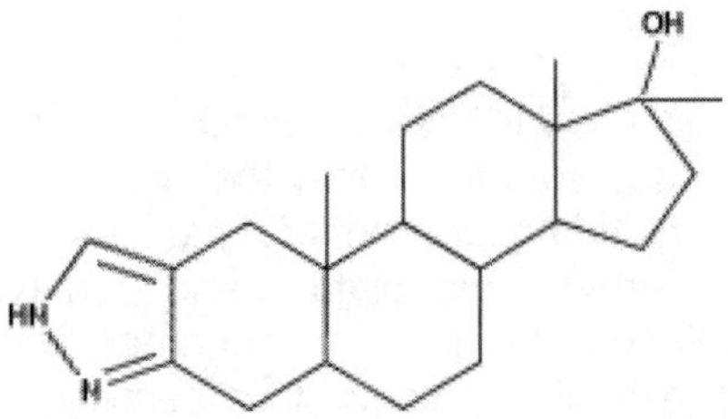

Stanozolol (+ 3,2 pyrazol; 17-alpha methyl)

Stanozolol is a potent anabolic steroid, owing to the fact that the 3-2 pyrazol group creates a stable configuration off the A-ring that allows for androgen receptor binding (this steroid is one of the few that does not possess an actual 3-keto group). As such, it is highly active in muscle tissue, unlike dihydrotestosterone.

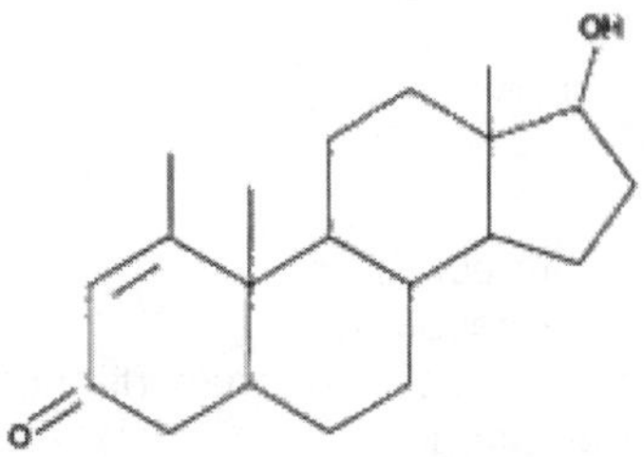

Methenolone (+ 1-methyl; 1-2 double bond).

Methenolone also is a potent anabolic steroid, due to the fact that the c1-2 double bond increases the stability of the 3-keto group. The 1-methyl group works to increase its oral bioavailability, making methenolone (as methenolone acetate) one of the few orally active non-17-alkylated orals. The c 1-2 bond may also help increase hepatic resistance (slightly) to 17-ketosteroid deactivation as well.

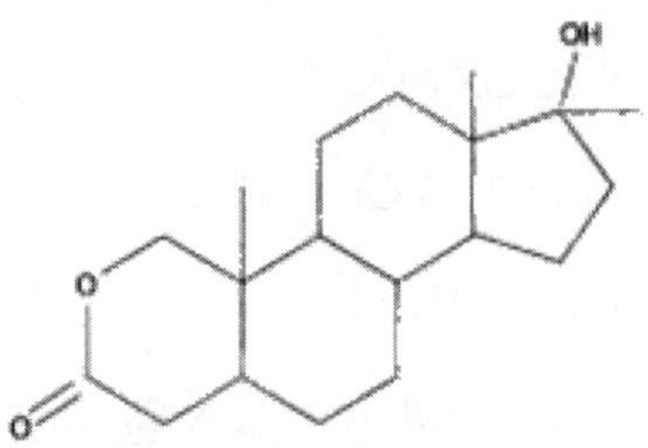

Oxandrolone (2-oxygen substitution; 17-alpha methyl)

Oxandrolone is an orally active derivative of dihydrotestosterone, due to its 17-methylation. It also differs from DHT by the substitution of its 2-carbon molecule with oxygen. This is the only commercial steroid to carry this group, and further, the only to have a modification to the base carbon structure of the Steran nucleus. The 2-oxo group increases resistance of the 3-keto group to metabolism considerably, making oxandrolone a potent anabolic.

Steroid Nomenclature

Perhaps not obvious at first glance, there is a naming convention in place that was used to create identities for the various anabolic/androgenic steroid hormones. This typically involves forming a root word to convey the structural base of the steroid, and signifying other unique structural characteristics by including appropriate prefixes or suffixes. Below, we will look at the common roots, prefixes and suffixes used in steroid nomenclature, and identify them, as they are used in the various commercial compound names. As you will see, the adoption of names like nandrolone, methandrostenolone and ethylestrenol were not as arbitrary as one might imagine. This section is also helpful if you wish to understand the deeper chemical designations for the various substances that one might find in the medical literature, which involve the exclusive use of this terminology (such as is the representation of methandrostenolone as 17b-hydroxy-17a-methylandrosta-1,4-dien-3-one).

Common prefixes and suffixes used in steroid naming:

Structural Property	Prefix	Suffix
Carbonyl (C=O)	oxo-; keto-	-one
Hydroxyl	hydroxy-	-ol
Double Bond (C=C)		-ene; -en
Methyl	meth-; methyl-	
Ethyl	eth-; ethyl-	

Common roots used in steroid naming:

Androstane	Base carbon structure of dihydrotestosterone (no double-bond)
Androstene	Base carbon structure of or similar to testosterone (one double-bond)
Androstadiene	Base carbon structure similar to methandrostenolone (two double-bonds; di-ene)
Estren; Estra *also: Norandrostene*	Base structure of nandrolone (19-norandrostene) and estrogen

Common Commercial Compound Names:

Name	***Taken From***	***Incorporated Into Name As***
Boldenone	[17b-ol, androstadiene, 3-one]	BOL DEN ONE
Ethylestrenol	[17a ethyl, estren, 17b-ol]	ETHYL ESTREN OL
Fluoxymesterone	[9-fluoro, 11b-hydroxyl, 17a-methyl, testosterone, 3-one]	FLU OXY ME STER ONE
Mesterolone	[1-methyl, dihydrotestosterone, 17b-ol, 3-one]	ME STER OL ONE
Methandienone	[1a-methyl, androstadiene, 3-one]	METH ANDIEN ONE
Methandrostenolone	[17a-methyl, androstadiene, 17b-ol, 3-one]	METH ANDROSTEN OL ONE
Methenolone	[1-methyl, c1-2 double bond (en), 17bol, 3-one]	METH EN OL ONE
Nandrolone	[norandrostene, 17b-ol, 3-one]	NANDR OL ONE
Norethandrolone	[19-nor, 17a-ethyl, (nor)androstene, 17b-ol, 3-one]	NOR ETH ANDR OL ONE
Oxandrolone	[2-oxy, androstane, 17b-ol, 2-one]	OX ANDR OL ONE
Oxymetholone	[2-hydroxymethylene, 17a-Methyl, 17b-ol, 3-one]	OXY METH OL ONE
Stanozolol	[Stanolone (androstanolone, DHT), 2-pyrazol, 17b-ol]	STANO ZOL OL
Trenbolone	[tri-en, 17b-ol, 3-one]	TREN BOL ONE

Steroid Side Effects

The action of testosterone can be both beneficial and detrimental to the body. On the plus side, this hormone has a direct impact on the growth of muscle tissues, the production of red blood cells and overall well being of the organism. But it may also negatively effect (among other things) the production of skin oils, growth of body, facial and scalp hair, and the level of both "good" and "bad" cholesterol in the body. In fact, men have a shorter average life span than women, which is believed to be largely due to the cardiovascular defects that this hormone may help bring about. Testosterone will also naturally convert to estrogen in the male body, a hormone with its own unique set of effects. As we have discussed earlier, raising the level of estrogen in men can increase the tendency to notice water retention, fat accumulation, and the development of female tissues in the breast (gynecomastia). Clearly we see that most of the "bad" side effects from steroids are simply those actions of testosterone that we are not looking for when taking a steroid. Raising the level of testosterone in the body will simply enhance both its good and bad properties, but for the most part we are not having "toxic" reactions to these drugs. A notable exception to this is the possibility of liver damage, which is a worry isolated to the use of c17-alpha alkylated oral steroids. Unless the athlete is taking anabolic/androgenic steroids abusively for a very long duration, side effects rarely amount to little more than a nuisance.

One could make a case that periodic steroid use might even be a healthy practice. Clearly a person's physical shape can relate closely to one's overall health and well being. Provided some common sense is paid to health checkups, drug choice, dosage and off-time, how can we say for certain that the user is worse off for doing so? This position is, of course, very difficult to publicly justify with steroid use being so deeply stigmatized. Since this can be a very lengthy discussion, I will save the full health, moral and legal arguments for another time. For now I would like to run down the list of popularly discussed side effects, and include any current treatment/avoidance advice where possible.

Acne

Rampant acne is one of the more obvious indicators of steroid use. As you know, teenage boys generally endure periods of irritating acne as their testosterone levels begin to peak, but this generally subsides with age. But when taking anabolic/androgenic steroids, an adult will commonly be confronted with this same problem. This is because the sebaceous glands, which secrete oils in the skin, are stimulated by androgens. Increasing the level of such hormones in the skin may therefore enhance the output of oils, often causing acne to develop on the back, shoulders, and face. The use of strongly androgenic steroids in particular can be very troublesome, in some instances resulting in very unsightly blemishes all over the skin. To treat acne, the athlete has a number of options. The most obvious is to be very diligent with washing and topical treatments, so as to remove much of the dirt and oil before the pores become clogged. If this proves insufficient, the prescription acne drug Accutaine® might be a good option. This is a very effective medication that acts on the sebaceous glands, reducing the level of oil secreted. The athlete could also take the ancillary drug Proscar®/Propecia® (finasteride) during steroid treatment, which reduces the conversion of testosterone into DHT, lowering the tendency for androgenic side effects with this hormone. It is of note however that this drug is more effective at warding off hair loss than acne, as it more specifically effects DHT conversion in the prostate and hair follicles. It is also important to note that testosterone is the only steroid that really converts to dihydrotestosterone, and only a few others actually convert to more potent steroids via the 5a-reductase enzyme at all. Many steroids are also potent androgens in their own right, such as Anadrol 50® and Dianabol. As such, they can exert strong androgenic activity in target tissues without 5a-reduction to a more potent compound, which makes Propecia® useless. One can also simply opt take primarily "anabolic" compoiunds, which impart comparable less androgenic activity. For sensitive individuals attempting to build mass, nandrolone would, therefore, be a much better option than testosterone.

Aggression

Aggressive behavior can be one of the scarier sides to steroid use. Men are typically more aggressive than women because of testosterone, and likewise the use of steroids (especially androgens) can increase a person's aggressive tendencies. In some instances this can be a benefit, helping the athlete hit the weights more intensely or perform better in a competition. Many professional powerlifters and bodybuilders take a particular liking to this effect. But on the other hand, there is nothing more unsettling than a grown man, bloated with muscle mass, who cannot control his temper. A steroid user who displays an uncontrollable rage is clearly a danger to himself and others. If an athlete is finding himself getting agitated at minor things during a steroid cycle, he should certainly find a means to keep this from getting out of hand. Remembering to take a couple of deep breaths at such times can be very helpful. If such attempts prove to be ineffective, the offending steroids should be discontinued. The bottom line is that if you lack the maturity and self-control to keep your anger in check, you should not be using steroids.

Anaphylactic Shock

Anaphylactic shock is an allergic reaction to the presence of a foreign protein in the body. It most commonly occurs when an individual has an allergy to things like a specific medication (e.g. penicillin), insect bites, industrial/household chemicals, foods (commonly nuts, shellfish, fruits) and food additives/preservatives (particularly sulfur). With this sometimes-fatal disorder the smooth muscles are stimulated to contract, which may restrict a person's breathing. Symptoms include wheezing, swelling, rash or hives, fever, a notable drop in blood pressure, dizziness, unconsciousness, convulsions or death. This reaction is not really seen with hormonal products like anabolic/androgenic steroids, but this may change with the rampant manufacture of counterfeit pharmaceuticals. Being that there are no quality controls for black market producers, toxins might indeed find their way into some preparations (particularly injectable compounds). My only advice would be to make every attempt to use only legitimately produced drug products, preferably of First World origin. When anaphylactic shock occurs, it is most commonly treated with an injection of epinephrine. Individuals very sensitive to certain insect bites are familiar with this procedure, many of whom keep an allergy kit (for the self administration of epinephrine) close at hand.

Birth Defects

Anabolic/androgenic steroids can have a very pronounced impact on the development of an unborn fetus. Adrenal Genital Syndrome in particular is a very disturbing occurrence, in which a female fetus can develop male-like reproductive organs. Women who are, or plan to become pregnant soon, should never consider the use of anabolic steroids. It would also be the best advice to stay away from these drugs completely for a number of months prior to attempting the conception of a child, so as to ensure the mother has normal hormonal chemistry. Although anabolic/androgenic steroids can reduce sperm count and male fertility, they are not linked to birth defects what taken by someone fathering a child.

Blood Clotting Changes

The use of anabolic/androgenic steroids is shown to increase prothrombin time, or the duration it will take for a blood clot to form. This basically means that while an individual is taking steroids, he/she may notice that it takes slightly longer than usual for a small cut or nosebleed to stop seeping blood. During the course of a normal day this is hardly cause for alarm, but it can lead to more serious trouble if a severe accident occurred, or an unexpected surgery was needed. Realistically, the changes in clotting time are not extremely dramatic, so athletes are usually only concerned with this side effect if planning for a surgery. The clotting changes brought about by anabolic steroids are amplified with the use of medications like Aspirin, Tylenol and especially anticoagulants, so your doctor should be informed of their use (steroids) if undergoing any notable treatment with these types of drugs.

Cancer

Although it is a popular belief that steroids can give you cancer, this is actually a very rare phenomenon. Since anabolic/androgenic steroids are synthetic version of a natural hormone that your body can metabolize quite easily, they usually place a very low level of stress on the organs. In fact, many steroidal compounds are safe to administer to individuals with a diagnosed liver condition, with little adverse effect. The only real exception to this is with the use of c17 alpha alkylated compounds, which due to their chemical alteration are somewhat liver toxic. In a small number of cases (primarily with Anadrol 50®), this toxicity has lead to severe liver damage and subsequently cancer. But we are speaking of a statistically insignificant number in the face millions of athletes who use steroids. These cases also tended to be very ill patients, not athletes, who were using extremely large dosages for prolonged periods of time. Steroid opponents will sometimes point out the additional possibility of developing Wilm's Tumor from steroid abuse, which is a very serious form of kidney cancer. Such cases are so rare however, that no direct link between anabolic/androgenic steroid use and this disease has been conclusively established. Provided the athlete is not abusing methylated oral substances, and is visiting a doctor during heavier cycles, cancer should not be much of a concern.

Cardiovascular Disease

As mentioned earlier, the use of anabolic/androgenic steroids may have an impact on the level of LDL (low density lipoprotein), HDL (high density lipoprotein) and total cholesterol values. As you probably know, HDL is considered the "good" cholesterol since it can act to remove cholesterol deposits from the arteries. LDL has the opposite effect, aiding in the buildup of cholesterol on the artery walls. The general pattern seen with steroid use is a lowering of HDL concentrations, while total and LDL cholesterol numbers increase. The ratio of HDL to LDL values is usually more important than one's total cholesterol count, as these two substances seem to balance each other in the body. If these changes are exacerbated by the long-term use of steroidal compounds, it can clearly be detrimental to the cardiovascular system. This may be additionally heightened by a rise in blood pressure, which is common with the use of strongly aromatizable compounds.

It is also important to note that due to their structure and form of administration, most 17alpha alkylated oral steroids have a much stronger negative impact on these levels compared to injectable steroids. Using a milder drug like Winstrol® (stanozolol), in hopes HDL level changes will also be mild, may therefore not turn out to be the best option. One study comparing the effect of a weekly injection of 200mg testosterone enanthate vs. only a 6mg daily oral dose of Winstrol® demonstrates this well[41]. After only six weeks, stanozolol was shown to reduce HDL and HDL-2 (good) cholesterol by an average of 33% and 71% respectively. The HDL reduction (HDL-3 subfraction) with the testosterone group was only an average of 9%. LDL (bad) cholesterol also rose 29% with stanozolol, while it actually dropped 16% with the use of testosterone. Those concerned with cholesterol changes during steroid use may likewise wish to avoid oral steroids, and opt for the use of injectable compounds exclusively.

We must also note that estrogens generally have a favorable impact on cholesterol profiles. For example, estrogen replacement therapy in postmenopausal women is regularly linked to a rise in HDL cholesterol and a reduction in LDL values. Likewise the aromatization of testosterone to estradiol may be beneficial in preventing a more dramatic change in serum cholesterol due to the presence of the hormone. A recent study investigated just this question by comparing the effects of testosterone alone (280 mg testosterone enanthate weekly), vs. the same dose combined with an aromatase inhibitor (250mg testolactone 4 times daily)[42]. Methyltestosterone was also tested in a third group, at a dose of 20mg daily. The results were quite enlightening. The group using only testosterone enanthate showed no significant decrease in HDL cholesterol values over the course of the 12-week study. After only four weeks, the group using testosterone plus an aromatase inhibitor displayed a reduction on average of 25%. The methyltestosterone group noted an HDL reduction of 35% by this point, and also noted an unfavorable rise in LDL cholesterol. This clearly should make us think a little more closely about estrogen maintenance during steroid therapy. Aside from deciding whether or not it is actually necessary in any given circumstance, drug choice may also be an important consideration. For example, the estrogen receptor antagonist Nolvadex® does not seem to exhibit antiestrogenic effects on cholesterol values, and in fact often raises HDL levels. Using this to combat the side effects of estrogen instead of an aromatase inhibitor such as Arimidex® or Cytadren® may therefore be a good idea, particularly for those who are using steroids for longer periods of time.

Since heart disease is one of the top killers worldwide, steroid using athletes (particularly older individuals) should not ignore these risks. If nothing else it is a very good idea to have your blood pressure and cholesterol values measured during each heavy cycle, making sure to discontinue the drugs should a problem become evident. It is also advisable to limit the intake of foods high in saturated fats and cholesterol, which should help minimize the impact of steroid treatment. Since blood pressure and cholesterol levels will usually revert back to their pre-treated norms soon after steroids are withdrawn, long-term damage is not a common worry.

Depression

Obviously steroid use will have an impact on hormone levels in the body, which in turn may result in a change in one's general disposition or mood. On the one hand, we might see very aggressive behavior. But for some people there is also, at times, the other extreme side, depression. This can occur in certain individuals, whom are psychologically sensitive to an imbalance in androgen and estrogen levels. This is most common with male bodybuilders, at times when anabolic/androgenic steroids are discontinued. Given a deeply suppressed endogenous testosterone level, it may take time for one's normal hormonal balance to return. During this period, estrogen levels may be more stable than testosterone, as our bodies can produce it from adrenal hormones. The result may be a protracted window of time where estrogen seems to be the more dominant sex hormone. For some, this window can be filled with feelings of emotional sensitivity, sadness, and lack of motivation (symptoms of depression).

Depression may also occur during the course of a steroid cycle, particularly with the sole use of anabolics. Although these compounds are mild in comparison to androgens, many can still suppress the endogenous production of testosterone. If the testosterone level drops significantly during treatment, the administered anabolics may not provide enough of an androgen level to compensate, and a marked loss of motivation and sense of well-being may result. The best advice when looking to avoid cycle or post-cycle depression is to closely monitor drug intake and withdrawal. The use of a small weekly testosterone dose might prove very effective if added to a mild dieting/anabolic cycle, warding off feelings of boredom and apathy to training. Of course a strong steroid cycle should always be discontinued with the proper use of ancillary drugs (Nolvadex®, Arimidex®, HCG, Clomid® etc.). Although tapering schedules are very common, they are not an effective way to restore endogenous testosterone levels.

Gynecomastia

Gynecomastia is the medical term for the development of female breast tissues in the male body. This occurs when the male is presented with an unusually high level of estrogen, particularly with the use of strong aromatizing androgens such as testosterone and Dianabol. The excess estrogen can act upon receptors in the breast and stimulate the growth of mammary tissues. If left unchecked, this can lead to an actual obvious and unsightly tissue growth under the nipple area, in many cases taking on a very feminine appearance. To fight this side effect during steroid therapy, many find it necessary the use some form of estrogen maintenance medication. This includes an estrogen antagonist such as Clomid® or Nolvadex®, which blocks estrogen from attaching to and activating receptors in the breast and other tissues, or an aromatase inhibitor such as Femara® or Arimidex®, which blocks the enzyme responsible for the conversion of androgens to estrogens. Aromatase inhibitors like this are currently the most effective options, but also the most costly.

It is worth noting however, that many believe a slightly elevated estrogen level may help the athlete achieve a more pronounced muscle mass gain during a cycle (see: Estrogen Aromatization). With this in mind many athletes decide to use anti-estrogens only when it is necessary to block gynecomastia. It is of course still a good idea to always keep an anti-estrogen on-hand when administering an aromatizable steroid, so that it is readily accessible should trouble become evident. Puffiness or swelling under the nipple is one of the first signs of pending gynecomastia, often accompanied by pain or soreness in this region (an effect termed gynecodynea). This is a clear indicator that some type of anti-estrogen is needed. If the swelling progresses into small, marble like lumps, action absolutely must be taken immediately to treat it. Otherwise, if the steroids are continued at this point without ancillary drug use, the user will likely be stuck with unsightly tissue growth that can only be removed with a surgical procedure.

It is also important to mention that progestins seem to augment the stimulatory effect of estrogens on mammary tissue growth. There appears to be a strong synergy between these two hormones here, such that gynecomastia might even be able to occur with the help of progestins, without excessive estrogen levels being necessary. Since many anabolic steroids, particularly those derived from nandrolone, are known to have progestational activity, we must not be lulled into a false sense of security. Even a low estrogen producer like Deca can potentially cause gyno in certain cases, again fostering the need to keep anti-estrogens close at hand if you are very sensitive to this side effect.

Hair loss

The use of highly androgenic steroids can negatively impact the growth of scalp hair. In fact, the most common form of male pattern hair loss is directly linked to the level of androgens in such tissues, most specifically the stronger DHT metabolite of testosterone. The technical term for this type of hair loss is androgenetic alopecia, which refers to the interplay of both the male androgenic hormones and a genetic predisposition in bringing about this condition. Those who suffer from this disorder are shown to posses finer hair follicles and higher levels of DHT in comparison to a normal, hairy scalp. But since there is a genetic factor involved, many individuals will not ever see signs of this side-effect, even with heavy steroid use. Clearly those individuals who are suffering from (or have a familial predisposition for) this type of hair loss should be very cautious when using the stronger drugs like testosterone, Anadrol 50®, Halotestin® and Dianabol.

In many instances, the renewal of lost hair can be very difficult, so avoiding this side-effect before it occurs is the best advice. For those who need to worry, the decision should probably be made to either stick with milder substances (Deca-Durabolin® most favored), or use the ancillary drug Propecia®/Proscar® (finasteride) when taking testosterone, methyltestosterone or Halotestin. Propecia® is a very effective hair loss medication, which inhibits the 5-alpha reductase enzyme specifically in the hair follicles and prostate. However, it offers us little benefit with drugs that are highly androgenic without 5alpha reduction, the most notable offenders being Anadrol

50® and Dianabol. We must also remember that all anabolic/androgenic steroids activate the androgen receptor, and can, likewise, all promote hair loss given the right dosage and conditions.

Headaches

Athletes sometimes report an increased frequency of headaches when using anabolic/androgenic steroids. This seems to be most common during heavier bulking cycles, when an individual is utilizing strongly estrogenic compounds. One should not simply take an aspirin and ignore this problem, as it is may indicate a more troubling side effect of steroid use, high blood pressure. Since high blood pressure invites a number of unwanted health risks, monitoring it on a regular schedule is important during heavy steroid use, especially if the individual is experiencing headaches. Some athletes choose to lower their blood pressure in such cases with a prescription medication like Catapres, but most find this an appropriate time to discontinue steroid use. Milder anabolics, which generally display little or no ability to convert to estrogen, are also more acceptable options for individuals sensitive to blood pressure increases. Less seriously, many headaches are due to simple strain on the neck and scalp muscles. The athlete may be lifting with much more intensity during a steroid cycle, and as a result may place added strain on these muscles. In this case, a short break from training, and some general rest, will often take care of the problem. Of course if anyone is experiencing a very serious or persistent headache, a visit to the doctor may be in order.

High Blood Pressure/Hypertension

Athletes using anabolic/androgenic steroids will commonly notice a rise in blood pressure during treatment. High blood pressure is most often associated with the use of steroids that have a high affinity for estrogen conversion, such as testosterone and Dianabol. As estrogen builds in the body, the level of water and salt retention will typically elevate and lead to increased blood pressure. This may be further amplified by the added stress of intense weight training and rapid weight gain. Since hypertension (high blood pressure) can place a great deal of stress on the body, this side effect should not be ignored. If it is left untreated, high blood pressure can increase the likelihood for heart disease, stroke or kidney failure. Warning signs that one may be suffering from hypertension include an increased tendency to develop headaches, insomnia or breathing difficulties. In many instances these symptoms do not become evident until BP is seriously elevated, so a lack of these signs is no guarantee that the user is safe. Obtaining your blood pressure reading is a very quick and easy procedure (either at a doctors office, pharmacy or home); steroid-using athletes should certainly be monitoring BP values during stronger cycles so as to avoid potential problems.

If an individual's blood pressure values are becoming notably elevated, some action should/must be taken to control it. The most obvious is to avoid the continued use of the offending steroids, or at least to substitute them with milder, non-aromatizing compounds. It is also of note that although aromatizing steroids are typically involved, nonaromatizing androgens like Halotestin® or trenbolone are occasionally also linked to high blood pressure, so these are perhaps not the ideal alternatives in such a situation. The athlete also has the option of seeking the benefit of high blood pressure medications such as diuretics, which can dramatically lower water and salt retention. Catapres (clonidine HCL) is also a popular medication among athletes, because in addition to its blood pressure lowering properties, it has also been documented to raise the body's output of growth hormone.

Immune System Changes

The use of anabolic/androgenic steroids has been shown to produce changes in the body that may impact an individual's immune system. These changes can be both good and bad for the user. For instance, during steroid treatment, many athletes find they are less susceptible to viral illnesses. New studies involving the use of compounds like oxandrolone and Deca-Durabolin® with HIV+ patients seem to support this claim, clearly showing that these drugs can have a beneficial effect on the immune system. Such therapies are, in fact, catching on in recent years, and many doctors are now less reluctant to prescribe these drugs to their ill patients. But just as a person may be less apt to notice illness during steroid treatment, the discontinuance of steroids can produce a rebound effect in which the immune system is less able to fight off pathogens. This most likely coincides with the rebound activity/production of cortisol, a catabolic hormone in the body, which may act to suppress immune system functioning. When the administered steroids are withdrawn, an androgen deficient state is often endured until the body is able to rebalance hormone production. Since testosterone and cortisol seem counter each other's activity in many ways, the absence of a normal androgen level may place cortisol in an unusually active state. During this period of imbalance, cortisol will not only be stripping the body of muscle mass, but may also cause the athlete to be more susceptible to colds, flu, etc. The proper use of ancillary drugs (anti-estrogens, testosterone stimulating drugs) is the most common suggestion for helping to avoid this problem, which will hopefully allow the user to restore a proper balance of hormones once the steroids are removed.

We also cannot ignore the other possibility that steroids could actually increase cortisol levels in the body during treatment. Termed hypercortisolemia, this effect is a common occurrence with anabolic/androgenic steroid therapy. This is because anabolic/androgenic steroids may interfere with the ability for the body to clear corticosteroids from circulation, due to the fact that in their respective pathways of metabolism these hormones share certain enzymes. When overloaded with androgens competing for the same enzymes, cortisol may be broken down at a slower rate, and levels of this hormone will in turn begin to build. Due to their strong tendency to inhibit the activity of the 3beta hydroxysteroid dehydrogenase enzyme, oral c17 alpha alkylated orals may be particularly troublesome in regards to elevated cortisol levels, as again this is a common pathway for corticosteroid metabolism. Though an elevated cortisol level is not a common concern during typical steroid cycles, problems can certainly become evident when these drugs are used at very high doses or for prolonged periods of time. This, of course, may lead to the athlete becoming "run-down" and more susceptible to illness, as well as foster a more over-trained and static (less anabolic) state of metabolism.

Kidney Stress/Damage

Since your kidneys are involved in the filtration and removal of byproducts from the body, the administration of steroidal compounds (which are largely excreted in the urine) may cause them some strain. Actual kidney damage is most likely to occur when the steroid user is suffering from severe high blood pressure, as this state can place an undue amount of stress on these organs. There is actually evidence to suggest that steroid use can be linked to the onset of Wilm's Tumor in adults, which is a rapidly growing kidney tumor normally seen in children and infants. However, such cases are so rare that no conclusive link has been established. Obviously the kidneys are vital to one's heath, so the possibility of any kind of damage (although low) should not be ignored during heavy steroid treatment. If the user is noticing a darkening of color (in some cases a distinguishable amount of blood), or pain/difficulty when urinating, kidneys strain might be a legitimate concern. Other warning signs include pain in the lower back (particularly in the kidney areas), fever and edema (swelling). If organ damage is feared, the administered steroidal compounds should be discontinued immediately, and the doctor paid a visit to rule out any serious trouble.

Since kidney stress/damage is generally associated with the use of stronger aromatizing compounds such as testosterone and Dianabol (which often raise blood pressure), individuals sensitive to high blood pressure/kidney stress should avoid such compounds until health concerns are safely addressed. If steroid use is still necessitated by the individual, it may be a good idea to avoid the stronger compounds and opt for one of the milder anabolics. Primobolan®, Anavar and Winstrol®, for example, do not convert to estrogen at all, and may be acceptable options. Also favorable drugs in this regard are Deca-Durabolin® and Equipoise®, which have only a low tendency to convert to estrogen.

Liver Stress/Damage

Liver stress/damage is not a side-effect of steroid use in general, but is specifically associated with the use of c17 alpha alkylated compounds. As mentioned earlier, these structures contain chemical alterations that enable them to be administered orally. In surviving a first pass by the liver, these compounds place some level of stress on the organ. In some instances, this has led to severe damage, even fatal liver cancer. The disease peliosis hepatitis is one worry, which is an often life-threatening condition where the liver develops blood-filled cysts. Liver cancer (hepatic carcinoma) has also been noted in certain cases. While these very serious complications have occurred on certain occasions where liver-toxic compounds were prescribed for extended periods, it is important to stress that this is not very common with steroid using athletes. Most of the documented cases of liver cancer have in fact been in clinical situations, particularly with the use of the powerful oral androgen Anadrol 50® (oxymetholone). This may be directly related to the high dosage of this preparation, as Anadrol 50® contains a whopping 50mg of active steroid per tablet. This is a considerable jump from other oral preparations, most of which contain 5mg or less of a substance. With one Anadrol 50® tablet, the liver will therefore have to process (roughly) the equivalent of 10 Dianabol tablets. This obvious stress is further amplified when we look at the unusually high dosage schedule for ill patients receiving this medication. With Anadrol 50®, the manufacturer's recommendations may call for the use of as many as 8 or 10 tablets daily. This is a far greater amount than most athletes would ever think of consuming, with three or four tablets per day being considered the upper limit of safety. It is also important to note that the actual number of cases involving liver damage have been few, and have not been a significant enough of a problem to warrant discontinuing this compound. Methyltestosterone, the first steroid shown to cause liver trouble, is also still available as a prescription drug in this country. The average recreational steroid user who takes toxic orals at moderate dosages for relatively short periods is therefore unlikely to face devastating liver damage.

Although severe liver damage may occur before the onset of noticeable symptoms, it is common to notice jaundice during the early stages of such injury. Jaundice is characterized by the buildup of bilirubin in the body, which in this case will usually result from the obstruction of bile ducts in the liver. The individual will typically notice a yellowing of the skin and eye whites as this colored substance builds in the body tissues, a clear sign to terminate the use of any c17 alpha alkylated steroids. In most instances, the immediate withdrawal of these compounds is sufficient to reverse and prevent any further damage. Of course, the athlete should avoid using orals for an extended period of time, if not indefinitely, should jaundice occur repeatedly during treatment. It is also a good idea to visit your physician during oral treatment in order to monitor liver enzyme values. Since liver stress will be reflected in your enzyme counts well before jaundice is noticed, this can remove much of the worry with oral steroid treatment.

Prostate Enlargement

Prostate cancer is currently one of the most common forms of cancer in males. Benign prostate enlargement (a swelling of prostate tissues often interfering with urine flow) can precede/coincide this cancer, and is clearly an important medical concern for men who are aging. Prostate complications are believed to be primarily dependent on androgenic hormones; particularly the strong testosterone metabolite DHT in normal situations, much in the same way estrogen is linked to breast cancer in women. Although the connection between prostate enlargement/cancer and steroid use is not fully established, the use of steroids may theoretically aggravate such conditions by raising the level of androgens in the body. It is, therefore, a good idea for older athletes to limit/avoid the intake of strong 5-alpha reducible androgens like testosterone, methyltestosterone and Halotestin, or otherwise use Proscar® (finasteride), which was specifically designed to inhibit the 5-alpha reductase enzyme in scalp and prostate tissues. This may be an effective preventative measure for older athletes who insist on using these compounds. However, drugs like Dianabol, Anadrol 50® and Proviron, which do not convert to DHT yet are still potent androgens, are not effected by its use. It is also important to mention that not only androgens, but also estrogens, are necessary for the advancement of this condition. It appears that the two work synergistically to stimulate benign prostatic growth, such that one without the other would not be enough to cause it. It has, therefore, been suggested that a non-aromatizable compound like DHT may be a safer option for older men looking for androgen replacement therapy than testosterone. Anti-estrogens might even turn out to be more effective at treating BPH than a drug like finasteride, which is used to lower androgenic activity in the prostate. Estrogen suppression is easier to accomplish in males, and should be accompanied with less side effects. It would also be very sound advice, regardless of steroid use, for individuals over 40 to have a physician check the prostate on a regular basis.

Sexual Dysfunction

The functioning of the male reproductive system depends greatly on the level of androgenic hormones in the body. Therefore, the use of synthetic male hormones may have a dramatic impact on an individual's sexual wellness. On one extreme, we may see a man's libido and erection frequency become significantly heightened. This is most commonly seen with the use of strongly androgenic steroids, which seem to have the most dramatic stimulating impact on this system. In some instances, this can reach the point of becoming problematic, although more often than not, the athlete is simply much more active and sexually aggressive during the intake of steroids.

On the other extreme, we may also see a lack of sexual interest, possibly to the point of impotency. This occurs mainly when androgenic hormones are very low. This will often happen after a steroid cycle is discontinued, as the endogenous production of testosterone is commonly suppressed during the cycle. Removing the androgen (from an outside source) leaves the body with little natural testosterone until this imbalance is corrected. The loss of its' metabolite DHT is particularly troubling, as this hormone may have a strong affect on the reproductive system that may not be apparent with other less androgenic hormones. Therefore, it is a very good idea to use testosterone-stimulating drugs like HCG and/or Clomid®/Nolvadex® when coming off of a strong cycle, so as to reduce the impact of steroid withdrawal. Impotency/sexual apathy may also occur during the course of a steroid cycle, particularly when it is based strictly on anabolic compounds. Since all "anabolics" can suppress the manufacture of testosterone in the body, the administered drugs may not be androgenic enough to properly compensate for the testosterone loss. In such a case, the user might opt to include a small androgen dosage (perhaps a weekly testosterone injection), or again reverse/prevent the androgen suppression with the use of a medication like HCG.

It is also interesting to note that it is not always simply an androgen vs. anabolic issue. People will often respond very differently to an equal dose of the same drug. While one individual may notice sexual disinterest or impotency, another may become extremely aggressive. It is, therefore, difficult to predict how someone will react to a particular drug before having used it.

Stunted Growth

Many anabolic/androgenic steroids have the potential to impact an individual's stature if taken during adolescence. Specifically, steroids can stunt growth by stimulating the epiphyseal plates in a person's long bones to prematurely fuse. Once these plates are fused, future linear growth is not possible. Even if the individual avoids steroid use subsequently, the damage is irreversible and he/she can be stuck at the same height forever. Not even the use of growth hormone can reverse this, as this powerful hormone can only thicken bones when used during adulthood. Interestingly enough, it is not the steroids themselves, but the buildup of estrogen that causes the epiphyseal plates to fuse. Women are shorter than men on average because of this effect of estrogen, and likewise the use of steroids that readily convert to estrogen can prematurely suppress/halt a person's growth. In fact, the use of steroids like Anavar, Winstrol® and Primobolan® (which do not convert to estrogen) can actually increase one's height if taken during adolescence, as their anabolic effects will promote the retention of calcium in the bones. This would also hold true for non-aromatizing androgens such as trenbolone, Proviron® and Halotestin®. It is still good common sense to advise adolescents to avoid steroid use, at least until their bodies are fully mature and steroid use will have a less dramatic impact.

Testicular Atrophy

The human body always prefers to remain in a very balanced hormonal state, a tendency known as homeostasis. When the administration of androgens from an outside source causes a surplus of hormone, it will cause the body to stop manufacturing its own testosterone. Specifically, this happens via a feedback mechanism where the hypothalamus detects a high level of sex steroids (including androgens, progestins and estrogens) and shuts off the release of GnRH (Gonadotropin Releasing Hormone, formerly referred to as luteinizing hormone releasing hormone). This, in turn, causes the pituitary to stop releasing luteinizing hormone and FSH (follicle stimulating hormone), the two hormones (primarily LH) that stimulate the Leydig's cells in the testes to release testosterone (negative feedback inhibition has been demonstrated at the pituitary level as well). Without stimulation by LH and FSH, the testes will be in a state of production limbo, and may shrink from inactivity. In extreme cases the steroid user can notice testicles that are unusually and frighteningly small. However, this effect is temporary, and once the drugs are removed (and hormone levels rebalanced) the testicles should return to their original size. Many regular steroid users find this side-effect quite troubling, and use HCG during a steroid cycle in order to try to maintain testicular activity (and size) during treatment. The more estrogenic androgens (testosterone, Anadrol 50® and Dianabol) are most dramatic in this regard, and are therefore poor choices for individuals who seriously want to avoid testicle shrinkage. Non-aromatizing anabolics would be a better option, however be warned that all steroids will have an impact on the production of testosterone if taken at an anabolically effective dosage (yes, even Anavar and Primobolan®).

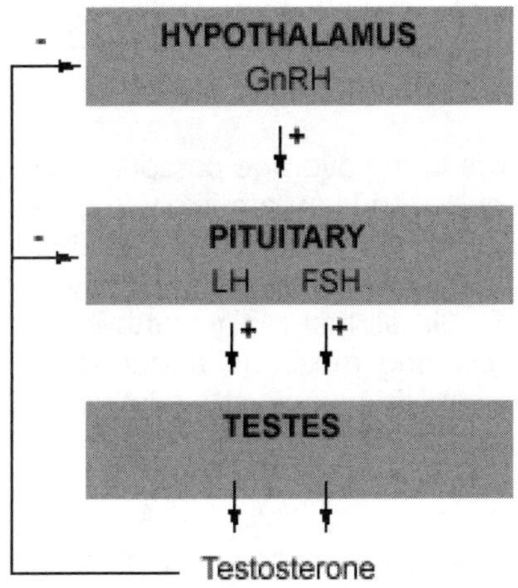

The Hypothalamic-Pituitary-Testicular Axis: The hypothalamus releases Gonadotropin Releasing Hormone, which stimulates the pituitary to release luteinizing hormone and follicle stimulating hormone. This promotes the release of testosterone from the testes. Testosterone, as well as estrogens and progestins, in turn cause negative feedback inhibition at the hypothalamus (and to some extent the pituitary).

Water and Salt Retention

Many anabolic/androgenic steroids can increase the amount of water and sodium stored in body tissues. In some instances, steroid induced water retention can bring about a very bloated appearance to the body (hands, arms, face etc.), which will also reduce the visibility of muscle features (loss of definition). Athletes often ignore this side effect, particularly during bulking cycles when the excess water stored in the muscles, joints and connective tissues will help to improve an individual's overall strength. With the use of many strong androgens, water retention can account for much of the initial strength and body weight gain during steroid treatment, with "water-weight" sometimes amounting to ten or more pounds.

Although water retention may not be the most unwelcome side effect during a bulking cycle (greater strength and mass), it can lead to dangerous problems such as high blood pressure and kidney damage. The body is clearly under more strain when dealing with an unusually high level of water, so athletes should not simply ignore this. Water retention is most specifically associated with the presence of estrogen in the body, and is therefore common with the use of aromatizing compounds (such as testosterone and Dianabol). If water retention becomes an obvious problem during a cycle, the use of an anti-estrogen (Nolvadex®, Proviron®) may help minimize it. An antiaromatase like Arimidex® is, in fact, the most effective option, a drug that inhibits the conversion of testosterone to estrogen. Sometimes the athlete will alternately opt to use a diuretic, which can rapidly shed the water so as to achieve a more comfortable/attractive physique in a short period of time. This is a common practice when preparing for a competition, as diuretic use allows the user a great level of control over water stores. Of course, discontinuing the offending compounds, or substituting them with a milder anabolic would be the simplest option for recreational steroid users.

Virilization

Since anabolic/androgenic steroids are synthetic male hormones, they can produce a number of undesirable changes when introduced into the female body. This includes the possibility of "virilization", which refers to the tendency for women to develop masculine characteristics when taking these drugs. Virilization symptoms include a deepening or hoarsening of the voice, changes in skin texture, acne, menstrual irregularities, increased libido, hair loss (scalp), body/facial/pubic hair growth and an enlargement of the clitoris. In extreme cases the female genitalia can become very disfigured, and may actually take on a penis-like appearance. Clearly, women must be very careful when considering the use of steroids, especially since most virilization symptoms are irreversible. The stronger androgenic compounds should be off-limits, with cautious female athletes restricting themselves to the use of only mild anabolics such as Winstrol®, Primobolan®, Anavar and Durabolin® (the shorter acting nandrolone). Nandrolone is actually the preferred hormone, as it displays the lowest level of androgenic to anabolic activity. Since even these milder anabolics have the potential to cause problems, users should additionally remember to be conservative with drug dosages and duration of intake. After each cycle a notable break from treatment would be a good idea as well, so that the body has sufficient time to reestablish a hormonal balance.

Steroid Safety: Studies with Real-World Dosages

If you so much as mention anabolic steroids to the average person, you usually get some cross looks in response. State that you are actually considering a cycle, and you are likely to be lectured about the tremendous heath risks you are about to undertake; how your hair might fall out and testicles disappear, or your body eaten away by cancer. Or maybe you will just lose you mind to uncontrolled fits of psychotic rage, or suffer a life-threatening heart attack. You'll probably hear something like, "Is all that really worth it... to build a little more muscle?" Clearly, the American public has been given a very strong message about steroids: stay far away from them, they are DEADLY! You can't convince too many people that smoking a joint will *REALLY* cause a 16-year-old kid to pull out his dad's gun and shoot his friend in the face, but, for some reason, the "over the top" anti-drug message with steroids seems to have worked. Most people are terrified of them.

Those actually taking anabolic steroids usually see things very differently. They believe the dangers are terribly exaggerated in the media. In fact, these athletes will routinely point out that the medical literature for the past 50 years fails to make much note of any serious consequences of steroid use, with most clinical studies looking quite favorably on these drugs. Steroid opponents, on the other hand, will still make sure you know that bodybuilders take much larger doses of steroids than those used in medical situations; therefore, in much greater danger than the patients using them. Who is right? Is that occasional cycle really a serious health risk? This month I would like to touch on this debate by looking closely at three medical studies that were published recently. They concern not small clinical doses, but a level of steroid usage that any recreational bodybuilder would recognize as sufficient for building muscle. Many markers of safety are assessed in these papers, giving us a fairly good indication of what dangers, realistically, are presented.

600mg/wk of Testosterone

The first is a testosterone dose-response study published in the American Journal of Physiology Endocrinology and Metabolism in July of 2001, which looked at the effects of various doses of testosterone enanthate on body composition, muscle size, strength, power, sexual and cognitive functions, and various markers of health[43]. 61 normal men, ages 18-35, participated in this investigation. They were divided into five groups, with each receiving weekly injections of 25, 50, 125, 300 or 600 milligrams for a period of 20 weeks. This treatment period was preceded by a control (no drug) period of 4 weeks, and followed by a recovery period of 16 weeks. Markers of strength and lean body mass gains were the greatest with larger doses of testosterone, with the 600mg group gaining slightly over 17 pounds of fat-free mass on average over the 20 weeks of steroid therapy. There were no significant changes in prostate-specific antigen (PSA), liver enzymes (liver stress), sexual activity, or cognitive functioning at any dose. The only negative trait noted was a slight HDL (good) cholesterol reduction in all groups except those taking 25mg. The worst reduction of 9 points was noted in the 600mg group, which still averaged 34 points after 20 weeks of treatment. All groups, except this one, remained in the normal reference range for males (40-59 points).

600mg/wk of Nandrolone

Next we look at a study conducted with HIV+ men, which charted the lean-mass-building effects of nandrolone decanoate[44]. 30 people participated in this investigation, with each given the same (high) weekly dose of this drug. Half underwent resistance training so that two groups (trained and untrained) were formed. The dosing schedule was quite formidable, beginning with 200mg on the first week, 400mg on the second, and 600mg for the remaining 10 weeks of peak therapy. Doses were slowly reduced from weeks 13 to 16 to withdraw patients slowly from the drug. Potential negative metabolic changes were looked at closely including cholesterol and lipid levels (including subfractions of HDL and LDL), triglycerides, insulin sensitivity and fasting glucose levels. Even with the high dosages used here, no negative changes were noted in total or LDL cholesterol, triglycerides, or insulin sensitivity. In fact, the group also undergoing resistance exercise noticed significant improvements in LDL particle size distribution, lipoprotein(a) levels, and triglyceride values, which all indicate improved cardiovascular disease risk. Carbohydrate metabolism was also significantly improved in this group. The only negative impact noted during this study was a reduction in HDL (good) cholesterol values similar to that noted with the testosterone study, with an 8-10 point reduction noted between both groups.

100mg/day of Anadrol

Lastly, we find a study looking at the potent oral steroid oxymetholone (Anadrol)[45]. This steroid is thought by bodybuilders to be one of the most dangerous ones around, who as a group seem to treat it with both a lot of respect and caution. It is not common to find them exceeding the doses and intake durations of this investigation, making it a very good representation of real-world Anadrol usage. This study involves 31 elderly men, between the ages of 65 and 80. The men were divided into three groups, with each taking 50mg, 100mg or placebo daily for a 12-week period. Changes in lean body mass and strength were measured, as well as common markers of safety including total, LDL and HDL cholesterol levels, serum triglycerides, PSA (prostate-specific antigen) and liver enzymes. Muscle mass and strength gains were again relative to the dosage taken, with the end results being similar to those noted with 20 weeks of testosterone enanthate therapy at 125mg or 300mg per week (about 6.4 and 12 lb of lean body mass gained for the 50mg and 100mg doses respectively). There were no significant changes in PSA, total or LDL cholesterol values, or fasting triglycerides; however, there was a significant reduction in HDL cholesterol values (reduced 19 and 23 points for the 50mg and 100mg groups respectively). Liver enzymes (transaminases AST and ALT) increased only in the 100mg group, but the changes were not dramatic, and were not accompanied by hepatic enlargement or the development of any serious liver condition.

Adding It All Up

One hundred and twenty one men participated in these three studies, which involved the use of high doses of steroids for periods of three to five months. It may be shocking to most of the staunch opponents of steroid use, but all of the men participating were still alive at the conclusion of their respective investigations. An unbiased assessment of the metabolic changes and health risks does not seem to reveal any short-term significant dangers. The main negative impact of steroid use in all three cases was a reduction in good (HDL) cholesterol values, which is a legitimate concern when it comes to assessing one's risk for developing cardiovascular disease. However, it is uncertain if a short-lived increase in this particular risk factor will relate to any tangible damage to one's health. It is also unknown how much, if any of this is offset by the other positive metabolic changes that were seen to accompany combined steroid use and exercise. Logic would seem to suggest that the very periodic use of steroids, under parameters similar to these studies, should entail relatively minimal risks to ones health overall. At the very least, it is extremely difficult to argue that an isolated cycle with a moderate drug dose, such as those used here, is tantamount to playing Russian roulette with your body, as most media campaigns against the use of these drugs would seem to suggest.

PART II

Practical Application

Steroid Cycles

With the wide variety of anabolic/androgenic steroids available, planning the most appropriate cycle may seem like a difficult task to the steroid novice. Even if we have settled on a particular drug or drug combination, it is still easy to question whether or not we are using them in the most effective manner. This is one of those topics which can get more confusing with research, as you will find the popular literature filled with various stacking, cycling, tapering and receptor response (upregulation/downregulation) theories. If you have purchased this book in the hopes it will provide you some new and unusual ways to take anabolic/androgenic steroids, you will probably be disappointed. I have actually developed the opinion that athletes usually place too much importance on cycle construction. Experimenting with fancy dosing patterns, rotation schedules and (especially) tapering routines, hoping they will bring about enhanced results, is, in my opinion, a very unreliable practice. Therefore, in this section I will be ignoring the more lavish intake regimens, and focus on the more fundamental aspects to using these drugs. This is obvious when you look at the sample cycles included, which you will notice display little fluctuation in drug dosages from start to finish. They are not fashioned as such due to laziness, but simply because my personal experience has led me to a place where picking a dosage and sticking with it (unless there is an obvious need to adjust) seems to make the most sense. It is ultimately up to the individual to find out what works best for him or her, as nobody can rightly claim that there is one "correct" way for everyone to use steroids. Here are a few things to think about when deciding on the right cycle for your needs.

Stacking

It is an extremely common practice for an athlete to take more than one individual steroid during a cycle. By taking a combination of steroids, the user is of course seeking to enhance the amount/quality of muscle mass gained from drug therapy. While I'm sure it is no surprise that stacking is generally an effective practice, you should probably give some thought to expected goals and side effects before simply combining steroids. For example, if you are looking to gain considerable mass, the use of two strong androgens like testosterone and Anadrol 50® would be one of the more potent cycles to attempt. But this combination would also lead to very harsh side effects, and may be too uncomfortable for some individuals. In this case it may be a good suggestion to combine a milder anabolic with a base androgen instead. A stack such as Deca-Durabolin® and Dianabol would still produce very formidable muscle mass gains, but would provide the user much less water/fat retention, gynecomastia, hair loss/growth, and acne than the former.

On the other hand, non-aromatizable anabolics are typically the favored class of steroids for cutting/dieting phases of training. This is because the lack of estrogen conversion makes them less apt to induce fat and water accumulation. It is important to remember, however, that these steroids can still suppress endogenous testosterone production during a cycle. Since the administered drug(s) may not provide the body enough androgen content to compensate for this loss, this type of cycle may sometimes interfere with aggression and libido (Deca is a common offender). In such a state the user might become depressed and unmotivated (see: side effects, depression), seriously reducing the quality (results and comfort) of the cycle. Therefore, it is usually a good idea to include some type of androgen during this type of cycle, especially if you have experienced such problems before. The preference would be a non-aromatizing androgenic compound like Proviron®, Halotestin® or trenbolone, which will not increase the likelihood for fat/water retention. In the absence of excess estrogen, the heightened androgen level brought about by these drugs can actually enhance the removal of body fat, and noticeably increase the look of hardness/density to the physique (provided the user's body fat percentage is low enough to make this visible). If such compounds were unavailable, perhaps a weekly (low dosage) shot of testosterone would prove sufficient to ward off any problems.

Finally, is also good to remember that it is not absolutely necessary to take more than one steroid at a time. The term you hear most often is synergy, which implies that two (or more) steroids used together will often compliment (and amplify) each other, and provide a greater muscle gain than if they had been used consecutively. Though not well understood, a number of studies do suggest that different modes of action might exist for steroids outside of the androgen receptor (which would seem to support the notion that cooperative or synergistic effects can be seen with different drug arrangements). Athletes also seem to know that certain drug combinations work extremely well together (Deca & Dianabol, testosterone and Anadrol 50®, trenbolone and Winstrol® etc.), which is a testament to the notion of drug synergy. But this should not be confused with the idea that you cannot make gains on one drug alone. For example, an athlete new to the world of steroids could make exceptional gains on a cycle of testosterone, Anadrol 50® or Dianabol, without ever needing to add a second drug. Heavily increased dosages and multi-drug stacks are likewise most prominent among those who are already very familiar with steroid use, and find they are necessary in order to continue to gain or maintain muscle mass.

Dosing and Megadosing

There are many different opinions as to exactly what dosage an individual should use of any particular drug in order to elicit optimal results. Some seem to find they make exceptional gains on relatively low dosages of most steroids, while others insist they need to administer very large amounts of androgens for the proper level of bulk. While I by no means claim to have the solution for everybody, I would say that most steroids seem to work best in a particular range of dosage, and usually fall short of expectations as we go higher or lower. On the one hand we may find that going below what is considered to be a normal dosage for a specific drug will result in very poor gains being achieved, the hormone level perhaps not rising enough above normal to stimulate a considerable response. For example, 200-800mg of testosterone enanthate per week is typically sufficient for a man to receive very formidable gains, while 50-100mg may not provide very noticeable results at all (this is all common sense). On the other extreme, athletes generally find that unusually large doses (let's say 1000-2000mg per week) will provide a relatively low quality increase over that of the normal dosage range. Yes, the amount of muscle mass may be considerably more than expected with a typical dose, but this will probably not be proportionate with the gain of new body fat and water weight. The user will typically be stuck with a much more noticeable level of side effects, while receiving a poor return (as in solid muscle mass) on his money. When steroids were abundant and cheap in the 1980', megadosing among recreational steroid users was not all that uncommon. No doubt paying $20 per week as opposed to $5 was not a very difficult decision to make. But today high prices will usually prevent the widespread practice of such excessive dosing, as such a cycle could cost hundreds of dollars each week. The side note to this is that one can reach an extreme level of development where year round high dosage steroid use is a necessity to maintain an anabolic state.

Cycle Duration

There are also many arguments as to how long one should stay on a steroid cycle before taking a break. Opinions range from those of cautious individuals, who are often vehement about short cycles and long off-periods, to the seriously hard-core user, who suggests year round use for optimal results. Since it is really up to the individual to choose the cycle that is best for him or her, I can only provide some general advice.

For starters, it is very important to watch your intake duration when on stronger or more toxic substances. This includes all c17 alpha alkylated orals, or high-dose cycles of easily aromatized steroids. These compounds place the most stress on your organs, and likewise should be utilized for only limited intervals (preferably less than 8 weeks). Afterwards a break of at least as much time (preferably more) should be taken to give the body ample time to rest/recover. For those who refuse to follow such advice, blood work and regular health checkups should be an absolute necessity.

When taking milder anabolics like Deca-Durabolin®, Primobolan® or Equipoise®, one might opt to take the drugs for a longer duration. This is due to the fact that these compounds do not act in an extremely dramatic manner, and instead promote a slow but consistent buildup of muscle tissue. With this understanding it is not unusual for an athlete to find a cycle of three, even four or more months, to be the most appropriate. If used for only a short duration, the individual might find the overall gains to be uninspiring.

Year round, on-all-the-time steroid use should be avoided if at all possible, as one should respect the natural hormonal balance your body strives for. The body really should be given time to regain a natural hormonal balance every so often, to ensure that there is little possibility for future problems. Although many believe the effects of these drugs to be 100% fully reversible, it is not impossible to see problems with virility, libido, etc. after the body had been overloaded with hormones for many years. The health risks associated with elevated cholesterol levels, high blood pressure or liver toxicity are important reasons the athlete should limit the duration of steroid intake.

Tapering

One of the most fundamental beliefs among steroid users is that tapering, or the practice of slowly reducing their drug dosage when discontinuing a cycle, is an absolute necessity when wishing to preserve your newly gained muscle mass. It is rare to find an athlete who does not religiously dedicate (at least) three or four weeks to a tapering schedule after every serious cycle. The belief is that the body will notice the lowering androgen level, and compensate by resuming the manufacture of testosterone. Unfortunately, you will see that this theory is, in fact, extremely flawed. This is because in order for the production of testosterone to be fully restored, the body will really need to recognize an androgen deficit, not just a drop in steroid dosage. For example, since even one Dianabol tablet could provide the equivalent of a full day's androgen supply for the average male, tapering from five, to four, to three, etc. will accomplish relatively nothing. In the three or four weeks the athlete will spend doing this, his body is still reading "androgen overload", and will not attempt to restore the output of testosterone. This will hold true for all anabolic steroids, not just the strong androgens. Anecdotal evidence suggests that even tapering with mild anabolics such as Primobolan® or Anavar (normally thought of as mild in terms of testosterone suppression) is enough to prevent or delay a hormonal rebound.

So, if tapering is useless, what should the athlete do in order to properly discontinue a steroid cycle? The obvious answer is to pay much closer attention to ancillary drug use than tapering. The proper application of testosterone stimulating compounds like HCG, Clomid®, Nolvadex® and/or cyclofenil are the most critical, as these can greatly aid in the balancing of body hormones. [The popular methods for using all the above medications are laid out under their individual profiles.] In the few cycles I have illustrated in this section, you will notice that I have not even bothered to lower the drug dosages before the ancillary drugs are added. Simply stated, there is no need to. In my opinion, going "cold turkey" is just the most logical option.

Sample Steroid Stacks

Sample steroid stacks are provided to demonstrate common and/or effective drug combinations in use by bodybuilders. For most of these cycles, the dosages used are in the moderate range. They are intended to represent a balance of peak effectiveness with tolerable side effects, and are also designed so that they can be assembled with very basic and common black market items. For most novice steroid users, stacks like these provide more than a sufficient level of steroid for very dramatic results. Some even find that they can make substantial progress on much less. These represent only common guidelines toward typical use, and by no means are intended to be the perfect cycles for everybody. You will also notice that I have not provided cycles geared towards women. This is simply because I think women should be extremely cautious with these drugs. Those absolutely determined to use them should certainly avoide multiple drug combinations, especially as a novice to these agents.

Beginner Stacks

Deca/D-bol (Mass Builder):

Ingredients: 100 tabs Methandienone 10mg, 10ml vial Deca 300mg/mL

Comments: This is a modified version of the Deca/Dbol stack printed in the first edition. The Deca dose has been increased, to reflect the purchase of one of the newer 300mg nandrolone decanoate products. 50mg versions of this steroid are now in extremely low demand due to the influx of new Mexican veterinary steroids. The Dbol dosage has been adjusted to reflect the use of 100 tablets of a 10mg product.

	Dianabol	Deca-Durabolin®
Week1		300mg
Week2		300mg
Week3		300mg
Week4	20mg/day	300mg
Week5	20mg/day	300mg
Week6	20mg/day	300mg
Week7	20mg/day	300mg
Week8	20mg/day	300mg
Week9	20mg/day	300mg
Week10	20mg/day	300mg

Non-Toxic Oral (Lean Mass Cycle):

Ingredients: 390 Caps (13 30 cap bottles of Mexican product) Andriol, 500 Tabs 5mg Primo

Comments: By far the most costly cycle of the group, this one is provided for the individual who does not want to use needles, nor liver toxic orals. More Primo could be used, to a dosage of 100-150 mg, if available.

	Andriol	Primobolan
Week1	8 caps/day	50mg/day
Week2	8 caps/day	50mg/day
Week3	8 caps/day	50mg/day
Week4	8 caps/day	50mg/day
Week5	8 caps/day	50mg/day
Week6	8 caps/day	50mg/day
Week7	8 caps/day	50mg/day

Proviron/Deca/Winny (Cutting/Lean Mass Cycle):

Ingredients: 140 tabs of Proviron, 10ml 200mg/mL Deca, 100 tabs 10mg stanozolol

Comments: This is an extremely effective lean mass building/cutting cycle. The Proviron adds good androgen content to the nandrolone base, which often too anabolic to use on its own. The Winstrol, added later, greatly enhances the fat burning and anabolic nature of the combination.

	Proviron®	Deca	Winstrol®
Week1		200 mg	
Week2	50 mg/day	200 mg	
Week3	50 mg/day	200 mg	
Week4	50 mg/day	200 mg	
Week5	50 mg/day	200 mg	20 mg/day
Week6	50 mg/day	200 mg	20 mg/day
Week7	50 mg/day	200 mg	20 mg/day
Week8	50 mg/day	200 mg	20 mg/day
Week9	50 mg/day	200 mg	20 mg/day
Week10	50 mg/day	200 mg	20 mg/day
Week11	50 mg/day		20 mg/day

Anavar/Primo (Cutting Cycle):

Ingredients: 200 tabs 5mg oxandrolone, 14 ampules 100mg Primobolan Depot

Comments: A basic but very efficient cutting stack. This combo provides zero estrogen, and is only moderately androgenic in nature. Low side effects and solid results.

	Anavar	Primobolan Depot
Week1	20 mg/day	200 mg
Week2	20 mg/day	200 mg
Week3	20 mg/day	200 mg
Week4	20 mg/day	200 mg
Week5	20 mg/day	200 mg
Week6	20 mg/day	200 mg
Week7	20 mg/day	200 mg

Tren/Winny (Cutting Cycle):

Ingredients: 2 (10ml) bottles Trenbolone acetate 75mg/mL, 20ml injectable stanozolol.

Comments: This is a potent cutting/hardening cycle. Do not let the low 300-375mg dose fool you. These are two very active steroids, and the combination is sure to provide quite a pronounced effect.

	Trenbolone Act.	Winstrol®
Week1	150 mg	
Week2	150 mg	150 mg
Week3	150 mg	150 mg
Week4	150 mg	150 mg
Week5	225 mg	150 mg
Week6	225 mg	150 mg
Week7	225 mg	150 mg
Week8	225 mg	100 mg

Tren/Test/Deca (Mass Builder):

Ingredients: 2 (10ml) bottles Trenbolone acetate 75mg/mL, 10ml bottle 200mg/mL cypionate (or enanthate), 10ml bottle 200mg/mL Deca

Comments: This is an excellent bulking cycle based on lower priced Mexican veterinary steroids. The trenbolone helps to harden up the gains, and the use of only 200mg of testosterone and Deca should keep estrogen levels from getting too far out of hand.

	Cypionate	Trenbolone Act.	Deca
Week1	200 mg		
Week2	200 mg		
Week3	200 mg	150 mg	
Week4	200 mg	150 mg	
Week5	200 mg	150 mg	200 mg
Week6	200 mg	150 mg	200 mg
Week7	200 mg	150 mg	200 mg
Week8	200 mg	150 mg	200 mg
Week9	200 mg	150 mg	200 mg
Week10	200 mg	150 mg	200 mg
Week11		150 mg	200 mg
Week12		150 mg	200 mg
Week13			200 mg
Week14			200 mg

Equipoise/Test (Mass Builder):

Ingredients: 50ml vial Equipoise® (50mg), 10 amps Testosterone Enanthate

Commends: This is a basic testosterone and Equipoise stack. The Equipoise allows for a lower overall dosage of testosterone, without sacrificing much in terms of expected gains. Estrogen buildup should be controllable with this stack, yet still should reach a point where it is aiding in the promotion of an anabolic state. A great beginners muscle-building stack.

	Equipoise®	Test. Enanthate
Week1	250 mg	
Week2	250 mg	250 mg
Week3	250 mg	250 mg
Week4	250 mg	250 mg
Week5	250 mg	250 mg
Week6	250 mg	250 mg
Week7	250 mg	250 mg
Week8	250 mg	250 mg
Week9	250 mg	250 mg
Week10	250 mg	250 mg
Week11		250 mg

Intermediate-Advanced Stacks

Short Anadrol/Test (Mass Builder):

Ingredients: 100 tabs Anadrol 50®, 20 amps/preloads/ML of Sustanon

Comments: This is the classic Anadrol/Test stack. If you are looking for sheer mass, you are not going to find a better mix. Be warned though, estrogenic side effects are likely to be intense. It is a good idea to have Nolvadex® close by.

	Anadrol 50®	Sustanon
Week1		750 mg
Week2	2 tablets/day	750 mg
Week3	2 tablets/day	750 mg
Week4	2 tablets/day	750 mg
Week5	2 tablets/day	750 mg
Week6	2 tablets/day	750 mg
Week7	2 tablets/day	500 mg
Week8	2 tablets/day	

Super Test Cycle (Mass Builder):

Ingredients: 112 tabs Proviron, 30 ml Sustanon, 100 tabs 10mg stanozolol

Comments: This cycle is designed to maximize the level of free testosterone in the body. Proviron competitively inhibits both estrogen aromatization and testosterone to SHBG binding, and Winstrol adds to the androgen-induced lowering of binding protein levels. Gains with this stack should be leaner than the Test and Anadrol cycle, as there is less of an estrogenic component.

	Proviron®	Sustanon	Winstrol®
Week1		500 mg	
Week2	50 mg/day	1,000 mg	10 mg/day
Week3	50 mg/day	1,000 mg	10 mg/day
Week4	50 mg/day	1,000 mg	20 mg/day
Week5	50 mg/day	1,000 mg	20 mg/day
Week6	50 mg/day	1,000 mg	20 mg/day
Week7	50 mg/day	1,000 mg	20 mg/day
Week8	50 mg/day	1,000 mg	20 mg/day
Week9	50 mg/day		20 mg/day

EQ/Suspensions Stack (Lean Mass Builder):

Ingredients: 3 (10ml) vials Equipoise (200mg), 1 (20ml) vial 100mg/ml T. Suspension, 1 (20ml) vial stanozolol (50mg)

Commends: This is an excellent RAPID lean muscle-building stack. Aromatase inhibitor may be needed during the first 6 weeks, otherwise the remaining 6 (unless you are very sensitive to estrogen) should entail low enough estrogen levels to dramatically increase hardness and definition. A combination building/cutting cycle.

	Equipoise	T. Suspension	Winstrol®
Week1	600 mg	100 mg EOD	
Week2	600 mg	100 mg EOD	
Week3	600 mg	100 mg EOD	
Week4	600 mg	100 mg EOD	
Week5	600 mg	100 mg EOD	
Week6	600 mg	100 mg EOD	
Week7	600 mg		50 mg EOD
Week8	600 mg		50 mg EOD
Week9	600 mg		50 mg EOD
Week10	600 mg		50 mg EOD
Week11			50 mg EOD
Week12			50 mg EOD

15-week Mass Builder:

Ingredients: 5 (10ml) bottles 250mg/ml T. cypionate, 2 (10ml) bottles 100mg/mL Durabolin, 300 5mg tabs stanozolol

Comments: This is an excellent lean bulking cycle, with only periodic use of c-17 alpha alkylated orals. Durabolin serves as a bridge between both treatment periods, giving the liver time to detoxify. This cycle pushes the limits of growth, but does so without pushing the limits of safety.

	Cypionate	Dbol	Durabolin	Winstrol
Week1	750 mg	40 mg		
Week2	750 mg	40 mg		
Week3	750 mg	40 mg		
Week4	750 mg	40 mg		
Week5	750 mg	40 mg		
Week6	750 mg		400 mg	
Week7	750 mg		400 mg	
Week8	750 mg		400 mg	
Week9	750 mg		400 mg	
Week10	750 mg		400 mg	
Week11	750 mg			40 mg
Week12	750 mg			40 mg
Week13	750 mg			40 mg
Week14	750 mg			40 mg
Week15	750 mg			40 mg

15-Week Cutting Stack:

Ingredients: 2 (10ml) bottle 200mg Equipoise, 200 tabs Proviron, 150 IU HGH, 420-640 tabs clen, 315 tabs Zaditen

Comments: This is an extremely potent cutting stack. Some may find a need to add in small doses of T-3. However, most will find the low GH dose and thermogenic adjunct products to work excellent for cutting alone. EQ is the only aromatizable steroid used, and adds little estrogen when accompanies by Proviron to inhibit aromatase.

	Equipoise	Proviron	HGH	Clen	Zaditen
Week1	400 mg	50 mg/day	1 IU/day	2 tabs/day	3 tabs/day
Week2	400 mg	50 mg/day	1 IU/day	3 tabs/day	3 tabs/day
Week3	400 mg	50 mg/day	1 IU/day	4 tabs/day	3 tabs/day
Week4	400 mg	50 mg/day	1 IU/day	4 –6 tabs/day	3 tabs/day
Week5	400 mg	50 mg/day	1 IU/day	4 –6 tabs/day	3 tabs/day
Week6	400 mg	50 mg/day	1 IU/day	4 –6 tabs/day	3 tabs/day
Week7	400 mg	50 mg/day	1 IU/day	4 –6 tabs/day	3 tabs/day
Week8	400 mg	50 mg/day	2 IU/day	4 –6 tabs/day	3 tabs/day
Week9	400 mg	50 mg/day	2 IU/day	4 –6 tabs/day	3 tabs/day
Week10	400 mg	50 mg/day	2 IU/day	4 –6 tabs/day	3 tabs/day
Week11		50 mg/day	2 IU/day	4 –6 tabs/day	3 tabs/day
Week12		50 mg/day	2 IU/day	4 –6 tabs/day	3 tabs/day
Week13		50 mg/day	2 IU/day	4 –6 tabs/day	3 tabs/day
Week14		50 mg/day	2 IU/day	4 –6 tabs/day	3 tabs/day
Week15		50 mg/day	2 IU/day	4 –6 tabs/day	3 tabs/day

22-Week Super-Blitz Lean Mass Cycle:

Ingredients: 5 (10ml) bottles 100mg T. Propionate, 48 amps Primobolan, 84 tabs Anadrol, 5 (10ml) bottles 100mg Durabolin, 160 tabs (10mg) dbol.

Comments: An excellent half-year lean-building stack. Focuses on the periodic use of c-17alpha alkylated orals, bridged with injectable compounds, to minimize chance for liver toxicity.

	T. Propionate	Trenbolone	Anadrol	Primobolan	Durabolin	Dbol
Week1	400mg		100 mg/day			
Week2	400mg		100 mg/day			
Week3	400mg		100 mg/day			
Week4	400mg		100 mg/day			
Week5	400mg		100 mg/day			
Week6	400mg		100 mg/day			
Week7		225 mg		400mg		
Week8		225 mg		400mg		
Week9		225 mg		400mg		
Week10		225 mg		400mg		
Week11		225 mg		400mg		
Week12		225 mg		400mg		
Week13					400mg	40 mg/day
Week14					400mg	40 mg/day
Week15					400mg	40 mg/day
Week16					400mg	40 mg/day
Week17					400mg	40 mg/day
Week18					400mg	40 mg/day
Week19	400mg	225 mg		400mg		
Week20	400mg	225 mg		400mg		
Week21	400mg	225 mg		400mg		
Week22	400mg	225 mg		400mg		
Week23	400mg	225 mg		400mg		
Week24	400mg	225 mg		400mg		

17 Week Pre-Contest Dual Phase (Pro Level)

The following is a 2-phase cycle used by an IFBB professional bodybuilder. He used this cycle leading up to a recent show, in which he placed in the top 5. The total use duration was 17 weeks, or approximately 4 months. This cycle dispels the myth that pros all need to take massive doses of steroids, or exotic and expensive compounds like IGF-1, to be competitive. The 1-2 gram per week range in this program is formidable, but not unreasonable given the level of performance of the athlete. The most exotic drugs taken in this 2-part stack are also insulin and GH, which are "basic" bodybuiulding drugs by any standard. It does, however, make use of c-17 alpha alkylated compounds for prolonged periods of time, which does legitimately add some level of risk. This bodybuilder was smart enough to have regular health checkups during his cycles, and tried to mitigate the negative cardiovascular side effects as best he could with diet and exercise. Although no adverse health effects were reported, it should be noted the pro level cycles are especially not recommended for beginners, and are definitely "use at your own risk" kind of programs.

Phase I/Bulking

Week	Enanthate	Deca	Dbol	Equipoise	GH	Insulin	Nolvadex
1	1000mg	500mg	50mg/d		4IU/3IU	14IU	20mg/d
2	1000mg	500mg	50mg/d		4IU/3IU	14IU	20mg/d
3	750mg	500mg	50mg/d		4IU/3IU	14IU	20mg/d
4	750mg	500mg	50mg/d		4IU/3IU	14IU	20mg/d
5	750mg		50mg/d	500mg	4IU/3IU	14IU	20mg/d
6	750mg		50mg/d	500mg	4IU/3IU	14IU	20mg/d
7	500mg		50mg/d	500mg	4IU/3IU	14IU	20mg/d
8	500mg			500mg	4IU/3IU	14IU	20mg/d

Insulin (Humalog) is taken 7IU in the morning and 7IU before training, with a loading of carbohydrates. Growth hormone is taken 4IU on training days, 3IU for non-training days.

Phase II/Cutting

Week	Propionate	Deca	Tren	Winstrol	Halotestin	Proviron	Arimidex
1	100mg/d	500mg				75mg/d	
2	100mg/d	500mg				75mg/d	
3	100mg/d	500mg				75mg/d	
4	100mg/d	500mg				75mg/d	
5	100mg/d	500mg				75mg/d	
6			225 mg	100mg/EOD	20mg/d		
7			225 mg	100mg/EOD	20mg/d		
8			225 mg	100mg/EOD	20mg/d		1tab/d
9			225 mg	100mg/EOD	20mg/d		1tab/d

Diet begins 7 weeks out from competition. Sodium is not cut. GH is added through much of the cutting phase at a dose of 2IU per day. Injectable Lasix is added the last 3 days, at a dose of 1 ampule twice daily. Arimidex is taken the last 2 weeks, at a dose of 1 tablet per day. Dyazide is taken 1 tablet twice during the last day (competition).

12-Week Serious-Bulk (Pro Level):

Comments: This pro-level bulking stack uses a formidable injectable base (mean dose of 1gram per week), a rotation of high-dosed orals, andd the new IGF-1 analog (IGF-1 Long R3). This is an extremely effective program, but again is not for novice bodybuilders. Arimidex or Nolvadex are alternated to combat estrogenic side effects, depending on the individual's sensitivity to them. Nolvadex is preferred to help keep HDL (good) cholesterol in check (at least from dropping into the toilet completely), but may not be strong enough with this much testosterone, boldenone and dianabol. The latter 2/3rds of the cycle should be somewhat less estrogenic due to the discontinuance of dianabol at week 5, so some may opt to start with Arimidex only. Insulin is also added in most cases, as a post-training anabolic (with carbohydrate loading).

	Sustanon	Dianabol	Primobolan Oral	IGF-1lr3	Equipoise	Winstrol
Week1	1,000mg	50mg/d			600mg/week	
Week2	1,000mg	50mg/d			600mg/week	
Week3	1,000mg	50mg/d			600mg/week	
Week4	1,000mg	50mg/d			600mg/week	
Week5	1,000mg		150mg/day		600mg/week	
Week6	1,000mg		150mg/day	30mcg/d	600mg/week	
Week7	1,000mg		150mg/day	30mcg/d	600mg/week	
Week8	1,000mg		150mg/day	30mcg/d	600mg/week	
Week9	1,000mg			50mcg/d	600mg/week	50mg/d
Week10	1,000mg			50mcg/d	600mg/week	50mg/d
Week11	1,000mg			50mcg/d	600mg/week	50mg/d
Week12				50mcg/d		50mg/d

12-Week Anabolic Rotation Cycle. Lean Mass and Cuts (Pro Level):

Comments: This pro-level cutting cycle was used for before a recent competition. This particular bodybuilder likes to use clenbuterol on and off, for 4 weeks at a time. He also felt that he didin't like to be on a lot of GH around show time, and preferred to use only 1IU during the last 5 weeks leading up to a show. When we examine the cycle we see no estrogenic steroid being used past week 6. To spite this, the bodybuilder would take an additional tablet of arimidex daily for the last half of the cycle. 100mg of injectable Winstrol is used every third day during weeks 7-8, and every other day during weeks 9-12.

	Primobolan	Parabolan	T. Propionate	Masteron	Winstrol	Clenbuterol	HGH
Week1	500mg	300mg	400mg			6tabs/d	2IU/d
Week2	500mg	300mg	400mg			6tabs/d	2IU/d
Week3	500mg	300mg	400mg			6tabs/d	2IU/d
Week4	500mg	300mg	400mg			6tabs/d	2IU/d
Week5	500mg	300mg	400mg				2IU/d
Week6	500mg	300mg	400mg				2IU/d
Week7	500mg			300mg	100mg/ETD		2IU/d
Week8	500mg			300mg	100mg/ETD		1IU/d
Week9	500mg			300mg	100mg/EOD	6tabs/d	1IU/d
Week10	500mg			300mg	100mg/EOD	6tabs/d	1IU/d
Week11	500mg			300mg	100mg/EOD	6tabs/d	1IU/d
Week12	500mg			300mg	100mg/EOD	6tabs/d	1IU/d

Andreas Munzer's Last Cycle:

Comments: This cycle was used leading up to the death of IFBB professional bodybuilder Andreas Munzer. The German magazine Der Spiegel first published Munzer's program shortly after his death, which was reportedly obtained by a source close to him. The death of Andreas Munzer was a shock to the bodybuilding world, and demonstrated well that the precontest regimen of the competitive bodybuilder, which can include heavy drug use, severe calorie and fluid restriction, and marked dehydration, can be a very dangerous undertaking. This is not to suggest that a cycle such as this is "normal" in the IFBB ranks. If you review the cumulative drug intake, you will see that Andreas Munzer was using staggeringly high dosages and a wide variety of drugs. Most professional bodybuilders would not use such high levels of steroids, however, there are indeed some that do. This cycle is too large to place into one chart, so it is divided into segments. It is provided for informational purposes only, and given the circumstances should not be attempted by anyone.

Other things of interest include the fact that Captagon is a trade name for fenethylline. This is an amphetamine-type stimulant. Captagon is a schedule I drug in the U.S., placed under the tightest controls and classified as a drug with no legitimate medical use. Munzer also reportedly used Cytadren in his contest preparations. There has been a lot of speculation that Cytadren, combined with amphetamines and severe dehydration, were key factors in his death. Since no official autopsy was released, we do not know the exact pathology of his death. With the amount of drugs he used, I doubt the exact cause is even possible to pinpoint.

Weeks 1-10:

Ephedrine
Aspirin
Clenbuterol
Valium
Captagon
Cytomel

Weeks 1-5:

500mg daily	Testosterone Enanthate
152mg daily	Parabolan
150mg daily	Dianabol
150mg daily	Halotestin
20IU daily	HGH
20IU daily	Insulin

Weeks 6-8:

300mg daily	Masteron
152mg daily	Parabolan
250mg daily	Winstrol Tab
150mg daily	Halotestin
50mg daily	Winstrol Inj.
24IU daily	HGH

Weeks 9-10:

200mg daily	Masteron
100mg daily	Winstrol Inj.
200mg daily	Halotestin
400mg daily	Winstrol Tab
24IU daily	HGH
Insulin - daily	
IGF-1 – daily	

Days 1-3 leading up to show:

Aldactone, Lasix to cut water.

Giving the Injection

All anabolic/androgenic steroid solutions were designed for deep intramuscular injection. The most common sites of injection are the upper outer quadrant of gluteus (buttock) and the outer side of the mid to upper thigh. This provides an ample area of thick muscle, facilitating the goal of a deep (typically 1 to 1 ½ inch) deposit of the steroid solution into muscle tissue. Occasionally these solutions are also injected into smaller muscles such as the deltoid, biceps or triceps.

The chosen site is not crucial, although there are some things to consider in deciding. For starters, the gluteus and thigh muscles are the best for larger injection volumes. They are sufficiently large in size that a 3ml deposit will not be extremely irritating. When using the shoulders and other small muscles, 1-1 ½ ml is the typical limit for comfort. Administering more may result in a deep soreness and possibly swelling to the muscle. The upper outer gluteus also has the lowest pain sensitivity to needle penetration, and is likewise an easy site to start with. The thickness and level of blood circulation given to a site also affect the rate of steroid release, although this does not amount to a great deal of variation. Technically a steroid deposit will remain in the gluteus muscle for the longest period of time, release slightly faster in the thigh or shoulder (most rapid). Over the course of a cycle the difference would probably not be noticeable to the athlete.

SYRINGE/NEEDLE SIZE

The gauge represents the size (diameter) of a needle. The larger the number, the finer the needle is in thickness. This measurement bears no relation to the size (capacity) of the syringe, which in many cases is sold separately from the needle. The type of needle used for steroid injections varies depending on the type/viscosity of solution (water/oil) and site of injection, ranging from the standard deep intramuscular oil needles of 21-22 gauge to a fine insulin needle of 27-28 gauge. Below are a few stock needle/syringe combinations and their corresponding use with anabolic/androgenic steroids.

3ml syringe, 22-gauge needle, 1 ½ inch in length
3ml syringe, 23-gauge needle, 1 inch in length

Standard needle sizes used for the injection of oil based compounds in the gluteus or thigh. Here you should limit injection volume to 3ml. Occasionally this size needle is also used for water-based compounds that contain steroid in the form of unusually large particles. For example, Winstrol-V and some Australian veterinary testosterone suspensions will jam in a needle any smaller. Having to use such a large size makes repeated injections extremely uncomfortable.

3 ml syringe, 25-gauge needle, 5/8 inch in length

Often referred to as a vitamin needle, this is a standard sized needle used for the thigh or deltoid injection of oil-based compounds. Water-based steroids are also commonly injection at the same sites with this needle, but solutions with finely ground steroid (Stanazolic and Winstrol from Zambon in Spain, for example) are more comfortably given with an insulin needle.

1ml syringe, 27-gauge needle, ½ inch in length
1ml syringe, 28-gauge needle, ½ inch in length
1ml syringe, 29-gauge needle, ½ inch in length

These are standard insulin needles used by athletes for the injection of water-based steroids, HCG, insulin, and growth hormone into smaller muscles such as the deltoid, biceps or triceps. These are also the only sized needles comfortable to use for the subcutaneous injection of insulin and growth hormone. In desperate situations insulin needles are sometimes also used for the injection of oil-based compounds in the deltoid. While extremely tedious, there is no immediate danger with such a practice provided normal protocol were followed.

Injection Protocol

1. Sanitize the intended area of injection with an alcohol swab, and wash hands thoroughly.
2. If using a multiple-dose vial, clean the stopper with alcohol also.
3. Remove the syringe's packaging, and fill with an equal amount of air in comparison to the intended dose. Inject the air into the vial, a practice that keeps a balance of internal/external pressure (making future withdrawal easier).
4. Draw solution into the syringe, and remove needle from the vial.
5. Holding it needle-side-upright, tap the side of the syringe, and expel any extra air bubbles (tiny bubbles are not a danger to health, but this is still correct practice).
6. Stretch the skin over the site of injection with the thumb and forefinger of your free hand, and penetrate the muscle with the needle.
7. Pull back on the stopper to make sure the syringe does not fill with blood. Should blood be present, the needle should be removed, and reinserted into another area (to avoid injecting into a blood vessel).
8. Press the stopper down firmly and steadily until all of the oil has been injected.
9. Remove the needle, and press down on the injection site with an alcohol swab.
10. Repackage and dispose of the needle. If it must be reused, it can be stored in the freezer to minimize contamination.

Chemical Analysis Report

Set ID # 411004-A

Set Description : 3 lots of tablets
Date Received : 11/01/04
Date(s) Analyzed : 11/15/04
Date Reported : 11/17/04

Company Name : Molecular Nutrition
Directed To : William Llewellyn
Address : 5500 Military Trail #308
Jupiter, FL 33458

Sample Preparation and Analysis Conditions :

For methandrostenolone, a weighed portion of a composite of ground tablets from each sample was dissolved/extracted in acetonitrile, filtered, and then analyzed under the following instrumental conditions:

Chromatograph : High performance liquid chromatograph (Hewlett Packard Model 1090 II / L)
Column : Synergi Hydro-RP, 150 x 3.0mm, 4μm, 80Å
Detector : Photodiode array, scanning from 190 to 600 nm; quantitation at 245 nm

Analytical Results

Reporting results to three significant figures is for statistical evaluation only and is not intended to be an indication of analytical precision

Sample Identification		Tablets	Methandrostenolone	
		ave. wt. g	mg/g	mg/tab
Laboratory ID# **Client ID#**	411004-1 Metavet QV Tablets Lot# QVTMTA 005	0.117	89.7	10.5
Laboratory ID# **Client ID#**	411004-2 Denkall D Bol Tablets Lot# TBD 012	0.116	83.6	9.70
Laboratory ID# **Client ID#**	411004-3 Reforvit Simple Tablets Lot# 1290603	0.117	187.	21.9

Analyzed ________ **Release Authorized** ____________________ ________________

By By Date

****

Steroid Lab Test Results

If we have learned anything over the past five or ten years, it is that counterfeit steroid manufacturers all around the world are working very hard to trick you out of money. The fake drugs of the 80's and 90's, with poorly printed labels, improperly sealed bottles, and obvious "basement-made" looks, are almost entirely things of the past. Nowadays, surreptitious manufacturers are investing tens, if not hundreds, of thousands of dollars on equipment that will allow them to duplicate their particular drugs of choice with previously unseen accuracy. In many cases they are using things like ampule sealing equipment, foil/plastic tablet sealers, even investing is custom pill dyes so they may duplicate a product down to its own unique tablet markings. Some of the fakes today are nearly impossible to spot if you do not know what to look for. I do the best job I can to keep you informed by staying up on global product availability, and comparing minute features of each new box I receive to known legitimate originals in an effort to spot inconsistencies. However, it is a battle that nobody, not even myself, is equipped to win every single time. The only true way of being 100% sure of the steroid content of your drug product is to have it analyzed and quantified in a laboratory. This section deals with exactly that.

Lab analysis also allows us to keep on top of which of the legitimate steroid manufacturers are truly honest. Mexico, for example, is the home of literally dozens of steroid manufacturing companies, and unfortunately is an area of the world where drug makers are much less actively scrutinized by government agencies, particularly in the field of veterinary medicine. For years we have been hearing reports of underdosing and underfilling from various Mexican veterinary manufacturers. This is probably owed to the fact that there is a very competitive market for steroids, and shaving a little off of your manufacturing costs can make a huge difference in the amount of profit brought home at the end of the day. Lately things have been changing, and more often than not companies are correctly dosing their steroid products. But things are still not perfect, as you will see. In an effort to help guide you to some of the better steroid makers in this and other countries I have, likewise, included this section of compiled independent lab analysis results.

The preceding page shows an actual report sheet on three anabolic steroid products I had sent in for analysis. All tests in this section were conducted by San Rafael Chemical Services in Utah, one of the most well known laboratories for anabolic steroid testing in the United States. For the sake of space I have included only the one report. For the rest I will display the results panel only, followed by a description of what the particular drug product was supposed to contain. I have sorted them by specific drug. Obviously, there is no guarantee even if you have one of the steroids listed that your lot contains the same amount of drug as was reported here. But, at the very least, it will allow you to take an up close look at what some of these companies are putting out, and perhaps may even change your mind as to what particular brand you will be shopping for next time.

Anavar (oxandrolone)

Product Name	Manufacturer	Lot Number	Label Claim	Actual Result
Oxandrolone	SPA (Milano)	N/a	2.5mg/tab	2.22mg

Comments: Italian Export version.

Product Name	Manufacturer	Lot Number	Label Claim	Actual Result
Oxanabol	British Dragon	MFG: 08 Mar 2004	10mg/tab	7.25mg

Product Name	Manufacturer	Lot Number	Label Claim	Actual Result
GS Anavar	Generic Supplements	261323	5mg/tab	4.33mg

Comments: Underground product, of European Origin.

Anadrol (oxymetholone)

Product Name	Manufacturer	Lot Number	Label Claim	Actual Result
Oxybolone	Genepharm	N/a	50mg/tab	51.3mg

Clenbuterol

Product Name	Manufacturer	Lot Number	Label Claim	Actual Result
Clenbuterol	Generic Supplements	261323	.04mg/tab	.0473mg

Comments: Underground product, of European Origin.

Deca-Durabolin (nandrolone decanoate)

Product Name	Manufacturer	Lot Number	Label Claim	Actual Result
Deca-Durabolin	Organon	93201 B	50mg/mL	56.1mg/mL

Comments: This is an ampule of Organon Deca-Durabolin from Egypt.

Durabolin (nandrolone phenylpropionate)

Product Name	Manufacturer	Lot Number	Label Claim	Actual Result
Nandrobolin	Luoyang Pharm	L04084	100mg/mL	112mg/mL

Dianabol (methandrostenolone)

Product Name	Manufacturer	Lot Number	Label Claim	Actual Result
Metavet QV	Quality Vet	QVTMTA 005	10mg/tab	10.5mg

Product Name	Manufacturer	Lot Number	Label Claim	Actual Result
D Bol	Denkall	TBD 012	10mg/tab	9.7mg

Product Name	Manufacturer	Lot Number	Label Claim	Actual Result
Reforvit Simple	Loeffler	1290603	25mg/tab	21.9mg

Product Name	Manufacturer	Lot Number	Label Claim	Actual Result
Dianabol Inj	Salud	SA4F020	25mg/mL	.187mg/mL

Comments: This test was a follow up from last year, shown below. There was barely a trace this time around, however.

Product Name	Manufacturer	Lot Number	Label Claim	Actual Result
Dianabol Inj	Salud	SA2B006	25mg/mL	20.3 mg/mL

Product Name	Manufacturer	Lot Number	Label Claim	Actual Result
Dianabol Tab	Salud	SA2D009	10 mg tab	8.84 mg

Product Name	Manufacturer	Lot Number	Label Claim	Actual Result
Reforvit-B	Loeffler	1320702	25mg/mL	24.2 mg/mL

Product Name	Manufacturer	Lot Number	Label Claim	Actual Result
Reforvit-B	Loeffler	1320702	25mg/mL	13.1 mg/mL

Comments: The above two samples represent an unusual situation. The bottom was sent in and tested for Anabolics 2004. One year later I ordered a second vial from the same supplier. The lot number was the same as the year before, but the result was significantly better than the first. I have no explaination for why one bottle would be so different from another of the same lot.

Product Name	Manufacturer	Lot Number	Label Claim	Actual Result
Methandrostenolone	Bioreactor	020201	5mg/tab	4.49mg

Product Name	Manufacturer	Lot Number	Label Claim	Actual Result
Methandrostenolone	Generic Supplements	261323	10mg/tab	9.75mg

Equipoise (boldenone undecylenate)

Product Name	Manufacturer	Lot Number	Label Claim	Actual Result
Bold QV 200	Quality Vet	QVB 013	200mg/mL	198mg/mL

Product Name	Manufacturer	Lot Number	Label Claim	Actual Result
Ultragan 100	Denkall	UB11	100mg/mL	106mg/mL

Product Name	Manufacturer	Lot Number	Label Claim	Actual Result
Equi-gan	Tornel	170	50mg/mL	56.2mg/mL

Product Name	Manufacturer	Lot Number	Label Claim	Actual Result
Equipoise	Fort Dodge	TL0203109	50mg/mL	53.9mg/mL

Product Name	Manufacturer	Lot Number	Label Claim	Actual Result
Boldabol	British Dragon	02 2009	200mg/mL	132mg/mL

Masteron (drostanolone propionate)

Product Name	Manufacturer	Lot Number	Label Claim	Actual Result
Mastabol	British Dragon	MAN: 02 2004	50mg/mL	38.7mg/mL

Primobolan Depot (methenolone enanthate)

Product Name	Manufacturer	Lot Number	Label Claim	Actual Result
Primobol	British Dragon	05 2009	100mg/mL	154mg/mL

Product Name	Manufacturer	Lot Number	Label Claim	Actual Result
Primobolan Depot	Generic Supplements	261324	100mg/mL	95.3mg/mL

Product Name	Manufacturer	Lot Number	Label Claim	Actual Result
Metabolin	Luoyang Pharm	L04075	100mg/mL	92.9mg/mL

Sustanon 250

Product Name	Manufacturer	Lot Number	Label Claim	Actual Result
Sustanon 250	Nile	093104	250mg/mL	224.2mg/mL

Testosterone cypionate

Product Name	Manufacturer	Lot Number	Label Claim	Actual Result
Cypiotest	Denkall	CYP 004	250mg/mL	238mg/mL

Product Name	Manufacturer	Lot Number	Label Claim	Actual Result
Teston QV	Quality Vet	QV 010	200mg/mL	166mg/mL

Product Name	Manufacturer	Lot Number	Label Claim	Actual Result
Anabolic TL	SYD Group	53902	200mg/mL	187mg/mL

Testosterone Enanthate

Product Name	Manufacturer	Lot Number	Label Claim	Actual Result
Testosterone Enanthate	Norma Hellas	0403015	250mg/mL	278mg/mL

Product Name	Manufacturer	Lot Number	Label Claim	Actual Result
Testosterone Enanthate	Generic Supplements	264323	250mg/mL	304mg/mL

Comments: Underground product, of European Origin.

Product Name	Manufacturer	Lot Number	Label Claim	Actual Result
Testosteronum Prolongatum	Jelfa	10402	100mg/mL	140mg/mL

Product Name	Manufacturer	Lot Number	Label Claim	Actual Result
Testosteronum Prolongatum	Jelfa	X10403	100mg/mL	139mg/mL

Comments: The above two samples are of testosterone enanthate, from Jelfa in Poland. Both tested out significantly overdosed.

Product Name	Manufacturer	Lot Number	Label Claim	Actual Result
Testosterone 200 Depot	Tornel	181MAY06	200 mg/mL	160 mg/mL

Product Name	Manufacturer	Lot Number	Label Claim	Actual Result
Testosteron-Depo	Galenika	3850	250mg/mL	264mg/mL

Product Name	Manufacturer	Lot Number	Label Claim	Actual Result
Testosteron-Depo	Galenika	0020	250 mg/mL	179 mg/mL

Comments: The above two samples are of Galenika's Testosterone Depot from Serbia. The bottom sample was taken last year, and published in Anabolics 2004. The top sample was sent in recently, and reflects a great improvement over the first test.

Testosterone propionate

Product Name	Manufacturer	Lot Number	Label Claim	Actual Result
Testone-E	MISR	20198	25mg/mL	23.2mg/mL

Comments: This is a testostosterone product from MISR in Egypt.

Product Name	Manufacturer	Lot Number	Label Claim	Actual Result
Testosterone Propionate	Generic Pharma	N/a	100mg/mL	98.4mg/mL

Comments: Underground product, of European Origin.

Product Name	Manufacturer	Lot Number	Label Claim	Actual Result
Testopro L/A	Loeffler	5701	250mg/mL	133 mg/mL

Comments: Product was significantly underdosed.

Product Name	Manufacturer	Lot Number	Label Claim	Actual Result
Testosterona 100	Brovel	3102	100mg/mL	71.9mg/mL

Trenbolone acetate

Product Name	Manufacturer	Lot Number	Label Claim	Actual Result
Trenabol	British Dragon	03 2003	100mg/mL	87.5mg/mL

Product Name	Manufacturer	Lot Number	Label Claim	Actual Result
Trenbolone Acetate	Generic Supplements	261323	100mg/mL	91.9mg/mL

Comments: Underground product, of European Origin.

Product Name	Manufacturer	Lot Number	Label Claim	Actual Result
Finaject	Australian Pacific	113	100mg/mL	120mg/mL

Comments: Underground product, of European Origin.

Paper Steroids

These are U.S. Customs' worst nightmare: Oral anabolic steroids that are sold in sheets of paper instead of the standard dosage units (pills and capsules) used for these drugs. I believe the idea originated from Dan Duchaine, and it is both simple and ingenious. The main point of interest is that these sheets of paper are easily mailed in regular envelopes, so as to attract little attention from the federal agents that screen international mail shipments. Let's face it; customs lacks the capacity to open most of the packages that are sent to this country from around the world. They are totally lost when it comes to being able to effectively deal with regular letters that contain steroids in sheets of paper.

The manufacturing process works like this. A steroid compound is mixed with alcohol, which is an excellent solvent for steroid hormones. The dissolved solution is placed in a flat tray, and a sheet of blotter paper is placed on it to absorb the liquid. We now have a sheet of blotter paper that is soaked in alcohol and steroid. Now if you leave it out to sit, the alcohol will evaporate pretty quickly, leaving the steroid behind in the process. The hormone is going to be left distributed throughout the blotter sheet, which is now officially serving as the drug carrier. The blotter sheet is usually made so that it is divided into a grid (typically 50 or 100 squares), with each edible square carrying a measured dose of steroid. This idea is actually used, routinely, in a laboratory setting, where you don't always have access to finished tablets or capsules. It is simply being exploited here for a very different purpose. Lab tests on PaperVar confirm the product contains active oxandrolone, however they do note some inconsistencies in dosing from one square to the next. This is likely due to some inherent imperfections in the process, as it is probably much harder to control for error or outside interference than when making tablets or capsules.

Currently PaperRoids are available in the following forms:

PaperVar	oxandrolone	10mg
PaperBol	methandrostenolone	10mg
PaperStrol	stanozolol	10mg
PaperDrol	oxymetholone	50mg

Feedback on the paper products, at least those from the main manufacturer that I have been in contact with, has been nothing short of remarkable. People are raving about these steroids, probably because they work as expected, and are so easy to get in the mail. This means a lot less anxiety for many customers, who would normally spend days worrying that their latest steroid order might get snagged in Customs (and their ass arrested for the attempt). Running down a current price sheet, we find that these products are also fairly affordable. The Dianabol and Winstrol version tend to run from about $.50 to $1.00 per dose, while the Anavar and Anadrol run about $2-$3 each. You'll pay about the same price for commercial versions of these steroids anyway, not to mention the added value in being able to avoid another lost shipment.

The current major manufacturer of these products is reporting an extremely high success rate in their mailings. According to them, 95% of the paper products sent from Thailand are making it to customers, while every item sent from the U.K. so far has arrived without a single seizure by customs. Other underground companies have started to follow suit by manufacturing their own paper products, probably owing to the fact that the design is so easy to copy, and the technology is currently in high demand. One manufacturer has even started making something they call a Flexi-Tab, which is more rigid, and less devious in appearance. I was able to see a sample of this recently, and was quite impressed. I expect to see a lot more of the standard blotter sheet "PaperRoids", as well as the new "Flexi-Tabs", in the future.

Underground Manufacturers

As the name would indicate, an underground steroid manufacturer is an operation that manufactures steroids specifically for sale to athletes on the black market, and not through legitimate pharmaceutical distribution channels. These firms are unlicensed, unregulated, and operate in a completely clandestine manner. An underground maker is different from a counterfeit steroid manufacturer only in that these operations *usually* produce real steroid products. They are not operating to outright steal money from customers with totally worthless products. Many clearly are trying to focus on building good reputations in the marketplace, operating for the most part on a small scale, and catering to tight-knit circles of Internet savvy steroid shoppers.

There has been an amazing explosion of underground steroid manufacturing companies in the past half decade. The Internet, a communications medium that has been able to put bodybuilders in the West in ready contact with bulk raw steroid manufacturers in the East, has no doubt fueled this. It is now quite easy to find places to sell you bulk raw materials, in multi-kilogram amounts. The raw steroid power is usually quite cheap given the amount of final product each kilo can produce. Bottling and encapsulating are usually done with inexpensive low volume manually operated machinery. Let's do a little math. 1kg of methandrostenolone will produce 2,000 bottles with 100 5mg tablets in each. The cost will come to roughly $2 per bottle for the actual steroid. Clearly there are very high profits to be made for anyone willing to do some "basement bottling". Judging by the sheer number of these firms in operation right now, it seems that everyone wants to run an underground steroid manufacturing business.

Below is a sample price list from a raw materials supplier in China. Note the high cost for drugs like oxandrolone, methenolone and trenbolone. We can see counterfeiters rarely use these actual steroids in their products.

Ethylestrenol	$9,900/kg
Methenolone	$18,000/kg
Methandriol	$2,100/kg
Methandrostenolone	$4,000/kg
Methyltestosterone	$1,150/kg
Nandrolone phenylpropionate	$4,000/kg
Nandrolone decanoate	$4,800/kg
Oxandrolone	$27,000/kg
Oxymetholone	$4,000/kg
Stanozolol	$4,600/kg
Testosterone	$1,900/kg
Testosterone Undecanoate	$3,000/kg
Testosterone Propionate	$2,500/kg
Trenbolone	$23,000/kg

There are things that must be taken into consideration when thinking about buying an underground steroid product. First, you need to remember that you never truly know what you are getting. These operations are clandestine, and nobody is looking over their shoulders making sure things are up to code. Second, almost none of them are making their drugs in a truly sterile environment either. Most, in fact, are probably made in someone's house. The only real exception this may be a handful of larger companies (such as International Pharmaceuticals, Eurochem, and Generic Supplements), which have their product manyufactured in a sterile (pharmaceutical quality) laboratiroes or contract manufacturers. IP, for example, has a long and solid history, and have been operating for decades. But given their nature as an illegal underground company, even the sterility and quality of their products cannot be verified all the time. You can ultimately never be sure your product is clean, or accurately dosed, if you are buying an underground version.

Even with the given risks and uncertainties, many bodybuilders still prefer to shop with underground companies, perhaps finding attraction in cheaper prices, higher doses, or easier availability. For whatever reason, these companies do exist, and many people do buy their products regularly. In the last edition, I tried to start keeping somewhat of a list of these operations, however, I quickly found that an exercise in futility. Due to the entirely secretive and unregulated nature of these companies, they are simply too elusive to keep tabs on. Half of the manufacturers listed in the last book have already gone out of business, and some of the rest have seen their own on and off issues with quality controls. Given the illegitimate nature of this market, I have decided the best thing to do was to simply advise on the potential risks associated with underground drugs, and refrain from rating these firms individually. Instead, I will display photographs, and when possible run lab tests. I believe the information presented in the lab testing section will be of much greater value than vague recommendations.

Counterfeit Steroids

Counterfeit steroids are products that are made by illegal underground operations, which resemble the packaging of legitimate steroid products. They are made specifically for sale to bodybuilders on the black market. Obviously we cannot verify the contents of these products, as real drug companies do not make them. Sometimes the counterfeit producers use real steroids in their preparations, but most often they do not. One must be aware that money should be a secondary concern when coping with the existence of counterfeit pharmaceuticals. Today we take for granted that the drug products we purchase are manufactured in a sterile environment, with filtered air that is free of contaminants. The illicit producers do not provide us this safety. Money is the issue to them, not safety. Injectables are especially of concern, as this method of delivery bypasses most of your natural defenses. Bacteria or toxins could prove very harmful if injected into your body. It is not uncommon to hear of stories in which an athlete had become very ill from using a counterfeit product. One must stay educated to protect not only money but also health.

Counterfeit steroids remain a significant problem on the black market. When you have product in high demand and limited availability, the market will usually fight to exist and meet demand. If need be and possible, this will include counterfeiting legitimate products. With steroids, this is a major problem because fakes are easily made, and the validity of each product difficult to ascertain without using it for a period of time. I would, however, like to report that things have been changing over the years in my observation, in terms of the magnitude of this problem. I think fake steroids became most problematic after two important events in the history of these compounds. The first was the removal of Dianabol in the late 1980's. This was an extremely popular product, and taking it off the market led many to scramble to cash in on the demand by bottling fake Dbol. From this point forward the term "counterfeit steroid" became woven into the fabric of the black market. I think the true counterfeit explosion occurred in the early 90's, specifically right after these drugs became controlled substances in early 1991. Before this, domestic anabolics were easily diverted toward illicit avenues. I remember seeing a ton of legitimate American pharmaceuticals in 1990 and 1991. Steris suspension, cyp, Deca, it was everywhere. But a year or two later, these had all but dried up and were replaced with loads of copies. Steris clones were everywhere, while the real thing was becoming almost impossible to obtain.

I think the mid to late 1990's was a transition time for the black market. Our domestic avenues for steroids were cut off, and it would take some time to solidify new sources for these drugs. This period of time was a perfect breeding ground for counterfeiters. If the drugs couldn't be located easily, many simply just made passable copies. Sure, as with any industry most people did business honestly and worked hard to find, even import legitimate products. But there is always a bad segment out there, and at that point in time they seemed to actually thrive on the manufacture of counterfeit goods. But we are in a new time now. The black market no longer needs to carry counterfeit products in order to meet an otherwise impossible demand. New, reliable avenues for these drugs have opened up. Most notably, our neighbor to the south, Mexico, has emerged as a world leader in steroid manufacture and sales. As a result, the U.S. black market is now bursting with Mexican products. I think the actual percentage of fakes on the market is much smaller today than 10 years ago, and your odds for buying a legitimate product are very good. Do not confuse me with saying that fakes have gone away. Far from it. They are still a big problem today, as they probably always will be.

If you do not obtain steroids via a doctor or N. American pharmacy, it is my hope this book will provide you with the skills you need to make intelligent purchases. The current situation is not that grim. Counterfeit marketers thrive on ignorance. Most people make purchases with little or no research beforehand, and that is what the counterfeiters are relying on. You will quickly realize that a little bit of research will go a long way when shopping for anabolics, as an educated consumer is much harder to swindle.

THE BASICS

This section deals with the most general attributes to look for when attempting to spot counterfeit anabolics. Before starting, it is important to stress the fact that underground manufacturers are much more advanced today than they were 15 years ago. The fakes of today are generally much better looking, and harder to recognize than they used to be. The methods mentioned in this section are mostly inadequate for counterfeit identification, as only the sloppiest of fakes will fail here. Marketers have recognized some years back that in order to be competitive, (and remain in business) they had to update equipment, and put together a nicer item. So, do not be overconfident if your items pass the following tests.

MATCHING LABELS:

15 years ago, many fakes were put together as the below suspension was. The counterfeiter used the same label for both the box and vial to save time and money. In general, be suspicious of any box that carries a sticker instead of print. There are only a rare few exceptions to this rule, and they tend to be products of Eastern or South East Asian origin.

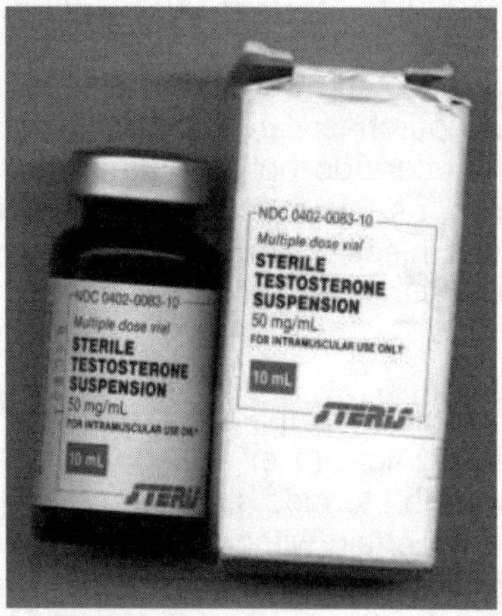

UNUSUAL AMPULES:

When underground manufacturers first began to duplicate ampules, many were quite unusual in appearance. Some leaked, contained air bubbles in the glass, or uneven. Some were so crooked, that they would fall over should you try to stand them on a desk. One would want to make sure all ampules are consistent in size and shape, do not leak, and look professional in appearance. Oil levels should be relatively even when they are lined up, and the solution clean (free of particulate) when drawn into a syringe. It should also be sized proportionately to the volume it contains. The below ampule is very odd, as it can hold about 4 or 5ml, but is a 1ml Sustanon clone. Definitely a fake.

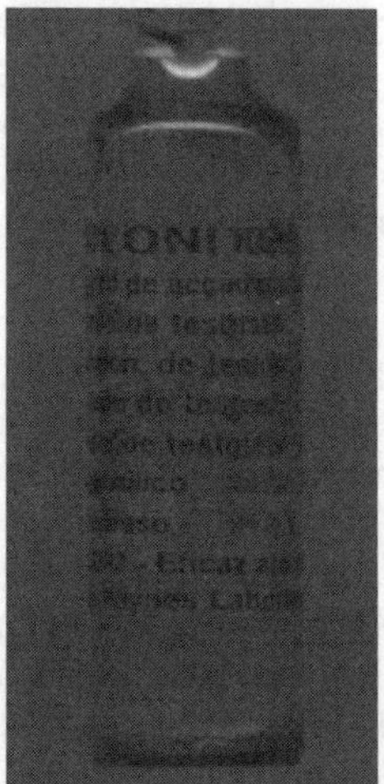

PILL BOTTLES:

Bottles of loose pills are the crudest of all steroid knockoffs. Very easy to assemble, just about anyone looking to produce a fake could find the resources to do this. In Anabolics 2000, I mentioned that you would not find many legitimate bottles with loose pills on the black market that are real. Most foreign (human) drug marketers package tablets in foil or foil and plastic strips. However, in the past five years, numerous legitimate veterinary firms have started producing steroid tablets in bottles. Many are legit, and good buys. However, it is still a very good ideal to avoid unknown products of this type to be safe.

EXPIRATION DATES:

One will want to examine the expiration date on the box/vial to determine if it was stamped or printed separately from the rest of the writing. Legitimate drug manufacturers print the boxes and labels in bulk, and then run the lot number/exp. dates at the time of packaging. Counterfeiters often include these dates with the rest of the printing on the box, avoiding the need for an extra piece of equipment. It is best to see some form of stamp or indent that would tell you for certain that it was added at a later time.

Machine stamping on Spanish Primobolan® and generic Clomid® from Greece.

Stamping on an Anabol Label.

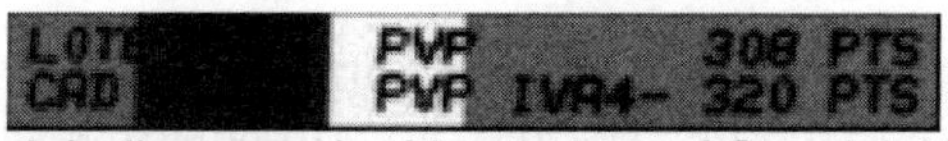

Computer labeling on a legitimate box of Spanish Winstrol®.

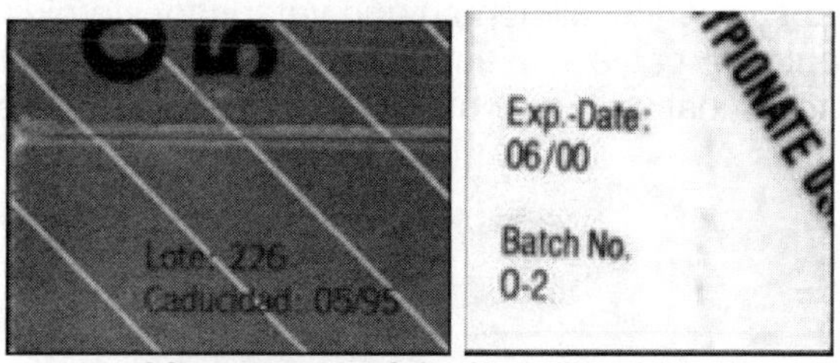

Many counterfeits look like this.

The above two counterfeits clearly have dates printed with the rest of the box. Although there are certainly expections to this, notably in areas of Eastern Europe, few legitimate drug manufacturers will use this method of coding their items. It is simply too cost ineffective, and inflexible. Seeing this is a fairly reliable indication you have a fake drug.

Non-Glossy Surfaces

Also take a minute to look at the area where the dates and lot codee are applied on your box and/or label. This is a particularly important thing to look at if your box is made out of glossy cardboard (it will have a shine to it). Many legitimate pharmaceutical companies will leave a small area on their boxes/labels that does not have a glossy surface. This is for the printing of the lot number and expiration date. Doing this prevents smearing of these vital numbers, which is often a problem when ink is applied directly to a glossy surface. You may have tried to jot a number down on a glossy sheet of paper at one time or another, and found that it rubs off easily. That is the same thing. Although certainy not done in enough frequency to consider this a rule to live by, finding a small non-gloss area on your product does show there is a little extra intricacy to it. Counterfeit drug makers will often overlook small features like this.

Country Specifics

In most countries, a pharmaceutical company is required to meet a specific set of regulations when manufacturing a drug product. This helps us when evaluating our black market anabolics, as counterfeiters often do not have the resources to keep up with these regulations (few do) and cut corners in order to release a product. Here, I will discuss some attributes to look for which will hold true for all of the drugs produced in the specified country.

United States:

First, it is very important to stress the fact that steroids are a controlled substance in the United States. If you think this makes little difference to the underground community, think again. Current controls are very effective at keeping American products off of the black market. It is much easier for the illicit dealers to import or manufacture their own products than it is to get any volume of legitimate American anabolics to distribute. Be leery of every American item you see too, it is in all probability a fake. The best rule is to avoid all American items unless you can personally trace them back to a pharmacy.

The FDA does provide us with a couple of strict requirements, which, to date, are not being met by most counterfeiters. The most predominant is that all legitimate American drugs cannot carry a label that will easily be removed from the vial/bottle. It is to be so saturated with glue that you would need a razor blade and saintly patience to remove it, small piece by small piece. This is to protect the public from the possibility of drug mislabeling. I have never seen a counterfeit in which the label could not be peeled off the bottle quickly, in one or a few large pieces. Underground labs just do not have the needed machinery, which provides us the most efficient method for spotting fake American drugs.

If you are unsure, you can also moisten your thumb and rub the expiration date on the box and label. Quite often the ink on the counterfeit will smear and rub off. The real item may streak slightly, but will remain relatively intact and legible.

Also, being a Schedule 3 controlled substance, all human and veterinary steroids are required to bear the following tag (CIII). The only exception would be cattle implant pellets, which are technically not controlled. Some lazy counterfeiters are still duplicating items that were manufactured before 1991, when this tag was not present.

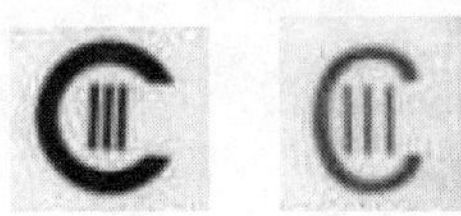

Italy:

All drugs produced in Italy will bear the pictured drug identification sticker. The sticker itself is white, with red and black print. It has also been recently modified, so that like Greek drugs it can be peeled off of a laminated surface. All new Italian drugs will have this peel-off sticker. Do not purchase an Italian drug if it is not present. Likewise, you can probably trust the product if you do see it. Drugs from Italy will also use abbreviations like Prep, Scad, and Del for the counterpart of Lot #, manufacture and expiration dates.

Greece:

Greece also has a drug ID sticker that must be present on all drugs sold. The sticker itself rests on a laminated surface, so that it can be peeled off of the box and affixed to paperwork when a prescription is filled. Do not purchase any Greek drug without the proper sticker attached. Also of note, drugs from Greece will use the abbreviations Lot, Man and Exp. for date stampings. Due to its inclusion in the European Union, all stickers will now display the retail price of the drug in Euros. You MUST look for the € symbol on all boxes manufactured after 2002. When looking at the coded numbers, note that two digits under AE reflect the year of manufacture, in this case 2003. More importantly, Greek stickers will show a hidden mark when placed under UV light (see: Security Stickers for more details). Some counterfeiters have copied these stickers with excellent accuracy, right down to the laminated surface. However, as of yet they have not been able to copy the hidden UV watermark.

Spain:

Spanish drugs do not bear a sticker, but have an area on the box that contains a bar code, and some drug information. This area will sometimes have indentations in the cardboard, so as to be removable if you tore the surface. At other times, the barcode is simply printed on the box. Spanish drugs also use the abbreviations Lote and Cad for lot number and expiration date. Recently, many drug boxes are also seen to carry Braille lettering on the box face. Although this is not yet mandatory for all drugs, finding this is certainly a good indicator of a real product. Also, due to recent inclusion in the European Union, all Spanish boxes manufactured after 2002 will display the price in both Pesetas (local currency) and Euros. Look for the € symbol somewhere on the box. Stickers are often seen affixed to boxes with this information, allowing companies to continue to use older boxes already in inventory.

Printed Only

Removable Barcode

Sticker with Euro Pricing

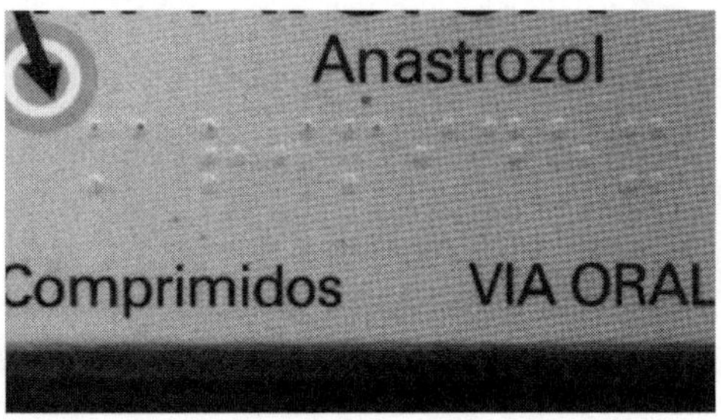

Braille lettering

Portugal:

Drug boxes from Portugal also contain a specific area to look for. It is rectangular, and contains a bar code along with some pricing information. This is sometimes found as a sticker, but most commonly is printed, not stamped, onto the surface. In many cases, the area is scored, so that it can be removed from the box. It is likely that a counterfeiter would have a little difficulty reproducing this, although it has been done before. Drugs from Portugal will also use the abbreviations "Lote:" and "Val. Ate:" for lot number and expiration date stampings. Again, be sure to find pricing in Euros in this area.

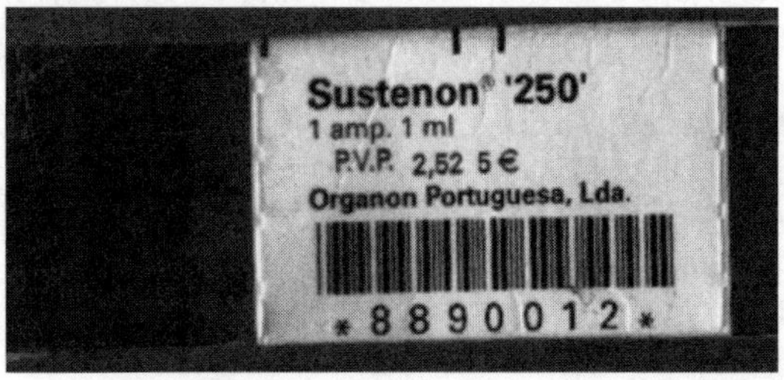

New area with price in Euros

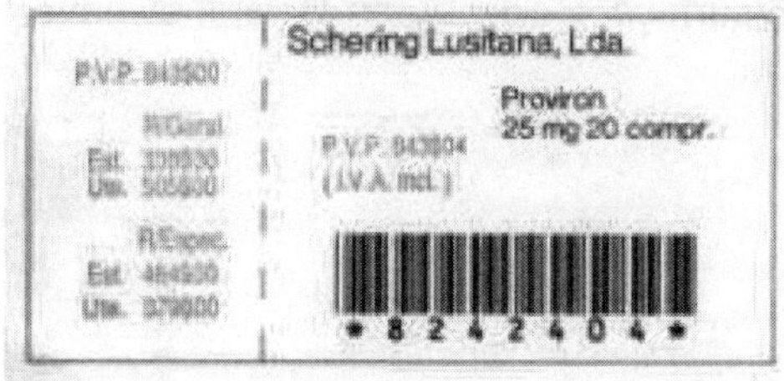

Old one without

France:

All legitimately produced French drugs will bear a rectangular sticker somewhere on the surface of the box. The text and format is often slightly different item to item, so do not rely on these as foolproof indicators of legitimacy. Also, packaging from this country always contains an area with a green and red box. In this case, it is in the lower left side of the Androtardyl box.

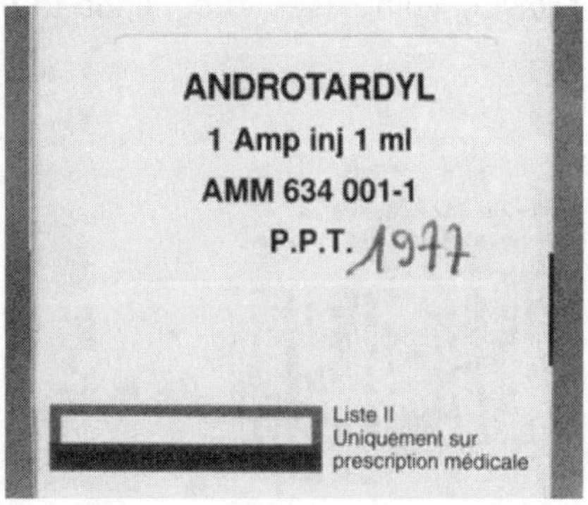

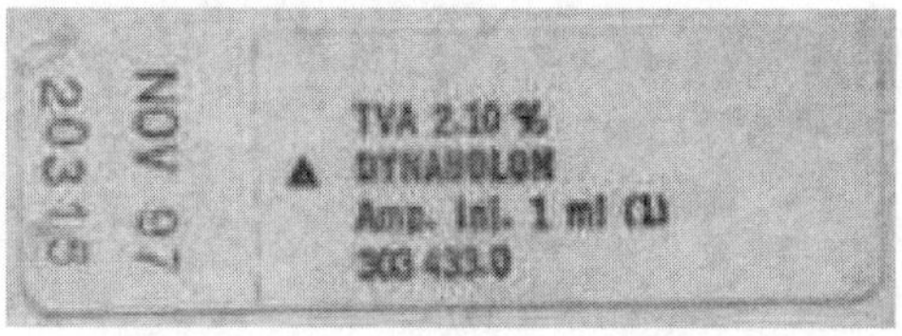

Security Stickers

In the multi-billion dollar international steroid business, counterfeit steroids are big money. They are also perhaps the number one financial concern for all parties involved. These drugs cheat consumers out of their hard-earned money, and chip away millions from the bank accounts of legitimate drug manufacturers. As a company owner you can work hard for years to build a recognizable line, just to have a bunch of crooks come in and devalue your products. It doesn't take much. Once enough fakes are dumped into the marketplace, people start waking away from your company and move on to products they can better trust. The more popular your company is in this business, the more you have to worry about it. The smart ones today are not taking this sitting down.

Numerous companies have invested in security features, which they hope the counterfeiters will not have the resources to copy. These include custom designed holograms, etched vials and bottles, watermarked printing, and other general security stickers. Although to this point counterfeiters have demonstrated the capability and willingness to duplicate just about anything, a number of companies have been very successful in their implementations thus far. In this section we will look at a variety of security features in use by popular steroid companies, so you know exactly what to look for when shopping. If you stay resolved to only purchase products with the features listed in this section, you should be able to make safe purchases for some time to come.

Greek Pharmacy Stickers

As I mentioned in "Country Specifics", Greek drugs all carry a particular pharmacy sticker. What most people do not know, however, is that these stickers show a hidden mark under ultraviolet light. In the "Security Stickers" section in the back of this book you will see several different stickers, from different years of use, taken under blacklight. If you don't have a blacklight, get one! This is an ultra reliable method for weeding out the best of Greek fakes at this time.

Animal Power (Mexico)

Animal Power is a new company in Mexico, and started operating right from the start with security in mind. In fact, they have among the most intricate set of anti-counterfeiting features in the industry. These include:

A) A hologram with the company name, "Paw" logo background, and the words "Animal Power Original Product" all included inside the holographic image.
B) Etched vials and bottles with the Animal Power Logo.
C) Custom printed flip caps for vial tops, with Animal Power "Paw" logo.

Brovel (Mexico)

Brovel uses a hologram sticker with "Securite" imbedded in the background of the holographic image, and the company logo printed in ink on the surface. These holograms appear on all boxes and vials. Note that these stickers are easier to duplicate than true custom made holograms, as someone might be able to obtain a similar looking generic hologram sticker and just print the Brovel logo on top of it. Even given that fact, fakes of this type are not yet a problem. Brovel also seals its boxes with tape printed with the company's "BL" logo in yellow ink.

Denkall (Mexico)

Denkall uses a small round hologram sticker on all of its products. This has the Denkall "DK" logo and "Securidad" imbedded in the holographic image. I have seen some good-looking copies of this hologram made out of a plain silver sticker. However, holding it to the light immediately reveals that there was no rainbow "prism effect", and thus it was not a real QV hologram.

Loeffler (Mexico)

Loeffler uses a generic hologram sticker, which bears no distinct markings like the company name. They are also inconsistent with its use, and do not seem to put it on all products.

Pet's Pharma (Mexico)

Pet's Pharma uses a small circular security sticker. It is half red, half blue (both metallic inks), and printed with the company logo. There is a weak hologram in the background, but it is difficult to see through the ink. It says something generic like "Securite". This logo appears on all products.

Quality Vet (Mexico)

Quality Vet uses a square hologram sticker on all products. This has the QV logo and "Securidad" both inside the holographic image.

SYD Group (Mexico)

SYD Group uses a small round holographic sticker with the company logo, "Securidad", and web address embedded in the holographic image. This sticker is affixed to all boxes, as well as the top of the vials.

Ttokkyo (Mexico)

Ttokyo used to use a rectangular hologram sticker, with the company logo imbedded (as both front image and background pattern) in the holographic image. This sticker would seal one of the flaps on each box, and was affixed to the back of all pill bottles. Ttokkyo has since gone out of business, however, so only leftover stock may be remaining on the black market at this time.

Xelox (Philippines)

Xelox uses a rectangular silver sticker (not a hologram) with the company logo printed on the surface. Once the sticker is peeled from the box, the word "VOID" appears. This stick seals one of the flaps on all product boxes.

British Dragon (Thailand)

British Dragon uses a small round hologram sticker on its oral products. It is a generic holographic sticker, with the company name and dragon logo are printed onto the surface in regular ink. The sticker itself is affixed to all tablet pouches, and was formerly placed on all vials. BD has since changed to using a red embedded metallic foil inlay on the vial labels only, which has the letters BD and company logo.

Unfortunately, the BD security sticker no longer provides 100% assurancy of a real purchase. This manufacturer is currently the victim of a sophisticated counterfeiting scheme, which includes the duplication of this sticker. They have not done a perfect job clonine the line, however. They incorrectly affixed a fake BD hologram to their vials, which is now only on their tablet pouches. They have also duplicated the foil inlay on the vial labels in a blue color instead of red. The fake vials also have plastic tops that say "FLIP OFF". The real BD uses a very specific vial top, which reads, "TEAR" (with an arrow to the left) and "FLIP UP" (with an arrow down). Note that this operation is also still duplicating the old pentagon shaped tablets as well, not the new square BD marked pills that the real company is producing.

British Dispensary (Thailand)

British Dispensary uses a small round hologram sticker, with the company snake logo and the words "British Dragon" as the background pattern. Both are imbedded in the image. BD has been the victim of numerous very sophisticated counterfeiting operations in the past. The hologram sticker has been doing a lot to help with this, and has not yet been duplicated. It is, therefore, still a reliable security check.

Serono (U.S.)

Serono, makers of Serostim recombinant human growth hormone (rHGH), have seen their share of counterfeiting. Their Serostim kits were being duplicated with such accuracy that they were actually being sold through some pharmacies. They have since adopted the use of a custom designed hologram sticker, which has the Serono logo imbedded into the graphic. The hologram sticker itself is further imbedded into the box.

PLEASE REFER TO APPENDIX F FOR DETAILED PHOTOGRAPHS OF ALL SECURITY STICKERS

Designer Steroids

There is a fatal flaw in the steroid detection methods used by the various sports agencies. That is, in order to test someone for anabolic steroids, you need to know exactly what you are looking for. You can't just look for "steroids" in the urine, but are forced to test for each specific compound individually. To make things even more complicated, you need to know more that just what these steroids look like chemically before they are administered. You need to know what they are going to look like by the time they appear in the urine, because the original steroids themselves will largely be metabolized into other compounds. For example, nandrolone use is most easily detected by looking for its major metabolites 19-norandrosterone and 19-noretiocholanolone[46], not nandrolone itself. With this in mind, you need to investigate each potential steroid of "misuse" very closely, and each plan of detection is going to be difficult, and timely, to develop. The past couple of decades have seen a lot of progress in identifying the metabolites unique to most commercially available synthetic steroids. As a result, they are almost all detectable in a urine sample now. In reality, this may still only be a drop in the bucket.

You see, several hundred, if not a thousand or more, different steroids were synthesized and investigated in various laboratories around the world during the heyday of steroid research. In most cases, their anabolic and androgenic potencies were measured, with the same methods that have been used on all of the popular steroids we know today. Only a minute fraction of these research compounds ultimately became commercially available drug products, leaving many potentially excellent steroids by the wayside. This is to be expected in any area of drug research though, as there would be no way for hundreds of similar drugs to exist in the same market. But the early research is still out there, and remains a very valuable source of information for the clever chemists of today.

Some of these old research steroids of the 50's and 60's still exist today, due to the diligence of underground chemists and researchers. We refer to these drugs collectively as "Designer Steroids", and they are here only for the purpose of defeating a drug screen. A true designer steroid is structurally unique next to the known anabolic/androgenic steroids, sharing no common metabolites, so as to be undetectable to even the most thorough steroid test. The thought of tracking down metabolites for all possible steroids compounds, to eliminate the designer steroids issue, seems like an impossible task to say the least. Even if somehow this old research were to be exhausted, and metabolites identified for all known steroids, there are still nearly limitless other ways to alter testosterone, nandrolone, or dihydrotestosterone to make unique new steroids. The designer steroid phenomena could obviously present an overwhelming problem to the sports organizations given present drug testing methods. The athletes can easily stay one or two steps ahead, and nobody on the sidelines is the wiser.

At this point in time, the fact that designer steroids exist is no secret to the sports agencies. It became painfully obvious to the IOC (international Olympic Committee) in March of 2002, when the UCLA Olympic Analytical Lab detected norbolethone, a potent c-17 alpha alkylated nandrolone derivative investigated back in the 1960's, in the urine samples from a female athlete[47] (see Drug Profiles: Norbolethone). It turned out to be Tammy Thomas, a 32-year-old cyclist from Colorado Springs. This was the second time she failed a drug test actually, which resulted in a lifetime ban from competition. One of the samples in question was actually flagged previously, with a group of others, because it had extremely low endogenous steroid concentrations (suggesting suppression from exogenous steroid administration). Don Catlin, who runs the UCLA Olympic Analytical Laboratory, would connect it to the designer steroid norbolethone much later. The fact that only one of these samples retroactively tested positive suggests that other designer steroids were being used by competitors in addition to norbolethone.

Catlin was able to obtain a sample of pure norbolethone from the drug company Wyeth, and must have been greatly aided by the fact that metabolites of this steroid had been identified in earlier studies[48]. The procedure for norbolethone detection has now been made available to all testing agencies, and unfortunately it is now unsafe for competition. Its value as a designer steroid has likewise vanished overnight. Perhaps it was a bad idea to use a steroid that actual made it all the way to the point of clinical trials in the U.S., as there is quite a bit of information to be found on it (not having the urinary metabolites study would have made things a lot harder on Catlin). Honestly, I can think of a number of more effective and safer compounds to use than this hideously progestational one (ooh, the water bloat). I don't think the chemist was really thinking this one through very thoroughly, and may want to get some help from someone that really knows these agents next time.

The norbolethone story quietly fell from the public conscience not long after it broke. The number of athletes that ultimately tested positive for the drug was minimal, so it really never evolved into the big scandal that was initially expected. The USADA thrives on negative media attention to steroids, because it leads to more government funding, so no doubt this lack of public outrage was a disappointment. I would suspect many involved were hoping for global story on par with what happened when Ben Johnson was stripped of his gold medal during 1988 summer Olympics. This would be of little matter by January 2004, however, because a much bigger doping scandal was about to hit. It involved the use of the designer steroid tetrahydrogestrinone (see Drug Profiles: THG), and this time would snare some of the biggest figures in amateur and professional sports. Not just Olympic competitors, but professional football and baseball players were being listed as potential violators. Many household names were being thrown around, including Jason Giambi, Barry Bonds and Gary Scheffield. Over 20 athletes ultimately tested positive for THG, or were specifically named for using it in the evidence. The investigation continues today, so this number may rise. Don Catlin was once again the scientist who helped identify this compound in the first place, as well as a method of its detection in urine. This time around, however, he had a lot more help then he did with norbolethone. THG was actually handed over to the IOC testing laboratory in a syringe, by an anonymous coach who did not approve of its use. With the help of an inside informant, USADA got their Ben Johnson story, and then some. THG was at the center of the biggest organized doping scandal in the history of competitive sports, and would come to spark a more vigorous government fight against steroid use than we had yet seen. The steroid-using community is only now beginning to feel the backlash.

I include these stories not because they illustrate victories for the IOC. Quite the contrary, I believe they underline the major failings in current steroid testing methods. These two incidents logically do not represent the only two designer steroids ever used in competitive sports. For one, we surely cannot expect a 100% success rate for the IOC when we know that THG use went completely unnoticed for months, if not years. Nobody knew anything about this steroid until a sample was handed over to the testing facility, which is the same facility that had unwittingly been passing urine samples containing the same steroid just days before. Were it not for the inside source, THG would probably still be in use today. The norbolethone and THG stories spit in the face of those on the sidelines, who insist that drug testing ensures their favorite athlete is drug free. The fact is, many other potent designer steroids are probably out there, either in the books, or in the gym bags, of many of the world's top competitors. It may take years for the next designer compound to be identified by the IOC labs, and perhaps only a matter of weeks for a new one to be synthesized once it is. It is a game the drug testers simply cannot win given the tools they have available to them now. We may see repeats of these scandals in the future, but such events will only exemplify the proficiency of those working against drug testing. They show the public the unshakable will of the athletes who are going to use these agents, not the testing agencies that police them.

Anabolic Steroids and the Law

If you live outside of the United States, chances are the country that you live in has a reasonable grasp on the how minimally anabolic steroids affect society as a whole. Your country is probably not sensing a public health crisis, nor locking up and persecuting bodybuilders for mere possession of these drugs. In the United States, however, things are very different. Here, it is a federal crime to possess anabolic steroids without a doctor's prescription. Get caught with some of the same hormones that your already have in your body naturally, and you could land yourself in serious trouble. The current federal penalty for the possession of anabolic steroids is up to one year in jail and a $100,000 fine for a first offense. The penalties for distribution are much more severe. If you live in the United States, and are not obtaining your drugs through a doctor's prescriptions, this section may be of particular relevance to you.

Although anabolic steroids have been classified as controlled substances in the U.S. since 1991, there was a recent expansion to this law called the Anabolic Steroid Control Act of 2004. It was signed into law by President George W. Bush in October of 2004. The new law is in effect as of January 20th, 2005. Of particular interest are the new compounds that have been added to the list of controlled drugs. They include most steroidal precursor hormones, such as androstenediol, norandrostenediol, and hydroxyandrostenedione (formestane), as well as many of the new synthetic agents, like methyl-1-testosterone, methyldienolone, and hydroxymethylnandrolone. Also added are some old commercial drugs that were missed the first time, including bolasterone, mestanolone (methylDHT), and oxabolone (Steranabol Ritardo). The new law also removes the legal requirement that a compound be proven anabolic in humans before it can be added to the list of controlled substances. This "promotes muscle growth" clause was the key roadblock to removing all of the "legal steroids" that have slipped through to market the past 8 years. The new law effectively eliminates the legal steroid loophole in the U.S.

The main body (drug listings) of the Anabolic Steroid Control Act of 2004 has been included for your review below.

`(A) The term `anabolic steroid' means any drug or hormonal substance, chemically and pharmacologically related to testosterone (other than estrogens, progestins, corticosteroids, and dehydroepiandrosterone), and includes--

`(i) androstanediol--
`(I) 3b,17b-dihydroxy-5a-androstane; and
`(II) 3a,17b-dihydroxy-5a-androstane;
`(ii) androstanedione (5a-androstan-3,17-dione);
`(iii) androstenediol--
`(I) 1-androstenediol (3b,17b-dihydroxy-5a-androst-1-ene);
`(II) 1-androstenediol (3a,17b-dihydroxy-5a-androst-1-ene);
`(III) 4-androstenediol (3b,17b-dihydroxy-androst-4-ene); and
`(IV) 5-androstenediol (3b,17b-dihydroxy-androst-5-ene);
`(iv) androstenedione--
`(I) 1-androstenedione ([5a]-androst-1-en-3,17-dione);
`(II) 4-androstenedione (androst-4-en-3,17-dione); and
`(III) 5-androstenedione (androst-5-en-3,17-dione);
`(v) bolasterone (7a,17a-dimethyl-17b-hydroxyandrost-4-en-3-one);
`(vi) boldenone (17b-hydroxyandrost-1,4,-diene-3-one);
`(vii) calusterone (7b,17a-dimethyl-17b-hydroxyandrost-4-en-3-one);
`(viii) clostebol (4-chloro-17b-hydroxyandrost-4-en-3-one);
`(ix) dehydrochloromethyltestosterone (4-chloro-17b-hydroxy-17a-methyl-androst-1,4-dien-3-one);
`(x) *1-dihydrotestosterone (a.k.a. `1-testosterone') (17b-hydroxy-5a-androst-1-en-3-one);
`(xi) 4-dihydrotestosterone (17b-hydroxy-androstan-3-one);
`(xii) drostanolone (17b-hydroxy-2a-methyl-5a-androstan-3-one);
`(xiii) ethylestrenol (17a-ethyl-17b-hydroxyestr-4-ene);
`(xiv) fluoxymesterone (9-fluoro-17a-methyl-11b,17b-dihydroxyandrost-4-en-3-one);
`(xv) formebolone (2-formyl-17a-methyl-11a,17b-dihydroxyandrost-1,4-dien-3-one);
`(xvi) furazabol (17a-methyl-17b-hydroxyandrostano[2,3-c]-furazan);
`(xvii) 13a-ethyl-17a-hydroxygon-4-en-3-one;
`(xviii) 4-hydroxytestosterone (4,17b-dihydroxy-androst-4-en-3-one);
`(xix) 4-hydroxy-19-nortestosterone (4,17b-dihydroxy-estr-4-en-3-one);
`(xx) mestanolone (17a-methyl-17b-hydroxy-5a-androstan-3-one);
`(xxi) mesterolone (1a-methyl-17b-hydroxy-[5a]-androstan-3-one);
`(xxii) methandienone (17a-methyl-17b-hydroxyandrost-1,4-dien-3-one);

`(xxiii) methandriol (17a-methyl-3b,17b-dihydroxyandrost-5-ene);
`(xxiv) methenolone (1-methyl-17b-hydroxy-5a-androst-1-en-3-one);
`(xxv) methyltestosterone (17a-methyl-17b-hydroxyandrost-4-en-3-one);
`(xxvi) mibolerone (7a,17a-dimethyl-17b-hydroxyestr-4-en-3-one);
`(xxvii) 17a-methyl-*1-dihydrotestosterone (17b-hydroxy-17a-methyl-5a-androst-1-en-3-one) (a.k.a. `17-a-methyl-1-testosterone');
`(xxviii) nandrolone (17b-hydroxyestr-4-en-3-one);
`(xxix) norandrostenediol--
`(I) 19-nor-4-androstenediol (3b, 17b-dihydroxyestr-4-ene);
`(II) 19-nor-4-androstenediol (3a, 17b-dihydroxyestr-4-ene);
`(III) 19-nor-5-androstenediol (3b, 17b-dihydroxyestr-5-ene); and
`(IV) 19-nor-5-androstenediol (3a, 17b-dihydroxyestr-5-ene);
`(xxx) norandrostenedione--
`(I) 19-nor-4-androstenedione (estr-4-en-3,17-dione); and
`(II) 19-nor-5-androstenedione (estr-5-en-3,17-dione;
`(xxxi) norbolethone (13b,17a-diethyl-17b-hydroxygon-4-en-3-one);
`(xxxii) norclostebol (4-chloro-17b-hydroxyestr-4-en-3-one);
`(xxxiii) norethandrolone (17a-ethyl-17b-hydroxyestr-4-en-3-one);
`(xxxiv) oxandrolone (17a-methyl-17b-hydroxy-2-oxa-[5a]-androstan-3-one);
`(xxxv) oxymesterone (17a-methyl-4,17b-dihydroxyandrost-4-en-3-one);
`(xxxvi) oxymetholone (17a-methyl-2-hydroxymethylene-17b-hydroxy-[5a]-androstan-3-one);
`(xxxvii) stanozolol (17a-methyl-17b-hydroxy-[5a]-androst-2-eno[3,2-c]-pyrazole);
`(xxxviii) stenbolone (17b-hydroxy-2-methyl-[5a]-androst-1-en-3-one);
`(xxxix) testolactone (13-hydroxy-3-oxo-13,17-secoandrosta-1,4-dien-17-oic acid lactone);
`(xl) testosterone (17b-hydroxyandrost-4-en-3-one);
`(xli) tetrahydrogestrinone (13b,17a-diethyl-17b-hydroxygon-4,9,11-trien-3-one);
`(xlii) trenbolone (17b-hydroxyestr-4,9,11-trien-3-one); and
`(xliii) any salt, ester, or ether of a drug or substance described in this paragraph.';

State vs. Federal

Things are also more complicated for citizens of the United States than just having to pay attention to Federal laws. Most criminal prosecutions for steroid possession actually take place at the State level, and in accordance with State laws. In many instances, the State law was written with compound names and penalties that are similar to the Federal statutes. Sometimes they are vastly different in structure. In some instances, the States have even enacted more encompassing laws than the Federal government, such as California and Nevada, which already had made some of the "legal steroids" and steroidal precursors illegal when their steroid laws were first enacted. The penalties for mere possession can also vary greatly from State to State, as does the way the dosage units are counted. In some States, 100 tablets of Dianabol is looked at as felony distribution weight, instead of just the personal-use cycle it would actually be. Possession of any steroid in many regions of the country can land you in jail for up to five years, sometimes more. Sometimes the State courts so misunderstand steroids, that they weigh the carriers in a pill or injectable vial when making prosecutions. In such jurisdictions, a single 30ml vial of testosterone can be interpreted as a 30-gram dealing dose of drug. Don't be surprised if you hear a prosecutor saying, "He is a drug dealer your honor. He had more than a full ounce in his trunk!" Two states actually do not have any laws against steroid possession at all. It is a big mess.

There is a tremendous amount of confusion over anabolic steroids in the United States, especially at the State level. Given the recent push from the Federal government for increased prosecutions, as well as heightened controls and expanding laws for possession, things are likely to get even tougher for steroid-using athletes here. If you are not obtaining your medications legally through a physician's prescription, it is a good idea to study the steroid laws closely, particularly those of your State. It is important to understand what particular risks you are taking, so you can make decisions accordingly. For example, the last thing you want to be doing in many of these States is driving around with your bottle of Dianabol in the glove compartment, just so you can pop a few tabs after you workout. The book "Legal Muscle: Anabolics in America" by lawyer Rick Collins [teamlegalmuscle.com] is an excellent review of the legal situation concerning steroids in the U.S., and provides invaluable eye-opening advice, including a detailed breakdown of all State steroid laws to sort out the mess described above. I advise everyone taking legal risks to use these drugs to pick it up. It could save you a great deal of time, money and grief.

Part III

Drug Profiles

Anabolic/Androgenic Steroids

Drug Profiles

1-Testosterone (dihydroboldenone)

Androgenic	Anabolic	Standard[49]
100	200	Testosterone propionate

Chemical Names:
17beta-hydroxyandrost-1-en-3-one
5alpha-androst-1-en-3-one,17beta-ol

Estrogenic Activity: None
Progestational Activity: n/a

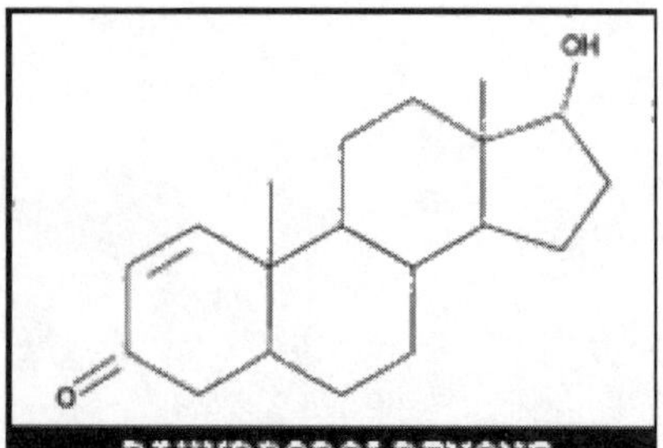

DIHYDROBOLDENONE

1-Testosterone is a dihydro (5-alpha reduced) form of boldenone, hence its chemical name dihydroboldenone. It is also structurally almost identical to Primobolan (methenolone), except that 1-testosterone lacks the additional 1-methyl group that was used to increase steroid oral bioavailability. There is a definite trade off in this. One the one hand, the lack of 1-methylation makes 1-Testosterone a much more powerful hormone than Primobolan. In standard assays, 1-testosterone exceeds Primobolan in potency by a factor of approximately 10. This is most certainly a good thing if you want a potent steroid, as the two are worlds apart in this regard. But on the other hand, lack of 1-methylation means that it will be more difficult to get 1-testosterone into your body via oral administration. With Primobolan, the 1-methyl group is really the only trait that significant slows hepatic metabolism. Without it, oral dosing is not going to be an easy option. Therefore, we need to be a little crafty in order to get the most out of 1-testosterone, as the traditional oral route would require very high daily doses to produce an anabolic effect.

In looking at its basic structural properties, we can point out a few obvious traits. For starters, as a 5-alpha reduced derivative of boldenone, 1-testosterone is unable to undergo 5-alpha reduction in the human body. Its activity is much more along the lines of a balanced anabolic than an androgenic steroid, as it is not potentiated in androgen-responsive target tissues such as the skin, scalp, and prostate like testosterone is. In terms of its ability to build muscle tissue, its anabolic potency is quite profound. The standard rat assays actually show it to be considerably more active than boldenone, nandrolone, dihydrotestosterone, Primobolan, and even the base androgen testosterone itself. 1-testosterone is without question the most potent naturally occurring steroid to be isolated. Only the synthetics, with their greatly extended half-lives and biological activities, begin to exceed 1-testosterone in milligram for milligram potency.

Being a 5-alpha reduced steroid, 1-testosterone is also incapable of being converted to estrogen. This means there is little chance for gynecomastia, bloating, or fat retention. Users of 1-test are more often than not reporting very lean gains in muscle mass, which are often accompanied by body fat reductions and an increased appearance of hardness to the physique (effects that would be characteristic of a strong non-aromatizing anabolic steroid). The only concern with this is that estrogen plays an important role in not only certain muscle-building (anabolic) processes, but also in the functioning of the central nervous system. One of the few common side effects to be reported with this steroid is tiredness and lethargy, something seen with aromatase inhibitors from time to time. For this reason, many will stack 1-testosterone with some form of aromatizable steroid, so as to bring estrogen back up to near physiologically normal levels.

As I mentioned, 1-testosterone is not intrinsically a very orally active hormone. Therefore, it is a little difficult to create a product of extreme potency with this method of administation. It is very much like taking a powerful hormone like testosterone, and trying to stuff it in a capsule. The liver is too efficient at breaking steroids down for this to be effective. When 1-testosterone was available as a supplement legally in the U.S., I had formulated the first oil-solubilized softgel using 1-testosterone tetrahydropyranyl ether. The design of this product was similar to that of Andriol, which dissolves an ester-modified form of testosterone (undecanoate) in oil to help deliver the steroid to the body via the lymphatic system (bypassing the destructive first-pass through the liver). I later switched to 1-testosterone hexyldecanoate, which was more oil soluble and allowed for a higher per capsule dosage and greater absorption. These are the only oral 1-testosterone products I would ever recommend. Some were also formulating this steroid in transdermal gels, which is another moderately effective method of getting this hormone in your body. Lastly, there were a few products that were made as 1-testosterone injectables (as 1-testosterone cypionate), which reportedly worked very well. This would be the preferred method of using 1-testosterone.

1-testosterone was legally sold on the sports supplement market in the U.S. starting in early 2002, and remained on the market in various forms until it was finally classified as a Class III controlled substance in January 2005. Old product will likely be found in black market circulation for the next couple of years, until "pre-ban" stockpiles dry up. Many have reported gains in lean mass exceeding 10-15 pounds in only a 6-8 week period with this steroid, which was phenomenal when 1-testosterone was a legal supplement. Unfortunately, 1-testosterone is now just another illegal steroid. Should you still find it, recommended dose for men is usually in the range of 100-250mg per day with oil-solubilized softgels, or roughly 100mg daily when applied transdermally. Injectable dosages would fall in the range of 100-200mg per week (as 1-testosterone cypionate). One must keep in mind that 1-testosterone is several times more potent than testosterone, so a 200mg injection might provide an effect one would expect with as much as 400-600mg of an injectable testosterone ester. 1-Testosterone is probably a little too strong to recommend to women, for fear of virilization symptoms. Should one risk it, it is usually advised to stick with a very low dose, and be sure to discontinue the product immediately if any unwelcome side effects become apparent. I have seen excellent results on a single 25mg 1-testosterone THP softgel capsule per day in women, but again find the steroid a little strong to recommend myself.

1-Testosterone remained lost in the steroid research books for decades before it finally came to market as a supplement. There are probably many reasons for its lack of prior introduction as a prescription drug. For one, there is simply no need to develop an endless catalog of steroid products. The drug market is a business after all, and with every new drug that is released to treat the same condition as existing drugs, the more diluted the market becomes. I could show you books with literally hundreds, if not a thousand or more, of anabolic/androgenic steroids that were researched but never sold as commercial drug products. This is how drug research typically goes. Another point of interest is that 1-testosterone is intrinsically irritating for some unexplained reason. This makes injection with the base hormone, even transdermal delivery at times, a little difficult to do comfortably. However, injections with 1-testosterone cypionate are reportedly much more comfortable. Some even tend to notice a burning sensation when urinating while taking any 1-testosterone product. To my knowledge, this side effect has never been a dangerous to anyone, and is looked at more as an inconvenience than dangerous. This trait is clearly not present in Primobolan, which perhaps explains why only the 1-methylated (and 2-methylated, see Drug Profiles: Anatrofin) form of this steroid really ever made it to market.

Anabolic DN (nandrolone cypionate)

Androgenic	Anabolic	Standard
37	125	Testosterone

Chemical Names:
19-norandrost-4-en-3-one-17beta-ol
17beta-hydroxy-estr-4-en-3-one

Estrogenic Activity: low
Progestational Activity: moderate

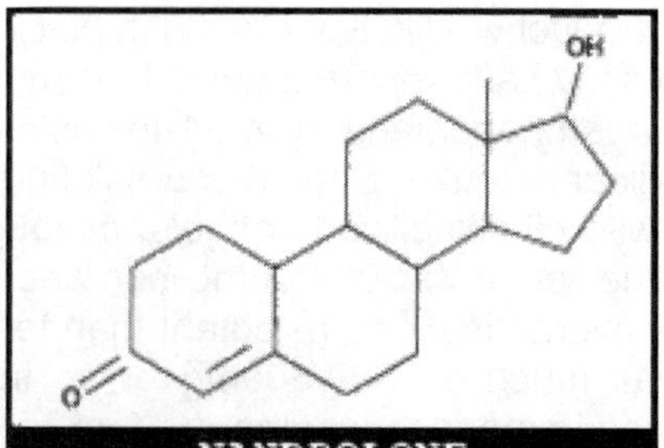

NANDROLONE

Anabolic DN is an Australian steroid, made by the international drug firm SYD Group. It contains the unique compound nandrolone cypionate. The Australian company Jurox also sold this steroid at one time under the brand name Dynabol, however they have since discontinued it and many of their other anabolic steroid products. At this time, the SYD Group item remains the only product in the world to use this nandrolone ester. Anabolic DN is very similar in effect to Deca-Durabolin®, allowing a slow release of the mild steroid nandrolone. The primary difference here is that cypionate will only sustain a notable release for about two weeks. Deca, on the other hand, is active in the body for up to one month. The shorter duration should, however, not really be looked to as an unfavorable characteristic. In this case it produces an extremely interesting steroid. Blood levels peak much faster, and gains will probably accumulate in a shorter time frame. This is supported by the fact that many bodybuilders in Australia swear this is one of the most favorable nandrolone preparations, often said to provide a stronger "kick" than Deca-Durabolin®.

Much of what can be said for Deca holds true for Anabolic DN. It is a strong anabolic, with a mild androgenic component. As with all nandrolones, this steroid has a relatively low affinity for estrogen conversion (estimated to be about 20% of the rate testosterone converts). Anabolic DN is noted as producing a bit more water retention than nandrolone decanoate, which of course is due to the fact that this ester acts so quickly in the body. It builds a substantial blood hormone concentration within the first few days, much more rapidly than the slower acting decanoate ester. Estrogen levels will also build quickly, more hormone being free to convert in the starting weeks. With Deca taking three of four weeks of repeated dosing in order to reaching peak levels, it will take a little bit longer to notice estrogen related trouble. But aside from timing, there is no real difference between the two compounds. Individuals very sensitive to gynecomastia may need to addition an antiestrogen like Clomid® or Nolvadex® when using this product, but otherwise ancillary drugs are usually not necessary for estrogen maintenance with a nandrolone.

Endogenous testosterone levels are likely to be effected by this drug however, especially after longer cycles. A testosterone stimulating drug such as (again) Clomid®/Nolvadex® and/or HCG may therefore be needed to avoid a post-cycle "crash", resulting in excessive muscle loss. HCG is typically used for only a week or two to help kick-start the testes, enabling them to respond normally to the resumed release of endogenous gonadotropins (this capacity may be diminished after a period of long inactivity). After this point Clomid® or Nolvadex® are continued for two to three more weeks in an effort to normalize testosterone production in the body, and minimize any estrogenic side effects until endogenous hormones stabilize.

Although these steroids are very mild, female athletes can sometime have problems with nandrolones. Conversion to DHT, in this case dihydronandrolone (milder then its parent nandrolone), makes androgenic buildup a much lower concern than with most other steroids. The activity of nandrolone is actually reduced somewhat in androgen target tissues, which gives this steroid a much more favorable ratio of anabolic to androgenic effect than most steroids. While virilization symptoms are not usually a pronounced problem with responsible use of a nandrolone, women may still wish to use a faster acting ester such as Durabolin®. This gives the user a greater level of control over blood hormone levels, and reduces the risk for inadvertent androgenic buildup.

Anabolic DN would be about as versatile as Deca-Durabolin®, the compound being well suited for both cutting and bulking cycles. Many however feel the more rapid effect and slightly faster onset of estrogenic side effects (sensitive individuals) causes this steroid to fit most appropriately into mass building phase of training (completely non-aromatizing steroids are often the preference for cutting). A weekly dosage of 200-600mg is most commonly used with this steroid, a range that should provide a very noticeable amount of quality muscle mass, without the heavy water bloat of a testosterone. Although higher doses may bring out a stronger anabolic effect, injections can become very uncomfortable with the volume of oil required each week. Anabolic DN will further mix well with almost any other steroid, including popular mass drugs such as testosterone, Dianabol or Anadrol 50®.

Although in Australia this steroid would have been found in a maximum strength of 50mg/mL (from Jurox), SYD Group has a 300mg/mL version manufactured for the Mexican drug market. It carries the **Anabolic DN** brand name, and a much more vibrant label than its Australian counterpart. The Mexican SYD Group products have a new colorful look and jacked-up Kangaroo mascot they call "Jim Anabolic", funny but effective marketing I would imagine. SYD is a reputable company, and itheir products are becoming extremely popular with bodybuilders in the U.S. This product is definitely recommended. The company apparently takes security more seriously than marketing, protecting all of its products from counterfeiting with a hologram sticker bearing the SYD logo. Provided a leigitmate hologram is present on the product, consumers can be confident they are making a safe purchase.

Anabolic NA (nandrolone/methandriol blend)

Anabolic NA is another one of those unique blended injectable veterinary steroid products that Australia is so famous for. It contains a mixture of methandriol dipropionate and nandrolone cypionate, the two steroids present in a concentration of 45mg/mL and 30mg/mL respectively. This adds up to a total of 75mg per milliliter of steroid, or 750mg total for the 10ml multi-dose vial it comes in. These two agents are primarily anabolic in nature, and tend to provide their users a very good ratio of muscle growth to androgenic/estrogenic side effects (for a more comprehensive discussion of these two steroids individually, please see their respective profiles). Anabolic NA is not quite a bulking drug, but its individual component should make it an excellent lean tissue builder.

For a long time Anabolic NA was sold by Jurox, a company with a 30-year history of manufacturing veterinary drugs in Australia. But not long ago Jurox scaled back its line of steroid products considerably, amidst a great deal of public controversy concerning their exportation of high volumes of steroids to Mexico (known to feed the American black market). Many of their discontinued products are currently being sold under the SYD Group label. SYD is technically a Mexican company, but their steroid products (most which were formerly made by Jurox) were all first manufactured, registered, and sold by their Australian parent company of the same name. SYD Group recently acquired Grupo Comercial Tarasco as well, a company that was formed several years ago specifically to import the Jurox products into Mexico. For a period of time all of these products were being sold in Mexico under the Grupo Comercial Tarasco label, however it appears that SYD is now the sole brand using the tradenamarks and formulations. They are even sporting a cartoon Kangaroo Mascot called Jim Anabolic to help them out (I am getting serious flashbacks of Joe Camel here). At this time it does not appear that Anabolic NA is among the products they continue to sell.

Although Anabolic NA uses the medium to long acting ester cypionate with its nandrolone base, which would typically need to be injected only once per week, this is complemented by a relatively fast acting methandriol dipropionate. As a result, this drug is probably best administered twice weekly to keep blood levels more uniform. Effective weekly doses for male bodybuilders would be in the range of 300-450mg, which would equate to 4-6cc of oil volume in total. Due to the relatively modest steroid concentration, most will opt to add Anabolic NA to a cycle based on other drug instead of using it in higher (uncomfortable) doses alone. With this in mind it is usually used at a dose of 2-3ml, or 150-225mg. Stacked with 200-300mg of testosterone per week, the user will likely find a favorable balance of anabolic and androgenic effect.

Anabolic NA is unavailable at this time. Since it has been so long sicne a real version of this drug was being made, no forms located on the black market should be trusted.

Anabolicum Vister (quinbolone)

Androgenic	Anabolic	Standard
50	100	Testosterone

Chemical Names:
1,4-androstadiene-3-one,17beta-cyclopentenyl
1-dehydrotestosterone cyclopentenyl

Estrogenic Activity: low
Progestational Activity: n/a (low)

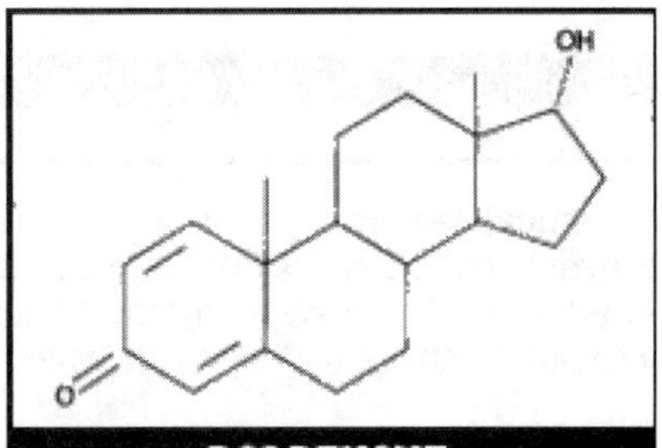

BOLDENONE

Anabolicum Vister is an oral anabolic steroid that was produced in the 1970's by the Parke Davis Company. Peculiarly this product was only sold in Italy, and never had much commercial success outside of this country. The active substance in this product is quinbolone, which is an oral form of the anabolic steroid boldenone. As such it is chemically identical to the veterinary steroid Equipoise® except in this case the boldenone base has a 17beta cyclopentenyl (enol) ether attached instead of an undecylenate ester. The ether functions very much like an ester however, increasing the fat solubility of the compound and protecting it from metabolism. While esterified boldenone was designed as an injectable medication, here the similarly structured ether was used as a means to increase the oral bioavailability of the hormone. The design of this steroid is likewise very similar to the testosterone product Andriol® (testosterone undecanoate), which is also an encapsulated, oil dissolved steroid intended for oral administration. Our experiences with Andriol® remind us that this type of steroid delivery is not very efficient however; but with frequent dosing a steady blood hormone level could be achieved with both of these compounds nonetheless.

The effects of this drug would likewise be characteristic of that reported with Equipoise®. Androgenic side effects are not very prominent when boldenone is taken in moderate doses, except among sensitive individuals. Anabolicum Vister would therefore not cause many problems in terms of estrogenic side effects, and gynecomastia would not be a big concern for the user. The hormone boldenone is able to convert to estradiol in the body, however it seems to do so with a relatively low affinity (about half that of testosterone). So while mild water retention is sometimes documented with this steroid it will usually be related to a more ambitious dosing pattern. Additionally Anabolicum Vister was one of only a few commercially available oral compounds that were not c17 alpha alkylated. Likewise this steroid is not liver toxic, even when used at higher doses for extended intervals. Overall it was one of the safest, most well tolerated oral steroids in production. It was said that in Italian medicine it was prescribed to elderly patients to enhance general health and well being, particularly after weakened from illness, and was even prescribed to postmenopausal Women who were feeling the effects of age. It is unfortunate that with the atmosphere surrounding anabolics in the U.S. such avenues are not more readily explored. One would think that in many instances a mild anabolic could be used to great benefit for an elderly patient. It is further unfortunate that in Italy it seems this unique oral form of boldenone has been discontinued in spite of its favorable design and clinical safety record. Since this was the only country making this steroid it can now be considered extinct.

The disappearance of this product from the black market seemed to go surprisingly unnoticed, probably because athletes usually considered this steroid too mild to warrant consideration. Even when taken in high doses, muscle mass gains would typically be very slight. Clearly this was not simply an alternative to injecting Equipoise®, no doubt due to the low bioavailability of this compound. Used in combination with other steroids it might have proven to have solid benefit as an anabolic, but the money would still have been better spent on a number of more cost-effective items. Men who have experimented with this compound generally found a dosage of 80-120mg (8-12 capsules) per day necessary for any noticeable results. It would obviously not have much use in a bulking cycle, but perhaps the added weak effect might have been welcome during cutting cycles. Women who were curious about steroid use might have found this steroid ideal to experiment with though, perhaps finding notable muscle growth and low side effects on 30-40mg (3-4 capsules) daily. Of course with its stop in production Women are still left with the orals oxandrolone, Primobolan or Winstrol® to fiddle with.

Anadrol 50 (oxymetholone)

Androgenic	Anabolic	Standard
45	320	methyltestosterone (oral)

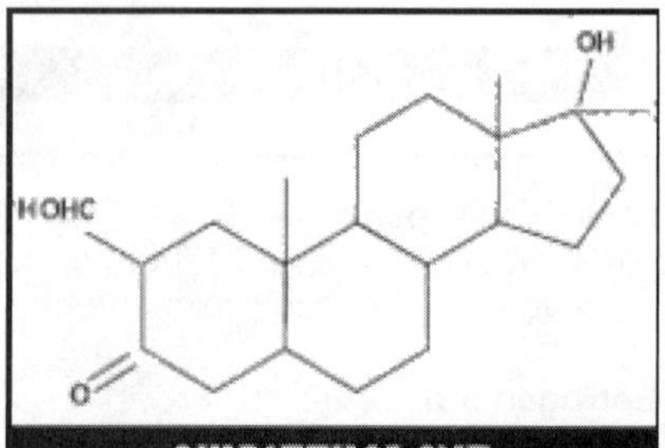

OXYMETHOLONE

Chemical Names:
2-hydroxymethylene-17a-methyl-dihydrotestosterone
4,5-dihydro-2-hydroxymethylene-17-alpha-methyltestosterone
17alpha-methyl-2-hydroxymethylene-17-hydroxy-5alpha-androstan-3-one

Estrogenic Activity: High
Progestational Activity: Not Significant

Anadrol 50® is the U.S. brand name for oxymetholone, a very potent oral androgen. This compound was first made available in 1960, by the international drug firm Syntex. Since oxymetholone is quite reliable in its ability to increase red blood cell production (and effect admittedly characteristic of nearly all anabolic/androgenic steroids), it showed particular promise in treating cases of severe anemia. For this purpose it turned out to be well suited, and was popular for quite some time. But recent years have brought fourth a number of new treatments, most notably the non-steroidal hormone Epogen (erythropoietin). This item is shown to have a much more direct effect on the red blood cell count, without the side effects of a strong androgen. Financial disinterest finally prompted Syntex to halt production of the U.S. Anadrol 50® in 1993, which was around the same time they decided to drop this item in a number of foreign countries. Plenastril from Switzerland and Austria was dropped; following soon was Oxitosona from Spain. Many Athletes feared Anadrol 50® might be on the way out for good. But new HIV/AIDS studies have shown a new light on oxymetholone. These studies are finding (big surprise) exceptional anti-wasting properties to the compound and believe it can be used safely in many such cases. Interest has been peaked, and as of 1998 Anadrol 50® is again being sold in the United States. This time we see the same Anadrol 50® brand name, but the manufacturer is the drug firm Unimed. Syntex continues to market & license this drug in a number of countries however (under a few different brand names).

Anadrol 50® is considered by many to be the most powerful steroid available, with results of this compound being extremely dramatic. A steroid novice experimenting with oxymetholone is likely to gain 20 to 30 pounds of massive bulk, and it can often be accomplished in less than 6 weeks, with only one or two tablets per day. This steroid produces a lot of trouble with water retention, so let there be little doubt that much of this gain is simply bloat. But for the user this is often little consequence, feeling bigger and stronger on Anadrol 50® than any steroid they are likely to cross. Although the smooth look that results from water retention is often not attractive, it can aid quite a bit to the level of size and strength gained. The muscle is fuller, will contract better and is provided a level of protection in the form of "lubrication" to the joints as some of this extra water is held into and around connective tissues. This will allow for more elasticity, and will hopefully decrease the chance for injury when lifting heavy. It should be noted however, that on the other hand the very rapid gain in mass might place too much stress on your connective tissues for this to compensate. The tearing of pectoral and biceps tissue is commonly associated with heavy lifting while massing up on steroids. There can be such a thing as gaining too fast. Pronounced estrogen trouble also puts the user at risk for developing gynecomastia. Individuals sensitive to the effects of estrogen, or looking to retain a more quality look, will therefore often add Nolvadex® to each cycle.

It is important to note however, that this drug does not directly convert to estrogen in the body. Oxymetholone is a derivative of dihydrotestosterone, which gives it a structure that cannot be aromatized. As such, many have speculated as to what makes this hormone so troublesome in terms of estrogenic side effects. Some have suggested that it has progestational activity, similar to nandrolone, and is not actually estrogenic at all. Since the obvious side effects of both estrogens and progestins are very similar, this explanation might be a plausible one. However we do find medical studies looking at this possibility. One such tested the progestational activity of various steroids including nandrolone, norethandrolone, methandrostenolone, testosterone and oxymetholone[50]. It reported no significant progestational effect inherent in oxymetholone or methandrostenolone, slight activity with testosterone and strong progestational effect inherent in nandrolone and norethandrolone. With such findings it starts to seem much more likely that oxymetholone can intrinsically activate the estrogen receptor itself, similar to but more profoundly than the estrogenic androgen methandriol. This means that we can only combat the estrogenic side effects of oxymetholone with estrogen receptor antagonists such as Nolvadex® or Clomid®, and not with an aromatase inhibitor. The strong anti-aromatase compounds such as Cytadren and Arimidex® would similarly prove to be totally useless with this steroid, as aromatase is not involved.

Anadrol 50® is also a very potent androgen, and tends to produce many pronounced, unwanted androgenic side effects. Oily skin, acne, and body/facial hair growth can be seen very quickly with this drug. Many individuals respond with severe acne, often requiring medication to keep it under control. Some of these individuals find that Accutaine works well, which is a strong prescription drug that acts on the sebaceous glands to reduce the release of oils. Those with a predisposition for male pattern baldness may want to stay away from Anadrol 50® completely, as this is certainly a possible side effect during therapy. And while some very adventurous female athletes do experiment with this compound, it is much too androgenic to recommend. Irreversible virilization symptoms may be the result and occur very quickly, possibly before you have a chance to take action.

It is interesting to note that Anadrol 50® does exhibit some tendency to convert to dihydrotestosterone, although this does not occur via the 5-alpha reductase enzyme (responsible for altering testosterone to form DHT) as it is already a dihydrotestosterone based steroid. Aside from the added c-17 alpha alkylation (discussed below), oxymetholone differs from DHT only by the addition of a 2-hydroxymethylene group. However, this grouping can be removed metabolically, reducing oxymetholone to the potent androgen 17alpha-methyl dihydrotestosterone (mestanolone; methyldihydrotestosterone)[51]. There is little doubt that this biotransformation contributes at least on some level to the androgenic nature of this steroid, especially when we note that in its initial state Anadrol 50® has a notably low binding affinity for the androgen receptor. So although we have the option of using the reductase inhibitor finasteride (see: Proscar®) to reduce the androgenic nature of testosterone, it offers us no benefit with Anadrol 50® as this enzyme is not involved.

The principle drawback to Anadrol 50® is that it is a 17alpha alkylated compound. Although this design gives it the ability to withstand oral administration, it can be very stressful to the liver. Anadrol 50® is particularly dubious because we require such a high milligram amount per dosage. The difference is great when comparing it to other oral steroids like Dianabol or Winstrol®, which have the same chemical alteration. Since they have a slightly higher affinity for the androgen receptor, they are effective in much smaller doses (seen in the 5mg and 2mg tablet strengths). Anadrol 50® has a lower affinity, which may be why we have a 50mg tablet dosage. For comparison, taking three tablets of Anadrol 50® (150mg) is roughly the equivalent of 30 Dianabol tablets or 75 Winstrol® tablets(!). When looking at the medical requirements, the recommended dosage for all ages has been 1 - 5 mg/kg of body weight. This would give a 220lb person a dosage as high as 10 Anadrol 50® tablets (500mg) per day. There should be little wonder why when liver cancer has been linked to steroid use, Anadrol 50® is generally the culprit. Athletes actually never need such a high dosage and will take in the range of only 1-3 tablets per day. Many happily find that one tablet is all they need for exceptional results, and avoid higher amounts. Cautious users will also limit the intake of this compound to no longer than 4-6 weeks and have their liver enzymes checked regularly with a doctor. Kidney functions may also need to be looked after during longer use, as water retention/high blood pressure can take a toll on the body. Before starting a cycle, one should know to give Anadrol 50® the respect it is due. It is a very powerful drug, and not always a friendly one.

When discontinuing Anadrol 50®, the crash can be equally powerful. To begin with, the level of water retention will quickly diminish, dropping the user's body weight dramatically. This should be expected, and not of much concern. What is of great concern is restoring endogenous testosterone production. Anadrol 50® will quickly and effectively lower natural levels during a cycle, so HCG and/or Clomid®/Nolvadex® are a must when discontinuing a cycle. The common practice of slowly tapering off your pill dosage is wholly ineffective at raising testosterone levels. Without ancillary drugs, a run away cortisol level will likely strip much of the muscle that was gained during the cycle. If HCG and/or Clomid®/Nolvadex® are used properly, the person should be able to maintain a considerable amount of new muscle mass. Before going off, some alternately choose to first switch over to a milder injectable like Deca-Durabolin®. This is in an effort to harden up the new mass, and can prove to be an effective practice. Although a drop of weight due to water loss is likely when making the switch, the end result should be the retention of more (quality) muscle mass with a less pronounced crash. Remember ancillaries though, as testosterone production will not be rebounding during Deca therapy.

Oxymetholone remains widely available on the black market. Although there are many counterfeits in circulation, there are also enough legitimate companies making the drug to make some good suggestions when shopping.

British Dragon is now selling **Oxydrol** 50mg. This is a square green pill, which is scored in the middle. It reads "BD" on one side and "50" on the other. The product is sold in foil lined white paper packets containing 100 tablets each. To deter counterfeiting, the company has added a hologram sticker. However, the sticker itself is a basic "security" hologram, with the company's dragon logo printed on the outer surface with blue ink. It is a fair method of protection, but not as effective as a hologram with an embedded logo. Generic security stickers would be easy to obtain and modify to look like these. Please also note that British Dragon is a Thai company. There are numerous fakes of this line being manufactured by a Russian counterfeiter. These items are reported to be excellent in appearance, and may even duplicate many of the small details of the real BD line. Be weary of any source for BD products of Russian origin. They are likely not from British Dragon.

Animal Power is a new company to fly onto the Mexican scene this past year, and they are getting a lot of interest. Their oxymetholone product is sold under the brand name **Metalon Tabs**. It comes in a strength of 75mg per tablet, with 100 tablets coming packaged to each glass vial. Animal Power uses several security features to deter counterfeiting, making them a very trusted brand name. Your bottle should come in its own cardboard box, and both will carry the Animal Power security hologram sticker. The company's logo is imbedded in the holographic image. The bottle itself will also have the Animal Power logo printed on the surface of the glass. All of the image, except the canine paw print, will be covered by the adhesive label (the paw print will stick out on the side). Feedback has been very good on the line thus far.

Oximetalon 75mg tablets from Denkall remain a hot commodity on the black market. The higher than normal dosage makes each 100-count bottle of Oximetalon equivalent to a bottle and a half of any standard oxymetholone product. The bottle itself is white, and comes with a child-resistant top. This product is a very reliable buy provided you look for Denkall security hologram sticker. Be sure it is a real hologram, and not just a close-looking substitute made from a standard silver sticker. Counterfeiters have been using these to copy the Denkall line. They are easy to spot when you hold them to the light, as you do not see the "prism" effect that you do with a real hologram.

Not to be outdone by Denkall, the Mexican veterinary firm Quality Vet released its own oxymetholone product this past year called **Oxivet QV**. It is also in the form of a 75mg tablet, packaged 100 tablets to a bottle. Each bottle is also boxed, and the standard QV security hologram sticker protects both from countefeiting. Be sure to look for this when shopping. QV is a very reputable company, and Qxivet a recommended product.

Ttokkko had still been operating on a very small scale in Mexico until very recently, however they have reportedly closed their doors for good very recently. Their **Oxymetolona** product may still be in circulation, but not for much longer. If you do find it, it should carry the Ttokkyo hologram.

Androlic continues to be readily sold in Thailand, manufactured by the drug firm British Dispensary. It comes in a dark plastic bottle with a silver cap and bright green label. No versions are currently circulating in pouches, as all such preparations have been discontinued. The tablets themselves are green, with a hexagon shape and company snake emblem stamped onto the surface.

Kanestron is a veterinary version of oxymetholone made in Mexico by the veterinary firm Loeffler. This product is legit, although I have not seen lab test results on this particular product yet. The line, in general, has been hit or miss in the past as far as dosing goes, so I wouldn't count on getting the full 50mg every time.

Anadrol 50® (U.S.): Unimed Anadrol 50® is rarely found on the black market. It is also going to be extremely expensive when it does, running nearly $15 per 50mg tablet at most pharmacies. With its high cost and tight controls, never purchase this product on the black market unless you can personally trace it to someone receiving it from a doctor.

Brovel started making its own oxymetholone product in Mexico recently, called **Anabrol**. It comes as a 50mg tablet, of which 100 are packaged in each white plastic container. A cardboard box further encloses the bottle. Be sure to look for the Brovel security hologram to assure legitimacy.

You may see a generic oxymetholone product from Israel circulating on the black market on rare occassion. It is a product by **Al-Havi**. One hundred 50mg tablets come in each dark amber bottle, which will be found packed in its own cardboard box.

Oxymetholone is available in Turkey under the **Anapolon** brand name. These are packaged in a foil & plastic push through strip of 20 tablets, 1 strip per box. The back reads Anapolon Tablet, Oksimetolon 50mg in black ink. Although a legitimate product, I have been getting very negative feedback on it as of late. There have been suggestions that the dosing is very off on this product. I have been unable to confirm this with lab testing as of yet.

At the present time this product is not being exported in the same volume that it was several years ago, so you are not likey to see tons of it.

Oxybolone from Greece is still circulating on the black market, and should be reliable provided you have the real thing. At this time counterfeits are easy to weed out, as the real item will carry a pharmacy sticker that will show a hidden image when placed under blacklight (see Security Stickers for more information).

Brazilian **Hemogenin** has been in and out of production in recent years. The version from Sarsa is no longer made, however, the brand is now being sold under the Aventis label.

Han Seo, Han Bul, Korea United, and Dongindang produce Oxymetholone in Korea. The product from Han Seo is most popular. There are numerous fakes of "Korean Anadrol", making them all a risky purchase.

Bratis Labs in Mexico may still be making **Oxitron 50**, which contains the standard 50mg tablet in 100 count bottles. I have not seen lab tests to confirm the contents, but do suspect, with the good feedback on this product, that it is accurately dosed.

Anapolon from the UK and **Oxitosona** from Spain are both long out of commerce now. Occassionally, counterfeiters still duplicate the packaging on these old time items. Don't be fooled. These products were discontinued so long ago that any product that one could theoretically find on the black market (if, for example, someone were to have stockpiled large amounts) would have long been expired already.

Body Research is making a 50mg oxymetholone in Thailand called **Bonalone**. It comes in white plastic bottles of 100 tablets each, similar in appearance to their Stanol (stanozolol) product. The Bonalone bottles have a yellow label instead of green, but they do carry the same metallic foil stamping of the Body Research logo in the center. Presently, looking for this is a good way to ensure a legitimate purchase.

Anadur (nandrolone hexyloxyphenylpropionate)

Androgenic	Anabolic	Standard
37	125	Testosterone

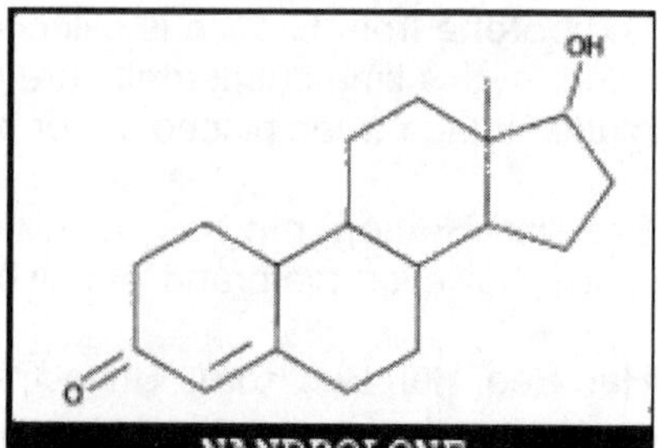

NANDROLONE

Chemical Names:
19-nortestosterone hexyloxyphenylpropionate
17beta-Hydroxyestra-4-en-3-one hexyloxyphenylpropionate

Estrogenic Activity: low
Progestational Activity: moderate

Anadur was a popular trade name for the injectable steroid nandrolone hexyloxyphenylpropionate. This is one of the longer acting nandrolones, similar in effect to the veterinary steroid Laurabolin. One injection would remain active in the body for approximately four weeks, again similar to that seen with nandrolone laurate. Although active for such a long time, athletes usually inject this steroid on a weekly basis due to its low dosage. Produced at a maximum strength of 50 mg/mL, one would most commonly inject 100-150mg (2-3 ml) two or three times weekly. This dosage is sufficient for the slow, even buildup of quality muscle mass associated with nandrolone esters. Since this drug has such a slow release, it may take a considerable amount of time for blood levels to reach a peak. Gains from Anadur are therefore likely to become pronounced only after three or four weeks have past. This characteristic makes it suited for longer cycles, often lasting more than 10 or 12 weeks.

The side effects of Anadur will be those associated with all nandrolones. Estrogen buildup is slight at best, so water retention and gynecomastia should only be a problem among sensitive individuals. The need to use an anti-estrogen like Nolvadex® is likewise not common with this drug. Additionally, this compound does undergo a change via the 5a-reductase enzyme, which is responsible for changing testosterone into DHT. But here the product is dihydronandrolone, a metabolite less androgenic than the parent nandrolone. Likewise androgenic side effects are much less pronounced with this drug. Women are particularly attracted to nandrolone preparations, as they encounter virilization symptoms very infrequently with these drugs if taken in low doses. Since androgenic activity can still become evident with use, even with nandrolone, a shorter acting version like Durabolin® would technically be the better choice for female athletes (allowing the user greater control over blood hormone levels). Those women who do use this product find a dosage of 50 to 100mg every 10 days sufficient.

Anadur is a good base steroid, and combines well with a variety of different compounds. For a mass cycle, the addition of a powerful oral such as Dianabol or Anadrol 50® should prove very effective. This should elicit exceptional muscle growth, while at the same time allowing the user to keep the oral dosage within limits. Three or four Dianabol tablets (15-20mg) or one to two Anadrol 50s (50-100mg) in combination with 200mg weekly Anadur is a very nice range to work in. Hopefully the result will be a more solid, quality muscle gain than when using these potent steroids alone. The low estrogen conversion rate of nandrolone also makes Anadur somewhat attractive for cutting purposes. Combining Anadur with Winstrol®, Primobolan® or Oxandrolone should result in a highly defined, quality look to the muscles without excess water. This combination should noticeably preserve the muscle density during times of calorie restriction, otherwise a destructive period of time to the muscles.

Anadur is not being produced at this time. Avoid all products bearing this trade name.

Anatrofin (stenbolone acetate)

Androgenic	Anabolic	Standard
107-144	267-332	Testosterone

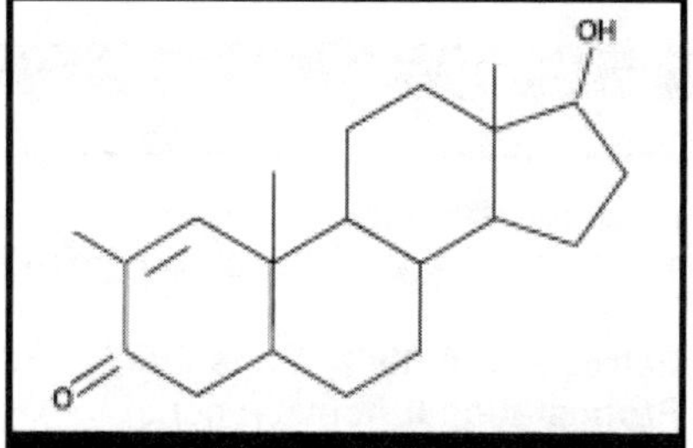

STENBOLONE

Chemical Names:
2-methyl-5a-androst-1-en-17b-ol-3-one

Estrogenic Activity: none
Progestational Activity: n/a

Stenbolone acetate is an injectable anabolic steroid that was introduced by Syntex in 1963. Syntex had sold this agent for a brief period of time in the United Kingdom and Mexico, under the brand name Anatrofin. It was also sold through license in Spain under the basic (generic) name Stenbolone. Stenbolone acetate has long since been discontinued, with the last commercial preparation reportedly withdrawn from market (voluntarily) in the early 1980's. This steroid was reported to have been developed by Syntex in an effort to find a less toxic alternative to Anadrol. Anatrofin was, likewise, looked at as a non-methylated injectable alternative to this powerful oral steroid, used in similar areas of clinical research and medicine (mainly in the treatment of Anemias). Its demise was likely financially driven, as Anatrofin disappeared at a time when many manufacturers were dropping their lesser-used steroids.

Structurally stenbolone is a 2-methylated derivative of 1-testosterone (dihydroboldenone). In this case, the resulting steroid remains very similar to its non-methylated parent, with only modest differences in anabolic and androgenic potency. On the tissue building side, stenbolone is probably a little weaker on a milligram for milligram basis than 1-testosterone. It is a little difficult to make direct comparisons, however, as the studies on these two steroids used different drugs as standards of comparison. As an androgen, stenbolone is also probably slightly weaker than 1-testosterone, when you are talking milligram for milligram dose. The anabolic/androgenic ratio, which is really the most relevant measure, remains roughly equal between the two steroids. Users will adjust the dosage of any steroid up or down to meet a desired level of growth, making these two steroids easily interchangeable. When compared to testosterone, stenbolone has roughly three times greater anabolic effect, and somewhere between 7% and 44% more androgenic activity.

As a 1-testosterone derivative, stenbolone also cannot aromatize into estrogen. This makes water retention and fat gain relatively a non-issue. There is always a chance that as a 1-testosterone derivative we will see some progestational activity (and therefore a possible intensification of the estrogenic side effects of other steroids); however, there seems little in the known history of this drug to support that. In fact, stenbolone always had a reputation for being an ideal cutting drug, helping athletes shed significant water and fat mass when stacked with a variety of other steroids. Common effective doses ranged from 100-250mg per week for men and 25mg per week for women. Being that Anatrofin uses stenbolone with the fast acting acetate ester, one would subdivide the total weekly dosage into two or three applications if wishing to keep blood levels steady. Stenbolone is not the least androgenic steroid, however, it does have a favorable enough anabolic/androgenic ratio to make it of interest to female athletes. They may be well served, however, to extend beyond the normal bi or tri-weekly injections. This will minimize androgenic buildup, and allow for a little time each week for steroid levels to settle down. Provided dosage is kept reasonable, this drug does seem to work well with female bodybuilders.

When Anatrofin was available, it was packaged in individual 1ml glass ampules. These came in three different strengths, containing 25, 50 or 100mg of steroid per ml. As with most injectables, oil was used as a solvent. European bodybuilders were disappointed when Anatrofin was removed from the market global market a couple of decades ago. Its loss was a hard felt one, very much like the old Primobolan acetate injectables. Old timers often claimed that the likes of this steroid were never replaced with the other popular non-aromatizable anabolics. Whether or not this is based on realistic experience or simple nostalgia remains to be seen. It is difficult today to say how different this agent ultimately is from 1-testosterone, a close chemical and pharmacological relative which we have much more modern experience with. Perhaps in the future we will get the opportunity to find out. Until then, stenbolone will remain nothing more than an elusive mystery drug, and an interesting chapter in the history of anabolic steroids.

Anavar (oxandrolone)

Androgenic	Anabolic	Standard
24	322-630	Methyltestosterone (oral)

Chemical Names:
17b-hydroxy-17a-methyl-2-oxa-5a-androstane-3-one

Estrogenic Activity: none
Progestational Activity: none

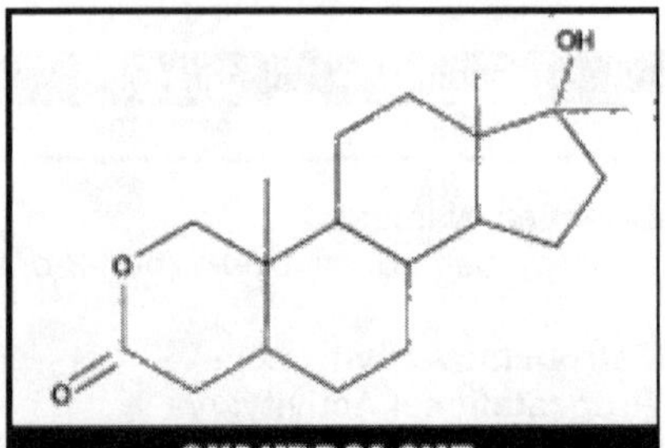

OXANDROLONE

Anavar was the old U.S. brand name for the oral steroid oxandrolone, first produced in 1964 by the drug manufacturer Searle. It was designed as an extremely mild anabolic, one that could even be safely used as a growth stimulant in children. One immediately thinks of the standard worry, "steroids will stunt growth". But it is actually the excess estrogen produced by most steroids that is the culprit, just as it is the reason why women stop growing sooner and have a shorter average stature than men. Oxandrolone will not aromatize, and therefore the anabolic effect of the compound can actually promote linear growth. Women usually tolerate this drug well at low doses, and at one time it was prescribed for the treatment of osteoporosis. But the atmosphere surrounding steroids began to change rapidly in the 1980's, and prescriptions for oxandrolone began to drop. Lagging sales probably led Searle to discontinue manufacture in 1989, and it had vanished from U.S. pharmacies until recently. Oxandrolone tablets are again available inside the U.S. by BTG, bearing the new brand name Oxandrin. BTG purchased rights to the drug from Searle and it is now manufactured for the new purpose of treating HIV/AIDS related wasting syndrome. Many welcomed this announcement, as Anavar had gained a very favorable reputation among athletes over the years.

Anavar is a mild anabolic with low androgenic activity. Its reduced androgenic activity has much to due with the fact that it is a derivative of dihydrotestosterone. Although you might think at first glance this would make it a more androgenic steroid, it in fact creates a steroid that is less androgenic because it is already "5-alpha reduced". In other words, it lacks the capacity to interact with the 5-alpha reductase enzyme and convert to a more potent "di-hydro" form. It is a simply matter of where a steroid is capable of being potentiated in the body, and with oxandrolone we do not have the same potential as testosterone, which is several times more active in androgen responsive tissues compared to muscle tissue due to its conversion to DHT. It essence oxandrolone has a balanced level of potency in both muscle and androgenic target tissues such as the scalp, skin and prostate. This is a similar situation as is noted with Primobolan and Winstrol, which are also derived from dihydrotestosterone yet not known to be very androgenic substances.

This steroid is known as a good agent for the promotion of strength and quality muscle mass gains, although the mild nature of this compound makes it less than ideal for bulking purposes. Among bodybuilders it is most commonly used during cutting phases of training when water retention is a concern. The standard dosage for men is in the range of 15-25mg (6-10 tablets) per day, a level that should produce noticeable results. It can be further combined with anabolics like Primobolan® and Winstrol® to elicit a harder, more defined look without added water retention. Such combinations are very popular and can dramatically enhance the show physique. One can also add strong non-aromatizing androgens like Halotestin®, Proviron® or trenbolone. In this case the androgen really helps to harden up the muscles, while at the same time making conditions more favorable for fat reduction. Some athletes do choose to incorporate oxandrolone into bulking stacks, but usually with standard bulking drugs like testosterone or Dianabol. The usual goal in this instance is an additional gain of strength, as well as more quality look to the androgen bulk. Women who fear the masculinizing effects of many steroids would be quite comfortable using this drug, as this is very rarely seen with low doses. Here a daily dosage of 5mg should illicit considerable growth without the noticeable androgenic side effects of other drugs. Eager females may wish to addition mild anabolics like Winstrol®, Primobolan® or Durabolin®. When combined with such anabolics, the user should notice faster, more pronounced muscle-building effects, but may also increase the likelihood of androgenic buildup.

Studies using low dosages of this compound note minimal interferences with natural testosterone production. Likewise when it is used alone in small amounts there is typically no need for ancillary drugs like Clomid®/Nolvadex® or HCG. This has a lot to do with the fact that it does not convert to estrogen, which we know has an extremely profound effect on endogenous hormone production. Without estrogen to trigger negative feedback, we seem to note a higher threshold before inhibition is noted. But at higher dosages of course, a suppression of natural testosterone levels will still occur with this drug as with any anabolic/androgenic steroid.

This makes clear that while estrogen is important in this regard, androgen action triggers feedback inhibition as well. In the context of the average bodybuilder using this steroid at a level to promote growth, we would probably expect that maintaining a normal level of endogenous testosterone release would likewise be very difficult.

Anavar is also a 17alpha alkylated oral steroid, carrying an alteration that is noted for putting stress on the liver. It is important to point out, however, that to spite this alteration oxandrolone is generally very well tolerated. While liver enzyme tests will occasionally show elevated values, actual damage due to this steroid is not a statistical problem. Bio-Technology General states that oxandrolone is not as extensively metabolized by the liver as other 17aa orals are; evidenced by the fact that nearly a third of the compound is still intact when excreted in the urine. This may have to do with the understood milder nature of this agent (compared to other 17aa orals) in terms of hepatotoxicity. One study comparing the effects of oxandrolone to other agents including methyltestosterone, norethandrolone, fluoxymesterone, and methandriol clearly supports this notion[52]. Here it was demonstrated that oxandrolone causes the lowest sulfobromophthalein (BSP; a marker of liver stress) retention among all the alkylated orals tested. 20mg of oxandrolone, in fact, produced 72% less BSP retention than an equal dosage of fluoxymesterone, which is a considerable difference being that they possess the same liver-toxic alteration. With such findings, combined with the fact that athletes rarely report trouble with this drug, most feel comfortable believing it to be much safer to use during longer cycles than most other orals with this distinction. Although this may very well be true, the chance of liver damage still cannot be excluded.

Like virtually all oral anabolic/androgenic steroids, oxandrolone does not have an extremely long half-life in the body. Although we do not have exact calculations on this, we can point to a study published in the Journal of Clinical Endocrinology and Metabolism investigating (among other things) blood levels of oxandrolone in response to oral dosing of the drug[53]. Researchers noted that measurements taken 10 hours after administration do show a steady elevation of drug in the bloodstream. Between the 10 and 18-hour mark, however, drug concentrations fell 73%. Such a drop in an 8-hour window indicates a pretty rapid metabolism of oxandrolone, and suggests that at least two oral doses would be needed per day if one wished to keep relatively steady blood concentrations over an entire 24-hour period.

At one time oxandrolone was looked at as a possible drug for those suffering from disorders of high cholesterol or triglycerides. Early studies showed it to be capable of lowering total cholesterol and triglyceride values in certain types of hyperlipidemic patients, which was thought to signify potential for this drug as a hypo-lipid (lipid lowering) agent[54]. With further investigation we find, however, that while use of this drug can be linked to a lowering of total cholesterol values, it is such that a redistribution in the ratio of good (HDL) to bad (LDL) cholesterol occurs, usually moving values in an unfavorable direction[55] [56]. This would, of course, negate any positive effect this drug might have on triglycerides or total cholesterol, and in fact make it a danger in terms of cardiac risk when taken for prolonged periods of time. Today we understand that as a group, anabolic/androgenic steroids tend to produce unfavorable changes in lipid profiles, and are really not useful in disorders of lipid metabolism. As an oral c17 alpha alkylated steroid, oxandrolone is probably even more risky to use than an injectable esterified injectable such as a testosterone or nandrolone in this regard.

Oxandrolone has always been a hot item on the black market. The past several years has brought forth many new oxandrolone containing products. This was right after a period of time when many drug manufacturers were dropping oxandrolone from their lines, due to low financial interest. Luckily, things have changed. Now there are numerous companies selling this steroid. Below, I will run down some of the more popular items on the black market.

Animal Power is a new and very active Mexican company, with a big interest in anabolics. They recently introduced their own oxandrolone product under the brand name **Oxandro Tabs**. It comes in 5mg tablets, with 100 packaged to each glass bottle. The bottle itself rests inside a cardboard box, and both carry the company's holographic security sticker. The bottle is further imprinted with the company logo, which rests mostly under the label. So far we have a lot of confidence in AP, given the good feeback on their line and the obvious attention to security.

Quality Vet, another popular Mexican company, threw its hat into the oxandrolone ring this past year as well. Their new product is called **Oxavet QV**. It comes in the form of 5mg tablets, with 100 packaged to each bottle. QV also uses a holographic security sticker to deter counterfeiting. Provided it is present on both the box and bottle, you should have a safe purchase. QV products are always in very high demand, due to their excellent reputation. This is definitely a recommended product if you are faced with a large selection.

Ttokkyo is no longer in business, but you may find their 5mg **Oxandrolone** product still in circulation at this time. If you do locate this product, be sure to look for the holographic security sticker on the plastic 100-count bottle. Note that in the past, counterfeiters had appropriated some of their stickers. Therefore, finding them may not be a 100% reliable check.

.

Oxandrovet by Denkall is another oxandrolone product circulating the black market in steady volume. It contains 5mg per tablet, and is found in bottles of 100 tablets each. The presence of a hologram security sticker should assure a legitimate purchase. This is a heavily sought after item right now, probably due to the fact that Denkall is amongst the most reputable labs operating in Mexico.

Bratis Labs, another new veterinary steroid manufacture in Mexico, has also been selling an oxandrolone product called **Oxandrol 10**. It is supposed to contain 10mg of steroid per tablet. I have no analysis of the product to confirm this. It has been my observation that Bratis has been very low key the past year. I'm not sure what that means in regards to the stability of this company.

Bonavar from Body Research in Thailand is another excellent oxandrolone product. It comes in 2.5mg tablets, 10 tablets to a plastic and foil strip. Feedback on the item has been extremely good so far, and I have seen lab test results confirming accurate dosing. Definitely a recommended item.

Loeffler has also started selling an oxandrolone product recently, called **Oxafort**. These are 5mg tablets, and come packaged in bottles of 100 tablets each. Loeffler recently began using hologram stickers on some of their boxes to assure a legitimate purchase; however, be warned they are plain generic stickers that just read "Securidad" (Security). Still, this product has a good reputation on the black market, and fakes do not yet appear to be a problem. Lab analysis on two separate lots has confirmed this product to contain the correct amount of oxandrolone. Keep in mind though that Loeffler has underdosed other products often in the past.

Oxanabol from British Dragon is another product to storm onto the global steroid market as of late. Formerly in a 5mg tablet dose, the manufacturer has since doubled the dose to 10mg. The product comes packed in sealed pouches of 100 tablets each. The tablets themselves are orange, and contain the same 5-sided shape as the British Dispensary Anabol tablets. BD is a reputable company. Be warned, however, that very good looking fakes of the BD line have been reported. BD is a Thai company. These fakes are of Russian origin.

Hubei Labs in China has recently decided to reuse Searle's old trade name, in their own new version of **Anavar**. These are 2.5mg blue tablets, sold in strips of 30 tablets each. Aside from this product, no other product anywhere in the world carries the name Anavar at this time. Trust no other product sold as such.

A generic is produced by **Planet Pharmacy** in Belize. This is a country with a very meager steroid market, which is otherwise fed by only a couple of Mexican products like Sustanon and Deca-Durabolin. Don't expect to find these products in Belizean pharmacies if you travel, as Planet Pharmacy seems to manufacture its products mainly for export.

Oandrolone is manufactured in the U.S. by BTG Pharmaceuticals. However, the exorbitant price they are asking for **Oxandrin** (2.5mg) precludes it from entering the black market. At the pharmacy, these tablets sell for anywhere from $3.80 to $4.50 each, a tremendous jump from the price Searle was selling it for a decade earlier. Even if someone were able to divert a large quantity to be sold on the black market, the price for it would be too high to justify next to other items now readily available. BTG released a 10mg tablet of Oxandrin two years ago, however, it offers little savings over the 2.5mg version. This is a high risk item, as real U.S. steroids rarely circulate the black market.

SPA Oxandrolone from Italy is still seen regularly on the black market. They come 30 tabs to a box, in 2 foil and plastic strips of 15 each. The tablets usually sell for $1-2 each, which is much more reasonable than the U.S. item. You should be aware of the fact that oxandrolone is officially off of the Italian drug market. If you plan on taking a trip to Italy, hoping to stock up on Oxandrolone, you are likely to be disappointed. This product is still sold for export though. Historically SPA made two different boxes of Oxandrolone, one for the Italian drug market and one (containing English writing) for export. Only the export item remains available at this time.

Andractim (dihydrotestosterone)

Androgenic	Anabolic	Standard
30-260	60-220	Testosterone, T. Propionate

Chemical Names:
5-alpha-androstan-3-one-17beta-ol
5-alpha-androstanolone

Estrogenic Activity: none
Progestational Activity: none

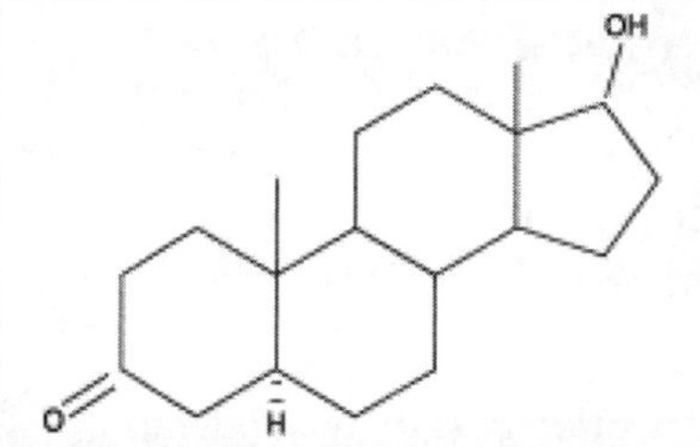

DIHYDROTESTOSTERONE

Andractim is a steroid preparation that contains the potent androgenic steroid dihydrotestosterone. This product comes in the form of a transdermal gel, typically containing 2.5% dihydrotestosterone by weight in an 80gram tube. As with Androgel, we can expect roughly 10% of the active steroid to make it into circulation with each application. This would equate to 80 doses of 25mg (each dose delivering approximately 2.5mg of steroid to the body). Dihydrotestosterone itself is the most active androgen in the human body, displaying an ability to bind and activate the androgen receptor at least three of four times greater than that of its parent steroid testosterone. It is a potently androgenic steroid, however this trait is not accompanied by equally powerful anabolic tendencies (as we often note with other highly androgenic steroids). In the case of Andractim, we have a steroid that is essentially a pure androgen.

Due to its non-aromatizing and anti-estrogenic nature, percutaneous dihydrotestosterone may be an effective option for the treatment of gynecomastia. Studies have reported a good level of success when treating certain forms of this disorder with Andractim, the drug affecting the ratio of androgenic to estrogenic action in the breast area enough that notable regression of mammary tissue has been achieved in many cases[57 58]. It has also been used successfully to treat gynecomastia triggered by HAART (Highly Active Antiretroviral Therapy) in HIV positive patients, a somewhat common problem with the powerful hormone-altering medications that are being used to treat this disease. Unimed, current maker of Anadrol-50 and Androgel in the U.S., has also been conducting clinical trails on Andractim, suggesting that it plans to release this drug on the U.S. drug market before long. Instead of using it to treat gynecomastia, however, they seem to be looking into this product to replace androgen levels due to Andropause. They are likely looking at the non-estrogenic nature of DHT to provide a safer alternative to testosterone-replacement therapy for those at risk for prostate hypertrophy (estrogen is involved in the pathology of this condition), and idea well supported by other medical research studies[59 60].

Dihydrotestosterone is a poor choice when it comes to building muscle. This is due to the fact that this steroid is extremely open to alteration by the 3-alpha-hydroxysteroid-dehydrogenase enzyme, which is responsible for breaking down active steroids like DHT into their inactive or less active metabolites. 3a-HSD is present in high quantities in muscle tissue, running interference between the outer cell membrane and the androgen receptors that all steroid hormones are trying to reach. In humans, little DHT ends up actually making its way to this receptor. Testosterone is very resistant to this enzyme however, which allows it to be a much more effective muscle-building agent. 3a-HSD steroid deactivation in muscle tissue causes the same problem with Proviron (1-methyl-dihydrotestosterone). Although Proviron is a very potent steroid due to its resemblance to dihydrotestosterone, binding to the androgen receptor with high affinity, it is a very poor muscle-building agent for the same reason. DHT and Proviron both have very effective uses in areas such as fat loss, hardening, increasing CNS activity and pure strength gain, but they do not hold up well as anabolic agents at all.

Andractim is not widely available, and is rarely seen on the black market. It is sold in several countries, but steroid dealers and consumers just do not pay enough attention to it for it to circulate here in any volume. Its effectiveness in treating conditions of gynecomastia and Andropause is rarely discussed, and to be honest most consumers really do not even know this product even exists. This is unfortunate, because all of the medical data on dihydrotestosterone seems to show it to be both safe and effective treatment option in many instances. Hopefully with the new attention Unimed is giving this drug, things will change. We can keep our fingers crossed that it will be FDA approved for the treatment of gynecomastia. However, I expect it will more than likely be prescribed for the limited use of replacing androgen levels in cases of Andropause.

Andriol (testosterone undecanoate)

Androgenic	Anabolic	Standard
100	100	Standard

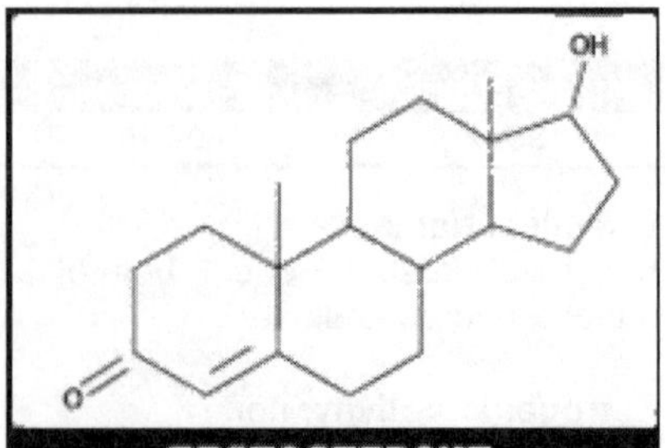

TESTOSTERONE

Chemical Names:
4-androsten-3-one-17beta-ol

Estrogenic Activity: moderate
Progestational Activity: low

Andriol is a unique oral testosterone product, developed by the international drug firm Organon. One of the more recently developed anabolic steroids, Andriol first became available in the early 1980's. This compound contains 40 mg of testosterone undecanoate, based in oil (oleic acid) and sealed inside a capsule. Subtracting the ester weight, this equates to a dosage of approximately 25mg of raw testosterone per cap. The design of this steroid is quite different from that of most oral steroids. Drugs administered orally generally enter the blood stream through the liver. When a steroid compound is given this way without some form of structural protection, it will be quickly broken down during the "first pass". This process leaves very little steroid intact, basically deactivating the drug. Adding a methyl group (c-17 AA) to the structure is one way to protect it from this process, however stress is also placed on the liver as a result. In some instances this stress can lead to actual damage to liver tissues, so the designers of this steroid sought another way to protect the testosterone molecule. With Andriol, this was accomplished by making a form of testosterone that would be absorbed through the lymphatic system. This is due to its high fat solubility brought about by the ester, and its suspension in oil. Having the compound absorbed this way was thought to be very advantageous, as it allows the steroid to bypass the destructive first-pass through liver. This should permit the compound to enter the blood stream intact, without the need for a harsh chemical alteration. The ester breaks off once it is in circulation of course, yielding free active testosterone. In design this steroid appears to be that of a completely liver safe and orally active form of testosterone.

Pharmacokinetics of Oral Testosterone Undecanoate

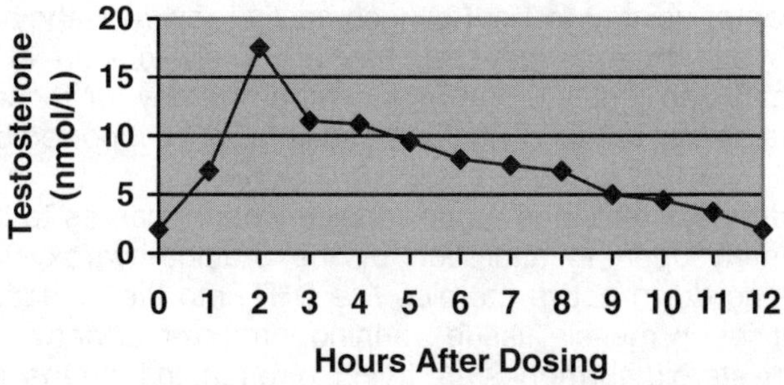

Figure 1. The graph to the right depicts the median response pharmacokinetics after oral administration of 40mg of testosterone undecanoate. As you can see, the testosterone peak is reached very quickly (approximately 2 hours). Levels subsequently decline, reaching baseline by 12 hours. Source: Which Androgen Replacement Therapy for Women? Buckler, Robertson and Wu. J Clin Endocrinol and Metab. 83 (1998) 3920-24

On paper this drug seems like an ideal oral testosterone product. Clean, safe and worlds apart from other oral testosterone derivatives like the crude methyltestosterone. But as we always hear in life, if it looks to good to be true, it probably is. And there are definitely some issues with Andriol®. The first problem is that bioavailability, although clearly worlds apart from trying to take straight testosterone orally, is probably not significant next to c17-alpha alkylated orals. Athletes typically find that in doses of less than 240mg per day (6 capsules) effects are generally not seen at all. 240mg of testosterone ester daily, the primary male androgen, and only a meager effect. When doses go higher, maybe 8-10 capsules (320-400mg), new muscle growth is slight to moderate at best, but no incredible bulky gains are ever reported. Logic leads one to think that only a little testosterone is making its way into circulation. Testosterone is a powerful hormone no matter what the ester or form of administration. If it were active in the blood stream, the results would have to be pronounced. When one injects an oil based testosterone ester like cypionate, a dosage of 400mg per week is more than sufficient. 400mg Andriol per day should be packing on an incredible amount of mass. Where does it all go?

Individual problems with absorption may play into things here. The graph above shows the median response noted when this drug was given to a group of women. It does not however depict the striking differences in individual metabolism that were noted in this experiment. If we look at results from each of the four subjects, the differences are dramatic to say the least. While one is off the scale with testosterone levels, another barely budges at all. What is even more confusing is that results were so inconsistent, that at times higher levels were achieved with a lower 20mg dose compared to the 40mg when given to the same subject. Clearly there is little to be said except that this drug is unpredictable in its ability to be absorbed and utilized by the body. While one day you might be getting great absorption, perhaps the next day you are getting very little. Studies with men were no better than with women, where again this drug was shown to be unpredictably absorbed and utilized with blood levels ranging from 11.5 to 60.1 nmol/L with 80mg twice daily[61].

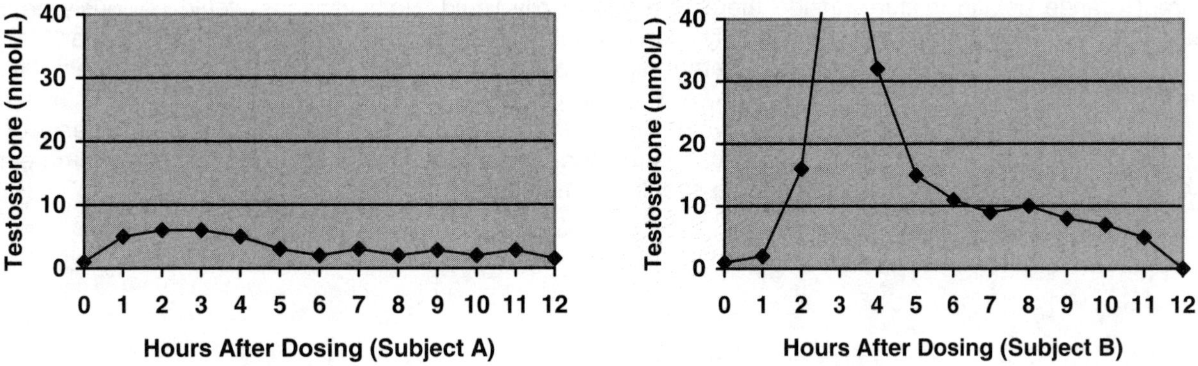

Figure 2. The graphs above illustrate the high and low responding subjects from the testosterone undecanoate dosing study discussed and referenced in Figure 1. As you see, the graph on the left shows a subject who received a very poor response in terms of testosterone increase, while the graph on the right shows another subject who went off the chart, peaking at 65 nmol/L of testosterone

One might also pay interest to the "mildness" of this compound as described by other bodybuilding materials. Andriol® is often spoken about as some type of magic product, which to spite being a form of regular testosterone somehow allows for only minimal estrogen conversion. You should know that the way a drug is administered includes a number of factors that can slightly alter its effect, the most predominant being the speed of release. This effects the time it takes for a peak blood level to be reached, and likely the length it takes to see results. The primary reason testosterone suspension seems more powerful than enanthate is because more drug is active on day one. At the same time, estrogen builds up faster and side effects become pronounced very quickly. The ester is also part of the total weight, and 100mg testosterone contains a much larger quantity of testosterone molecules that testosterone plus ester, another reason for varying effect. But these changes do not amount to all that much. The structure of testosterone is what allows it to break down into estrogen. The only way we can really prevent an androgen from converting to estrogen is to change the base molecule, not the ester. Once free in the blood stream we cannot prevent testosterone from being aromatized without interfering with the aromatase enzyme itself. The lack of results and side effects often reported with Andriol® must be going hand in hand with poor absorption.

Most athletes today consider Andriol a very poor buy. I know other references do find use for this drug, which is defendable because some amount of steroid clearly does enter the blood stream intact. Technically it is still an oral testosterone, and definitely does not carry the same liver-toxicity risks associated with most steroids designed for this type of administration, so all is not lost. Those specifically looking for a mild oral at times do purchase this product, and are occasionally even satisfied with their results. But for most its high price and required high daily dosages usually causes them to avoid it when coming across it on the black market. Besides, if we want a mild steroid the last thing we really should shop for is a testosterone.

It is of note that Organon has started reformulated Andriol in some markets, replacing the old Andriol® brand with the new Andriol® Testocaps®. The new Testocaps® contain the same dose of testosterone undecanoate, however, it is dissolved in a different carrier base. Instead of oleic acid, a blend of caster oil and propylene glycol laurate is used. I am actually unclear in the purpose for the change. An investigation published in the Journal of Pharmacology and Experimental Therapeutics in 2003 looked at the relative lymphatic absorption and systemic distribution of testosterone, testosterone undecanoate, and DHT undecanoate after oral administration of both formulations, and found no significant differences between the two[62]. They close their paper in reporting, "*The results from the current study demonstrate conclusively that the therapeutic advantage associated with oral TU [testosterone undecanoate] administration is a consequence of lymphatic transport of TU to the systemic circulation. Furthermore, the study demonstrated conclusively that there is no difference in the systemic exposure of T, or TU, resulting from the oral administration of Andriol or Andriol Testocaps.*" Regardless of the reason, at this point in time we can look at new Andriol® Testocaps® as completely interchangeable with the old product athletes are long familiar with.

Andriol® and Andriol® Testocaps® are both very difficult items to duplicate, so your odds are good when purchasing them. Available in a number of countries, they can be found packaged in both bottles (30 and 60 capsules) and foil strips of 10 (all foil, no plastic). With legit Andriol® we are looking for a brown/red colored capsule that contains oil inside. It is completely sealed and does not pull apart. DV3 and ORG are printed on the surface of the capsule. The Testocaps® are also soft oval glossy capsules, but these are made out of a transparent orange gelatin mixture. Inside there is a yellow oily liquid. Both versions would obviously be very difficult to copy, which is probably why I have only seen one fake (of the original Andriol® version) thus far. Easy to identify, it was a generic strip that contains 10 unmarked red pull-apart capsules. Inside the capsule one will find a very strong smelling powder, not oil. It is unknown what the powder actually is but it is definitely not a legitimate preparation of testosterone undecanoate, so avoid. Since all of the legitimate capsules are sold under a brand name (Andriol®, Andriol® Testocaps®, Androxon, Panteston, Restandol, Undestor or Virigen), any item bearing only the generic name testosterone undecanoate should be immediately considered a fake.

Androderm (testosterone)

Androgenic	Anabolic	Standard
100	100	Standard

Chemical Names:
4-androsten-3-one-17beta-ol

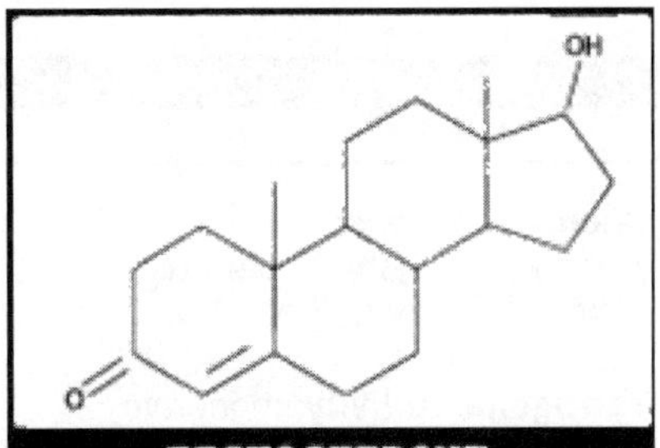
TESTOSTERONE

Estrogenic Activity: moderate
Progestational Activity: low

Androderm® is a recently developed testosterone product, which delivers the hormone transdermally. This product is quite different from previous testosterone patches, which were designed for application on the shaved scrotal area (obviously not a comfortable practice). The new Androderm® patches are designed to give the patient much more freedom. They can be applied almost anywhere, but are generally placed on the abdomen, back, thigh or upper arm. The area must be free of excess hair, but this is clearly a much easier place to work. This product is being used primarily by older men who have reached an age in which there body no longer produces sufficient amounts of testosterone ("Andropause"). When testosterone levels start to diminish, one can notice a severe lack of motivation, sex drive and an overall lost sense of well-being. Restoring an acceptable androgen level is often critical to reviving the person's previous quality of life.

These patches are designed to release testosterone in a varying level, over a 24 hour period. This is to mimic the natural (uneven) pattern of a health young man, with peaks and lows throughout the duration. Each patch contains 12.2mg of testosterone, but according to the paperwork only about 2.5mg is dispersed during each 24-hour application. Since the average healthy male will produce between 2.5 and 11 milligrams of testosterone per day, two patches are generally used daily for an approximate dose of 5mg. Athletes would no doubt find the dosage of this product much too low, as quite a number of patches would have to be used simultaneously to elicit the strong anabolic effect sought after by this group. It would be much easier, and cheaper, to use an injectable testosterone. Those who may consider using this drug (perhaps due to unexpected availability) would be better served adding another steroid with it than loading their body up with patches.

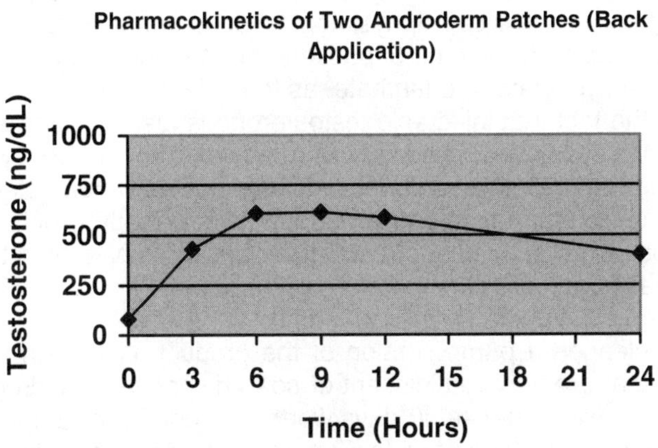

Figure 1. Mean serum testosterone concentrations (ng/dL) measured during single-dose applications of two Androderm 2.5 mg systems applied at night to the back. The figures reflect the greatest response in a study comparing four different sites of application (abdomen, back, thigh and upper arm) in 34 hypogonadal men. Source: Androderm® prescribing information. Watson Pharma, Inc.

Androgel (testosterone)

Androgenic	Anabolic	Standard
100	100	Standard

Chemical Names:
4-androsten-3-one-17beta-ol
17beta-hydroxy-androst-4-en-3-one

Estrogenic Activity: moderate
Progestational Activity: low

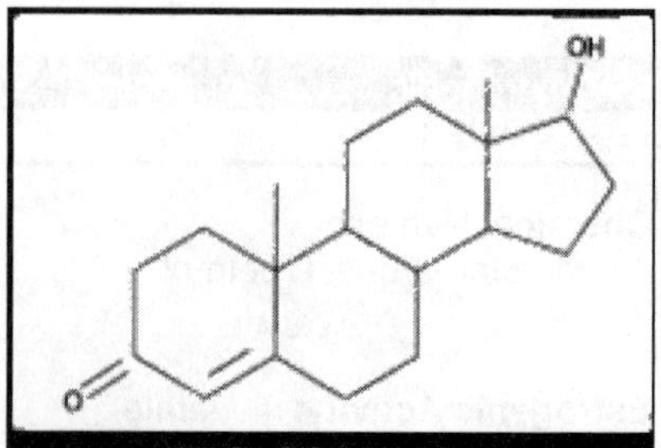

TESTOSTERONE

Androgel is the newest steroids to make its way to the drug market in the United States. This product is being made by UniMed Pharmaceuticals (a division of Solvay Pharmaceuticals), and was approved by the FDA for sale by prescription in February of 2000. As its name suggests, Androgel comes in the form of a transdermal gel that contains a 1% concentration of testosterone. It is being prescribed by doctors to restore normal androgen levels in men who are noticing a decline due to age, a job that it accomplishes both comfortably (no injections) and effectively (the product boasts a clinical success rate of 87%). It is quite ironic that this new testosterone-containing drug is being heralded by the media as a great achievement in the field of medicine and endocrinology, yet it contains one of the same steroids that has been vilified over and over again as a great danger to the public.

As mentioned, Androgel contains 1% testosterone by weight. It is packaged in both 2.5 gram and 5-gram packages, equating to a total per-application dose of 25mg or 50mg. The data available on Androgel suggests a transdermal bioavailability of approximately 10%. This means that each dose delivers 2.5mg or 5mg systemically (respectively). Although you might think a transdermal to be pretty slow acting, studies do show that testosterone levels begin to elevate 30 minutes after applying the gel to the body. Within 4 hours, most have dramatic elevations in serum androgen levels. Newly elevated levels of testosterone do tend to remain elevated for a full 24-hour period, which means that the drug only need be applied once per day. As you will see in the included graph, regular dosing will provide a relatively steady hormone balance over each 24-hour period.

In terms of bodybuilding, Androgel is not going to offer a whole lot. The highest dosed packet delivers only 5mg of testosterone to the body per day, which is not really that much when you are trying to pack on serious muscle mass. Were a person planning on getting a supraphysiological dose of testosterone with this drug, even say 25mg daily, it would require the regular daily use of 5 packets of the 5gram product. Try to use Androgel as a replacement for say testosterone cypionate or enanthate, as the sole drug in a cycle, and you would probably need even more. Combine this with the fact that injectable testosterone is just so much easier and cheaper to use, and we can see why Androgel doesn't circulate on the black market very often. At best you tend to find it being used by males who has been prescribed the drug by a doctor for Andropause treatment, stacked with other drugs that their doctors don't know they are using. Being a strong androgen, it is of course difficult to recommend Androgel to women. At best, a very low dose (maybe ¼ to ½ of a 2.5gram packet) would be attempted, which would be taken for a very brief period (a few weeks).

Androgel® has also recently released a pump version of the product, called simply Androgel® Pump. It comes white plastic pump containers that are very reminiscent of soap dispensers. Androgel Pump is currently available in one formulation only. Each box will dispense 30 days worth of medication (at the starting 5g daily dosage). The box actually provides two pumps, each which provide 60 pumps of 1.25grams each. 4 squirts per day will give the 5gram dose. Over the past several years we have also seen many new testosterone gels have come to market, owing to the tremendous popularity of Androgel in the U.S. market. All of these products are of the same basic design as U.S. Androgel. Testim is a particualy popular brand in Europe, which is formulated as a comparable 1% gel of testosterone. It comes in single application foil packets of 2.5g and 5g of gel each, the same as Androgel®. Given the current lack of interest counterfeiters seem to be paying to these drugs, which are rarely used outside of legitimate channels due to their low delivered dose, all can probably be considered real should they be located on the black market.

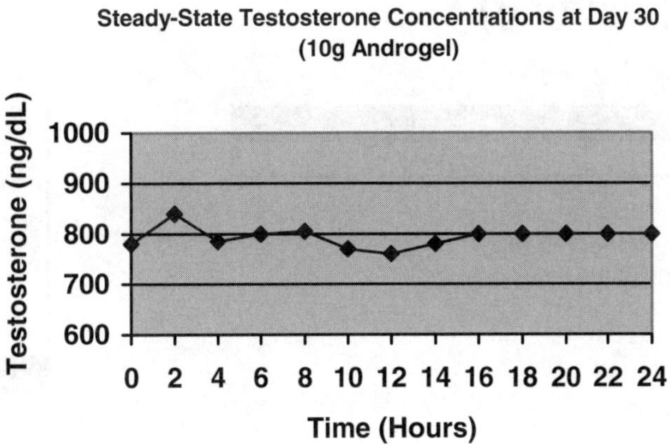

Figure 1. Steady-State Testosterone concentrations in blood, measured 30 days after beginning therapy with Androgel (10g application). Drug was applied to the body once daily.

Cheque Drops (mibolerone)

Androgenic	Anabolic	Standard
250	590	Methyltestosterone (oral)

Chemical Names:
7,17-dimethyl-19-norandrost-4-en-3-one-17b-ol
17beta-Hydroxy-7alpha,17-dimethylestr-4-en-3-one

Estrogenic Activity: low
Progestational Activity: high

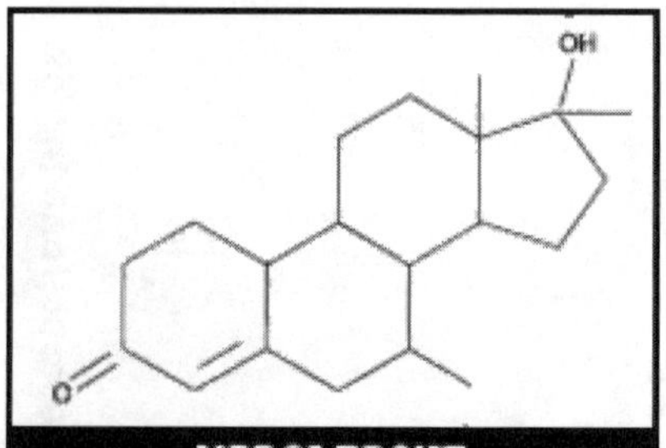

MIBOLERONE

Cheque Drops is a powerful anabolic steroid that is used in veterinary medicine to prevent female dogs from going into heat. This product was originally manufactured in the United States by Pharmacia & Upjohn, however it has since been discontinued. It remains an approved veterinary drug in the U.S., and can still be found in the form of a privately compounded medicine. Cheque Drops contain the synthetic nandrolone derivative mibolerone. This is an extremely strong steroid, so much so that it is effective in microgram, not milligram, amounts. Upjohn's product contained an oral solution with only 100mcg of steroid per milliliter, packaged in a 55ml vial. This means that each bottle contained only, yes you are reading this correctly, 5.5 milligrams of active steroid! Yet to spite this low steroid concentration, Cheque Drops gained a reputation amongst many bodybuilders as being one of the strongest steroids ever made.

Mibolerone is specifically a 7,17-dimethylated derivative of nandrolone. This means that they took the base steroid nandrolone, and added a methyl group at both the 7 and 17 positions. The addition of C-17 alpha alkylation serves an obvious purpose; it makes the steroid orally active. The addition of a methyl group at C-7, however, does something very different; it prevents 5-alpha reduction of the steroid[63]. This means that although mibolerone is based on nandrolone in structure, it will not convert to a weaker (dihydro) metabolite in androgen responsive target tissues like nandrolone does. It is more androgenic in nature, a trait most bodybuilders who have used the product will attest to. The combined efforts of C-7 and C-17 do something else though, they allow the steroid to exist in an almost entirely free state in the blood. Mibolerone simply does not like to bind to proteins like SHBG and albumin. This, combined with a slow rate of metabolic clearance and high relative affinity for the androgenic receptor, and we can understand why they would make a bottle of steroid that only contained 5.5mg of steroid.

Don't get the idea that it is all roses with mibolerone. This can be one nasty steroid. For one, neither the C-7 nor C-17alpha methyl groups prevent estrogen conversion. And since this steroid is a synthetic dimethylated androgen with high biological potency, it likely converts to an extremely active estrogen. One thing is for sure; estrogenic side effects can be intense when taking this drug. But then the progestational activity of mibolerone is documented to be extreme as well, so it is a little difficult to know how much to attribute to what. Just know that it is an extremely problematic steroid when it comes to gynecomastia, water retention (often to the point of heavy bloating) and increased fat buildup. Being such a potent, C-17 alpha alkylated compound, it will also present some level of toxicity to the liver. For this reason cycles need to be kept to a minimum length, preferably no longer than 4-6 weeks in length. Otherwise, you are just playing with fire.

Athletes usually take Cheque Drops by placing the solution under the tongue, in the hopes that it will be absorbed sublingually. This is not really necessary however, owing to the fact that the compound is already highly resistant to hepatic breakdown because of the synthetic alterations it carries. The typical daily dose was 500mcg (5ml) or less. Some profess to have taken 1mg per day or more, however at that level side effects are expected to be extremely problematic for most. It effects tend to be more androgenic than anabolic, offering more by way of strength gain and aggression than actually body mass increases; definitely too strong to recommend safely to women. Since mibolerone is effective in such low doses, it does have the added benefit of being difficult to detect in a drug screen. One could stop much closer to the urinalysis date with this drug than with most others, perhaps only a few days, feeling confident that the extremely small doses of total steroid needed to see an effect would be at an undetectable level by the time the sample were given.

As mentioned above, Pharmacia & Upjohn no longer makes this product. It is still being sold as a compounded veterinary medicine by at least one pharmacy, but obtaining it is easier said than done. Don't plan on just ordering it through a veterinary catalog; it is a controlled substance. You would need nothing less than a licensed veterinarian, able to prescribe controlled substances, to send a prescription directly to the compounding pharmacy. Unless you have a close friend that is a vet, I wouldn't expect having a chance to use this drug any time soon. Perhaps some other drug companies will find an interest in the drug in the future, allowing it to once again emerge on the black market. But for now, real Cheque Drops are gone.

Danocrine (danazol)

Chemical Names:
17alpha-Pregna-2,4-dien-20-yno[2,3-d]isoxazol-17-ol

Although steroidal in structure, danazol is technically an anti-gonadotropin agent. This means that its main function is to suppress the body's release of sex hormones like testosterone and estrogen, not to build muscle. In a medical setting it is used to treat a number of disorders where sex steroids are involved in the pathology, such as endometriosis and fibrocystic breast disease. Danazol appears to have little if any anabolic effect, and at best slight androgenic activity. Due to that fact that its main activity is that of an anti-gonadotropic agent, and not as an anabolic steroid, it was deemed there would be little chance for abuse with this drug. It was likewise never registered as a controlled substance in the United States.

Danazol is structurally a c-17-alpha-alkylated compound, which means that it will display some level of toxicity on the liver. This usually becomes problematic in doses of 400mg per day or above, or when used for very long periods of time. Its toxicity is not to be endured for much reward, however. In a bodybuilding setting there is simply little need to even think about using this compound. I guess a case can be made that if you are suppressing your testosterone output with other steroids, there would be no concern over the anti-gonadotropic effects of danazol. In such case its weak anabolic/androgenic effect would be welcome; at whatever intensity it is present. But even in doses of 600mg or above, the effect will be meager, and the expense great. This makes one question if there is ever a circumstance that would warrant buying this odd steroidal compound. Clearly any price is difficult to justify when there are so many other (better) anabolic/androgenic agents readily available to use.

Danocrine, and generic copies of this steroid, typically come in capsules of 50mg, 100mg, and 200mg strength. The 200mg brand name capsules from Sanofi usually sell in the U.S. for about $4.50 per capsule, and the generic equivalent for about $3.00. This drug can be obtained for a slightly lower cost from some overseas sources, and at this time is legal to import under the current "personal-use" loophole for international drug purchasing. And since bodybuilders have little interest in this steroid, counterfeiters do not either. You are unlikely to come across Danocrine on the black market, but if you do, you can bet it will be real. This is one of those products that you probably will never see a fake box of. But then again, even if it is real, do you really want it?

Deca-Durabolin (nandrolone decanoate)

Androgenic	Anabolic	Standard
37	125	Testosterone

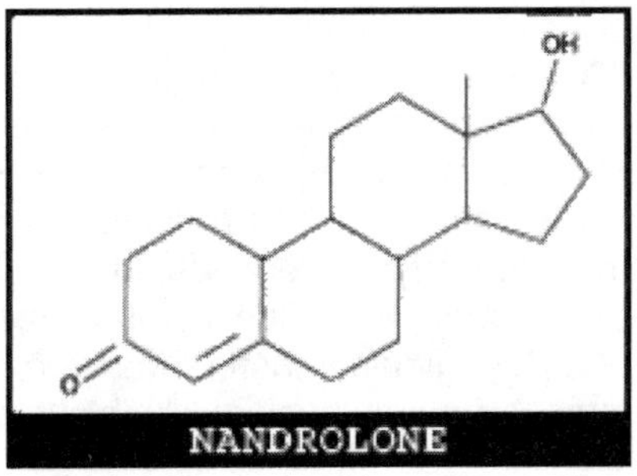

Chemical Names:
19-norandrost-4-en-3-one-17beta-ol
17beta-hydroxy-estr-4-en-3-one

Estrogenic Activity: low
Progestational Activity: moderate

Deca-Durabolin® is the Organon brand name for the injectable steroid nandrolone decanoate. This compound came around early in the wave of commercial steroid development, first being made available as a prescription medication in 1962. This steroid is an extremely long acting compound, with the decanoate ester said to provide this drug a slow release time of up to three or four weeks. While perhaps true in a technical sense, what we find with further investigation is that the release parameters after a single injection are such that a strong release of nandrolone is really only maintained for one to two weeks. This figure admittedly fails to take into account drug buildup that may occur after multiple injections, which may allow a longer duration of good effect to be seen. Figure 1 is provided to illustrate the release dynamics of a single 200mg injection. As you will see, by the end of the second week levels are already approaching baseline.

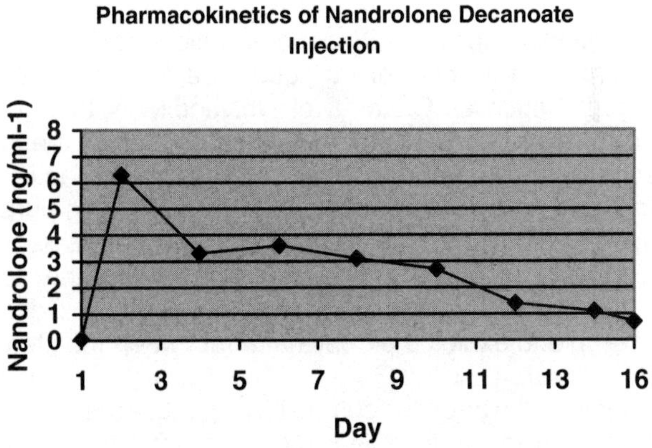

Figure 1. Pharmacokinetics of 200mg Nandrolone Decanoate injection. Source: Pharmacokinetic parameters of nandrolone (19-nortestosterone) after intramuscular administration of nandrolone decanoate (Deca-Durabolin®) to healthy volunteers. Wijnand H, Bosch A, Donker C. Acta Endocrinol 1985 supp 271 19-30.

World Wide "Deca" is one of the most widely used anabolic steroids. Its popularity is due to the simple fact that it exhibits many very favorable properties. Structurally nandrolone is very similar to testosterone, although it lacks a carbon atom at the 19th position (hence its other name 19-nortestosterone). The resulting structure is a steroid that exhibits much weaker androgenic properties than testosterone. Of primary interest is the fact that nandrolone will not break down to a more potent metabolite in androgen target tissues[64]. You may remember this is a significant problem with testosterone. Although nandrolone does undergo reduction via the same (5-alpha reductase) enzyme that produces DHT from testosterone, the result in this case is dihydronandrolone. This metabolite is weaker than the parent nandrolone[65], and is far less likely to cause unwanted androgenic side effects. Strong occurrences of oily skin, acne, body/facial hair growth and hair loss occur very rarely. It is however possible for androgenic activity to become apparent with this as any steroid, but with nandrolone higher than normal doses are usually responsible.

Nandrolone also show an extremely lower tendency for estrogen conversion. For comparison, the rate has been estimated to be only about 20% of that seen with testosterone[66]. This is because while the liver can convert nandrolone to estradiol, in other more active sites of steroid aromatization such as adipose tissue nandrolone is far less open to this process[67]. Consequently estrogen related side effects are a much lower concern with this drug. An antiestrogen is likewise rarely needed with Deca, gynecomastia only a worry among sensitive individuals. At the same time water retention is not a usual concern. This effect can occur however, but is most often related to higher dosages. The addition of Proviron® and/or Nolvadex® should prove sufficient enough to significantly reduce any occurrence. Clearly Deca is a very safe choice among steroids. Actually, many consider it to be the best overall steroid for a man to use when weighing the side effects and results. It should also be noted that in HIV studies, Deca has been shown not only to be effective at safely bringing up the lean body weight of patient, but also to be beneficial to the immune system.

It is of note however that nandrolone is believed to have some activity as a progestin in the body[68]. Although progesterone is a c-19 steroid, removal of this group as in 19-norprogesterone creates a hormone with greater binding affinity for its corresponding receptor. Sharing this trait, many 19-nor anabolic steroids are shown to have some affinity for the progesterone receptor as well[69]. This can lead to some progestin-like activity in the body, and may intensify related side effects. The side effects associated with progesterone are actually quite similar to those of estrogen, including negative feedback inhibition of testosterone production, enhanced rate of fat storage and possibly gynecomastia. Many believe the progestin activity of Deca notably contributes to suppression of testosterone synthesis, which can be marked despite a low tendency for estrogen conversion[70].

Deca is not known as a very "fast" builder. The muscle building effect of this drug is quite noticeable, but not dramatic. The slow onset and mild properties of this steroid therefore make it more suited for cycles with a longer duration. In general one can expect to gain muscle weight at about half the rate of that with an equal amount of testosterone. A cycle lasting eight to twelve weeks seems to make the most sense, expecting to elicit a slow, even gain of quality mass. Although active in the body for much longer, Deca is usually injected once per week. The dosage for men is usually in the range of 200-600mg. If looking to be specific, it is believed that Deca will exhibit its optimal effect (best gain/side effect ratio) at around 2mg per pound of bodyweight/weekly. Deca is also a popular steroid among female bodybuilders. They take a much lower dosage on average than men of course, usually around 50mg weekly. Although only slightly androgenic, women are occasionally confronted with virilization symptoms when taking this compound. Should this become a concern, the shorter acting nandrolone Durabolin® would be a safer option. This drug stays active for only a few days, greatly reducing the impact of androgenic buildup if withdrawal were indicated.

As mentioned earlier, endogenous testosterone levels can be a concern with Deca-Durabolin®, especially after long cycles. It is therefore a good idea to incorporate ancillary drugs at the conclusion of therapy. An estrogen antagonist such as Clomid® or Nolvadex® is therefore commonly used for a few weeks. These both provide a good level of testosterone stimulation, although they may take a couple of weeks to show the best effect. HCG injections could be added for extra reassurance, acting to rapidly restore the normal ability of the testes to respond to the resumed release of gonadotropins. For this purpose one could administer three injections of 2500-5000I.U., spaced five days apart. After which point the antiestrogen is continued alone for a few more weeks in an effort to stabilize the production of testosterone. Remember to begin the ancillaries after Deca has been withdrawn for a few weeks, not the first week after the last shot. Deca stays active for quite some time so the ancillary drugs will not be able to exhibit their optimal effect when the steroid is still being released into the bloodstream.

The major drawback for competitive purposes is that in many cases nandrolone metabolites will be detectable in a drug screen for up to a year (or more) after use. This is clearly due to the form of administration. As discussed earlier in this book, esterified compounds have a high affinity to stay stored in fatty tissues. While we can accurately estimate the time frame it will take for a given dose to enter circulation from an injection site, we cannot know for sure that 100% of the steroid will have been metabolized at any given point. Small amounts may indeed be stubborn in leaving fatty tissue, particularly after heavy, longer-term use. Some quantity of nandrolone decanoate may therefore be left to sporadically enter into the blood stream many months after use. This process may be further aggravated when dieting for a show, a time when body fat sores are being actively depleted (possibly freeing more steroid). This has no doubt been the cause for many unexpected positives on a drug screen. The fact that nandrolone has been isolated as the "hands-off" injectable for the drug tested athlete is most likely due to its popularity (and therefore common appearance on drug screens). The same risk would of course hold true for other long chain esterified injectables such as Equipoise®, Parabolan and Primobolan®.

On the other hand, the use of oral nandrolone precursors norandrostenedione and norandrostenediol (now considered controlled substances in the U.S.) can allow the drug-tested athlete the benefit of an injectable nandrolone, without the same risk for a positive result. A recently published French study demonstrates this. During this investigation, it was shown that trace levels of the nandrolone metabolites norandrosterone and noretiocholanolone could be found in human urine up to eight months after a single 50mg injection of nandrolone undecanoate[71]. This time frame shrank to only 8 days with norandrostenediol (50mg) and norandrostenedione (100mg). I have also had the opportunity to speak with an amateur bodybuilder recently, who was unexpectedly subject to a drug screen and now strongly supports the use of oral precursor hormones. He was using up to 3 grams norandrostenedione daily not very far from the date of the show, and to his amazement did not test positive for steroid use. Although not currently available, the possibility does exhist that an Andriol®-type drug could be developed with a nandrolone base, which would allow for much closer use to tested events.

Those not subject to a drug screen are likely to find the low water retention and good effect of this drug favorable for use in pre-contest cutting stacks. A combination of Deca and Winstrol® during the weeks/months leading up to a show for example, is noted to greatly enhance the look of muscularity and definition. A strong non-aromatizing androgen like Halotestin® or trenbolone could be further added, providing an enhanced level of hardness and density to the muscles. Being an acceptable anabolic, Deca can also be incorporated into bulk cycles with good results. The classic Deca and Dianabol cycle has been a basic for decades, and always seems to provide excellent muscle growth. A stronger androgen such as Anadrol 50® or testosterone could also be substituted, producing greater results. When mixed with Deca, the androgen dosage can be kept lower than if used alone, hopefully making the cycle more comfortable. Additionally one may choose to continue Deca for a number of few weeks after the androgen has been stopped. This will hopefully harden up some of the bloat produced by the androgen, giving a more quality appearance. Remember that endogenous testosterone production will not resume during Deca therapy, and ancillaries are likewise still needed.

Deca-Durabolin is one of the most widely duplicated steroids in the world, with fakes taking on many different forms. Since this drug is marketed in so many countries throughout the world, it will no doubt always be a tricky buy. In an effort to help you pick out some of the best products, I will start by running down some of the more popular items currently found on the U.S. black market.

Animal Power is a new Mexican steroid manufacturer, with a number of interesting products. Their Deca clone is called **Deca 300**, and is a high dosed fomulation containing 300mg/mL of steroid. Animal Power uses security hologram stickers on all products, which display the company logo as an integral part of the holographic image. These stickers are very difficult to duplicate, and at the present time offer an excellent counterfeit detection method. So far feedback on this company has been excellent, definitely making them worthy of a recommendation.

Pet's Pharma is another relatively new company to enter the Mexican steroid market. They produce a nandrolone decanoate called **Decandrol 300**. It comes in a 10ml vial, with a concentration of 300 mg/mL of steroid. This firm uses a security sticker to deter counterfeiting, however it is not holographic. It is a circle that is half red and half blue, and both inks are a very shiny metallic color (see Security Stickers). Fakes at this time do not appear to be a big problem.

Quality Vet produces both a 200mg/mL and 300mg/mL nandrolone decanoate product. They are called **Deca QV200 and Deca QV300** respectively. The 200mg product comes in both 10ml and 50ml vials, while the 300mg version is currently sold in a 10ml vial only. QV uses a hologram sticker to deter counterfeiting, and has recently started using logo imprinted tops on their injectable vials. Feedback on this line is consistently excellent, and their products are highly recommended.

Denkall makes a 200mg/mL Deca product called **Decanandrolen**. It comes packaged in 10ml vials, each affixed with a holographic sticker to deter counterfeiting. This product has always had a good reputation on the black market, and represents a good buy provided a real hologram is affixed to the bottle.

Brovel makes a brand in Mexico called **Norandren**, which comes in 50mg/mL and 200mg/mL dosage strengths. This company has been around for decades now, and is well regarded by athletes for providing fair quality items at better than fair prices. The line has a reputation for being a bit underdosed (20-30%), but the price usually makes up for this drawback.

Tornel makes a generic in Mexico as well, **Decanoato de Nandrolona** to be specific. This product is a safe buy, although you may expect the steroid dosage to be 20% or so under the label claim of 200mg/mL.

Ttokkyo is no longer in business, but you may find their 300mg/mL **Nandrolona 300 L.A.** in circulation. Be sure to look for the company's holographic security sticker before buying. Note that in the past these stickers have been appropriated by counterfeiters, so be sure to investigate other features, such as the company's custom printed flip tops (with "Ttokkyo" on them).

Bratis also makes a 250mg/mL product in Mexico, called **Decatron 250**. This firm has been fairly quiet as of late. However, this product does seem to garner good feedback when you hear about it.

British Dragon makes another highly regarded nandrolone decanoate in Thailand, called **Decabol**. It carries 250mg/mL of steroid in a clear 10ml vial. Current product should not carry a hologram sticker, but will have a bright shiny area on the label that is inlayed metallic foil. Also, make sure your product has a cap that reads, "TEAR (with a left arrow)" and "FLIP UP (with a down arrow)". A very popular fake right now uses a copy of the BD hologram sticker (which shouldn't be on the injectable vials) and a top that only reads, "FLIP OFF".

Copies of the Greek **Extraboline** may still be circulating, and can be identified by an overlapping label placed on the vial, and a box that is devoid of the proper Greek Drug ID sticker. As with all Greek drugs, only buy this when properly boxed so you can place the peel-off pharmacy sticker under UV lighting to look for the hidden watermark.

Norma Hellas Deca (100 mg/mL nandrolone decanoate in 2ml vials) from Greece is a good product, but also widely counterfeited. The most reliable way to spot the real thing is to only purchase this steroid when packaged in a box with paperwork. This way you can put the Greek drug ID sticker under UV light. It should reveal a hiffen mark (see Security Stickers). If your box does not have this sticker, it is not real. The vial itself should also have a tightly printed label. By that I mean it will have the blue box in the center going all the way to the edge; no margin. Many of the fakes in circulation have distinct white borders above and below the text. Take note also that the real vial lists the Lot number first, above the expiration date. If your vial lists them in reverse, it is a fake. Norma also started printing their name directly on the glass, underneath the label. Peel it off, and you should see either NORMA or NORMA HELLAS, in blue or red, underneath. This company is run by a bunch of indecisive people when it comes to their packaging, as it seems to change in small ways every other month. Therefore, the Greek drug ID sticker will be the most reliable counterfeit detection method.

Greek **Deca-Durabolin** from Organon is another widely counterfeited product. It is one of only a handful of European nandrolone injectables to be found in multi-dosed vials, making it an easy target for counterfeiters that lack the capacity to produce glass ampules. Again, knowing what to look for is key in avoiding the rip-offs. To begin with, make sure you purchase this product only when it comes in a box with the proper Greek drug ID sticker. As with all Greek drugs, the sticker should show a hidden mark under UV light. This is currently the most reliable method of detection, with all Greek drugs. The box itself will carry three or five vials, depending on the date of manufacture (the 5 vial boxes are newest). If you are looking at the vials themselves, note that the labels on the real product do not have rounded corners. Half of the fakes in circulation carry rounded labels, and immediately standout trait, as the product is never made this way. Also check that the lot number and expiration date are printed with black ink, not blue or purple. Lastly, make sure the ink is not too deep of a black. The real thing sort of looks grayish in color, not really a deep crisp black. Photo comparisons are included in the picture section.

BM Pharmaceuticals in India makes **Deca-Dubol 100**, a 100mg/mL nandrolone decanoate injectable. It is packaged in 2ml multi-dose vials, similar in its format to the 200mg Deca vials from Greece. Feedback on the BM line has been very good so far, although their products do not seem to make their way into the U.S. in very high volume.

Organon sells brand name **Deca-Durabolin** in the United States. This item is such a rare find on the black market, however, that I wound not trust it if located. Fakes must outnumber the real by at least 20 to 1. Should you want to risk it, make sure first that your product is in a maximum dose of 200mg/mL in a 1ml vial. Fakes are often made as 2ml vials, due to the higher selling price for 400mg. Also, make sure the label does not peel easily off the vial. Real U.S. drugs are made with strong glues so this does not happen. Lastly, look for legitimate date/lot stamping on the box and vial. These should be visibly computer printed (box) and stamped (vial label). Still, there may be many sophisticated fakes that will pass on all counts. Be careful.

Both **Watson** and **Schein** Pharmaceuticals have generic nandrolone decanoate products in the U.S. The most commonly dispensed versions for both companies are the 1ml dark glass vials containing 200mg of steroid. Watson is also known to make a 100mg/mL product as well. Both of these items are also sold in pharmacy packs of 25 vials, if you are lucky enough to locate one. As with Organon Deca, these items are extremely rare finds on the black market. When located, the odds are greatly in favor of the product being a fake. As this product is subject to the strict requirements of the FDA, you should investigate for similar labeling and lot/date stamping traits to Organon Deca-Durabolin. This means computer printing on the box, and hard stamping on the label.

Deposterona (testosterone blend)

Androgenic	Anabolic	Standard
100	100	Standard

Chemical Names:
4-androsten-3-one-17beta-ol
17beta-hydroxy-androst-4-en-3-one

Estrogenic Activity: moderate
Progestational Activity: low

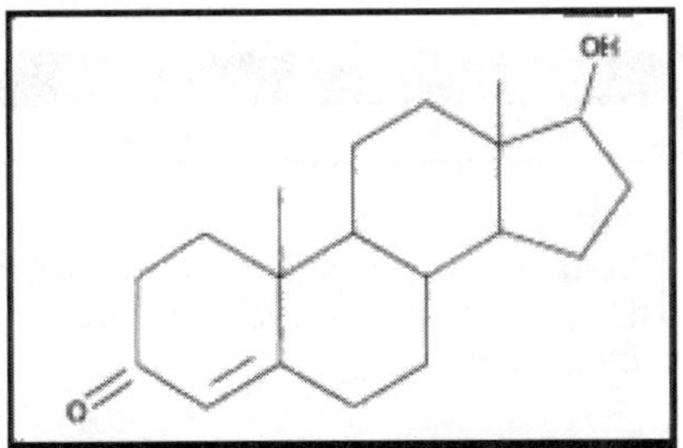

TESTOSTERONE

Deposterona is an injectable veterinary steroid from Mexico, which contains a blend of various esters of testosterone. This product has been around for many years, first sold under the Syntex label and more recently Fort Dodge, who acquired the Syntex Animal Health Company in the mid 1990's. Each milliliter of Deposterona specifically contains 12mg of testosterone acetate, 12mg of testosterone valerate, and 36 milligrams of testosterone undecanoate, for a total steroid concentration of 60 mg/mL. Each multi-dose vial contains 10ml of steroid, and 12 vials are packed together in a master box. This is the first compound I have seen to ever contain testosterone valerate. If you are unfamiliar, this is a medium to long acting ester, with a whole body half-life measured to be approximately double that of testosterone propionate in animal models[72].

With its blend of slow and fast acting esters, Deposterona is sort of a low-dosed alternative to Sustanon. Mind you its shortest ester (acetate) is a little faster acting than the propionate in Sustanon, and its longest ester (undecanoate) a tiny bit slower acting than Sustanon's decanoate. But it is a pretty close comparison nonetheless. As such, it will be an excellent mass and strength builder (for a more complete discussion, please see Sustanon). The main disadvantage to Deposterona is its low steroid concentration. If you were planning on using a "standard" dose of testosterone (400-600mg per week), be prepared to do a lot of injecting. In such instances it would require injecting 8-10ml, up to a full bottle of steroid, each week. Since it is usually not too pricey of a product a cycle like this shouldn't break you. But the oil volume would most certainly be uncomfortable, unless of course you have a sick fondness for injecting yourself. For this reason it is most often used as an adjunct steroid to other compounds (maybe to add an extra hundred milligrams or two of testosterone), and not as the main focus of a steroid cycle.

Because it contains such a low concentration of steroid, Deposterona is in pretty low demand among athletes. There are plenty of more useful testosterone products to be found in Mexico. As such, this product is not readily smuggled into the U.S. After all, a 12 vial box takes up quite a lot of valuable space, and doesn't net a whole lot of money. This space could be filled with much more profitable items such as ampules or high-concentration veterinary steroids. This does, however, also make Deposterona low on the radar when it comes to counterfeiting, which is a good thing. I wouldn't be too worried about fakes if you have just purchased some. There are many other products to duplicate in Mexico, almost all of which would make a counterfeit manufacturer a lot more money on a per unit basis.

Dianabol (methandrostenolone)

Androgenic	Anabolic	Standard
40-60	90-210	Methyltestosterone (oral)

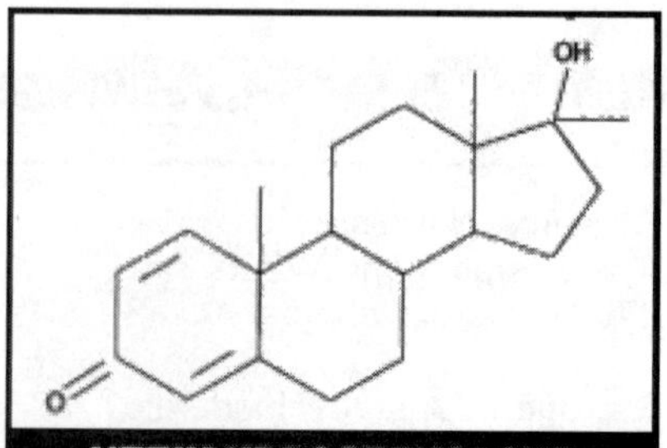

METHANDROSTENOLONE

Chemical Names:
17a-methyl-17b-hydroxy-1,4-androstadien-3-one
1-Dehydro-17a-methyltestosterone
methandienone

Estrogenic Activity: moderate
Progestational Activity: not significant

Dianabol is the old Ciba brand name for the oral steroid methandrostenolone. It is a derivative of testosterone, exhibiting strong anabolic and moderate androgenic properties. This compound was first made available in 1960, and it quickly became the most favored and widely used anabolic steroid in all forms of athletics. This is likely due to the fact that it is both easy to use and extremely effective. In the U.S. Dianabol production had meteoric history, exploding for quite some time, then quickly dropping out of sight. Many were nervous in the late 80's when the last of the U.S. generics were removed from pharmacy shelves, the medical community finding no legitimate use for the drug anymore. But the fact that Dianabol has been off the U.S. market for over 10 years now has not cut its popularity. It remains the most commonly used black market oral steroid in the U.S. As long as there are countries manufacturing this steroid, it will probably remain so.

Similar to testosterone and Anadrol 50®, Dianabol is a potent steroid, but also one which brings about noticeable side effects. For starters methandrostenolone is quite estrogenic. Gynecomastia is likewise often a concern during treatment, and may present itself quite early into a cycle (particularly when higher doses are used). At the same time water retention can become a pronounced problem, causing a notable loss of muscle definition as both subcutaneous water and fat build. Sensitive individuals may therefore want to keep the estrogen under control with the addition of an antiestrogen such as Nolvadex® and/or Proviron®. The stronger drug Arimidex® (anti-aromatase) would be a better choice, but can also be quite expensive in comparison to standard estrogen maintenance therapies.

In addition, androgenic side effects are common with this substance, and may include bouts of oily skin, acne and body/facial hair growth. Aggression may also be increased with a potent steroid such as this, so it would be wise not to let your disposition change for the worse during a cycle. With Dianabol there is also the possibility of aggravating a male pattern baldness condition. Sensitive individuals may therefore wish to avoid this drug and opt for a milder anabolic such as Deca-Durabolin®. While Dianabol does convert to a more potent steroid via interaction with the 5-alpha reductase enzyme (the same enzyme responsible for converting testosterone to dihydrotestosterone), it has extremely little affinity to do so in the human body[73]. The androgenic metabolite 5-alpha dihydromethandrostenolone is therefore produced only in trace amounts at best. The benefit received from Proscar®/Propecia® would therefore be insignificant, the drug serving no real purpose.

Being moderately androgenic, Dianabol is really only a popular steroid with men. When used by women, strong virilization symptoms are of course a possible result. Some do however experiment with it, and find low doses (5mg) of this steroid extremely powerful for new muscle growth. Whenever administered, Dianabol will produce exceptional mass and strength gains. In effectiveness it is often compared to other strong steroids like testosterone and Anadrol 50®, and it is likewise a popular choice for bulking purposes. A daily dosage of 4-5 tablets (20-25mg) is enough to give almost anybody dramatic results. Some do venture much higher in dosage, but this practice usually leads to a more profound incidence of side effects. It additionally adds well with a number of other steroids. It is noted to mix particularly well with the mild anabolic Deca-Durabolin®. Together one can expect an exceptional muscle and strength gains, with side effects not much worse than one would expect from Dianabol alone. For all out mass, a long acting testosterone ester like enanthate can be used. With the similarly high estrogenic/androgenic properties of this androgen, side effects may be extreme with such a combination however. Gains would be great as well, which usually makes such an endeavor worthwhile to the user. As discussed earlier, ancillary drugs can be added to reduce the side effects associated with this kind of cycle.

In order to withstand oral administration, this compound is c17 alpha alkylated. We know that this alteration protects the drug from being deactivation by the liver (allowing nearly all of the drug entry into the bloodstream), however it can also be toxic to this organ. Prolonged exposure to c17 alpha alkylated substances can result in actual damage, possibly even the development of certain kinds of cancer. To be safe one might want to visit the doctor a couple of times during each cycle to keep an eye on their liver enzyme values. Cycles should also be kept short, usually less than 8 weeks long to avoid doing any noticeable damage. Jaundice (bile duct obstruction) is usually the first visible sign of liver trouble, and should be looked out for. This condition produces an unusual yellowing of the skin, as the body has trouble processing bilirubin. In addition to the skin, the whites of the eyes may also yellow, a clear indicator of trouble. Should this occur the drug should be discontinued immediately and a doctor visited. This is usually a point where further, permanent damage can be avoided.

It is also interesting to note that methandrostenolone is structurally identical to boldenone, except that it contains the added c17 alpha alkyl group discussed above. This fact makes clear the impact of altering a steroid in such a way, as these two compounds appear to act very differently in the body. The main dissimilarity seems to lie in the tendency for estrogenic side effects, which seems to be much more pronounced with Dianabol. Equipoise® is known to be quite mild in this regard, therefore, users commonly take this drug without the need to add an antiestrogen. Dianabol is much more estrogenic not because it is more easily aromatized, as in fact the 17 alpha methyl group and c1-2 double bond both slow the process of aromatization. The problem is that methandrostenolone converts to 17alpha methylestradiol, a more biologically active form of estrogen than regular estradiol[74]. But Dianabol also appears to be much more potent in terms of muscle mass compared to boldenone, supporting the notion that estrogen does play an important role in anabolism. In fact boldenone and methandrostenolone differ so much in their potencies as anabolics that the two are rarely thought of as related. As a result, the use of Dianabol is typically restricted to bulking phases of training while Equipoise® is considered an excellent cutting or lean-mass building steroid.

The half-life of Dianabol is only about 3 to 5 hours, a relatively short time. This means that a single daily dosage schedule will produce a varying blood level, with ups and downs throughout the day. The user, likewise, has a choice, to either split up the tablets during the day or to take them all at one time. The usual recommendation has been to divide them and try to regulate the concentration in your blood. This however, will produce a lower peak blood level than if the tablets were taken all at once, so there may be a trade off with this option. The steroid researcher Bill Roberts also points out that a single-episode dosing schedule should have a less dramatic impact on the hypothalamic-pituitary-testicular axis, as there is a sufficient period each day where steroid hormone levels are not extremely exaggerated. I tend to doubt hormonal stability can be maintained during such a cycle however, but do notice that anecdotal evidence often still supports single daily doses to be better for overall results. If this is the better option, I am more inclined to think it has to do with higher peak dosages vs. lower more even blood concentrations. Since we know the blood concentration will peak about 1.5 to 3 hours after administration, we may further wonder the best time to take our tablets. It seems logical that taking the pills earlier in the day, preferably some time before training, would be optimal. This would allow a considerable number of daytime hours for an androgen rich metabolism to heighten the uptake of nutrients, especially the critical hours following training.

Athletes are also often asking how to go about cycling 100 tablets (5mg) when that is the only amount available to use. Although most strongly prefer to cycle at least 200 tablets, half this amount can be used successfully for a small "mini" cycle. The goal should be to intake an effective amount, but also to stretch it for as long as possible. We can do this by taking four tablets daily during the week (Monday to Friday) and abstaining on the weekend. This gives us a weekly total of 20 tablets, 100 tabs lasting the user five weeks. This should be a long enough time to receive noticeable gains from the drug, particularly if you have not used steroid extensively before. Although unconventional, it is not necessary to vary the pill dosage throughout a cycle. This method should provide a much more consistent gain than attempting an intricate pyramid schedule, which can eat up most of your pills during dosage adjustments. As discussed earlier in this book, tapering the dosage toward the end would offer us no real benefit.

Dianabol is one of the most popular steroids in the world, and consequently one can find a variety of such preparations on the black market. You must be warned though. This drug is also amongst the most widely counterfeited. You need to do some educated shopping to avoid getting ripped off. One of the first things you need to remember is that most of the Western world has completely done away with this steroid. In medical circles here it is thought to hold no real value anymore. Its potential existence is viewed as supporting doping/performance-enhancement only. Therefore, you are not going to come across legitimate Dbol from the U.S., Canada, or Western Europe. This drug is made exclusively in ares such as Asia, South America (limited), Mexico, and

Eastern Europe. Ignore anything labeled as Italian or Spanish etc. They will not be legitimate. In regards to some of the most popular legitimate brands on the black market, here is what to look for.

Animal Power has recently introduced its **Methan Tabs** to Mexico. This is a 10mg methandrostenolone tablet product, which comes packaged 100 tablets per glass bottle. Animal Power has taken counterfeiting seriously from the start, and as such has included hologram stickers on all of their boxes, bottles, and vials (see Security Stickers). Methan Tabs will also carry the company logo written directly on the glass, of which most will be obscured by the label until peeled off. Do not buy the product if either feature is missing. Feedback has been excellent on the AP line thus far, making them easy to recommend.

Pet's Pharma is another new firm in the Mexican steroid scene. They sell two versions of methandrostenolone, one an injectable and another the standard oral. The injectable is called **Metandiol 60**, and carries 60mg/ml of steroid in a 10ml vial. The oral is **Metandiol 25**, and comes as a 25mg tablet in bottles of 100. Both products will carry the Pet's Pharma security sticker (see Security Stickers). At the present time counterfeits of this line are not a big issue.

Among the more popular today are the **D-Bol** preparations from **Denkall** in Mexico. D-Bol comes in three distinct forms: 10mg tablets, 10mg capsules, and a 25mg/mL injectable. The injectable uses oil to dissolve the steroid instead of propylene glycol, making it much more comfortable to inject compared to Reforvit, if that is your intention. All versions are to be considered top quality. To date I have never seen a lab test from Denkall that had unfavorable results; making this a definite recommended buy.

Reforvit is a Mexican veterinary methandrostenolone product from Loeffler. It is prepared in both oral and injectable forms. The injectable contains 25mg/mL of steroid, with each 50ml bottle containing the equivalent of 250 tablets. A 10ml vial is also produced, but not commonly seen in the U.S. due to general disinterest (it contains only 50 tablets worth of drug). Note that the product uses propylene glycol instead of oil as a solvent, which makes for very painful injections. Most users opt the take it orally for this reason. It tastes like ass though (big time!), so you may want to buy some '00' size empty gelcaps at the healthfood store and fill them with your dose. You can inject the assembled caps by piercing the tip.

The now more popular oral Reforvit tablets (called **Reforvit Simple**) carry 25mg of steroid each, and are sold in bottles of 100 and 1,000 tablets in total. Loeffler uses a hologram sticker to deter counterfeiting, however, thus far it has been only a generic one with no specific markings for Loeffler. It is, therefore, not going to be highly reliable as a security feature (see Security Stickers for more detail). Also, this manufacturer has a history of underdosing their products, sometimes significantly. You may find yourself taking higher doses to compensate for expected shortages.

Salud in Mexico sells methandrostenolone under the **Dianabol** brand name. Like Denkall and Pet's Pharma, they produce it in both oral and injectable forms. The injectable comes in a 10mL, 50mL, or 100mL multi-dose vial, and carries 25mg/mL of steroid. It uses an oil carrier instead of propylene glycol, which makes injections much more tolerable than Reforvit. Their Dianabol tablets contain 10mg of drug each, and are packaged in very small plastic bottles of 100 tablets each. This product has passed lab testing before, and represents a very cost effective buy on the Mexican market right now.

Norvet in Mexico makes oral and injectable forms of this steroid. The injectable is sold as **Anabol-Jet**, and it contains 25mg/mL of methandrostenolone in 10ml, 30ml, 100ml, and 250ml sizes. They also make a variant called Anabol-Jet ADE. This has 30mg/mL of steroid with some added vitamins, and comes in 100ml and 250ml sizes. Their oral is sold as **Anabol Pet's**, and comes in 10mg and 25mg dosage strengths. Two hundred tablets are included per bottle. All of the Norvet products can probably be trusted when located, as they are still low on the radar for counterfeiting. I have not seen any lab test results yet, so I cannot confirm that they are accurately dosing these products.

Although no longer in business, you may still find **Ttokkyo's** generic from Mexico on the black market in small volume. If you do come across this product, it should bear a security hologram sticker and a plastic bottle with "Ttokkyo" imprinted in the bottom. Note that in the past, counterfeiters had appropriated some of their stickers so, finding them may not be a 100% reliable.

British Dispensery **Anabol** tablets from Thailand are still very popular. Due to rampant counterfeiting, the manufacturer has instituted three security guards. One is a hologram sticker, which is affixed to each 1,000 count tub of tablets. Second, the tablets themselves are imprinted with the company's snake emblem. Do not buy any blank Anabol at this time, as the tabs will be fake. Lastly, the 1,000 count tub bears the company logo formed into the plastic top (there are fakes with this too). Make sure your product matches on all three counts, and you should have a safe purchase. Otherwise, Thai "pinks" are a risky item to buy. Note also that the latest reiteration has the word "promotion" misspelled as "pormotion" on the label. This is a typographical error, not a counterfeit.

The Thai company British Dragon is also selling its own brand of methandrostenolone. It is called **Methanabol**, and comes prepared in both 10mg and 50mg(!) tablets. The 10mg version comes 500 to a pouch, while the 50mg dosed tablets are sold in lots of 100. The tablets are square and are marked "BD" on one side and the dosage on the other. All oral products from BD will carry a security hologram sticker to deter counterfeiting, however, this has been duplicated before. Thus far the new square tablets have not been copied.

British Dragon also recently introduced an injectable methandrostenolone called **Averbol 25**. It contains 25mg/mL of steroid in a 20ml vial. This product never carried a hologram sticker, but does have a bright shiny area on the label that is inlayed red metallic foil. Also, make sure your product has a cap that reads, "TEAR (with a left arrow)" and "FLIP UP (with a down arrow)". A very popular fake right now uses a copy of the BD hologram sticker (which shouldn't be on the injectable vials) and a top that only reads, "FLIP OFF".

Generic "Russian D-Bol" (**METAHAPOCTEHOROH**) is still being produced in Russia by **Akrikhin** (the name looks like **Akpnxnh** in Cyrillic). The current box is purple in color, and carries 10 strips of 10 tablets each. This has always been a highly regarded form of Dbol. As such, it has also been a regularly counterfeited one. Most of the fakes have been poor copies of the original, however, often coming as bottles of loose tablets instead of proper foil and plastic push-through strips. That is not to say locating the current production version assures a safe purchase, however, this brand is somewhat less risky than many of the other brands on the market.

Another generic popular in Europe is the Russia **Bioreaktor (Peaktop)** brand. The packing of this drug has recently changed, and now reflects a more modern looking white/black/green design. Some of the older boxes may still be in circulation at this time. There have been a handful of very adept fakes of this product in the past (of the previous design), which means the new item is likely to be targeted as well. Note also that in 2000 court battle with Akrikhin, Peaktop lost the right to use the trade name **METAHAPOCTEHOROH**. They have since changed it to (roughly) **METAHANEHOH.** This involved a change in the barcode as well. Prior to two thousand, the strips would each carry a barcode number that ended in 000359. After 2000, they end in 000700. Several counterfeits have been seen that still carry the old barcode number, beware.

Naposim from Rumania has just changed the look of its packaging also. The new white box reflects a much more modern design when placed next to the old orange colored packaging. The older version has been heavily counterfeited in recent years, with exceptional accuracy. Since old lots may still be in circulation, it is worth offering the following tips on the orange box product. The foil strip on real Naposim has date and lot number stampings on both ends, while the current popular fake has them on one side. The machine that seals the foil backing on the real product also uses a pattern of dots, while the fake is seen to have a waffle pattern. Additionally, there is a little nipple in the center of each pill bubble on the real Naposim strip, while the fake pill bubbles are just smooth plastic. The new product may very likely be the subject of a similar counterfeit scheme, as the former producer finds it hard to push off outdated copies. This has not been a problem as of yet, so the new product is still a good buy.

Danabol DS is a 10 mg version of Dianabol from Body Research/March Pharmaceutical Company in Thailand. It comes in bottles of 500 very distinct blue tablets, formed in the shape of hearts. To spite the cheap appearance of the bottle, this product is legit, and can be trusted when found. Fakes are not yet known to be a problem.

Methandon and **Melic** from Thailand are both legit items, and come packed in containers of 1,000 tablets each. Both of these products have been relatively nonexistent on the black market as of late. My sources in Thailand have not been able to find either in a single pharmacy this year. One or both may have been dropped from market.

Bionabol from Bulgaria is another legitimate methandrostenolone preparation. Please note that the packaging should reflect that Balkanpharma sells the product, and it should be prepared in foil and plastic strips of 10 tablets. There are numerous counterfeits that come as bottles of loose tablets. At one time Bionabol was sold like this, but it was too long ago to trust any such product on the black market today.

Anabolex 3mg tabs from the Dominican Republic are still a safe buy. Note that each pill contains an added 1.5mg of Periactin, used as an appetite stimulant. It's an antihistamine and may cause drowsiness. Make sure your product is packaged in the modern style blue pouches, not the older plain white ones. These are long off the market at this point.

Bratis Labs in Mexico is making a 10mg tablet under the name **Metandrol 10**. There has been good feedback on this product in the past; however, I haven't been hearing much from them lately. I cannot confirm they are still producing at the time of writing this update.

Metanabol from Poland is another legit brand, but be sure to purchase these only in strips of 20 tabs, as shown in the picture library.

Nerobol from Hungary is no longer being manufactured. Avoid all products bearing this brand name.

The Sulfuric Acid test

One of my contributing researchers, Ronny Tober, recently informed me about a home test kit that was being used by European bodybuilders to help spot fake Dianabol tablets. It is called "EZ-Test", and it is sold in various alternative lifestyle ("head-shop") stores to help recreational drug users identify fake Amphetamine or Ecstasy products. The method, however, also seems to work for steroid tablets. EZ-Test contains a simple sulfuric acid solution (which can be obtained as a raw chemical with a little effort), which is a strong reactive agent that cleanly breaks down and dissolves the inert binders and fillers used in the making of most tablets. The sulfuric acid will produce a strong visible reaction when it comes into contact with the active agent however, enabling you to identify if you have a real drug product. In the case of methandrostenolone, the tablets will produce a strong reddish/brown color almost immediately upon being dropped into the acid solution. A lack of this reaction would obviously indicate that your tablets are worthless, and contain nothing but inert ingredients. The "sulfuric acid test" is not 100% reliable though, as it could easily be fooled by substitute steroid ingredients or under-dosing. But with the many totally bogus zero-steroid-containing products that circulate the black market every day, it can still be a valuable tool to make use of.

Dinandrol (nandrolone blend)

Androgenic	Anabolic	Standard
37	125	Testosterone

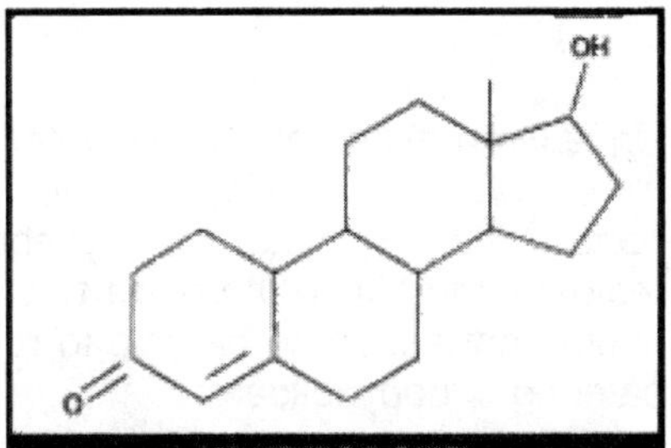
NANDROLONE

Chemical Names:
19-norandrost-4-en-3-one-17beta-ol
17beta-hydroxy-estr-4-en-3-one

Estrogenic Activity: low
Progestational Activity: moderate

Dinandrol is to nandrolone what Sustanon is to testosterone, well sort of. This product is an injectable anabolic steroid from the Philippines that contains a blend of one short and one long acting ester of nandrolone. The intent, as with Sustanon, is to provide the user more of a sustained-release effect compared to that obtained with single-ester injectables. Each ml of Dinandrol contains 60mg of nandrolone decanoate and 40mg of nandrolone phenylpropionate, for a total steroid concentration of 100mg per ml (200mg per 2ml vial). Although this product lacks the propionate and isocaproate esters that would make it a true nandrolone equivalent of Sustanon, I suspect it still provides a release profile very similar to this drug. After all, the difference in steroid release time between propionate and phenylpropionate esters are not that great, and with a good dose of decanoate it is difficult to think the isocaproate will be tremendously missed. It is about as close as we can get to a real "Sustanon", and with a product like this there would seem little added benefit in actually developing one.

As with all nandrolone products, Dinandrol offers a moderate anabolic effect with only mild androgenic or estrogenic side effects (for a more comprehensive discussion, please see the Deca-Durabolin profile). Although designed as a long and steady acting product, bodybuilders are not looking for a nandrolone replacement drug that is injected once a month. With this in mind Dinandrol is most often injected on a weekly basis. The dose, as with regular Deca-Durabolin, would be in the range of 200-600mg per application. If anything, one would only be noticing a difference between Dinandrol and Deca when first starting a cycle (due to the faster onset of action), and only if they tended to notice the benefits of steroid therapy very quickly. Otherwise the drug will build to pretty significant and "steady-state" levels within a few injections, making it impossible to distinguish from regular Deca-Durabolin. For the bodybuilder it is, therefore, not any type of "must have" steroid to go run out and start searching for, but most certainly is an acceptable option if found at a fair price.

Dinandrol is one of those odd steroid products that are rarely found in an actual pharmacy. This is because it is not registered as a prescription drug in the country in which it is made (so don't expect to take any home if you visit). Instead, it is an export only item, sold to importers in other countries who likely are quick to divert it to the black market. Although you may not have the benefit of obtaining it through legitimate channels, it is not that difficult to recognize real Dinandrol when one crosses this item on the black market. Its packaging is unique, and would seemingly be difficult and costly to duplicate. Well, maybe the multi-dose vials are not that unique, three of which are packaged in a blue shaded box that is also pretty easy to copy. But you do open the box to find the vials sitting nicely in a clear-plastic tray that bears the firm's name (Xelox). It is not printed on the tray but molded directly into the plastic, which would obviously be some task for an underground manufacturer to duplicate. Being that this item is rarely even heard of at this time, I do not expect fakes to be a problem very soon.

Drive (boldenone/methylandrostenediol blend)

Drive is an extremely unique veterinary steroid, available only in Australia. This is actually a very interesting place for steroids, possessing a number of unusual compounds. Strange methandriol mixes, unusual esters (such as nandrolone cypionate, see Dynabol) and probably the only place in the world that produces 500ml bladders of testosterone. Quite the place to visit. Laws regarding steroids have become stricter in recent years, so travelers should not expect to be able to run into a veterinary shop to load up. There is of course an active black market catering to bodybuilders.

This particular item is an oil based injectable, containing 25mg boldenone undecylenate and 30mg methandriol (methylandrostenediol dipropionate) per ml. Boldenone is familiar to us as the preparation Equipoise®, but methandriol is very rarely seen on the U.S. black market. It is a strong anabolic with a notable androgenic component. Methandriol can come in one of two forms actually, there is a 17-methylated compound designed for oral administration, or the methylated & esterified (dipropionate) version commonly seen as an injectable in Australian vet compounds. Methandriol produces notable muscle mass and strength gains, usually without accompanying water retention. In this mix it works nicely when mixed with the anabolic boldenone. Together the two compounds produce exceptional gains in strength and muscle mass.

As with almost every effective steroid, Drive can produce a noticeable set of side effects. While the boldenone is only mildly androgenic, methandriol shows slightly more pronounced activity. Androgenic side effects like oily skin, acne and increased aggression are all possible with this product. Women may want to stay away from Drive, fearing the androgen content will produce virilization symptoms. Estrogen can sometimes become troublesome with this drug, presumably from the aromatization of boldenone which is slight. Methylandrostenediol itself cannot directly aromatize, however it has been shown to display some low affinity for the estrogen receptor (possibly enhancing estrogenic activity as well). Sensitive individuals may therefore opt for the addition of an antiestrogen such as Nolvadex® and/or Proviron®, in an effort to avoid any chance of developing gynecomastia and to minimize any slight smoothness due to subcutaneous water retention. In comparison to stronger stacks however, water bloat is usually not a major problem with Drive. This combination is in fact often noted for producing a very hard, quality physique.

Since methandriol is a c17 alpha alkylated compound, liver toxicity can be a concern. The injectable dipropionate does offer us less toxicity however, as your liver will not have to process the entire dosage at once during the first pass. It is therefore the preferred form of administration among bodybuilders, on those rare instances that both might be available. Of course the possibility of liver damage cannot be excluded with the injectable though. It is also interesting to note that once the esters have been removed, we see that structurally methandriol is just a methylated form of 5-androstenediol. This is clear when we look at the chemical name (methyl-androstenediol) or a methylated form of this hormone (which is of course a popular pro-hormone supplement).

Drive is rarely smuggled into the U.S. in noticeable quantity, but can be found on occasion. The packaging of many Australian vet compounds, Drive included, is quite simple and easy to duplicate, so beware should an abundance of any particular substance begin to circulate.

Durabolin (nandrolone phenylpropionate)

Androgenic	Anabolic	Standard
37	125	Testosterone

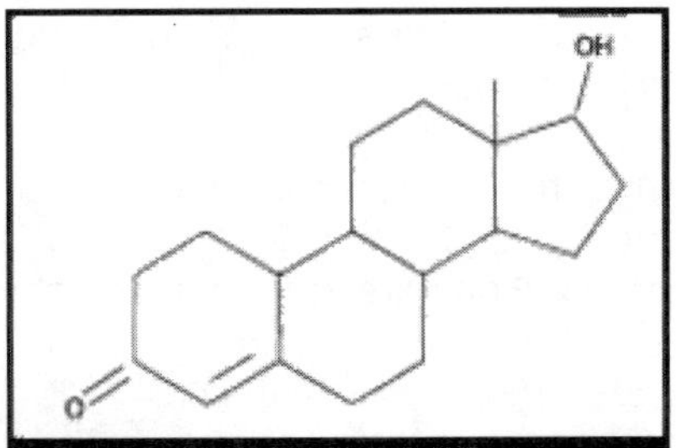

NANDROLONE

Chemical Names:
19-norandrost-4-en-3-one-17beta-ol
17beta-hydroxy-estr-4-en-3-one

Estrogenic Activity: low
Progestational Activity: moderate

Durabolin® is the Organon brand name for the injectable steroid nandrolone phenylpropionate. As one could guess, the properties of this drug are very similar to that of Deca-Durabolin®. Both contain the anabolic hormone nandrolone and are produced by the same drug firm (Organon). The primary difference between these two preparations is the speed in which the drug is released. While Deca provides the extremely slow release duration of up three or four weeks, Durabolin® is active for only a few days. In clinical situations Deca can thus be injected once every two or three weeks, while Durabolin® is usually administered every few days.

As with Deca, estrogen buildup is not a typical worry when using this drug. Some feel the fast action of Durabolin® is associated with slightly less water retention than Deca-Durabolin®, but this observation is probably just due to a lower blood concentrations during typical use. There is no difference between the nandrolone which is released into the body by each drug, so we cannot assign Durabolin® any unique set of properties. Nandrolone is generally not noted to cause estrogen trouble in any event, so the chance of developing gynecomastia and water bloat is slight, even among sensitive individuals. Likewise an antiestrogen is usually not necessary when using this steroid. Durabolin® is also the preferred nandrolone product during dieting and contest preparation phases of training when estrogen and water retention are a major concern. This is just due to the fact that blood hormone levels are easier to control with a faster acting substance.

We also know that nandrolone is not an extremely potent androgen. This is because it will reduce to a less active metabolite (dihydronandrolone) in many androgen target tissues, due to interaction with the 5-alpha reductase enzyme. This is of course the same enzyme that potentates the action of testosterone by transforming it to a more active form (dihydrotestosterone). Related side effects such as oily skin, acne, body/facial hair growth and aggravated male pattern hair loss likewise occur much less frequently with these drugs compared to testosterone and many other anabolic/androgenic steroids, making Durabolin a very favorable steroid for those concerned.

While the level of such side effects is low with this anabolic, so may be the gain of strength and muscle mass. This is to be expected, as nandrolones are noted as being slow but quality builders instead of mass drugs. They are however noted to allow for the retention of a higher percentage of new body weight gain after a cycle is over, the user not having to endure a dramatic loss of stored water due to estrogen buildup. Although the buildup of estradiol is not marked, this drug can still notably affect endogenous testosterone levels. One may therefore still need to use an ancillary drug like HCG and/or Clomid® when coming off a cycle. This should ensure the lowest chance for suffering a hormonal crash when the steroid has been removed.

Due to its rapid rate of release from the injection site, Durabolin® is usually administered every two or three days. The dosage of each given shot is usually in the range of 50-100mg, equating to 1ml or 2ml when using the 50mg version. To keep injection volume to a comfortable level men will typically use a slightly lower weekly dosage than with Deca, generally 200-300mg (2 or 3 injections of 100mg). As discussed earlier, the buildup of muscle tissue resulting from Durabolin® is slow and even. This combined with a low incidence of side effects makes it an ideal steroid to use for longer periods of time, so that gains are given time to accumulate. It is likewise not unusual to see someone utilizing a nandrolone such as this in cycles greater than three months in length.

The short action of this drug is highly attractive to female athletes. Although usually more expensive, Durabolin® should be the preference if both it and Deca are available. While all nandrolone are generally well tolerated, blood hormone levels are more difficult to control with a long acting ester such as decanoate. Should virilization symptoms become evident, the rapid metabolism of Durabolin® would be a very welcome trait. Here it would only take a matter of days for most of the active hormone to leave the body. The chance for more serious side effects would of course be heightened with Deca, the female athlete left with a highly elevated hormone level for weeks after ceasing use. The preferred administration schedule for women would also be a single injection weekly, at a dosage no more than 50 to 75 mg. This level is sufficient for a quality gain, yet low enough to feel safe from most side effects.

In general, Durabolin® will produce the same side effects seen with Deca, but they may be slightly less pronounced if the dosage used is lower (and/or more controlled, with less peaks) in comparison. Nandrolone preparations are among the most well tolerated steroids in manufacture, causing a very low incidence of unwanted side effects.

The only real problems with this drug are availability and price. Although produced in a fair number of countries, **Durabolin®** in particular is not commonly found in the U.S. This may be due to the high selling price and low strength of the Organon preparations. A single 50mg ampule could cost as much as $15 when sold on the black market, which is a high price for such a low dosage of steroid. Quite often the only strength available is the 25mg version, which can be even less cost effective. At the same time the injections may be too frequent or too large a volume for most to tolerate. These factors make Organon's Deca-Durabolin® much more abundant on the black market.

This steroid does occasionally find its way here in volume from India, where you can find **Dubol** by **BM Pharmaceuticals** in addition to the Organon brand-name product. Dubol is made in both 50mg/mL and 100mg/mL dosage strengths (Dubol-50 and Dubol-100 respectively), and is considerably more cost effective than its Organon-manufactured counterpart. For a while, Dubol was being sold as a generic from the former company name **Haryian Biologicals**, however enough time has passed now that you should expect to see mostly the BM product on the black market.

British Dragon in Thailand also makes **Durabol**, which comes in the form of a 100mg/mL 10ml vial. BD is a reputable lab, and the product should be accurately dosed. New vials no longer carry a security hologram sticker. Instead the labels are inlayed with a red foil stamping, which has the letters "BD" and the company's Dragon logo. Also, make sure the top on your vial says "TEAR" and "FLIP UP". A common fake of the BD line has tops that read "FLIP OFF".

Superanabolon from Spofa in the Czech Republic also circulates from time to time, although not very abundantly in the U.S. (it is much more common in Europe). This is a legitimate product, although it only contains 25mg of steroid per 1ml ampule.

Dynabolon (nandrolone undecanoate)

Androgenic	Anabolic	Standard
37	125	Testosterone

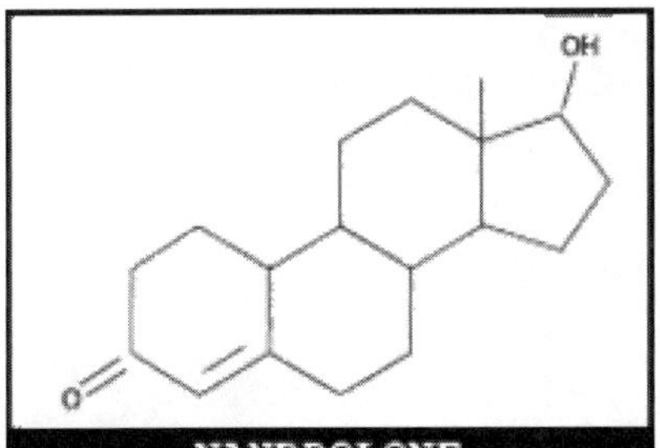

NANDROLONE

Chemical Names:
19-norandrost-4-en-3-one-17beta-ol
17beta-hydroxy-estr-4-en-3-one

Estrogenic Activity: low
Progestational Activity: moderate

Dynabolon is a very unique nandrolone ester, produced only in Italy (the French version was recently discontinued). This particular compound is nandrolone undecanoate, the same ester that Organon uses for their testosterone preparation Andriol. Here the compound is obviously not intended for oral administration however, instead the design being that of a long acting, oil based injectable. The undecanoate provides an active duration of approximately three to four weeks, very similar than what is expected with Deca-Durabolin®. The undecanoate ester is actually one carbon atom longer, making Dynabolon slightly slower to release than Deca. Athletes however, usually inject both in weekly intervals.

This steroid is obviously quite similar in appearance to Deca. It is noted for being an effective anabolic, while not giving the user an excessive level of side effects. Estrogen conversion is slight with nandrolone; so related side effects should be minimal. While water retention is sometimes reported when taking this drug, an actual smoothness and bloating to the muscles would be very uncommon, just as we expect with Deca-Durabolin®. Gynecomastia is also a rare concern, but can be a problem with individuals very sensitive to the effects of estrogen. In order to minimize such side effects, an ancillary drug like Nolvadex® and/or Proviron® could be added if absolutely necessary.

It is also of interest that nandrolone undergoes the same conversion process that changes testosterone into dihydrotestosterone, a more potent androgenic metabolite. But the result with nandrolone is dihydronandrolone, a much milder hormone. DHN is in fact miler than its parent nandrolone, which means that the activity of the steroid will actually be reduced in tissues with a high concentration of 5-alpha reductase. Androgenic side effects will therefore be much less pronounced than if we were using a stronger compound such as testosterone enanthate. Oily skin, acne, body/facial hair growth and hair loss are all uncommon with nandrolone esters, making them very well tolerated. These preparations are also considered safe for women (at low doses), as virilization symptoms are not a common occurrence. It is important to note however, that there is always the possibility of developing virilization symptoms with this steroid (as with all anabolic/androgenic steroids). To be safest, the faster acting Durabolin® would make a better choice. This faster acting preparation allows the athlete much greater control over blood hormone levels, and is much easier to withdrawal from if problems become evident.

As an anabolic, Dynabolon would be quite similar in effect to Deca-Durabolin®. Again, this drug may display a slightly slower rate of release, with a peak blood concentration being reached slightly later. This may technically equate to a more delayed effect, however this should not be discernible to the user. The most common dosage is 3-4 ampules (241.5 to 322mg) per week, a level that should elicit a very acceptable gain of new muscle mass. Since 4ml is a large injection to administer at one time, this can be further divided into two biweekly injections to avoid discomfort. A higher dosage could be used to elicit a more pronounced anabolic response, however injection volume and frequency will likely become uncomfortably above 6-8 ml weekly.

Nandrolone injectables such as Dynabolon are most commonly incorporated into bulking cycles, although many find that they fit very comfortably in cutting stacks as well. Of course drug testing will limit its use in many such cases however, leaving only the oral nandrolone precursors norandrostenedione and norandrostenediol open to use. Dynabolon can be used alone for a quality mass gain, or in combination with a number of stronger androgens for a heavier gain. Together with testosterone or Anadrol 50®, the growth achieved can be quite formidable. This drug could obviously replace Deca-Durabolin® in the classic Deca/Dbol stack so loved by many. Going back to cutting, we find combining Dynabol with non-aromatizing compounds such as Winstrol® or Anavar helps to dramatically increase the look of hardness and definition. A stronger nonaromatizing androgen such as

Halotestin®, Proviron® or trenbolone would provide even more dramatic effect, however related side effects may also become much more pronounced.

Equilon 100 (boldenone blend)

Androgenic	Anabolic	Standard
50	100	Testosterone

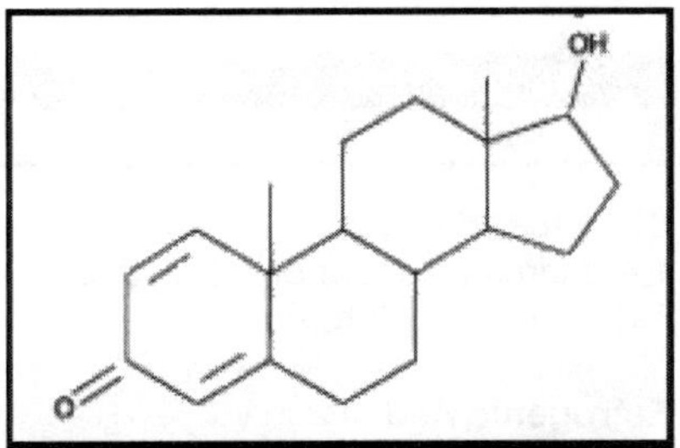

BOLDENONE

Chemical Names:
1,4-androstadiene-3-one,17beta-ol
1-dehydrotestosterone

Estrogenic Activity: low
Progestational Activity: n/a (low)

Equilon is an extremely interesting new steroid to hit the black market in recent years. This product is manufactured by WDV Pharma, a veterinary steroid manufacturer based in Myanmar. This is the same company that makes the very unique seven-ester blend of testosterone called Equitest. Equilon could be considered the Equipoise counterpart to that product, containing a sustained-release blend of four different esters of boldenone. These specifically include boldenone acetate, propionate, cypionate and undecylenate. They add up to a steroid concentration of 100mg/mL, with each multi-dose vial of Equilon containing 6ml of steroid in total. One vial is found in each box.

Each ml of Equilon contains:

Boldenone Acetate	10 mg
Boldenone Propionate	30 mg
Boldenone Undecylenate	40 mg
Boldenone Cyclopentylpropionate (cypionate)	20 mg

Equilon is the first multi-component boldenone product ever to be developed. In this regard, it is quite an innovative product. On the one side it has the early kick-in power of boldenone acetate and propionate, the two fastest acting esters available. This is definitely going to sit well with bodybuilders who love Equipoise, yet prefer to kick off their cycles with faster acting injectable esters like testosterone propionate or nandrolone phenylpropionate. On the other side it has the long-lasting effectiveness of cypionate and undecylenate, which allows a once-per-week injection schedule to be more than sufficient for maintaining steady hormone concentrations. Although ultimately slow and fast acting forms of the same drug release *the same drug*, we can still see some clear value in a blended product like this.

Equilon is a boldenone product, providing a strong anabolic effect with only moderate androgenic/estrogenic activity (for a more comprehensive discussion, please refer to the Equipoise profile). Equipoise has always been a drug of relatively high demand because of its favorable properties, and I expect this new blended product to be no exception. If anything, it sits in relative obscurity at this time, as WDV is not a major manufacturer and they operate in an area of the world fairly isolated from the international underground steroid market. Once bodybuilders begin to learn of this products existence, however, I expect demand for it to skyrocket. It is a decently dosed, very innovated new blend of a hormone long-favored by bodybuilders. Provided it can be consistently obtained for a reasonable price, what else could we possibly expect?

Equipoise (boldenone undecylenate)

Androgenic	Anabolic	Standard
50	100	Testosterone

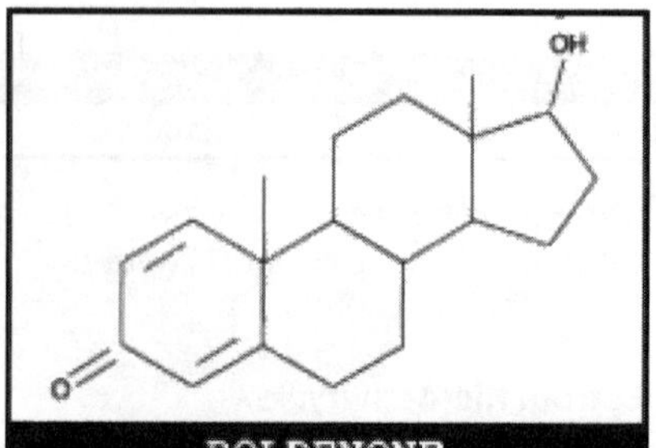

Chemical Names:
1,4-androstadiene-3-one,17beta-ol
1-dehydrotestosterone

Estrogenic Activity: low
Progestational Activity: n/a (low)

Equipoise® is the popularly referenced brand name for the veterinary injectable steroid boldenone undecylenate. Specifically it is a derivative of testosterone, which exhibits strong anabolic and moderately androgenic properties. The undecylenate ester greatly extends the activity of the drug (the undecylenate ester is only one carbon atom longer than decanoate), so that clinically injections would need to be repeated every three or four weeks. In veterinary medicine Equipoise® is most commonly used on horses, exhibiting a pronounced effect on lean bodyweight, appetite and general disposition of the animal. This compound is also said to shows a marked ability for increasing red blood cell production, although there should be no confusion that this is an effect characteristic of nearly all anabolic/androgenic steroids. The favorable properties of this drug are greatly appreciated by athletes, Equipoise® being a very popular injectable in recent years. It is considered by many to be a stronger, slightly more androgenic Deca-Durabolin®. It is generally cheaper, and could replace Deca in most cycles without greatly changing the end result.

The side effects associated with Equipoise® are generally mild. The structure of boldenone does allow it to convert into estrogen, but it does not have an extremely high affinity to do so. To try and quantify this we can look toward aromatization studies, which suggest that its rate of estrogen conversion should be roughly half that of testosterone[75]. The tendency to develop a noticeable amount of water retention with this drug would therefore be slightly higher than that with Deca-Durabolin® (with an estimated 20% conversion), but much less than what would be expected with a stronger agent such as Testosterone. While one does still have a chance of encountering an estrogen related side effect as such when using this substance, it is not a common problem when taken at a moderate dosage level. Gynecomastia might theoretically become a concern, but is usually only heard of with very sensitive individuals or (again) those venturing high in dosage. Should estrogenic effects become troublesome, the addition of Nolvadex® and/or Proviron® should of course make the cycle more tolerable. An anti-aromatase such as Cytadren® or Arimidex® would be stronger options, however probably not indicated with a mild drug as such.

Equipoise® can also produce distinct androgenic side effects. Incidences of oily skin, acne, increased aggression and hair loss are likewise all possible with this compound, although will typically be related to the use of higher doses. Women in fact find this drug quite comfortable, virilization symptoms usually unseen when taken at low doses. Boldenone does reduce to a more potent androgen (dihydroboldenone) via the 5alpha reductase enzyme (which produces DHT from testosterone), however its affinity for this interaction in the human body is low to nonexistent[76]. We therefore cannot consider the reductase inhibitor Proscar® to be of much use with Equipoise®, as it would be blocking what is at best an insignificant path of metabolism for the steroid. And although this drug is relatively mild, it may still have a depressive effect on endogenous testosterone levels. A combination of HCG and Clomid®/Nolvadex® may likewise be needed at the conclusion of each cycle to avoid a "crash", particularly when running long in duration.

Although it stays active for a much longer time, Equipoise® is injected at least once per week by athletes. It is most commonly used at a dosage of 200-400mg (4-8 ml, 50mg version) per week for men, 50-75 mg per week for women. Should a 25mg version be the only product available, the injection volume can become quite uncomfortable. The dosage schedule can be further divided, perhaps injections given every other day to reduce discomfort. One should also take caution to rotate injection sites regularly, so as to avoid irritation or infection. Should too large an oil volume be injected into one site, an abscess may form that requires surgical draining. To avoid such a problem, athletes will usually limit each injection to 3ml and reuse each site no more than once per week, preferably every other week. With Equipoise® this may require using not only the gluteus, but also the outer thighs for an injection site. Of course all problems associated with 25mg and 50mg dosed products are eliminated with the newer 100mg and 200mg/mL versions of this steroid, which clearly give the user much more dosage freedom and injection comfort.

Not a rapid mass builder, instead Equipoise® will be looked at to provide a slow but steady gain of strength and quality muscle mass. The most positive effects of this drug are seen when it is used for longer cycles, usually lasting more than 8-10 weeks in duration. The muscle gained should not be the smooth bulk seen with androgens, but very defined and solid. Since water bloat is not contributing greatly to the diameter of the muscle, much of the size gained on a cycle of Equipoise® can be retained after the drug has been discontinued. It is interesting to note that structurally Equipoise® and the classic bulking drug Dianabol are almost identical. In the case of Equipoise® the compound uses a 17beta ester (undecylenate), while Dianabol is 17 alpha alkylated. Aside from this the molecules are the same. Of course they act quite differently in the body, which goes to show the 17-methylation effects more than just the oral efficacy of a steroid.

As discussed earlier, Equipoise® is a very versatile compound. We can create a number of drug combinations with it depending on the desired result. For mass, one may want to stack it with Anadrol 50®(oxymetholone) or an injectable testosterone such as Sustanon 250. The result should be an incredible gain of muscle size and strength, without the same intensity of side effects if using the androgen (at a higher dose) alone. During a cutting phase, muscle hardness and density can be greatly improved when combining Equipoise® with a non-aromatizable steroid such as trenbolone acetate, Proviron® (mesterolone; 1-methyl DHT), Halotestin® (fluoxymesterone), or Winstrol® (stanozolol). For some however, even the low buildup of estrogen associated with this compound is enough to relegate its use to bulking cycles only.

Equipoise® is not an ideal steroid for the drug tested athlete. This drug has the tendency to produce detectable metabolites in the urine months after use, a worry most commonly associated with Deca-Durabolin®. This is due to the high oil solubility of long chain esterified injectable steroids, a property which enables the drug to remain deposited in fatty tissues for extended periods of time. While this will reliably slow the release of steroid into the blood stream, it also allows small residual amounts to remain present in the body far after the initial injection. The release of stubborn stores of hormone would no doubt also be enhanced around contest time, a period when the athlete drastically attempts to mobilize unwanted body fat. If enough were used in the off-season, the athlete may actually fail a drug screen for boldenone although many months may have past since the drug was last injected.

Getting to black market availability, counterfeit bottles of the veterinary injectable are quite common in the U.S. Again, knowing which preparation to buy can save you a lot of hassle. For starters, the most common fakes are still of the brand name **Equipoise®,** which used to be produced by Solvay in the U.S. and Canada. This steroid is now produced by the Fort Dodge Company, so avoid all products bearing the Solvay name. The Fort Dodge products are sold readily in Mexico, and afterwards smuggled back into the U.S. in high volume, so expect to see Equipoise on the black market quite frequently. Legitimate vials are made of clear glass, and carry a label with a shiny metallic surface on the under side.

Animal Power has just introduced a new Equipoise clone to the Mexican veterinary drug market. It is called **Bold 200**, and it contains 200 mg/mL of steroid in a 10ml vial. This company uses a detailed hologram sticker to deter counterfeiting (see Security Stickers).

Anabolic BD from SYD Group in Mexico is another popular product, and comes in a dosage of 200mg/mL (in a 10ml vial). This is a reputable company, with top quality products. Definitely recommended. Be sure to look for a security hologram sticker bearing the SYD Group logo, which will assure a safe purchase.

Pet's Pharma in Mexico also released a boldenone undecylenate product. It is called **Boldenona 200**, and carries 200mg/mL of steroid in a 10ml vial. This product should come with a security sticker. Though not holographic, it uses a specific type of red and blue metallic inks (see Security Stickers). At this time fakes of the Pet's Pharma line do not appear to be a big problem.

Ultragan 50 and **Ultragan 100** from Denkall are very reputable Mexican products. These come in 10 and 50ml vials, and provide a nice increase from the old 50mg products the market used to be stuck with. They have yet to upgrade to a higher dose, however, although the product remains popular. Be sure to look for the Denkall security hologram sticker on each box and vial. Note that fake QV clones have been found using a plain silver sticker instead of a real hologram. Be sure to examine it closely, and shift it in the light to see the prism (rainbow) effect.

Quality Vet's **Bold QV 200** is also popular in Mexico. This is a 200mg/mL version, and comes packaged in a 10ml vial. Like the previous companies, QV products carry security hologram stickers to deter counterfeiting. Provided you locate this when shopping, you should be making a safe purchase.

Denkall purchased the rights to the Mexican brand name product **Maxigan** from Inpel recently. This item was made in the low dose of 50mg/mL, and came in 10ml and 50ml vials. However, Denkall has since discontinued the product. It makes you wonder if they lucked onto a bankruptcy sale and got the remaining lot for a steal, or perhaps just wanted to buy and dump the brand to take over its market share. For whatever reason, this low dose Equipoise clone is gone, and will probably not be sorely missed. Since the release of 100mg/mL and 200mg/mL versions, companies with 50mg/mL products are finding that they move very slowly. You may find old vials of Maxigan in circulation, but probably not for much longer.

Equi-gan from Tornel (10ml and 50ml vials) is still found on the black market, but not as abundantly as it used to. This probably has to do with the dose, which remains at the low concentration of 50mg/mL. The 100mg/mL and 200mg/mL far outsell the 50's these days. I have not tested the Tornel boldenone product yet, but did notice about 20% underdosing in their testosterone enanthate in a recent test. This means that the already low dose may actually be a little lower still. You may want to factor an under-dosing like this in when calculating the cost.

Ttokkyo, by all indications, is no longer in business, but you may find their **Boldenon 200** still floating around Mexico. Be warned, counterfeit manufacturers have been able to get security hologram stickers bearing the Ttokkyo logo. Therefore, these alone are no longer indicative of a safe purchase, so be careful when shopping.

The Thai company British Dragon makes a boldenone undecylenate injectable called **Boldabol**. It contains 200mg/mL of steroid in a 10ml vial. This is a reputable brand, with consistently good feedback. In recent tests the dosing on this product has been slightly off. I believe this is due to recent and persistent manufacturing issues with raw material in China. This means that most of the veterinary steroid makers using Chinese raw material (probably all) are noticing dosing issues this year. The BD product is still fairly dosed, and a very good buy. Reportedly the company has decided to switch to different compounds altogether (tentatively a boldenone acetate/propionate mix), instead of passing along the inconsistencies to consumers. Note that the current packaging will not carry a hologram sticker. BD has replaced it with a red metallic foil inlay on the vial label, which reads BD and displays the company logo. Also, make sure your tops read "TEAR" and "FLIP UP". There is a large scale counterfeiting operation that uses tops that read only "FLIP OFF". BD has plans to revamp their packaging again this year, so we may see a new packaging style come to market, again using holograms.

Ganabol, produced in a number of South American countries, is still a popular brand found in the States as well though. Seen in two strengths (25mg/mL and 50mg/mL) and in five sizes (10, 50, 100, 250 and 500ml). The manufacturer recently gave the product a cosmetic overhaul. The new Ganabol is a lot more modern looking. Too bad the company was not able to modernize the dosage.

The **Legacy** brand name product from Tecnoquimicas in Argentia seems to be reaching to U.S. as of late, at least in small volume. This product carries 50mg/mL of steroid in a 50ml vial. At this time the Legacy product is very low on the radar, and probably can be trusted when located.

The brand name **Boldenona 50** from Gen-Far is also popular in South America, and occasionally smuggled into the United States. This is another low dose (50mg/mL) preparation. Like Ganabol, it comes in a variety of vial sizes. Counterfeits of this brand do not appear to be a big issue at this time, making this product a fairly trustworthy item when located on the black market.

Equitest 200 (Testosterone blend)

Androgenic	Anabolic	Standard
100	100	Standard

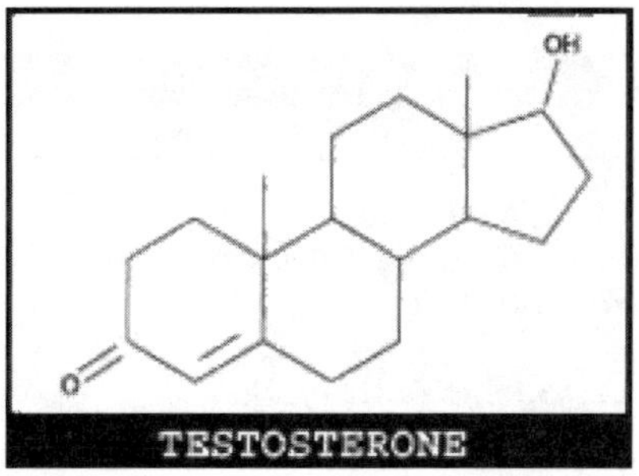

Chemical Names:
4-androsten-3-one-17beta-ol
17beta-hydroxy-androst-4-en-3-one

Estrogenic Activity: moderate
Progestational Activity: low

When it comes to blended steroid products (ones that contain more than just a single steroid), Sustanon is usually thought of as king. After all, it has a whopping four different esters of testosterone. Well, it is time for Sustanon to move over. Equitest just took the prize for the highest number of different steroid ingredients in a single product. This multi-ester injectable testosterone leaves the four-ester-blend of Sustanon in the dust, containing no less than seven different esters of testosterone. Specifically these are testosterone acetate, propionate, phenylpropionate, caproate, enanthate, cypionate and decanoate. The concentration of steroid is 200mg/mL (hence the name Equitest 200), with each vial containing 6ml of steroid in total.

Equitest is a product of WDV Pharma, a veterinary drug manufacturer out of Myanmar. This obscure company has been operating for a decade now, and offers a full line of veterinary drug products (only three are anabolic steroids). The size (small) and remoteness of this company would normally have allowed it to stay low on the "steroid radar", however the few products they do make are unusual enough to catch one's eye. Well, maybe not the 50mg/mL trenbolone acetate product. But Equitest certainly is, as well as their 4-component boldenone injectable called Equilon 100. I believe the sheer uniqueness of these products has earned WDV some attention in the bodybuilding world. Their products may not be abundant on the black market, but at one time or another you may very well come across them.

Each ml of Equitest 200 contains:

Testosterone Acetate	10 mg
Testosterone Propionate	30 mg
Testosterone Phenylpropionate	20 mg
Testosterone Caproate	20 mg
Testosterone Heptanoate (enanthate)	40 mg
Testosterone Cyclopentylpropionate (cypionate)	20 mg
Testosterone Decanoate	60 mg

So does all this make Equitest an unbeatable testosterone? Probably not. This seven-ester blend really offers no advantages over the 4-component blend in Sustanon, or any testosterone for that matter once it is used in the context of bodybuilding (repeated frequent dosing negates any real need to use a sustained-release formulation). Even if you were specifically looking for a "sustained-release testosterone" that you didn't have to inject often, it would have no greater appeal than Sustanon. The two products are essentially the same, with the same ultimate release duration of 3-4 weeks (max). The seven esters are good for marketing though, as many buyers will simply look at it like seven different steroids in one. Regardless, Equitest is still just as powerful a testosterone product as Sustanon for our purposes, and does come packaged in a nice big 6ml bottle. Provided it is located for a good price, it may most certainly blow Sustanon away – in terms of getting the most for your money, anway. For a more comprehensive discussion of Equitest 200's potential benefits, side effects and common dosing, please refer to the Sustanon profile).

Esiclene (formebolone)

Androgenic	Anabolic	Standard
N/a	N/a	-

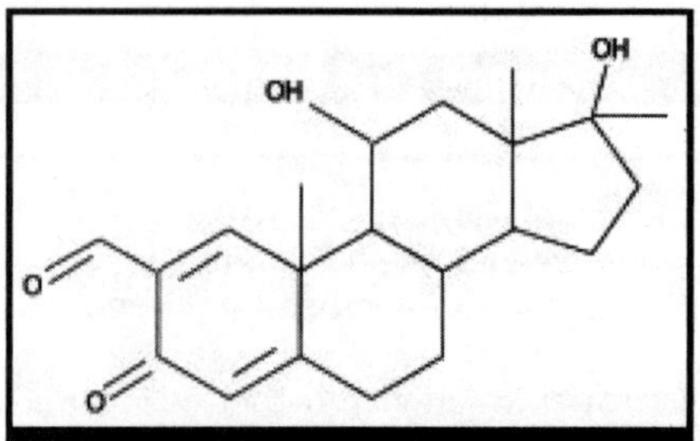

FORMEBOLONE

Chemical Names:
11alpha,17beta-Dihydroxy-17-methyl-3-oxoandrosta-1,4-dien-2-carboxaldehyde
Formyldienolone

Estrogenic Activity: None
Progestational Activity: n/a (low)

Esiclene is the brand name for the steroid formebolone, a compound that was (when available) almost exclusively utilized (non-legitimate use) in the world of professional bodybuilding. It was produced both in oral and injectable form, the injectable solution containing only 2mg per milliliter of steroid. The compound itself shows little anabolic or androgenic activity, and is not highly useful for building muscle. It is however effective in one very novel way. When given by injection, the drug formebolone irritates the muscle tissue at the site of administration. The body will respond to this with a localized inflammation, the muscle tissues storing fluid in reaction. This will cause an increase in the overall diameter of the affected muscle, obviously a desired result for bodybuilders. This irritation can be uncomfortable however, so each ampule contains 20mg of added lidocaine (a local painkiller) to make the injection less painful. While this does compensate somewhat, Esiclene is still relatively uncomfortable to use. The procedure is of course endured for the results, which can be dramatic in a very short period of time.

The swelling produced by this drug is only temporary. It will usually take only five days after the last injection was given for the swelling to subside, the muscle returning to its usual dimensions. For this reason injectable Esiclene is really only used during the last week or two before a competition, offering us little off-season benefit. When used for contest purposes, it is usually to be injected daily into each muscle site. Those trying to stretch out the dosage schedule may opt to inject every other day, but no longer an interval. When stretched too many days apart, the accumulated swelling will likely not reach a desirable point. In order to keep this procedure more comfortable, the full dosage is not to be given from the onset of the regimen. Instead, the user will begin with half of an ampule, or 1ml (2mg) per muscle. After a number of days the dosage is increased to 2ml, or a full ampule for each individual injection site. After continuing at this dosage for a week or two, one can possibly see an increase of 1 or 1.5 inches in their arm and calf measurements. This is clearly a tremendous improvement for only two weeks use. In addition, those who have used this steroid often report the drug produces an increase in overall muscle hardness. This is an added benefit when preparing for a contest as a large, hard and defined muscle is the obvious goal. Over the years a large number of male and female competitors have relied heavily on this drug for their exceptional show physiques. Esiclene has no doubt been the difference between winning and losing for many competitors.

Esiclene does not work this way for every muscle though. Bodybuilders experimenting with this compound have found that it is most effective with the smaller muscle groups such as the biceps, deltoid and calf. The resultant swelling will equate to a very favorable size increase in these small muscles, looking much larger and fuller. But when we try to inject Esiclene into larger muscles like the chest, back and legs we run into trouble. The result in this case can be a very uneven look, producing lumps in the muscle body and not an overall size increase. For this reason the large muscle groups are usually off limits.

Although an extremely mild steroid, the oral form (delivering a much higher dose of steroid) may offer some benefit to athletes. It seems to exhibit some level of anti-catabolic activity, shown in studies to interfere with the protein degenerative effects of synthetic corticosteroids. It also does not seem to aromatize, at least in it's initial state, so estrogenic side effects are not a major concern with use. If not a strong base steroid for muscle growth, it certainly has potential as a secondary steroid used in cycles for added effect. The compound however is c-17 alpha alkylated, and carries with it the same risk for liver toxicity we see with similar oral steroids. This risk of course is not isolated to the oral use of this drug, however the relatively low dose used with the injectable makes serious liver strain very unlikely.

In all forms of Esiclene have been discontinued, and are no longer available on the black market.

Genabol (norbolethone)

Androgenic	Anabolic	Standard
17	350	Testosterone Propionate

Chemical Name:
13-ethyl-17-hydroxy-18,19-dinor-17a-pregn-4-en-3-one

Estrogenic Activity: Low
Progestational Activity: Moderate

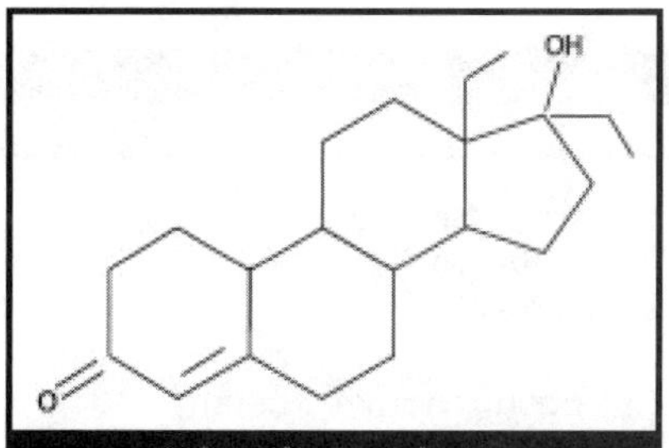

NORBOLETHONE

Norbolethone is an obscure anabolic steroid that was developed by the drug manufacturer Wyeth in the mid 1960's. It is an orally active derivative of nandrolone, displaying a high ratio of anabolic to androgenic effect. This drug was reviewed favorably during early investigations with children, however it was never released as a commercial prescription agent. It remained lost in steroid journal obscurity until just very recently, when it was revealed that athletes were using it during drug-tested competitions. Because norbolethone was never sold as a commercial steroid, the athletic bodies were not looking for it during their tests. A private chemist realized this, and manufactured it for the specific purpose of beating the drug screen. The norbolethone doping scandal was the first modern reappearance of the ages old "designer steroid" phenomenon. These are non-commercial steroids that do not show up on a drug screen by virtue of their anonymity. For as long as they remain anonymous, drugs like norbolethone are highly valued commodities among competitive athletes.

As a primarily anabolic agent, norbolethone fits in well among the nandrolone family. Although we have no study examining this, it is reasonable to think that this agent does aromatize to some degree, similar to its parent nandrolone. Estradiol (or in this case 17alpha-ethyl estradiol) levels should be increased somewhat at higher levels, but estrogenic side effects should not be as measurable as a testosterone based compound of similar structure would produce. Norbolethone should also display some moderate progestational activity, making it less than ideal for quality lean mass gains. It is likely to produce some measurable water retention in its user, which may also be accompanied by fat gain. However, it should not be excessive in either regard. Clinical tests have shown norbolethone to be effective as an anabolic in doses of approximately 7.5mg daily[77], which suggests that on the outside, maybe 10-15mgs per day would be recommended as a starting point for a male bodybuilder. Women would want to start off with much less, maybe 2.5--5mg, for fear of virilizing side effects. Even though this is more of an anabolic than an androgenic agent on paper, women should still be careful with its use. All steroids can be virilizing at the right dose, and often the dosage threshold is a lot lower than you originally think.

The commonplace side effects associated with norbolethone as likely to be similar to most anabolic/androgenic steroids. Oily skin and acne should occur to some degree, but depending on the dose should be much less pronounced than with a more androgenic steroid like Dianabol. Although the 20 to 1 anabolic to androgenic ratio cited in the studies is probably an overly optimistic paper analysis (it will undoubtedly not hold true to real-world human use), we can still expect a pretty favorable balance of effect based on its nandrolone-type structure. Its anabolic to androgenic propensities are probably going to be on par with milder anabolic agents such as oxandrolone, Winstrol or Primobolan, much more favorable than something like (again) Dbol. It is also probably easier on the hairline than even these others anabolics, falling closer to injectable Deca in this regard. As a C17-alpha alkylated oral, however, it is still going to present some level of liver toxicity. This will probably be similar mg for mg to most common commercial alkylated oral steroids. It is therefore worthy of keeping an eye on liver functioning, with regular blood tests during each cycle.

As suggested in the opening of this profile, norbolethone no longer holds any value as an undetectable designer steroid. It has been "discovered" so to speak, and is now being actively screened for during standard steroid urinalysis tests. There is little doubt that most of the athletes that were using this compound have long since abandoned it. The scandal surrounding the use of this compound broke in the media in mid 2002, when it was announced that Dr. Don Catlin of the UCLA Analytical Laboratories had discovered that athletes were using this drug to beat the drug screens being conducted at his facility. Catlin promptly devised and released a method for the detection of norbolethone metabolites in the urine. Several world-class athletes were ultimately suspended for using this drug during competition, including U.S. Olympic Cyclist Tammy Thomas. Although there is still no commercial source for this agent, I suspect it will be available again sooner or later in the ever-expanding global steroid market.

Halotestin (fluoxymesterone)

Androgenic	Anabolic	Standard
850	1,900	Methyltestosterone (oral)

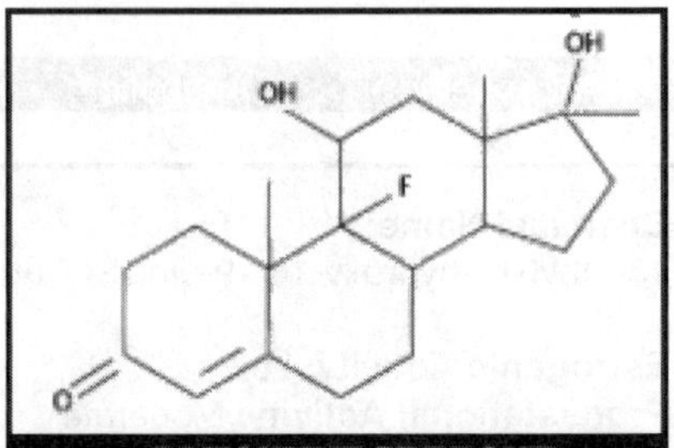
FLUOXYMESTERONE

Chemical Names:
9a-fluoro-11b,17b-dihydroxy-17a-methyl-4-androsten-3-one
9a-fluoro-11b-hydroxy-17a-methyltestosterone

Estrogenic Activity: none
Progestational Activity: n/a (low)

Halotestin® is the Pharmacia & Upjohn brand name for the steroid fluoxymesterone. Structurally fluoxymesterone is a derivative of testosterone, differing from our base androgen by three structural alterations (specifically 17alpha-methyl, 11beta-hydroxy and 9-fluoro group additions). The result is a potent orally active steroid that exhibits extremely strong androgenic properties. This has a lot to due with the fact that it is derived from testosterone, and as such shares important similarities to this hormone. Most importantly, like testosterone Halotestin® appears to be a good substrate for the 5-alpha reductase enzyme. This is evidenced by the fact that a large number of its metabolites are found to be 5-alpha reduced androgens[78], which coupled with its outward androgenic nature, suggests it is converting to a much more active steroid in androgen responsive target tissues such as the skin, scalp and prostate.

The 11beta-hydroxyl group also inhibits aromatization, making estrogen production impossible with this steroid. Estrogenic side effects such as water retention, fat fain and gynecomastia are similarly not a concern when taking this substance. Strong androgenic side effects are to be expected though, and in many cases are unavoidable. Oily skin and acne a very common for instance, at times requiring sensitive individuals to seek some form of topical or even prescription drug treatment to keep it under control. Hair loss is an additional worry, making Halotestin® a poor choice for those with an existing condition. Aggression may also become very pronounced with this drug. This effect is often desired by users looking to "harness" this in order to increase the intensity of workouts or a competition. Clearly Halotestin® is a strong androgen, and definitely one female athletes should stay away from. Masculinizing side effects can be intense, and may occur very rapidly with this substance. Even women daring enough to take Dianabol should think twice about this compound, as virilization symptoms are most often permanent.

Although Halotestin® appears to be more androgenic than testosterone, the anabolic effect of it is not very strong. This makes it a great strength drug, but not the best for gaining serious muscle mass. The predominant effect seen when taking Halotestin® is a harder, more dense look to the muscles without a notable size increase. It is therefore very useful for athletes in weight-restricted sports like wrestling, powerlifting and boxing. The strength gained from each cycle will not be accompanied by a great weight increase, allowing most competitors to stay within a specified weight range. Halotestin® also makes an excellent drug for bodybuilding contest preparation. When the competitor has an acceptably low body fat percentage, the strong androgen level (in absence of excess estrogen) can elicit an extremely hard and defined ("ripped") look to the muscles. The shift in androgen/estrogen ratio additionally seems to bring about a state in which the body may be more inclined to burn off excess fat and prevent new fat storage. The "hardening" effect of Halotestin® would therefore be somewhat similar to that seen with trenbolone, although it will be without the same level of mass gain. Clearly non-aromatizing androgens such as Halotestin® and trenbolone can play an important role during contest preparations.

The main concern with this steroid is that it can be a very toxic drug. This is due to the fact that fluoxymesterone is a 17 alpha alkylated compound, its structure altered to survive oral administration. As we discuss throughout this book, 17alpha alkylation can be very harsh to the liver. The possibility of damage is therefore a legitimate concern with Halotestin®, especially when used at higher doses or for prolonged periods of time. The total daily dosage is likewise best kept in the range of 20-40mg, used for no longer than 8 weeks. After which an equally long break (at a minimum) should be taken from all c17-AA orals. One should also resist the temptation to stack this drug with other alkylated orals if possible, and instead opt for orals without this alteration or esterified injectable compounds (which will not add to the strain on the liver).

In cutting phases a mild anabolic such as Deca-Durabolin® or Equipoise® might be a good addition, as both provide good anabolic effect without excessive estrogen buildup. Here Halotestin® will provide a well needed androgenic component, helping to promote a more solid and defined gain in muscle mass than obtained with an anabolic alone. Perhaps Primobolan® Depot would even be a better choice, as with such a combination there is no buildup of estrogen (and likewise even less worry of water and fat retention). For mass we could alternately use an injectable testosterone. A mix of 400-800mg testosterone enanthate and 20-30mg Halotestin® for example, should prove to be an exceptional stack for strength and muscle gain. This however would be accompanied by a more significant level of side effects, both compounds exhibiting strong androgenic activity in the body.

Fluoxymesterone also seem to depress endogenous testosterone levels rather quickly with use, despite its complete lack of estrogen conversion. One therefore should consider ancillary drug use at the conclusion of each cycle in order to help restore the normal release of androgens in the body. Using a combination of HCG and Clomid®/Nolvadex® is of course the best option, the two drugs working well together to restore normal hormonal functioning. Although estrogen is not a problem with Halotestin®, the use of an antiestrogen such as Nolvadex® or Clomid® is still indicated when discontinuing a cycle. Since HCG stimulates aromatase activity in the Leydig's cells, here Nolvadex®/Clomid® help by blocking the activity of any excess estrogen that may be produced. Afterward they will also block the inhibitory effect of endogenous estrogens on the hypothalamus, stimulating the enhanced release of gonadotropins and supporting the normal biosynthesis of testosterone.

Since Halotestin® is only used for a few specific purposes, it is not in high demand among athletes. Likewise it is not a very popular item on the black market. Investing in the manufacture of a counterfeit version would probably not pay off well, no doubt the reason we haven't seen much yet. All of the various forms of Halotestin® could therefore be assumed legitimate when found in circulation. Currently the most popular item found on the black market is the Stenox brand from Mexico, sold in boxes of 20 tablets. Although the dosage of these tablets is only 2.5mg, the low price usually asked for this preparation more than compensates. Overall, Halotestin® is an effective steroid for a narrow range of uses, and is probably not the most ideal product for the recreational user.

Hydroxytestosterone (4-hydroxytestosterone)

Androgenic	Anabolic	Standard
25	65	Testosterone

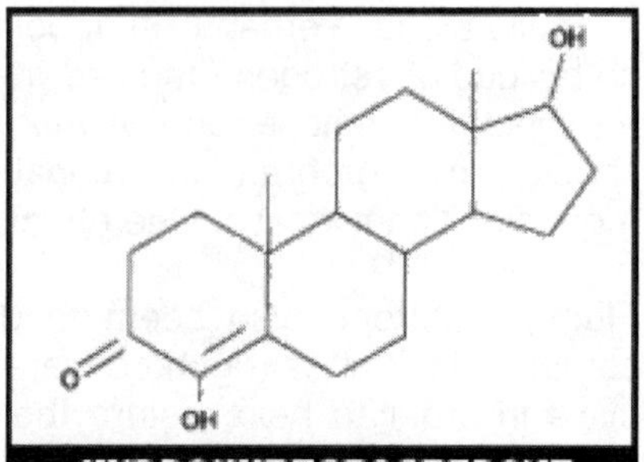

HYDROXYTESTOSTERONE

Chemical Names:
4-hydroxy-androsten-3-one-17beta-ol
4,17-dihydroxyandrost-4-en-3-one

Estrogenic Activity: none
Progestational Activity: n/a (low)

Hydroxytestosterone is an anabolic steroid that is, as its name would indicate, a close structural relative of the primary androgen testosterone. Specifically, it is testosterone with an added 4-hydroxl group, an alteration that makes this an extremely interesting steroid. In action it is only moderately anabolic and androgenic, ultimately bearing little resemblance to the androgen (testosterone) that it is so closely related to on a molecular level. Hydroxytestosterone was originally developed by the pharmaceutical manufacturing giant Searle back in the 1950's, however, it never did make it to the shelf as a commercial prescription steroid product. To spite having several unique and favorable characteristics, it lay lost in the research books for decades, the manufacturer and patent holder probably finding little financial incentive to market it next to the many other anabolic agents available. This steroid was sold legally as a sports supplement in the U.S. until January 2005, when it became a Schedule III controlled substance.

In regards to structure, the first thing we can point out about hydroxytestosterone is that the 4-hydroxyl group prevents aromatization. As such, this steroid is totally incapable of converting to estrogen. Not only that, this alteration also gives hydroxytestosterone strong aromatase inhibiting activities. You see, hydroxytestosterone differs from the suicide aromatase inhibitor formestane (4-hydroxyandrostenedione) only in that it is the active form of the steroid (17-beta hydroxysteroid) instead of the inactive dione (17-ketosteroid). Both types of steroid hormone will interact with the aromatase enzyme. In a clinical setting, formestane would be the obvious choice, as you would usually want to lower estrogen without presenting the often-female patients with unwanted androgenic side effects. So I can understand why hydroxytestosterone was never explored for this use. But this active steroid is still very much a potent aromatase inhibitor. This all means that with hydroxytestosterone, there is not only no need to worry about estrogenic side effects such as gynecomastia, water retention, or fat buildup, but that the agent can even be used to counter such side effects caused by the aromatization of other steroid compounds. It is therefore a dual-purpose anabolic/aromatase-inhibiting agent.

As with all naturally occurring (non-methylated) steroid hormones, hydroxytestosterone is not intrinsically very orally active. This has been the problem with the "legal steroid/prohormone" market from the beginning. These natural steroidal hormones work, some of them extremely well, *if you can get them into your body first.* As you may know, I found and publicized the research showing the natural occurrence of 4-hydroxysteroids like hydroxytestosterone, and eventually sold it through my supplement company (Molecular Nutrition) as an oil-solubilized softgel (as hydroxytestosterone hexyldecanoate). This is about the only type of oral product I would have recommended. Otherwise, it could have been used in a transdermal formula, or homebrewed injection. The latter would be the preferred in terms of bioavailability, not really for safety. In any event, the product is now illegal to sell in the U.S., so any version produced now would have to be of black market or international pharmaceutical origin.

Effective daily doses for most male bodybuilders would be in that range of 200-400mg per week by injection, or 100-300mg if taking an oil-solubilized oral product. Maximum aromatase inhibition is reached by 250mg per week when given by injection, or 100-200mg per day when taking oral softgels. One could obviously keep the doses limited to this range if estrogen minimization is the main focus of use. Hydroxytestosterone and formestane may not be quite as potent as the selective third generation non-steroidal aromatase inhibitors Arimidex or Femara in terms of estrogen minimization, but they do seem to do a much better job here than the "standard issue" estrogen receptor antagonists Nolvadex and Clomid (especially when it comes to shedding water and producing the tight "high androgen" look). As with all effective aromatase inhibitors, its estrogen lowering action is likely to be accompanied by a negative lowering of HDL (good) cholesterol levels. For this reason hydroxytestosterone should never be used for long periods of time, and regular doctor's checkups are recommended during use.

Laurabolin (nandrolone laurate)

Androgenic	Anabolic	Standard
37	125	Testosterone

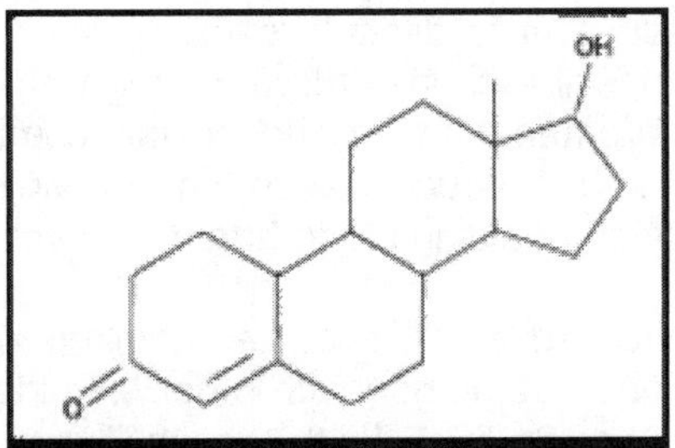

NANDROLONE

Chemical Names:
19-norandrost-4-en-3-one-17beta-ol
17beta-hydroxy-estr-4-en-3-one

Estrogenic Activity: low
Progestational Activity: moderate

Laurabolin is a popular trade name for the oil based injectable steroid nandrolone laurate. This steroid is a pronounced anabolic, with only moderately androgenic properties. As this is a nandrolone product, the effect is comparable to that of Deca-Durabolin® (nandrolone decanoate). Aside from releasing the same steroid hormone, the two products also stay active in the body for a very similar period of time. Both compounds are extremely long acting, the decanoate ester sustaining a notable release of nandrolone for about three to four weeks while Laurabolin should remain active the full four (the laurate ester is only two carbon atoms longer). The main difference between these two compounds is really the field in which they are applied. Deca-Durabolin® is generally a human use item while Laurabolin is exclusively used in veterinary medicine. This of course is of little concern to athletes, finding Laurabolin a welcome, and often reasonably priced substitute for Deca. Since veterinary items are usually held in a slightly lower regard however, Deca is usually the preference if both steroids are available.

Nandrolone is similar in structure to testosterone, although it lacks a carbon atom at the 19th position (which explains its other given name 19-nortestosterone). This feature causes it to exhibit much weaker androgenic properties than testosterone. This is primarily due to the fact that unlike testosterone, nandrolone does not break down into the harsh metabolite dihydrotestosterone. Although it is altered by the same enzyme (5a-reductase), the product here is a much milder hormone, dihydronandrolone (less active than the parent nandrolone). Side effects like oily skin, acne, body/facial hair growth and hair loss therefore occur much less frequently than if using an androgen such an injectable testosterone. Androgenic effects can still become apparent with nandrolone (as with all anabolic/androgenic steroids) however, but usually only when high dosages are used. Laurabolin (and Deca) is also not the ideal steroid for female athletes. The much faster acting Durabolin® (nandrolone phenylpropionate) should be preferred, as with it blood hormone levels are easier for the user to control (you don't have to wait 3 or 4 weeks to get it out of your system if there is a problem).

Laurabolin also display a relatively low tendency for estrogen conversion. The rate in which nandrolone converts has been estimated to be roughly 20% of that seen with testosterone, quite a considerable difference. This is because in many active sites of aromatase activity such as adipose tissue, nandrolone interacts poorly with this enzyme. The liver remains as the primary site of aromatization for nandrolone, as tissues here are shown to aromatize both it and testosterone with similar efficacy. Consequently estrogen related side effects are generally not a major concern with this steroid. The possibility for gynecomastia cannot be excluded however, but is usually only seen among very sensitive individuals or those taking very large doses. Water retention may appear with this steroid to some extent, but again, is usually only a mild occurrence when the drug is taken at normal therapeutic levels. In the unlikely event that estrogen related side effects become too pronounced during a cycle, the addition of Proviron® and/or Nolvadex® should prove to be more than a sufficient remedy.

In general, all of the side effects associated with androgen use will be greatly reduced with a nandrolone. Likewise Laurabolin, and other nandrolones, are extremely well tolerated by their users. This clearly makes these compounds an exceptional choice for the athlete who wants to gain muscle mass, yet is conscious about possible health effects. Although new muscle growth is likely going to be less pronounced than what is seen with an equal dose of testosterone, it will no doubt be of a higher quality (greater definition). One can also expect to retain a larger percentage of gained weight after the cycle is concluded, not having the same water loss of a testosterone to deal with. Nandrolone injectables can still interfere with endogenous testosterone production however, to spite the fact that estrogen conversion is not pronounced. The use of a testosterone stimulating compound like Clomid®/Nolvadex® and/or HCG may therefore still be necessary when discontinuing a cycle however, especially after taking the drug for longer periods.

Although active for much longer, most users opt to inject this drug at least weekly. For men, the ordinary dosage each week is in the range of 200-400mg. Although the anabolic effect would likely be amplified at a slightly higher dose, it is difficult to inject this much if you are using a product in the strength of 50mg/mL. Some do find it possible to inject 500-600mg with the Intervet product, but I cannot imagine this practice being very comfortable. Women who do choose this compound will generally keep to the dosage range of 50 to 100mg per week. To further reduce the chance for virilization symptoms, the interval between injections can be expanded to prevent high peaks in blood hormone level.

Just as with Deca, Laurabolin is quite versatile. Although it is a strong enough anabolic to use alone, it is most often combined with other steroids. For bulking, it fits comfortably with androgens like Dianabol, testosterone, or Anadrol 50®. In this case it can allow the user exceptional mass gains, while at the same time keeping the androgen dosage to an effective but comfortable level. For cutting we can add an oral anabolic like Winstrol® or Primobolan®. Here we are looking to minimize the water and fat retention usually associated with excess estrogen. We can further add a non-aromatizing androgen like Halotestin®, Proviron® or trenbolone. This should further enhance the level of hardening and fat loss attained during the cycle, making for a harder and more defined physique.

U.S. bodybuilders were recently taken aback with the release of a 250mg version of nandrolone laurate (**Laurdrol 250**) from the Mexican veterinary drug firm Loeffler. This is five times the strength of all preceding products, and similarly is the only nandrolone laurate product athletes are really looking for right now. I have not run lab tests to confirm Loeffler is accurately dosing the product; however, this has been an issue in the past with this company. Still, even if underdosed you should still be assured to get a much higher concentration of steroid than Intervet will ever provide you. Loeffler has released several products lately in this high strength in fact, which is clearly representative of the new trend in this country to produce newer and ever more potent anabolic compounds.

The Intervet brand name **Laurabolin** product from Mexico is still circulating, and can usually be trusted. Note that Intervet has started shipping vials of Laurabolin to Mexico that come without sealed caps (the rubber stopper is exposed). This presents a problem to the buyer, as you may not be able to tell if someone had adulterated the contents of the vial before it reached your hands. It would be quite easy to use a high gauge needle to remove some or all of the contents, leaving a mark in the rubber that is so small it will be difficult to spot with the naked eye. Therefore, it may be best to purchase Laurabolin only from a vet pharmacy in Mexico directly, and not on the open black market.

In the past, **Fortabol** was found on very rare occasion in the U.S. This product includes 20mg nandrolone laurate with an added amount of Vitamin A. Since the dosage is so low, this brand is really only beneficial to women. This brand has been very quiet as of late, and may have discontinued the product.

Although even less common than other brands, Intervet sells Laurabolin in a couple of European countries. These are, of course, of similar reliability to Mexican Laurabolin.

Libriol (nandrolone/methandriol blend)

Libriol is a blended injectable veterinary steroid preparation that is made by RWR (Nature Vet) in Australia. This is primarily an anabolic agent, containing a mixture nandrolone phenylpropionate and methandriol dipropionate. These two steroids are present in a concentration of 30mg/mL and 45mg/mL respectively, equating to a total steroid concentration of 75mg/mL. Both agents in this product are considered pretty mild in terms of side effects and overall effectiveness, and are looked at more so for their abilities to promote lean tissue gain than bulk mass (for a more comprehensive discussion on the individual components, please refer to their respective drug profiles). This makes Libriol a great lean tissue builder, but far removed from drugs like testosterone, Dianabol or Anadrol in its ability to pack on sheer weight, size and strength.

Since both of the steroids present in Libriol are modified with fast acting esters, blood hormone concentrations will not stay steady for very long after each injection. It would therefore be most effective to inject this drug at least twice per week, three times if you want to be meticulous about dosing. The total concentration of steroid is not remarkably high in this product either, so you better get used to quite a bit of injecting if you plan on using this as the sole drug in your next cycle. A weekly total dose of 6cc would probably be most appropriate (adding up to 450mg), perhaps even 8cc (600mg). This would mean two to three injections would be given each and every week, with a full 3cc's of oil volume needed almost each time (not too comfortable). For this reason most use a bottle or two of Libriol to add some potency to an already existing stack, rather than relying on this drug alone.

Libriol is currently sold only in 10ml multi-dose vials, which means that you are getting only 750mg of steroid in total in each. This is not a lot of steroid, and likely the vial will not be dirt-cheap to purchase either. As a result, it is probably not one of the most cost effective steroids available. Plus, its packaging is pretty simple, and well suited for counterfeiting. This means that any abundance of Libriol, especially in the U.S. where Aussie steroids do not circulate very often, should be looked at with extreme suspicion. Aside from the above concerns, there is little else to criticize about this product. It is a very simple blend of two effective and mild anabolic agents, which do exactly what you would expect them to do (provide fair gains with minimal side effects). If you have a real bottle, and you paid a fair price for it, I suspect you will find it is a very good addition to your next cycle.

Masteron (drostanolone propionate)

Androgenic	Anabolic	Standard
25	62	Testosterone

Chemical Names:
2alpha-methyl-androstan-3-one-17beta-ol
2alpha-methyl-dihydrotestosterone

Estrogenic Activity: none
Progestational Activity: n/a (low)

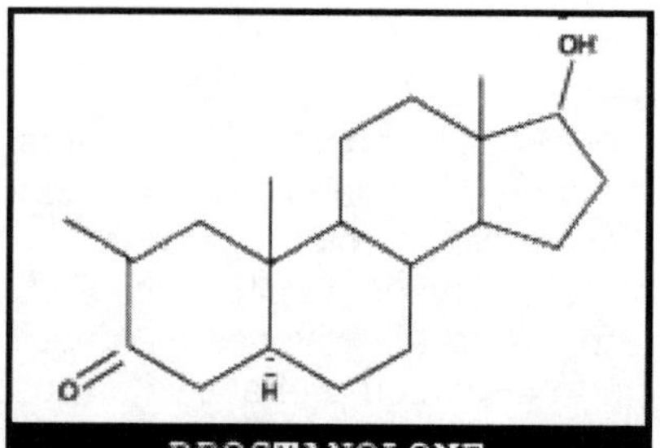

DROSTANOLONE

Masteron is an injectable preparation containing the steroid drostanolone propionate. Drostanolone is a derivative of dihydrotestosterone, most specifically 2alpha-methyldihydrotestosterone. As a result, the structure of this steroid is that of a moderate anabolic/potent androgen which does not aromatize to estrogen. Water retention and gynecomastia are therefore not a concern with this compound; as of course here estrogen is usually the culprit. Masteron may in fact exhibit antiestrogenic activity in the body, competing with other substrates for binding to aromatase. This would reduce the conversion rate of other steroids, Masteron acting in the same manner as the oral steroid Proviron®.

Bodybuilders have a strong appreciation for non-aromatizing androgens, and find Masteron very useful as a cutting agent. It is likewise generally used a number of weeks prior to a competition, in an effort to bring out an improved look of density and hardness to the muscles. For this purpose Masteron should work exceptionally well so long as the body fat percentage is low enough. Provided everything fits as if should, the user can achieve that "ripped" look so popular to professional bodybuilding. The androgenic effect can also be crucial during this period, a time when caloric intake is drastically lowered. The user is provided added "kick" or "drive" to push through the grueling training sessions leading up to the show. Drostanolone was once also popular with athletes subject to drug testing, as for a period of time this compound was not screened for during competition. The urinary metabolites of drostanolone were recognized by the early 90's however, and this drug now adjoins a long list of anabolic/androgenic steroids identifiable during urinalysis testing. Although some bodybuilders claim they can safely use Masteron if discontinued three to four weeks before a test, there are always uncertainties with the use of esterified injectable steroids. This perhaps makes the oral DHT Proviron® (1-methyldihydrotestosterone) a slightly better choice, as orals offer much better control.

Recreational users might also be interested in Masteron. Although dihydrotestosterone is not highly active in muscle tissue, the 2 alkylation present on drostanolone considerably intensifies its anabolic effect. It can therefore be used somewhat effectively as bulking agent, providing a consistent gain of high quality muscle mass. It can also be successfully combined with other steroids for an enhanced effect. Mixing drostanolone with an injectable anabolic such as Deca-Durabolin® (nandrolone decanoate) or Equipoise® (boldenone undecylenate) can prove quite useful for example, the two providing notably enhanced muscle gain without excessive water retention. For greater mass gains, one can alternately addition a stronger androgen such as Dianabol or an injectable testosterone. The result here can be an extreme muscle gain, with a lower level of water retention & other estrogenic side effects than if these steroids were used alone (usually in higher doses). Masteron could of course be used during cutting phases of training as well. A cycle of this drug combined with Winstrol®, Primobolan® or Oxandrolone should provide great muscle retention and fat loss, during a period which can be very catabolic without steroids. It is an added benefit that none of these steroids aromatize, and therefore there is no additional worry of unwanted water/fat retention.

The propionate ester used with this compound will extend its activity for only a few days. With such a short duration of effect, injections need to be repeated at least every 3 or 4 days in order to maintain a consistent level of hormone in the blood. Factoring this in with its low strength (50mg/mL), men will generally inject a full 2ml ampule of Masteron (100 mg) every two or three days. The weekly dosage therefore lands in the range of 200-350mg, a level more than sufficient to receive good results. We also should mention that while some women do profess to using this item before a show, it is much too androgenic in nature to recommend. Virilization symptoms can result quickly with its use, making Masteron a very risky item to experiment with. If attempted, the dosage should be limited to no more than 25 to 50mg each week. The female athlete would be further served by increasing the number of days between injections to prevent buildup of steroid in the body. In this case, Masteron can perhaps be administered once every 7 days.

Since estrogen offers us no trouble, side effects are generally mild with this steroid. As discussed earlier, gynecomastia and water retention go unseen. So are problems controlling blood pressure, again usually associated with estrogen. Masteron is also not liver toxic, so there is little concern stress will be placed on this organ, even during longer cycles. The only prominent side effects stem from the basic androgenic properties of dihydrotestosterone. This includes oily skin, acne, body/facial hair growth, aggression, and accelerated hair loss. Since this compound is already a synthetic DHT, Proscar® would have no impact on the level of androgenic effects. Men with a receding hairline (or those with a known familial predisposition for baldness) may therefore wish to stay away from Masteron completely, as the potent androgenic effect of this steroid can easily exacerbate such a condition.

The original Syntex Masteron is now unavailable on the black market. It was discontinued in Europe several years ago. No old lots should still be circulating, meaning that there is no legitimate source for brand name product "Masteron" anywhere. Those consumers who highly regarded the former European product will be happy to learn that there are other versions to be found. British Dragon has introduced **Mastabol** this past year. This Masterone close first came in a 50mg/mL dosage, but this was later replaced by a stronger 100mg/mL concentration. You will notice in the Lab Testing section that I had tested Masteron before the printing of this book, and it came out very favorably. This is the first drostanolone propionate product I was able to conclusively verify, although there are a few other underground labs reportedly selling their own version. With the BD product, make sure it has a vial top that reads "TEAR" and "FLIP UP". There are fakes in circulation that use tops that read, "FLIP OFF" only. Also, BD is not currently putting a hologram sticker on its vials. Instead, the red area on all injectable labels (where the logo is) will be made of a shiny metallic foil inlay.

Also found on the black market currently is a version of drostanolone sold in Myanmar by the Xelox Company called **Dromostan**. It contains base drostanolone only, not drostanolone propionate. Although unconfirmed by lab testing, this is a legit company, hopefully making a legit product. If so, it would be only the second real drostanolone currently sold worldwide. Due to the lack of an ester, injections would best be given every two days with this product, just short of the 3-4 typically used with Masteron.

Megagrisevit-Mono (clostebol acetate)

Androgenic	Anabolic	Standard
25	46	Testosterone

Chemical Names:
4-chloro-testosterone
4-chloro-androsten-3-one-17beta-ol

Estrogenic Activity: none
Progestational Activity: n/a (low)

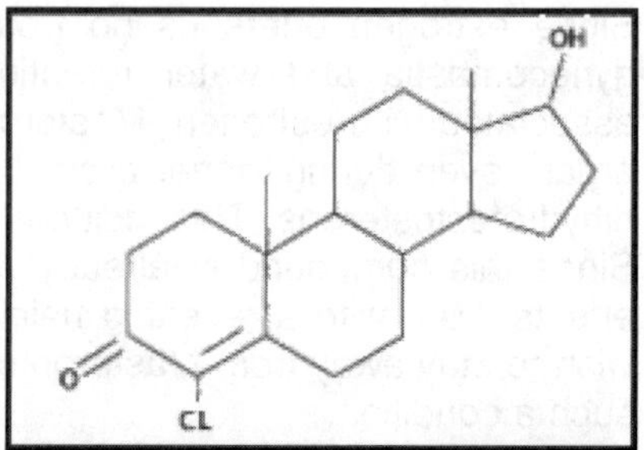

CLOSTEBOL

Megagrisevit-Mono is the old German trade name for the steroid clostebol acetate, a derivative of testosterone (most specifically 4 chloro-testosterone acetate). Clostebol is a low strength anabolic compound, which exhibits minimal androgenic potency. While side effects are possible with any anabolic/androgenic steroid, this compound overall is extremely mild. Due to 4-chloro substitution in the A ring this form of testosterone additionally does not aromatize, so there is little worry of developing noticeable water retention or gynecomastia during use. The substance is also not c-17 alpha alkylated, so those experimenting with the oral need not fear liver toxicity. The hydrogen substitution at the 4 position does not greatly enhance the oral efficacy of this drug however, and therefore the injectable is much more potent on a milligram for milligram basis.

As mentioned, the androgenic activity of this steroid is also very low. Related side effects such as oily skin, acne, body/facial hair growth and male pattern hair loss are therefore not commonly associated with use unless higher doses than normal of the drug are taken. Likewise Women have little risk of developing virilization symptoms provided they remain reasonable with the dosage. The fact when it was being made Megagrisevit-Mono was commonly used with geriatric patients makes clear the real mildness of this anabolic. The side effects of anabolic/androgenic steroid use seem to become much more pronounced in patients as they age, so typically very weak androgens are shown to be the most tolerable in such cases. Although a derivative of the potent androgen testosterone, clostebol is certainly far removed from its parent steroid in action.

The anabolic effect of this drug is also very weak, so clostebol is really only utilized in combination with other steroids. The general application is to use it for contest preparations with other non-aromatizing anabolics such as Winstrol® or oxandrolone. Here a daily dose of 20mg (2 vials) of the old Megagrisevit-Mono would be added in with an average dose (20-30mg) of the oral anabolic, which together should provide the user a nice muscle building effect without any water retention. Here the effect of clostebol would be somewhat similar to that seen with the old Primobolan® acetate ampules, although Megagrisevit-Mono is admittedly weaker in effect (injectable Primobolan® acetate being a sorely missed product). We could also use this compound in addition with strong non-aromatizing androgens such as trenbolone, Halotestin® or Proviron®. Here the result can be an even more pronounced effect of muscle definition, although this will be accompanied by a much stronger set of side effects. As discussed women will also find this drug favorable, of course here a lower dosage would apply. This would perhaps mean using no more than one 10mg per day (1.5ml of the old German remedy), perhaps even every other day to help avoid any buildup of steroid in the blood.

Overall we can say that while this compound can provide benefit to many cycles, it's effect is clearly too weak to warrant using it alone. This is really a moot point though, as Megagrisevit-Mono, the last remaining injectable to contain clostebol acetate, is no longer available. The only products left anywhere containing clostebol appear to be a couple of topical products still left on the Italian market, namely Alfa-Trofodermin and Trofodermin. Transdermal delivery is less than efficient with steroids, making this already weak drug even harder to get into the body. We can understand why these products don't seem to circulate on the black market.

Mestanolone

Androgenic	Anabolic	Standard
78-254	107	Testosterone

Chemical Name:
17a-methyl-4,5a-dihydrotestosterone

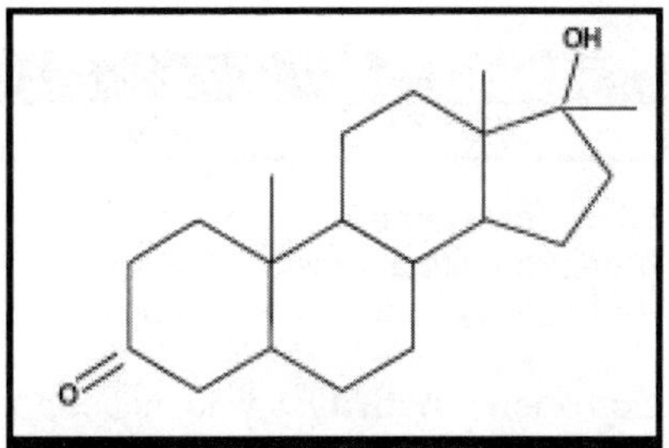

MESTANOLONE

Estrogenic Activity: None
Progestational Activity: None

Long since removed from the commercial drug market, mestanolone is a synthetic oral derivative of dihydrotestosterone. This steroid is a 17-alpha methylated form of this potent endogenous androgen, being essentially (in structure) to DHT what methyltestosterone is to testosterone. Overall this new oral androgen has an activity profile not very dissimilar to the natural steroid used to make it. For starters, since no further structural modification was added to protect the 3-ketone group, this steroid will be rapidly broken down in skeletal muscle tissue by the 3-alpha hydroxysteroid dehydrogenase enzyme. This means that just like DHT, mestanolone will offer minimal direct anabolic activity. Its effect is almost purely androgenic instead. Both DHT and mestanolone are also devoid of estrogenic activity, which eliminates the chance for estrogenic side effects like water retention, fat deposition and gynecomastia. In fact, both should be measurably anti-estrogenic in effect, inhibiting the aromatase enzyme in a competitive and dose-dependant manner.

Mestanolone is one of the oldest secret drugs of the East German doping machine, the infamous State sponsored doping program of the 1960's and 70's that developed advanced systematic techniques designed to assist drug-tested athletes avoid detection. This program allowed East German athletes to evade countless urine tests and become a dominant force in Olympic sports throughout much of the Cold War era. Mestanolone, itself, was valued not for its potency as a muscle builder, but for its ability as a pure and powerful androgen. Its effect was thought to be largely focused on the central nervous system and neuromuscular interaction. Athletes would routinely comment that while the drug would not make you huge, it was very capable of improving speed, strength, aggression, endurance, and resistance to stress. Drug tested or not, mestanolone remains intrinsically valuable today as a fast acting oral capable of providing tangible benefits unique from other anabolic agents. While it might not make an ideal agent to base an entire steroid cycle on, it seems that it would make an exceptional compound to stack with other anabolics.

An effective oral daily dosage for most males would be in the range of 10-15mg. At this level mestanolone should impart considerable strength gains, and may also aid in the speed performance of competitive athletes. Provided diet is adequate, this androgen should also promote fat loss, and will increase muscular definition by reducing the level of water retention. This steroid is, likewise, a very effective option for pre-contest use. In such a role, it would make a good, albeit not perfect, substitute for Masteron. Being such a potent androgen, mestanolone should never be recommended to women. The chance for virilizing side effects is too great to risk using it, even in low dosages. General side effects for males would be in line with what you would expect from injectable dihydrotestosterone, including oily skin, acne, potential hair loss, and increased aggression. Since mestanolone is a methylated steroid, it may impart some level of liver toxicity. This would be amplified if combined with other oral steroids, or if unnecessarily high doses or drug duration were used. As with all liver-toxic orals, it is best to limit intake to no longer than 6-8 weeks, after which point an equally long break at a minimum should be taken.

Being that mestanolone is no longer in commercial production, finding a trustworthy human prescription version of this drug is not going to be a possibility. Five years ago that would have meant that you were likely to never see this steroid again; however, that does not appear to be the case today. The thriving steroid business this past decade has given a lot of financial incentive for the overseas bulk materials manufacturers to start producing old steroids that were popular thirty years ago. In what has become a very competitive market, a variety of underground and Third World manufacturers are buying these obscure compounds up, so they can release “new” (previously unavailable) steroids, gaining market share and attention in the process. Several underground laboratories have already released Mestanolone, and it should not take long for some of the popular veterinary manufacturers to follow suit. So far as this agent is able to regain its cult status it had in the 60's and 70's, it may very well become a pre-contest androgen of interest in the months and years to come.

Methandriol (methylandrostenediol)

Androgenic	Anabolic	Standard
30-60	20-60	Testosterone propionate

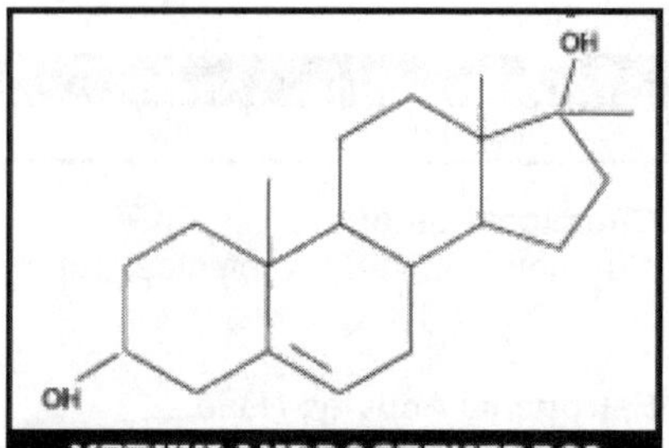

METHYLANDROSTENEDIOL

Chemical Names:
4-chloro-testosterone
4-chloro-androsten-3-one-17beta-ol

Estrogenic Activity: low to moderate
Progestational Activity: n/a (low)

The steroid Methandriol is manufactured in two very distinct forms. Unesterified (straight) methylandrostenediol is most commonly used when making an oral medication with this steroid (although an injectable once existed in the U.S.), and esterified methylandrostenediol dipropionate is usually prepared as an injectable. The added propionate esters in the injectable form extend the activity of the drug for several days. Basically methandriols are altered forms of the "pro-hormone" 5-androstenediol. This is clear when we look at the chemical structures, as they simply have a methyl group or methyl plus two propionate esters added to the compound (hence the name methyl-androstenediol). Yes, the injectable methandriol does carry both 17alpha methylation and two propionate esters (one at carbon 17, the other at carbon 3). Methandriol was first produced in the United States during the early 1980's. Powerlifting and bodybuilding circles caught on to it quickly, and Methandriol enjoyed a period of great popularity. This did not last very long however, and Methandriol preparations have been unavailable in the states for many years now. Today this steroid is not common on the black market, and is almost exclusively used in Australian veterinary preparations.

Methandriol is thought of as a strong anabolic with notable androgenic properties. It does sometimes display a level of estrogenic activity, so related side effects such as water and fat retention may be of concern (but this is usually dose related). Most of this is due to the fact that 5-androstenediol displays a low affinity to bind and activate the estrogen receptor. There is actually no direct estrogen conversion with this steroid, although since one of its known active metabolites is methyltestosterone we must assume that some aromatization does take place. The properties of this drug are therefore most appropriately suited for the buildup of strength and muscle mass, where any slight estrogenic effect will be less of a concern. For this purpose a typical dosage would be in the range of 25-50mg daily for the oral form, and 200-400mg per week with the injectable. In order to keep blood levels more even with the injectable, it is best administered at least every three to four days.

This compound is clearly strong enough to be used alone for muscle building purposes, although methandriol is most often combined with other anabolics for a stronger effect. A cycle of methandriol and Deca-Durabolin® or Equipoise® (anabolic) for example can produce an exceptional gain of hard, muscle mass, without an extreme level of water retention. This is the general composition of most Australian vet blends that include methandriol. Since the aforementioned drugs do aromatize to some degree however, sensitive individuals may wish to add an antiestrogen such as Nolvadex® and/or Proviron® to keep related side effects to a minimum. When looking for a more pronounced gain in mass, a stronger androgen such as Dianabol, Anadrol 50® or testosterone could of course be added. The resulting growth can be quite exceptional, but the user will also have to deal with a much stronger set of estrogenic side effects. Likewise the new muscle mass will be accompanied by considerable smoothness due to water retention. Again, the already mentioned antiestrogens could prove very useful. The strong antiaromatase Arimidex® may be more applicable in this circumstance, effectively halting estrogen production. This compound is quite expensive however (see: Arimidex®).

For contest preparations this steroid can sometimes prove quite useful. With a sufficiently low body fat percentage, the androgenic nature of methandriol can help bring out a look of hardness and density to the muscles. It also combines well with other non-aromatizing anabolics such as Winstrol®, Primobolan® and oxandrolone. The result here should be an even more pronounced effect on muscle hardness, while at the same time subcutaneous water is kept to a minimum. One may further addition a strong non-aromatizing androgen like Halotestin® or trenbolone, but then increases the risk for notable androgenic side effects.

Side effects associated with Methandriol use are generally considered mild. Although estrogenic side effects are sometimes reported with this drug, they do not seem to be a very common problem. One therefore will probably no be faced with heavy water bloat, gynecomastia, increased blood pressure or body fat gain during a cycle unless a very high dosage is used. The most common trouble is likely to come in the form of general androgenic side effects. Oily skin, Acne, body/facial hair growth and hair loss are likewise all possible with methandriol. Since such effects are probably not stemming from the conversion of 5-androstenediol to methyltestosterone and ultimately methyl-DHT (it appears to have a low tendency for this) Proscar® would offer us no benefit. Men with a predisposition for male pattern baldness may likewise want to be very cautious when administering this compound. Women should also probably avoid this steroid, as virilization symptoms can occur quickly with the more strongly androgenic drugs.

Since methandriol is a 17-alpha alkylated compound, we do have some additional worries in regard to liver stress. In order to reduce the damaging effect of this substance, cycles are best kept to a minimum. It may also be a good idea to monitor liver values during treatment, particularly if other oral steroids are being used at the same time. The same level of liver stress is not present with the injectable form of course, the body not having to process the 17-methylation all at once. While we cannot exclude the possibility of liver damage with the injectable however, it is still the preferred form of administration if both were available

As discussed earlier, this steroid is not a common inside the U.S. The only place it can be found in abundance is unfortunately Australia. There, a number of veterinary preparations still include methandriol in their blends. These occasionally do reach the U.S., often selling for a high price. The Mexican firm Denkall was selling **Denkadiol** for some time, however I am unable to confirm they are still manufacturing it. The firm was importing it into Mexico from Australia, where they originally purchased it iun Bulk from Ilium. Ilium and Jurox cut off all direct exports to Mexico a couple of years ago, and we have since not seen much from Denkadiol. Old lots may still be on the market, so there is a chance you will see this drug. Remember to look for the Denkall security hologram if you do, which should assure you are getting the real thing (although I have never heard, nor would expect, to see much interest in a fake Methandriol).

Methyl-1-testosterone

Androgenic	Anabolic	Standard
100-220	910-1600	Methyltestosterone (oral)

Chemical Name:
17alpha methyl-17beta-hydroxy-androst-1-ene-3-one

Estrogenic Activity: none
Progestational Activity: moderate

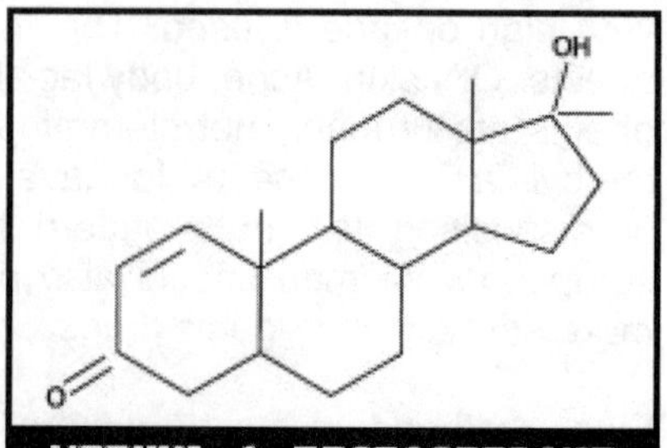

METHYL-1-TESTOSTERONE

Methyl-1-testosterone (or 17alpha-methyldihydroboldenone) is an orally active derivative of the potent anabolic/androgenic steroid 1-testosterone. M1T for short, this compound was first investigated back in the 1950's, during they most active days of steroid research. However, it was not developed as a commercial steroid product and lay dormant on the books for decades until only very recently. This agent can be looked at some kind of bastard amalgamation of Primobolan, Winstrol, and trenbolone. It has the basic 1-ene structure of Primobolan, the bioavailability of a methylated oral steroid like Winstrol, and the high potency of a strong receptor binding of an agent like trenbolone. Truth be told, the potency of methyl-1-testosterone exceeds that of every prescription anabolic steroid currently sold.

As a Primobolan derivative, methyl-1-testosterone does not aromatize. It lacks the 4-ene group necessary for aromatization. Normally this would suggest a very lean tissue building anabolic, with no significant water retention. However, that does not appear to be the case with M1T. A good number of users report noticeable water retention when taking this steroid, even in moderate doses. This would suggest a moderate progestational activity inherent in this steroid, and activity that can sometimes mimic the effects of estrogen. Progestational steroids can actually intensify the biological actions of estrogen, so care should be taken when stacking this agent with other aromatizable steroids. Side effects like bloating and gynecomastia might easily result. Even when used alone, many will opt to stack an anti-estrogen like Nolvadex with this steroid, just to make it a little cleaner of an anabolic.

Other things to expect include the typical androgenic side effects like oily skin, acne, and aggravated hair loss. M1T does not appear to be particularly androgenic in the grand scheme of things, however, these side effects are all possible with every anabolic steroid. Since this compound lacks a 4-ene group, there is no chance it will metabolize into a stronger "dihydro" derivative in androgen responsive tissues. Therefore, it is a balanced steroid, and more of an "anabolic" than an "androgen". As a c-17 alpha alkylated (methylated) oral, liver toxicity should be taken seriously with this steroid too. Being so potent, this is going to be more intense than most of the other commercially available orals. It would probably not be wise to assume that 20mg of M1T would offer the same stress to your liver as 20mg of Dianabol. It may very well be significantly more at the same dose. Bodybuilders will usually find it advisable to monitor their liver enzymes during each cycle, and limit drug duration to 6-8 weeks.

A typical effective oral dose for men will be in the range of 5-10mg per day, with 20mg really being on the extreme end for the recreational bodybuilder. He would probably be better served with a 10mg daily dose, and stacking it with an injectable like testosterone cypionate. This would minimize the chance for liver toxicity, and would also provide a more balanced cycle in terms of anabolic vs. androgenic effect. A common complaint when M1T is taken alone is lethargy, which may be due, in part, to its low androgenic component. Stacking it with an androgen like testosterone will usually alleviate this problem quickly, making for a very good compliment to methyl-1-testosterone. A combination of 400mg of cypioante, and 10mg daily of methyl-1-test, would be quite an effecting mass building stack. Of course, these are what fall in the realm of "recreational doses". I do not have to tell you that many exceed such recommendations, and take as much as 40mg per day of this steroid. While probably far in excess of what you need, some seem to really swear by high-dose cycles of this steroid. One thing is for certain, even 20mg per day is a very serious dose, and is not to be taken lightly, either for its effectiveness or toxicity. Like Anadrol, M1T is not necessarily a friendly steroid, but it is definitely an effective one.

Although this agent was once sold legally as a nutritional supplement (due to the fact that it was unknown when the 1991 law was written, and therefore not included), methyl-1-testosterone is controlled as an illegal anabolic steroid in the United States as of January 20, 2005. Therefore, it carries the same penalties for possession and distribution as all anabolic steroids. Due the once abundant and legal supply of this steroid in the U.S., many leftover bottles of product from supplement stores are likely to find their way to the black market in the months and years to come, where they will likely sell for a premium. Given the high potency of this steroid, we might also expect some of the underground or veterinary drug manufacturers to add it to their lines before long. This would be great to see, as it would ensure that this very powerful and formerly unknown anabolic steroid does not disappear into research oblivion once again.

Methyldienolone

Androgenic	Anabolic	Standard
200-300	1000	Methyltestosterone (oral)

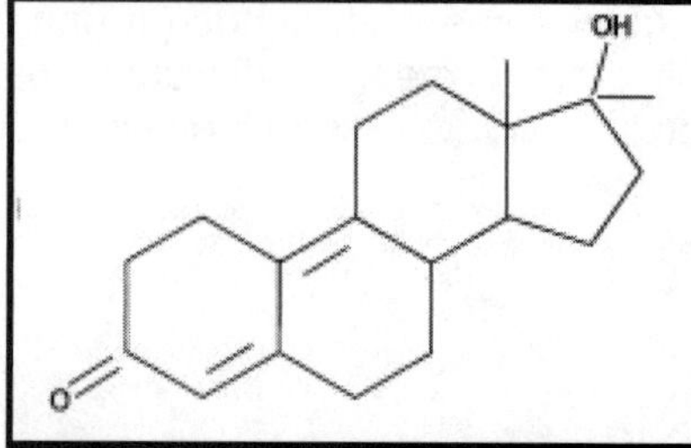

METHYLDIENOLONE

Chemical Name:
17a-methyl-17beta-hydroxyestra-4,9(10)dien-3-one

Estrogenic Activity: none
Progestational Activity: moderate

Methyldienolone (MD) is a synthetic oral anabolic steroid that was researched in the 1960's but never sold as a prescription drug. It is fundamentally a nandrolone-based compound, modified from this base hormone in two ways. First, it has been c-17alpha-alkylated (methylated) to protect against hepatic breakdown. This alteration, in of itself, turns the mild-mannered nandrolone into the formidable oral agent methylnandrolone. Next, it has been given a second double-bond at the 9 position, which considerably increases its anabolic and androgenic potency. Methyldienolone actually differs from methyltrienolone, the most potent steroid profiled in this book, only by the lack of a third double-bond (hence the "di" part). Although not actually #2 in the book, methyldienolone is 5 times more potent than Dianabol, 10 times more potent than methyltestosterone, and 13 times more potent than Primobolan®.

Other characteristics of note include an inability to be converted into estrogen, which limits this steroid's potential for related side effects like fat gain, water retention, and gynecomastia. This trait makes it a drug more ideally suited for cutting cycles than bulking ones. However, as a nandrolone based compound, it may have some progestational activity, which can work to intensify the effects of estrogen. Therefore, it may not be the ideal steroid to use with other aromatizable (estrogen producing) compounds, if fat loss and muscle definition are key concerns. Methyldienolone is also only moderately androgenic, with just a modest propensity to trigger oily skin and acne when used in reasonable dosages. Overall, this agent is classified as an "anabolic", and should fall somewhere between the milder nandrolone derivatives and more androgenic orals like Dianabol and Anadrol.

Effective oral daily doses are going to fall in the range of 2-10mg per day for men, and under 1mg daily for women. At this level, one should expect measurable strength and lean tissue gains, which should be accompanied by decent fat loss and minimal side effects. When determining dosage one also needs to respect the fact that methyldienolone is a c-17alpha-alkylated compound, and presents some liver toxicity to its user. For optimal safety it is usually recommended to limit drug duration to no longer than 8 weeks, after which a break is taken from all methylated or ethylated steroids. One might also want to avoid stacking this drug with other liver toxic orals, and instead opt to use an injectable base instead. 5mg per day of methyldienolone combined with 400mg weekly of testosterone cypionate/enanthate or Equipoise® would make an excellent lean-mass stack, while trenbolone (225mg) or Primobolan® (300-400mg) could be used instead for cutting.

Availability of methyldienolone is going to be limited over the next couple of years, due to the recent scheduling of this agent as a class III controlled substance. This agent was manufactured as a nutritional supplement for a brief period of time before the 2004 amendment to the anabolic steroid act was passed, which means there should be a fair amount of leftover supplement available as people take advantage of its increasing value and sell off their pre-ban "stockpiles". The long-term future of this agent remains uncertain, however, as no legitimate drug company has yet to take an interest in it. It is unfortunate to think that this drug may no longer be available in a couple of years. This is a very powerful agent though, and may very well peak the interest of some of the companies looking for a "different" oral to sell. That is, of course, if the consumer market can get over the fact that this drug was once "legal". Although sold openly for a while, MD is indeed still one very powerful, and one very real, steroid.

It is important to note that there may be an issue with methyldienolone "counterfeits". I was made aware that the compound 3,17-dimethyldiendiol (a 3-methylated diol analog of MD) was being manufactured and sold as methyldienolone to various U.S. supplement companies. This was apparently done because of manufacturing troubles, and with the knowledge of some of the buyers, who felt it was "essentially the same thing". Other companies may have been selling this material as MD unwittingly, given the rarity of true "quality control" in the supplement industry (few independently lab test their products). Therefore, those who have noticed poor results from this steroid may not have been using the real thing. I do believe that early manufacturing issues were resolved, and raw methyldienolone has made its way to the market before the passing of the law. Provided you are buying legitimate methyldienolone, you can feel good knowing you have a very rare, structurally unique, and extremely powerful steroid, that few in history were given an opportunity to use.

Methylhydroxynandrolone

Androgenic	Anabolic	Standard
281	1304	Methyltestosterone (oral)

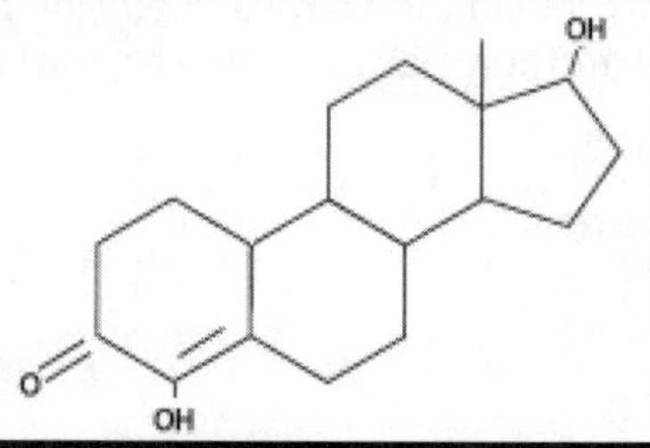

METHYLHYDROXYNANDROLONE

Chemical Name:
4-Hydroxy-17alpha-methyl-hydroxyestra-4-ene-3-one

Estrogenic Activity: none
Progestational Activity: moderate

Methylhydroxynandrolone, or MHN for short, is a potent derivative of the anabolic steroid nandrolone. It differs from this base steroid structurally in two ways. First, it has been c-17alpha alkylated (methylated), a modification that allows this steroid to be orally active. Next, an additional hydroxyl group has been added at its 4 position, similar to hydroxytestosterone. Together these two alterations have created a potent orally active and non-aromatizable anabolic steroid, with a profile somewhat similar to that of Winstrol or Anavar – a primarily anabolic agent with no discernable estrogenic activity. This anabolic was investigated back in the 1960's, and to spite its effective nature was never released as a prescription drug. Its properties make it of obvious interest as a designer steroid, and I would not be surprised if numerous athletes have used it for this purpose over the years. However, since we have not seen a MHN scandal in the media, this remains a matter for speculation.

Although this steroid is a nandrolone derivative, it acts quite differently from its chemical parent. For starters, while nandrolone is a relatively mild steroid, MHN is an exceedingly potent synthetic agent. According to assay results published in Hormonal Steroids (Academic Press, 1964), methylhydroxynandrolone is 13 times more potent than methyltestosterone. This is clearly something of interest for this makes MHN stronger than any prescription steroid known currently. MHN is also quite potent as an androgen, behaving more like trenbolone than nandrolone in this regard. The relative androgenicity of this steroid is likely intensified by its 4-hydroxyl group, a modification that prevents its 5-alpha reduction to weaker "dihydro" metabolites in the skin, scalp and prostate. MHN cannot interact with the reductase enzyme, therefore, it retains its original level of potency in these same tissues. This steroid is still technically more of an "anabolic" than an "androgen", but it is definitely not the mild nandrolone you are familiar with.

Due to its displaying such a high level of milligram for milligram potency, the typical effective daily dosage for men is going to be comparatively much lower than one would expect with other agents. For example, while Dianabol might warrant using 25-35mg daily to notice a pronounced benefit, methylhydroxynandrolone users will likely be working in the range of only 2-5mg per day. At this level MHN should provide very solid gains in muscle mass and strength, with no water retention or increased fat deposition. If anything the user is likely to lose body fat at the same time, one of the reasons why athletes will often spend the extra money on an anabolic like Winstrol, instead of simply taking cheap testosterone or Dbol. This drug is also versatile for stacking, and mixes well with most other anabolics (for cutting) or androgenic (for bulking phases). Women should probably stay away from this steroid altogether, and instead opt for an agent known to be less androgenic (and friendlier to women). Something like Primobolan, Winstrol or Anavar would be a much better choice than MHN, with less chance for permanent masculine side effects.

Methylhydroxynandrolone is not available as a prescription agent at this time, in any part of the world. This agent was merely investigated as a drug, and never sold as one. It has appeared on the U.S. supplement market very recently, sold legally and openly as a nutritional product. This was due primarily to the fact that it was never regulated as a drug in this country, and, barring a direct listing on the 1992 steroid law, could not be covered by it. MHN has since been included in the most recent expansion of our nation's steroid laws, and is formally a controlled anabolic steroid in the U.S. as of January 20, 2005. Possession of this agent after this date carries all the same legal risks and consequences as other popular and illegal steroids. Due to the fact that it is not a prescription drug, we also run the risk of watching it become extinct in the very near future. At best we can hope one of the enterprising veterinary drug makers in Mexico will take an interest in it. Otherwise, MHN may very well disappear right back to the library shelves where it sat for decades.

Methyltestosterone

Androgenic	Anabolic	Standard
94-130	115-150	Testosterone

Chemical Names:
17b-hydroxy-17a-methyl-4-androsten-3-one
17alpha-methylandrost-4-en-3-one-17b-ol

Estrogenic Activity: high
Progestational Activity: not significant

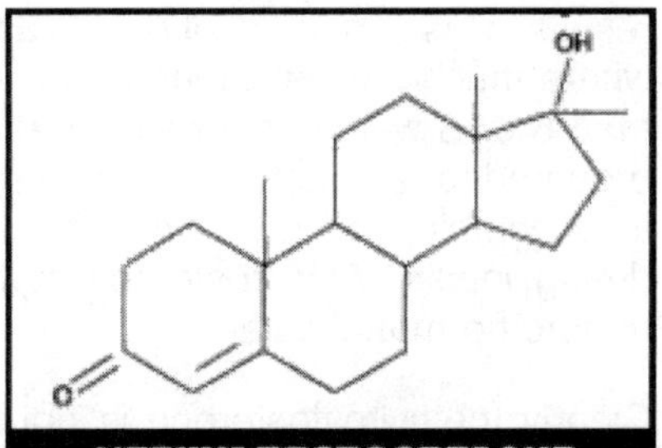

METHYLTESTOSTERONE

Methyltestosterone is an orally available form of the primary male androgen testosterone. Looking at the structure of this steroid, we see it is basically just testosterone with an added methyl group at the c-17 alpha position (a c-17 alpha alkylated substance). Alkylation such as this is necessary when administering testosterone (and other steroids) orally, as without it the liver will destroy most of the steroid during the "first pass". The resultant compound "methylated-testosterone" was among the first functional oral steroids to be produced. This field of research has consequently improved greatly over the years, and today methyltestosterone is quite crude in comparison to many of the other orals that were subsequently developed.

The action of this steroid is somewhat androgenic, with a moderate anabolic effect. As is typically seen with 17 alpha methylation, the resulting steroid has lower anabolic activity than its parent testosterone. Additionally it is extremely estrogenic, another property that seems to be enhanced when this alteration is present (when the steroid is receptive to the aromatase enzyme). The problem seems to be its conversion to the more biologically active estrogen 17-alpha methylestradiol. 17-alpha methylation in fact slows aromatization, however the potent nature of 17-methylestradiol more than compensates for this. Additionally it has a very short half-life in the body, so the drug needs to be administered several times daily if a consistent blood level is to be obtained. All of this heightens the ratio of side effects to muscle growth enough to make methyltestosterone a very inefficient muscle-building drug. In order to administer an effective amount of hormone, the user simply must deal with too many estrogenic side effects, including water retention and gynecomastia, which can be very troublesome with this steroid. One may choose to addition an anti-estrogen such as Nolvadex® and/or Proviron® to combat related side effects, which should effectively minimize their intensity enough to make a cycle tolerable. The powerful antiaromatase Arimidex® is a notably more effective option when dealing with aromatizable steroids, as it shows great ability to stop the conversion of androgens to estrogens. Using this drug with methyltest would be somewhat ironic however, spending up to $10 per day for an ancillary drug and at most a couple of dollars for the actual steroid.

Just as we see with its parent testosterone, methyltestosterone has a high rate of conversion to DHT (in this case 17alpha-methyldihydrotestosterone). This metabolite is of course more active than methyltestosterone, and likewise responsible for many of the unwanted androgenic side effects encountered with use. Oily skin, acne, body/facial hair growth and hair loss are likewise all common with this steroid, and may present themselves very early into a cycle. Also seen with use of this compound is an increased level of aggression, an effect commonly associated with testosterone and other strong androgens. The addition of Proscar® could quite prove useful with this steroid, inhibiting the conversion of methyltestosterone into methyl-DHT in many target tissues and lowering the impact of related side effects. Avodart®, a newer and more effective reductase inhibitor, would be even better. But again, these ancillary drugs are considerably more expensive than the steroid they would be used to treat.

A strong androgen such as methyltest obviously has little to offer female athletes except virilization symptoms. In this arena, methyltestosterone should be strictly avoided. The only time females should really be taking this potent steroid is when indicated for a specific medical application. While not a new concept, using an androgen to treat the symptoms of menopause has been catching on in recent years nonetheless. An example is the product Estratest, which contains esterified estrogens and a small amount of added methyltestosterone. This proves beneficial not only to the energy, sex drive and overall wellness of the patient, but can effectively combat osteoporosis. While estrogen replacement can only halt calcium loss in the bones, testosterone can actually rebuild stores. This effect can restore much of the lost strength in the bones, something estrogen alone just cannot accomplish.

Being a c-17 alpha alkylated compound, methyltestosterone also places notable stress on the liver. This is further amplified when looking at the amount of drug necessary to see an anabolic effect. Those willing to use this drug for actual muscle growth ordinarily find that a daily dosage of 40-50mg is necessary (at a minimum) for acceptable results. This is quite a lot of c-17aa steroid for the liver to process, especially when comparing it to the effect seen with a much smaller amount of Dianabol or Winstrol®. One should therefore limit a cycle of this drug to no more than 6 or 8 weeks, after which a longer break should be taken from all "toxic" oral steroids. One should also be prepared for a substantial loss of mass and bodyweight at the conclusion of each cycle with methyltest. This is due to a combination retained water being excreted, and the suppression of endogenous testosterone production during intake. A testosterone stimulating drug such as Clomid®/Nolvadex® and/or HCG is therefore used to restore hormonal balance.

Clearly methyltestosterone is not a very advanced compound. While it is close derivative of testosterone, with potential as such, it offers us little benefit in practice. The short activity and high rate of estrogenic activity generally make this product too troublesome to use for performance enhancement. The only commonly accepted application for methyltestosterone is to stimulate aggression in the user. Powerlifters, bodybuilders and competitive athletes often attempt to "harness" this aggression, looking for extra intensity in a training session or competition. Additionally, many methyltest tabs are designed for sublingual administration, or to be placed under the tongue and left to dissolve. These tabs can generally be identified by a pleasant tasting citrus flavor, which is most often included. Sublingual intake is an added benefit for aggression stimulating purposes, providing fast (albeit incomplete) absorption of the drug. A couple of tablets placed under the tongue before a visit to the gym can make for an intense, and possibly more productive, workout session. Aside from this methyltest offers little except side effects. It is quite toxic, elevating liver enzymes and causing acne, gynecomastia, aggression and water retention quite easily. Were one to tolerate these side effects, methyltest will offer little more than poor quality (but bulky) gains. One looking for quality muscle building steroid should likewise look elsewhere.

Methyltestosterone is produced by a large number of pharmaceutical manufacturers. It is likewise found in wide variety countries, usually selling for an extremely low price (especially in bulk). Methyltestosterone is therefore a popular ingredient in many counterfeit (oral) preparations. An inexperienced buyer can easily mistake the effect of this drug for whatever is written on the label, unaware of the cheap, crude steroid actually being administered. As crude as it may be, methyltestosterone is still a controlled substance in the United States. The practice of substituting methyltestosterone is therefore much more common now outside of the U.S., where bulk purchases of raw steroid are still possible.

Metribolone (methyltrienolone)

Androgenic	Anabolic	Standard
6000-7000	12,000-30,000	methyltestosterone

Chemical Names:
17alpha-methyl-17beta-hydroxyestra-4,9,11-triene-3-one
17alpha-methyl-trenbolone

Estrogenic Activity: None
Progestational Activity: n/a

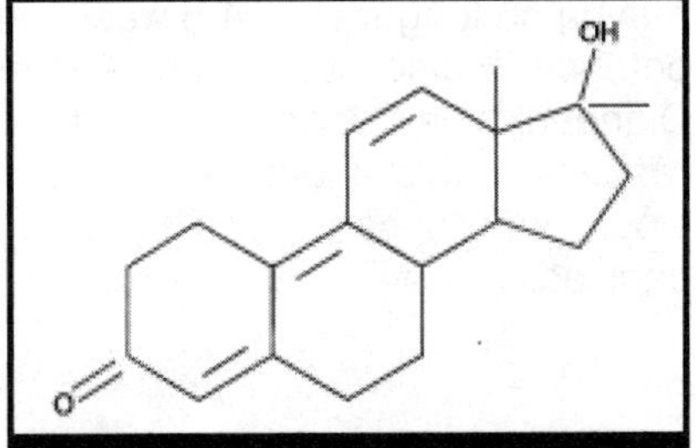

METHYLTRIENOLONE

Methyltrienolone is an extremely powerful anabolic steroid, perhaps one of the strongest ever produced in a laboratory. But it is also one that remains in the laboratory, far outside of commercial circles. This is therefore not a "clinical-use" steroid, but an obscure research material rarely discussed outside of the science journals. Methytrienolone is specifically a derivative of the anabolic steroid trenbolone (trienolone), methylated to allow for oral administration. Like trenbolone, it will not aromatize, and does not have "estrogenic" properties to speak of. But this is really where the similarities between these two compounds end. Methyltrienolone may chemically differ from trenbolone only by the addition of one methyl group at C-17, as we have discussed before, this alteration changes the activity of a steroid considerably. It would be a big mistake to simply consider it "oral trenbolone".

Fundamentally, methyltrienolone is a significantly stronger and more toxic steroid than its non-methylated cousin. Its potency has been measured in animal assays to be anywhere from 120-300 times greater than that of methyltestosterone, with greater dissociation between anabolic and androgenic effects[79 80] (both traits are very pronounced). If we were to look at trenbolone as the high school bully amongst steroids, methyltrienolone would be its badass older brother that just got released from a long prison stretch. Basically, it is one tuff steroid that you really don't want to fuck with. To begin with, this steroid was built to be exceedingly resistant to breakdown by the liver. This trait does admittedly leaves methyltrienolone with a level of anabolic potency that is hard to match in a synthetic anabolic. Mg for Mg it exceeds every steroid on the market, by far, in its effectiveness, requiring doses as little as 1 milligram per day to notice a strong effect. But such high resistance to hepatic metabolism also makes this steroid terribly liver toxic. Studies published from the University of Bonn Germany back in 1966 make this very clear[81]. In fact, at this time researchers had deemed this the most liver toxic steroid to ever be studied in humans, summing up their findings well when stating:

> "Methyltrienolone... which is orally active as an anabolic agent in a dose less than 1.0 mg per day in normal adults, has been tested with regard to its influence on liver function. As measured by multiple parameters (BSP retention; total bilirubin; activities of transaminases, alkaline phosphates and cholinesterase in serum; activity of proaccelerin in plasma) methyltrienolone turned out to be very active as to causing biochemical symptoms of intrahepatic cholestasis. ...thus methyltrienolone at present being the most "hepatotoxic" steroid."

High hepatotoxicity (liver toxicity) precludes methyltrienolone from being sold as a prescription agent at this time, in any part of the world. At least amongst legitimate channels, it is used solely as a research chemical. For this purpose the agent is very well suited. Its sheer potency makes it an excellent in-vitro receptor-biding standard to compare other agents to, and being so resistant to metabolism, active methyltrienolone metabolites are not going to greatly interfere with the results of most experiments. This is somewhat of a logical problem when you think about it. Body tissues can metabolize most steroids fairly easily, which means that even incubation studies can be complicated with the question of what is causing a particular effect, the steroid or one of its unidentified metabolites. This is much less of an issue with methyltrienolone. But outside of the laboratory, it is not an agent anyone would want to recommend for human use. Being so liver toxic, it is actually one of the last steroids you'd want to take. There are many more drugs worthwhile to look at, so the risks of something like this are probably not going to be warranted.

Initially I was going to include this profile only as a matter of curiosity. It is an odd but interesting steroid, and worthwhile of some academic discussion at least. However, the rapid expansion of underground steroid manufacturers over the past few years, and the potential release of this agent already as a black market designer compound, make this profile more practical than I had initially anticipated. Those considering the use of an underground form of methyltrienolone should keep a few things in mind. For starters, it is being released for human use in such channels without any government approval or even common sense contemplation. The liver toxicity of this agent needs to be taken very seriously, and at the very least, routine blood tests should be conducted to ensure the agent is not imparting damage. Drug duration should likewise be very limited in scope, maybe no longer than 4-6 weeks at a time. After this point all methylated steroids should be avoided for a while. Its potency is also not a joke, and the agent will legitimately work in doses of as little as 1-2 milligrams per day. Dianabol-type doses of 20-30mg daily are completely unthinkable, and should never be attempted. If absolutely respected, this agent can be used to one's benefit. But again, this is one hardcore steroid, and all good advice would say to pass on it instead. Any one of the many commercially available steroids would be much safer choices.

Miotolan (furazabol)

Androgenic	Anabolic	Standard
73-94	270-330	Methyltestosterone

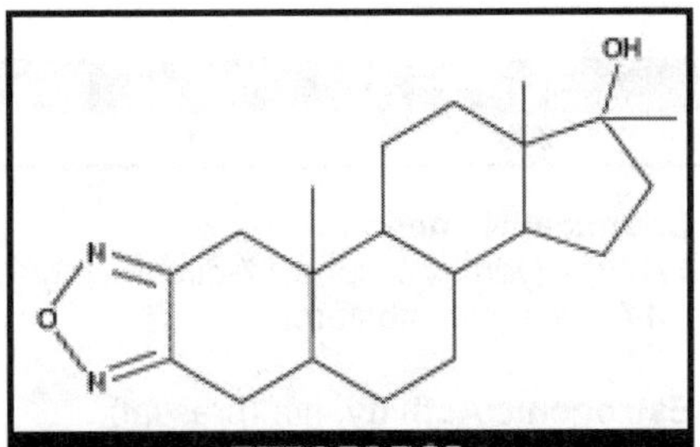

FURAZABOL

Chemical Names:
17-Methyl-5alpha-androstano[2,3-c]furazan-17beta-ol

Estrogenic Activity: none
Progestational Activity: n/a (low)

Miotolan is the trade name for the steroid furazabol, which was at one time produced in Japan. Furazabol is a derivative of dihydrotestosterone, but only moderately androgenic in nature. Being DHT based this compound will also not aromatize, so estrogen related side effects such as water retention and gynecomastia are of no concern with use. It also seems to be potent as an anabolic, much more so than dihydrotestosterone. This is no doubt due to alterations in the A ring, which presumably allows the steroid structure to remain stable and bind receptors in muscle tissues long enough to provide an anabolic benefit. The gain received is reportedly not extreme however, and would more closely resemble the hard/quality growth of a non-aromatizing androgen like Masteron.

Furazabol is also shown to have little effect on endogenous testosterone levels when taken in low therapeutic doses. This is likely due to a lack of estrogen conversion; a hormone that we know produces more dramatic inhibition of testosterone production. Of course, all anabolic/androgenic steroids can interfere with normal androgen production given the right dosage, so it is doubtful this tendency will hold true at a performance-enhancing amount. There will probably still be a need for ancillary drugs such as HCG and/or Clomid®/Nolvadex® at the conclusion of a heavy cycle, used to help reestablish a balance of endogenous hormone levels.

The only prominent side effects with furazabol are those associated with its androgenic characteristics. Oily skin, acne, body/facial hair growth, aggression, and hair loss are therefore all possible. Those with a familial predisposition for male pattern baldness should probably look toward nandrolone or Primobolan before this one. Although Proscar® is used effectively to prevent the conversion of testosterone to DHT, it will offer us no benefit with this steroid. Miotolan is already derived from DHT, so its androgenic activity is not intensified by interaction with the 5alpha-reductase enzyme. We should additionally mention that furazabol is a c-17 alpha alkylated compound, and may therefore place unwanted stress on the liver. For this reason it is only to be used for limited periods, typically no longer than 6 or 8 weeks in length.

The main application for this drug is to use it when cutting or preparing for a bodybuilding competition. Here the high androgen content can help bring out an enhanced look of hardness and density to the muscle, especially in the absence of excess estrogen/body fat. Its muscle building activity could be further enhanced by the addition of a mild anabolic such as Deca-Durabolin® or Equipoise®. In this case, the combined androgen/anabolic stack should provide a noteworthy gain of solid, quality muscle mass without a loss of definition due to water bloat. We could alternately use the more potent androgen trenbolone, although here androgenic side effect will be greatly intensified. An acceptable dosage for men, regardless of application, would be in the range of 10-20mg daily (equating to 10-20 tablets). Women might tolerate Miotolan, however, its somewhat prominent androgenic side might make nandrolone a safer option in comparison.

Miotolan has not been manufactured in Japan for years, so there is little chance you will find even residual stock on the black market. With that being said, there is at least one underground manufacturer who claims to be selling legitimate generic furazabol at this time. It is, therefore, very possible this agent is on the black market again. If so, it also means the drug is being made in a legitimate manufacturing facility somewhere. This is good news to Miotolan fans, because it opens the door for other legitimate drug companies to start selling it. This is especially of interest in the West, where we have had minimal, if any, access to the former Japanese product. Until this happens, however, furazabol will remain at best an underground product, and at worst a memory. Therefore, this profile is written more out of interest than practical application.

Myagen (bolasterone)

Androgenic	Anabolic	Standard
300	575	Methyltestosterone (oral)

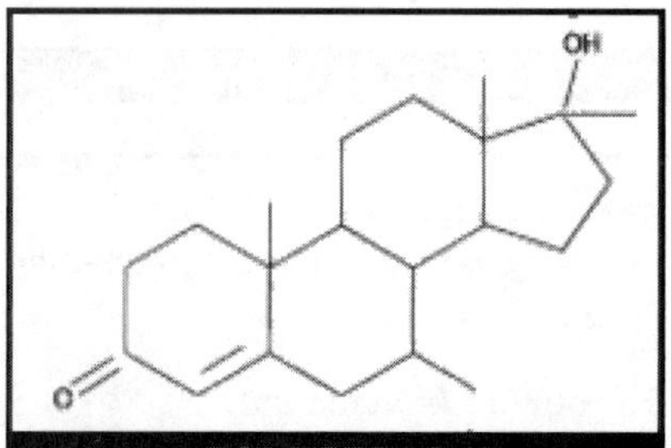

BOLASTERONE

Chemical Names:
17beta-Hydroxy-7alpha,17-dimethylandrost-4-en-3-one
7,17-dimethyltestosterone

Estrogenic Activity: n/a (present)
Progestational Activity: n/a

Bolasterone is a close structural relative to methyltestosterone, differing only by the addition of another methyl group at C-7. This would, of course, account for its chemical name, dimethyltestosterone. This added C-7 methyl group, however, makes the activity of this steroid so far removed from that of methyltestosterone that a comparison in any form is difficult to justify. For starters, the dual methyl groups give the steroid the ability to avoid SHBG to a tremendous extent – in the blood it exists largely in an unbound (active) state. You may remember that this is one of the same reasons mibolerone (Cheque Drops) is so potent, and effective in microgram (not milligram) doses. The C-7 methyl group also interferes with the ability of the steroid to interact with 5-alpha reductase, so to spite being a testosterone derivative, bolasterone should not convert to its "dihydro" derivative in the body. This means that the steroid is technically much more anabolic than androgenic in nature. The only real similarity between the two is like methyltestosterone, bolasterone probably converts to estrogen in the body. This is evidenced by studies with 7-methyl-nandrolone, which have demonstrated that, at least in this case, the addition of C-7 methylation did not interfere with aromatization[82].

I cannot give you much information about finding the most appropriate dose to use, as I don't know anybody that has actually used this drug. With the potency of the anabolic/androgenic index data though, I suspect you would not need all that much to see a good effect. If I had to guess I would think that a dose in the range of 10-30 mg daily would probably outperform most oral steroids on the market. In terms of safety, it is difficult to think that this steroid will present any unique hazard to the user. Early clinical studies seemed to report very favorably on this compound, with no mention of specific dangers or toxicity[83]. It is a C-17 alpha alkylated (methylated) oral anabolic steroid though, and as such needs to be respected for the stressful nature that all such compounds display toward the liver.

Bolasterone was discontinued worldwide long before I knew what anabolic steroids even were, and not too many people speaking about the subject today are going to be able to give you firsthand information about the drug. The few people who think they have used it are likely confusing it with a counterfeit steroid called Bolasterone (purportedly made in East Germany but actually made in a U.S. underground lab) that was circulating in the 1980's. This product was labeled to contain the real thing, but in fact turned out to be little more than an overpriced mixture of readily available and cheap injectable steroids. I do expect, however, that this ages old steroid will emerge again. The supply list from at least one Chinese steroid manufacturing company has started to include bolasterone as a bulk chemical. With the ever-growing underground steroid manufacturing business, fueled by the manufactures in China, it is only a matter of time before some enterprising individual sees the value in producing a bolasterone tablet for the black market. Perhaps it has even been done already, at least on a smaller scale. The United States Anti-Doping Agency has added bolasterone to its list of prohibited anabolic steroids, along with norbolethone, just this year (2003). This may suggest that the USADA believes bolasterone is already being used as an undetectable designer steroid.

Neotest 250 (testosterone decanoate)

Androgenic	Anabolic	Standard
100	100	Standard

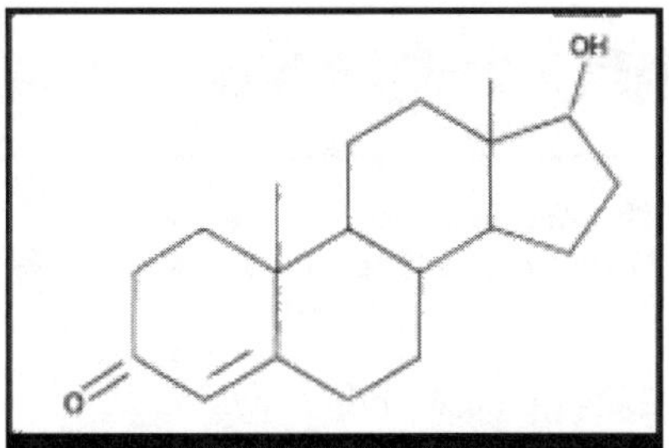

TESTOSTERONE

Chemical Names:
4-androsten-3-one-17beta-ol
17beta-hydroxy-androst-4-en-3-one

Estrogenic Activity: moderate
Progestational Activity: low

Neotest 250 is a relatively new injectable preparation, which uses the decanoate ester of testosterone. It is essentially the testosterone equivalent to Deca-Durabolin, at least as far as its release pattern goes. Neotest is made by Loeffler, the same Mexican veterinary drug manufacturer that produces the popular injectable methandrostenolone product Reforvit-B. Although testosterone decanoate is not a new compound, as it is of course the same slow acting ester used in Sustanon, this is the first commercial preparation ever to use this ester exclusively. This is the slowest acting single ester of testosterone available on the black market at this time, providing a gradual release of testosterone from the site of injection for approximately a two to three week period (See: Deca-Durabolin® for pharmacokinetics).

Neotest offers an ideal alternative to Sustanon for those who like a less frequent injection schedule yet find this four-component testosterone too painful to use. The propionate content in Sustanon® is largely to blame, as this is a notoriously painful compound to use due to the irritating nature of the short chain carboxylic acid propionate. Neotest could similarly be injected every ten days or so, and the pain of the propionate would not have to be endured. The decanoate ester is extremely well tolerated with injection in fact, even more so than testosterone enanthate in many individuals. Provided Loeffler has created a pain-free product in other regards such as using a tolerable alcohol content and clean materials, this product will probably grab the attention of many individuals sensitive to other testosterone injectables. Those in Southern boarder states who like the concept of crossing over to Mexico every other week to inject a slow acting product (as a way to avoid illegally possessing anabolics in the U.S.) might also find Neotest appealing, as it should again be a much easier product to inject in a higher volume than Sustanon®. Even the moderate soreness most feel from Sustanon would certainly be multiplied, possibly to an intolerable point, if 4+ milliliters were attempted in a single day.

Other than injection comfort, Neotest will likely be indistinguishable in effect from other esterified testosterone injectables such as cypionate, enanthate or Sustanon®. With athletes typically injecting all on a weekly basis, we cannot expect any significant differences in the testosterone release pattern to be noted. Gains and side effects would likewise be similar to all esters of testosterone. This hormone is an extremely effective bulking agent, and in fact is one of the best muscle-builders known. One could expect marked gains in size and strength at a dosage of 500mg every week to ten days, but they may be accompanied noticeable side effects. This includes estrogen related water retention, fat buildup and possibly even the onset of gynecomastia. Androgenic side effect such as oily skin and acne are often unavoidable when taking a testosterone as well, and are usually just dealt with using topical treatments and endured as a clear indicator the drugs are working. As we exceed 500mg per shot gains will probably be more pronounced, but side effects can be expected to become much more problematic. Water retention may begin to hide muscle definition in a very noticeable way at this dosage, and often is even noticed in the face. If gynecomastia were not developing before, it should certainly be a concern now. One should be cautious when taking testosterone in a high dose, and certainly be ready to use ancillary drugs if problems start to occur. Having a drug like Nolvadex® on hand is especially important with Neotest, as it is such a long acting agent. If gyno starts to develop, you may be stuck with several more weeks of high estrogen levels even after your last shot.

Nilevar (norethandrolone)

Androgenic	Anabolic	Standard
22-55	100-200	Methyltestosterone (oral)

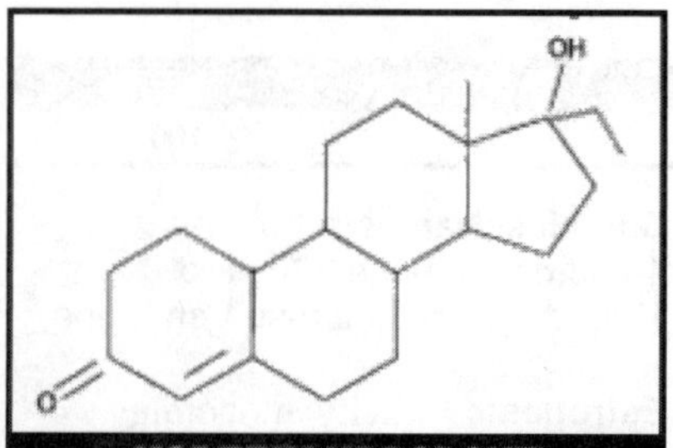

NORETHANDROLONE

Chemical Names:
17alpha-Ethyl-17beta-hydroxyestr-4-en-3-one
17a-ethyl-19-nortestosterone

Estrogenic Activity: low
Progestational Activity: high

Nilevar is a trade name for the oral steroid norethandrolone, developed by the pharmaceutical firm Searle in the mid 1950's. Norethandrolone is a derivative of nortestosterone (nandrolone), containing an added c17 alpha ethyl group so the molecule can withstand oral administration. The activity of this steroid is that of a mild to moderate anabolic, which is accompanied by an equally distinguishable androgenic and estrogenic component. This item was the predecessor to Anavar (oxandrolone), which was introduced to the US drug market about a decade later. When comparing the quality and overall effect of the two substances, oxandrolone is considered to be notably superior to the more androgenic and estrogenic norethandrolone. This is probably why we do not see this steroid much anymore. It has been off U.S. shelves for many years now, and is currently marketed only in Australia, France and Switzerland.

Although structurally nandrolone and norethandrolone are very similar, they seem to behave quite differently in the body. For starters, androgenic side effects such as oily skin, acne and body/facial hair growth seem to be slightly more pronounced with this drug. In this regard Nilevar is usually thought to more closely resemble a steroid such as Dianabol than a mild anabolic like Deca. And since the 5-alpha reduced metabolite of norethandrolone is weaker than its parent (just as we see with nandrolone), Proscar® would offer us no benefit in reducing such symptoms (this drug is really only applicable with testosterone compounds). One might even run the risk of developing (or aggravating) a male pattern hair loss condition with Nilevar, although this steroid is admittedly still much less potent here than many stronger androgens including testosterone and Anadrol 50®. Those with a familial predisposition for baldness would still be much better served with an injectable nandrolone preparation such as Deca-Durabolin®, which is in all respects a better steroid.

And while we see a very low tendency for estrogen conversion with nandrolone, unfortunately again norethandrolone seems to have a reputation as a much more estrogenic steroid. This is likely due to the fact that it converts to a more biologically active form of estradiol, 17alpha-ethyl-estradiol, instead of regular estrogen. A similar problem is noted with Dianabol, which is much more troublesome than its non-alkylated cousin boldenone. Excessive water retention is the usual result with norethandrolone, producing an unsightly smoothness and loss of definition to the physique. In addition, the extra estrogen can also lead to the development of gynecomastia very quickly. It may therefore be advisable to include an antiestrogen such as Nolvadex® and/or Proviron® from the start of a cycle, in order to keep these side effects to a minimum. We also have the option of using the antiaromatase Arimidex®, which is a much more effective remedy. It will efficiently stop the compound from converting to estrogen, essentially halting related side effects. The high selling price for this product makes it quite costly to use however, especially when we are taking it to treat the effects of what is considered to be a cheap and crude oral steroid.

Norethandrolone will also suppress endogenous testosterone production quite readily with use. This may be a result of not only its androgenic and estrogenic activity, but its action as a progestin as well. As mentioned when discussing Deca-Durabolin®, 19-norandrogens are often shown to exhibit some affinity for the progesterone receptor. This tendency seems to be notably heightened in Nilevar, and contributes not only to its ability to suppress testosterone production, but also its propensity to induce fat storage and gynecomastia (side effects normally associated with estrogen). In order to help restore hormonal balance after each cycle a combination of HCG and Clomid®/Nolvadex® may prove very useful. While HCG is not always indicated with many of the milder anabolics, the strong suppressive nature of norethandrolone makes having this drug on-hand almost a necessity (especially for those inclined to notice testicular atrophy during steroid intake).

Clearly Nilevar cannot be looked at as an oral alternative to Deca-Durabolin®, as this compound is much more troublesome. The increased tendency for estrogen conversion (when possible) and lowered anabolic effectiveness that results when a steroid is 17-alpha alkylated make norethandrolone very inefficient for building muscle. In administering an effective amount of steroid in terms of muscle growth, the user has to deal with much more in terms of side effects compared to nandrolone. The accumulation with norethandrolone is also going to be bloated mass, and not the quality muscularity we associate with Deca. A notably more pronounced strength increase may result with this substance, not doubt partly due to the extra fluid retention. The androgenic component also makes this steroid a less than ideal choice for women, who would be better served by an injectable nandrolone such as Durabolin® (nandrolone phenylpropionate).

Those who find an interest to take Nilevar most commonly find a daily dosage of 30-40mg (3-4 tablets) is needed to receive an anabolic effect. In order to keep blood levels more constant, the tablets are also taken in divided doses (spread evenly throughout the day). As mentioned, norethandrolone is a c-17 alpha alkylated steroid in order to make oral dosing possible. Although a methyl group is typically used for this purpose with anabolic/androgenic steroids, in this case the steroid carries an ethyl substitution (just as we see with Orabolin). This is just as stressful to the liver of course, so the length of each cycle best kept to a minimum to avoid any serious damage. A logical duration would probably be no longer than 6 to 8 weeks, after which a longer break (from all related oral compounds) should be taken.

Although this steroid is sometimes circulated in Europe, it is not commonly found in the U.S. The demand for it is quite low, so large volume steroid dealers are not very interested in importing it. The only exception as of late seems to be the Jurox item **Anaplex** from Australia. This has been readily exported from Australia to Mexico, and thereafter has been reaching the States. As a result many athletes have been experimenting with this steroid recently, but admittedly it still does remain relatively unpopular on the black market. Although Anaplex is quite inexpensive compared to the older French Nilevar, one should not be tempted to use excessive dosages for a stronger anabolic effect. The level of estrogenic side effects and strain placed on the liver are certainly to be compounded as the dosages go up, making such a practice less than worthwhile in terms of gain vs. side effects. Dianabol is clearly a better alternative as far as orals go, and as already mentioned Deca-Durabolin® is a much more tolerable option in terms of a nandrolone.

Omnadren (testosterone blend)

Androgenic	Anabolic	Standard
100	100	Standard

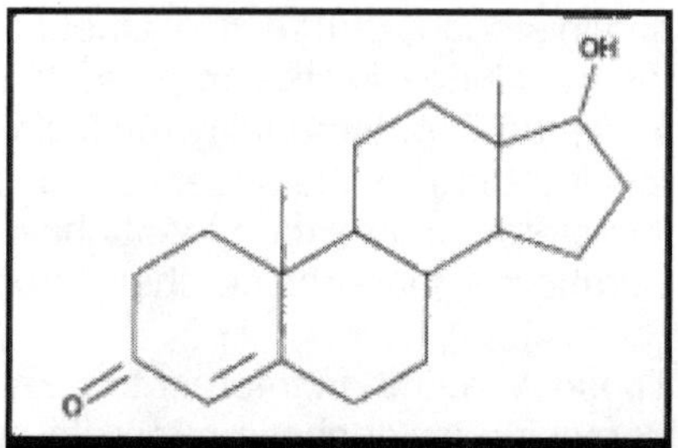

TESTOSTERONE

Chemical Names:
4-androsten-3-one-17beta-ol
17beta-hydroxy-androst-4-en-3-one

Estrogenic Activity: moderate
Progestational Activity: low

Contains:
30mg testosterone propionate
60mg testosterone phenylpropionate
60mg testosterone isocaproate
100mg testosterone caproate

Omnadren 250 is an oil-based injectable containing a blend of four different testosterone esters: testosterone propionate, phenylpropionate, isocaproate and caproate. Being a four-component testosterone, Omnadren is most commonly compared to Sustanon. While it does contain testosterone propionate, testosterone phenylpropionate and isocaproate in the same strength as Sustanon, the last ester is different. Please note however, that the older versions of Omnadren list isohexanoate and hexanoate as the final two ingredients. Hexanoate is simply another work for caproate, so the last ester (decanoate) is the only Sustanon constituent missing from Omnadren.

One of the only noticeable differences between Sustanon and Omnadren seems to be the speed in which estrogen buildup occurs. In comparison, the process appears to be slightly more pronounced with Omnadren. This is of course just a matter of timing, as the slowest releasing ester in Omnadren (caproate) is a little faster acting than enanthate. Blood testosterone levels will therefore peak much faster with this compound, not having the same gradual release time imposed by testosterone decanoate. Users likewise report water retention much earlier into a cycle. While water retention may lead to a more rapid buildup of size and strength, it can become pronounced enough to cause a very smooth and watery look to develop (hiding muscle definition). In addition, the excess estrogen is likely to cause the development of gynecomastia. This effect is especially pronounced with Omnadren, usually presenting itself quickly after a cycle has been started. Estrogen can also be responsible for increases in body fat storage during treatment, resulting in a further loss of definition. Individuals who are sensitive to the effects of estrogen, yet still seek the power of a testosterone, would therefore need to addition an antiestrogen such as Nolvadex® and/or Proviron®. Arimidex®, a powerful antiaromatase, is another option available to us. Although very costly, this drug works much more efficiently than any other antiestrogen in use by athletes. It would have great use with such a strong item as Omnadren, as the standard remedies would not be quite as effective.

Being a testosterone, one can also expect the typical set of androgenic side effects. Oily skin, acne, body/facial hair growth and increase aggression are all very common with this product. It can also bring out or aggravate a condition of male pattern baldness. Men with a familial predisposition for hair loss should probably avoid this item. We do however, have the option to addition Proscar® (finasteride). This is a drug that can effectively prevent testosterone from converting into DHT (dihydrotestosterone) in certain androgen target tissues. Since DHT is the primary culprit with testosterone's androgenic side effects, adding Proscar® to the cycle should allow it to be much more comfortable. Omnadren is also likely to suppress endogenous testosterone production rather quickly. It is therefore almost a necessity to add a testosterone stimulating drug like HCG and/or Clomid®/Nolvadex® when concluding therapy. This way we can prevent a retracted period of unbalanced hormone levels, hopefully avoiding a "crash" after the steroids have been removed.

Being a powerful, long acting testosterone blend, the effect of Omnadren is of course quite comparable to that of Sustanon (except that its release time is closer to cypionate or enanthate). It is similarly a powerful androgen, capable of providing great gains in mass and strength. Due of the high level of water retention associated with testosterone, Omnadren is really only applicable for bulking purposes. While it is very effective alone, it is also combined often with a number of other steroids depending on the desired result. Many athletes prefer to combine Omnadren with a strong anabolic like Deca-Durabolin® or Equipoise® for example, in an attempt to lower the overall testosterone dosage and run a more quality mass building cycle. On the other hand, power-lifters and those looking for dramatic gains in mass and strength (regardless of quality) may stack Omnadren with heavy orals such as Anadrol 50® or Dianabol. Here of course the strength and weight gain should be even more extreme, although androgenic/estrogenic side effects are expected to be as well.

Although Omnadren stays active in the body for about two weeks, it is generally injected on a weekly basis. A dosage of 250-750mg (1-3 ampules) per week is more than sufficient to achieve great results. Some take advantage of the very low price of Omnadren (Europe) and take excessively large amounts. Beyond 750mg or 1000mg weekly added side effects will no doubt be greatly outweighing growth, so there is usually little need for such excess. With this drug we really don't want to mistake water bloat for muscle growth. And while a number of adventurous women do experiment with testosterone products, Omnadren is probably not a good choice. The long action of this compound, mixed with the highly androgenic nature of testosterone, makes a poor combination. Virilization symptoms can develop quite easily with a strong androgen, making a long acting product like Omnadren notably dangerous should problems become evident. Testosterone propionate is a much better choice should an androgen like this be absolutely necessary, as it will give the user much greater control over her blood testosterone level.

Due to the extremely low price for this drug in Poland, Omnadren is made readily available on the black market. Among bodybuilders, Omnadren is generally considered to be inferior to Sustanon however. Price may have something to do with this belief, as this drug is generally much cheaper than Sustanon on the black market. It is likewise usually pushed when availability of (or money for) Sustanon is short. Realistically the two are interchangeable, and I would suggest going for whatever one is providing the most testosterone per dollar. In most cases this will turn out to be testosterone enanthate, and not a blended product. Still, Omnadren remains a good product, and is usually found for a good price. At this point counterfeits are not a major concern, but they are definitely out there. Best advice would be to purchase this product only when it is properly packaged in its box. This will weed out a good majority of the fake loose ampules in circulation.

Take note to look for the newer style packaging, which has a pink box that opens up in the front to reveal a row of ampules neatly sitting inside. Be careful though, as there are already fakes of the newer style boxes in circulation, and these fakes are extremely difficult to spot. All basic details are the same on the counterfeit, barring only a couple of slight inconsistencies. For starters, the real box has a barcode that ends in the numbers 9312. The fake incorrectly ends in 931P. When looking at the ampules, you notice that the fake has the **&** symbol stamped on the label. Real Omnadren ampules always carry letters from the end of the alphabet like **v**, **w**, **x** or **y**. Pictures of both the real and fake ampules have been provided. You can see in looking at them that the fake is first-rate. If you didn't know to look for these minute details, you'd never know the product were counterfeit until using it.

Orabolin (ethylestrenol)

Androgenic	Anabolic	Standard
20-400	200-400	Methyltestosterone (oral)

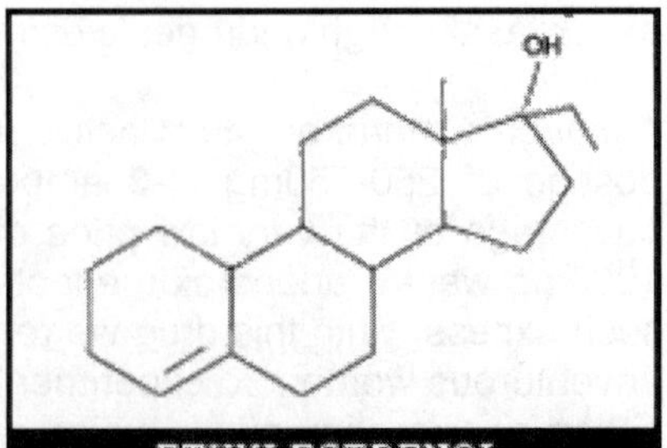
ETHYLESTRENOL

Chemical Names:
19-Nor-17alpha-pregn-4-en-17b-ol
17alpha-ethly-estr-4-en-17b-ol

Estrogenic Activity: low
Progestational Activity: low to moderate

Orabolin® is a trade name for the oral anabolic steroid ethylestrenol. This compound is manufactured by the international drug firm Organon, and was once available in the United States under the name Maxibolin. This drug was phased out many years ago however, in a wave of growing disinterest toward anabolic steroids. Today this steroid is a rare find, as it is only manufactured a few countries. The compound ethylestrenol is structurally similar to the anabolic steroid nandrolone (19-nortestosterone), although here the design is that of an oral steroid. This is the reasoning behind its given trade name of Orabolin, as this is the compressed appearance of "Durabolin®-Oral". It was first marketed (obviously) as an oral alternative to the injectable compound Deca-Durabolin®.

Similar to Deca, Orabolin is classified as an anabolic with mild androgenic properties. It aromatizes only slightly, so estrogen related side effects are rarely a concern. Water retention and gynecomastia are likewise not common occurrences, even when sensitive individuals take this drug. Androgenic side effects are also extremely slight with Orabolin, so one should not be concerned with hair loss and acne (etc.) unless unusually high doses are taken. This compound is actually well tolerated by women, who were actually a main focus of its design. Virilization symptoms are therefore highly unlikely, again barring the use a high daily dosage. Also of note is that ethylestrenol is a c17 alpha alkylated compound, containing the same ethyl substitution we see with the oral steroid Nilevar. Administration may therefore place some level of strain on the liver, particularly when it is taken for longer periods of time. Those who take this compound would be best served by remaining conservative with the daily dosage, and limiting intake to no more than 6 to 8 weeks.

The comparison of Orabolin to Deca-Durabolin® is really not a fair one in a practical sense. While clinically the relationship is clear, athletes find the action of Orabolin to be worlds apart from Deca. The fundamental difference is that the activity of ethylestrenol is tremendously weaker in comparison. When we look at Deca, we see a drug with a distinct anabolic and (lesser) androgenic tendency. It is likewise an efficient compound for muscle buildup. But the extreme mildness of Orabolin makes its anabolic activity very slight. This is clearly not due to poor bioavailability, as c17 alpha alkylation will efficiently protect the structure from first-pass metabolism. Ethylestrenol simply has a low tendency to bind with the androgen receptor, and therefore requires higher amounts to receive any type of notable anabolic response. In fact structurally ethylestrenol much more closely resembles Nilevar (norethandrolone) than nandrolone. The two differ only by the absence of an oxygen atom at the c3 position of ethylestrenol, and in the body Orabolin actually has some affinity to convert to Nilevar[84]. This path of metabolism may be responsible for some of the androgenic activity, and estrogenic buildup, we see with this compound.

Overall the level of muscle growth obtained with ethylestrenol should be much less noticeable than that expected with either Nilevar or Deca-Durabolin®. It is even weaker than both Winstrol® and oxandrolone on a milligram for milligram basis, this drug likewise gathering little attention with athletes. The only group that usually finds an appreciation for Orabolin is female athletes, who find the mild nature of this drug quite favorable when wishing to avoid the virilizing side effects of steroid use. Here it may actually be a better option than an injectable nandrolone preparation, as blood hormone levels are obviously much easier to control with an oral steroid. While Nilevar may be too androgenic to recommend for this purpose, Orabolin seems to fit the build quite nicely.

Experienced steroid users (especially men) will again most likely be disappointed with the effect of Orabolin. Those who have experimented with this compound have generally found that a considerable amount of tablets are needed for a noticeable benefit. The recommended dosage for an athlete is therefore in the range of 20-40mg (10-20 tablets) per day for men and 12-16mg (6-8 tablets) for women. Men can up this dosage a bit more (supply provided) for added effect, but it will be accompanied by an increased intensity of estrogenic side effects (and of course level of strain placed on the liver). As with most milder steroids, it is usually much easier to just addition a second steroid to enhance the effect of therapy than it is to keep raising the dosage. For men, the effect of Orabolin is really two week for it to be used alone effectively, so stacking is probably a very good recommendation. Women can use it alone to good benefit, but should begin to worry about androgenic activity if the dosage goes above 8 tablets.

Since the demand for Orabolin is so low, it does not make its way to the black market very often. When found it is usually not the Organon brand name, which may even be nonexistent at this point, but one of a couple Australian veterinary preparations. The only solid tablet from this country is in fact the .5mg Nandoral, made by Intervet. When found this can probably be considered a safe buy, but then again its pitiful dose would make it a very poor choice next to just about any other available steroid. The cost just to use en effective amount would have to be absurd. The oral paste, Nitrotain by Nature-Vet, would be a much better choice (if you don't mind eating a mouthful of paste every day). It should also be noted that in Mexico, the drug preparation Maxibol is sometimes confused with the old American preparation Maxibolin. This is purchased in the belief that it is a steroid, a notion commonly enforced by unscrupulous pharmacy workers. Mexican Maxibol is in fact a vitamin supplement, containing only a coenzyme of vitamin b12.

Oral Turinabol (4-chlorodehydromethyltestosterone)

Androgenic	Anabolic	Standard
N/a	>100	Methyltestosterone (oral)

Chemical Names:
4-chloro-17a-methyl-17b-hydroxyandrosta-1,4-dien-3-one

Estrogenic Activity: none
Progestational Activity: n/a (low)

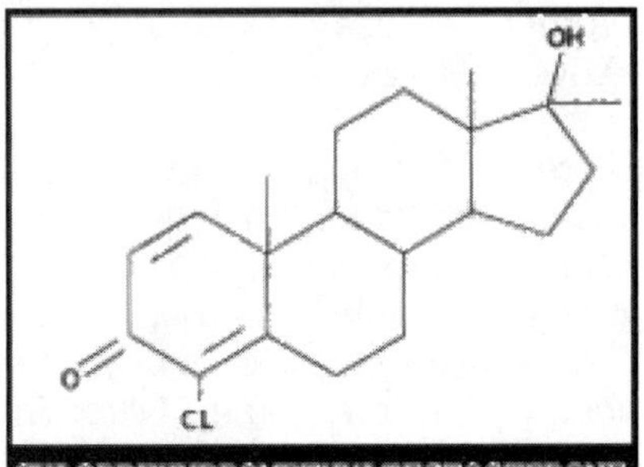

CHLORDEHYDROMETHYLTESTOSTERONE

Oral Turinabol is an anabolic steroid developed and made famous by scientists in East Germany years ago. Actually, this is more a steroid of infamy actually, as it was one of the closely held secrets inside the "East German Doping Machine". I am referring to a state sponsored doping program, called "State Plan 14.25", that operated in East Germany for a period of time between the 1960's and 80's. It was an aggressive anabolic steroid administration program, designed with one goal in mind: cheating the Olympic drug test. In many cases, the Olympic athletes, both male and female, were unwitting participants, simply told by their trainers and coaches that they were being given "vitamins". Many of these blue vitamins turned out to be Oral Turinabol, a potent and undetectable (at the time) anabolic steroid. As many as 10,000 unsuspecting athletes were given anabolic steroids during the time the program was active. For a more in-depth look at this dramatic historic event, including the trials of several former East German officials for their participation, I recommend you look at the book "Faust's Gold: Inside the East German Doping Machine" by Steven Ungerleider.

OT, as it is called, is a potent derivative of Dianabol. It is structurally a cross between methandrostenolone and clostebol (4-chlorotestosterone), having the same base structure as Dianabol with the added 4-chloro alteration of clostebol. This makes OT a "kindler gentler Dianabol", the new steroid displaying a much lower level of androgenic activity in comparison to its more famous counterpart. Its anabolic activity of chlorodehydromethyltestosterone is somewhat lower than that of Dianabol as well, but it does maintain a much more favorable balance of anabolic to androgenic effect overall. This means that at any given level of muscle-building activity, OT will be much less likely to produce the classic androgenic side effects such as oily skin, acne, aggression, and male-pattern hair loss (if genetically prone) than would Dianabol.

The 4-chloro attachment used with this steroid also inhibits its ability to be aromatized. Therefore, OT is not going to present its user with unwanted estrogenic side effects like water retention, increased fat deposition, or gynecomastia. While Dianabol tends to produce puffiness and a little fat retention in its users, which hides muscle definition, the exact opposite effect usually happens with OT. OT tends to promote gain in lean tissue mass, accompanied by an increased look of density, hardness, and definition due to the intensified androgen to estrogen ratio. For bodybuilding purposes, this makes OT a great pre-contest or cutting steroid, not really a bulking agent of choice. Athletes in sports where speed tends to be a primary focus would also find favor in OT, obtaining a strong anabolic benefit without having to carry around any extra water or fat weight.

When this drug was available in Western Europe, the typical daily dosages used by men were in the rage of 20mg to 40mg. Women would get by on less, usually a single 5mg tablet. That is, unless you were an East German female Olympic swimmer, in which case you could have been swallowing as many as 30 tablets per day (we can understand why long-term virilizing side effects were reported over and over again in the "doping trails"). When used in the recommended dosing levels, OT definitely proves itself as a potent lean tissue builder. Again, it will provide less overall muscle bulk than Dianabol, but with its lack of estrogen conversion, the gains obtained with OT, even if smaller in total, are visibly of better quality. Although there is a clear relationship between OT and Dianabol when it comes to molecular structure, ultimately it would be much more appropriate to be comparing the activities of this steroid to those of other mild, non-aromatizing anabolics like stanozolol, oxandrolone or methenolone.

For a long time the only known preparation of OT to ever circulate on the black market was the 5mg tabs from Jenapharm in Germany. It was one of the fringe benefits of the post-Berlin Wall reunification. This product was sold in foil and plastic strips of 10 small blue oval shaped tablets each. Twenty tablets (2 strips) came packed in each box. The Jenepharm product lasted a little longer than the public doping scandal over its use in the former

East Germany, and for more than a decade chlorodehydromethyltestosterone was officially extinct. Recently, British Dragon in Thailand started producing this steroid again, to the amazement of most of the steroid market. They sell it under the old brand name of **Turanabol**. The product comes in the form of 10mg small pink square tablets, with “BD” stamped into one side and “10” in the other. They are sold in pouches of 500 tablets each. The pouches themselves should carry a BD security hologram sticker (see Security Stickers). There were a couple of underground manufacturers who were purportedly selling this steroid shortly before BD, however they are the first established company to add it to their line (I think you known my views on underground steroids). Feedback on the product has been excellent thus far, and although I have been unable to lab test it, I am confidant it is the real thing. British Dragon actually directly challenged me to test it, but the lack of a “standard” (a purified sample known to be pure drug from a laboratory source) has made absolute quantification difficult. I tend to doubt they would have done so, however, unless they knew ahead of time what the results were going to look like.

Oranabol (oxymesterone)

Androgenic	Anabolic	Standard
50	330	Methyltestosterone (oral)

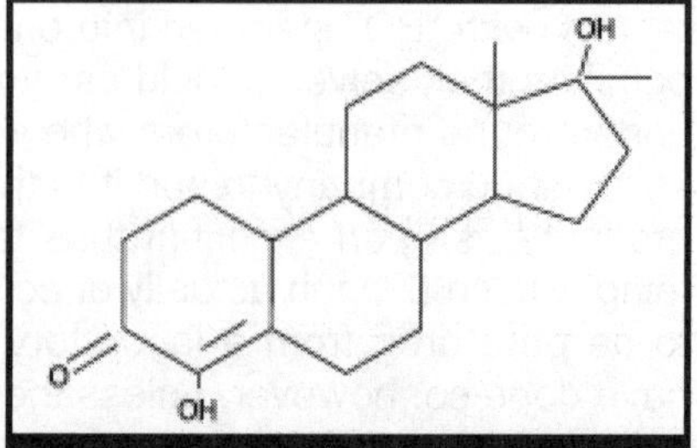

OXYMESTERONE

Chemical Names:
4-hydroxy-17a-methyltestosterone
4,17-dihydroxyandrost-4-en-3-one

Estrogenic Activity: none
Progestational Activity: none

Oranabol (oxymesterone) is a potent synthetic derivative of the anabolic steroid 4-hydroxytestosterone. The then well-known Italian drug manufacturer Societa Farmaceutici Italia first investigated it back in the late 1950's. They filed patent for this compound around the same time, in at least three countries including the United Kingdom, the United States, and Italy[85]. This drug saw limited clinical use as a prescription agent under the Oranabol brand name in Spain and Italy, and under the names Anamidol, Balnimax, and Theranabol in other countries including Japan and the UK. Oxymesterone has been unavailable as a prescription drug worldwide for more than three decades now, and was never released in the United States. At very best I would guess that only a small handful of U.S. athletes have been lucky enough to experiment with this obscure anabolic steroid over the years, and certainly very few in recent times.

By the 1990's, oxymesterone had already become a forgotten relic of early steroid development. If you asked around, nobody would probably have been able to remember what this drug was, let alone how well it worked with bodybuilders and athletes. In all this time there was only one isolated mention of its use in the medical literature. The drug showed up in a report released in 1993 by the department of Clinical Pharmacology and Toxicology at St. Vincent's Hospital in New South Wales, concerning two young football players who died of cardiac events in 1988 and 1990. The two men, whom had unobstructed arteries and were only 18 and 24 years of age[86], died during routine training sessions. To spite never being offered for sale in Australia, and having been removed from the global market long before 1988, oxymesterone had been detected in the men during autopsy. No conclusive link between the drug and their deaths was established. There is nothing else in the medical literature to suggest that this steroid is of any particular danger, and little that we can infer from this paper except that oxymesterone was likely being used widely as a designer steroid in the Australian Football league. Although steroid abuse may have been a contributing factor in the deaths of these men, it seems illogical to conclude that Oranabol was the cause.

In regards to its structure, oxymesterone differs from 4-hydroxytestosterone only by the addition of a c-17 alpha methyl group. This essentially makes Oranabol the "methyltest of hydroxytestosterone". This analogy may not be 100% fair, however. The word methyltestosterone conjures up some fairly negative impressions. It is looked upon as sort of the rotten stepchild of testosterone, with behavior that is quite offensive compared to its non-methylated parent. It is always causing trouble with water bloat, gynecomastia, and a poor overall ratio of results to side effects. For many it is nothing more than a failed attempt to make an oral testosterone. Oxymesterone, fortunately, does not share in methyltestosteroene's failures. Just like its non-methylated analog hydroxytestosterone, oxymesterone remains an effective lean-tissue-building steroid with only a minimal to moderate androgenic component. It has no estrogenic or progestational activity, and no ability to cause side effects related to these female hormones. Overall, Oranabol is a "clean" drug amongst oral steroids: potent, non-aromatizable, and primarily anabolic in nature.

As mentioned already, oxymesterone does not convert to estrogen. The 4-hydroxyl group present on this steroid inhibits the process of aromatization. In fact, when applied to testosterone (as in hydroxytestosterone) a suicide aromatase inhibitor is created, capable of significantly suppressing serum estrogen levels. It is unknown if this property exists in Oranabol, as this potential aspect of its behavior has never been investigated. Its non-estrogenic and non-progestational profile would support, at the very least, this being a steroid for increasing muscle density and visibility, regardless of a related aromatase inhibiting effect. This steroid's 4-hydroxylation also prevents 5-alpha reduction, an activity that otherwise would allow this steroid to be considerably androgenic. Oxymesterone is a lot milder than its monstrosity of a chemical name (4-hydroxy-17-alpha-methyltestosterone) might at first suggest. Again, this is ultimately a cutting anabolic much more than it is a bulking androgen like testosterone, Dianabol, or Anadrol, ideal for precontest use or incorporation into lean-mass building stacks. Of course as a potentially active aromatase inhibitor, this agent may stack well with other aromatizable "bulking" steroids as well.

When it comes to other safety issues, we need to remember that oxymesterone is going to behave in many regards like a typical methyated oral anabolic steroid. It carries some risk of liver toxicity due to the c-17 alpha alkylation, and should be respected as such. Drug duration of alkylated orals is usually kept under eight weeks or so, in an effort to minimize the chance that a significant level of liver toxicity will be reached. This steroid also has the same potential to cause androgenic side effects found in all steroids, and as such is not immune from causing oily skin, acne, or aggravated hair loss (if you are genetically prone). It may be milder than many other steroids, but it is not completely benign in this regard. No agent is. As a steroid that potentially has an intrinsic aromatase-inhibiting effect, women should also take extreme caution with its use. If this trait holds true, oxymesterone might act as more than just a mild anabolic. It may indeed precipitate the uncomfortable menopausal-type side effects that can befall women when they suppress their estrogen levels.

According to the standard laboratory assays, methylhydroxytest is over three times more anabolic than methyltestosterone on a milligram for milligram basis. This is a considerable difference, but not quite the extreme potency we see with some of the other recent methylated steroids we've seen released like methyl-1-testosterone, methyldienolone, and methylhydroxynandrolone. Therefore, we would see more "normal" doses used by male bodybuilders with this drug, who would typically find 10-20mg per day to provide a very measurable benefit. At this level one should be seeing formidable strength gains, increased fat loss, increased muscle definition, and an overall increase in lean tissue mass. This drug would further stack well with a variety of other steroids, especially a 400-600mg per week dose of an injectable base like testosterone or Equipoise® during bulking phases of training, or a milder anabolic like Deca-Duraboln® or Primobolan® for cutting and defining. All of these stack combinations should work extremely well, and would not add to the moderate liver toxicity already present in oxymesterone.

To spite being an effective steroid, oxymesterone has just never been a widely available one. This agent has not been available as a prescription drug in over 30 years, so there is little chance you are going to run into one of the old European products. It is possible that one of the international steroid manufacturing companies might decide to add it to their lines one day, given the recent trend of searching out novel old compounds for re-release. Personally, I think this would be very interesting to see, given how extremely rare this drug is, and how decent it looks on paper. Perhaps over the next few years we will see a number of old steroids make a comeback on the international steroid market. If so, there are not a large number of drugs that I would place in front of this one as compounds of great interest. However, short of this happening, oxymesterone will remain a drug of myth and conjecture for today's steroid user.

Parabolan (trenbolone hexahydrobenzylcarbonate)

Androgenic	Anabolic	Standard
500	500	Nandrolone acetate

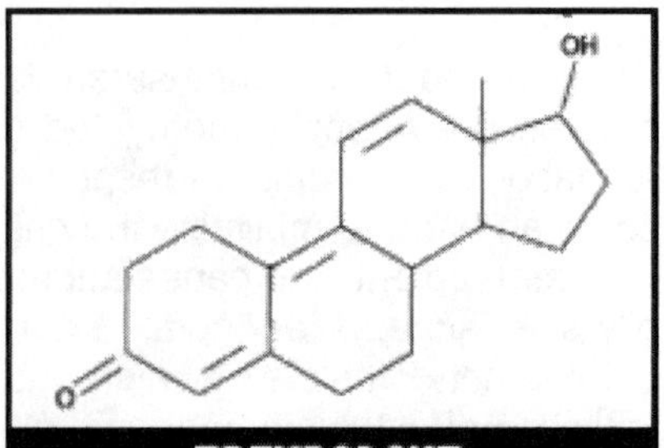

TRENBOLONE

Chemical Names:
17beta-Hydroxyestra-4,9,11-trien-3-one

Estrogenic Activity: none
Progestational Activity: low to moderate

Parabolan® is the former French brand name for trenbolone hexahydrobenzylcarbonate, a rarely seen injectable ester of the anabolic steroid trenbolone. Negma in France produced Parabolan until its voluntary discontinuance in 1997. For some time after, there was no real Parabolan preparation to be found on the black market (although to this day you can still find counterfeits of the former French product). That, however, is no longer the case, and this steroid is indeed being sold again through other manufacturers. You may associate the base steroid in this product, trenbolone, with the long deceased Finajet. Finaject was a veterinary steroid that was popular in the United States during the 1980's, which contained trenbolone acetate. This is a much faster acting form of trenbolone than we have present in Parabolan, but otherwise they are the same (see: trenbolone acetate). Parabolan contains the long acting ester hexahydrobenzylcarbonate instead, which extends the activity of the drug for more than two weeks. This form has always been thought of as more suitable design for human use, due to the need for less frequent injections. Original French Parabolan was packaged only in ampules of 1.5ml, one ampule per a box. Each ampule contained 76mg of trenbolone hexahydrobenzylcarbonate, which is equivalent to 50mg of trenbolone base (French drugs commonly make this calculation). Since it is no longer available, however, it is pointed out for reasons of interest only.

Trenbolone is a very potent androgen with strong anabolic activity. It is well suited for the rapid buildup of strength and muscle mass, usually providing the user exceptional results in a relatively short time period. The anabolic effect of this drug is often compared to popular bulking agents such as testosterone or Dianabol, with one very important difference. Trenbolone does not convert to estrogen. This is indeed a very unique compound since mass drugs, almost as a rule, will aromatize (or cause other estrogen related troubles) heavily. When we think of taking milder (regarding estrogen) steroids we usually expect much weaker muscle growth, but not so with Parabolan. Here we do not have to worry about estrogen related side effects, yet still have an extremely potent mass/strength drug. There is no noticeable water retention, so the mass gained during a cycle of Parabolan will be very hard and defined (providing fat levels are low enough). Gynecomastia is also not much of a concern, so there shouldn't be any need to addition an antiestrogen if trenbolone is the only steroid administered.

The high androgen level resulting from this steroid, in the absence is excess estrogen, can also accelerate the burning of body fat. The result should be a much tighter physique, hopefully without the need for extreme dieting. Parabolan can therefore help bring about an incredibly hard, ripped physique and is an ideal product for competitive bodybuilders. This is of course no secret, and when available on the market, Parabolan was the most sought after contest preparation drug. Now this it is no longer produced, acceptable substitutes for this purpose include of course veterinary trenbolone acetate preparations, as well as Halotestin®, Proviron® and Masteron.

Trenbolone is notably more potent than testosterone, and has an effect that is as much as three times as strong on a milligram for milligram basis. Likewise we can expect to see some level of androgenic side effects with use of this compound. Oily skin, aggressive behavior, acne and hair loss are therefore not uncommon during a cycle with this steroid. The androgenic nature of this drug of course makes it a very risky item for women to use, the chance for virilization symptoms extremely high with such a potent androgen. And since the hexahydrobenzylcarbonate ester will extend the activity of this drug for weeks, blood levels can be very difficult to control. Since many of the masculinizing side effects associated with steroid use can be permanent, women considering the use of this compound should take extreme caution. It can be weeks before blood levels decline should a problem become evident.

Trenbolone is also much more potent than testosterone at suppressing endogenous androgen production. This makes clear the fact that estrogen is not the only culprit with negative feedback inhibition, as here there is no buildup of this hormone to report here. There is, however, some activity as a progestin inherent in this compound, as trenbolone is a 19-nortestosterone (nandrolone) derivative (a trait characteristic of these compounds). However, it seems likely that much of its suppressive nature still stems from its powerful androgen action. With the strong impact trenbolone has on endogenous testosterone, of course the use of a stimulating drug such as HCG and/or Clomid®/Nolvadex® is recommended when concluding steroid therapy (a combination is preferred). Without their use it may take a prolonged period of time for the hormonal balance to resume, as the testes may at first not be able to normally respond to the resumed output of endogenous gonadotropins due to an atrophied state.

Those who have used Parabolan regularly would often claim it to be indispensable. A weekly dosage of 3 ampules (228mg) was the most popular range when running a cycle, however, many did find it highly effective in lesser amounts. Although a weekly administration schedule would prove sufficient, athletes usually injected a single ampule per application, the total amount spread evenly throughout the week. While Parabolan is quite potent when used alone, it was generally combined with other steroids for an even greater effect. Leading up to a show one could successfully add a non-aromatizing anabolic such as Winstrol® or Primobolan®. Such combinations will elicit a greater level density and hardness to the build, often proving dramatic for a stage appearance. We could also look for bulk with this drug, and addition stronger compounds like Dianabol or Testosterone. While the mass gain would be quite formidable with such a stack, some level of water retention would probably also accompany it. Moderately effective anabolics such Deca-Durabolin® or Equipoise® would be somewhat of a halfway point, providing extra strength and mass but without the same level of water bloat we see with more readily aromatized steroids.

The main problem with Parabolan historically was that it had always been extremely difficult to obtain, even when the original brand was still being manufactured in France years ago. The demand for this drug was always much greater than the supply, leading to many many counterfeits over the years. Some fakes of the old French drug were of such superb accuracy that the untrained eye would miss the details every time. However, too many years have past to hope you will ever see even a single old ampule of this brand on the black market. Some of those good-looking counterfeits are still being made today. Don't be fooled. Although real French Parabolan is long gone now, the steroid itself is not. Body Research in Thailand has recently started selling trenbolone hexahydrobenzylcarbonate under the name **Danabolan**. This product is an exact copy of the original Parabolan formulation, even down to the 1.5ml ampule. Body Research is a reputable firm, making this item one I'd be more likely to trust than not.

The Thai firm British Dragon is also selling this steroid. They have formulated it into a 100mg/mL product called **Trenabol Depot**. This is also the first Parabolan clone to come in a large multi-dose vial, in this case 10ml in total. This is a rare product, and will lilely be a high profile target for counterfeiters within a short period of time. Be sure your vial 1) does not carry a hologram sticker (BD now uses these on tablet products only) 2) The label has a shiny metallic red strip, not just red ink and 3) your top reads, "TEAR" and "FLIP UP" (BD uses a very specific top). British Dragon has also added this steroid to their blended trenbolone product called **Trinabol 150**. This product includes equal amounts of trenbolone acetate and trenbolone enanthate (see Drug Profiles: Trinabol 150).

Primobolan (methenolone acetate)

Androgenic	Anabolic	Standard
44-57	88	Testosterone

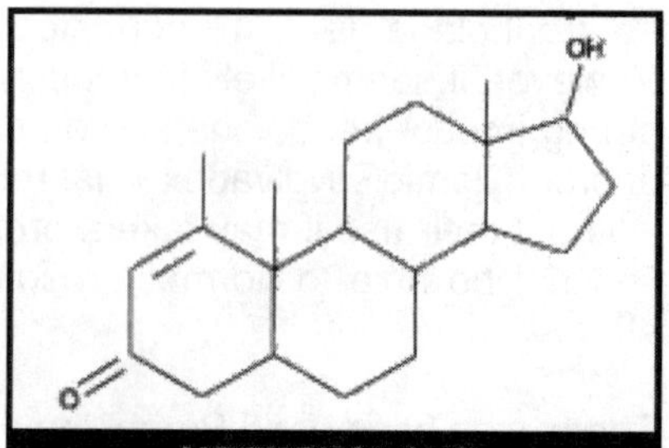

METHENOLONE

Chemical Names:
17beta-Hydroxy-1-methyl-5alpha-androst-1-en-3-one
1-methyl-1(5-alpha)-androsten-3-one-17b-ol
1-methyl-1-testosterone (informal)

Estrogenic Activity: none
Progestational Activity: n/a (low)

This section refers to the oral Primobolan® preparation, which contains the drug methenolone acetate. It is very similar in action to the injectable Primobolan® Depot (methenolone enanthate), but obviously here the drug is designed for oral administration. At one time Schering was in fact also manufacturing an injectable methenolone acetate (Primobolan® acetate, out of manufacture since 1993), which proved to be very useful for pre-contest cutting purposes. This steroid is now gravely missed, as it was once a favorite among European competitors. Although we still have the acetate in oral form, it is a close, but not equal substitute (injection is a much more efficient form of delivery for this steroid).

Methenolone regardless of the ester is a very mild anabolic steroid. The androgenic activity of this compound is considerably low, as are its anabolic properties. One should not expect to achieve great gains in muscle mass with this drug. Instead, Primobolan® is utilized when the athlete has a specific need for a mild anabolic agent, most notably in cutting phases of training. It is also a drug of choice when side effects are a concern. A welcome factor is that Primobolan® is not c17 alpha alkylated as most oral steroids are. Due to the absence of such an alteration, this compound is one of the few commercially produced oral steroids that are not notably stressful to the liver. While liver enzymes values have been affected by this drug in some rare instances, actual damage due to use of this substance is not a documented problem. Unfortunately the 1 alkylation and 17-beta esterification of Primobolan® do not protect the compound very well during first pass however, so much of your initial dose will not make circulation. This is obviously why we need such high daily dose with the oral version of Primobolan®.

Primobolan® will also not aromatize, so estrogen related side effects are of no concern. This is very useful when leading up to a bodybuilding contest, as subcutaneous water retention (due to estrogen) can seriously lessen the look of hardness and definition to the muscles. Non-aromatizing steroids are therefore indispensable to the competitor, helping to bring about a tight, solid build the weeks leading up to a show. And of course without excess estrogen there is little chance of the athlete developing gynecomastia. Likewise there should never be a need for antiestrogen use with this steroid. Primobolan® is also said to have a low impact on endogenous testosterone production. Although this may well be true in small clinical doses, it will not hold true for the bodybuilder. For example, in one study more than half of the patients receiving only 30-45 mg noted a suppression of gonadotropin levels of 15% to 65%[87]. This is a dose far less than most bodybuilders would use, and no doubt increasing it would only lead to worse suppression. One would therefore still need a testosterone stimulating drug like HCG or Clomid®/Nolvadex® when concluding a low-dose Primobolan® cycle, unless a deliberately small dose were being used.

It is also important to note that although the androgenic component of Primobolan® is low, side effects are still possible. One may therefore notice oily skin, acne and facial/body hair growth during treatment. Men with a predisposition for hair loss may also find it exacerbates this condition, and wish to avoid this item (nandrolone injectables are a much better choice). While always possible, side effects rarely reach a point where they interfere with the progress of cycle. Primobolan® is clearly one of the milder and safer oral steroids in production. Female athletes, older or more sensitive individuals and steroid beginners will no doubt find this a comfortable steroid to experiment with.

The dosage for men is somewhere in the range of 75-150mg daily. A mild anabolic such as Primobolan® is often used in conjunction with other steroids for optimal effect, so some users find a slightly lower dose effective when stacking. During a dieting or cutting phase, thought to be its primary application, a non-aromatizing androgen like Halotestin® or trenbolone can be added for example. Such combinations would enhance the physique without water retention, and help bring out a harder and more defined look of muscularity. Non-aromatizing androgen/anabolic stacks like this are in fact very popular among competing bodybuilders, as they prove to be quite reliable for rapidly improving the contest form. This compound is also occasionally used with more potent androgens during bulking phases of training. The addition of testosterone, Dianabol or Anadrol 50® would prove effective for instance, although the gains are likely to be accompanied by some level of smoothness due to the added estrogenic component.

Among women, Primobolan® is one of the most popular steroids in use. At a dosage of 50-75mg daily, virilization symptoms are extremely uncommon. One would of course not expect a tremendous amount of muscle mass with this drug, and instead should expect a slow and steady (quality) increase. Some women choose to further add-in other anabolics such as Winstrol® or oxandrolone, in an effort to increase the muscle building effectiveness of a cycle. While both of these compounds are quite tolerable, one must be sure not to use too high an accumulated dosage. Troublesome androgenic side effects are always a possibility with steroid use, even with very mild substances. Taken at too high a dosage, these weak anabolics can become a formidable danger to femininity. It would, therefore, be the best advice not to use the normal dosage range of both, but instead start with a much lower dosage of each steroid to compensate for the other.

Over the past several years, oral Primobolan tablets have become increasingly more difficult to find on the black market. It seems that Schering, the first and almost only company to ever manufacture this drug, has been aggressively discontinuing production in most of the markets around the world. About a decade ago we could find Primobolan orals in nearly two-dozen different countries, and in three different dosage strengths (5mg, 25mg, and 50mg). Now, only two of Schering's oral Primobolan preparations remain, sold only in Japan (5mg) and South Africa (25mg). It seems likely that Schering is no longer finding the drug very profitable, or perhaps is finding few legitimate (medical) reasons to continue selling it. With the medical community largely steering away from anabolic steroids these days, it would seem likely that bodybuilders have been the main block of consumers of Primobolan for some time now. Perhaps the company simply doesn't feel the minimal profits are worth the potential long-term PR disaster if they continue to support this market of customers.

Thankfully there are a few other legitimate firms to come out with this steroid in recent years, making the loss of the Schering product not a fatal one. The most recent is the Brisith Dragon product **Primobol**, which carries a whopping 50mg per tablet dose. It is sold in foil-lined paper pouches of 30 tablets. Since the demise of the old French 50mg product more than 10 years ago, we had not seen such a high dose of this steroid for a long time. The Primobol product is, therefore, likely to catch the attention of counterfeiters very quickly (BD has had numerous issues with counterfeiters already), so make sure you inspect the product closely when shopping. First, the tablets are square and are imprinted with "BD" on one side and "50" on the other. So far none of the bogus operations have been able to copy this new pill dye. Also, be sure you see the BD security hologram sticker on the pouch (see Security Stickers).

Quality Vet in Mexico also released **Metenol QV** this pass year, which is another high dosed 50mg tablet of methenolone acetate. The product comes in bottles of 50 tablets, each of which is packaged in its own box. Both the box and bottle will carry the company's security hologram sticker. Be sure to look for this when shopping.

The Mexican veterinary drug firm Ttokkyo laboratories introduced an oral version of Primobolan at one time, named **Primo-Plus**. This product, as with the full Ttokkyo line, is no longer in production. The company had been hanging on the past couple of years, to spite the arrest of owner Dr. Molina; however, it does appear they finally closed their doors recently.

Bratis Labs, another veterinary drug manufacturer in Mexico, was also selling a product called **Metabolon 25**. This product is made in 25mg tablets, and is packaged in bottles of 100 tablets each. However, I have not seen much of this product lately, nor the firm. I cannot confirm this product is still being made, nor have I been able to lab test it for its contents.

Overall, oral Primobolan is an extremely scarce item today. Since we do not find many steroids on the black market that originate from Japan or South Africa (likely due to tighter controls on these drugs), you can probably expect not to find the name brand Primobolan product ever again. At best, you can rely on the British Dragon product for now, and hope that the next couple of years bring about new manufacturers willing to invest in this very expensive pharmaceutical. There is still a clear demand for it out there, as one of the few effective non-toxic orals to ever be produced commercially.

Primobolan Depot (methenolone enanthate)

Androgenic	Anabolic	Standard
44-57	88	Testosterone

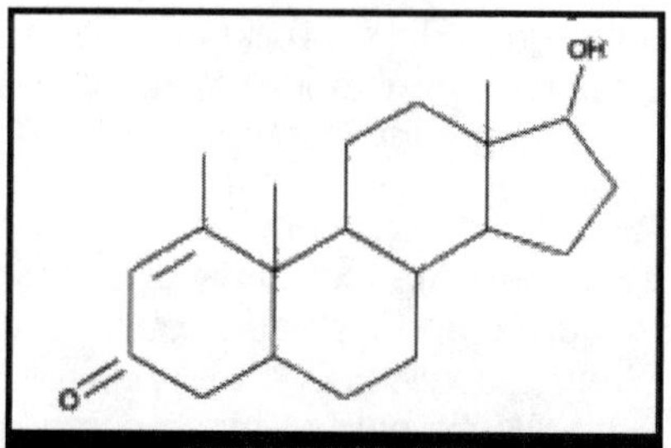

METHENOLONE

Chemical Names:
17beta-Hydroxy-1-methyl-5alpha-androst-1-en-3-one
1-methyl-1(5-alpha)-androsten-3-one-17b-ol
1-methyl-1-testosterone (informal)

Estrogenic Activity: none
Progestational Activity: n/a (low)

Primobolan® Depot is the injectable version of the steroid methenolone. This of course is the same constituent in Primobolan® Orals (methenolone acetate), both produced by the firm Schering. In this preparation, an enanthate ester is added to the steroid, which causes a slow and gradual release from the site of injection. Its duration of activity would thus be quite similar to testosterone enanthate, with blood levels remaining markedly elevated for approximately two weeks. Methenolone itself is a long acting anabolic, with extremely low androgenic properties. On the same note the anabolic effect is also quite mild, its potency considered to be slightly less than Deca-Durabolin® (nandrolone decanoate) on a milligram for milligram basis. For this reason, Primobolan® is most commonly used during cutting cycles when a mass increase is not the main objective. Some athletes do prefer to combine a mild anabolic like "Primo" with bulking drugs such as Dianabol, Anadrol 50® or testosterone however, presumably to lower the overall androgen dosage and minimize uncomfortable side effects. When choosing between Primobolan® preparations, the injectable is preferred over the oral for all applications, as it is much more cost effective.

Primobolan® displays many favorable characteristics, most which stem from the fact that methenolone does not convert to estrogen. Estrogen linked side effects should therefore not be seen at all when administering this steroid. Sensitive individuals need not worry about developing gynecomastia, nor should they be noticing any water retention with this drug. The increase seen with Primobolan® will be only quality muscle mass, and not the smooth bloat which accompanies most steroids open to aromatization. During a cycle the user should additionally not have much trouble with blood pressure values, as this effect is also related (generally) to estrogen and water retention. At a moderate dosage of 100-200mg weekly, Primobolan® should also not interfere with endogenous testosterone levels as much as when taking an injectable nandrolone or testosterone. This is very welcome, as the athlete should not have to be as concerned with ancillary drugs when the steroid is discontinued (a less extreme hormonal crash). At higher doses strong testosterone suppression may be noticed however, as all steroids can act to suppress testosterone production at a given dosage. Here of course an ancillary drug regimen may be indicated.

Side effects in general are usually not much of a problem with Primobolan® Depot. There is a chance to notice a few residual androgenic effects such as oily skin, acne, increased facial/body hair growth or an aggravation of male pattern baldness condition. This steroid is still very mild however, and such problems are typically dose related. Women will in fact find this preparation mild enough to use in most cases, observing it to be a very comfortable and effective anabolic. If both the oral and injectable were available for purchase, the faster acting oral should probably be given preference however. This is simply due to the fact that blood hormone levels are more difficult to control with a slow acting injectable, the user also having to wait many days for steroid levels to diminish if side effects become noticeable.

Overall, Primobolan® Depot is actually considered to be one of the safest anabolic steroids available. Steroid novices, older athletes or those sensitive to side effects would undoubtedly find it a very favorable drug to use. The typical "safe" dosage for men is 100-200mg per week, a level that should produce at least some noticeable muscle growth. In European medicine it is not uncommon for Primobolan® to be used safely at such a dosage for extended periods of time. Among athletes, men may respond to weekly doses of 200mg but regular users will often inject much higher doses looking for a stronger anabolic effect. It is not uncommon for a bodybuilder to take as much as 600 or 800mg per week (6 to 8 100mg ampules), a range which appears to be actually quite productive. Of course androgenic side effects may become more pronounced with such an amount, but in most instances it should still be quite tolerable.

In addition, it is most popular for male bodybuilders to stack Primobolan® with other (generally stronger) steroids in order to obtain a faster and more enhanced effect. During a dieting or cutting phase, a non-aromatizing androgen like Halotestin® or trenbolone can be added. The strong androgenic component should help to bring about an added density and hardness to the muscles. On the other hand (or in addition), we could add Winstrol®, another mild anabolic steroid. The result of this combination should again be a notable increase in muscle mass and hardness, but in this case the gain should not be accompanied by greatly increased side effects. As mentioned earlier, Primobolan® Depot is also used effectively during bulking phases of training. The addition of testosterone, Dianabol, or Anadrol 50® would prove quite effective for adding new muscle mass. We would, of course, have to deal with estrogenic side effects, but in such cases Primobolan® should allow the user to take a much lower dosage of the more "toxic" drug and still receive acceptable results.

Women respond well to a dosage of 50-100mg per week, although (as stated above) the oral should usually be given preference. Additionally, some choose to include Winstrol® Depot (50 mg per week) or Oxandrolone (7.5-10mg daily) and receive a greatly enhanced anabolic effect. Remember though, androgenic activity can be a concern and should be watched, particularly when more than one anabolic is used at a time. If stacking, it would be best to use a much lower starting dosage for each drug than if they were to be used alone. This is especially good advice if you are unfamiliar with the effect such a combination may have on you. A popular recommendation would also be to first experiment by stacking with oral Primobolan®, and later venture into the injectable if this is still necessary.

All forms of Schering Primobolan® Depot will be packaged in 1ml glass ampules. They will contain 100mg of the drug in Europe, and 50mg in Mexico. A single 100mg ampule will generally sell for around $15 to $20 in the United States. The 50mg ampule was usually a bit cheaper, perhaps $10 on average. However, as of late, we have not seen this steroid in Mexican pharmacies. It is possible that Schering has dropped Primobolan® from production in this country too. This was not a very cost cost effective product anyway, as it would usually sell for at or near the price of the 100mg version.

The situation with injectable **Primobolan® Depot** is similar to that of the oral Primobolan® tablets. The drug is available, but not as abundantly as it was a few years ago. Schering has been actively discontinuing this drug in most of the markets around the world, and only a few countries still carry it at this time. Most notably, Greek Primobolan ampules have been discontinued, as have German, French, and Italian versions of the drug. The only major source countries for genuine Schering Primobolan Depot right now are Spain and Turkey. The way things are going, it will only be a matter of time before the drug is discontinued in these areas of the world as well.

Note that Schering has recently changed the look of their packaging on the **Spanish** and **Turkish** ampules. The new version looks very similar to the ampule of Sustanon from the UK, clear glass with a paper label. The new Primo has three rings on the ampule tip, one yellow and two red. The older dark-glass ampules will no longer be found in circulation, so avoid these. One should also be very cautious when buying Schering Primobolan, especially when the ampules are loose. I'd trust only boxes with accompanying paperwork, and even then you are not out of the woods.

To further differentiate real Turkish Primobolan® Depot from the many counterfeits, here are a couple of things to look at. First, open the bottom flap of the box. It should be cut at an unusual angle, and will not be even left to right like a normal box flap. Many of the more popular fakes missed this, probably for lack of a proper cutting dye. However, at least one counterfeiter has correctly copied this. Therefore, you need to keep looking. Another good point of detail to look at is the Schering logo, which is found on the box and product insert. The counterfeiters tend to show the ribbon in the center of the Schering logo as one filled block < symbol. The correct logo has this ribbon with a small cut where the top and bottom lines intersect, as if to show that the top ribbon is resting on the second one under it. Most often this small detail is lost when the box and insert are scanned into a computer. Now with the ampule, first take a look at the lot number and manufacture date (not the expiration date). The first number in the lot always corresponds with the year the drug was made. Many of the fakes thus far have missed this trait, and these digits do not match.

In regards to the Spanish counterpart, this item is also a high profile item for counterfeiters. There have been many fakes of circulating the past several years, often in large numbers. We've tested a couple of the more popular fakes of recent, and both came back with no steroid ingredients. Spanish Primo is, likewise, a high-risk item. Also, note that Schering is now operating under the name Scherimed in Spain. Many sophisticated copies of the old Schering item are likely to circulate for a while, until counterfeiters update their items. Make sure any new product you purchase reflects the new packaging change. .

The Thai company British Dragon also released its own Primobolan injectable recently, called **Primobol**. It comes in a 10ml vial and provides 100mg/mL of steroid. Actually, I had a chance to lab test this product recently (see Lab Testing), and the lot I sent in was approximately 50% overdosed. This is a significant plus given the relative expense of this rare anabolic. Of course that is not to suggest that BD does this as a matter of practice, but it does bode well in regards to the quality of this company's products. They certainly aren't trying to cut corners. Note that BD does not place a hologram on its injectable vials anymore, but instead uses a red metallic foil inlay on the label (see Security Stickers). Also, the top of a real BD vial should read, "TEAR" and "FLIP UP". A current popular fake reads "FLIP OFF" only.

SYD Group released an injectable Primobolan product in Mexico last year as well, called **Suprimo 100**. It contains the standard dosage strength of 100mg/mL, and comes packaged in a 10ml vial. SYD Group is a very reputable company, so I trust this will be a very popular product on the black market in the months and years ahead. Just be sure your vial carries the SYD Group security hologram sticker, which should assure a legitimate purchase.

Ttokkyo had reportedly introduced **Primo-Plus** not that long ago, which was a 10ml 100mg/mL vial of the drug. At best it was available for a few months, around the time that the company's owner was arrested and extradicted to the U.S. on narcotics distribution charges. Ttokkyo operated for much longer than expected after that, however, have since closed down by all reports. Do not expect to find real old vials of this product on the black market.

Protabol (thiomesterone)

Androgenic	Anabolic	Standard
61	456	Methyltestosterone (oral)

Chemical Names:
1,7-bis(acetylthio)-17b-hydroxy-17-methylandrost-4-en-3-one

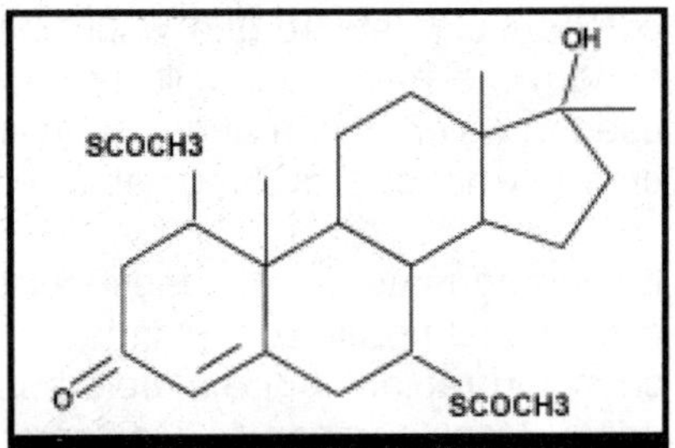

THIOMESTERONE

Estrogenic Activity: none
Progestational Activity: n/a

Protabol (thiomesterone) is an oral anabolic steroid that is derived from methyltestosterone. This drug was sold back in the 1960's by AB Drago in Sweden, and under the Emdabolin brand name by Chugai Labs in Tokyo Japan. It saw an extremely limited period of use in Europe, and has gone practically unseen in the United States. Thirty years ago American athletes were treated to rumors of thiomesterone, and how this rare and highly coveted steroid was the holy grail of anabolics. The problem is, nobody could obtain a cycle to very its effect. Little was even known about the compound itself. To date I have never even seen its chemical structure disclosed in any of the bodybuilder's steroid reference books. Dan Duchaine made the single note of this steroid I could find, and wrote of it in his Underground Steroid Handbook II only, *"This is the elusive thiomesterone, always written up in the research as the most promising, most potent anabolic with no androgenic side effects. Let me know if you ever find any."*

Although there is no real-world feedback on this steroid to make reference of, it was possible to locate its chemical structure and some basic research into its pharmacological properties. We have enough to look at now to say that thiomesterone is certainly no magic steroid, however it does indeed appear to display very favorable properties. To spite being a derivative of the potent oral methyltestosterone, thiomesterone is far more anabolic than it is androgenic. In fact, standard laboratory assays show that its anabolic potency exceeds its androgenic by a factor 7.5. Milligram for milligram it is also about 4.5 times more anabolic than methyltestosterone, while having only about 60% of its androgenic component. Perhaps not quite the "pure" anabolic that it was rumored to be thirty years ago, in regards to potency and anabolic/androgenic separation, thiomesterone is still very much in the same class as the popular anabolics stanozolol and oxandrolone.

As mentioned, thiomesterone is a derivative of methyltestosterone. It differs from this base steroid by the addition of two acetylthio groups, one at carbon 1 and the other at carbon 7. This creates a hormone with significantly different behavior than methyltestosterone. For one, occupation of a bond at C-1 by the first acetylthio group prevents aromatization. This eliminates any tendency for estrogen-linked side effects like water retention, increased fat deposition and gynecomastia. The second acetylthio modification at C7, furthermore, inhibits 5-alpha reduction. As this is a testosterone analog, one would expect its 5-alpha reduced "dihydro" metabolite to be significantly stronger. This accounts for the stronger androgenic activity of testosterone-based drugs in general. No such increase in potency is possible with thiomesterone, however. The C7 acetylthio group contributes, at a very significant level, to the high anabolic to androgenic ratio of this agent.

Since thiomesterone has a similar level of anabolic potency to stanozolol and oxandrolone, we would expect that oral effective daily dosages for men would fall in the range of 15-25mg. Here we should see effective lean tissue gains, modest strength gains, increased muscle definition and heightened vascularity. The fact that estrogen levels will be kept low definitely helps this agent when it comes to tightening up or contest preparations. Thiomesterone is a very versatile steroid in general, and should stack well with other mild injectable anabolics like Primobolan or Deca-Durabolin for cutting cycles, or stronger androgens/aromatizable steroids like testosterone or boldenone for bulking phases. Being that this steroid is a c-17 alpha alkylated (methylated) compound, it will present some level of liver toxicity. It would therefore be best not to stack it with other c-17aa orals, so that this toxicity is kept to a minimum.

Thiomesterone is a steroid of low androgenic side effects. Sensitive individuals would probably notice some oily skin or acne, but should not be responding with heightened aggression and mood elevations the same way they would with something stronger like testosterone or Dianabol. It might also be one of the few orals that those worried about hair loss might experiment with in low doses. Its low androgenic and estrogenic component may put many of this drug's more sensitive users at risk for incurring a loss of libido and even lethargic side effects, however. This would be readily corrected by the addition of some other aromatizable or more androgenic compound (testosterone would be the preferred remedy). One might want to be prepared by having some on hand. As a highly anabolic agent, thiomesterone would also be a preferred agent among women, and would be used in a versatile manner very similar to Primobolan or Anavar. Doses would be kept low, of course, and would probably not exceed 5mg per day.

It is unfortunate that thiomesterone is not a steroid we have available on the global steroid market today. With its exceptional profile and high level of potency, it certainly would be a popular product if it were. Things have been changing rapidly in the steroid business though, and if current trends continue we may very well see this steroid again. Many companies are searching out old steroids in an effort to provide their customers something new. For now, at the very least, we can say it is no longer an agent of myth and legend. We have pulled back the curtain, and seen thiomesterone for the steroid that it is. It is nothing magic, but an excellent steroid nonetheless. Even if it is not possible to put this information to practical use right now, I suspect many readers will still find this profile of interest as rare look into a very poorly known and understood drug. Perhaps it may even spark an interest in the right person, who will be responsible for resurrecting thiomesterone one day. We can hope, anyway.

Proviron (mesterolone)

Androgenic	Anabolic	Standard
30-40	100-150	Testosterone propionate

Chemical Names:
17beta-hydroxy-1alpha-methyl-5alpha-androstan-3-one
1-methyl-5alpha-dihydrotestosterone

Estrogenic Activity: none
Progestational Activity: not significant

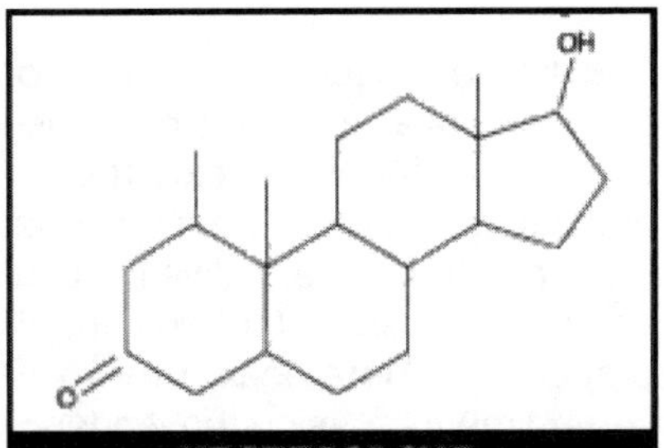

MESTEROLONE

Proviron® is the Schering brand name for the oral androgen mesterolone (1methyl-dihydrotestosterone). Just as with DHT, the activity of this steroid is that of a strong androgen which does not aromatize into estrogen. In clinical situations Proviron® is generally used to treat various types of sexual dysfunction, which often result from a low endogenous testosterone level. It can usually reverse problems of sexual disinterest and impotency, and is sometimes used to increase the sperm count. The drug does not stimulate the body to produce testosterone, but is simply an oral androgen substitute that is used to compensate for a lack of the natural male androgen.

Although this steroid is strongly androgenic, the anabolic effect of it is considered too weak for muscle building purposes. This is due to the fact that Proviron® is rapidly reduced to inactive metabolites in muscle tissue, a trait also characteristic of dihydrotestosterone, The belief that the weak anabolic nature of this compound indicated a tendency to block the androgen receptor in muscle tissue, thereby reducing the gains of other more potent muscle building steroids, should likewise not be taken seriously. In fact due to its extremely high affinity for plasma binding proteins such as SHBG, Proviron® may actually work to potentate the activity of other steroids by displacing a higher percentage into a free, unbound state.

Among athletes Proviron® is primarily used as an antiestrogen. It is believed to act as an antiaromatase in the body, preventing or slowing the conversion of steroids into estrogen. The result is somewhat comparable to Arimidex® (though less profound), the drug acting to prevent the buildup of estrogen in the body. This is in contrast to Nolvadex®, which only blocks the ability of estrogen to bind and activate receptors in certain tissues. The anti-aromatization effect is preferred, as it is a more direct and efficient means of dealing with the problem of estrogenic side effects. A related disadvantage to Nolvadex® is that if discontinued too early, a rebound effect may occur as high serum estrogen levels are again free to take action. This of course could mean a rapid onset of side effects such as gynecomastia and water retention. Most athletes actually prefer to use both Proviron® and Nolvadex®, especially during strongly estrogenic cycles. With each item attacking estrogen at a different angle, side effects are often greatly minimized.

The anti-estrogenic properties of Proviron® are not unique to this compound. A number of steroids have in fact demonstrated similar activity. Dihydrotestosterone and Masteron (2methyl-dihydrotestosterone) for example have been successfully used as therapies for gynecomastia and breast cancer due to their strong anti-estrogenic effect. It has been suggested that nandrolone may even lower aromatase activity in peripheral tissues where it is more resistant to estrogen conversion (the most active site of nandrolone aromatization seems to be the liver). The anti-estrogenic effect of all of these compounds is presumably caused by their ability to compete with other substrates for binding to the aromatase enzyme. With the aromatase enzyme bound to the steroid, yet being unable to alter it, and inhibiting effect is achieved as it is temporarily blocked from interacting with other hormones.

Many bodybuilders also favor this drug during contest preparation, when a lower estrogen/high androgen level is particularly sought after. This is especially beneficial when anabolics like Winstrol®, oxandrolone and Primobolan® are being used alone, as the androgenic content of these drugs is relatively low. Here Proviron® can supplement a well-needed androgen, and bring about an increase in the hardness and density of the muscles. Many experienced bodybuilders are now swearing by it in fact, incorporating it effectively in most any cycles that require upward adjustments to the androgen/estrogen ratio. Many women even find a single 25mg tablet to efficiently shift the hormone balance in the body, greatly impacting the look of definition to one's physique. Since this is such a strong androgen however, extreme caution should be taken with administration. Higher dosages clearly have the potential to cause virilization symptoms quite readily. For this reason, females will rarely take more than one tablet per day, and limit the length of intake to no longer than four or five weeks. One tablet used in conjunction with 10 or 20mg of Nolvadex® can be even more efficient for muscle hardening, creating an environment where the body is much more inclined to burn off extra body fat (especially in female trouble areas like the hips and thighs). Again, extreme caution should be taken.

The typical dosage for men is one to four 25 mg per tablets per day. This is a sufficient amount to prevent gynecomastia, the drug often used throughout the duration of a strong cycle. As mentioned earlier, it is often combined with Nolvadex® (tamoxifen citrate) or Clomid® (clomiphene citrate) when heavily estrogenic steroids are being taken (Dianabol, testosterone etc.). Administering 50mg of Proviron® and 20mg Nolvadex® daily has proven extremely effective in such instances, and it is quite uncommon for higher dosages to be required. And just as we discussed for women, the androgenic nature of this compound is greatly welcome during contest preparation. Here again Proviron® should noticeably benefit the hardness and density of the muscle, while at the same time increasing the tendency to burn off a greater amount of body fat.

Proviron® is usually well tolerated and side effects (men) are rare with dosages under 100 mg per day. Above this, one may develop an excessively high androgen level and encounter some problems. Typical androgenic side effects include oily skin, acne, body/facial hair growth and exacerbation of a male pattern baldness condition, and may occur even with the use of a moderate dosage. With the strong effect DHT has on the reproductive system, androgenic actions may also include an extreme heightening of male libido. And as discussed earlier, Women should be careful around Proviron®. It is an androgen, and as such has the potential to produce virilization symptoms quite readily. This includes, of course, a deepening of the voice, menstrual irregularities, changes in skin texture and clitoral enlargement.

Proviron® is also not a c17 alpha alkylated compound, an alteration commonly used with oral anabolic/androgenic steroids. Not using this structure in the case of Proviron® removes the notable risk of liver toxicity we normally associate with oral dosing. We therefore consider this a “safe” oral, the user having no need to worry about serious complications with use. This steroid in fact utilizes the same 1-methylation we see present on Primobolan® (methenolone), another well tolerated orally active compound. Alkylation at the one position also slows metabolism of the steroid during the first pass, although much less profoundly than 17 alpha alkylation. Likewise Proviron® and Primobolan® are resistant enough to breakdown to allow therapeutically beneficial blood levels to be achieved, although the overall bioavailability of these compounds is still much lower than methylated oral steroids.

All versions of the drug are manufactured or licensed by Schering at this time, and should cost about $1-$2 per 25 mg tab. In many instances this item is obtained via mail order, and here can sell for less than .50 per tab. This drug is packaged in both push-through strips and small glass vials, so do not let this alarm you. There is currently no need to worry about authenticity, as no counterfeits are known to exist. If money and availability does not prevent it, Arimidex® is actually a much better choice than Proviron® though, at least as far as aromatase inhibitors go (Arimidex offers no androgenic action). But due to much lower costs, drugs like Nolvadex® and Proviron® remain the “standard” antiestrogen treatments among athletes, even if they are not quite the most effective agents.

Sanabolicum (nandrolone cyclohexylpropionate)

Androgenic	Anabolic	Standard
37	125	Testosterone

Chemical Names:
19-norandrost-4-en-3-one-17beta-ol
17beta-hydroxy-estr-4-en-3-one

Estrogenic Activity: low
Progestational Activity: moderate

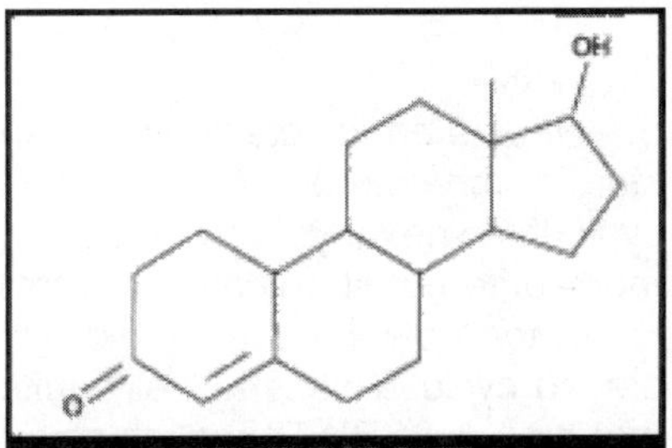

NANDROLONE

Sanabolicum is an injectable nandrolone compound, specifically using the long-acting ester cyclohexylpropionate. The most recent products known to use this steroid are Sanabolicum by the Nile Company in Egypt, and Sanabolicum-Vet by Werfft-Chemie in Austria. Other products existed that used this steroid at one time as well, however, to my knowledge they have been off the market for a very long time now. The cyclohexylpropionate ester used here, incidentally, was also used with testosterone in the French product Testosterone CHP Theramex (also off the market at this time). This ester is long enough acting that products using it can be injected on a less frequent basis (in a medical setting anyway), however, in the context of bodybuilding the standard once weekly schedule is usually adhered to.

In both the Egyptian and Austrian product, the maximum steroid concentration used is only 50 mg/mL. We also need to take into account that the cyclohexylpropionate ester is large, taking up nearly a third of the total steroid weight. As such, each 50mg dose delivers less than 34 milligrams of actual nandrolone. To say this steroid was not a powerhouse would be an understatement. In the dosages provided these products are too weak to consider using alone. Well, unless you are a masochist, and go out of your way to find low dosed steroids that need to be injecting in large volumes each week. If so, this steroid may be for you (you might want to look for the Egyptian 25mg ampules though). Otherwise, your best bet would be to use 100-200mg per week, and stack it with other anabolics (which ones would of course depend on your goals). Women would find the dosage strength fine, however it would be advisable to opt for a faster acting ester such as nandrolone phenylpropionate, which allows for a better level of control over blood levels.

I am unsure of the current production status of this steroid. The Sanabolicum compounds never seem to circulate, even years ago when their existence was a confirmed fact. I, therefore, cannot give you much by way of advice on spotting fakes. I think these two steroids are so rarely even heard of, and available in such low doses, that counterfeiters have little interest in trying to duplicate them. Since Sanabolicum is essentially interchangeable with Deca-Durabolin anyway, you are probably much better off opting for a 100 mg/mL or 200 mg/mL version of this steroid instead, especially if you are sure of its legitimacy.

Spectriol (testosterone/nandrolone/methandriol blend)

Spectriol is an injectable veterinary steroid preparation from Australia, which contains a blend of several different steroid ingredients. More specifically, it contains five components: three testosterone esters (propionate, cypionate, hexahydrobenzoate), nandrolone phenylpropionate and methandriol dipropionate. To spite having so many different steroids in the same vial, we are only looking at a total steroid concentration of 65 mg/mL. Spectriol is not the powerhouse steroid by any means, but can still most certainly be a value item to include in your next steroid cycle. This is actually quite an unusual steroid product, but then again this is Australia, and the company that makes it (RWR) makes several oddball steroids like this (many of which are blends that include methandriol dipropionate).

Each ml of Spectriol contains:

Methandriol Dipropionatye	20 mg
Nandrolone Phenylpropionate	15 mg
Testosterone Propionate	10 mg
Testosterone Cypionate	10 mg
Testosterone Hexahydrobenzoate	10 mg

This product seems to be designed so that it will provide a fairly good balance of anabolic and androgenic effect for its user. Of the 65mg present in each milliliter of solution, about 30mg are esters of the strong androgen testosterone. The remaining 35mg is a combination of methandriol and nandrolone, two steroids which are much more anabolic in nature. The two sides complement each other very well, allowing for greater muscle growth, and less androgenic and estrogenic side effects, than if taking an injectable testosterone exclusively (for a more comprehensive discussion of these individual steroids, please refer to their respective drug profiles). The only main issue with this steroid is its relatively low dosage strength, which makes it difficult to run a full cycle on Spectriol alone. Were one to attempt this, the weekly dosage would probably have to be in the range of 260-520mg, which equates to a total oil volume of 4-8ml. This is quite a bit of oil to inject each week, especially when many other steroid products are available that come in a strength of 200mg/mL or more.

Spectriol is found only in 10ml multi-dose vials, and is made only by RWR (Nature Vet Pty) in Australia. This item does not circulate on the international black market in much volume, as Australia is no longer considered a major source country for steroids. Australian prescription drugs are definitely not as easy to divert to the black market in high volumes as they are in some other countries, and the steroid market especially has been scrutinized in recent years. Add this to the fact that the packaging on most Australian veterinary products, Spectriol included, is pretty easy to duplicate, and I would not consider this to be an item I'd immediately trust when coming across it. Be especially suspicious of anyone that suddenly has a whole lot of it. But provided you can verify the source, and are obtaining it at a good price, it most certainly can be a good steroid to have in your toolbox. Unfortunately, not many people find themselves in such a situation, and should be rightly suspicious of this and all Australian veterinary products with unverifiable authenticity.

Sten (testosterone cypionate & propionate)

Androgenic	Anabolic	Standard
100	100	Standard

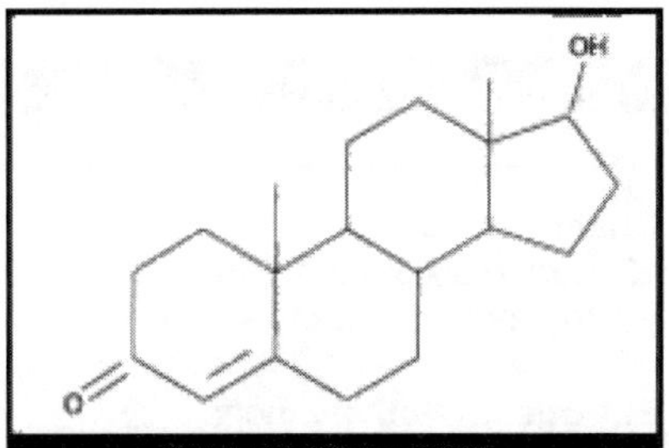
TESTOSTERONE

Chemical Names:
4-androsten-3-one-17beta-ol
17beta-hydroxy-androst-4-en-3-one

Estrogenic Activity: moderate
Progestational Activity: low

Sten is a two-component testosterone blend that is made only in Mexico. It is manufactured by the firm Atlantis, and Sten is one of Mexico's more inexpensive human-use testosterone products. The two active steroids in this product are testosterone propionate (25mg), testosterone cypionate (75mg). Each ampule also contains an added 20mg of DHEA (dehydroepiandrosterone). Some references incorrectly list it to contain 20mg DHT or dihydrotestosterone (another androgen). This is just a confusion of the Spanish word for DHEA (dehidroisoandrosterona), which at a quick glance looks similar to DHT. Holding the DHEA irrelevant at the moment, this steroid basically contains 50mg of testosterone per ml.

Many compare this item to Sustanon, but consider it to be a low budget alternative. While it does contain two testosterone esters with a "sustained release" effect, Sten is active for a much shorter duration. The testosterone propionate does provide a fast effect, as with Sustanon, but the blood levels from the testosterone cypionate will drop about two weeks after each injection. This far short of the duration seen with Sustanon, so clearly there is a noticeable difference between the two compounds. Of course they are both strong testosterone products, and the end result difference would not be very great between the two.

If we used these two testosterone esters separately, a cumulative dosage of 200-400mg per week would be the most common. Therefore, 2 to 4 ampules of Sten are usually injected each week. To reduce the volume of each injection, this amount is usually broken up into two to four separate shots, each consisting of 2ml or one full ampule. Even with this separation we are taking 4 to 8 ml per week, which is quite a bit when compared to other products like Sustanon. It makes it additionally difficult to add in another injectable steroid, as the volume would no doubt be quite uncomfortable. For this reason Sten is not in high demand, and generally used only when other testosterone preparations are unavailable.

The effect of this steroid would be comparable to that seen with all injectable testosterone products. It is well suited for a quick mass and strength gain, accompanied by a number of androgenic and estrogenic side effects. Water retention of course is common, as is the development of gynecomastia. Sensitive individuals may find an antiestrogen necessary when taking this drug, as is common with virtually all testosterones. Androgenic side effects like oily skin, acne, facial/body hair growth and premature hair loss are also likely. The addition of Proscar/Propecia® may prove useful to minimize such effects, especially for those noticing the onset male pattern baldness. And although some female bodybuilders do occasionally utilize testosterone propionate, the cypionate present in this substance (being much longer acting) makes for poor company. An unlucky female athlete would have to wait a couple of weeks for testosterone levels to significantly drop, which is obviously much too long when virilization symptoms are developing.

In Mexico, 2 ampules are packaged in a box and sells for about $5. Here on the U.S. black market, a single loose ampule of Sten can sell for as much as $10. There are currently no fakes.

Steranabol Ritardo (oxabolone cypionate)

Androgenic	Anabolic	Standard
20-60	50-90	Testosterone

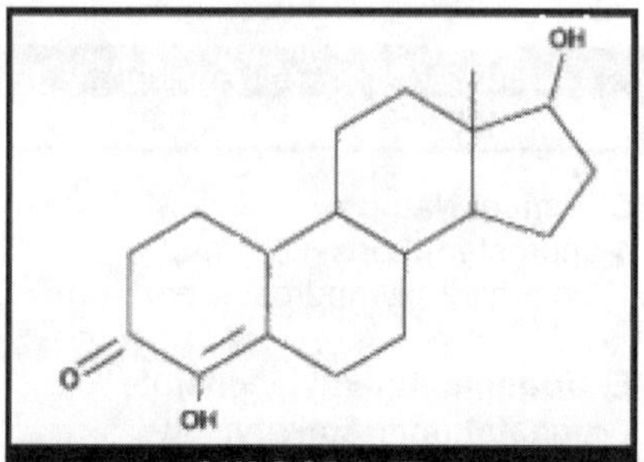

OXABOLONE

Chemical Names:
19-norandrost-4-en-4,17b-ol-3-one
4,17beta-dihydroxyestr-4-en-3-one

Estrogenic Activity: none
Progestational Activity: n/a (low)

Steranabol Ritardo is an injectable steroid product that was being produced by Pharmacia & Upjohn in Italy until fairly recently (it has been discontinued for several years now). This product specifically contains the obscure anabolic steroid oxabolone cypionate. Oxabolone is a close structural derivative of 19-nortestosterone (nandrolone). It differs from this mild anabolic agent only by the addition of a 4-hydroxyl group, the same alteration that is used to make hydroxytestosterone (oxabolone is 4-hydroxynandrolone) from testosterone. This compound is present in Steranabol Ritardo in a dosage concentration of 12.5 mg per ml, with each 2ml ampule carrying only 25mg of steroid in total. This low dosage was always an unfortunate trait of this product, as hydroxynandrolone is otherwise a fairly effective steroid.

As a nandrolone based compound, oxabolone is more anabolic than androgenic in nature. However, it does seem to have some unique traits that make it stand out next to nandrolone, such as an inability to convert to estrogen (blocked by the addition of 4-hydroxylation). Hydroxynandrolone even seems to exhibit strong anti-aromatase activities, at least the best I can tell anecdotally without a formal study. This probably makes sense, given that it is the 4-hydroxyl group that makes formestane (hydroxyandrostenedione) and hydroxytestosterone both potent suicide substrates for the aromatase enzyme. This means not only that estrogenic side effects are not likely with the use of this drug, but also that it may even be useful in countering side effects caused by the conversion of other steroid hormones to estrogen.

Studies with hydroxyandrostenedione show that (in this case) the 4-hydroxy group seems to interfere with 5-alpha reduction, at least to some extent. This may explain another trait of oxabolone, namely that it seems to not have the same dramatic dissociation between anabolic and androgenic affects that we see with nandrolone. This steroid, although more anabolic than androgenic, is a little more balanced in this regard. It may therefore be, at least slightly, less likely to interfere with libido in the same way that Deca-Durabolin tends to (at least in terms of a direct head-to-head comparison, oxabolone is still primarily anabolic in nature, and such libido interfering traits tend to be present in many of the "anabolic" compounds for certain users).

It terms of muscle-building potency, it would be a mistake to simply equate oxabolone with nandrolone. Oxabolone is actually a moderately weaker steroid, at least according to the standard assays that we use to evaluate steroid compounds. However, that does not mean it is a useless agent, as indeed this is an interesting steroid to say the least. In my experience it seems to help you produce a much harder, tighter look than nandrolone, probably owing to the fact that it probably delivers an anti-estrogenic effect instead of a slight estrogenic one. For those who find nandrolone to be a failure during cutting/hardening cycles, this nandrolone derivative may be worth looking at.

Being that it came in such a low concentration (12.5mg/mL), Steranabol Ritardo was a little difficult to use as an anabolic. If you are a male bodybuilder, had this item, and wanted to use it alone for your next cycle, all I could say is: good luck. It is less potent than nandrolone, which means you are probably going to need at least 200-300mg weekly. At 25mg per 2ml ampule, reaching this dose would be a painful and arduous task. Just do the math. 300mg per week, with a dose of 25mg per ampule, would equate to 12 ampules. With each ampule containing 2ml of solution, that is a full 24cc of oil to inject each week (8 full 3cc needles full). You certainly would not catch me trying it. Instead, I would look at this steroid as more of an adjunct to an already running stack. 3-4 ampules per week, or 75-100mg in total, should be sufficient to notice some level of hardening and fat loss. Provided it did not get lost in a plethora of other drugs, you should be able to notice it working at this dose. All this is really academic anyway, as Steranabol Ritardo is no londer available. The base steroid hydroxynandrolone was sold in the U.S. as a supplement for a short time, however officially became a controlled substance in 2005.

Sustanon (testosterone blend)

Androgenic	Anabolic	Standard
100	100	Standard

Chemical Names:
4-androsten-3-one-17beta-ol
17beta-hydroxy-androst-4-en-3-one

Estrogenic Activity: moderate
Progestational Activity: low

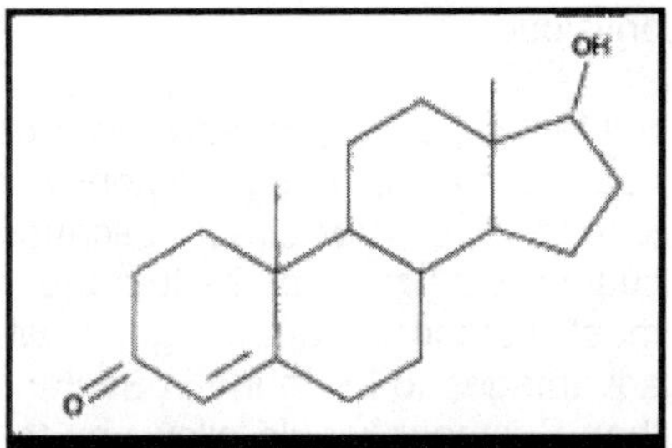

TESTOSTERONE

Sustanon 250® is an oil-based injectable testosterone blend, developed by the international drug firm Organon. It typically contains four different testosterone esters: testosterone propionate (30 mg); testosterone phenylpropionate (60 mg); testosterone isocaproate (60mg); and testosterone decanoate (100 mg), although a lower dosed version is also produced. An intelligently "engineered" testosterone, Sustanon is designed to provide a fast yet extended release of testosterone. The propionate and phenylpropionate esters in this product are quickly utilized, releasing into circulation within the first four days. The remaining esters are much slower to release, staying active in the body for about two and three weeks (respectively). This is a big improvement from standard testosterones such as cypionate or enanthate, which provide a much shorter duration of activity, and a more variable blood level. A slightly shorter acting Sustanon 100, which uses only three esters, is also made by Organon in certain areas.

Sustanon '100'	Sustanon '250'
20mg testosterone propionate	30mg testosterone propionate
40mg testosterone phenylpropionate	60mg testosterone phenylpropionate
40mg testosterone isocaproate	60mg testosterone isocaproate
	100mg testosterone decanoate

As with all testosterone products, Sustanon is a strong anabolic with pronounced androgenic activity. It is most commonly used as a bulking drug, providing exceptional gains in strength and muscle mass. Although it does convert to estrogen, as is the nature of testosterone, this injectable is noted as being slightly more tolerable than cypionate or enanthate. As stated throughout this book, such observations are only issues of timing however. With Sustanon, blood levels of testosterone are building more slowly, so side effects do not set in as fast. For equal blood hormone levels however, testosterone will break down equally without regard to ester. Many individuals may likewise find it necessary to use an antiestrogen, in which case a low dosage of Nolvadex®(tamoxifen citrate) or Proviron®(mesterolone) would be appropriate. Also correlating with estrogen, water retention should be noticeable with Sustanon. This is not desirable when the athlete is looking to maintain a quality look to the physique, so this is certainly not an idea drug for contest preparation.

Being a strong androgen, we can expect the typical side effects. This includes oily skin, acne body/facial hair growth and premature balding. The addition of Proscar®/Propecia® should be able to minimize such side effects, as it will limit the testosterone to DHT (dihydrotestosterone) conversion process. Sustanon will also suppress natural testosterone production rather quickly. The use of HCG (human chorionic gonadotropin) and/or Clomid® (clomiphene citrate)/Nolvadex® (tamoxifen citrate) may be necessary at the conclusion of a cycle in order to avoid a hormonal crash. Remember though, Sustanon will remain active in the body for up to a month after your last injection was given. Beginning you ancillary drug therapy immediately after the steroid has been discontinued will not be very effective. Instead, HCG or Clomid®/Nolvadex® should be delayed two or three weeks, until you are near the point where blood androgen levels are dropping significantly.

Although Sustanon remains active in the body for approximately three weeks, injections are taken at least every 10 days. An effective dosage ranges from 250mg (one ampule) every 10 days, to 1000mg (four ampules) weekly. Some athletes do use more extreme dosages of this steroid, but this is really not a recommended practice. When the dosage rises above 750-1000mg per week, increased side effects will no doubt be outweighing additional benefits. Basically you will receive a poor return on your investment, which with Sustanon can be substantial. Instead of taking unnecessarily large amounts, athletes interested in rapid size and strength will usually opt to addition another compound. For this purpose we find that Sustanon stacks extremely well with the potent orals Anadrol 50® (oxymetholone) and Dianabol (methandrostenolone). On the other hand, Sustanon may work better with trenbolone or Winstrol® (stanozolol) if the athlete were seeking to maintain a harder, more defined look to his physique.

Sustanon 250 is probably the most sought after injectable testosterone. I must, however, emphasize that this is not due to an unusual potency of this testosterone combination (remember esters only effect the release of testosterone), but simply because a "stack" of four different esters is a very good selling point. To the naïve customer it "*must*" be better; after all, there are *four* different steroids in there, not just one! But the reality is that in most instances you will get a whole lot more for your money with testosterone enanthate or cypionate. The advantages to be found in Sustanon are for the medical user only. If you tied to your doctor for regular injections, than Sustanon would allow you to visit the doctor on maybe a monthly basis, whereas you would need to fork up the cash and time for an office visit every two weeks with one of the other esters. This equates to a clear and dramatic improvement in patient comfort. But if you are a bodybuilder injecting the drug every week anyway, there is simply no advantage to be found in Sustanon at all. Blood levels will build to the same extremes either way. Don't let the fancy stack fool you - Sustanon is just overpriced testosterone.

To spite being much more costly than other esters, Sustanon remains very abundant on the U.S. black market. In fact, the high demand for this steroid has stirred new interest in its manufacture, particularly by veterinary companies in Mexico. As a result, we now have a lot more than the Organon brand name to choose from.

Old lots of Ttokkyo's **Testonon 250** may still in circulation, however, the company is no longer in operation. This item did carry a security hologram sticker when produced, so be sure to locate this on your product should you come across it.

Loeffler's **Testosterona IV L/A** is still around, which contains the same steroid blend in a 10ml vial. Lab tests on Loeffler's Reforvit-B and testosterone propionate did not fair well during the publication of Anabolics 2004, so I can't make any guarantee about the quality of this product.

Tornel makes a version of this steroid called **Supertest-250**. This Mexican vet firm has a long-standing reputation as a *fair quality* company. It always seems to deliver a good dose of steroid, but by most accounts it is typically a little less than what is listed on the label. Tests on their 200mg/mL enanthate in Anabolics 2004 showed about 20% underdosing. That may be the case here, so keep this in mind when calculating cost. Tornel is usually a cheaper product than most competitive brands, so it may still be a better deal even with modest underdosing.

Norvet makes **Testo-Jet LA** in Mexico, which is another 10ml veterinary product. This is a new lab on the steroid scene, although they have a long history of making other vet drugs. Currently the line is not very popular, but will likely catch on if their quality is good.

Bratis, a quasi-legit Mexican manufacturer, was making a version called **Testron 4**. This first has been very quiet as of late, so I cannot confirm they are still producing this item.

Intervet, makers of Laurabolin, manufactures a 5ml vial in Australia called **Durateston**. Don't expect it to circulate the black market very much though, as these drugs are tightly controlled in Australia these days.

BM Pharmaceuticals in India just started producing **Sustaretard 250**, which is in the form a 1ml ampule. This product is very reminiscent of Russian Sustanon by Infar (see below) in its packaging. Pictures are included in the steroid photo section of the book.

Russian Sustanon, manufactured under license by **Infar in India** (for export to former Soviet countries), is still found in the U.S. with some frequency. This product comes packaged in plastic strips that hold five ampules, sealed on the face with white paper label. Each ampule is enclosed in a separate compartment, and the packaging is scored so as to break off individual ampule sections. One standout characteristic is that the ampule labels and packaging bear a big green "250" imprint under the lettering.

Organon Sustanon is marketed directly in Russia now. The product looks very much like European forms of Sustanon, with clear glass ampules, colored bands, and paper labels. Note that the product name is written in Cyrillic as "CYCTAHOH".

Sostenon 250 redi-jects manufactured by Organon in Mexico are also still found, although much less commonly in recent years in light of the less expensive products now coming out of this country. The price for a Sostenon redi-ject is about $7-8 in Mexico, $10 in some more expensive tourist areas. In the United States they can sell for as high as $25 each. Note that even though Organon never had any problems with counterfeit Redi-Jects, they still decided to update their packaging recently with a new security feature. Specifically, they have embedded watermarks of the Organon logo all around the surface of the box. This is a difficult trait to copy without spending quite a bit of money, although probably unnecessary given that the syringes and foil sealed trays are already too costly for underground labs to consider duplicating. If you want a guaranteed safe buy, the Mexican "Pre-load" has always been one.

Less common, but still seen on the US black market, are the **European** versions of **Sustanon** from countries like Italy, Portugal, Belgium, and England. All of these products use ampules that are scored, carry colored (yellow and red) rings on the tip, and have white paper labels.

Durateston, the brand name Organon uses to market this multi-component testosterone blend in Brazil, is also seen in the U.S. on occassion, and should be a reliable buy.

Two versions of this steroid are being made in Egypt by the Nile Co. The first is called **Testonon,** and the second **Sustanon**. The fact that two different versions exist may have to do with licensing issues with Organon, as only the latter product is seen to bear the Organon logo. Fakes are known to exist, so be careful when shopping. In particular, make sure the Nile logo is genuine on the box, which will help you identify one of the most common fakes in circulation at this time (see photo section for comparison photographs).

Sustanon 250 from **Karachi** Pakistan is also popular as of late. These ampules are clear glass with yellow silk-screen printing. This is one of the few versions of this steroid product sold by Organon globally that does not carry a paper label. Fakes are circulating in high volume at this time, so be careful. Note that the current real product has its lot numbers printed on with electronic equipment, and are not silk-screened on the glass at the same time as the rest of the lettering.

Synovex (testosterone propionate & estradiol)

Androgenic	Anabolic	Standard
100	100	Standard

Chemical Names:
4-androsten-3-one-17beta-ol
17beta-hydroxy-androst-4-en-3-one

Estrogenic Activity: moderate
Progestational Activity: low

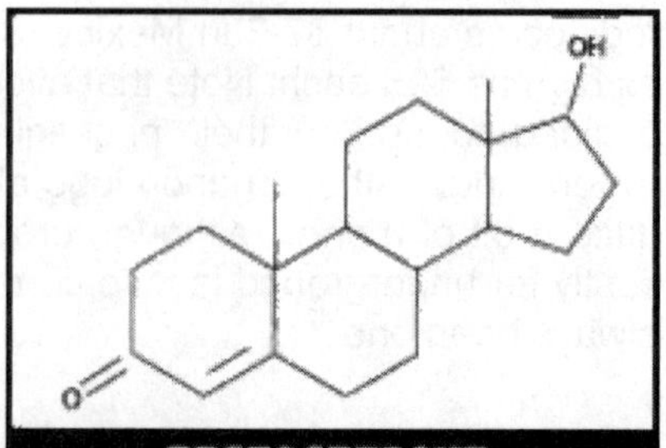

TESTOSTERONE

Synovex is a steroid implant preparation, which is available only as a veterinary item for use in cattle (livestock). The implant comes in the form of small pellets, which are pushed into the ear of an animal with a large implant gun. Here they slowly dissolve and provide an extended release of steroid, lasting for many weeks. The hormone content of Synovex is mixed, with each pellet containing 25mg testosterone propionate and 2.5mg Estradiol Benzoate. The number of pellets in each cartridge will also vary depending on the intended target. Implants denoted "H" for heifer carry the most; in the case of U.S. Synovex-H it is 80 pellets (10 doses consisting each of 8 pellets). We will see a slightly lower pellet count in the "S" implants (steer) and "C" (calf) cartridges.

The combination of estrogen with testosterone (in a 10:1 ratio) has proven to provide an added anabolic/weight gaining effect in feed animals. Athletes have long been aware that strong androgens like testosterone, which aromatize into estrogen quite readily, are the strongest anabolics. It is also observed that antiestrogen drugs like Nolvadex® can decrease the muscle and strength gains received from androgen therapy. It has been therefore theorized that the added estrogen level is in some way responsible for increasing the anabolic effect of androgens. Perhaps this is accomplished by somehow increasing the number of available receptor sites or receptor sensitivity.

With this understanding one might think the estrogen combination in Synovex would prove to be a powerful mix for athletes. But those who have experimented with it have been generally disappointed with the results, as the estrogen in this product is very likely to produce many unwanted side effects. This includes severe gynecomastia, noticeable body fat accumulation and water retention. In many cases the water retained will lead to an unsightly bloated look (extreme loss of definition). Synovex is clearly a good cattle item, but not the ideal steroid for humans. I really think athletes have only become attracted to this product out of sheer desperation for legitimate anabolics. Here in the U.S., cattle implants like this are not controlled substances to spite their steroid content. Synovex is often easy to purchase directly from Agricultural or Veterinary supply stores, as no paperwork is required.

An athlete will typically grind up these pellets, and either rub them on the skin mixed with DMSO and water for transdermal delivery, or mix up his own injection. One should remember that the practice of preparing this for injection would obviously not be very sterile and could be potentially dangerous. Others feel that simply snorting the Synovex powdered is a sufficient delivery method. Some have additionally worked out methods of removing the estrogen from the pellets, to make the drug much more comfortable to use. While this is possible, I think such procedures are generally much more trouble than they are worth. They involve the use of highly flammable materials, and take a number of different steps to complete. All of the estrogen will likely not be removed after all is done, and I cannot see the end product as being the most sanitary thing to administer. In addition to the U.S. version made by Syntex, Synovex is also available in other countries but is never imported due to lack of demand. No counterfeits currently exist, nor are they likely to show up in the future.

Test 400 (testosterone propionate/cypionate/enanthate)

Androgenic	Anabolic	Standard
100	100	Standard

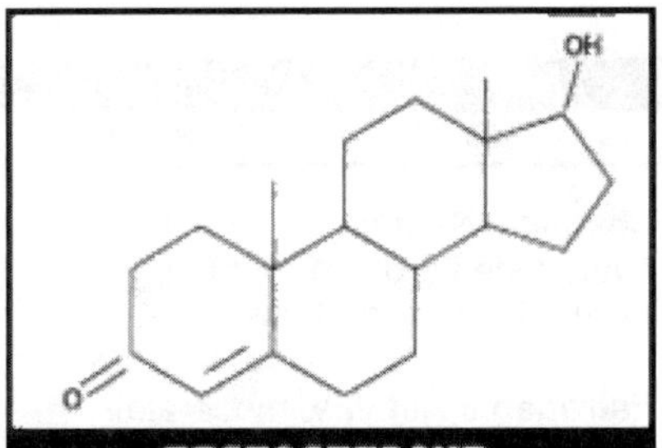

TESTOSTERONE

Chemical Names:
4-androsten-3-one-17beta-ol
17beta-hydroxy-androst-4-en-3-one

Estrogenic Activity: moderate
Progestational Activity: low

Denkall's Test 400 wins the prize for the absolute highest concentration for any steroid in one milliliter of oil. Measuring in at an unheard of 400 milligrams, this product is nothing short of a shocking new addition to the high-dosed veterinary steroid market in Mexico. Test 400 is a blended product, with each milliliter containing 25 milligrams of testosterone propionate, 187 milligrams of testosterone cypionate and 188 milligrams of testosterone enanthate. In order to achieve such a high concentration of steroid it appears that the amount of alcohol used in the solution has been markedly increased. Without increasing the alcohol level 400 milligrams of steroid would simply be too much for the solution to dissolve. The steroid hormone is more soluble in an oily solution with heightened amounts of alcohol, which allows us to achieve a dosage otherwise not possible. The drawback however is that the alcohol makes for an irritating, almost caustic solution to inject. Users commonly report strong irritation and pain at the site of injection, in many instances requiring the user to dilute the steroid with lower dosed oil based products if Test 400 is to be continued. But for those solely interested in maximum dosage, or those willing to later dilute a steroid in order to purchase the most steroid in single vial possible, Test 400 looks like an instant winner.

The design of this steroid most closely resembles that of Testoviron, containing a mix of rapid and medium/slow acting esters. In fact the only difference between the enanthate/propionate blend Testoviron and Test 400 are the dosages of the esters, and the addition of testosterone cypionate. I see no real advantage in stacking testosterone cypionate with enanthate though, as the pharmacokinetics of these two esters are literally identical. Testosterone levels peak and drop in parallel with these two agents, with no visible distinction. Upon closer investigation we see that the only advantage to adding cypionate appears to be a marketing one, as we have a product with three steroids instead of two. At least with Sustanon the release parameters are different with each ester, such that an attempt is made to integrate the four and support the balanced release of testosterone. But with test 400, having propionate and all cypionate would be totally indistinct from having propionate and all enanthate.

The effects of Test 400 would be similar to that of all testosterones. Testosterone is one of the best mass-building agents, so users can expect substantial gains with this product. Testosterone is also strongly estrogenic and androgenic however, so one should expect these gains to be accompanied by equally strong side effects. This includes water retention, possible fat increases and even gynecomastia is estrogenic levels get too high, and acne, oily skin and possible hair loss from the androgenic component of this steroid. As you will see throughout this book and our discussions with testosterone, side effects can be minimized with ancillary drugs such as anti-estrogens like Nolvadex®, Clomid® or Arimidex®, and/or the 5-alpha reductase inhibitor Proscar®. However, most refrain from these drugs, enduring minor side effects unless they become a problem so as to maximize potential tissue gains (both anti-estrogens and Proscar are believed to lower the anabolic potency of a cycle based on testosterone).

Be sure to look for the Denkall security hologram sticker when shopping. This is placed on the packaging to deter duplication, and provides an immediate check that you are getting a legitimate product. Be very careful when you examine the stickers though. If you hold the real hologram up to the light, you will see the image change colors (sort of a prism effect). Counterfeits of Test 400 have been located that carry fake stickers, which are not actually holograms at all. These are just plain silver stickers with faded white printing, but at first glance they look very much like the real thing. Don't be fooled by them.

Testolent (testosterone phenylpropionate)

Androgenic	Anabolic	Standard
100	100	Standard

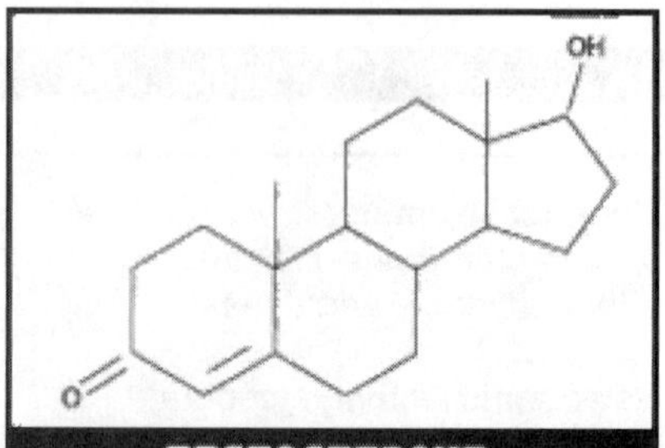

TESTOSTERONE

Chemical Names:
4-androsten-3-one-17beta-ol
17beta-hydroxy-androst-4-en-3-one

Estrogenic Activity: moderate
Progestational Activity: low

Testolent is testosterone's answer to Durabolin (nandrolone phenylpropionate). This product contains testosterone phenylpropionate, the same rapidly deploying ester that makes Durabolin such a fast acting nandrolone injectable. Although testosterone phenylpropionate is one of the constituents in the widely distributed and favored steroid Sustanon, this is the only time it has been made available as a stand-alone product. When it comes to nandrolone, Deca-Durabolin and Durabolin are the standards. One is fast acting; the other quite slow. The need for a fast acting version like nandrolone phenylpropionate (if nandrolone decanoate was the only ester available) is quite clear, as there are indeed times when you need a drug that will get into the system fast. But when it comes to testosterone, we already have testosterone propionate. Is there really any need for a testosterone phenylpropionate?

For the average person, the activity of Testolent will be very difficult, if not totally impossible, to discern from testosterone propionate. For starters, the release duration with phenylpropionate will only be slightly longer than propionate, causing testosterone levels to build in the blood almost as quickly. By the time the second shot is due, blood levels of testosterone should be pretty comparable with both products. Being so fast acting, this drug must obviously be administered on a regular basis if maintaining steady blood levels is desired. Although we would be best served to inject propionate every third day, phenylpropionate can likely be stretched out to an injection every fourth day. While not a major difference, over the course of a full cycle it does save the discomfort of an extra couple of injections.

As an injectable testosterone, Testolent will be an effective strength and mass builder (for a more comprehensive discussion of results and side effects, see testosterone propionate). But aside from requiring fewer shots, and perhaps the chance that some users will notice injection pain with propionate and not phenylpropionate (propionate is notoriously painful at the site of injection), there is really no great advantage to using it. Ultimately testosterone is testosterone regardless of the ester that aids its release into the body, so it is usually difficult to say any one is really superior to another in terms of building muscle. Over the course of a normal cycle one should usually just go with what provides the most amount of base steroid for the least amount of money. If you specifically feel you need a fast acting drug for some reason, either testosterone propionate or phenylpropionate will do the trick. In the end there is no reason to specifically seek out Testolent. However, if it is available for a good price next to propionate, it most certainly will be an acceptable substitute.

Testolent was manufactured until very recently by the Rumanian drug firm Sicomed. It was packaged in 1ml ampules, with each containing 100mg of steroid. However, this product is now discontinued, so only residual stock will be left in circulation at this time. This is expected to dry up rather quickly of course, so do not plan on finding Testolent circulating the black market for very long. This product is not all that unique though, so its loss will not be a hard felt one. Testosterone propionate will likewise work as an effective, almost indistinguishable, substitute for this steroid for all applications.

Testosterone buciclate

Androgenic	Anabolic	Standard
100	100	Standard

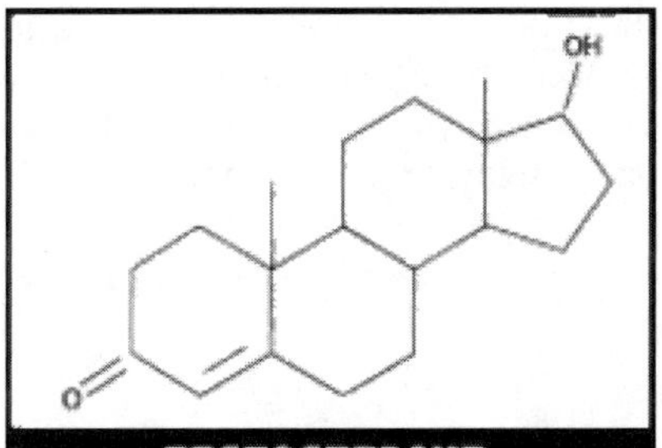

TESTOSTERONE

Chemical Names:
4-androsten-3-one-17beta-ol
17beta-hydroxy-androst-4-en-3-one

Estrogenic Activity: moderate
Progestational Activity: low

Buciclate is one of the newest esters of testosterone to catch the attention of the medical world, entering clinical trials in the early 1990's. This is quite late in the world of steroids. Nearly all of the drugs we have available to us today were identified and studied back in mid 20th century. This drug was created by a group of scientists focused on finding a form of injectable testosterone that would be longer acting and steadier in its day-to-day release than the esters normally in use. The compound they developed utilizes the extremely long, highly oil soluble, and slow acting buciclate ester, which is 20 carbon atoms in length. Being that ester chain length usually correlates well to the duration of release, we can see how different buciclate is next to the other testosterone drugs. This ester is about seven times longer than propionate and three times longer than enanthate. In fact, it is even double the size of testosterone decanoate, the longest acting testosterone ester used as an injectable prescription medication prior. Although testosterone buciclate has seen extensive study at this point, it has yet to be adopted as a prescription drug for widespread use.

To examine the pharmacokinetics of this drug, we can take a look at a study published in the journal of Clinical Endocrinology and Metabolism in November 1992. Here, a group of male patients suffering from primary hypogonadism (low endogenous testosterone output) were given single injections of 200 or 600milligrams. Various markers of health were examined on a regular basis for several months after the shot was given. The 600mg dose was able to restore normal androgen levels rapidly in the treated men, and maintain a therapeutically effective level for an amazing 12 weeks. 200mg was not a sufficient enough dose to return androgen levels back to their normal range, which could have been expected given the level of hormone we know is normally produced by the body. No significant peaks were noted in testosterone levels in either group, which are normally observed with esters like enanthate and cypionate. There were also no significant elevations in estrogen levels, or any side effects of merit. DHT levels did exceed normal in the 600mg group, however there were no unfavorable changes in urine flow, PSA (prostate specific antigen) values, or prostate volume. This investigation seems to suggest that testosterone buciclate holds great promise as a slow acting injectable androgen, with potential to replace other esters for use in areas of androgen replacement and male contraception.

In the context of bodybuilding, testosterone buciclate will be an effective drug, but it is probably not going to win any awards. For one, a cycle based on this compound would be very slow to start. It will take time and numerous injections for peak blood levels of testosterone to be reached. For the same reason it is going to be a drug for long cycles (greater than 4 months in length) only. The slow acting nature of this testosterone ester might cause it to impart its most prominent effects after your other drugs are finished otherwise. There would clearly be no sense in using it during a 6-week cycle of testosterone and dbol, for example. Testosterone buciclate will end up offering its greatest value in cycles lasting more than 6 months, where its slow acting nature may be a benefit by allowing for less frequent injections and greater user comfort. In short cycles this same trait will just be a hindrance, preventing the rapid achievement of optimal blood hormone levels and delay the anabolic effect. In all applications we must also remember that this is a testosterone product, and ultimately offers the same hormone, anabolic benefit and side effects as all other injectable testosterone esters. Aside from its release duration, there is nothing magic about testosterone buciclate.

Most effective use of this compound in a bodybuilding sense is difficult to estimate, but would probably entail the injection of several full doses of 600mg (men) in the first two weeks of a cycle. After this point another full dose can be given every 5 to 15 days, depending on the desired potency or other steroids used. The drug could be discontinued 6-9 weeks before the cycle is going to be concluded, and may even cause androgen levels to remain elevated for as long as 12 weeks after the last dose is given. Post-cycle therapy should be planned accordingly.

Women should never attempt using this agent, even those adventurous enough to meddle with injectable testosterones. This ester is simply too long acting to take the risk. Should you find yourself encountering virilizing side effects, you'd be stuck in a bad cycle for months waiting for the last shots to wear off. It is much safer (if you must take testosterone) to use a fast acting drug, where you have more control over blood levels in the short term. As testosterone buciclate is still really a research drug in Europe, it is not readily available to athletes at this time. It will not be seen on the black market until it is adopted for prescription use in a steroid source country, or the various underground labs decide to take an interest in it. Until then, it remains a drug of academic interest only.

Testosterone butyrate

Androgenic	Anabolic	Standard
100	100	Standard

Chemical Names:
4-androsten-3-one-17beta-ol
17beta-hydroxy-androst-4-en-3-one

Estrogenic Activity: moderate
Progestational Activity: low

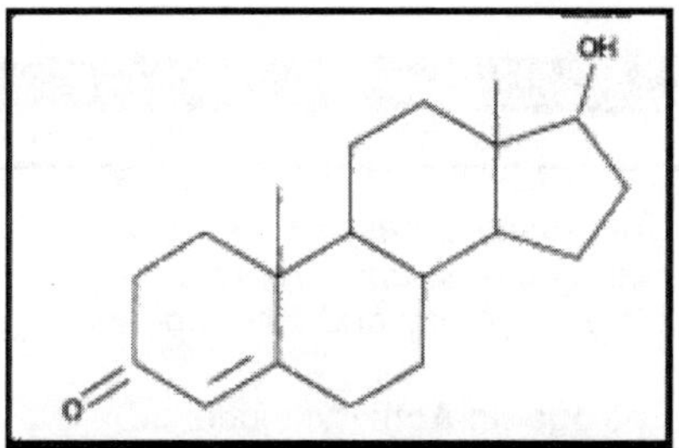

TESTOSTERONE

Testosterone butyrate is a rare ester of testosterone that you are not likely to see in a prescription drug product. It is one of the many steroid esters that had seen a period of investigative interest back in the heyday of steroid research, but ultimately never made its way to commercial production. This is not surprising, as the number of investigated steroids that were never marketed probably exceeds those that were by a factor of 50. There just isn't room for hundreds of different steroid products on pharmacy shelves, which means that many effective compounds are going to be left to sit in research obscurity. Testosterone butyrate is definitely one of them, although it is difficult to call this drug anything special. Its structure is extremely similar to testosterone propionate, with the butyrate ester being only one carbon atom longer. The level of oil solubility and release patterns for these two steroids are, therefore, going to be very close to each other, with the drugs maintaining strong testosterone elevations for only a few days.

Due to the short acting nature of testosterone propionate, it is typically injected every 2nd or 3rd day in order to maintain consistent blood testosterone levels. Since butyrate is ever so slightly longer acting, you could maybe stretch it to every 4th day. We must keep in mind, however, that in the context of taking higher than normal doses for bodybuilding purposes, the different properties of the various agents become immediately blurred. It all comes down to how much hormone you are getting per day, with the esters serving only to prolong the time it takes for each injection to dissipate. Milligram-for-milligram of hormone, they are all the same thing. Therefore, I cannot say much about testosterone butyrate that you haven't heard before. As a testosterone it will be prone to producing both considerable mass gains and normal androgenic/estrogenic side effects of a testosterone product. Should you come across this drug, for all intents and purposes, it can be included in all of your normal cycles in place of testosterone propionate.

Since this drug is not a "commercial" steroid, you cannot buy a legitimate prescription version at this time. It does appear, however, that some of the underground steroid manufacturers are selling this compound, perhaps in an effort to offer their customers something new and different. In reality, there is nothing you can say about this drug that you really couldn't say for propionate. It is a fast acting testosterone product, which provides a relatively low dose of steroid per mg compared to the more oil soluble drugs like testosterone enanthate or cypionate. You can admittedly exceed the 100mg/ml mark pretty easily by adding a lot of alcohol to the product, but that really doesn't make for comfortable injections. The shorter acting butyrate ester itself may also be irritating to many, just as testosterone propionate is. With all this in mind, I see little incentive to risk using an underground product just to experiment with testosterone butyrate. There are just too many other legitimately manufactured esters of testosterone available to choose from, which will work equally well.

Testosterone cyclohexylpropionate

Androgenic	Anabolic	Standard
100	100	Standard

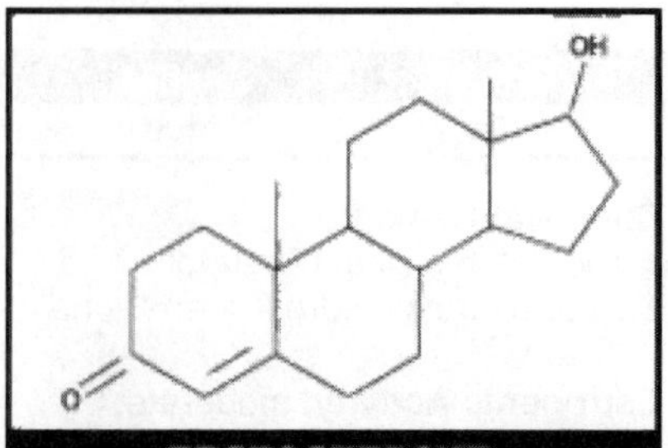

TESTOSTERONE

Chemical Names:
4-androsten-3-one-17beta-ol
17beta-hydroxy-androst-4-en-3-one

Estrogenic Activity: moderate
Progestational Activity: low

Testosterone cyclohexylpropionate, or CHP for short, is a long acting testosterone ester formerly manufactured in France by Theramex. It was made with a steroid concentration of 296, 148 and 37 mg/mL, which equates to 200, 100 and 25 mg of active testosterone respectively. Each dosage-strength of Testosterone CHP was manufactured in 1 ml glass ampules, with two ampules being packaged per box. This steroid lasted for about 17 years on the French drug market, first appearing back in 1974 and discontinued by the manufacturer in 1991. Today, no residual stock of Testosterone CHP is left anywhere, and to the best of my knowledge other versions of this steroid were removed from market long before the Theramex product.

When this steroid was available, the 296 mg/mL version would be the most popular one located on the black market, for obvious reasons. Although one could get by administering the steroid on a less frequent basis, it was most common to inject 2-3 ampules (equating to 400 to 600mg of free testosterone) once each week. At this dose, Testosterone CHP was about as effective as any other ester of testosterone (we certainly cannot attribute any unique properties to this drug). Now that it is gone, any long acting ester of testosterone will serve as a replacement. For example, its former manufacturer, Theramex, continues to produce Testosterone Heptylate Theramex (testosterone enanthate), a steroid that would be indistinguishable from Testosterone CHP for the average user.

Although no longer available, this steroid is really not sorely missed. I say that not because Testosterone CHP was a bad compound, but simply because there are many other esters of testosterone available that work just as well. Should this steroid resurface one day under another manufacturer, it would most definitely be an acceptable testosterone compound to use. It just would not be anything special, and definitely not worth spending more money on than other esters like cypionate, enanthate or decanoate.

Testosterone cypionate

Androgenic	Anabolic	Standard
100	100	Standard

Chemical Names:
4-androsten-3-one-17beta-ol
17beta-hydroxy-androst-4-en-3-one

Estrogenic Activity: moderate
Progestational Activity: low

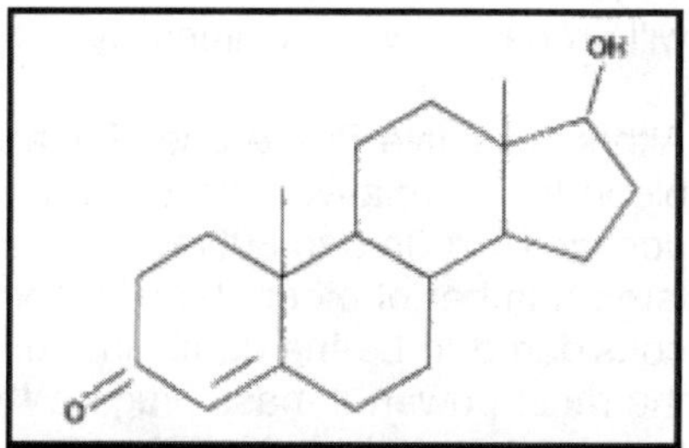

TESTOSTERONE

American athletes have a long a fond relationship with Testosterone cypionate. While testosterone enanthate is manufactured widely throughout the world, cypionate seems to be almost exclusively an American item. It is therefore not surprising that American athletes particularly favor this testosterone ester. But many claim this is not just a matter of simple pride, often swearing cypionate to be a superior product, providing a bit more of a "kick" than enanthate. At the same time it is said to produce a slightly higher level of water retention, but not enough for it to be easily discerned. Of course when we look at the situation objectively, we see these two steroids are really interchangeable, and cypionate is not at all superior. Both are long acting oil-based injectables, which will keep testosterone levels sufficiently elevated for approximately two weeks. Enanthate may be slightly better in terms of testosterone release, as this ester is one carbon atom lighter than cypionate (remember the ester is calculated in the steroids total milligram weight). The difference is so insignificant however that no one can rightly claim it to be noticeable (we are maybe talking a few milligrams per shot). Regardless, cypionate came to be the most popular testosterone ester on the U.S. black market for a very long time.

Pharmacokinetics of Testosterone Cypionate Injection

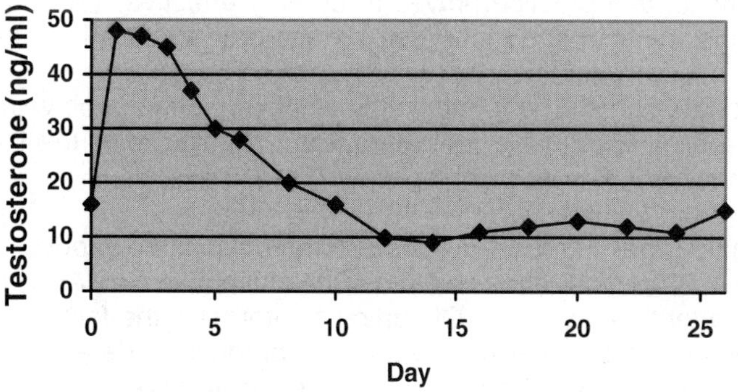

Figure 1. Pharmacokinetics of 200mg testosterone cypionate injection. Source: Comparison of testosterone, dihydrotestosterone, luteinizing hormone, and follicle-stimulating hormone in serum after injection of testosterone enanthate or testosterone cypionate. Schulte-Beerbuhl M, Nieschlag E. Fertility and Sterility 33 (1980) 201-3.

As with all testosterone injectables, one can expect a considerable gain in muscle mass and strength during a cycle. Since testosterone has a notably high affinity for estrogen conversion, the mass gained from this drug is likely to be accompanied by a discernible level of water retention. The resulting loss of definition of course makes cypionate a very poor choice for dieting or cutting phases. The excess level of estrogen brought about by this drug can also cause one to develop gynecomastia rather quickly. Should the user notice an uncomfortable soreness, swelling or lump under the nipple, an ancillary drug like Proviron® and/or Nolvadex® should probably be added. This will minimize the effect of estrogen greatly, making the steroid much more tolerable to use. The powerful antiaromatase Arimidex® is yet a better choice, but the high price tag prevents it from being more popularly used. Those who have a known sensitivity to estrogen may find it more beneficial to use ancillary drugs like Nolvadex® and Proviron® from the onset of the cycle, in order to prevent estrogen related side effects before they become apparent.

Since testosterone is the primary male androgen, we should also expect to see pronounced androgenic side effects with this drug. Much intensity is related to the rate in which the body converts testosterone into dihydrotestosterone (DHT). This, as you know, is the devious metabolite responsible for the high prominence of androgenic side effects associated with testosterone use. This includes the development of oily skin, acne, body/facial hair growth and male pattern balding. Those worried that they may have a genetic predisposition toward male pattern baldness may wish to avoid testosterone altogether. Others opt to add the ancillary drug Propecia®, which is a relatively new compound that prevents the conversion of testosterone to dihydrotestosterone (see: Proscar®). This can greatly reduce the chance for running into a hair loss problem, and will probably lower the intensity of other androgenic side effects.

Although active in the body for a much longer time, cypionate is injected on a weekly basis. This should keep blood levels relatively constant, although picky individuals may even prefer to inject this drug twice weekly. At a dosage of 200mg to 800mg per week we should certainly see dramatic results. It is interesting to note that while a large number of other steroidal compounds have been made available since testosterone injectables, they are still considered to be the dominant bulking agents among bodybuilders. There is little argument that these are among the most powerful mass drugs. While large doses are generally unnecessary, some bodybuilders have professed to using excessively high dosages of this drug. This was much more common before the 1990's, when cypionate vials were usually very cheap and easy to find in the states. A "more is better" attitude is easy to justify when paying only $20 for a 10cc vial (today the typical price for a single injection). When taking dosages above 800-1000mg per week there is little doubt that water retention will come to be the primary gain, far outweighing the new mass accumulation. Therefore, the practice of "megadosing" is inefficient, especially when we take into account the typical high cost of steroids today.

It is also important to remember that the use of an injectable testosterone will quickly suppress endogenous testosterone production. Therefore, it may be good advice to use a testosterone stimulating drug like HCG and/or Clomid®/Nolvadex® at the conclusion of a cycle. This should help the user avoid a strong "crash" due to hormonal imbalance, which can strip away much of the new muscle mass and strength. This is no doubt the reason why many athletes claim to be very disappointed with the final result of steroid use, as there is often only a slight permanent gain if anabolics are discontinued incorrectly. Of course we cannot expect to retain every pound of new bodyweight after a cycle. This is especially true whenever we are withdrawing a strong (aromatizing) androgen like testosterone, as a considerable drop in weight (and strength) is to be expected as retained water is excreted. This should not be of much concern; instead the user should focus on ancillary drug therapy so to preserve the solid mass underneath. Another way athletes have found to lessen the "crash", is to first replace the testosterone with a milder anabolic like Deca-Durabolin®. This steroid is administered alone, at a typical dosage of 200-400mg per week, for the following month or two. In this "stepping down" procedure the user is attempting to turn the watery bulk of a strong testosterone into the more solid muscularity we see with nandrolone preparations. In many instances, this practice proves to be very effective. We must still remember to administer ancillary drugs at the conclusion, as endogenous testosterone production will not be rebounding during the Deca therapy.

Cypionate can still be found on the black market in good volume. In fact, its availability is actually much better right now than it was just a few years ago. In going over the list of common products, you should be aware of the following:

Animal Power introduced a testosterone cypionate product in Mexico recently. It is called **Cypiotest 250**, and it carries 250mg/mL of steroid in a 10ml mulit-dose vial. AP is a hot new company in Mexico, and has been getting a lot of attention as of late. Of particular interest is the fact that this line takes counterfeiting very seriously. They use a number of security checks on this product to deter illicit duplication, the least effective of which is not the holographic sticker the company affixes to all boxes and vials (see Security Stickers). Also make sure the top on your vial has a paw print in it, which is part of the corporate logo.

The veterinary drug maker Quality Vet has one of the more popular cypionates on the Mexican drug market. It is called **Teston QV 200**, and it carries 200mg/mL of steroid in a 10ml vial. QV uses a security hologram sticker to deter counterfeiting, so be sure to look for this when shopping.

Denkall makes a similar product in Mexico, called **CypioTest 250.** This item also comes in a 10ml multi-dose vial. Denkall is a top-notch company; just be sure your vials are protected with the appropriate security hologram stickers.

The Aussie company Jurox has scaled back its steroid manufacturing business considerably, and many of their former products have been discontinued. **Testo LA** is one of them. It used to be exported to Mexico in some frequency. Note that there have been a lot of fake Jurox products on the market lately. One counterfeiter is producing an entire line of very good-looking fakes, all complete with boxes and intricate Jurox security hologram stickers. The Jurox logo is imbedded in the holographic image, making for a sticker that looks absolutely top notch. Problem is, Jurox never used a hologram!

SYD Group of Mexico has been selling a copy of the former Jurox product, called **Anabolic TL**. It comes in two strengths, 100mg/mL and 200mg/mL. Both are supplied in 10ml multi-dose vials. SYD Group is a very reputable company, and their product definitely trustworthy. Recent tests on this product showed that it was farily dosed (see Lab Testing). Just be sure your product carries the SYD group circular hologram sticker.

Ttokkyo used to make a cypionate in Mexico, called **Testosterone Cypionate L.A.** It came in both 100mg/mL and 200mg/mL strengths. Both forms were packaged in 10ml multi-dose vials. By all accounts Ttokkyo has closed shop, however, so I would not expect to see much of this on the black market.

Loeffler sells **Cypriotest L/A** in Mexico, which should not be confused with Denkall's Cypiotest. This product also comes in a dosage of 250 mg/mL, and is packaged in a similar 10 ml multi-dose vial. Dosing on Loeffler's testosterone propionate and Reforvit products tested out significantly off for Anabolics 2004, and I have not tested this product yet. Quality Control is likely going to be hit or miss with Loeffler.

Xelox Pharmaceuticals, an export-only company operating in the Phillippines, also released a testosterone cypionate product very recently. This product is called **Vironate**. Xelox also uses a security sticker to deter counterfeiting, although it is not a holographic one. Make sure you look for this when shopping.

The Thai firm British Dragon has introduced a cypionate product called **Testabol Depot**. It carries 200mg/mL of steroid, and comes prepared in a 10ml multi-dose vial. BD discontinued using hologram stickers on their injectable products recently, and instead has started using a red metallic foil inlay on all of its vial labels. Counterfeits of BD, thus far, have used either just ink for this area of the label, or a blue metallic foil. Also, make sure your vial top reads, "TEAR" and "FLIP UP". A current popular fake reads "FLIP OFF" only.

Body Research in Thailand makes **Cypionax**, another cypionate injectable for the steroid black market in fair volume. So far feedback on this line has been very positive, making this product a definite "thumbs up". Body Research recently had a run-in with the Thai authorities, and reportedly had large quantities of its steroid inventory seized because they were not registered for sale with the State. From what my sources are telling me, this is not going to put Body Research out of business, but may slow supply for a couple of months.

The **U.S. generics,** such as **Steris, Schein and Geneva,** are long gone. Don't be fooled. You will still see tons of these fakes. There is only one cypionate product left on the U.S. drug market at this time, **Depo-Testosterone** from Pharmacia (formerly Upjohn). This is a high profile target of counterfeiters, whos products will outnumber the real thing on the black market by as much as 10 to 1. Be careful to examine the packaging closely and compare it to the photos in the picture library. One trait to look at in particular is the opening flap on the box. As you will notice in the real vs. comparison shot of the older Upjohn product (in the photo section), the flap on the legitimate item comes to a blunt point at the tip. The fake is perfectly curved at the tip. The new Pharmacia packaging still has the same blunt tip. To date, I have not seen a counterfeit that had correctly copied this trait.

There are a few pharmacies **privately labeling** drugs for doctors that specialize in androgen replacement therapy, but these products rarely circulate on the black market. Some photos were included in the picture library for your reference.

Spanish **Testex** from Spain can stil be located on the black market. This product is made by Altana Pharma (formerly Byk Leo), and is packaged in 2ml dark glass ampules with yellow silkscreen lettering. It comes in two doses, containing a total of 100mg or 250mg of steroid. Testex has always been a high-risk item on the black market, so be careful when shopping. Although the newer version of this product has not yet been subject to counterfeiting, it no doublt will be, just like the old Leo brand.

Deposteron is also still made by Novaquimica in Brazil, and makes its way to the U.S. from time to time. Note that they are now using dark amber glass for the ampules instead of clear. Due to the fact that plain ampules are very easy to duplicate, it would be best to trust this product only when it is packaged in the appropriate box.

Miro Depo from Korea is still found in the U.S. from time to time, but not abundantly. Note that this product uses multi-dose vials, which sit in a foil topped plastic tray. Obtaining this item with the full packaging is the best way to guarantee authenticity, although fakes of this item have not been a problem so far. The box has been updated recently, to reflect a more modern design.

Testosterona Ultra from Uruguay has been scare as of late, perhaps because it is much easier to find and bring in testosterone cypionate from Mexico now. I cannot confirm this drug is still in manufacture.

Testosterone enanthate

Androgenic	Anabolic	Standard
100	100	Standard

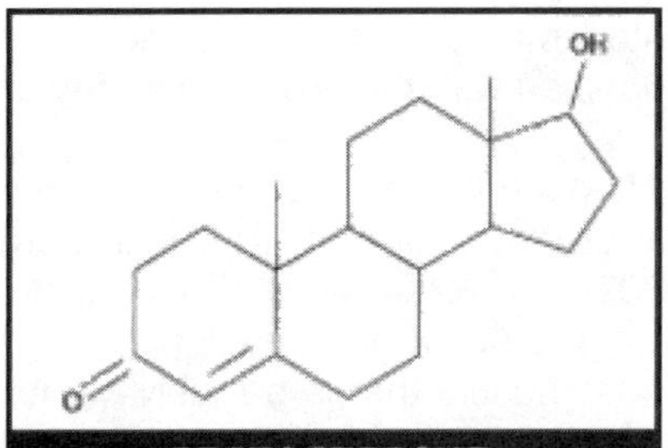

TESTOSTERONE

Chemical Names:
4-androsten-3-one-17beta-ol
17beta-hydroxy-androst-4-en-3-one

Estrogenic Activity: moderate
Progestational Activity: low

Testosterone enanthate is an oil based injectable steroid, designed to release testosterone slowly from the injection site (depot). Once administered, serum concentrations of this hormone will rise for several days, and remain markedly elevated for approximately two weeks. It may actually take three weeks for the action of this drug to fully diminish. For medical purposes this is the most widely prescribed testosterone, used regularly to treat cases of hypogonadism and other disorders related to androgen deficiency. Since patients generally do not self-administer such injections, a long acting steroid like this is a very welcome item. Therapy is clearly more comfortable in comparison to an ester like propionate, which requires a much more frequent dosage schedule. This product has also been researched as a possible male birth control option[88]. Regular injections will efficiently lower sperm production, a state that will be reversible when the drug is removed. With the current stigma surrounding steroids however, it is unlikely that such an idea would actually become an adopted practice.

Figure 1. Pharmacokinetics of 194mg testosterone enanthate injection. Source: Comparison of testosterone, dihydrotestosterone, luteinizing hormone, and follicle-stimulating hormone in serum after injection of testosterone enanthate or testosterone cypionate. Schulte-Beerbuhl M, Nieschlag E. Fertility and Sterility 33 (1980) 201-3.

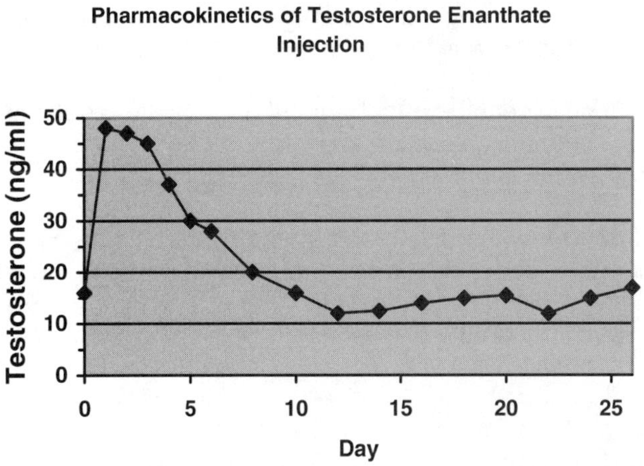

Testosterone is a powerful hormone with notably prominent side effects. Much of which stem from the fact that testosterone exhibits a high tendency to convert into estrogen. Related side effects may therefore become a problem during a cycle. For starters, water retention can become quite noticeable. This can produce a clear loss of muscle definition, as subcutaneous fluids begin to build. The storage of excess body fat may further reduce the visibility of muscle features, another common problem with aromatizing steroids. The excess estrogen level during/after your cycle also has the potential to lead up to gynecomastia. Adding an ancillary drug like Nolvadex® and/or Proviron® is therefore advisable to those with a known sensitivity to this side effect. As discussed throughout this book, the antiaromatase Arimidex® is a much better choice. The expense of this drug unfortunately stops its use from becoming a widespread practice however. It is believed that the use of an antiestrogen can slightly lower the anabolic effect of most androgen cycles (estrogen and water weight are often thought to facilitate strength and muscle gain), so one might want to see if such drugs are actually necessary before committing to use. A little puffiness under the nipple is a sign that gynecomastia is developing. If this is left to further develop into pronounced swelling, soreness and the growth of small lumps under the nipples, some form of action should be taken immediately to treat it (obviously quitting the drug or adding ancillaries).

Being a testosterone product, all the standard androgenic side effects are also to be expected. Oily skin, acne, aggressiveness, facial/body hair growth and male pattern baldness are all possible. Older or more sensitive individuals might therefore choose to avoid testosterone products, and look toward milder anabolics like Deca-Durabolin® or Equipoise® which produce fewer side effects. Others may opt to add the drug Proscar®/Propecia®, which will minimize the conversion of testosterone into DHT (dihydrotestosterone). With blood levels of this metabolite notably reduced, the impact of related side effects should also be reduced. However, with strong bulking drugs, the user will generally expect to incur strong side effects and will often just tolerate them. Most athletes really do not find the testosterones all that uncomfortable (especially in the face of the end result), as can be seen with the great popularity of such compounds.

Although this particular ester is active for a much longer duration, most athletes prefer to inject it on a weekly basis in order to keep blood levels more uniform. The usual dosage would be in the range of 250mg-750mg (200mg-800mg U.S. strength). This level is quite sufficient, and should provide the user a rapid gain of strength and body weight. Above this level, estrogenic side effects will no doubt become much more pronounced, outweighing any new muscle that is possibly gained. Those looking for greater bulk would be better served by adding an oral like Anadrol 50® or Dianabol, combinations which prove to be nothing less than dramatic. If the athlete wishes to use a testosterone yet retain a level of quality and definition to the physique, an injectable anabolic like Deca-Durabolin® or Equipoise® may prove to be a better choice. Here we can use a lower dosage of enanthate, so as to gain an acceptable amount of muscle but keep the buildup of estrogen to a minimum. Of course, the excess estrogen that is associated with testosterone makes it a bulking only drug, producing too much water (and fat) retention for use near contest time.

It is also important to remember that endogenous testosterone production is likely to be suppressed after a cycle of this drug. When this occurs, one runs the risk of losing muscle mass once the steroid is discontinued. HCG and/or Clomid® are in most cases considered to be a necessity, used effectively to restore natural testosterone production and avoid a post-cycle “crash”. The user should always expect to see some loss of body weight when the steroid is discontinued, as retained water (accounting for considerable weight) will be excreted once hormone levels regulate. This weight loss is to be ignored, and the athlete should be concerned only with preserving the quality muscle that lies underneath. With the proper administration of ancillary drugs, much of the new muscle mass can be retained for a long time after the steroid cycle has been stopped. Those who rely solely on a fancy tapering-off schedule to accomplish this are likely to be disappointed. Although a common practice, this is really not an effective way to restore the hormonal balance.

Worldwide, enanthate is the most abundantly produced ester of testosterone, and consequently is also the one most commonly found on the black market. It would be impossible to describe every product that you may come across when shopping in detail here, but I can give you some advice concerning products most popular right now.

Delatestryl is the only brand of enanthate sold by a major manufacturer in the U.S. at this time. It comes in both 1ml pre-loaded syringes and 5ml multi-dose vials, the latter being the only form really found on the black market (and rarely at that, due to strict controls). Note that the vials are short, and carry a label with metallic backing you can see through the glass. Looking for this will help assure you are getting the real thing, if somehow you luck out and come across a vial.

Animal Power, a new veterinary manufacturer in Mexico, has a testosterone enanthate product called **Enantest 250**. It contains 250mg/ml of steroid in a 10ml multi-dose vial. So far feedback on this line has been very favorable, suggesting that this is the new company on the block to look at in Mexico. Fakes are not yet known to be a problem on the black market. Be sure your product carries the company's holographic sticker (see Security Stickers), and you should be assured of a safe buy.

Pet's Pharma is another Mexican drug manufacturer to enter the steroid ring. They are selling an enanthate product called **Enantato 350**, and it is supposed to carry a whopping 350mg/mL dose. This would exceed the normal limit of comfortable dosing in oil, suggesting that if they do indeed have this much steroid, higher than normal levels of alcohol accompany it. The high concentration and alcohol content may make for more painful injections. Enantato 350 comes prepaired in 10 ml multi-dose vials, each of which will carry a security sticker to deter counterfeiting. The sticker is not holographic, however, although it does use uncommon metallic red and blue inks. Be sure to locate this sticker when shopping. Right now fakes are not reported to be a problem.

Quality Vet is still producing **Enantat QV 250**, which is amongst the more trusted testosterone enanthate preparations in Mexico right now. It comes in both 10ml and 50ml vials, and provides a nice 250mg/mL steroid concentration. The whole QV line is protected with hologram stickers to deter counterfeiting. Be sure to look for these when shopping.

The 200mg/mL generics from the veterinary firms Brovel and Tornel are also still common in Mexico. They are called **Testosterona 200** and **Testosterone 200 Depot** respectively, and are both packaged in 10 ml multi-dose vials. These products offer an excellent value for the amount of steroid included, often selling for about $20 or so in Mexico. Previous lab tests on Tornel's product showed it to be underdosed by about 20%. Although I did not have a chance to test the Brovel product, their testosterone propionate was tested, and came back similarly underdosed. Keep in mind though that these products are very inexpensive. Even with a slight underdosing, you are still offered a good value. Just keep the dosing a little higher during your cycles and you should be fine. With Brovel, be sure to look for the hologram sticker when shopping, to assure that you have the real thing (there are a lot of Brovel and Tornel fakes, so be careful).

Loeffler offers its own testosterone enanthate in Mexico, called **Testoenan 250 L/A**. This is another 250mg/mL version of this steroid, in a 10ml multi-dose vial. Having not had a chance to lab test this particular item, I cannot give you any details as to the exact dose contained in a recent lot. Loeffler does have a reputation for underdosing their products, but then again, the selling price also tends to be very favorable, which might make up for it.

Primoteston from Schering in Mexico is also still circulating, although not abundantly at this time. It seems that Sustanon, Deca-Durabolin, and Sten are the most popular injectables in the Mexican pharmacies right now, although you can find this item if you look for it hard enough.

Norma Hellas in Greece, famous makers of Norma Hellas Nandrolone, recently added a generic 250mg/mL enanthate injectable to their product offerings. It comes in a single dark amber 1ml glass ampule, and is packaged 1 ampule per box. Be sure to look at the Greek Pharmacy sticker under UV light to assure you have a legitimate product

Testoviron® from Schering in Spain is also still found in abundance. Note that Schering has recently changed the packaging. Testoviron has dropped the drab silk-screened amber ampules, and replaced them with clear glass amps with paper labels. The new look is very similar to the new Schering Primobolan, as would be expected. Note that many fakes are known to exist at this time, even of the newer style ampules.

The French product **Testosterone Heptylate Theramex** also circulates on the black market. Note that heptylate is not a unique ester of testosterone as described by other writers. It is simply another word for enanthate. Make sure to buy this item only when in the proper box, sitting (in pairs) in a foil lined plastic tray. You are much more likely to get a fake product if buying loose ampules.

Androtardyl is also produced in France, and occasionally circulates on the black market. Again, be sure to look for the proper box before buying.

Testo-Enant is another brand in Europe, this one being made by Geymonat in Italy. These ampules contain 250mg of steroid, either in 1ml or 2ml of oil. Currently fakes are not a problem; however, this steroid is not found on the black market in high volumes either. Italy has been tightening up its regulations in regards to steroid sales, making this land, once of abundant supply, a very inhospitable place for athletes as of late.

Galenika makes **Testosteron Depo** in Serbia (formerly Yugoslavia). These 1ml ampules contain 250mg/mL of steroid, and are extremely cheap at the retail level in their country of origin. In the last update this product tested out fairly underdosed. I decided to retest this manufacturer this year, and came back with a much more favorable result. At present, Galenika seems to be correctly (actually over) dosing their product, making an already excellently priced product even better of a deal. Note that the up and down tested could indicate quality control issues, so this appraisal is no guarantee.

Jelfa in Poland is still making **Testosteronum Prolongatum**, a 100 mg/mL enanthate product. Each box contains five 1ml ampules, which are themselves made of clear glass and carry a paper label. Fakes of this product do not appear to be an issue at this time. Lab tests on two lots of this product came back very favorably, also making this a best buy amongst the ampule products on the European black market.

BM Pharmaceuticals in India is making **Testen 250**, a 250mg/mL product in 2ml multi-dose vials. Testen is becoming relatively popular in some areas. Currently, fakes are not a problem.

Testosterone propionate

Androgenic	Anabolic	Standard
100	100	Standard

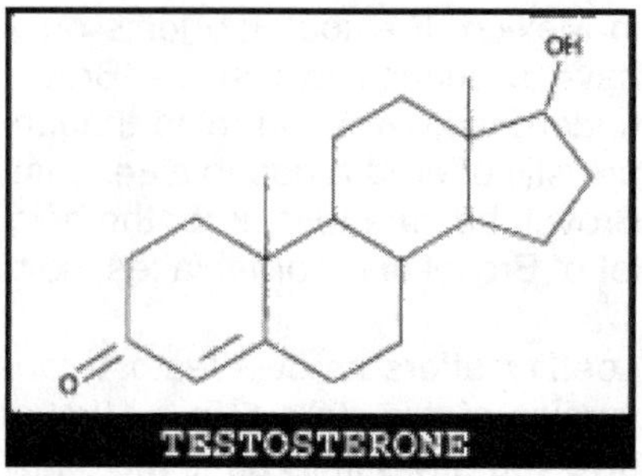

Chemical Names:
4-androsten-3-one-17beta-ol
17beta-hydroxy-androst-4-en-3-one

Estrogenic Activity: moderate
Progestational Activity: low

Testosterone propionate is a commonly manufactured, oil-based injectable testosterone compound. The added propionate ester will slow the rate in which the steroid is released from the injection site, but only for a few days. Testosterone propionate is therefore comparatively much faster acting than other testosterone esters such as cypionate or enanthate, and requires a much more frequent dosing schedule. While cypionate and enanthate are injected on a weekly basis, propionate is generally administered (at least) every third day. Figure one illustrates a typical release pattern after injection. As you can see, levels peak and begin declining quickly with this ester of testosterone. To make this drug even more uncomfortable to use, the propionate ester can be very irritating to the site of injection. In fact, many sensitive individuals choose to stay away from this steroid completely, their body reacting with a pronounced soreness and low-grade fever that may last for a few days. Even the mild soreness that is experienced by most users can be quite uncomfortable, especially when taking multiple injections each week. The "standard" esters like enanthate and cypionate, which are clearly easier to use, are therefore much more popular among athletes.

Pharmacokinetics of Testosterone Propionate Injection

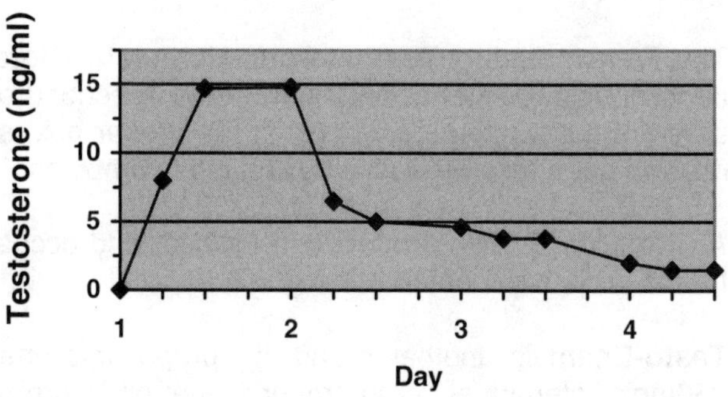

Figure 1. Pharmacokinetics of 25mg labeled testosterone propionate injection. Source: Pharmacokinetic properties of testosterone propionate in normal men. Fujioka M, Shinohara Y, Baba S. et. Al. J Clin Endocrinol Metab 63 (1986) 1361-4.

Those who are not bothered by frequent injections will find that propionate is quite an effective steroid. As an injectable testosterone it is, of course, a powerful mass drug, capable of producing rapid gains in both much size and strength. At the same time the buildup of estrogen and DHT (dihydrotestosterone) will be pronounced, so typical testosterone-related side effects are to be expected. Bodybuilders generally consider propionate to be the mildest testosterone ester, and the preferred form of this hormone for dieting/cutting phases of training. Some will go so far as to say that propionate will harden the physique, while giving the user less water and fat retention than one typically expects to see with a testosterone like enanthate, cypionate or Sustanon. Realistically however, this is nonsense. The ester is removed before testosterone is active in the body, and likewise the ester cannot alter the activity of the parent steroid in any way, only slow its release. It all boils down to how much testosterone you are getting into your blood with each particular compound – otherwise there is no difference between them.

During a typical cycle one will see action that is consistent with other forms of testosterone. Users sensitive to gynecomastia may therefore need to addition an antiestrogen. Those particularly troubled may find that a combination of Nolvadex® and Proviron® works especially well at preventing/halting this occurrence (Arimidex or Femara are even more effective options, but are also more costly). Also unavoidable with a testosterone are androgenic side effects like oily skin, acne, increased aggression and body/facial hair growth. Those who may have a predisposition for male pattern baldness may also find that propionate will aggravate this condition. To help combat this we also have the option of adding Propecia®/Proscar® or Avodart®, which will reduce the buildup of

DHT in many androgen target tissues. This will help minimize related side effects (particularly hair loss), although it offers us no guarantees. And as with all testosterone products, propionate will suppress endogenous testosterone production soon into the cycle. The use of a testosterone stimulating regimen of HCG and Nolvadex/Clomid® is, therefore, almost a requirement at the end of the cycle, in order to avoid enduring the dreaded hormonal crash.

The most common dosage schedule for this compound (men) is to inject 50 to 100mg, every 2nd or 3rd day. As with the more popular esters, the total weekly dosage would be in the range of 200-400mg. As with all testosterone compounds, this drug is most appropriately suited for bulking phases of training. Here it is most often combined with other strong agents such as Dianabol, Anadrol 50®, or Deca-Durabolin®, combinations that prove to be quite formidable. However, Propionate is sometimes also used with non-aromatizing anabolics/androgens during cutting or dieting phases of training, a time when its fast action and androgenic nature are also appreciated. Popular stacks include a moderate dosage of propionate with an oral anabolic like Winstrol® (15-35 mg daily), Primobolan® (50-150mg daily), or oxandrolone (15-30mg daily). Provided the body fat percentage is sufficiently low, the look of dense muscularity can be notably improved (barring any excess estrogen buildup from the testosterone). We can further add a non-aromatizing androgen like trenbolone or Halotestin®, which should have an even more extreme effect on subcutaneous body fat and muscle hardness. With the added androgen content any related side effects will become much more pronounced.

Women who absolutely must use an injectable testosterone should only use this preparation. This is simply because blood levels are easier to control with it compared to other long-acting esters. Should virilization symptoms develop, one would not wish to wait the weeks needed for testosterone concentrations to fall after a shot of enanthate. The dosage schedule should also be more spread out, with injections coming every 5 to 7 days at most. Obviously, the dosage would be lower as well, generally in the range of 25mg per injection. Androgenic activity should be less pronounced with this schedule, giving blood levels time to sufficiently decrease before the drug is administered again. In order to further reduce any risks, the duration of this cycle should not exceed 8 weeks. Should a stronger anabolic effect be needed, a small amount of Durabolin® (Deca-Durabolin® if unavailable), Oxandrolone, or Winstrol® could be added. Of course, the risk of noticing virilizing effects from these drugs may increase, even with the addition of a mild anabolic. Since many of the masculinizing side effects of steroid use can be irreversible, it is very important for the female athlete to monitor the dosage, duration and incidence of side effects very closely.

Testosterone propionate is very abundant on the black market right now, perhaps more so than it was a couple of years ago. This probably has a lot to do with the fact that it is a very cheap steroid to manufacture next to some of the longer acting esters. In going over some of the more popular items circulating the black market at this time, I can offer the following observations.

Animal Power has released a propionte product in Mexico called **Propiotest 100**. This is a 100mg/mL steroid, which comes in a 10ml multi-dose vial. Animal Power is a new company in Mexico, but they are getting a lot of attention as of late. Most attention grabbing is their focus on counterfeit prevention. Animal Power uses several security checks on its injectable products, including a security holographic sticker with the company logo embedded in the image (see Security Stickers).

Quality Vet is making **Propionat QV 100** in Mexico, which is another 100mg/mL preparation in a 10ml multi-dose vial. Just be sure to look for their holographic security sticker when shopping, which should assure a safe purchase.

Testosterona from Brovel in Mexico is still abundant, the 100mg version (**Testosterona 100**) much more so than the 50mg one (**Testosterona 50**). Brovel has been around for a long time, and has always delivered a fair quality product for an excellent price. I conducted a lab test on Testosterona 100 recently, which revealed it to be underdosed by almost 30%. This is not great, but then again, Brovel products have always been amongst the most affordable on the Mexican market. Even if you take into account that your getting 30% less than what is listed on the label, it is still going to be a very good buy in most cases. Remember to look for the Brovel Hologram sticker to be sure you are getting the real thing, as there are a lot of fakes of this line floating around (not this product in particular though).

By all reports **Ttokkyo** has ceased operations in Mexico. This comes in the wake of the arrest of Ttokkyo's owner, Dr. Molina. The firm had been holding on for some time after this; however, I am hearing their doors are finally closed. Note that this firm used a security hologram sticker, however, a counterfeit manufacturer was able to appropriate a quantitiy of these. I have seen poor looking copies on the black market that carried a perfect Ttokkyo sticker. Old lots of the Ttokkyo may still be in circulation, so just keep in mind that a sticker does not provide 100% assurance you are getting the real thing.

Testopro L/A from Loeffler in Mexico contains a whopping 250mg/mL, at least according to the label on this 10ml multi-dose vial. Loeffler products seem to have been hit or miss in quality lately though, and a previous test of this item in particular showed it to have a bit over 133mg of testosterone propionate in each ml. This is a little better than half of the label claim, which leaves us wondering if Loeffler has ever produced a true 250mg/mL testosterone propionate. Hopefully, I will have the opportunity to test some lots in the future to find out.

Testolic from Body Research in Thailand also circulates from time to time. This product comes in the form of 2ml glass ampules, with each ml containing 50mg of steroid. Body Research ran into some trouble recently, when Thai authorities seized a large amount of their steroid stock. Apparently, some of their formulations are not registered with the State, and were being pushed through the pharmacies. My sources are telling my that Body Research will continue to operate and export these items; however, they may have some problems in the immediate future with inventory.

British Dragon also makes **Testabol Propionate** in Thailand, another export only item (you will not find it is pharmacies when shopping on vacation). The BD line is very hot right now, with a very good reputation. Note that the have stopped using hologram stickers on their injectable products. Instead, they are using a red metallic foil inlay on their labels. A current popular fake inforrectly still carries a hologram. Also, this fake has a top that reads, "FLIP OFF" only. The real manufacturer purchases very specific vial tops, which read "TEAR" and "FLIP UP".

BM Pharmaceuticals in India makes a brand of testosterone propionate called **Testopin-100**. As the name indicates, it contains 100mg/mL of steroid. It is packaged in both 1ml glass ampules and 2ml multi-dose vials. Currently, fakes of this line are not much of a problem.

Jelfa makes **Testosteronum Propionicum** in Poland, which makes its way most often to the European black market (rarely to the U.S.). However, it only contains 25mg of steroid in each 1ml ampule, so it doesn't stack up much to the more popular 100mg/mL products here in the States.

Virormone is still manufactured in the U.K., most recently by the firm Nordic. These 2ml 100mg ampules are not extremely popular in the U.S., but do circulate here from time to time. The UK has been taking steroid distribution more seriously as of late, limiting greatly the supply of domestic drugs making it to the international black market.

No testosterone propionate products are being manufactured in the **U.S.** at this time, so avoid all such products on the black market.

Testosterone Suspension

Androgenic	Anabolic	Standard
100	100	Standard

Chemical Names:
4-androsten-3-one-17beta-ol
17beta-hydroxy-androst-4-en-3-one

Estrogenic Activity: moderate
Progestational Activity: low

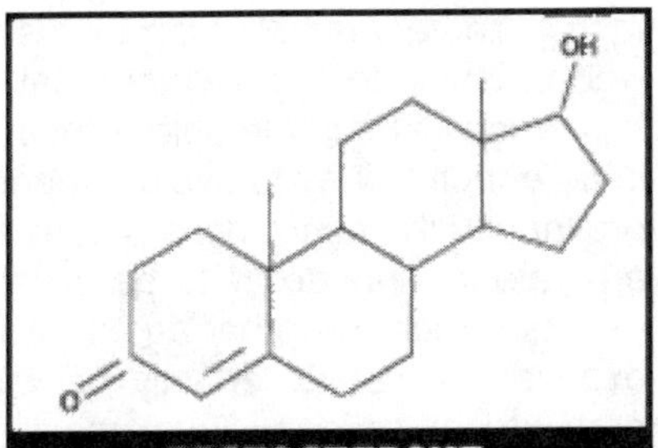

TESTOSTERONE

Testosterone suspension is an injectable preparation containing testosterone (no ester) in a water base. Since testosterone is not highly water soluble, the steroid will noticeably separate from the solution when the vial is left to sit. A quick shake will temporarily place the drug back into suspension, so that the withdrawn dosage should always be consistent. Many reference materials have not given this steroid the proper credit, stating it to be a very crude and ineffective product. Although it may contain testosterone without the benefit of an ester, the micro-crystal design of this injectable will in fact sustain an elevated testosterone release for 2-3 days. The suspension we see today is clearly not the basic water plus testosterone design used in the 1940's. And since the drug will not leave circulation in a matter of hours, it is obviously useful. This is not news to the many Americans bodybuilders who have had a chance to experiment with this item, and regard it very highly.

Among bodybuilders, "suspension" is known to be an extremely potent mass agent. Most often it is ranked as the most powerful injectable steroid available, producing an incredibly rapid gain of muscle mass and strength. This is largely due to the very fast action of this drug, as the water-based steroid will begin to enter the blood stream almost immediately after an injection is given. When using a slow acting oil based steroid like Sustanon, it can take weeks before a peak testosterone level is reached. With suspension it is just a matter of days. This will usually result in the athlete noticing a size and strength gain by the end of the first week. By the time the athlete is 30 days into a cycle of suspension, the length it will usually take for a Sustanon cycle to really begin to work consistently, the mass gains are already (generally) very extreme. Clearly the anabolic effect of this testosterone will be realized much more quickly than we would expect with an oil based (esterified) preparation.

It is also important to remember that 100mg of a testosterone ester is not equivalent to 100mg testosterone of pure testosterone (as in suspension). When an ester is present, its weight is obviously included in the preparation's milligram total. Looking at testosterone enanthate, 100mg of this compound equates to only 72mg of raw testosterone. So the bodybuilder who uses 400mg of enanthate weekly is really getting about 288mg of testosterone into his body each week. This is clearly a great increase over the endogenous testosterone level of the average male, which is in the range of 2.5 to 11mg per day. But the general point is that during a cycle of testosterone suspension we will often see a much more dramatic intake of testosterone on average than is typically utilized with oils. Following common advice, the athlete will commonly inject a full 100mg of testosterone daily, a total of 700 milligrams per week. This is up to 40 times the amount produced by a normal male. Those who have attempted such a cycle are rarely disappointed with the results, as such heavy doses of this hormone will produce nothing less than a dramatic weight gain.

The most popular practice with testosterone suspension is to inject the drug at least every two or three days. The dosage will vary greatly depending on the needs of the individual, but is most often in the range of 50mg to 300mg per shot. Athletes looking to achieve an extremely rapid bulk gain will inject the already mentioned dose of 100mg daily. In most cases this cycle can be amazing, the user seeming to just "inflate" with bloated muscle mass in a short period of time. Back when they were being manufactured, the U.S. 30ml vials (100mg/mL) were always the most sought after for this procedure, as each would run the cycle for about a month. Although this drug does require a frequent injection schedule, it will pass through a needle as fine as 27 gauge (insulin). This allows the user more available injection sites, hitting the smaller muscle groups such as the deltoid, triceps and calves. Although some users do complain about discomfort when injecting water-based steroids, it has been my experience that suspension is generally well tolerated. In fact, many bodybuilders find the speed of drawing and administering a water based solution to be quite a welcome change from oils, which as you know can be a lengthy procedure.

As would be expected with a strong androgen, suspension can produce a number of unwelcome side effects. For starters, with a testosterone product, we will expect to see a high rate of estrogen conversion. Estrogen levels, in fact, build very quickly with testosterone suspension, which is actually reputed to be the worst testosterone to use when wishing to avoid water bloat. Gynecomastia can also develop very rapidly during a cycle, and in many cases, this drug will be intolerable without additionally taking an antiestrogen. A combination of Nolvadex® and Proviron® is an effective way to avoid experiencing such side effects, and is often taken from the onset of a cycle in order to prevent such occurrences before they become a problem. Sensitive individuals may find an investment in the anti-aromatase Arimidex® to be wiser. While this drug is very costly, it is also much more effective at controlling estrogen than the other agents which are currently being used by athletes. If there were ever a time to justify this expense, it would certainly be with a drug like suspension. It is also important that the athlete monitor blood pressure and kidney functions closely during a heavy cycle, a trouble area as water retention becomes more pronounced. Although testosterone puts very little strain on the liver, this drug can be harsh to the kidneys as the dosage increases. Of course, if the athlete is encountering noticeably high blood pressure or trouble urinating (pain or darkening of the urine), the cycle should probably be discontinued and the doctor paid a visit.

Conversion to DHT (dihydrotestosterone) will, of course, potentiate the action of testosterone in certain tissues, making this steroid quite androgenic. Therefore, one can expect to endure oily skin, acne, increased aggression, and body/facial hair growth during a typical cycle. Propecia®/Proscar® or Avodart® may be a requirement for those with a familial predisposition for male pattern hair loss, as suspension is known to aggravate this condition quite easily. Men with an existing hair loss problem may actually prefer to stay far away from this steroid altogether, finding it to be just too strong an item to take risks with. The slower acting oil based injectables like Propionate and Sustanon would be a much better place to start experimenting if the individual still desires the power of an injectable testosterone.

Also, endogenous testosterone production will be quickly and efficiently reduced when using suspension. This can often reach the point of severe testicular shrinkage (atrophy). Some athletes will periodically take HCG while on a cycle, in an effort to try and keep endogenous testosterone suppression and testicular atrophy to a minimum. However, this practice isn't always extremely effective, and if overused can even be counterproductive. Even if nothing is used during the cycle, a combination of HCG and Clomid®/Nolvadex® should always be used as the cycle is discontinued to minimize the post-cycle hypoandrogenic (low androgen) window. When used correctly, these drugs can be very effective at stimulating natural production, hopefully allowing the athlete to avoid an otherwise strong post-cycle crash. It is important to mention that in addition to stimulating the release of testosterone, HCG also acts to enhance the rate of aromatization in the testes. The risk for enhanced estrogen buildup makes concurrent anti-estrogen use very important, especially when the athlete had been taking large doses of testosterone.

Overall, testosterone suspension is an extremely powerful drug, but also one that is prone to causing many uncomfortable side effects. Those looking for only a potent mass agent need not look for a better substitute; this product will certainly do the trick. But those athletes who want not just quantity but quality are likely to be disappointed with suspension, as the muscle mass gain is not going to be a hard, dense one. In fact, the user must constantly fight fat and water bloat when building his new physique, and will often seek the benefit of cutting agents soon afterwards. The only exception to this would be cases where the drug is used for very short periods of time (pre-contest), to rapidly raise the androgen level and harden up the body. When estrogen is not given time to wreak havoc on the physique, the rapid androgen increase can certainly be beneficial. Of course, it will only take a few days for the newly elevated levels of estrogen to start having an unfavorable effect on the physique.

Testosterone suspension is not abundant on the black market at this time. American products have been gone for years, leaving only a few available versions of this steroid left to purchase.

Denkall in Mexico recently started selling **Aquatest**, a 100mg/mL testosterone suspension. Denkall is highly regarded for the quality of its products, with buyers rarely questioning the accuracy of their dosing (all of the lab tests I have ever seen on the line were very good). This is a very nice suspension, passing smoothly through a 25-gauge vitamin needle. It is definitely a recommended product, and, in fact, probably the highest quality suspension being sold anywhere in the world at this time. Just be sure to look for the Denkall hologram sticker.

Anabolic-TS is another popular testosterone suspension in Mexico, sold by the international veterinary drug company SYD Group. SYD purchased Grupo Comercial Tarasco recently, which used to sell Anabolic-TS under its own label. Currently, they are still pushing old stock of the Grupo Tarasco labeled product. This is a great quality product in terms of dosing, but the particle size of the steroid inside is a little large for the comfort of most (you will need a 21 gauge to inject it).

Univet **Uni-test** suspension from Canada is also found on the black market at times, and is reportedly even worse than the SYD product in terms of particle size. There are also numerous fakes of this product in circulation. The current popular knock-off uses a gold cap, and has an error that sticks out on the ingredients list. The legitimate item lists Benzyl Alcohol in the amount of 0.01g (10mg, or about 1% - a standard amount), while the fake incorrectly puts 0.01mg in the same location; far too little benzyl to offer any value.

Aquaviron from Nicholas in India is still being sold, and occasionally makes its way to the U.S. and European black markets (although not widely). This product comes in the form of 25mg ampules, with each dose mixed in 1ml of solution. 12 ampules are packed in each box, all side-by-side in a flat cardboard tray. Fakes are not a problem at this time.

Czech **Agovirin** is still being manufactured as well. To be correct, this is not actually "testosterone suspension", but a testosterone isobutyrate suspension. Still, this is a very rapid acting water-based injectable testosterone, so it seems most appropriate to discuss in this section (the casual user will not be able to distinguish between the two). Agovirin is a trusted item when located; however, it does not appear on the black market in the United States very often. It does appear to be the dominant form of testosterone suspension on the European black market, though.

Testoviron (testosterone propionate/enanthate blend)

Androgenic	Anabolic	Standard
100	100	Standard

Chemical Names:
4-androsten-3-one-17beta-ol
17beta-hydroxy-androst-4-en-3-one

Estrogenic Activity: moderate
Progestational Activity: low

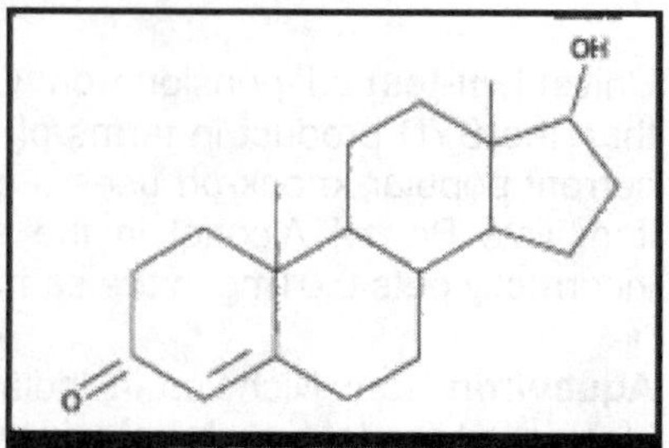

TESTOSTERONE

Testoviron® is a mixed testosterone injectable (propionate/enanthate), produced by the firm Schering in a few different parts of the world. Since Schering also uses the Testoviron® brand name to market pure testosterone enanthate, one should not confuse all such items with this mixed preparation. In fact, most preparations found circulating with this brand name are actually the pure enanthates, which are vastly more popular among athletes. When locating the Testoviron® blends, we notice they are prepared in a number of different strengths. All will contain a base of testosterone enanthate, with a lesser amount of testosterone propionate added in. Being much faster acting, the propionate gives us a quick effect while the enanthate is slowly reaching circulation. The result is an injectable that will increase the testosterone level very quickly; yet sustain an elevation for approximately two to three weeks. The design of this steroid is therefore similar to that of the testosterone blend Sustanon, although Testoviron® will remain active in the body for a noticeably shorter duration.

This steroid is clearly not an unusual compound, as it would obviously have an effect similar to other blended testosterone products such as Sten and Sustanon. One can expect to see a rapid buildup of strength and muscle mass during a cycle of this drug, as is to be expected with all injectable testosterones. This will likely go hand in hand with a noticeable level of water retention, as testosterone converts into estrogen quite readily. A loss of muscle definition is likely to result, as subcutaneous water and fat stores reduce the visibility of muscle features. For this reason Testoviron® is not the ideal item for cutting phases of training. The added estrogen level may also cause the development of gynecomastia. In order to reduce this possibility, sensitive individuals may need to add an antiestrogen like Nolvadex® and/or Proviron® during each cycle. Testosterone preparations will also suppress endogenous androgen levels, so a stimulating drug like HCG and/or Clomid®/Nolvadex® may be needed to avoid a post-cycle crash. Since this effect is particularly pronounced with testosterone, a combination of both drugs may prove to be the most useful in many cases

Testosterone also converts to the more potent steroid DHT (dihydrotestosterone) in many areas of the body, a process that is responsible for the strong androgenic activity of this hormone. Testoviron® is therefore likely to produce a number of unwanted androgenic side effects, including oily skin, acne, body/facial hair growth and male pattern hair loss. Those who have an existing male-pattern hair loss condition, or believe they may be prone to this problem, may wish to stay away from testosterone products for this reason. Strong androgens can easily aggravate cases of hair loss, a side effect of steroid use that is pretty much irreversible once noted. Others may simply opt to include a daily dosage of Proscar®/Propecia®, which will greatly reduce the buildup of DHT and lighten the androgenic nature of testosterone. We must remember however, that while Proscar® offers us help, it is no assurance this side effect will not develop during a cycle all androgenic effects are mediated by the same receptor as anabolic. Deca-Durabolin® would still be a much safer choice in this regard however.

Testoviron® is clearly an acceptable alternative to standard testosterone preparations. These ampules are not commonly found on the black market however, but are certainly a good choice if located.

Here in the U.S., **Testoprim-D** ampules are the most likely to show up. This is not a counterfeit item as other steroid references may list, but is in fact a legitimately manufactured Mexican pharmaceutical. Counterfeits of this item have never been located, so Testoprim will probably remain to be a safe buy for some time. When looking for this item in Mexico, we see a single light resistant ampule that is packaged in a red box bearing white print. With the ampule, we also note that the writing is printed directly on the glass surface. The ink used is a white/grayish color that does not smear with a good thumb rub. By the time this item is found in the United States, these boxes have usually been discarded (the ampules are easier to smuggle loose).

Aratest from Mexico has also been circulating. However, early unconfirmed reports have been that it is a markedly underdosed product, so be careful.

BM Pharmaceuticals in India makes **Testenon**, which contains a 135mg/mL Testoviron blend in a 2ml multi-dose vial. I have not had the opportunity to lab test any of their products yet, but the feedback has been very good on the whole BM line thus far.

Schering has discontinued manufacture of its blended Testoviron product in many parts of the world. The only common steroid source countries still producing this steroid right now are Italy (Testoviron 135mg) and the Dominican Republic (Testoviron 135mg), and it is probably only a matter of time before they are discontinued there as well. Spanish Testoviron (the blend), the main source of this steroid for the international steroid black market, is long gone now.

THG (tetrahydrogestrinone)

Androgenic	Anabolic	Standard
N/a	N/a	-

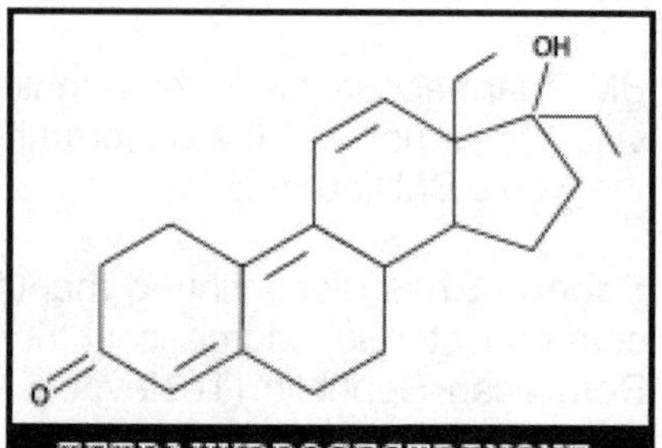

Chemical Name:
18a-Homo-pregna-4,9,11-trien-17b-ol-3-one

Estrogenic Activity: None
Progestational Activity: Very High

Tetrahydrogestrinone (THG) is a unique designer steroid that was recently brought to light in what was called "the biggest organized bust for steroid use in the history of competitive sports". These were the words of Terry Madden, Chief Executive Officer of the U.S. Anti-Doping Agency (USADA), when addressing a group of newspaper and television reporters in a press conference disclosing the new international doping scandal. His accompanying press release spoke of an anonymous Olympic coach, who turned over a syringe containing this designer steroid and implicated Victor Conte of BALCO Labs in California as the source for the agent. The anonymous source was later identified as top track coach Trevor Graham. Conte is credited with coaching many of the world's top athletes. USADA was soon amidst a media frenzy, with many big names fingered for testing positive for the use of THG. Criminal charges have been filed against Conte, and as of the release of Anabolics 2005, the case is still pending. THG arose from the doping scandal fallout as the world's famous superstar of designer steroids, and its existence a constant reminder that the determination of athletes to utilize all available tools to win goes far beyond the abilities of the governing athletic bodies to police them.

Upon closer inspection of this odd designer steroid, we see that THG is similar in structure to the European prescription anti-gonadotropic agent gestrinone[89]. Gestrinone does have an obvious structural relationship to trenbolone, however, it is not an active anabolic steroid. This is due to its 17-alpha ethynyl modification, a trait that prevents this agent from binding to the androgen receptor. With anabolic steroids we typically see methyl or ethyl groups used to increase oral bioavailability, never ethynyl modifications. But when we add four hydrogen atoms to the ethynyl group of gestrinone, we break it down to a new ethylated derivative (THG) capable of strong anabolic/androgenic action. THG is simply 17-alpha-ethylated gestrinone, a novel ethylated offshoot of the powerful anabolic steroid trenbolone, made from a readily available and unregulated intermediary chemical. For a while, THG was an ideal steroid for athletes in drug-tested sports, being both extremely effective and undetectable on a urine screen. It was also technically legal, being that it was unknown to lawmakers at the time the Anabolic Steroid Control Act was written. But with the international doping scandal that would come to surround BALCO Laboratories, any value that THG held as a "designer steroid" has since disappeared. This steroid has also been added to the U.S. controlled substance list as of January 2005.

For those athletes who use THG, the results should be measurable improvements in strength, muscle size and performance. Lack of estrogen conversion allows this steroid to impart relatively lean muscle tissue gains, not the sheer water-retaining mass we would expect from bulking agents like testosterone, Dianabol, or Anadrol. At least in this regard, it is more along the lines of Winstrol or Anavar. We can say with some certainty that milligram for milligram it is much more potent than any of the standard commercially available anabolics. Methyltrienolone is its closest chemical relative, and known to be effective in doses lower than 1mg per day. THG should also require very small doses, perhaps in the range of 2-5mg per day. We can also note that THG minus its delta-11 modification (a di-ene instead of a tri-ene) has been documented to be over 14 times more active than methyltestosterone[90]. There is no reason to think that the jump to full-blown THG would be anything but an improvement. Although I can't give exact figures, this designer steroid should be far more potent than any anabolic steroid commercially available, and would probably fall short only of methyltrienolone in this book.

THG is extremely potent in one other regard. This steroid is an extremely active progestin. This was elucidated in a recent investigation published in Journal of Clinical Endocrinology and Metabolism, which looked at the androgen, estrogen, and progestin receptor binding potency of this unusual designer steroid[91]. Researchers compared the agent to the popular anabolic steroids nandrolone and trenbolone, two 19-norsteroids with known progestational activity. The results of their experiments were both expected and shocking at the same time. On the one hand, THG was more progestational in nature than the two nandrolone-based steroids of reference. THG is also a 19-nor compound, so similar activity is not extremely surprising. But the difference between these three drugs was considerable. In fact, not only was THG more progestational than Deca and trenbolone, it was 7 times more potent than progesterone itself! Even gestrinone, a synthetic progestin many times more potent than endogenous progesterone, was less active than THG. THG turned out to be the most potent progestin in the experiment (the shocking part). The transformation from gestrinone to THG, which increases androgen receptor binding, made a more potent progestin at the same time.

THG's progestational side needs to be taken into consideration before use, especially if other aromatizable steroids are being considered at the same time. This steroid could easily exacerbate the estrogenic side effects of other drugs. Even when taken alone, THG still might not guarantee quality lean mass gains, so be warned. Aside from this, basic androgenic side effects such as oily skin, acne, and male pattern hair loss should also be looked out for, and should be somewhat dose related. Liver toxicity is perhaps the biggest concern with this drug. THG would be on the more extreme end of liver toxicity, standing well in front of the more popular commercial steroids like Anadrol, Halotestin, Winstrol, and Dianabol due to its very high milligram for milligram potency. In this regards, it would rate more along the lines of methyltrienolone (see: Drug Profiles, Methyltrienolone), a steroid sold only as a research chemical and deemed too hepatotoxic to be given clinically to humans. That is not to say that THG is outright dangerous, but extreme care (and routine blood work) should be taken if one were to consider using this drug for performance enhancement. THG is presently unavailable, however I suspect it will re-emerge on the underground or veterinary drug market as soon as some enterprising company realizes the value of releasing such a novel and talked about compound.

Trenbolone acetate

Androgenic	Anabolic	Standard
500	500	Nandrolone acetate

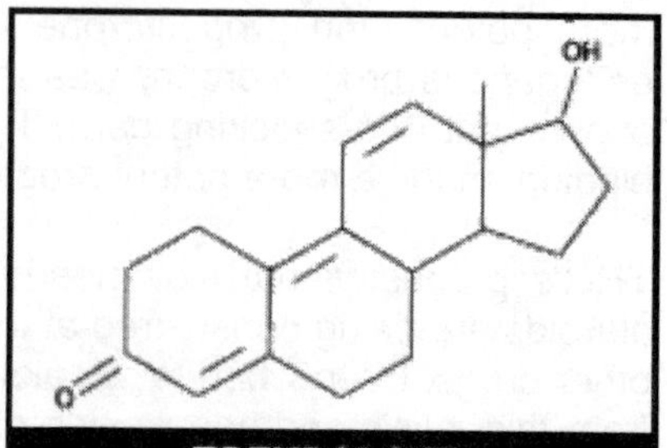
TRENBOLONE

Chemical Names:
17beta-Hydroxyestra-4,9,11-trien-3-one

Estrogenic Activity: none
Progestational Activity: low to moderate

Trenbolone is a strong androgen that is devoid of estrogenic activity. The first preparation containing this steroid to catch the attention of the American bodybuilding community was Finajet, a veterinary preparation introduced in the 1980's in U.S. and Europe (as Finaject) by the drug firms Hoechst and Roussel. This product contained 30mg/mL of this fast acting acetate ester of trenbolone, and came packaged in a whopping 50ml vial. Finajet made a strong showing for a short period in the 80's, where this androgen became a sought after cutting steroid. The strong androgenic and non-estrogenic properties of this steroid made it ideal for increasing muscle hardness, definition and strength without water retention, and consequently Finajet became popular with competitive bodybuilders. Hoechst removed the product from the market by 1988 however, the European version soon followed, and the U.S. source for trenbolone quickly dried up. It had disappeared from the market for quite some time, earning cult status as some type of unobtainable super-steroid. After some time however trenbolone acetate had reemerged in the U.S., first in the form of Finaplix® cattle implant pellets and more recently as the injectable Trenbol 75 introduced in and imported from Mexico. Its old reputation stuck, and these products are now in very high demand on the U.S. market.

Structurally trenbolone is a 19-nor steroid, being derived from the anabolic nandrolone. Its additional two alterations however (c9 and c11 double bonds) make trenbolone very different in appearance than its parent nandrolone. First, as mentioned estrogenic activity has been eliminated. This is a result of the c 9-10 double bond, which occupies a bond that would be necessary for aromatization of the A ring to be possible. This bond does not appear to be removed metabolically, which is the only way estrogen conversion would be possible with this compound. Although nandrolone is rarely thought of as an estrogenic steroid, conversion to estradiol is still possible to a low extent. The fact that trenbolone does not convert to estradiol therefore remains to be a significant difference between the two steroids.

Its lack of estrogenic activity has made trenbolone very appealing for competitive athletes looking to shed fat, while at the same time trying to avoid water retention. Likewise "tren" can give us the high androgen content needed in order to elicit a very hard, defined physique. While it is a noteworthy hardening agent, this is certainly not the only benefit to this steroid however, it also a noteworthy anabolic. The muscle building properties of this steroid are often compared to strong drugs such as testosterone and Dianabol, said to be very similar just without the same level of water retention. This may be a little generous of a description however. Its lack of estrogenic activity does seem to hurt this agent in its abilities to promote muscle mass gains. For many, it is similarly still relegated to cutting cycles. Of interest is the fact that while tren is often recommended as a great addition to a good mass cycle, it is rarely reported to be such a powerful agent when used alone. When taken without another estrogenic steroid, results are most often reported as good lean tissue growth accompanied by exceptional hardening and fat loss. Although perhaps it is not quite as potent as the more estrogenic bulking agents if sheer mass is the goal, I think we can still safely say that trenbolone is a better builder milligram for milligram than nandrolone, and likely the most anabolic of all the non-estrogenic steroids.

The androgenic activity of this drug is also much stronger than that of its parent nandrolone. This is due to two interesting traits. First, trenbolone does not appear to undergo 5-alpha reduction in humans[92]. As such, it does not display the strong anabolic/androgenic dissociation noted with nandrolone. It retains the same level of potency when entering cells of various androgen target tissues as it does when entering muscle tissues, and does not get weaker. This in of itself makes trenbolone far more androgenic in appearance. Furthermore the induction of double bonds at c9 and c11 seems to increase androgen receptor binding[93]. This represents a second way that the potency of trenbolone is increased. Side effects like acne, body/facial hair growth and hair loss are therefore all possible during use of this steroid. To spite the base structural similarities of the two steroids, we should clearly not confuse trenbolone in any way with nandrolone in regards to its ability to induce such side effects. Tren is simply much more androgenic.

Trenbolone will also suppress natural testosterone production very quickly, making clear that estrogen is not the only culprit in this regard. This would necessitate the use of a testosterone stimulating drug like Clomid®/Nolvadex® and/or HCG in order to avoid a pronounced "crash" as the drug is discontinued. This may have something to do with its progestational activity. Although listed as non-progestational in other steroid literature, studies clearly show trenbolone to bind with this receptor[94 95]. Since we know that all sex steroids promote negative feedback inhibition of testosterone production, including progestins, this mechanism cannot be excluded. We also know that the effects of estrogen seem to be augmented by heightened progestin levels[96], with this hormone capable of inducing side effects that might not otherwise be apparent with a given level of estrogen in the body. However, while we do notice that estrogenic side effects do not seem to be reported with trenbolone, it may still be reasonable to conclude that some caution should be taken with this compound (particularly when using this steroid with other estrogenic steroids). Logic leads one to think that without heightened estrogen levels, the slight progestational nature of trenbolone may fail to induce side effects, while it would have the potential of lowering ones threshold to side effects when other estrogenic steroids are used concurrently by enhancing the actions of this hormone. This theory cannot be proven at this time.

Trenbolone is a very versatile steroid, working exceptionally well for both bulking and cutting purposes. It seems to mix well with just about any type of steroid. For a lean, hard build, one can add a mild anabolic like Winstrol® or Primobolan®. Without extra water beneath your skin, the androgen/anabolic mix will elicit a very solid, well-defined build. For a good mass gain, still without excessive bloat, Deca-Durabolin® or Equipoise® are popular additions. Here again, the tren will greatly enhance and solidify the new muscle growth. When looking purely for mass, trenbolone pairs well with testosterone, Anadrol 50® or Dianabol. The result will no doubt be an incredible gain of (somewhat solid) muscle mass. In some rural areas where anabolics are hard to obtain, Finaplix® (discussed below) is commonly used in conjunction with Synovex pellets (testosterone propionate/estradiol benzoate). Although the slight estrogen content of Synovex does give us some unwanted bloat, the testosterone propionate adds in very well. A very cheap, easy to obtain combination which is still technically legal since cattle implants are excluded from U.S. controlled substance laws.

Finaplix® is a veterinary cattle implant that contains trenbolone acetate. It was the first commercial product to contain trenbolone acetate after its long hiatus following the withdrawal of Finajet and Finaject in the late 80's. Its release has garnered a lot of attention with athletes, to spite being in the form of an implant pellet. What is so unusual about all of these products is the fact that, remarkably, they are all exempt from U.S. controlled substance laws. They are totally and perfectly legal to buy with no license or prescription, albeit for the use of implanting cattle and not self-consumption. I assume this is to make it easy for livestock owners to have access to growth promoting agents. If a veterinarian were needed every time these products were to be used, they might be too troublesome or cost prohibitive to consider. Admittedly, since these products come in the form of pellets they are not in a form suitable for human consumption either, making their exemption seem a little more reasonable than at first glance.

Currently, the most popular product is still the original Finaplix® brand name, although it is currently being marketed by Intervet instead of the Hoechst-Roussel Agri-vet Company. This product comes in two forms, Finaplix-H and Finaplix-S, which denotes if the product was intended for a Heifer or a Steer respectively. The total dosages of both products are different, with the "H" version containing 100 20mg TA pellets (2,000 mg) and the "S" version only 70 (1,400 mg). Ivy Animal Health has introduced two competing products of equivalent makeup, sold as Component-TH and Component-TS. There are also the Revalor and Synovex+ brands that contain trenbolone acetate with an added dose of estrogen. However, these are much too troublesome for the athlete to consider using and should never be purchased.

Since the drug comes in the form of a cattle implant, administration is a bit difficult. Most commonly one or two implant pellets are ground up and mixed with a 50/50 water/DMSO mix and applied to the skin daily. This home-brew transdermal mix is effective, but the user is forced to walk around bearing the ripe scent of garlic (an effect of the DMSO). Others simply grind up one or two pellets with the back of a spoon and inhale (snort) them. Here the drug enters the blood stream through the mucous membrane, a poor, but still effective means of delivery for steroid hormones. Those who have tried this often claim it is not as irritating as they had imagined it would be. One, however, does always run the risk of wearing away at the lining of your nose after time, so it would be best not to make this a regular habit. More adventurous individuals make a practice of mixing their own injections. The pellets are ground into a fine powder (usually anywhere from 2 to 6 pellets), and then they are added to sterile water, propylene glycol, or an oil-based injectable steroid (or veterinary vitamin). This is usually repeated twice weekly, although some do manage to undergo this practice more frequently. Since this is not being done in a controlled sterile environment, one is obviously taking a risk. I do not doubt that infection is a common result. Some have actually started selling kits that contain all the necessary ingredients to separate the binders from the active steroid and brew a pure sterile injectable right in your kitchen. Most of the kits sold at this time are very thorough in their designs, and feedback on them has typically been excellent. I prefer not to mention actual product names, as it would probably not be a good idea to draw attention to the companies selling them. But they are not that hard to find right now. It is also of note that trenbolone acetate implant pellets are the active ingredients in a number of black market preparations, including the once popular Finabolan. Make no mistake; this is an underground product, to spite the fact that it now carries a very official looking hologram sticker.

Finaplix® and competing trenbolone acetate pellets are available through many veterinary suppliers. This is the least expensive way to locate this steroid, as an agricultural store will typically sell a single Finaplix-H cartridge (2,000mg) for approximately $35. On the black market this same amount can easily sell for as much as $75 or $100. Since many vet/agricultural suppliers have become aware that athletes are ordering these products, you should know that many are reluctant to sell. It is also rumored that the FDA gets a report of the sales of this product, however, this has not been confirmed. There is also talk of athletes being visited by the DEA and postal inspectors after ordering the pellets through the mail. At this time, Finaplix is still fully legal to possess, however, the DEA may be paying an unwelcome interest in companies that market or support its sale to bodybuilders. One would be best advised to be careful.

Moving on from Finaplix pellets, legitimate pharmaceutical preparations using trenbolone are not as scarce today as they were 5 years ago. In reviewing the popular, legitimate products to be found on the black market, here is what you should expect.

Animal Power, one of the new veterinary manufacturers in Mexico, is selling a 75mg/mL trenbolone acetate injectable called **Trenbo 75**. AP products are probably going to be amongst the most difficult for counterfeiters to duplicate accurately, as this manufacturer has a very strong focus on security measures. Most notable is the Animal Power holographic sticker, which is affixed to all product packaging (see Security Stickers).

Pet's Pharma is another new drug company in the Mexican steroid scene. They produce a trenbolone acetate injectable called **Trenbolon 75**. This product comes packed in both 10ml and 20ml multi-dose vials, and carries the company's (non-holographic) security sticker to deter counterfeiting. Pet's Pharma has not been a big target of counterfeit manufacturers, as of yet, making them a fairly safe company to shop.

Quality Vet's **Trembolona QV 75** is still one of the most popular in Mexico. It also contains a 75mg/mL dose of trenbolone acetate, packaged in a 10ml multi-dose vial. QV is an extremely reputable company, and to deter counterfeiting the line is protected by hologram stickers.

Ttokkyo's **Trenbol 75** is off the market now, given the recent closing of the company. Ttokkyo was at one time the hottest new firm in the Mexican scene. It is unfortunate they had to close shortly after, and I hope the principles continue in the steroid market. They were amongst the first companies to start using holographic security stickers to deter counterfeiting, and to cater directly to the needs of athletes... I mean athletic pets.

Loeffler makes an oral trenbolone acetate product in Mexico called **Acetenbo 50**. This may not be as crazy as you think, as the synthetic and hard-to-metabolize nature gives this steroid a fair level of oral bioavailability. The product, however, is extremely expensive for what it provides, so it is not extremely popular right now. Note that Loeffler has recently started using hologram stickers itself, although at this time they say only "Securidad" (security). Still, be sure to look for them when shopping.

British Dragon makes **Trenabol** in Thailand, containing 75 mg/mL of steroid in a 10ml vial. BD is a reputable company, and feedback on this product specifically has always been excellent. Note that they are no longer using holographic stickers on their injectable products. Instead, they use a red metallic foil inlay as part of all vial labels. Also, make sure the vial top reads, "TEAR" and "FLIP UP". A popular fake at the moment has tops that read, "FLIP OFF" only. BD additionally licensed an oral 25mg tablet called **Parabolan Tablets** to an Eastern European exporter; however, this relationship has since been discontinued (along with the product).

Trenol 50 is manufactured in Myanmar by WDV Pharmaceuticals. This 50mg/ml 6ml multi-dose vial provides a decent amount of steroid, although it does not make its way to the U.S. very often. WDV products seem most popular in areas of Eastern Europe, and to a lesser extent Western Europe.

Trenbolone enanthate

Androgenic	Anabolic	Standard
500	500	Nandrolone acetate

Chemical Names:
17beta-Hydroxyestra-4,9,11-trien-3-one

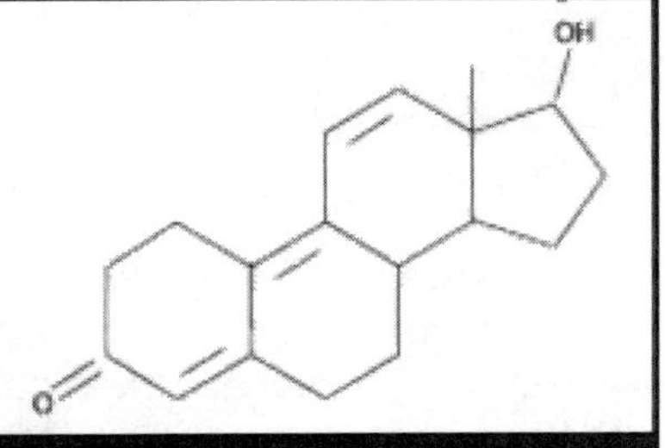

TRENBOLONE

Estrogenic Activity: none
Progestational Activity: low to moderate

Trenbolone enanthate is the most recent form of trenbolone to be developed, appearing on the market in mid-2004. This agent is essentially a new form of Parabolan, which uses the ubiquitous enanthate ester instead of the hexahydrobenzylcarbonate of the "old" product. Trenbolone enanthate is both unique and incredibly obvious at the same time. On the one hand, attaching an enanthate ester to trenbolone seems like a simple idea at best. After all, we are all familiar with testosterone and methenolone enanthate. But on the other hand, trenbolone enanthate had not been made commercially until now. With the loss of Parabolan, and only recent reemergence of a legitimate clone, the market was left with trenbolone acetate as its only readily available form of "tren". This ester of trenbolone is effective, but also very fast acting. Trenbolone enanthate is a much slower releasing drug, and offers a great alternative to the frequent injections of trenbolone acetate.

The pharmacokinetics of trenbolone enanthate should mirror those of testosterone enanthate, with peak hormone levels maintaining itself for approximately two weeks after each injection. Its action would be difficult to differentiate from Parabolan, as both of these agents use medium to long acting injectable steroid esters capable of releasing trenbolone from the site of injection for periods well in excess of the weekly intervals in which they are normally administered. The differences between the various esters of a particular steroid are going to be most noticeable in clinical medicine, where the relative speed of release controls the injection schedule of the patient. However, with athletic use high doses and regular injection schedules blur the different release patterns. Therefore, we really cannot attribute any special characteristics to this steroid, aside from saying that it is an excellent and well-conceived replacement for Parabolan.

The base steroid trenbolone is well understood at this point, and holds no real surprises. As a non-aromatizable compound, estrogenic side effects are not expected to be a problem. However, this drug is a nandrolone derivative, so it may exhibit some weak progestational activity. This means that while trenbolone alone should not cause side effects like water retention or gynecomastia, it may intensify the estrogenic traits of other steroids. Anti-estrogens are usually kept close at hand when trenbolone is taken with other aromatizable compounds. In regards to its androgenicity, trenbolone does not seem to fit well in with the nandrolone family of compounds. This steroid isn't metabolized into a weaker compound by 5-alpha reductase like most nandrolones are, which makes it quite androgenic. It is, therefore, very likely to produce such side effects as oily skin, acne, and aggravated hair loss (for those genetically prone).

We can expect to see new doors open with trenbolone enanthate, mainly those surrounding drug dosage. The poor oil solubility of trenbolone acetate limits the amount of steroid you can comfortably dissolve into solution around 75-100 milligrams per milliliter. And while the ester in Parabolan is much more oil soluble, most clones mimic the 50mg/ml dosage of the original French preparation. Therefore, we have yet to see high-dose forms of trenbolone on the drug market. Trenbolone enanthate will change this. We will likely see a number of trenbolone enanthate preparations released on the Mexican veterinary market over the next couple of years, formulated in a dosage range of 150-200mg/ml. Not only will such concentrations allow the adventurous athlete to experiment with high doses more easily, they will also give the average recreational user, who consumes only 2 or 3 different products during the average cycle, much more trenbolone per bottle/cycle.

The results from a cycle of trenbolone enanthate should include considerable increases in mass and strength, with great emphasis on muscle quality. This is often combined with notable fat loss, the desirable lean-gain and cut combination that has made Parabolan so talked about for all these years. To spite the potential for high doses with the new trenbolone enanthate compound, it may not actually be necessary. This is a steroid that is understood to work well on comparatively low doses. The average male bodybuilder will find that 150-250mg per week will provide a very strong effect, such that higher doses are probably not necessary in the average stack. This means that a 10ml vial with 200mg/ml of steroid could last for a full 10 weeks or longer. It should be no surprise to most readers to see such a low recommended dosage range. You will remember that Parabolan garnered a worldwide cult following while providing only 76mg/ml of steroid per 1.5ml ampule (50mg/ml). Women should not be advised to experiment with the series of trenbolones. These agents are significantly androgenic, and present too great a risk for permanent virilizing side effects.

All forms of pure trenbolone enanthate currently available on the black market are made by underground manufacturers. They are unverifiable for quality, as is the nature of "underground medicine" (although feedback on at least one product has been consistently very positive thus far). This is going to change very soon, however. Do not be surprised if you see legitimate drug companies start selling this agent shortly after Anabolics 2005 is published. If so, I would suggest trusting products sold by known companies with reliable security measures to deter counterfeiting, like hologram stickers. There is already talk that one of the veterinary drug firms in Mexico will be selling this material very shortly, which is welcome news. More companies are sure to follow suit as soon as word of this new drug gets out. If the popular companies all start adding this steroid to their lines en masse, availability will be great, as will the chance for this compound dominating the trenbolone market in the very near future.

Tribolin (nandrolone/methandriol blend)

Tribolin is a blended veterinary steroid product, produced by the Ranvet Company in Australia. Not quite doing its name justice, Tribolin contains two different steroid compounds instead of three (it really should have been called something like Dibolin if you ask me). This product specifically contains a blend of methandriol dipropionate and nandrolone decanoate, in a dose of 40mg/mL and 35mg/mL respectively. This adds up to a total steroid concentration of 75mg/mL. Tribolin is certainly not a high-dosed steroid, but is not a 25mg/mL steroid either. Incidentally, Ranvet makes a second product called Filybol, which is exactly the same as Tribolin except the nandrolone decanoate dose is 5mg/mL lower. I am not sure why they would make two seemingly identical products, but they are available nonetheless.

With its blend of methandriol and nandrolone, Tribolin is clearly an anabolic steroid in nature. Androgenic effects of this steroid would, likewise, only be slight for the average user. Its estrogenic effect should also be minimal, barring the methandriol content, which is intrinsically a bit estrogenic. Still, this product will not elevate estrogen levels itself very much, and unless the user is very sensitive to nandrolone, he should not be noticing gyno during a cycle. In many regards this product is like the Aussie vet steroid Drive, which contains a similar blend, but with boldenone instead of nandrolone. Typical dosing schedule for the male athlete would be in the range of 225mg (3cc's) to 450mg (6cc's) per week, a rage which should provide quality lean mass gain without bloat or much body fat retention (for a more comprehensive discussion of the individual steroids, please refer to their respective profiles).

Both Tribolin and Filybol come packaged in 10 and 20ml multi-dosed vials. Unfortunately, due to tight controls on drug products in Australia, these steroids do not make it to the U.S. very often. To make things worse, the packaging is pretty plain on both items. They obviously do not require a whole lot of ingenuity to duplicate. For these reasons I would be suspicious of any glut of Tribolin or Filybol (or any Australian vet steroids for that matter) that is found in the United States. It is just highly uncommon for volume sales of this product to be made. Unless you can personally trace these back to a legitimate supplier in Australia, I would consider them of unverified authenticity, and probably avoid.

Trinabol 150 (trenbolone blend)

Androgenic	Anabolic	Standard
500	500	Nandrolone acetate

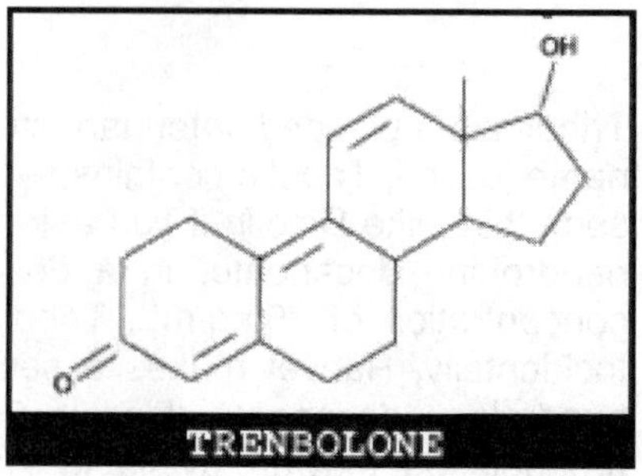

Chemical Names:
17beta-Hydroxyestra-4,9,11-trien-3-one

Estrogenic Activity: none
Progestational Activity: low to moderate

Each 1 ml contains:

Trenbolone acetate	50 mg
Trenbolone hexahydrobenzylcarbonate	50 mg
Trenbolone enanthate	50 mg

Trinabol is an injectable blend of three different trenbolone esters: trenbolone acetate, trenbolone hexahydrobenzylcarbonate, and trenbolone enanthate. These compounds are provided in equal parts, 50mg each. The total steroid concentration is 150mg/mL, and this product comes prepared in a 10ml vial. The formulation is intended to provide more of a sustained release effect than what is achieved with single ester products, and as such represents the first product of its type on the market. With a mix of both fast and slow acting components, it is essentially the trenbolone equivalent of Sustanon. This product is made by British Dragon, a Thai company with roots to British Dispensary in the same country (makers of Anabol and Androlic). British Dragon was formed by one of the principles of British Dispensary, with the intent to branch off and sell a wider variety of products, which they have successfully done. British Dragon now carries a full line of over a dozen items, and is one of the most talked about new companies on the international steroid market.

As a trenbolone injectable, Trinabol 150 is a potent lean mass building and cutting agent. Trenbolone itself has always been a favorite pre-contest drug, regardless of the ester used in its delivery. It is favorable here because it is strongly anabolic and androgenic, and at the same time structurally incapable of converting to estrogen. The gains produced by this drug tend to be of very high quality, often accompanied by fat loss instead of gain. Typical dosages for men are going to be in the range of 1-2ml per week, or 150-300mg of trenbolone ester. Being that trenbolone is significantly more potent than testosterone on a milligram for milligram basis, the 2cc weekly injection will provide a very substantial benefit. At this dosage one might even be able to make significant progress without the addition of other drugs. In most cases, however, trenbolone is combined with another base steroid. You will commonly see stacks with testosterone or boldenone during bulking phases of training, or Winstrol, Primobolan, or Anavar during cutting cycles. In such situations, a single 150mg dose per week will usually be enough on the trenbolone side. Women should probably avoid this drug altogether, due to both its strong androgenicity and long duration of action.

As a mixed ester product with mostly long-acting compounds, Trinabol provides a total duration of effect very similar to what we would see with Parabolan. The short-acting acetate ester, however, allows blood levels to peak much more quickly. In crude terms it is a form of Parabolan that kicks in faster than normal. In regards to bodybuilding, for all intents and purposes, this product is interchangeable with regular Parabolan, as weekly injections will blur any sustained-release properties the mixed esters might provide. However, this formulation is a big improvement over trenbolone acetate injectables, as the 2-3 times per week injection schedule needed for these products can be very uncomfortable. Trinabol also carries 150mg/mL of steroid, double the concentration of what most standard acetate-based products are going to provide.

Trinabol 150 is currently the only blended trenbolone injectable being produced by a commercial steroid manufacturer. BD is using specific security checks to deter counterfeiting, so be sure to pay attention to these when shopping. For starters, BD stopped using hologram stickers on its injectables some time ago. They now use them only on orals, and Trinabol came out after this switch (no old lots with stickers can be found). A current popular Russian counterfeiter is using duplicate labels, so be careful. Next, they have added a shiny red metallic foil inlay in their labels. Lastly, be sure your vial cap reads, “TEAR” and “FLIP UP”. British Dragon uses a very specific vial top, that to date the counterfeiters have not picked up on. The fakes typically read, “FLIP OFF” only. Provided your vial matches on these points, you should be assured of a legitimate purchase.

Triolandren (testosterone blend)

Androgenic	Anabolic	Standard
100	100	Standard

Chemical Names:
4-androsten-3-one-17beta-ol
17beta-hydroxy-androst-4-en-3-one

Estrogenic Activity: moderate
Progestational Activity: low

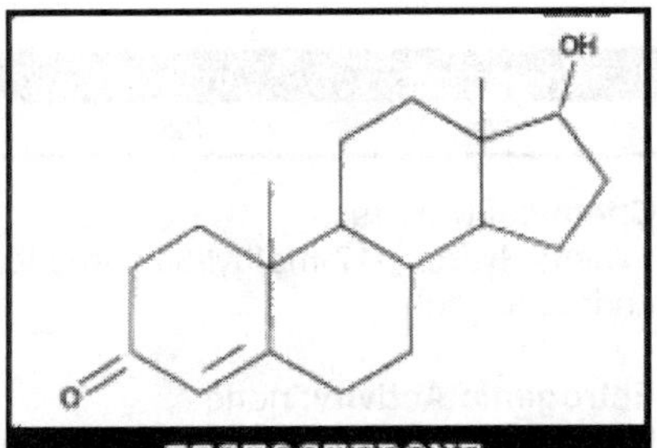

TESTOSTERONE

Triolandren is an injectable testosterone blend, produced by Novartis. More specifically, this product contains a mixture of testosterone propionate, n-valerianate, and undecylenate, for a total steroid concentration of 250mg/mL. With its mix of fast and long acting esters, Triolandren is very much like Sustanon in design. The intention in both cases was clearly to create a product that will deliver testosterone, slowly, evenly and comfortably, to a patient over a period of three to four weeks. In this case, the slowest releasing ester used was undecylenate, whereas Sustanon uses decanoate. This would make Triolandren ever so slightly the longer acting agent between the two.

Each 1 ml ampule of Triolandren contains:

Testosterone Propionate	20 mg
Testosterone-n-valerianate	80 mg
Testosterone Undecylenate	150 mg

As a testosterone injectable, Triolandren is a powerful strength and size builder. Really effective mass-building cycles almost always include some form of testosterone for this reason. That is not to say you *must* use testosterone. But it is cheap, and works better than just about anything else available for this purpose. The positive anabolic properties of this hormone, of course, are accompanied by equally strong androgenic and estrogenic properties. Side effects, at some level, are almost unavoidable as a result. If you are particularly sensitive to the effects of estrogen, you may want to have some form of anti-estrogen or aromatase inhibitor on-hand should side effects become problematic (for a more comprehensive discussion about the benefits and potential drawbacks to using a sustained-release testosterone product like this, please refer to the Sustanon profile).

Although much longer acting, in the context of using them for bodybuilding purposes, drugs like Triolandren and Sustanon are usually injected on a weekly basis. Such a schedule eliminates any real advantage in using a sustained-release blend of testosterone. After all, the main reason these drugs were designed is so that you don't have to inject them every week. If you are going to do this anyway, you are probably much better off purchasing a cheaper product that contains testosterone enanthate or cypionate. You'll get a lot more testosterone for your money, and a cycle that is utterly indistinguishable from one using Triolandren.

Triolandren is a rare find on the black market. To the best of my knowledge it is only manufactured in two countries currently, Egypt and Taiwan. Novartis is the manufacturer in both cases. Since these two countries are really not major source countries for steroids, you probably should not expect to see Triolandren very often. If you do find it, can verify its legitimacy, and are offered it for a fair price, it should most certainly be as acceptable for use as any other slow acting testosterone injectable. Unless you like giving money away, I'd base the decision on a simple calculation of how much testosterone are you getting for your money: cheapest product wins.

Winstrol (stanozolol)

Androgenic	Anabolic	Standard
30	320	Methyltestosterone (oral)

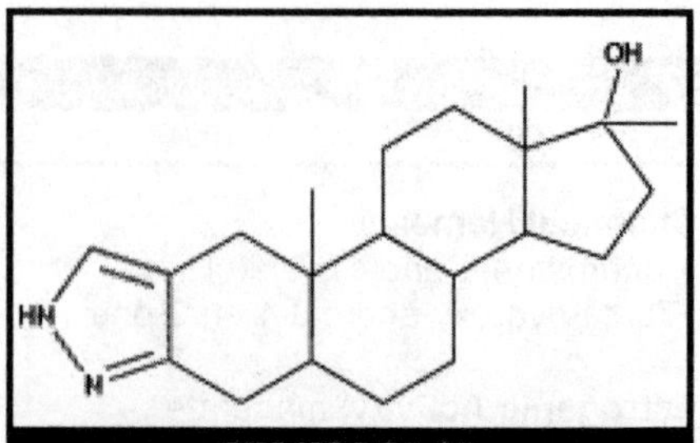

STANOZOLOL

Chemical Names:
17beta-Hydroxy-17-methyl-5alpha-androstano[3,2-c]pyrazole
androstanazol

Estrogenic Activity: none
Progestational Activity: not significant

Winstrol® is a popular brand name for the synthetic anabolic steroid stanozolol, first patented in U.S. by Sterling back in 1962 (patent # 3,030,358). The compound itself is a derivative of dihydrotestosterone, although its activity is much milder than this androgen in nature. It is technically classified as an anabolic steroid, shown to exhibit a slightly greater tendency for muscle growth than androgenic activity in early studies. While dihydrotestosterone really only provides androgenic side effects when administered, stanozolol instead provides quality muscle growth. Admittedly the anabolic properties of this substance are still mild in comparison to many stronger compounds, but it is still a reliable builder. Its efficacy as an anabolic could even be comparable to Dianabol, however Winstrol® does not carry with it the same tendency for water retention. Stanozolol also contains the same c17 methylation we see with Dianabol, an alteration used so that oral administration is possible. To spite this design however, there are many injectable versions of this steroid produced.

Structurally stanozolol is not capable of converting into estrogen. Likewise an antiestrogen is not necessary when using this steroid, gynecomastia not being a concern even among sensitive individuals. Since estrogen is also the culprit with water retention, instead of bulk Winstrol® produces a lean, quality look to the physique with no fear of excess subcutaneous fluid retention. This makes it a favorable steroid to use during cutting cycles, when water and fat retention are a major concern. It is also very popular among athletes in combination strength/speed sports such as Track and Field. In such disciplines one usually does not want to carry around excess water weight, and may therefore find the raw muscle-growth brought about by Winstrol® quite favorable over the lower quality mass gains of more estrogenic agents.

As mentioned Winstrol® is prepared in two distinct forms, as an oral tablet and an injectable solution. Although they are chemically identical, the injectable usually allows the user to take much higher dose of the steroid. This is of course because the injectables are much more cost effective, and therefore usually the preferred form of administration. You may find big differences in the appearance of one injectable product to another however. In particular there are big discrepancies in the size of the steroid particles used to manufacture the various stanozolol suspensions. For example, the European human use product Zambon uses a fine powder, capable of being comfortably injected through a 25-27 gauge needle. The Mexican veterinary product Stanazolic is even better, so refined that it can pass easily through an ultra-fine 29 gauge insulin needle. Many other veterinary products on the other hand use steroid in a much larger particle size, such as Winstrol®-V in the U.S., and Anabolic-ST from Australia and Mexico. In many instances jams and difficulty injecting have been noticed when trying to administer these products, even when using a large 22-gauge needle. But there are both advantages and disadvantages to each type of product. On the one hand the large particle size would form a longer acting deposit (depot) while the steroid dissolves, giving us the option of fewer injections. A larger shot every three to four days would likely be sufficient to keep blood levels within limits, which is a favorable schedule for a water-based product. On the other hand we are forced to use a standard size oil needle (21 gauge) for the injection, uncomfortable for regular administration. Products made with a finer substance do not allow for as slow acting a depot, and therefore are usually injected every other day to keep blood levels steady. But shots can be given with a much more comfortable sized needle, opening up many new injection sites. Although you can jam a big "oil pipe" into your shoulder, that is really not the place for it.

For men, the usual dosage of Winstrol® is 15-25mg per day for the tablets and 25-50mg per day with the injectable (differences based solely on price and quantity). It is often combined with other steroids depending on the desired result. For bulking purposes, a stronger androgen like testosterone, Dianabol or Anadrol 50® is usually added. Here, Winstrol® will balance out the cycle a bit, giving us good anabolic effect with lower overall estrogenic activity than if taking such steroids alone. The result should be a considerable gain in new muscle mass, with a more comfortable level of water and fat retention. For contest and dieting phases, we could alternately combine Winstrol® with a non-aromatizing androgen such as trenbolone or Halotestin®. Such combinations should help bring about the strongly defined, hard look of muscularity so sought after by bodybuilders. Older, more sensitive individuals can otherwise add compounds like Primobolan®, Deca-Durabolin®, or Equipoise® when wishing to stack this steroid. Here we should see good results and fewer side effects than is to be expected with standard androgen therapies.

Women will take somewhere in the range of 5-10mg daily, or two and a half to five 2mg tablets. Although female athletes usually find stanozolol very tolerable, the injectable is usually off limits. They risk androgenic buildup, as a regular 50mg injection will provide much too high a dosage. Here, the tablets are the general preference. It is obviously much easier to divide up pills than it is to break up a 1cc ampule into multiple injections. Those who absolutely must experiment with the injectable would be most comfortable dividing each 50mg ampule into at least two separate injections. At this point the dosage will adjusted by the number of days separating each shot. 25mg every third or fourth day should be a comfortable amount for most. More ambitious (and risk taking) females would take 25mg every second day, although this is not recommended. Although this compound is only moderately androgenic, the risk of virilization symptoms should remain a definite concern.

With the structural (c17-AA) alteration, the tablets will also place a higher level of stress on the liver than the injectable (which avoids the "first pass"). During longer or higher dosed cycles, liver values should, therefore, be watched closely through regular blood work. Although less common, the possibility of liver damage cannot be excluded with this injectable however. While it does not enter the body through the liver, it is still broken down by it, providing a lower (but more continuous) level of stress. Such stress would, of course, be amplified when adding other c17-AA oral compounds to a cycle of Winstrol®. When using such combinations, cautious users would make every effort to limit the length of the cycle (preferably 6 to 8 weeks). It is also of note that both versions of Winstrol® have been linked to strong adverse changes in HDL/LDL cholesterol levels. This side effect is common with anabolic steroid therapy, and can become a health concern as the dose/duration of intake increase above normal. The oral version should have a greater impact on cholesterol values than the injectable due to the method of administration, and may, therefore, be the worse choice of the two for those concerned and this side effect.

As discussed in the opening section of this book, the oral use of stanozolol can also have a profound impact on levels of SHBG (sex hormone-binding globulin). Admittedly, this is characteristic of all anabolic/androgenic steroids, however, its potency and form of administration make Winstrol® particularly noteworthy in this regard. Since plasma binding proteins such as SHBG act to temporarily constrain steroid hormones from exerting activity, this effect would provide a greater percentage of free (unbound) steroid hormone in the body. This may amount to an effective mechanism in which stanozolol could increase the potency of a concurrently used steroid. To further this purpose we could also add Proviron® (1methyl-dihydrotestosterone), which has an extremely high affinity for SHBG. This affinity may cause Proviron® to displace other weaker substrates for SHBG (such as testosterone), another mechanism in which the free hormone level may be increased. Adding Winstrol® and Proviron® to your next testosterone cycle may, therefore, prove very useful, markedly enhancing the free state of this potent muscle building androgen.

Winstrol is an extremely popular steroid, and the fact that it is found in abundance on the black market reflects this. It is also a popular target for counterfeit steroid manufacturers, so you need to be careful when shopping. If you know what to look for, you should be able to keep yourself safe. In going over the popular brands circulating right now, I can offer the following observations and advice.

The new Mexican firm Animal Power has release a pair of stanozolol products, one oral and one injectable. The oral product is called **Stan Tabs**, and carries 10mg of steroid in a 100-count bottle. The injectable is called **Stan 50**, and contains 50mg/mL of steroid in a 10ml multi-dose vial. Both products are packaged for sale in individual boxes, and all components (boxes, vials, and bottles) will carry the company's security hologram sticker. Although counterfeits of this line have not yet been a problem, be sure to still look for this hologram when shopping, as it should assure a safe purchase (see Security Stickers).

Denkall's **Stanazolic** is an excellent product, and highly recommended. It is found is four distinct forms, a number greater than any competing brand. You can find it as a 50mg/mL injectable, a 100mg/mL injectable, a 10mg tablet, and a 6mg capsule. All forms are to be considered of excellent quality, and are photographed in this book. As mentioned above, they have one of the most refined injectables on the market. Just be sure to look for the Denkall hologram sticker on each bottle/vial, which should assure you are purchasing the real thing.

Quality Vet produces a 50mg/mL and a 100mg/mL injectable called **Stan QV**. These products, and company, are also highly regarded. Again, look for the hologram sticker and you should be fine. This is definitely a recommended buy.

Anabolic-ST from SYD Group is also popular in Mexico. With this one, however, you need to use a large 21-gauge needle, as the particle size is not as refined as the European Zambon or Denkall Stanazolic products. Again, look for the hologram sticker to assure legitimacy.

Stanol-V by Ttokkyo is no longer being made in Mexico. The owner of Ttokkyo ran into legal trouble a couple of years ago, and although the company had been hanging on for some time after, all reports are now that the company is closed.

Bratis is another Mexican company, with roots in Eastern Europe and quasi-legal status in Meico. They have been selling a 50mg/mL injectable called **Stanol 50**, as well as a 10mg tablet called **Stanol 10**. Feedback on these products have been very good, thus far.

Norvet's **Estano-Pet's** is another new stanozolol product in Mexico, delivering either 10mg or 25mg of steroid per tablet. Both forms come in 100 tablet bottles. I have not had a chance to see lab test results, but if they indeed are making a 25mg tablet, it will go over very well on the black market.

Chinfield makes a 50mg/mL injectable stanozolol in Argentina called **Nabolic Strong**. This is the same firm that makes regular Nabolic, a very low dosed (2mg/mL) version of the same drug. This new product is now much more popular on the black market than the first, due to the more useable dosage. Note that Chinfield prints their logo on the inside of the vial carton, which offers somewhat of a simple security check (obviously one very easy to duplicate). Your box is definitely counterfeit if it is blank on the inside.

The Thai firm British Dragon has reworked its stanozolol offerings recently. They are now selling their **Stanabol** brand in two tablet strengths, 10mg and 50mg(!). Both versions are sold in foil-lined paper pouches of 100 tablets each. The tabs themselves are not longer pentagonal shaped, and are now square with the letters "BD" formed into one side and the dosage ("10" or "50") in the other. Note that BD oral products will carry a security hologram sticker to deter counterfeiting. This sticker has been copied before, however, so pay closer attention to the shape of the tablets and you should be fine.

The **Stanol** brand name is also used in Thailand, where the manufacturer, Body Research, uses it to sell 5mg stanozolol tablets and a 50mg/mL injectable. The tablets are packed in bottles of 200 tablets each, and the injectable in the form of 1ml glass ampules. Both products are highly regarded on the black market, and fakes do not appear to be a problem thus far.

Acdhon in Thailand makes **Stanozodon**, a relatively low dose today with the industry-old standard of only 2mg of steroid tablet. The fact that it is packaged in bottles of 1000 does make up for this, at least a little bit. This product is safe, but not extremely popular on the black market. It is possible Acdhon has discontinued steroid sales, as we have not seen much of this product as of late.

Xelox, an export company from the Phillippines, sells a brand of stanozolol called **Anazol**. It comes in both an oral and injectable form. The injectable, **Anazol Depot**, carries 50mg/mL of steroid in a 5ml multi-dose vial. The formulation includes 5mg/mL of added lidocaine, to reduce injection discomfort. The oral comes as a 2mg tablet, with 100 coming per plastic bottle. Both forms of the drug will carry the Xelox security sticker to deter counterfeiting.

Winstrol®-V, the multi-dose injectable produced in America and Canada, is the stanozolol product duplicated most by counterfeiters. With tight controls you will likely not see the real thing anymore, so avoid all such products on the black market. If you want to risk it, at least make sure the steroid crystals separate deeply when the bottle is at rest. The particles in real Winstrol®-V are also too large to be drawn into the finer gauge needles (25-27 gauge should jam quickly).

Zambon Winstrol® tablets and injectable ampules are still produced in large quantities in Spain as well. In fact, this remains the most popular stanozolol injectable in Europe. Note that the packaging on this product has changed again, now coming in the form of reddish colored boxes (see pictures section). However, the **Italian** Zambon products are no longer being made. Avoid all such items on the black market.

The Greek generic by **Genepharm** is also circulating, but not abundantly in the U.S. It does not appear to be a big target for counterfeiters as of yet, and can therefore be trusted. Remember to look for a Greek drug ID sticker on the box to assure legitimacy. This will show a hidden mark under UV light, and provides a very reliable detection method.

Aside from those products listed above I would trust no other stanozolol tablet unless you are absolutely sure of the source.

ANABOLIC AGENTS (NON-STEROID)

DRUG PROFILES

Arachidonic Acid

Arachidonic acid is the body's principle "anabolic fat". More specifically, it is an omega-6 fatty acid that serves as the principle building block for the synthesis of dienolic prostaglandins (such as PGE2 and PGF2α). These prostaglandins are integral to protein turnover and muscle accumulation, and have such activities as increasing blood flow to the muscles (pumps), increasing local testosterone sensitivity (androgen receptor levels), and increasing overall protein synthesis. Arachidonic acid is the body's core regulator of prostaglandin turnover in skeletal muscle tissue, and as such is responsible for initiating many of the immediate biochemical changes during resistance exercise that will ultimately produce anabolism. Among the large variety of nutrients we take into our bodies each day, arachidonic acid is among the most integral to muscle growth. It is, likewise, one of the most important to pay attention to when it comes to diet and supplementation.

Arachidonic acid begins to display its anabolic activity immediately during exercise. This nutrient is released from your muscle fibers as they are damaged during intense exercise, controlling the intensity of the body's inflammatory (and anabolic) response. This is the same process that causes you to be sore a day or two following a good workout, and reminds us that the old adage "no pain, no gain" is a fundamentally true one. Arachidonic acid liberation from damaged muscle fibers is, similarly, the very first anabolic trigger, in a long cascade that will control the rebuilding and strengthening of muscle tissue after exercise[97 98 99]. Among other things, by increasing local androgen receptor density[100], arachidonic acid allows testosterone to increase protein synthesis rates and start repairing the damaged tissue. This nutrient supports the anabolic actions of testosterone not by increasing hormone levels, but by giving this hormone more receptor sites to attach to (making the process both faster and more intense). As a crude explanation, arachidonic acid directs the body to where it needs muscle tissue repair, and opens the door for testosterone to do its job.

The availability of arachidonic acid, and our ability to liberate it during exercise, is vital to the productivity of our workouts. We also need to be aware of the fact that regular exercise significantly lowers the content of arachidonic acid in skeletal muscle tissue[101 102 103]. Since dienolic prostaglandin synthesis is inextricably tied to the amount of available arachidonic acid, lower levels result in less arachidonic acid being release with the stretching and damage of exercise. This means a less dramatic increase in androgen receptor density, and a lower rate of muscle protein synthesis. The depletion of arachidonic acid in skeletal muscle tissue is one of the key reasons we find it harder and harder to get sore the longer we have been working out. With lower levels of arachidonic acid, you need to work more vigorously to receive the same level of anabolic stimulation. On the other hand, when you change up your routine, and hit your muscles from new angles, arachidonic acid is the reason you'll find yourself more sore than usual. You have called upon new muscle fibers, and they have higher (untapped) stores of this vital nutrient to work with.

To support the pro-inflammatory/anabolic actions of prostaglandins, arachidonic acid can be taken in high levels. Typically, one would take a dosage of 800-1000mg daily, which is administered for a period of 7-8 weeks (it is cycled on and off in the same way anabolic steroids are). Short-term diets very rich in arachidonic acid like this are well documented to cause a high retention of arachidonic acid in body tissues[104 105 106 107], and also to significantly increase the output of prostaglandin metabolites. They will essentially overload the body's ability to regulate normal tissue levels, cause the retention of arachidonic acid in the muscles above what you would have been experiencing before. This will mean easier arachidonic acid liberation during exercise, greater PG output, greater tissue androgen sensitivity, and elevated protein synthesis rates. When you load arachidonic acid like this, early on you should be seeing an increase in pumps during your workouts, sometimes so profound that it can interfere with your range of motion. Within the first couple of weeks you should also start noticing that you are getting a lot sorer in the days following your training. I often hear comments like, "I haven't been this sore in years" or "I feel like I did when I first started training". By the third or fourth week this should all start equating to very measurable and welcome increases in size and strength. These gains also tend to be associated with modest losses in body fat, making arachidonic acid a versatile "lean mass" building agent.

Arachidonic acid is a supplement of interest to both steroid and non-steroid using athletes. For example, some people find it harder to get their muscles really sore when taking a lot of steroids, and what comes doesn't last as long as it did when off-cycle. The body just seems to recover so quickly when taking hormonal anabolics, sometimes too quickly to feel like you are damaging them enough during training. The greater intake of arachidonic acid during a steroid cycle like this will allow for much greater day to day stimulus from your training.

Your body will be able to "respond" to the lifting as if you were putting in much more effort, or have not been training as long (as if you haven't depleted your arachidonic acid stores as much). On the other hand, arachidonic acid is an effective anabolic agent in its own right. In my experience, a daily dosage of 800mg (under 200lbs) or 1,000mg (200lbs+) can consistently put an average of 1-2lbs of lean muscle on per week, with nothing more that heavy training and a high protein diet to support its anabolic activities. These are very significant numbers, making arachidonic acid by far most effective natural supplement for building muscle I've yet had the ability to work with.

Although arachidonic acid can produce a very weak androgenic effect by allowing testosterone to be more active in the body, this should not be significant enough to concern females about virilizing side-effects. At best, this effect usually causes mild oily skin in a small number of users. For most, it is entirely unnoticeable. There is also no hormonal disruption with arachidonic acid supplementation, which means no "post cycle" crash. The retention of gains after the product is discontinued, likewise, seems to be extremely high. While gains stop abruptly when arachidonic acid loading is discontinued, they do not tend to reverse. That is not to say there are zero side- effects to be concerned with when it comes to arachidonic acid. This is a "pro-inflammatory" supplement. If you suffer from injury, any type of an inflammatory condition, or other conditions where the intake of omega 6 fatty acids should be limited (such as cardiovascular disease, asthma or high blood pressure), then you should not be running out to take arachidonic acid. If you are healthy, however, and have no medical conditions requiring you to limit omega 6 intake (this nutrient is found largely in red meat), this supplement can be used with exceptional safety and benefit.

In case you were unaware, I am the pioneer of the arachidonic acid loading concept. I have been very excited about this discovery, and the progress I have made over the past couple of years while working with this nutrient. I have ultimately been granted patent on the concept, and have since released a supplement form of arachidonic acid called **X-Factor** (sold through my company, Molecular Nutrition). Each capsule provides 200mg of arachidonic acid, roughly what you'd get after a full day of eating the normal red-meat-rich Western diet[108]. When using this supplement to enhance muscle-growth, however, four to five capsules are recommended each day for a period of 50 days, which supplies levels of arachidonic acid far beyond what diet alone could possibly ever provide you (in this regard arachidonic acid levels are "overloaded", very much in the same way that creatine is loaded). At this point I can say with certainty that arachidonic acid holds remarkable power as a legal and non-hormonal muscle-building agent when used in this manner, more so than anything I have had the opportunity to experiment in this industry over the past decade and a half. I am positive it will become a staple anabolic nutrient in the years to come. Just remember where you heard about it first.

Kynoselen

Kynoselen is an injectable veterinary drug from France, produced by the firm Vetoquinol. It contains a mixture of Heptaminol, AMP (adenosine monophosphate), Vitamin B-12, Sodium Selenite, Magnesium Aspartate & Potassium Aspartate. This blend makes for a restorative "tonic" type drug, administered to protect an animal's muscle mass and overall wellness after illness, injury, or trauma. For example, it may be used as an anticatabolic after a strenuous race, or to help get an animal on its feet after a debilitating infection. At other times it is simply used to support the vitality of an animal that is otherwise healthy, but at the moment less than vigorous in its daily activities. In some cases it is even used for the very basic purpose of remedying a deficiency in vitamin B-12 or selenium intake.

Bodybuilders are attracted to Kynoselen for its mild anabolic and lipolytic properties. The principle active ingredient in the product is heptaminol, an inotropic compound that increases contractile strength, and minimizes fatigue, of the muscles[109]. It has also demonstrated a specific ability to increase the differentiation of satellite muscle cells[110], a process that helps generate new muscle tissue (skeletal muscle growth). This same ingredient is also known to affect the release and uptake of norepinephrine (noradrenalin), increasing levels of this hormone/neurotransmitter in the blood[111]. Since noradrenalin is an important regulator of lipolysis in humans, this allows heptaminol to impart a fat-loss effect. Admittedly, however, both its anabolic and lipolytic properties are not dramatic. But being that this drug is totally legal, it remains an attractive alternative to anabolic steroids for many. Even when used alone it can impart measurable increases in strength, muscle mass, fat loss and vascularity, which no doubt explains why Kynoselen is relatively popular drug these days.

The usual recommended dosage is around 1ml weekly for every 25 pounds of bodyweight. This would mean that a 200lb bodybuilder would use around 8ml per week, not a small injection volume by any means. For this reason, some opt to take a lower dosage, injecting at the very least a 2ml three times per week. At this dose, a single 100ml vial would last about 16 weeks. At 8-10ml per week the bottle would still last for ten to twelve weeks. It is best to use up the entire bottle once it has been opened, even if you didn't need that much drug for your cycle. As with all injectable drugs packaged in multi-dosed vials, contaminants will be introduced into the solution immediately once the seal is broken for the first injection. Being that it is water-based medication, it is not expected to keep very well. You most certainly do not want to leave a half used bottle of Kynoselen on the closet shelf for later use.

Because it tends to increase noradrenalin levels, Kynoselen is a mild stimulant. It is likely for this specific reason that its use has been banned by certain horseracing organizations. This means that one can expect certain stimulant-related side effects, especially when taking this drug in higher dosages. This includes rapid heartbeat, sweating, jitters, restlessness, increased blood pressure or insomnia. A good rule of thumb used by bodybuilders to try and keep such side effects from becoming a problem is never to inject more than 2ml per day. They may also want to start with an amount lower than the recommended dosage (determined by body weight), perhaps even half of this. The dose is then slowly increased, so that the peak level is reached only after three to four weeks of slow incremental increases.

Kynoselen will usually run you about $75 to $100 per bottle. It is not a controlled substance, and is likewise pretty easy to obtain locally or via mail order. Currently no fakes are known to exist. Given its abundance and low cost, I do not think we should expect counterfeits anytime soon. It is also important to note that legitimate Kynoselen is a veterinary drug only, and has never been manufactured for human use.

Lutalyse (diniprost)

Lutalyse is a synthetic form of prostaglandin F2alpha. Prostaglandins are a series of natural oxygenated unsaturated cyclic fatty acids, which have a variety of hormone like actions in the body. Among other things, prostaglandins are involved with pain, inflammation and the development of fever. They affect ovulation and the female reproductive system, alter gastric motility and fluid absorption in the gastrointestinal tract, and effect the respiratory system by constricting or dilating blood vessels in the lungs and smooth muscles lining the bronchial tubes. In the circulatory system they constrict and dilate blood vessels as well, often as a way of effecting blood pressure, and in the kidneys they affect the excretion of water and electrolytes. Of note is that prostaglandins also affect the buildup of fat and muscle protein synthesis.

Lutalyse is used in veterinary medicine for the purposes of controlling breeding. When used correctly with a series of other hormones, it can successfully stimulate ovulation and allow for a successful, timed impregnation. Athletes of course use it for a very different purpose, namely the strong thermogenic and anabolic potency of the compound. We see this combination a lot, but this prostaglandin may indeed live up to this goal. For starters, PGF2a has been shown in studies to stimulate protein synthesis[112]. Reports from athletes who have experimented with it often support this compound being an excellent site growth agent, and they occur with enough frequency to be believable. And it is supposed to be a very fast acting drug, with many claiming it has caused incredible pumps and noticeable increases in actual muscle tissue size after being injected in the site for only a couple of weeks. Data also supports it being a possible fat-loss drug, with PGF2a shown in studies clearly to inhibit the stimulation of lipogenesis in fat cells[113]. Again we have a lot of anecdotal support for this use as well, with many claiming they notice a slight temperature elevation and marked fat loss with use of this agent.

The main problems with diniprost are its side effects, which can be extremely severe. This includes pronounced soreness at the site of injection; often beginning with a dull burning pain almost immediately after the shot is given. Chills and flu-like feelings are also commonly reported during cycles, as occasionally are bouts of shortness of breath. Those with asthma should definitely not be taking this drug for fear it may induce a full-blown attack. Injections are also followed in many cases by uncontrollable urges to urinate and defecate, including strong spasmodic contractions of the muscles involved in the control of these functions. Nausea and vomiting have also been reported. For many, the cramping, diarrhea and general feelings of upset stomach, malaise and discomfort make PGF2a a drug they experiment with only shortly. Others however endure the intense side effects, and often do report that they become somewhat more tolerable as their use of the drug continues. For this group favorable results are consistently reported, with many claiming incredible site growth and marked fat loss.

Use of this drug typically involves starting with a low dosage, perhaps .5 milligram per injection site. Common target sites are the shoulders, biceps, triceps, calves, even chest, back and legs. The user will typically do only one site in a day to begin with as well, but may increase the number of shots given as they become more accustomed to the drug. If the first shot was event free, the next injection will be one milligram. This is slowly increased each time, with a typical target being 1 milliliter or 5mg. Injection sites are also rotated, so that several days separate injections in the same muscle group. It is also up to individual sensitivity how you schedule injections with your training routine. For some, the pain is too much to allow for training of the injected muscle for at least a few days post administration. In such a case you would want to work out a schedule of injecting in the right window of time during your post-training recovery and before your next workout targeting that muscle group.

ANALGESICS

DRUG PROFILES

NSAIDs (Non-Steroidal Anti-Inflammatory Drugs)

Non-Steroidal Anti-Inflammatory Drugs (NSAIDs) are a group of medications that exert analgesic (pain-relieving) actions in the body by inhibiting the release of inflammatory prostaglandins. They do a job very similar to that of cortisol, which also exerts its anti-inflammatory actions by blocking prostaglandin biosynthesis. A comparison to cortisol is even made in the term "non-steroidal anti-inflammatory", as cortisol is, of course, a steroidal hormone while these drugs are not. As a group NSAIDs are amongst the most widely used pain medicines in the world, and can be found in a variety of prescription and over-the-counter forms. The most popular OTC NSAIDs in the United States are Advil/Motrin (ibuprofen) and Aleve (naproxin sodium), while Celebrex (celecoxib), Indocin (indomethacin), Vioxx (rofecoxib) and Mobic (meloxicam) are all available by prescription. Although aspirin and Tylenol (acetaminophen) are technically not classified as non-steroidal anti-inflammatory drugs, they inhibit prostaglandin biosynthesis as well, and are therefore equally relevant to our discussion.

Although NSAIDs are effective analgesic medications, they are NOT good bodybuilding drugs. They should not be used to help you "work through the pain", and they will not enhance your rate of recovery. In fact, they can be very detrimental to muscle growth. This is because the inflammatory response that is mediated by prostaglandins is absolutely vital to protein synthesis. In March 2002 a study was published that made this fact very clear[114]. It involved a group of 24 recreationally active young male subjects, who were given maximum OTC doses of ibuprofen (1,200mg/day) or acetaminophen (4,000mg/day) and subjected to resistance training. Amino acid turnover was measured for 24 hours following the bout of exercise, which allowed the investigators to determine what effect, if any, these drugs would have on protein breakdown and synthesis. It turned out that both ibuprofen and acetaminophen effectively blunted the normal post-exercise rise in protein synthesis, which was increased 76% above baseline in the group taking only the placebo. A follow up investigation demonstrated that both drugs were specifically blocking the normal post-exercise rise in PGF2α[115]. These studies show us just how strongly prostaglandins actually support the basic process of muscle growth; they are the last things in the world we would want to inhibit when trying to build muscle.

This is not an outright crucifixion of anti-inflammatory drugs. Certainly if you have pain, these drugs are amongst your safest options for dealing with it. I am also not trying to suggest that if you take these drugs regularly you will be totally unable to grow. I'm sure many guys out there would disagree with this notion. I myself have taken these drugs regularly during my training at times, and have been able to make progress while doing so. But I can definitely feel the difference when they are not in my body; growth is much less restrained in comparison. The bottom line is that you should take these drugs if you need to take them. If pain is stopping you from being able to function, you need to treat this first and foremost. But if you don't need to take these drugs, definitely stay the hell away from them. NSAIDs are most certainly not going to offer you any muscle-building benefit!

Nubain (nalbuphine HCL)

Nubain is a trade name for the painkiller nalbuphine HCL. Specifically, it is an injectable opiate-based analgesic (narcotic) with mixed agonist/antagonist properties. The analgesic action is roughly the equivalent of morphine on a milligram for milligram basis, although the overall action of the two drugs is quite different. The main distinction stems from the opiate antagonist activity of Nubain. There are three classes of opioid receptors in the human body, labeled mu, delta and kappa. Nubain blocks activation of mu receptors, the primary target of morphine and other related opiates. It is the mu receptor that produces the strong euphoria, analgesia and respiratory depression we see with these drugs. Instead, Nubain induces analgesia through interaction with Kappa receptors.

The mixed properties of this drug give it a number of unique qualities. For starters, Nubain has a much lower abuse potential than we see with pure opiates. In fact, individuals dependent on an opiate drug like heroin will generally experience withdrawal symptoms when administering Nubain. This mixed action also makes overdosing on this drug more difficult. While an average dose (10-30mg) will have a depressive effect on the respiratory system, depression is not appreciably increased with higher doses. The possibility of overdose and dependency cannot be excluded with Nubain however, but does require a considerable level of use. In the United States Nubain is not considered a drug with much abuse potential, as can be seen by its classification as a standard prescription drug (not a controlled substance).

Clinically, Nubain is used (generally) for the treatment of moderately severe pain, as a component of surgical anesthesia, and as an analgesic during labor. It has the welcome characteristic of causing only a minimal decrease in the level of oxygen consumption (a problem associated with most pure opiates). It is particularly effective at lowering the cardiac workload, and is commonly used during treatment of myocardial infarction cases. The dosage given is adjusted according to severity of pain and physical status of the patient, but is generally in the range of 10 - 20 mg for 70 kg of bodyweight. This substance can be administered as an intravenous, subcutaneous or intramuscular injection, depending on the speed of release desired. The action of Nubain is evident within 2 to 3 minutes IV administration, and less than 15 minutes following a "SubQ" or I.M. injection. The half-life of nalbuphine is measured to be approximately 2-3 hours, and it is usually administered to the patient every four to six hours.

Athletes will most often utilize this drug for the treatment of exercise induced pain and soreness, after or during a workout. And since opiate drugs have been shown in some instances to lower cortisol levels and raise the output of growth hormone, the idea of Nubain being used as an anabolic/anti-catabolic is often thrown in as well. For this purpose Nubain is not only useless however, it may also turn out to be counterproductive. This is because suppressed cortisol levels and enhanced output of GH are effects mediated by mu receptors. You will remember Nubain is a mu antagonist, and as such may actually work to increase serum cortisol and lower growth hormone secretion.

Those who do take this compound will most commonly inject 1 or 1 1/2 ml (equivalent to 10-15mg) after a workout, in order to relax and unwind (recreational use). Or possibly 1/2 ml (5mg) before a workout, the analgesic effect sought after to lessen muscle soreness while lifting. The theory is that Nubain will allow you to push through extra sets, or workout at an intense schedule that would otherwise be too uncomfortable. Although a case can be made for the therapeutic use of Nubain, realistically it is just a recreational drug. When administered by an opiate naive individual, it will certainly produce a narcotic high. Its peculiar availability as a black market item is only a result of easy availability in Mexico (and lack of US controls). The volume steroid suppliers simply found another item that may be of interest in the States. Nubain is of course not new, and has been available as a prescription item in the US for quite a long time.

Opiate Analgesics

Opiates are amongst the world's oldest and most effective painkilling drugs. This class of medications originates with the opium poppy, a plant that produces morphine. Morphine is a potent natural analgesic, which has received its name from the Greek god of dreams, Morpheus, due to its ability to produce warm euphoric "dreamy" feelings of comfort. Morphine is considered the standard opiate analgesic by which all other opiate derivative drugs are measured. In the United States pure opiate drugs are highly controlled, due to their high potential for abuse. Opiates are narcotic drugs (heroin is an opiate), and undoubtedly a problem for many law enforcement agencies that deal with crime problems associated with opiate addiction on a daily basis.

Pharmaceutical manufacturers in the United States produce a number of opiate drugs, including morphine, hydromorphone, fentanyl, oxycodone, hydrocodone, dihydrocodone and codeine. Most pure opiate drugs are placed under the controlled substances lists as schedule II medications, believed to have a very high potential for abuse. Oxycodone is an example of a schedule II drug, and also of a medication with an extremely high problem with abuse (Oxycontin is the new oxycodone brand of choice, as it contains high doses of pure oxycodone in a tiny tablet, and is easy to crush and administer in a rapid-acting oral, intranasal, or even injectable form). It is very difficult to get most doctors to prescribe Schedule II medications. You may get a small script if you are ever in serious intractable pain from injury, or are recovering from surgery, but do not expect them to just be handing out Oxycontin tablets for no reason.

Many mixed analgesics, such as hydrocodone formulations with APAP (acetaminophen) or Ibuprofen, are listed as Schedule III controlled substances. You may recognize such popular brand names as Vicodin, Vicoprofen, Norco or Lortab. Hydrocodone is a potent opiate analgesic, not far behind oxycodone. The fact that it is a mixed product somewhat interferes with abuse potential, because an addict needing high doses of the drug to get "high" is likely to run into trouble with the acetaminophen or ibuprofen content before overdosing on the actual narcotic drug itself. Vicodin addiction, for example, usually entails the user running into liver trouble from taking toxic doses of acetaminophen (the daily short term limit is 4,000mg, or 8 tablets) on a continual basis. The mixture also allows for a lower total dose of opiate drug, as some analgesia will be produced by the adjunct medication. As it is a schedule III medication, Vicodin is usually easier to get than schedule II medications like oxycodone. Doctors are placed under less scrutiny, and the requirements for documentation and federal review are less strict. Mixed formulations are also available with oxycodone (Percodan, Percocet), however they remain on the list of Schedule II products due to the more potent and longer-acting nature of this drug.

In addition to the chance for addiction, opiate drugs have a number of other potential side effects including constipation, drowsiness, mental confusion, lethargy, impaired motor reflexes, anxiety, itching, rash or mood changes. There also seems to be odd occurrences of hearing loss in some patients abusing high doses of hydrocodone/APAP, specifically. Physical dependency occurs very quickly with opiates (please note that physical dependency and addiction are two separate things), producing abstinence syndrome when the drug is no longer given. This is often characterized by restlessness, sweating, nervousness, aches, nausea, flu-like symptoms, headaches, diarrhea or insomnia. Doctors are typically advised to slowly lower a patents daily dosage when discontinuing opiate therapy after any prolonged duration, so as to minimize discomfort. An accidental overdose of these drugs may also be life threatening, as opiates suppress the rate of respiration.

As you may have noticed by reading the profile for non-steroidal anti-inflammatory drugs, by blocking prostaglandin production acetaminophen and ibuprofen can notably interfere with protein-synthesis. This is somewhat of a problem for bodybuilders looking to use an opiate pain-medication, as they are likely to have the easier access to mixed Schedule III formulations. These should not be taken for long periods of time if avoidable. On top of the potential for physical dependency, which occurs quickly with all opiates, the anti-inflammatory properties of acetaminophen and ibuprofen will work against muscle growth. You will often hear people claim that Vicodin is a great bodybuilding tool, enabling them to workout harder and deal with the intense soreness that strenuous lifting brings. This is just bad thinking. You may be lifting harder, but as far as your muscle are concerned, you are doing less, not more. Pure opiates drugs might alternately be available to you, such as morphine, oxycodone (Oxycontin, Roxicodone), fentanyl or hydromorphone (Dilaudid), which are free of anti-inflammatory compounds. This might be looked at as a benefit, but at the same time you need to understand that these are amongst the most serious narcotic medications available. Tolerance, physical dependence, and the chance for developing an addiction are things that need to be taken very seriously.

There is no doubt that pain management with opiates can be a life-altering benefit for those suffering with chronic pain. For this reason I am a strong supporter of allowing doctors to prescribe them with as little government intervention as is necessary. I feel that too many doctors probably hold back on opiate therapy these days, for fear their patients may become addicts or that they might one day find themselves in a lawsuit, or even under arrest, for over-prescribing. But that aside, there is no place for narcotics outside of a medical setting. I would disagree wholeheartedly with any notion that these drugs have any purpose in the bodybuilding arena. Too many people have lost money, health, even their lives to addictions to narcotics, which many times began with seemingly innocent intentions of just using the drug for a temporary “edge”. Even playing around with these drugs is definitely not recommended.

ANTI-ESTROGENS

DRUG PROFILES

Arimidex (anastrozole)

Arimidex® (generic name is anastrozole) is a very new drug developed for the treatment of advanced breast cancer in women. It is manufactured by Zeneca Pharmaceuticals and was approved for use in the United States at the end of December 1995. Specifically, Arimidex® is the first in a new class of third-generation selective oral aromatase inhibitors[116]. It acts by blocking the enzyme aromatase, subsequently blocking the production of estrogen. Since many forms of breast cancer cells are stimulated by estrogen, it is hoped that by reducing amounts of estrogen in the body the progression of such a disease can be halted. This is the basic premise behind Nolvadex®, except this drug blocks the action and not production of estrogen. The effects of Arimidex® can be quite dramatic to say the least. A daily dose of one tablet (1 mg) can produce estrogen suppression greater than 80 % in treated patients. With the powerful effect this drug has on hormone levels, it is only to be used (clinically) by post-menopausal women whose disease has progressed following treatment with Nolvadex® (tamoxifen citrate). Side effects like hot flushes and hair thinning can be present, and would no doubt be much more severe in pre-menopausal patients.

For the steroid using male athlete, Arimidex® shows great potential. Up to this point, drugs like Nolvadex® and Proviron® have been our weapons against excess estrogen. These drugs, especially in combination, do prove quite effective. But Arimidex® appears able to do the job much more efficiently, and with less hassle. Its use is only now catching on, but early reports have been excellent. A single tablet daily, the same dose use clinically, seems to be all one needs for an exceptional effect (some even report excellent results with only ½ tablet daily). When used with strong, readily aromatizing androgens such as Dianabol or testosterone, gynecomastia and water retention can be effectively blocked. In combination with Propecia® (finasteride, see Proscar®), we have a great advance. With the one drug halting estrogen conversion and the other blocking 5-alpha reduction (testosterone, methyltestosterone and Halotestin® only), related side effects can be effectively minimized. Here the strong androgen testosterone could theoretically provide incredible muscular growth, while at the same time being as tolerable as nandrolone. Additionally the quality of the muscle should be greater, the athlete appearing harder and much more defined without holding excess water.

There are some concerns with using an aromatase inhibitor such as this during prolonged steroid treatment however. While it will effectively reduce estrogenic side effects, it will also block the beneficial properties of estrogen from becoming apparent (namely its effect on cholesterol values). Studies have clearly shown that when an aromatase inhibitor is used in conjunction with a steroid such as testosterone, suppression of HDL (good) cholesterol becomes much more pronounced. Apparently estrogen plays a role in minimizing the negative impact of steroid use. Since the estrogen receptor antagonist Nolvadex® is shown not to display an antiestrogenic effect on cholesterol values, it is certainly the preferred from of estrogen maintenance for those concerned with cardiovascular health.

Arimidex® has another principle drawback, namely the great price of this drug. Tablets can easily sell for $7-$10 each, becoming quite costly with regular use. I am currently looking at the product list of a reliable European anabolics dealer, who sells Arimidex® in packages of 28 tablets for $250. In a U.S. pharmacy 30 tablets will currently run you about $190. Clearly the price of an ancillary drug can be much greater than the steroids themselves, a situation destined not to be popular with recreational bodybuilders. Competitors on the other hand are likely to welcome this item. It can ward off the side effects of strong androgen therapy much better than Nolvadex® and/or Proviron®, making heavy cycles much more comfortable. As the number of countries manufacturing this drug increases, we may be able to look forward to a reduction in price. On a list from a Greek supplier (a country where drugs are government subsidized) for example, the price was nearly $100 better per box. Privately compounded versions of "liquid Arimidex" have also been formulated "for research purposes" and are currently circulating the black market. They contain a high concentration of anastrozole (1mg to 4mg/mL) in a liquid solution, which can be used orally, and represent very cost-effective alternatives for buying the brand name drug (typically selling for $5 per milligram or less).

Aromasin (exemestane)

Aromasin is a steroidal suicide aromatase inhibitor, extremely similar in structure and action to formestane. The agents, of course, work to lower estrogen production in the body by blocking the enzyme responsible for synthesizing these hormones. Aromasin is approved by the FDA for the treatment of breast cancer, specifically in post-menopausal women whose cancer has progressed following therapy with a first line agent such as tamoxifen. Aromasin is being advertised as the only "aromatase inactivator" available. That, of course, excludes the fact that we are able to sell formestane as an over-the-counter nutritional supplement in the U.S. (formestane is not approved as a drug here), at least for the time being. Although both of these agents essentially do the same thing in the body, Aromasin definitely seems to do the job much more efficiently. At this time it is the anti-estrogen of choice amongst bodybuilders.

Aromasin may perhaps be the most effective aromatase inhibitor available to date. While Femara and Arimidex boast of estrogen suppression around the 78-80% in their packaging inserts, Aromasin reports it can lower estrogen as much as 85% on average[117]. Feedback from bodybuilders tends to support the preference for Aromasin over other anti-estrogens, so this may very well be the case. Regardless of which one is the true "king" aromatase inhibitor, all of the newer pharmaceutical agents, Arimidex, Femara, and Aromasin, should be looked at as extremely effective for reducing estrogen synthesis in the body. A possible 10% difference in inhibition between the weakest and the strongest of the three is really not going to amount to all that much during your next cycle. If you are looking at one of these agents to prevent gynecomastia and help you lose fat and water on your next cycle, they are all going to do a good job for you. If you absolutely *need* the best agent, my money would be on this one.

It is important to point out that there are some disadvantages to using an aromatase inhibitor over mixed estrogen agonist/antagonists (anti-estrogen) like Nolvadex and Clomid, the most notable being unwanted (negative) alterations in serum cholesterol values. This is because estrogen is tied to HDL (good) cholesterol synthesis and LDL (bad) cholesterol metabolism, and aromatase inhibitors block total estrogenic action. Clomid and Nolvadex, on the other hand, tend to exert a positive influence on cholesterol values, as they are both active estrogens in the liver. If you are just trying to prevent estrogenic side effects like gynecomastia, bloating and excess water retention in general, these agents are probably better choices (they do the same job and are safer on your cholesterol levels).

At the pharmacy, 30 tablets of Aromasin will run you about $200. This makes it about at expensive as Arimidex or Femara on a per tablet basis, not cheap by any means. The good thing is that like Arimidex and Femara, Aromasin is potent enough to be used at lower doses than the recommended 25mg daily. In fact, studies have shown maximum estrogen suppression in some patients with as little as 2.5mg[118] per day. That is not a recommendation to smash each tablet into 10 little pieces, but it does make the current armchair advice of taking ½ a tablet every day or two seem well justified. This brings the cost of Aromasin down to about $50-100 per month, a much more reasonable figure for most. Then again, if maximum suppression is important to you, and you want to be sure you are getting the strongest effect you can, you may want to spring for the full 1 tablet per day dosage. One thing is for certain; you will not walk away feeling the money was wasted if you do.

Clomid (clomiphene citrate)

Clomid® is the commonly referenced brand name for the drug clomiphene citrate. It is not an anabolic steroid, but a prescription drug generally prescribed to women as a fertility aid. This is due to the fact that clomiphene citrate shows a pronounced ability to stimulate ovulation. This is accomplished by blocking/minimizing the effects of estrogen in the body. To be more specific Clomid® is chemically a synthetic estrogen with both agonist/antagonist properties, and is very similar in structure and action to Nolvadex®. In certain target tissues it can block the ability of estrogen to bind with its corresponding receptor. Its clinical use is therefore to oppose the negative feedback of estrogens on the hypothalamic-pituitary-ovarian axis, which enhances the release of LH and FSH. This of course can help to induce ovulation.

For athletic purposes, Clomid® does not offer a tremendous benefit to women. In men however, the elevation in both follicle stimulating hormone and (primarily) luteinizing hormone will cause natural testosterone production to increase. This effect is especially beneficial to the athlete at the conclusion of a steroid cycle when endogenous testosterone levels are depressed. If endogenous testosterone levels are not brought back to normal, a dramatic loss in size and strength is likely to occur once the anabolics have been removed. This is due to the fact that without testosterone (or other androgens), the catabolic hormone cortisol becomes the dominant force affecting muscle protein synthesis (quickly bringing about a catabolic metabolism). Often referred to as the post-steroid crash, it can quickly eat up much of your newly acquired muscle. Clomid® can play a crucial role in preventing this crash in athletic performance. As for women, the only real use for Clomid® is the possible management of endogenous estrogen levels near contest time. This can increase fat loss and muscularity, particularly in female trouble areas such as this hips and thighs. Clomid® however often produces troubling side effects in women (discussed below), and is likewise not in very high demand among this group of athletes.

Male users generally find that a daily intake of 50-100 mg (1-2 tablets) over a four to six week period will bring testosterone production back to an acceptable level. This raise in testosterone should occur slowly but evenly throughout the period of intake. Since an immediate boost in testosterone is often desirable, many prefer to combine Clomid® with HCG (human chorionic gonadotropin) for the first week or two after the steroids have been removed. The kick-start from HCG also helps to restore the normal ability for the testes to respond to endogenous LH, which may be hindered for some time after the cycle is ended due to a prolonged state of inactivity. Once the HCG is stopped, the user continues treatment with Clomid® alone. HCG should not be used for longer than two or three weeks though, as the resulting increased testosterone and estrogen levels may again initiate negative feedback inhibition at the hypothalamus. When planning your ancillary drug program, it is also important to remember that injectable steroids can stay active for a long duration. Using ancillary drugs the first week after a long acting injectable like Sustanon has been stopped may prove to be wholly ineffective. Instead, the athlete should wait for two to three weeks, to a point where androgen levels will be diminishing. Here the body will be primed and ready to restore testosterone production.

Clomid® and HCG are also occasionally used periodically during a steroid cycle, in an effort to prevent natural testosterone levels from diminishing. In many instances this practice can prove difficult however, especially when using strong androgens for longer periods of time. There is also no exact method for using the two drugs in this manner. Some have experimented by periodically administering small doses of HCG along with one or two tablets of Clomid®, perhaps for a few days at a stretch followed by a longer break. An on/off schedule would be implemented; for fear that this combination may lose some effectiveness if used continuously for this purpose. This method of intake may prove to be effective, although it is really much more feasible to stimulate testosterone production after the cycle than to try and maintain it for the long duration during.

In addition to helping with the post-cycle testosterone crash, this drug can also help with elevated estrogen levels during a steroid cycle. A high estrogen level puts an athlete in serious risk of developing gynecomastia, which is an obvious unwanted side effect. With the intake of Clomid®, the athlete can hopefully reduce his risk for developing gynecomastia. The estrogen "blocking" properties of Clomid® appear to be slightly weaker than Nolvadex® in comparison however, which is why it is not usually thought of as an equal substitute for estrogen maintenance. Of course both drugs have similar actions in the body, and are relatively interchangeable for this purpose. Clomid® can likewise also be used as a maintenance anti-estrogen throughout the duration of steroid intake with good confidence, just as is done with Nolvadex®. In most instances this will prove equally sufficient, the drug effectively minimizing the activity of estrogen in the body and warding off gyno and excess water/fat retention. Unfortunately just as with Nolvadex® this is not always the case however, and many find it necessary to addition another antiestrogenic drug. The most common adjunct is Proviron®, an oral DHT used to competitively lower aromatase activity and raise the androgen to estrogen ratio. The Clomid/Nolvadex and Proviron® combination is extremely effective, although we could alternately replace them both with a more specific aromatase inhibitor such as Arimidex® or Cytadren®. While stronger at combating estrogen in most cases, these drugs are also typically much more costly

As for toxicity and side effects, Clomid® is considered a very safe drug. Bodybuilders seldom report any problems, but listed possible side effects do include hot flashes, nausea, dizziness, headaches and temporarily blurred vision. Such side effects usually only appear in females however, as they feel the effects of estrogen manipulation much more readily than men. While female athletes can clearly gain some benefit from this substance, estrogen manipulation is probably not the most comfortable way to go about cutting up. Should it still be used for such purposed and side effects do become pronounced, the drug of course is to be discontinued and (at least) a break taken from it.

Clomiphene citrate is widely available on the black market in a variety of brand names. This substance can be expensive, often as high as $2-$4 per 50 mg tab. Generics such as Clomiphene citrate by Anfarm in Greece are frequently seen on the black market, and can sell for a considerably lower price. In the U.S., Omifin from Mexico appears to be most popular. Since there are no counterfeits known to exist, Clomid® is considered a safe buy on the black market. Many athletes prefer to purchase this item only from foreign mail-order sources, always shopping for the lowest available tablet price.

Cyclofenil

Cyclofenil is a non-steroidal ancillary drug used by athletes, very similar in action to Clomid® and Nolvadex®. All three act strongly as estrogen receptor antagonists, which gives them the ability to stimulate ovulation in Women and increase testosterone production in men. For athletic purposes this drug is of most benefit to males, typically used for the purpose of increasing endogenous testosterone levels at the conclusion of a steroid cycle. This is in an attempt to avoid a strong hormonal "crash" while waiting for testosterone levels to be restored. HCG is also commonly used for this purpose, but this drug works by mimicking the action of luteinizing hormone, a much different approach. The effect of HCG is very quick, leading it most often to be the first ancillary drug used after steroids are removed. But drugs like cyclofenil, Clomid® and Nolvadex® are better suited for the following weeks, usually continued for some time after HCG has been withdrawn. Women do occasionally find a use for antiestrogens, most often around contest time when the management of endogenous estrogens can help increase fat loss and definition. The side effects that can be brought about by a lowering of estrogen activity in the female body, however, make this approach less than ideal.

Cyclofenil (like Clomid® and Nolvadex®) is technically that of an estrogen agonist/antagonist. In the body it displays antiestrogenic properties, affecting the binding efficacy of estrogen receptors in certain target tissues. This is in fact how cyclofenil stimulates the release of testosterone. The hypothalamus is one target site, and here it acts to block the negative feedback inhibition brought fourth by estrogen. The enhanced release of gonadotropin releasing hormone (GnRH) results, which in turn stimulates the pituitary to heighten the release of luteinizing hormone. LH is the primary signal for the testes to increase the production of testosterone, so its increased release leads to an elevation in the androgen level. The antiestrogenic effect of this drug in breast tissue has also led to it during a steroid cycle to prevent gynecomastia, similar to how Nolvadex® might be used. Cyclofenil however, is reported to be somewhat weaker than Nolvadex® in comparison, and therefore is not usually the preferred estrogen maintenance drug if both were available.

When used after steroids to increase natural testosterone production it can be effective. A dosage of 400-600mg per day is the most common, generally used for the 4 to 5 weeks following a steroid cycle. It can take a few weeks before cyclofenil exhibits a noticeable effect, and therefore HCG is usually combined with it for the first week or two. HCG also helps to rapidly restore the ability of the testes to respond to endogenous gonadotropins, which may be notably diminished due to a period of long inactivity. Cyclofenil is continued alone afterwards, with the total duration of ancillary drug use lasting about five or six weeks. It should also be noted that some athletes have experimented with using cyclofenil not as a post-cycle ancillary drug, but alone as an anabolic. They are hoping that testosterone levels could be raised significantly enough for it to provide some extra muscle mass. Some have reported this approach does work, but results are not extremely significant. Anyone familiar with anabolics would likely be disappointed when using cyclofenil for this purpose, which is clearly not an equal to injecting testosterone.

Side effects associated with this drug are usually very minimal, and most often are felt my female recipients. The main side effect seen by females tends to be hot flashes due to hormonal changes. In males, the testosterone boosting properties can result in some androgenic effects like oily skin, acne, increased aggression and libido. These are not usually dramatic, as androgen levels will not reach the level seen with most steroids. With cyclofenil these effects are more welcome than anything, showing the user the drug is having some effect. Here in the U.S., cyclofenil is not an overly popular item. It is carried on occasion by dealers, but is much less common here than Clomid® or Nolvadex®. When located in the U.S. it is usually in the form of Fertodur, made by Schering in Europe and (formerly) Mexico.

Cytadren (aminoglutethimide)

Cytadren®, the U.S. brand name for the drug aminoglutethimide, is an interesting non-steroidal compound first brought to our attention several years ago by the late Dan Duchaine. It is popular with some competitive athletes who are drug tested, as in many disciplines this substance is currently not banned or tested for. Cytadren® inhibits the production of cortisol (by blocking the conversion of cholesterol to pregnenolone, this first step in its biosynthesis), the aromatization of androgens to estrogens and to a lesser degree the production of adrenal androgens. Its effect on cortisol production is what first brought Cytadren® to the attention of athletes. For someone with normal cortisol levels, it is thought that a little less could actually be a good thing. This is because while androgens give your muscle cells a message to increase protein synthesis, cortisol (a catabolic hormone) gives the exact opposite message (to breakdown amino acids). Obviously this is a process we would wish to avoid, so the use of this drug was proposed. But since Cytadren® also inhibits androgen production (to some extent), it was typically recommended that it be used by athletes with some form of testosterone. Together with even a relatively small dose, it was thought one could shift the ratio of anabolic to catabolic hormones well in favor of the former, the goal of course being new muscle growth. Cytadren® is also known to inhibit the aromatase enzyme, giving it a very separate second use as an effective antiestrogen to use during heavier steroid cycles. As you will see, this trait may in fact prove to be the most important one to the athlete. Its action in this regard is course very similar to that of the new antiaromatase Arimidex®, although Arimidex® seems to do the job a bit more efficiently (however it is also the more costly option).

Medically Cytadren® is used to treat estrogen dependent breast cancer as well as Cushing's syndrome, a condition in which the body overproduces cortisol. In these arenas effective dosing regimens are well documented. When first looked at in the realm of athletics however, research was bare as to the best way to use it as a cortisol lowering anti-catabolic. It was suggested after some thought that when used for this purpose a schedule of 2 days on and 2 days off would be effective. One thing is for certain, Cytadren® cannot be taken daily if prolonged cortisol suppression were desired. Dubbed the adrenal escape phenomenon, it was shown that after a short period of regular use your body would react to the lowered cortisol levels and release increased amounts of another hormone, ACTH (adrenocorticotropic hormone), in response. Increased ACTH will overcome the activity of Cytadren®, resulting in your body resuming normal cortisol production (basically making the drug useless)[119]. When used medically a moderate amount of hydrocortisone is often supplemented to avoid this reaction. For athletes however, it was assumed that this would probably be a counterproductive practice. Thus the 2-day on 2 day off regime was implemented as another way to delay or even avoid this response. This is only a suggested practice, and as you will see is only relevant to its use as an anti-catabolic.

In seeing exactly how an athlete might and might not benefit from this drug, we can look at studies demonstrating that the main mechanism in which this drug benefits breast cancer patients (inhibition of peripheral aromatase activity) is different from that which interferes with corticosteroid production[120]. We also see that the dosage is important in triggering each particular response. It appears that aromatase inhibition is achieved at a much lower dose than is needed to block steroid production by the adrenal gland[121]. While a daily dosage of 1000mg is typically needed to inhibit the demolase enzyme (the enzyme responsible for converting cholesterol to pregnenolone, and the target when reduced adrenal output is needed), maximum suppression of aromatase and estrogen levels is achieved at a dosage between 250 and 500mg (a point where adrenal steroid blockage should not be noted). There also seems to be no added benefit by adding cortisol in terms of survival/response rate among breast cancer patients, pointing to the fact that the “adrenal escape phenomenon” bears no relation at all to its abilities as an aromatase inhibitor. We find that not only do we need a very high dose (4 tablets per day) to really inhibit cortisol production, but also that there is no need for an athlete to implement a rotating dose schedule if the drug is being used as an anti-estrogen.

In effectiveness as an estrogen maintenance agent this compound rates highly. Studies have shown it capable of decreasing aromatase activity as much as 92% after administration of only 250mg, and patient response rates show aminoglutethimide to be at least as effective as tamoxifen therapy in treating estrogen dependent cancer cells, more so under certain conditions. However, due to its discussed broad range of activity, including the potential inhibition of not only estrogens, but corticosteroids, aldosterone and androgens as well, it is not regarded as highly in terms of patient comfort. This is not to give the impression that complaints are very common though, as aminoglutethimide still has an extremely good safety record. It has simply been pushed aside in many cases for more recently developed and selective agents. Athletes can however still consider it to be an extremely effective remedy for estrogenic side effects should it be available on the black market, at least as much so as Nolvadex. As for the daily dosage when taking Cytadren® to minimize estrogenic side effects, most experiment with anywhere from 1/2 a tablet to 2 tablets per day, with one tablet of 250mg probably being the most common dosage selected.

Although many believe they have used this drug as such, few ever reach the discussed necessary four tablets per day to notice true cortisol suppression. This drug is very rarely used as an anti-catabolic in a correct manner, and those who do venture this high commonly report fatigue and discomfort, stating that the drug is intolerable for any type of prolonged use. Sadly, we are starting to realize that its original proposed use of Cytadren® as a non-steroidal muscle-building agent does not seem a plausible one. The only instances I really have heard of this drug ever being used at such doses with any type of positive response were competitive bodybuilders partaking in high-dosed Cytadren shortly before a show. They claimed the short-term rise in androgen to corticosteroid ratio greatly aided in their abilities to bring out a show-ready hard and dense physique, and credit the drug as genuinely being a very effective pre-contest agent. In speaking with the late Paul Borresen he summed up the pre-contest use of Cytadren nicely:

"I have had considerable experience with the high dose use. It makes athletes sleepy and weak. It seems to help the last ten days before a show, and this is tried and tested."

Cytadren® is not without its side effects and warnings which are numerous. To be very succinct, these include, but are not limited to, the already mentioned possibility of fatigue, as well as dizziness, sleep disorder, apathy, depression, nausea/vomiting, stomach upset, thyroid dysfunction and liver disease. The few athletes to take it at a dosage high enough to promote cortisol suppression additionally note that reduced levels of this hormone will bring about more aches and pains in your joints when trying to lift heavy. It seems logical that this could even lead to a greatly increased susceptibility to injury, so one should be careful not to overexert during the short periods in which this drug is used in high doses. Most of the listed side effects listed here are in fact related only to high dosed regimens that inhibit the adrenal production of cortisol, and are rarely ever reported with athletes taking one or two tablets per day in an effort to use the drug as an anti-estrogen.

Cytadren® is an expensive pharmaceutical, selling for approximately $2 per tablet on the black market. This is probably the reason its use has not become more widespread. This price is however still considerably less than what would be spent on the more recently developed antiaromatase Arimidex®, which sells for as much as $10 per tablet. Since Cytadren® is not currently being counterfeited, all preparations seen on the black market could be considered a safe buy. Although manufactured in the United States, the black market will generally carry the Orimeten brand name from Europe.

Evista (raloxifene)

Evista (raloxifene) is a second-generation Selective Estrogen Receptor Modulator (SERM) of the benzothiophene family. This anti-estrogenic drug is similar in effect to tamoxifen, exhibiting estrogen receptor antagonist (blocking) properties in some tissues while acting as an estrogen receptor agonist (activator) in others. The main point of variation between these two agents is their tissue selectivity. While raloxifene is a strong anti-estrogen in breast and uterine tissues, it appears to be estrogenic in bone. This allows it to protect bone density, mimicking the beneficial effects of endogenous estradiol. This is quite different from tamoxifen, which is anti-estrogenic in both breast and bone. In a role that is completely novel for an anti-estrogen, raloxifene is approved by the FDA for the prevention and treatment of osteoporosis in post-menopausal women. It is also being investigated for several other potential uses, including the treatment and prevention of cardiovascular disease, breast cancer, gynecomastia, prostate cancer, acromegaly, and uterine cancer.

As an anti-estrogen, bodybuilders will be attracted to this compound for eliminating the side effects caused by aromatizable steroids. The principle among these is gynecomastia, a purpose for which raloxifene seems better suited than tamoxifen. We saw this in a July 2004 study in the Journal of Pediatrics, which looked at how these two agents compared in treating persistent pubertal gynecomastia[1]. The investigation involved a group of 38 patients, averaging 15 years of age and suffering from gynecomastia for a little over 2 years. Treatment for 3 to 9 months with either agent had a high success rate for seeing "some improvement" (91% for raloxifene and 86% for Nolvadex). However, a significant reduction of gynecomastia was seen in more than twice as many patients with raloxifene (86% compared to 41%). Raloxifene seems to have a much stronger effect in breast tissue, giving it a remarkable ability to treat even long-standing cases of hard-tissue gynecomastia. This drug may offer an effective and long overdue alternative to invasive mammary gland removal surgery, long thought of as the only reliable treatment option by most bodybuilders.

Typical of an anti-estrogen, raloxifene should also offer some benefit as a testosterone-stimulating compound. We see this effect demonstrated in studies on a group of older men (aged 60-70 years), where daily doses of 120mg were able to increase serum and bioavailable (unbound) testosterone by 20%[2]. Though these figures are not startling, they do clearly demonstrate an anti-estrogenic effect instead of an estrogenic (negative) one when it comes to testosterone production. This drug may, therefore, be of some value when utilized as an adjunct to HCG injections during a post-cycle testosterone recovery program. This same study above also showed raloxifene to have at least a partial estrogenic effect on serum lipids, exhibiting a trend toward decreases in all cholesterol values (total, LDL and HDL). It is difficult to discern if there are any real benefits to male bodybuilders when it comes to using raloxifene to counteract the negative cardiovascular side effects of steroid use. You will note when we discuss Nolvadex that this is a particularly welcome benefit to this first-generation agent.

There are some negatives to inhibiting the actions of estrogen that we need to talk about. For one, estrogen is a beneficial hormone when it comes to IGF-1 levels. In studies with acromegaly patients that suffer from GH hypersecretion, 60mg of raloxifene twice daily was able to reliably suppress IGF-1 levels by an average of 16%[3]. This is in line with what we expect with virtually all anti-estrogenic drugs. Estrogen is also understood to exert positive anabolic effects in regards to increasing androgen receptor concentrations, and enhancing enzyme levels involved in the utilization of glucose for tissue growth and repair. This is further support for the belief that anti-estrogens should not be used unless there is a clear defined reason for doing so. When used for simple side-effect prevention (without visible side effects occurring), the drug may inadvertently be hindering the total anabolic potency of a cycle. It is, therefore, good advice to include raloxifene during your next cycle only if there is a specific need to do so.

Price may also be of concern with this drug, as raloxifene is a bit more expensive than many of the anti-estrogens bodybuilders are accustomed to. A look at a recent mail-order pharmacy price list, 4-weeks worth of drug (28 tables) at 60mg daily will run about $60. That is a little more than $2 per dose/day. 100 tablets of generic tamoxifen (20mg) at the same pharmacy, is only around $54. This is about 50 cents per dose, or 1/4th the price of raloxifene. It can be found for even less if you shop around. This means that to spite many of the newer, more desirable drugs to hit the market in recent years, raloxifene will be used less frequently than the older anti-estrogens until the price drops. It may just be too expensive for a "simple anti-estrogen" in the eyes of consumers. For those not discouraged by its price, 60mg daily of raloxifene may offer a much stronger alternative in the prevention and treatment of gyno than first generation drugs like Nolvadex or Clomid, and also present less danger in terms of negative cardiovascular side effects than potent aromatase inhibitors. If gyno is a serious concern of yours, it should be money well spent.

Fareston (toremifene citrate)

Fareston is an estrogen receptor antagonist with mixed agonist/antagonist properties (specifically it is classified as a SERM: Selective Estrogen-Receptor Modulator). It is a nonsteroidal triphenylethylene derivative, similar in structure and action to both Nolvadex (tamoxifen citrate) and Clomid (clomiphene citrate). Fareston is used for the treatment of breast cancer in postmenopausal women with estrogen-receptor positive or estrogen-receptor unknown (unsure if the cancer is estrogen responsive) tumors. It works by attaching to the estrogen receptor in various tissues, blocking endogenous estrogen from exerting biological activity. This agent in the newest mixed estrogen receptor agonist/antagonist to get our attention in the bodybuilding world, and was approved by the FDA in 1997.

Anti-estrogenic drugs like Fareston are popular with bodybuilders because they help us deal with many of the “negative” aspects of high estrogen levels. Estrogen can work to hide muscle definition by increasing water retention and fat buildup for example, and can also promote gynecomastia (the development of female breast tissue) if levels get too high. Since androgens and estrogens play opposing roles on the disposition of body fat and the growth of mammary tissues, maximizing the ratio between these two hormones is also often an important objective, particularly at times when dieting and cutting are key goals or gynecomastia is a worry because strongly aromatized hormones such as testosterone are being supplemented. A drug like Fareston can be a key asset here.

But there are also some “positive” attributes to estrogen that need to be taken into account as well. This includes the support of "good" high-density cholesterol synthesis, increased muscle glucose utilization for tissue growth and repair, and even increased androgen receptor concentrations in various tissues. It is now understood that estrogen serves many useful purposes in men, particularly if we are looking for rapid muscle mass gain. If bulk is the goal, it is, therefore, usually advisable to hold off on estrogen maintenance compounds until there is a clear need for them.

All of the triphenylethylene compounds (Fareston, Nolvadex and Clomid) do have an added benefit of being somewhat intrinsically estrogenic in the liver. This means that while they can block estrogenic activity in areas where we do not want it, like the breast, they replace estrogenic action in this key area of the body where we do. Estrogenic action in the liver is, of course, important in the regulation of serum cholesterol (it tends to support HDL synthesis and LDL reductions). Since steroid-using bodybuilders are already dealing with the negative cardiovascular effects of these drugs, compounding the issue with aromatase inhibitors is not always the best option. Using a drug that blocks estrogen, while at the same time supporting cholesterol values, seems much more ideal. In terms of which agent is best in this regard, evidence does suggest that the positive lipid altering benefits of toremifene are stronger than those of tamoxifen[122]. If this is important to you, than Fareston may very well be your anti-estrogenic agent of choice.

At the pharmacy, thirty 60mg tablets of Fareston sell for about $100. The typical daily dose used is one tablet per day. Unfortunately, due to its rapid metabolism and less than maximum potency, it is not a good idea to split the dose into an every other day schedule. At 60mg per day you should notice estrogenic minimization at least on par with 20mg of tamoxifen, combined with a stronger positive effect on ones cardiovascular risk profile.

Faslodex (fulvestrant)

Faslodex is one of the newest weapons in the war on estrogen, approved by the FDA in 2002 for the treatment of estrogen receptor positive breast cancer. This product is not another highly selective aromatase inhibitor however, which has, of course, been an extremely popular area of medical exploration lately. It is, instead, a highly selective estrogen receptor antagonist (also classified as an estrogen receptor downregulator). This means that it does not target the production of estrogen, but prevents it from exerting activity in the body by blocking available estrogen receptors. It mode of action is very much along the same lines as Nolvadex (tamoxifen citrate) and Clomid (clomiphene citrate), not Arimidex or Femara. This agent also stands out as the first injectable anti-estrogen to catch our attention in the bodybuilding world, Nolvadex and Clomid of course being oral medications.

Unlike Nolvadex, Faslodex does not have mixed agonist/antagonist properties; it is a pure estrogen receptor antagonist. This makes it quite different from Nolvadex or Clomid, drugs that actually offer estrogenic activity in certain tissues. But the mixed action of Nolvadex and Clomid can be a benefit to bodybuilders, by supporting good (HDL) cholesterol biosynthesis in particular (due to their inherent estrogenic agonistic activities in the liver). Although I have been unable to find studies looking at cholesterol levels in response to Faslodex, knowing how closely tied estrogen is to the synthesis of HDL cholesterol, I can only assume it will have a strong negative influence here. This is an added concern for bodybuilders, who in most cases already have to deal with negative cholesterol alterations due to steroid administration. In this regard Faslodex may not be the “next best thing” when it comes to estrogen control, sharing the same negative cholesterol altering effects that are noted with strong aromatase inhibitors.

The product comes in a preloaded syringe of 5ml, with each ml containing 50mg of the anti-estrogen. There is also a version with 2.5ml, but two syringes are packed in the same box for the same total 5ml dose. This is an extremely potent and long acting anti-estrogen, requiring only one 5ml preloaded syringe (250mg) to be injected each month. At this dose it seems well equipped to compete with even some of the newer aromatase inhibitors. One study, for example, shows Faslodex to be as effective in Arimidex in treating breast cancer patients who have already failed with first line endocrine treatments[123]. Another shows the drug to prevent tumor cell turnover and growth significantly more effectively than tamoxifen citrate[124]. Studies investigating the physiological response to Faslodex made note that its strong actions allow it to downregulate estrogen receptor concentrations, and progesterone receptor concentrations as well[125]. Clearly when it comes to anti-estrogens, Faslodex is far more advanced than the “standard-issue” agents we have been using in the bodybuilding world for years.

Faslodex is not a cheap drug by any stretch of the imagination. In fact, it is one of the most expensive drugs I have ever seen. It almost makes growth hormone look like it is free in comparison. According to a current U.S. pharmacy price list that I am looking at right now, a single 5ml injection of Faslodex runs $936.70. Yes, you read that correctly. A single shot costs nearly one thousand dollars. I guess when you make a medicine that people are only going to need once per month, you aren’t going to make millions on it if you sell it for $50. Mind you I have no knowledge of how costly this drug is to manufacture, but if I had to guess I would think the price has much more to do with how much the company thinks they should get from a patient on a monthly basis than how troublesome it is to produce. Being so expensive, of course, there is little chance this drug will catch on with the bodybuilding public.

Femara (letrozole)

Letrozole is a non-steroidal selective third generation aromatase inhibitor, which is being sold under the brand name Femara by the international drug-manufacturing firm Novartis. It is used to treat postmenopausal women with estrogen receptor-positive or estrogen receptor-unknown (unsure if the cancer is responsive to estrogen) breast cancer. The structure and activity of this compound are very similar to that of Arimidex (anastrozole), which is approved in the U.S. for the same purpose. Femara is typically used as a second line of treatment, after an estrogen-receptor antagonist like tamoxifen has failed to elicit a desirable response (although at times it is used as a first line option as well).

Femara and Arimidex represent the newest achievements in a long line of drugs targeting aromatase inhibition. These are amongst the most potent estrogen-lowering drugs made to date, working far more effectively than the non-selective first generation aromatase inhibitors, like Teslac and Cytadren, to come before them. The dosage of each tablet of Femara is 2.5 milligrams, which according to the product insert was sufficient to lower estrogen levels by 78% during clinical trails. The drug, however, appears to still be extremely effective in much lower doses. The package insert for the product itself comments that during clinical studies doses of .1 and .5 milligram produced 75% and 78% estrogen inhibition, respectively. When it comes to a product like this, typically the recommended dose reflects what seems to work for almost everyone who takes it. A large number of people may respond extremely well to lower doses, however, to make sure each patient is receiving the proper benefit of the drug a standard effective dosage unit is ascertained and used.

It is important to point out that there are some disadvantages to using an aromatase inhibitor over mixed estrogen agonist/antagonists (anti-estrogen) like Nolvadex and Clomid, the most notable being unwanted (negative) alterations in cholesterol values (strong HDL suppression in particular). This is because estrogen is tied to HDL cholesterol synthesis and LDL metabolism, and aromatase inhibitors block total estrogenic action. Clomid and Nolvadex, on the other hand, tend to produce an estrogenic increase in good cholesterol values, as they are active estrogens in the liver. If I you are just trying to prevent estrogenic side effects like gynecomastia, bloating and excess water retention in general, these agents are probably better choices (they do the same job and are safer on your cholesterol levels). But if you want that really tight, dry, defined look that is often so sought after when you are cutting, Nolvadex or Clomid are not quite going to cut it (excuse the unintentional pun). In such cases, I think you will find Femara to serve you well.

At the pharmacy, 30 tablets will cost you a little under $200. This comes out to about $6.50 each tablet, roughly the same price you are going to pay for Arimidex. Like Arimidex, each tablet can be broken up if you desire to stretch out the value of the drug. In fact, with studies showing maximum inhibition in some patients with doses as low as ½ milligram, each 2.5 milligram tablet can be broken up in to as many as 5 separate doses (perhaps even more). But the typical use amongst bodybuilders is to cut the tabs in half, and take one every other day (unless needed daily). In terms of overall power, Femara seems to be a little bit more potent the Arimidex, at least by most peoples' estimations. If both agents were available for the same price, Femara would probably be the one I would go for.

Lentaron (formestane)

Formestane is a potent steroidal suicide aromatase inhibitor, sold by Novartis under the brand name Lentaron Depot. This agent is structurally a derivative of androstenedione, differing from this well known prohormone only by the addition of a 4-hydroxyl group. This group, however, is responsible for causing an irreversible attachment between formestane and aromatase when the two come into contact with each other. This means that formestane will bond with the enzyme, and never let it go, totally deactivating it as a result. The enzyme will actually need to be replaced, through normal attrition, before the body will recover its lost estrogen synthesizing capacity. This is how we get the classification of a suicide inhibitor, as formestane essentially sacrifices itself in the process of blocking estrogen conversion.

Because of its potent estrogen-suppressing action, 4-hydroxyandrostenedione has been successfully used on breast cancer patients in a number of countries including England, Germany, Switzerland, Spain, Australia, New Zealand, Italy and Malaysia [126] [127] [128] [129] [130] [131] [132] [133]. It has been shown to be an effective option as a second line of defense after tamoxifen, an estrogen receptor antagonist, has failed to elicit a positive response with patients, and to produce an overall response statistically similar to tamoxifen when administered as the first-line therapy[134]. Lentaron Depot, which is an injectable version of formestane, is typically given in a dosage of 250-500mg every two weeks (this produces a maximum level of effect in most patients and bodybuilders alike). Studies have demonstrated that a similar level of estrogen suppression can also be achieved with oral use of this drug, but due to poor bioavailability the dose needed is around 250mg per day[135]. Formestane is not actally sold as a drug in the U.S. It is legally considered an over-the-counter nutritional supplement, due to the fact that it is a naturally occurring compound. In early 2003 I uncovered an old German study demonstrating this fact, and with the information my company (Molecular Nutrition) started selling formestane in the U.S. under the brand name Formastat.

In terms of overall potency, formestane is not quite on the level of the new selective third generation inhibitors like Arimidex (anastrozole) or Femara (letrozole). One study, for example, notes a 79% level of suppression of estrogen levels with 4 weeks of Arimidex 1mg daily (on par with levels noted with Femara use), but only a 58% level of suppression with intramuscular formestane injections (250mg every two weeks)[136]. But next to estrogen receptor antagonists like Clomid (clomiphene citrate) and Nolvadex (tamoxifen citrate), formestane definitely proves itself the best agent. Mind you there are almost always some disadvantages to using an aromatase inhibitor over drugs like Nolvadex or Clomid, the most notable being an unwanted (negative) alterations in serum cholesterol values (both Clomid and Nolvadex tend to increase HDL and lower LDL). But if you want that really tight, dry, defined look so sought after when you are cutting, Nolvadex is not quite going to do the same job. I personally love to use formestane, but only at times when developing such tight definition is a concern of mine. If I were just trying to prevent estrogenic side effects like gynecomastia, bloating and excess water retention in general, I would go with Nolvadex. It works, and is probably going to be safer on your cholesterol levels in comparison.

Nolvadex (tamoxifen citrate)

Nolvadex®, a trade name for the drug tamoxifen citrate, is a non-steroidal agent that demonstrates potent antiestrogenic properties. The drug is technically an estrogen agonist/antagonist, which competitively binds to estrogen receptors in various target tissues. With the tamoxifen molecule bound to this receptor, estrogen is blocked from exerting any action, and an antiestrogenic effect is achieved. Since many forms of breast cancer are responsive to estrogen, the ability of tamoxifen citrate to block its action in such cells has proven to be a very effective treatment. It is also utilized successfully as a preventative measure, taken by people with an extremely high familial tendency for breast cancer. While Nolvadex® is effective against estrogen, it is not our strongest available remedy. We now have the drug Arimidex® (see: Arimidex®) available to us, which notably prevents estrogen from being manufactured in the first place. Altering the effect of estrogen in the female body can cause a level of discomfort, so antiestrogens are most bearable when used after the point of menopause. Since Nolvadex® is milder in comparison, it is more widely applicable and usually the first treatment option.

As discussed earlier in this book, an enzyme in the male body (aromatase) is capable of altering testosterone to form estradiol. The structure of estrogen is actually quite similar to testosterone, so its presence in the male body is not all that remarkable. Since this same enzyme can also aromatize many anabolic/androgenic steroids, the buildup of estrogens can be an important concern during intake. High levels can cause a number of unwanted side effects, a primary worry being gynecomastia or the development of female breast tissue in men. This can be first noticed by the appearance of swelling or a small lump under the nipple. If left to progress it can turn into a very unsightly development of tissue, often an irreversible occurrence without surgery. Estrogen can also lead to an increase in the level of water retained in the body. The result here can be a notable loss of definition, the muscles beginning to look smooth and bloated due to the retention of subcutaneous fluid. Fat storage may also be increased as estrogen levels rise. This hormone is in fact the primary reason women have a higher body fat percentage, and different fat distribution (hips/thighs) than men. Individuals sensitive to the effects of estrogen will usually be sure to have an antiestrogen on hand when taking problematic steroids, so as to minimize the impact of related side effects. It is also of note that when estrogen and body fat levels are normal, administering Nolvadex® (both Men and Women) can increase the look of hardness and definition the muscles.

This drug also shows the ability to increase production of FSH (follicle stimulating hormone) and LH (luteinizing hormone) in the male body. This is accomplished by blocking negative feedback inhibition caused by estrogen at the hypothalamus and pituitary, which fosters the release of the mentioned pituitary hormones. This of course is also the function of Clomid® and cyclofenil. Since a higher release of LH can stimulate the Leydig's cells in the testes to produce more testosterone, Nolvadex® can have a positive impact on one's serum testosterone level. This "testosterone stimulating" effect is an added benefit when preparing to conclude a steroid cycle. Since most anabolic/androgenic steroids will suppress endogenous testosterone production, Nolvadex® can help restore a balance in hormone levels. Nolvadex® should be preferred over Clomid for this purpose in fact, as side by side it is clearly the stronger agent. It has also been shown to increase LH responsiveness to Gonadotropin Releasing Hormone after time, while Clomid® slightly lowers this sensitivity as the drug is used for several weeks[137].

In some instances the use of only an estrogen antagonists such as Nolvadex® or Clomid® may be sufficient for testosterone stimulating purposes, particularly when halting the use of a milder or shorter steroid program (which should have a less pronounced impact on the hormonal system). With stronger cycles most option to enhance the stimulating effect of these drugs with HCG, a hormone that mimics the action of LH. HCG use provides an excessive level of stimulation to the testes, which in essence may shock them out of a prolonged state of inactivity. In such a condition the Leydig's cells may not be producing a normal amount of testosterone, even though the normal release of gonadotropins has been achieved. Nolvadex® can be tricky at this point. Remember it only blocks the effect of estrogen that is present in the body. If it is removed at a time when estrogen levels are still unusually high, related side effects can quickly become a pronounced problem. Since HCG not only increases the production of testosterone but also enhances the rate of aromatization in the testes, anti-estrogens should not be discontinued until at least a couple of weeks after HCG is discontinued. The result otherwise of course could be many unwanted side effects that were previously under control. When using Nolvadex® to ward off the effects of estrogen during the cycle, it should similarly not be removed until the user is confident that hormone levels are well under control. With a drug such as Sustanon, this may mean continuing it for several weeks after the last shot.

A typical daily dosage for men is in the range of 10 to 30mg, the chosen amount obviously dependent on the level of effect desired. It is advisable to begin with a low dosage and work up, so as to avoid taking an unnecessary amount. The time in which Nolvadex® is started also relies on individual needs of the user. If an athlete with a known sensitivity to estrogen is starting a strong steroid cycle, Nolvadex® should probably be added soon after the cycle had been initiated. If estrogen is probably not going to be a major problem during the cycle (but will likely be after), Nolvadex® is administered around the time exogenous steroid levels will drop. It will be continued for some weeks after, until the point when natural testosterone is thought to be at an acceptable level. As mentioned HCG is often used at this point as well (see related profile for more detail). Women have also utilized Nolvadex® in an effort to reduce the effect of their own endogenous estrogens. This can lower body fat concentrations, especially in stubborn areas like the hips and thighs. This is of course risky, as manipulating the effect of estrogen can become uncomfortable in women. Side effects like hot flashes, menstrual irregularities and a variety of complications with the reproductive system are all possible.

When looking for a stronger antiestrogenic effect, Proviron® can make a good adjunct to Nolvadex®. Although this compound is technically an androgen, it may have a pronounced effect on the production of estrogen in the body. Its mode of action is therefore very different than that of Nolvadex®. While Nolvadex® only blocks the binding ability of free-floating estrogen, Proviron® can minimize the creation of it. With each drug attacking estrogen via a different mechanism, we have a very synergistic combination. A daily intake of 20-30mg Nolvadex® and 25-50mg Proviron® can be extremely effective when dealing with a strong estrogenic cycle. Women often avoid adding Proviron® to Nolvadex® treatment (thought often it is still used to enhance fat loss), for fear of developing virilization symptoms (Proviron® is an oral DHT). Virilizing effects can occur very quickly once there has been a dramatic rise in the activity of androgens (intensified by a decrease in estrogen activity), so at a minimum women should be careful with such a combination.

Of great interest also is that Nolvadex is an estrogen agonist in the liver, capable of activating the estrogen receptor and mimicking the actions of this sex hormone in this region of the body. As such it can have a markedly positive impact on HDL (good) cholesterol values[138], as does estrogen. Many similarly use this drug to counter some of the negative consequences of steroid use in regards to cholesterol values and cardiac risk, as steroids often suppress HDL and raise LDL levels considerably. In some instances I have heard an athlete being able to maintain a very favorable HDL/LDL cholesterol ratio, to spite the use of a moderate dosage (400mg weekly) of an injectable like testosterone or nandrolone. It would probably be foolish to think however that Nolvadex® would be a sufficient remedy with the heavy use of c-17alpha alkylated orals or extremely high dosed cycles in general.

It has been reported by many however that Nolvadex® seems to slightly reduce to gains made during a steroid cycle. It appears that many androgenic/anabolic steroids will exhibit their most powerful anabolic effect when accompanied by a sufficient level of estrogen (See: Estrogen Aromatization). This may be one reason why gains made with a strong androgen like testosterone are usually much more pronounced than when using an anabolic that aromatizes to a lower degree. It therefore seems like good advice to be aware of how much Nolvadex® is actually needed before committing to it during a cycle. Many people in fact find it unnecessary, even when utilizing problematic compounds such as testosterone or Dianabol. Others however find they are troubled by water retention and gynecomastia, even with milder anabolics like Deca-Durabolin® and Equipoise®. The estrogenic response to steroid use is very individual, and may be influenced by factors such as age and body fat percentage (adipose tissue is a primary site of aromatization).

Nolvadex® is certainly the most popular antiestrogen used by athletes today, no doubt because it is simply an effective product. It is also widely manufactured, and easy to obtain on the black market. Since there never seems to be a lack of supply, there is little incentive to manufacture a counterfeit product. All of the various generics forms of this drug located are no doubt trustworthy. Nolvadex® tablets generally sell for approximately $1-2 each, depending on the dosage and source of the drug. Women should remember to be very cautious when considering the use of Nolvadex®, as they are usually very sensitive to changes in the activity of estrogen. Men looking for a stronger antiestrogenic effect may consider using Arimidex® (introduced earlier), a powerful new antiaromatase compound. It is much more effective for estrogen control, although it is also more costly than our other ancillary drugs. A single tablet of Arimidex® will generally cost close to $10, obviously some expense as the days drag on.

Teslac (testolactone)

Teslac is a first generation non-selective steroidal aromatase inhibitor, used clinically to treat estrogen-dependent breast cancers. This agent has been around for over 30 years now, and was first approved as a prescription drug by the FDA back in 1970. Its exact mode of action is unknown, but it is believed to inhibit the aromatase enzyme in a noncompetitive and irreversible manner, somewhat similar to formestane. This would explain why cessation of the drug does not provide an immediate restoration of normal estrogen production. Like formestane, it takes several days after ceasing use for the body to recover its normal estrogen synthesizing capacity.

Although testolactone is technically steroidal in structure, it offers no anabolic effect to its user. This is because it does not posses the traits necessary to bind and activate the androgen receptor, namely an active 17-beta-hydroxyl group. In fact, its D ring is an unusual 6 membered lactone ring, and not the normal 5 membered carboxylic ring that testosterone and its derivatives normally possess. This is, of course, where testolactone got its name (testo-lactone). Studies actually suggest this drug even has some level of anti-androgenic action, with an ability to interact with the androgen receptor enough to block testosterone and other steroids from attaching to it[139]. Regardless of this, testolactone has still been included in the U.S. controlled substance laws as an anabolic steroid.

The recommended dosage for maximum estrogen suppression is 250mg (five tablets) per day. Those bodybuilders experimenting with it usually report that an effective range is reached between 3 and 5 tablets daily, which is a level that is usually sufficient to prevent gynecomastia and keep off the extra water weight. The level of inhibition you will receive from this drug is not that dramatic however, at least compared to what the newer selective third generation inhibitors are able to accomplish. For example, one study conducted back in 1985 showed that 1,000mg per day given to nine normal men for a period of ten days suppressed serum estradiol levels by only 25%[140]. Another using the same 1,000 mg dose noted a 50% reduction after 6 days of use[141]. Clearly this falls short of the 80%+ levels of inhibition noted with the third generation agents of today.

In 1999 the FDA officially added "malaise" to the list of possible side effects from this drug, reflecting something we have been noticing as bodybuilders for some time: low estrogen levels can lead to lethargy, as this sex hormone plays an important role in the functioning of the central nervous system. This, of course, joins a list of other potential drawbacks to the suppression of estrogen production in men, including unfavorable alterations in serum cholesterol (strong HDL (good) cholesterol suppression in particular), interference with libido, and a slight dampening of the anabolic potency of a steroid cycle. But then again, if you want that really hard, ripped, dense look, aromatase inhibitors can be key in helping you achieve your goals here. Teslac is not the most effective option available to you however, and today is almost always brushed aside for one of the more potent, and less troublesome, agents like Aromasin, Femara or Arimidex.

APPETITE STIMULANTS

DRUG PROFILES

Periactin (cyproheptadine HCL)

Periactin® (cyproheptadine hydrochloride) is a first-generation prescription histamine and serotonin antagonist. It is also sold under such brand names as Ciplactin, Peritol, and Practin. This drug is most often given in the U.S. for the treatment of allergy-related symptoms, including hay fever, runny nose, irritated eyes, hives, and swelling. It is also FDA approved for the treatment of anaphylactic reactions caused by allergens, often as an adjunct to injectable epinephrine (adrenalin). The serotonin inhibiting effect of this drug also gives it a unique ability to increase appetite. This has led to a considerable amount of "off-label" use as a weight-gain medication, particularly with patients who are suffering from a lean tissue wasting associated with AIDS infection, cancer, or other debilitating diseases. Periactin is also used on occasion as an adjunct to growth hormone therapy in children, to foster greater nutrient uptake and increases in linear growth beyond what is normally achieved with rHGH alone[142].

References to the appetite stimulating properties of Periactin are easy to find in the medical literature. One of the more detailed papers compares the appetite increasing effects of Periactin to megestrol acetate[143] in a group of 14 men with weight loss associated with HIV infection. The other agent, megestrolm, is a progestin that was approved by the FDA in 1993 for the treatment of anorexia, cachexia, or weight loss in patients with AIDS. In this investigation, Periactin was shown to have a similar level of benefit to FDA approved agent megestrol, with patients consuming about 500 extra calories per day, and gaining a moderate amount of weight with either medications. While the benefits were similar, the side effects were not. The investigators reported that more than 50% of the patients taking megestrol suffered impotence during the investigation, while the cyproheptadine HCL group had no such side effects. Periactin may offer an effective alternative to megestrol therapy for many patients, especially those prone to negative side effects associated with this type of hormone manipulation.

That is not to suggest Periactin is free of concerns. As a first-generation anti-histamine, it may be prone to producing a number of side effects in its users. The most common of which is sedation, as this drug produces the classic "anti-histamine lethargy" we have come to expect from this class of drugs. For some users, the tiredness that the drug will produce will outweigh any potential as a weight-gaining/performance-enhancing agent. For most, this side effect of Pericatin is not very noticeable, and perhaps a nuisance (not strong enough to necessitate discontinuation) at best. Other less common side effects of concern include, but are not limited to, dizziness, disturbed coordination, muscular weakness, nausea, vomiting, diarrhea, constipation, dryness of the mouth, difficulty urinating, vertigo, blurred vision, tightness of the chest, wheezing, stuffed nose, sweating, early period, headaches, and faintness. Obviously, any strong incidence of unwelcomed side effects would immediately warrant discontinuing the drug, or even seeking immediate medical attention if severe.

The typical recommended dose for Periactin as an appetite stimulation is 4mg, which is taken 3 times per day. Above this level, side effects may start to become problematic (most notably sleepiness), interfering with the benefit of the drug. For those who tolerate this anti-histamine's side effects (mainly tiredness), Periactin is often highly valued as an appetite stimulant during weight gaining cycles. Considering the value of a high calorie, high protein diet for building muscle, as well as the difficulty many people have with eating enough to gain optimal weight, it is very understandable why. In fact, I am quite surprised that this drug is not more popular, given the rarity of effective appetite stimulants. It is interesting to note also that the Dominican steroid product, Anabolex, actually includes 1.5mg of cyproheptadine HCL in each 3mg methandrostenolone tablet, which was clearly added by its developers to facilitate increased caloric intake and weight gain during anabolic therapy. The 2:1 ratio provided is optimal for a daily dose of 24mg Dianabol (a very common amount), as it would provide 12mg of Periactin (the recommended daily dose). To my knowledge this is the only anabolic steroid product that includes cyproheptadine HCL as an ingredient.

Diuretics

DRUG PROFILES

Aldactazide (spironolactone/hydrochlorthiazide)

Aldactazide® is a trade name (Searle) for an oral, combination diuretic. Specifically it contains a mixture of spironolactone (Aldactone) and hydrochlorthiazide (Hydrodiuril). Aldactone® is a milder, potassium sparing diuretic while Hydrodiuril is a more potent compound from the thiazide family. The combination produces a diuretic with potency comparable to that seen with a doubling in thiazide dosage (when used alone), but without the same level of calcium and potassium excretion. While a potassium supplement is often required with thiazide treatment, the balance of the two drugs in Aldactazide® virtually eliminates this need. Medically this drug is used to treat cases of hypertension (high blood pressure) and edemas (swelling due to excessive water retention). When administered, diuresis (water excretion) becomes pronounced within a couple of hours. It may actually take three to four hours for the peak effect to be noticed, and the drug will remain active in the body for a total duration of approximately twelve hours.

Athletes use diuretics in order to shed extra water retained in the body. This practice is popular in competitive bodybuilding situations, as a drop in subcutaneous water storage can result in an increase in the level of definition to the physique. Competitors in weight class sports like boxing and wrestling also make use of diuretics, administering them to manipulate their body weight for category adjustments. Since the "weigh-in" procedure is generally done a day or days before a competition, the athlete has a clear window of opportunity to drop body weight and lower his/her weight class assignment. The hours or days after the weigh-in gives the competitor more than ample time to rehydrate, and compete at a weight well above that which is dictated by their category. This could certainly be considered an (extremely) unfair advantage, if it were not balanced out by the fact that "dropping weight" (either pharmaceutically or otherwise) is an almost universal practice within such disciplines.

The dosage of the two constituents does vary somewhat among the different preparations, so one should be cautious to notice the actual dosage of both drugs before administering Aldactazide®. The user, depending on individual needs, will need to judge the timing of his diuretic use in relation to the weigh-in or show. The whole intake/preparation schedule should also not run longer than a few days, so as to minimize potential health risks. It is also much more effective when the athlete is familiar with the process well before actually needing to do so. This way frantic last minute diuretic use can be avoided, as the user should be fully prepared. When administered haphazardly, it is very easy to achieve too great a diuretic effect. The result in this case might not be a defined look, but a flat, deflated appearance brought about by severe dehydration.

The most common practice among athletes is to administer a single 50mg/50mg tablet in the morning (with a meal), and to wait and judge the diuretic effect. After a number of hours, this is repeated if a stronger effect is needed. Usually 2-3 tablets will be taken by the days end. Remember that this compound, hydrochlorthiazide in particular, can remain active for many hours. Overlapping dosages will certainly amplify any diuretic effect. Without a large enough gap between tablets, the active dosage/effect may be difficult to judge. The accumulated effect, of course, has the potential to reach a dangerous point.

This diuretic (as all) can present a number of unwanted side effects to the user. This includes, but is not limited to, dehydration, cramping, diarrhea, dizziness, headache, anxiety, unrest, weakness, numbing of extremities and cardiac irregularities. One also risks severe dehydration, with potential to result in coma or death. Unfortunately athletes will too often push their diuretic use to the limits of personal health. The line between a desired effect and serious complications is, in many instances, very fine. While serious side effects appear less frequently with this class of diuretic (than say Lasix (furosemide)), it should still remain a constant concern. Additionally, spironolactone can lower serum androgen levels due to its interference with the biosynthesis of testosterone. This combined with a weak ability to inhibit androgen receptor binding give this drug notable anti-androgenic properties. Since athletes use this compound for only short periods of time however, this effect should not be much of a worry.

Aldactone (spironolactone)

Aldactone® (spironolactone) is a mild diuretic, manufactured widely throughout the world. Medically this class of drug is used to treat high blood pressure, efficiently lowering the retention of water and salt. Aldactone® acts by reducing the amount of aldosterone secreted by the adrenal gland, which is the hormone primarily responsible for water regulation in the body. This effect is beneficial to competitive bodybuilders, who need to shed subcutaneous water before a showing. Specifically this compound is a potassium-sparing diuretic, much weaker in effect than both Dyazide and Lasix. As can be surmised, potassium levels are not greatly reduced with Aldactone®. This is much unlike many stronger diuretics that can increase the rate of potassium excretion considerably. It is therefore very important that the user does not take any additional potassium supplement while using this compound. Too high an increase in potassium levels can prove to be life-threatening.

Using diuretics can present a number of unwanted side effects to the user. This includes, but is not limited to, dehydration, cramping, diarrhea, dizziness, headache, anxiety, unrest, weakness, numbing of extremities and cardiac irregularities. Such side effects seem much less common with this class of diuretic, but should still be of concern. Additionally, this compound exhibits notable anti-androgenic properties. This is because spironolactone is both a weak inhibitor of androgen/receptor binding, and a strong inhibitor of testosterone biosynthesis. Since athletes generally use Aldactone® for a very short period of time, interference with androgen levels should not be much concern however.

Male competitors generally find a dosage of 100mg per day, in a single Morning application, effective for subcutaneous water excretion. This is continued for 3 to 5 days prior to a showing and should result in a harder, more defined appearance to the muscles. Overuse of diuretics can result in notable dehydration, producing the unwanted look of "flattened" muscles. This is not a common occurrence with potassium-sparing diuretics, but is still possible. Many competitors in fact find Aldactone® too mild, and require stronger drugs like Lasix and Hydrodiuril, also with increased risks. Women are occasionally attracted to this product for its effect as an anti-androgen. It can be used at a point when androgen levels have become problematic during a cycle, hopefully reducing the risk of virilization symptoms. A dosage of 25-75mg daily for 1 to 2 weeks may be enough to ward off side effects while androgen levels decline (the steroid regimen terminated). Since spironolactone is more effective at lowering endogenous androgen levels than inhibiting androgen action, it is certainly not to be considered a cure-all remedy for the adventurous steroid-using female.

Since this compound is one of our safest (prescription) options, it is an obvious starting point for a beginning competitor. Once familiar with Aldactone® and wishing for a stronger effect, the addition of a thiazide or furosemide (Lasix) can prove successful. Here the overall dosage is to be reduced than if using either substance alone, and should provide strong water excretion with less calcium/potassium loss. If mixing with hydrochlorthiazide, we can cut the Aldactone® dosage in half (from 100mg) and add an equal mg amount of the thiazide. The 50mg/50mg combination should noticeably increase water excretion without dramatic side effects. The potassium re-absorption seen with Aldactone® should be balanced out with the thiazide, so potassium levels should not be greatly affected. On the other hand, Lasix (furosemide) makes a much stronger addition to Aldactone®. In this case, dropping the Aldactone® dosage to 50mg and adding 20mg oral Lasix is a popular place to start, hopefully providing the water-shedding effect of a 40mg Lasix tablet. Again, the potassium depleting effect of Lasix will likely be balanced out by the Aldactone®, so no additional supplement should be needed. In Europe many such combination diuretics are available and appear to be well liked among competitors.

Dyazide (triamterene and hydrochlorothiazide)

Dyazide® is an oral diuretic/antihypertensive drug, It containing a mix of the two commonly prescribed agents hydrochlorthiazide and triamterene. The hydrochlorothiazide component is a strong thiazide diuretic, noticeably increasing the rate of sodium excretion. The triamterene is a potassium sparing diuretic, increasing the rate water & sodium are excreted but interfering with the loss of potassium. This combination results in a pronounced diuretic effect without the calcium and potassium loss seen with thiazides alone. The need for potassium supplements is therefore (generally) eliminated with the use this preparation.

Clinically, these drugs are most commonly used to treat cases of edema and high blood pressure (hypertension). Athletes however, use them to shed subcutaneous water during bodybuilding competitions and for weight class adjustments in certain competitive sports. Bodybuilders in particular rely heavily on the definition that results when excess water is reduced. The highly defined, super hard and shredded look so common today is nearly impossible to achieve without diuretics. At the same time diuretics are the reason weight class competitors like wrestlers often appear much heavier during a meet than they do at the weigh-in. A considerable amount of bodyweight (in the form of water) can be removed with diuretic use, often resulting in a drop of one or more weight categories. The user of course will rehydrate after the weigh-in, and will be much heavier that his/her weight class dictates during competition. When everyone is expecting to be matched against someone considerably heavier than his or her class weight dictates, this method of cheating becomes almost mandatory for a "fair" competition.

Among athletes, Dyazide is considered a moderately effective diuretic for such purposes. The water loss is stronger than that of a potassium-sparing agent like Aldactone®, but much weaker than that seen with a loop diuretic like Lasix. It could be most closely compared to the effect seen when a thiazide like Hydrodiuril (hydrochlorthiazide) is used alone, but again without the same level of calcium and potassium loss. Dyazide is therefore used when one wants to receive a good diuretic effect without needing to worry much about potassium supplementation. The diuretic activity following a single dose is usually evident within one hour. It will reach peak effect at approximately 2 to 3 hours and taper off during the next 7 to 9 hours. The athlete will generally use this drug for only the four days prior to a competition, adjusting the dosage to elicit the best level of effect. Since it has a long lasting effect, it is generally administered only once per day. One tablet is usually taken the first thing in the morning with a meal, and the effect judged. The dosage is increased one tablet per day (for perhaps 2 or 3 days at most) until the user is noticing the proper water loss. It is generally thought much more advantageous to prepare the few days before a show instead of loading up on diuretics that morning. The difference between a highly defined physique and a flat smooth dehydrated look is most often just a slight adjustment in dosage.

There is little doubt that diuretic use poses the greatest risk to an athlete. The dangers of this practice are much more pronounced than that of steroids, and are usually the cause when an ambitious professional is sacrificed to drug use. These compounds are very powerful, and should be respected as such. One should be well aware of the many potential side effects associated with diuretics like Dyazide. Muscle cramps, weakness, dizziness, headache, dry mouth, rash, diarrhea, constipation and severe dehydration are all common occurrences. Symptoms of nausea and vomiting can be seen as well, often indicative of an electrolyte imbalance. Administering the drug only after meals can usually prevent nausea. In severe instances, dehydration has resulted in coma or death. Athletes often walk a fine line between obtaining an optimal show physique and severely dehydrating themselves. This is clearly a risky practice, one should be very cautious.

Hydrodiuril (hydrochlorthiazide)

Hydrodiuril® is a trade name for the drug hydrochlorthiazide. This is a diuretic from the thiazide family, used medically for the treatment of edemas and hypertension. This drug acts by reducing the reabsorption of electrolytes, thereby increasing the excretion of sodium, potassium, chloride, and consequently water. In comparison to other diuretics, Hydrodiuril is stronger than the potassium sparing agent Aldactone® (spironolactone), but weaker then the loop agent Lasix (furosemide). While potassium excretion is much less pronounced than that seen with Lasix, the use of a potassium supplement (or a potassium rich diet) may still be necessary with this product. The necessity for this is usually dependent on the dose and duration in which the drug is administered. Calcium excretion may also be pronounced with thiazides, but again, are weaker in this regard than Lasix.

The use of diuretics has been increasingly popular in a number of athletic disciplines. For starters, these drugs are very popular among bodybuilders who use them to shed subcutaneous water before a competition. The ability to have a winning physique often relies heavily on the definition that can result from diuretic use. The highly defined, super hard and shredded look so common today is nearly impossible to achieve without the use of these drugs. Diuretics are also utilized by athletes who compete in weight categories, using them to drop water weight and make category adjustments. They can allow competitors such as wrestlers and boxers to compete at a much heavier weight during an event than dictated by the “weigh-in” measurement. This is due to the fact that the weight-in is usually done the day before a competition. This allows the athlete to come in light due to diuretics, yet gives enough time to restore fluids and bodyweight before the meet. The result is often a drop of one or more weight categories, a formidable advantage in these types sports. And professional athletes are not the only offenders, as this practice is common in collage sports (sometimes even high schools!). Until the weight-in procedure is placed immediately before the competition, some form of “dropping weight” will always be entertained by such competitors.

The main concern with diuretic use is that it can be a very risky practice. There should be little doubt that diuretics involve a much greater risk to the athlete than that associated with steroid use. Using these drugs incorrectly can produce a dangerous level of dehydration, sometimes to a life threatening point. And unfortunately the line between a shredded physique (or the proper weight class adjustment) and dangerous dehydration is often fine. Sadly, a number of athletes are lost each year when self-administering these drugs, for nothing more than a competitive edge. One should be very careful when using diuretics, hopefully taking time to objectively evaluate the practice. Even when seemingly used correctly, Hydrodiuril can present a number of unwanted side effects to the user. These include, but are not limited to, dehydration, cramping, diarrhea, dizziness, headache, anxiety, unrest, weakness, numbing of extremities and cardiac irregularities. These side effects are generally less pronounced with this class of diuretic (in comparison to loop agents), but should still be a concern. One should take caution by discontinuing this drug should side effects become uncomfortable.

Athletes generally use Hydrodiuril for a short period of time, obviously only needing it for brief water level adjustments. The usual practice is to administer this drug once per day, after the morning meal. The athlete will monitor the level of water lost throughout the day, and adjust the dosage for the following day accordingly. The usual starting dosage is one or two 50mg tablets. The user will adjust the effect by adding a 25 or 50mg tablet each subsequent day, with the total dosage not exceeding 200mg (four 50mg tablets). This practice is only followed for three or four days, as the user calculates an optimal dosage. If the application of Hydrodiuril is not producing the desired effect, one may choose to addition another diuretic (mild) before moving to the stronger loop agents. A combination of a potassium sparing diuretic like Aldactone® (spironolactone) and Hydrodiuril would prove extremely useful, balancing out the calcium and potassium loss of the thiazide. The dosage of each agent would be reduced considerably, perhaps starting with a 50mg/50mg application and working upwards. Be careful not to overuse these drugs, as too much water loss will produce a flat, “deflated” looking muscle. More diuretic certainly does not always equate to more definition. It is the best advice to become familiar with this practice well before competition time. Otherwise the user may be left to make frantic dosage adjustments at the last minute, which can be a dangerous practice.

Lasix (furosemide)

Lasix is a brand name for the drug furosemide, a very potent diuretic. Technically it belongs to a class of drugs known as loop diuretics, which will cause the body to excrete water as well as potassium, sodium and chloride. Loop diuretics are among the strongest such drugs available, having an extremely dramatic effect on fluid levels in the body. Potassium levels need to be particularly watched, Lasix greatly increasing the amount excreted. The use of a prescription potassium supplement therefore is often required to keep levels in balance, otherwise a serious heart complications might develop. Mistakes in potassium dosage have equally serious consequences, so Lasix is clearly a risky item to use. But when an athlete needs to shed water, it is very difficult to find something that works better.

Athletes use diuretics for a couple of specific purposes. Competitive athletes use these drugs to drop water weight, in an effort to make adjustments in their weight class standings. Since the weigh-in is most often a day or days before a competition/match, one can drop their bodyweight considerably and be back to normal within hours after rehydration. This logically seems to provide an unfair advantage, the athlete competing at a much heavier weight than believed. This advantage is only offset by the now near universal nature of this practice. Bodybuilders also rely heavily on diuretics when preparing for a contest. It can efficiently lower subcutaneous water concentrations, helping to produce that super-ripped look so common on stage today. Make no mistake; a winning look is extremely difficult to obtain without some form of diuretic.

This drug is prepared as both an oral tablet (usually 20-40mg per tablet) or IM/IV injection solution, the injection being much more rapid in effect. The dosage and method of administration is tailored to the individual, dependent on the desired goals and condition of the athlete. Tablets are the most common form of administration. Each oral Lasix tablet becomes effective about 1 hour after ingesting and will remain active for an additional 3 or 4 hours. The athlete will usually start with a mild dose, and add to this amount accordingly later in the day. The initial dosage is usually 20 to 40mg, with the maximum amount usually not to exceed 80mg. The user will attempt to calculate the optimal dosage, and determine the best intake schedule in relation to the show or competition. In order to minimize the side effects associated with this drug, it is generally used for no longer than a few days.

Since Lasix has such a strong effect on electrolyte and potassium levels, it is much safer to addition a potassium sparing agent like Aldactone® (spironolactone) than it is to keep increasing the amount of Lasix used. A combination of 50mg Aldactone® and 20mg Lasix would be a good starting point, having roughly the effect of a 40mg Lasix tablet without the notable potassium loss. This dosage is repeated 2-3 times during the day and the effect judged to determine the optimal dosage. It is important to remember that these drugs can be active for many hours. It can become difficult to control the dehydrating effect with an overlapping schedule, so one should be careful not to administer such diuretics too frequently.

The injectable is a much more powerful version of the drug. It can be administered both intramuscularly and intravenously, depending on the intensity the user is looking for. The IV method is extremely fast, the strong effect of the drug felt in a matter of minutes. Since the injection is much more powerful than the oral, the dosage is to be considerably reduced in comparison. The injected dosage is usually in the range of 10-40mg, rarely going any higher. Drug testing for Lasix at bodybuilding competitions has increased the popularity of last minute IV diuretic use, a very dangerous practice. Instead of slowly shedding water the few days prior, the user is forced to wait until after the "piss-test". Then in a frantic rush to remove subcutaneous water before the show, the drug is administered. The user often has little time to adjust the dosage, resulting in a number of fatal mistakes in recent years. The effect of Lasix is actually easier to control with the injectable under normal conditions. When there is room to experiment, adjustments in dosage are much easier to make (the user not having to wait very long to see an effect). And the optimal dosage is certainly less trouble to calculate for a later time as well, the user having fewer variables to worry about. But again, when used in a rush this drug can be extremely dangerous.

Lasix is no doubt one of the most dangerous drugs a competitor will use. This can be seen on occasion when severe dehydration and electrolyte imbalance takes the life of an ambitious athlete. Warning signs that Lasix may be causing severe dehydration include (not limited to) dizziness, cramping, vomiting, diarrhea, fainting and circulatory disturbances. Potassium depletion can be marked as well, so as discussed users often opt to take a prescription potassium supplement, also with its own set of dangers. One should use extreme caution when considering using Lasix or other diuretics; they are certainly not needed for recreational users.

This product is widely available. It is manufactured and sold under many different brand names, in many countries. No version of Lasix (or any other diuretic) is currently being counterfeited. When found on the black market it can therefore be trusted. Although it is doubtful these will circulate, make sure never to purchase the 500mg tablets. These are used only in severe medical conditions, and contain a dosage that could prove fatal to a healthy person.

Lasilactone (spironolactone/furosemide)

Lasilactone is the Hoechst trade name for an oral, combination diuretic. Specifically, it contains a mixture of spironolactone (Aldactone®) and furosemide (Lasix). Aldactone® is a much milder, potassium sparing diuretic while Lasix is a notably potent compound from the family of loop agents. The combination of these two diuretics creates a drug with potency comparable to that seen with a much higher Lasix dosage (approximately double if used alone), but without the extreme level of calcium and potassium excretion. While a potassium supplement is often required with Lasix treatment, the balance of the two drugs in this compound will usually make this unnecessary. Medically, Lasilactone is used to treat cases of high blood pressure and edemas (swelling). When administered, diuresis (water excretion) becomes pronounced within an hour, and will remain notable for approximately four hours.

Like many patients, Athletes are attracted to diuretics because of their ability to remove stored water from the body. This effect is highly sought after by competitive bodybuilders, as a drop in subcutaneous water storage can increase the visibility of muscle features (increased definition). In sports where the competitor is restricted to a weight class (such as boxing and wrestling), diuretics are also extremely popular. They can be used to manipulate the bodyweight, in order for the athlete to make weight category adjustments. Since the “weigh-in” procedure is completed (generally) a day or days before the competition, the user has a clear window of opportunity to drop their bodyweight with a diuretic before hitting the scale. The long stretch of time after the weight in gives the user ample time to rehydrate, and as a result compete in a lower weight class than his/her bodyweight would dictate.

When administering this drug, the user will need to adjust the dosage in order to fit his or her individual needs. The most common practice is to administer a single 50mg/20mg tablet in the morning (with a meal), and to wait and judge the level of water loss. After a number of hours, this is repeated if a stronger diuretic effect is required. Usually no more than 2 or 3 tablets will be taken by the end of the day. This is perhaps repeated for a couple of more days, as the athlete looks to obtain the optimal result. So as to minimize any potential health risks, it is good advice to limit the use of such compounds to no more than a few days. It is also much more effective when the athlete is familiar with the whole process before using such drugs for a show/competition. Frantic, last minute diuretic use (due to poor planning) can easy lead to a troubling level of dehydration. The difference between a flat, deflated appearance and the all-important defined (ripped) look is in many cases only a small dosage adjustment.

This diuretic (as all) can present a number of unwanted side effects to the user. This includes, but is not limited to, dehydration, cramping, diarrhea, dizziness, headache, anxiety, unrest, weakness, numbing of extremities and cardiac irregularities. One also risks severe dehydration, which has the potential to result in coma or death. Unfortunately athletes will too often take great risks, pushing their diuretic use to the limits of personal health. The line between a desired effect and serious complications is, in many instances, very fine. While serious side effects appear less frequently with compound diuretics as such, it should still remain a constant concern. Lasix in particular can be a very powerful compound and should be respected as such.

ENDURANCE & ERYTHROPOIETIC AGENTS

DRUG PROFILES

Aranesp (darbepoetin alfa)

Aranesp is an erythropoiesis-stimulating drug, very similar in structure and action to the body's own endogenous erythropoietin. It is manufactured by Amgen, the world's largest biotechnologies company. In fact, it is also the same company that first brought recombinant erythropoietin (epoetin alfa) to the market in 1984. In structure darbepoetin alfa differs from human erythropoietin only slightly, and has all the same biological activity. Human erythropoietin is normally released by the kidneys in response to hypoxia, or low blood oxygen levels. It in turn triggers bone marrow to increase red blood cell production, and is likewise vital to the regulation of normal red blood cell concentrations. Darbepoetin alfa can likewise be used to augment erythropoiesis when the body is not maintaining adequate red blood cell levels on its own. It is approved by the FDA for the treatment of anemias (low red blood cell count) specifically associated with chronic renal failure or chemotherapy.

Aranesp differs from the recombinant human erythropoietin in Epogen (epoetin alfa) mainly in its duration of activity. This new protein maintains its levels in the blood for approximately three times longer, which is an extremely significant difference. This means that with Aranesp, patients are required to administer the product much less frequently. While Epogen is usually given on a schedule of three times a week, Aranesp requires only one injection each week. This course enhances patient comfort quite a bit, and is especially useful when the patient is visiting the doctor for drug administration. Studies comparing this form of therapy to the use of standard recombinant erythropoietin note that users need approximately the same amount of drug, it is just given in larger doses with more time between applications.

Erythropoiesis stimulating drugs are very popular in endurance sports, such as long distance running and cycling. In these sports maximum oxygen carrying capacity is of paramount importance to the performance of the athlete. We are all too familiar with the decades old practice of manually removing and later reinfusing blood plasma for the sake of increasing red blood cell count and endurance capacity for a sport, commonly referred to as "blood doping". Drugs like Aranesp and Epogen accomplish the same thing as this decades old practice, and are essentially just new forms of "chemical blood doping". In practice they can be just as effective as their antiquated counterpart, even more so. These agents are also used at times in bodybuilding circles, where the erythropoiesis stimulating effect may help bring out a greater look of vascularity when the body fat percentage is sufficiently low. It is likewise more of a "pre-contest" drug.

While Aranesp and Epogen can be just as effective as the practice of blood doping, be warned that these drugs can also be just as dangerous. A number of athlete deaths have been attributed to the use of these agents over the past several years, caused by an over-thickening of the blood due to abnormally high red cell concentrations. One must take extreme caution when using these drugs, making sure to meticulously measure red blood cell counts to be sure that the drug is not having an effect that could turn out to be life threatening. For a more comprehensive discussion on the uses, mechanisms, and dangers of erythropoiesis stimulating drugs, please refer to the Epogen drug profile. Take note also that Aranesp is now detectable during urinalysis, making it unsafe for drug-tested sports.

Aranesp comes in the dosage strengths of 25, 40, 60, 100, 200 and 300 mcg/mL. When shopping, you will quickly learn that this not a cheap drug. At a U.S. pharmacy, a four-vial pack of the 100mcg/mL dose will run you approximately $1,700. Due to the high cost for the new erythropoiesis stimulating agents, they are often the targets of counterfeit drug manufacturing operations. But these operations cater not to the black market like underground steroid makers, but push their drugs through legitimate channels - into the pharmacies where they are sold to unsuspecting consumers, often with diluted dosages. This has been a big issues as of late, suggesting that it may be a good idea to get your scripts filled (if you get them) thorough the larger pharmacy chains, which are unlikely to purchase their drugs through pharmaceutical wholesalers.

Epogen (epoietin alfa)

Erythropoietin (EPO) is a primary growth factor involved in regulating red blood cell formation in the human body. Isolation and manufacture of this hormone for medical purposes has proved extremely beneficial. This hormone is used to treat many forms of anemia, effectively stimulating and maintaining erythropoiesis in a large percentage of patients treated. The efficiency of this drug quickly made it a ready replacement for older (less effective) therapies such as Anadrol 50®. The structure of recombinant human erythropoietin (epoetin alfa, r-HuEPO) is a purified single chain polypeptide hormone, 165 amino acids in sequence. The compound is produced from animal cells, into which the gene coding for human erythropoietin has been inserted. The biological activity and structure of r-HuEPO are indistinguishable from that of human erythropoietin.

Endurance athletes are highly attracted to EPO for the effect it has on red blood cell production. It is no secret that the practice of "blood doping" is popular with endurance sports. This procedure involves removing and storing a quantity of blood from your body, to be later replaced. By adding this stored blood before an event (by then the body has restored the lost blood volume), the athlete has a much greater number of red blood cells. The blood can therefore transport oxygen more efficiently, and the athlete is given a noticeable endurance boost. This has no doubt been the difference between winning and losing for many individuals. This procedure however, carries with it a great number of risks. Blood is a difficult thing to store and administer, not to mention the problems that can occur with the extra cell volume. Some of these risks are reduced with EPO, a drug that basically equates to "chemical blood doping". While one does not have to worry about storing and injecting blood, problems with cell volume can still be very dangerous with this drug. Cell concentration can reach a life threatening point if this drug is incorrectly used, resulting in heart attach, stroke, seizure or death.

There are also a number of side effects associated with general use of this substance. Most notable, blood pressure can begin to rise are cell volume changes. This can reach the point of headaches and high blood pressure, obviously an unwanted effect. Additionally, flu-like symptoms, aching bones, chills and injection site irritations are also possible. Since athletes are not using this product for a medical condition, a strong incidence of side effects should be an indicator to discontinue using the drug. Clearly one should not wish to compromise their health for an athletic push.

Erythropoietin is available in an injectable solution, to be given subcutaneously (between the skin and muscle) or intravenously. The two paths of administration have greatly different effects on the blood level of the drug. When given as an IV injection, peak blood levels of the drug are reached very quickly. The half-life is also short, approximately 4 or 5 hours long. When administered "SubQ", the drug will take 12 to 18 hours to reach a peak level. Given an equal dose, this concentration will also be much lower than the intravenous method. The half-life also greatly extended, estimated to now be approximately 24 hours. When used clinically, the starting dosage range is 15-50U/kg of bodyweight, given three times per week. By this guideline a 176lb athlete would take a maximum of 4000U per injection, or .4 ml., every two or three days. This would be done in the days/weeks prior to a competition, the peak effect hopefully reached near the day of the event.

The user would be best served by familiarizing him/herself with this drug long before using it competitively. This way a specific intake schedule could be devised, the athlete knowing how best to administer it each time. This will also help to avoid any complications brought about by last minute dosing adjustments due to inexperience with this compound. The discussed dosage range is also adjusted upwards of 100U/kg per application in many clinical cases, however athletes should be very careful when tinkering with this drug. The potential side effects are very serious, and certainly not to be ignored. Remember that it is also very important to monitor blood cell counts during the intake of EPO. Watching that your red blood cell count stays within limits is the surest way to avoid any serious complications.

Due to the intricate manufacturing process, EPO is a very expensive compound. Since it is additionally a drug specific to certain athletic fields, it is not common on the black market. Those looking to purchase EPO will instead generally find it (obviously) within circles of endurance athletes. It is also easy to obtain via a number of foreign mail-order sources. Since this is not a controlled substance, it does not carry the same import restrictions that are placed on anabolic steroids.

Provigil (Modafinil)

Modafinil, known chemically as benzhydrylsulphinylacetamide, is a relatively new stimulant-type drug developed by Lafon Laboratories in France. It is sold in the U.S. under the brand name Provigil®, and internationally under such names as Modiodal®, Vigil®, Alertec®, and Modasomil®. Modafinil is specifically characterized as a psychostimulant, and is FDA approved for the treatment of narcolepsy (a disorder characterized by sudden and uncontrollable attacks of deep sleep), mental fatigue, or excessive sleepiness. It is being investigated for a number of other uses, including the treatment of Alzheimer's disease, depression, and attention deficit disorder. Modafinil belongs to a class of drugs known as Eugeroics ("good arousal"), designed to promote a mental state of vigilance and alertness. Modafinil is specifically an alpha 1 adrenoceptor agonist, and exerts its mood and energy enhancing effects through the increased release of dopamine in the CNS, as well as alterations in local GABA and glutamate levels.

The use of Modafinil as a stimulant has been shown to be very advantageous over amphetamines. Modafinil is believed to have a much lower potential for abuse (less euphoria), lower peripheral CNS stimulation (less side effects), minimal effects on blood pressure, no interruptions in normal sleeping patterns (no hangover or needing "catch-up sleep), and an overall greater safety record during clinical trials. This drug is of interest even to the U.S. military, which is looking at it as an energy enhancer for pilots and combat soldiers that need to operate for long periods of time without sleep. This is not as unusual as it may seem at first, as military combat pilots and soldiers have used Dexedrine (an amphetamine) extensively in the past when sleep was difficult. This drug does have its drawbacks, including jitters, jumpiness, poor judgment, and "crashes". However, soldiers on Modafinil report they maintain excellent cognitive functioning for a full 40 hours straight without sleep, with none of the side effects of Dexedrine. Modafinil has been tested in combat situations as recently as Afghanistan and Iraq, and seems poised for official acceptance as a battlefield drug.

Recently, modafinil has become a popular drug amongst competitive athletes. They use it not simply to "stay awake", but as a performance enhancing agent with both stimulant and endurance-increasing properties. This type of use probably comes as a surprise to those who developed this drug, as early reports suggested that this was a "mild" alertness drug, without strong stimulant properties that would improve athletic performance. Apparently, that is not the case. A study conducted just recently in Canada shows a very strong athletic benefit inherent in modafinil[144]. During this double-blind investigation, a dose of 4mg per kg of bodyweight (this equates to 200mg for a 220lb man) of modafinil, or placebo, was given to a group of fifteen male volunteers. Three hours after ingestion, aerobic exercise was conducted on a cycle ergometer at 85% V02max (maximum aerobic power), and time until exhaustion. While taking modafinil, the men were able to exercise for significantly longer (~30%), and had greater oxygen intake at exertion. They also reported lower subjective ratings of perceived exertion (RPE), which suggests that the increased performance was in part due to a significantly less pronounced sensation of fatigue during exercise.

The typical effective dose for both men and women is in the range of 100-400mg, which is given 2-3 hours prior to athletic competition. As the dosage increases, side effects may start to become an issue, including headache, nausea, nervousness, and anxiety. It is a good idea to start on the low end of the range, and increase by 50-100mg per application until the optimal level is determined. The arenas in which this drug can be applied are vast, and essentially include any sport focused on aerobic activity or endurance. It may also work well with those who are forced to repeat short bursts of strength or speed many times during competition, such as shot putting, pole vaulting, or long jumping. Here, it could help the athlete continue performing at optimal levels as the day of competition stretches on. Modafinil is not going to be the most popular drug amongst bodybuilders, as it holds little direct value for building muscle or cutting fat. It may, however, be an effective pre-workout stimulant, helping you spend more time in the gym, and allowing you to attack the weights with more ferocity during the time you spend there.

Although modafinil has an excellent safety record and profile, it is still considered a drug of potential abuse in the United States. As such, it has been classified as a schedule IV controlled substance, in the same category as Valium and Xanax. This limits its availability somewhat, and also places considerable legal penalties on its possession and importation. Therefore, it is probably not a good idea to order this drug freely from international pharmacies on the Internet. Instead, it would be advisable to seek a legitimate domestic prescription for this agent. Since Modafinil has been approved by the FDA for some general uses, including the treatment of metal fatigue, this should not be all that difficult. It is quite common for doctors to prescribe this agent to someone who finds him or herself in the middle of a particularly stressful time at work, perhaps suddenly covering a late shift or putting in longer-than-usual hours. Such “excuses” would probably afford a modest supply of the drug fairly easily.

Modafinil was very popular amongst competitive athletes for a brief period of time before the IOC became aware of its use and banned it. Some readers may incorrectly be operating under the assumption that this drug is still not being tested for. That is, unfortunately, no longer the case. The use of modafinil as a performance-enhancing agent was revealed to the public during the designer steroid (BALCO) doping scandal of 2004. It was disclosed that many of the same athletes who tested positive for THG also used the drug. Since then, the IOC has developed a methodology for detecting this chemical, and have implemented it during all standard urine screens. Most of the other international athletic bodies have followed the IOC’s lead. Modafinil has since lost all appeal as an “invisible” performance-enhancing drug. Although no longer of great value on the Olympic playing field, in the months and years to come, Modafinil is likely to become popular with bodybuilders and those athletes not subject to drug testing, who may find it an excellent addition to their regular pre-competition pharmaceutical toolbox.

FAT LOSS AGENTS - SYMPATHOMIMETIC

DRUG PROFILES

Albuterol

Albuterol is a selective beta-2 adrenergic agonist, very similar in structure and action to clenbuterol. Unlike clenbuterol, albuterol is readily available as a prescription drug in the United States. It is also sold as salbutamol in a number of other countries, which is simply another generic name for the drug. Albuterol is found most commonly in the form of a rescue inhaler, which is designed disperse a measured amount of the drug immediately and directly to the bronchial tubes in times of crisis (asthma attack). This form provides the least amount of systemic drug activity possible, which is great for minimizing unwanted cardiovascular side effects. But for the purpose of fat loss this will not do at all, as we need high levels of the drug to reach adipose tissues. The user is likewise forced to seek out one of the less popular, but still available, albuterol oral tablets, which work relatively well for this purpose when used correctly (For a more comprehensive discussion of the benefits, activities and side effects of beta-2 agonist drugs please refer to the clenbuterol drug profile).

Effective doses of albuterol usually start in the range of one to two 4mg tablets per day (1 tablet X 1-2 applications). This is often increased a little as the user becomes accustomed to the drug, perhaps to 4mg 3-4 times per day. Individuals very sensitive to the stimulant side effects of beta agonists might wish to start with the lower-dose 2mg tablets first, as albuterol is indeed a potent medication. Whatever the starting dosage, the administration intervals are always spread out as evenly as possible, so as to prevent overlap and sustain active concentrations in the blood for as much of the day as possible. We are looking to find a slight elevation in body temperature (a degree, give or take a little) with use of the drug, which is a good indicator that lipolysis (the removal of stored fatty acids in adipose tissue) is being effectively stimulated.

As is noted with all beta agonists, tolerance to the thermogenic benefits of this drug will tend to develop quickly. This is usually noted by a drop in body temperature, returning back to normal pretreated levels. Due to the potential side effects of these drugs, it is not advised to continually increase the dosage taken in order to chase down a diminishing effect. Instead, the user will usually opt to discontinue the drug for some time (4 weeks or so) to let the body restore its normal receptor concentrations. More recently, the antihistamine Zaditen (ketotifen) has become popular, which is a potent upregulator of beta-adrenergic receptors, especially beta-2 receptors. Taking Zaditen alongside albuterol should greatly enhance the thermogenic potency of this beta agonist, preventing receptor downregulation from cutting your cycle short.

As a beta agonist, albuterol possesses strong stimulant properties. This can lead to a number of unwelcome side effects including, but not limited to, restlessness (inner unrest), shaky hands, tremors, sweating, nausea, increased heart rate, heart palpitations and increased blood pressure. To minimize the occurrence of such side effects, the user is typically instructed to start with a very low dose at first, and slowly work up to a more effective range. You are looking to find a range where thermogenesis is effectively stimulated, but side effects are not so uncomfortable as to interfere with your rest and daily activities. Of course the strong incidence of any unwelcome side effects would warrant discontinuing the drug immediately.

Albuterol is not an expensive drug by any means. In the U.S. sixty 4mg tablets will run you only about $11. In Canada, 100 generic 4mg tablets (salbutamol) will run you only about $38. With a price of roughly 20-40 cents per tablet, this drug is definitely much less expensive than clenbuterol on average. But then again, in the real world it doesn't seem to offer quite the same level of potency. Given that clenbuterol is not really that much more costly in most cases (it usually runs $1 per tablet or less), is more abundantly found, and seems to be the most effective thermogenic agent in the beta-agonist class, this would be preferred over albuterol if both were available.

Clenbuterol

Clenbuterol is a widely used bronchodilator in many parts of the world. The drug is most often prepared in 20mcg tablets, but it is also available in syrup and injectable form. Clenbuterol belongs to a broad group of drugs knows as sympathomimetics. These drugs affect that sympathetic nervous system in a wide number of ways, largely mediated by the distribution of adrenoceptors. There are actually nine different types of these receptors in the body, which are classified as either alpha or beta and further subcategorized by type number. Depending on the specific affinities of these agents for the various receptors, they can potentially be used in the treatment of conditions such as asthma, hypertension, cardiovascular shock, arrhythmias, migraine headaches and anaphylactic shock. The text Goodman and Gillman's The Pharmacological Basis of Therapeutics 9th Edition does a good job of describing the diverse nature in which these drugs affect the body:

"Most of the actions of catecholamines and sympathomimetic agents can be classified into seven broad types: (1) peripheral excitatory action on certain types of smooth muscles such as those in blood vessels supplying the skin, kidney, and mucous membranes, and on the gland cells, such as those of the salivary and sweat glands; (2) a peripheral inhibitory action on certain other types of smooth muscle, such as those in the wall of the gut, in the bronchial tree, and in blood vessels supplying skeletal muscle; (3) a cardiac excitatory action, responsible for in increase in heart rate and force of contraction; (4) metabolic actions, such as an increase in the rate of glycogenolysis in liver and muscle and liberation of free fatty acids from adipose tissue; (5) endocrine actions, such as modulation of the secretion of insulin, rennin, and pituitary hormones; (6) CNS actions, such as respiratory stimulation and, with some of the drugs, an increase in wakefulness and psychomotor activity and a reduction in appetite; and (7) presynaptic actions that result in either inhibition or facilitation of the release of the neurotransmitters such as such as norepinephrine and acetylcholine."

The drug clenbuterol is specifically a selective beta-2 sympathomimetic, primarily affecting only one of the three subsets of beta-receptors. Of particular interest is the fact that this drug has little beta-1 stimulating activity. Since beta-1 receptors are closely tied to the cardiac effects of these agents, this allows clenbuterol to reduce reversible airway obstruction (and effect of beta-2 stimulation) with much less cardiovascular side effects compared to non-selective beta agonists. Clinical studies with this drug show it is extremely effective as a bronchodilator, with a low level of user complaints and high patient compliance[145]. Clenbuterol also exhibits an extremely long half-life in the body, which is measured to be approximately 34 hours long[146]. This makes steady blood levels easy to achieve, requiring only a single or twice daily dosing schedule at most[147]. This of course makes it much easier for the patient to use, and may tie in to its high compliance rate. To spite that clenbuterol is available in a wide number of other countries however; this compound has never been approved for use in the United States. The fact that there are a number of similar, effective asthma medications already available in this country may have something to do with this, as a prospective drug firm would likely not find it a profitable enough product to warrant undergoing the expense of the FDA approval process. Regardless, foreign clenbuterol preparations are widely available on the U.S. black market.

In animal studies clenbuterol is shown to exhibit anabolic activity[148 149 150], obviously an attractive trait to the athlete. This compound is additionally a known thermogenic[151], with beta-2 agonists like clenbuterol shown to directly stimulate fat cells and accelerate the breakdown of triglycerides to form free fatty acids. Its efficacy in this area makes clenbuterol a very attractive, and today almost mandatory, pre-contest drug. Those interested in this drug are most often hoping it will impart a little of both benefits, promoting the loss of body fat while imparting strength and muscle mass increases. But as was well pointed out by a review published in the August 1995 issue of Medicine and Science in Sports and Exercise, the possible anabolic activities in humans are very questionable, and based only on animal data using much larger doses than would be required for bronchodilation[152]. With such reports there has been a lot of debate lately as to whether or not clenbuterol is really anabolic at all. Some seem to swear by the fact that it builds muscle regardless, firmly sticking by "clen" as a great off-season or adjunct anabolic. To others such reports are confirmation that athletes have wasted valuable time and money on drugs that do not work as they are intended to by the user.

This debate continues today, with many still using clenbuterol as a potential anabolic. With this in mind athletes will tailor their dosage and cycling of this product individually depending on which of the two "possible" results are more desired, and how much side effects are to be tolerated. The possible side effects of clenbuterol include those of other CNS stimulants, and include such occurrences as shaky hands, insomnia, sweating, increased blood pressure and nausea. These side effects will generally subside after a week or so of use however, once the user becomes accustomed to the drug. One would typically start a cycle by gradually increasing the dosage each day until a desired range is established. This process will minimize the unwanted side effects seen from the drug;

which otherwise might be dramatic if a large dose is administered from the onset. Men generally end up in the range of 2-8 tablets per day, although some people do claim to tolerate even higher dosages. Women get by on less, generally 2-4 tablets daily. Very quickly, the drug will elevate the body temperature. The rise is not usually dramatic, perhaps a half of a degree or so, sometimes a little more. This elevation is due to your body burning excess energy (largely from fat) and is usually not uncomfortable.

Now that it is working, the number of consecutive days clenbuterol can be used is believed to be dependent on the goal of the individual. To be clear, the athletic benefits of this drug will only last for a limited time and then diminish, largely due to beta-receptor downregulation. When using it for fat loss, the primary effect of the drug, it seems to work well for approximately 4-6 weeks. During this period, users will want to constantly monitor their body temperature. We are assured clenbuterol is working by the temperature elevation. Once the temperature drops back to normal, clenbuterol is no longer exhibiting a thermogenic effect. At this point increasing the dosage would not be very effective, and a break for at least a few weeks should be taken before it is used again effectively. If one is looking for strength gains, clenbuterol appears to be effective for a much shorter period of time, around 3-4 weeks. This may be due to an absence of real anabolic effect, with the strength gain seen with clenbuterol possibly due only to the stimulant properties of the drug (similar to the strength boost seen by ephedrine users). Again however, this is still debated.

Many competitors also find the fat burning effect of clenbuterol can be further enhanced by additional substances. When combined with thyroid hormones, specifically the powerful Cytomel®, the thermogenic effect can become extremely dramatic. This can be to a point that the athlete could shred exceptional amounts of extra fat during contest preparations, without a dramatic restriction in calories. Such a mix can be further used during a steroid cycle, eliciting a much harder look from the anabolics. These cutting agents can often greatly inhibit extra fat storage during the cycle, even when using strong aromatizing androgens. A clenbuterol/thyroid mix is also common when using growth hormone, further enhancing the thermogenic and anabolic effect of this therapy. Ketotifen has also been an extremely popular adjunct to clenbuterol therapy as of late, which is an antihistamine that exhibits the peculiar and extremely welcome side effect of upregulating beta-2 receptor density. It seems capable of not only increasing the potency of each dose of clenbuterol, but also preventing the rapid drop in thermogenic effectiveness that is attributed to receptor downregulation (see the Ketotifen profile for a more comprehensive discussion).

On the black market real clenbuterol is readily available. A street price for 100 tablets of can run as high as $100-150 however, due to the large demand seen recently. A number of European mail order firms will commonly sell clenbuterol to Americans for approx. $.75 or so per tablet though, which is a much more reasonable figure. Clenbuterol has been counterfeited over the past few years, but not to the same extent that most anabolics have. Legitimate versions of clenbuterol are cheap and supplies abundant so the black market has not really needed to manufacture a large volume of fake product. If you know what not to purchase you will likely be able to protect yourself without much difficulty.

Clenbuterol is not produced in the **U.S.**, so avoid anything bearing a U.S. company name.

Clenbuterol should only be trusted when found with a proper brand name from a foreign drug maker. **Spiropent**, **Novegam** and **Oxyflux** from Mexico are the most common products here in the U.S., and all are safe buys.

From Europe, one should look for the popular brand names of **Spiropent**, **Broncoterol**, **Clenasma**, **Monores**, **Contraspasmin** and **Ventolase**.

Bulgarian Clenbuterol is also found commonly, but so are fakes. Look to be sure your box does not have too much English writing on it.

Ephedrine (ephedrine hydrochloride)

Ephedrine is a stimulant drug, belonging to a group of medicines known as sympathomimetics. Specifically it is both an alpha and beta adrenergic agonist (you may remember clenbuterol is a selective beta-2 agonist). In addition, ephedrine enhances the release of norepinephrine, a strong endogenous alpha agonist. The action of this compound is notably similar to that of the body's primary adrenergic hormone epinephrine (adrenaline), which also exhibits action toward both alpha and beta receptors. When administered, ephedrine will notably increase the activity of the central nervous system, as well as have a stimulatory effect on other target cells. This will produce a number of effects beneficial to the athlete. For starters, the user's body temperature should rise slightly as more free fatty acids are produced from the breakdown of triglycerides in adipose tissue (stimulating the metabolism). This should help the user shed subcutaneous body fat stores, enhancing the look of definition in the physique. The anabolic effectiveness of steroids may also be increased with this substance (mildly), as the metabolic rate is a measure of fat, protein and carbohydrate conversion by the body. An enhanced metabolic state could clearly hasten the deposit of new muscle mass.

This stimulant effect of this drug will also increase the force of skeletal muscle contractions. For this reason ephedrine is commonly used by powerlifters before a competition, as the resultant (slight) strength and energy increase can clearly improve the weight totals on major lifts. It may also provide a notable mental edge, as the user is more energetic and better able to concentrate on the tasks ahead. Many recreational weight lifters find this effect particularly welcome, and use 25-50mg of this stimulant as a regular adjunct to their training sessions. The user often feels capable of attacking the weights with much more intensity while taking ephedrine, and leaves the gym knowing they will have had a more productive workout. It is important that this compound not be used continuously for this purpose, as its effect will diminish as the body becomes accustomed to the drug. In most instances the user will take the drug only two or three times per week, usually on those days personally "important" (like chest day). The athlete is also wise to take a break (one to two months) from ephedrine treatment after several weeks have past, so as to continue receiving the optimal effect from this drug.

While the strength boosting effect of this drug is noteworthy, the primary application for ephedrine remains to be as a cutting agent. The athlete will generally take this drug a few times daily during dieting phases of training, at a dosage of 25 to 50mg per application. The widely touted stack of ephedrine (25-50mg), caffeine (200mg) and aspirin (300mg) is shown to be extremely potent for fat loss. In this combination, the ephedrine and caffeine both act as notable thermogenic stimulants. The added aspirin also helps to inhibit lipogenesis by blocking the incorporation of acetate into fatty acids. The athlete will be sure this stack is working by noticing an increase in body temperature, usually a degree or so (not an uncomfortable raise). This combination is taken two to three times daily, for a number of consecutive weeks. It is discontinued once the user's body temperature drops back to normal, a clear sign these drugs are no longer working as desired. At this point increasing the dosages would not prove very efficient. Instead a break of several weeks should be taken, so that this stack may once again work at an optimal level.

Ephedrine can produce a number of unwelcome side effects that the user should be aware of. For starters, the stimulant effect can produce shaky hands, tremors, sweating, rapid heartbeat, dizziness and feelings of inner unrest. Often these effects subside as the user becomes more accustomed to the effect of this drug, or perhaps the dosage is lowered. In general, those negatively impacted by caffeine would probably not like the stronger effects of ephedrine. The mental and physical state produced by this drug is also quite similar to that seen with clenbuterol, so those who find little discomfort with this treatment should (presumably) be fine with this item (and vice versa). While taking this drug one may also endure a notable loss of appetite, usually a welcome effect when dieting. Ephedrine is in fact a popular ingredient in combination (prescription) appetite suppressants. The user may further notice headaches and an increase in blood pressure with regular use of ephedrine. Those suffering from thyroid dysfunctions, high blood pressure or cardiac irregularities should also not be taking this drug, as it will certainly not mix well with such conditions.

As of late there is much discussion about the future availability of ephedrine. This is due to that fact that ephedrine tablets are used as the primary base for the manufacture of methamphetamine. This is you know is an illegal drug, made and sold illicitly. The structure of these two compounds is notably similar, as only a few chemicals are needed to change ephedrine into "meth". Since ephedrine is currently an over-the-counter product, underground manufacturers can easily obtain it. A trend involving large volume retail purchases for OTC ephedrine products has been developing, and many states are taking notice of it. With the widespread increase of amphetamine addiction (and related crime) ephedrine may soon join the list of federally controlled substances. While some states have already taken action to restrict the sale of this stimulant, federal action would probably be required in order have a major impact on availability. Even if a particular state is aggressively preventing the sale of these products, a thriving mail-order market still exists to fill the demand. Thumbing through the back pages of many national magazines should make this clear, as we notice advertisements for companies which ship ephedrine tablets out by the thousand.

HELIOS (clenbuterol/yohimbine hcl blend)

HELIOS is a new drug product that was developed for the spot reduction of stubborn areas of adipose (fat) tissue. The name HELIOS stands for Hyper Thermal Lipolytic System, and there is no question it is made solely for the bodybuilding drug market. It is produced by Generic Supplements, which is a popular underground steroid (and related drug) manufacturing operation located somewhere in Europe. Generic Supplements produces a full line of injectable and oral medications, ranging from standard bodybuilding drugs like testosterone suspension, methandrostenolone, oxymetholone and stanozolol, to clenbuterol, even obscure designer products Helios. To spite the relatively cheap appearance of the packaging, products from Generic Supplements are held in high regard among athletes at this time.

Helios specifically contains a mixture of clenbuterol hcl and yohimbine hcl, a potent beta agonist and alpha antagonist respectively. These two drugs are present in a concentration of 40mcg/mL (clenbuterol) and 5.4mg/mL (yohimbine), a balanced and appropriately dosed mixture for bodybuilding use. Clenbuterol and yohimbine work to promote fat loss through the same system (adrenergic), however they exert their effects through very distinct (but complementary) mechanisms. Clenbuterol, of course, is a potent beta-2 agonist, which directly and strongly stimulates lipolysis very much in the same way ephedrine does (though it is more selective in its actions). Yohimbine hcl is an alpha-2 receptor antagonist, which also promotes fat loss mainly by blocking the activity of other chemicals in the body. For a more comprehensive discussion of the side effects, dosing and actions of both pharmaceuticals, please refer to their respective drug profiles.

Helios spits in the face of anyone who claims that spot reduction is impossible. You see, some theorize that no agent can truly cause a localized reduction in adipose tissue, because all such drugs will ultimately reach circulation instead of remaining concentrated and active in the local region in which it was injection. If you follow this logic, nothing will ever be more than marginally effective at spot reduction until we can keep the drug isolated to one small region of the body. If you have used Helios, however, I doubt you will agree with this line of thinking. Most people are reporting excellent local fat removal with the use of this product; even to the point of swearing that the drug could quickly produce fat loss in areas that were stubborn and exceedingly difficult to get off with the use of conventional (oral) clenbuterol or yohimbine products.

This drug is obviously only found on the black market, so do not expect to find it being sold through the plethora of overseas Internet pharmacies catering to American athletes. You are going to have to find someone that deals strictly to bodybuilders. When located, a single 50ml vial will run you anywhere from $100-200, depending on how far up the chain (or greedy) your particular contact is. Currently fakes of this underground product are not known to exist, so it can be considered a reliable purchase when you do find it. As we have seen time and time again with underground labs that earn a good reputation on the black market (such as International Pharmaceuticals) however, this could quickly change at any time. It is also of note that an earlier version of Helios was being sold not that long ago, which was made as a two-part system (two bottles) that included T3 in addition to the clenbuterol and yohimbine. It was being made by QFS, an underground manufacturer operating out of Canada. Only the European version is being produced at this time. Generic Supplements apparently copied the product from QFS (minus the T3), however the idea of using clen and yohimbine injections for spot reduction ultimately came from Dan Duchaine[153].

Meridia (sibutramine HCL)

Meridia (sibutramine HCL) is a selective serotonin and noradrenaline re-uptake inhibitor, used for the medical management of obesity. This pharmaceutical was developed by Abbott Laboratories, who also sells it in many international markets under the brand name Reductil. Meridia is one of the more recent weight loss medications to reach the commercial drug market in the U.S., receiving Food and Drug Administration approval in 1998. This pharmaceutical is intended to be an adjunct to a reduced calorie diet, which will help increase weight loss compared to that achieved with modifying food intake alone. Meridia is not advertised as a rapid acting drug, but instead one that fosters slow, safe, and steady losses in fat mass, which are maintained long-term.

Sibutramine HCL exerts a weight-loss effect through two distinct mechanisms. On the one side, it has a marked ability to suppress appetite. During some studies, patients would reduce their daily energy intake by as much as 1300 calories while taking this drug.[154] In addition to its effects on caloric intake, sibutramine also stimulates metabolism and daily caloric expenditure. A single 10mg dose has been demonstrated to increase basal metabolic rate by up to 30%, an effect that is maintained for at least six hours. This thermogenic action is known to occur via the adrenergic system, mainly through the indirect support of beta 3 receptor activation. With the use of this drug, we are specifically seeing a strong increase in brown adipose tissue thermogenesis (BAT), which is accompanied by body temperature increases of .5 – 1 degree Celsius[155]. Elevated body temperature is a good indicator that thermogenesis is being triggered, which you may recall as one of the key things we are looking for when taking clenbuterol.

To get a better idea of exactly how well Meridia works, we can take a look at some of the recent clinical studies on this agent. One such investigation was conducted at the Kansas Foundation for Clinical Pharmacology in 2001. Here, a group of 322 obese patients were given either 20mg of sibutramine or placebo once daily for 24 weeks. By the conclusion of this study, 42% of patients in the sibutramine group lost 5% or more of their initial body weight, while 12% noticed a 10% or greater loss in body weight. Sibutramine was also associated with significant improvements in serum triglyceride and HDL cholesterol levels, which were displaying poor values at the onset of the study. Another detailed report emerged from the Department of Endocrinology for Rui-jin Hospital in China this same year, which involved giving only 10mg per day of sibutramine to a group of 120 men and women[156]. This investigation also faired extremely well, with patients losing an average of 15 pounds by the 24th week of use.

In what seems to be a rule for all prescription weight loss medications, sibutramine is not without its potential side effects. The most common is an increase in blood pressure, a trait that is strong and consistent enough to contraindicate the use of this drug in patents with high blood pressure or other cardiovascular issues. Other common side effects include dry mouth, sleeplessness, irritability, back pain, stomach upset, and constipation, all of which tend to become reduced in magnitude as the user becomes accustomed to the drug. Meridia should be discontinued immediately if any of the more serious side effects or symptoms of toxicity occur, including excitement, restlessness, loss of consciousness, confusion, agitation, weakness, shivering, clumsiness, rapid heartbeat, large pupils, vomiting, difficulty breathing, chest pains, swelling of feet, ankles or legs, fainting, disorientation, depression, high fever, eye pain, tremor, or excessive sweating.

Meridia comes in three strengths, 5, 10 and 15mg per capsule. The recommended starting dosage for most patients is 10mg once daily, which is to be adjusted upwards after 4 weeks if weight loss has not been sufficiently initiated. Once established, we commonly see the effective running dosage fall between 10 and 20mg per day. Meridia is classified as a schedule IV controlled substance in the United States, which imparts some legal consequences for distribution or possession. However, that is not to say the drug is extremely difficult to obtain. Being that obesity is a ubiquitous problem in the United States, the numbers of prescriptions written for this drug every year are quite high. Searching around for a short period of time will probably uncover a number of clinics that specialize in this type of therapy quite easily, some of which will likely dispense the drug through the mail. The drug is not currently extremely popular with athletes, although it does show up in related circles from time to time. Warranted or not, most tend to look at this as more of an appetite suppressant than a serious thermogenic, and will usually opt for any number of more potent drugs first.

Yohimbine hydrochloride

Yohimbine hcl is a sympatholytic agent, which means that its main function is to oppose stimulation of the sympathetic nervous system. In this case, it is a specific antagonist (blocker) of alpha-2 adrenergic receptors[157]. Yohimbine hcl is a prescription drug in many countries, and is used, among other things, to increase low blood pressure, to dilate the pupil of the eye, treat male impotence and stimulate fat loss. Common brand names include Aphrodyne, Viritab, Yocon and Yohimex. Due to the fact that yohimbine occurs naturally, it is in somewhat of a gray area in the U.S., where it is being tolerated as on OTC supplement ingredient at this time. It is likewise readily available here, and is a very common ingredient in the enormously crowded market for fat loss products.

To understand how yohimbine works, you need to first understand that adrenergic lipolysis (fat loss stimulated by adrenergic or sympathomimetic hormones) in human adipose tissue is regulated in a dual nature by adrenoceptors (the receptors that respond to these hormones). Most notably, activation of the beta-1, beta-2 or beta-3 subtype increases the process of lipolysis; while activation of alpha-2 receptors diminishes it. Fat cells appear to be the only type of cells in the human body that exhibit such dual regulation by adrenoceptors[158]. By antagonizing alpha 2 receptors, yohimbine can shift the balance of sympathetic activity to a place that measurably stimulates lipolysis[159]. This is further enhanced by an intrinsic ability to increase synaptic norephinephrine release[160], one of the body's own natural lipolytic hormones. In effect, it serves both beta stimulating and alpha blocking properties, an ideal combination if we want to stimulate fat loss.

The typical dose used for fat loss is around 15-20mg, which is taken the first thing in the morning on an empty stomach. Some may opt to take a second dose later in the day, but this is an individual decision based on desired effect and tolerance to the drug's effects. Levels do build in the body over time, so it often takes a few weeks before you really notice any effect. When used at the recommended doses yohimbine is usually well tolerated. This is supported by not only anecdotal data but medical studies, which have shown single doses as high as 21.6mg, or daily cumulative doses as high as 43.2 mg, to have no significant impact on blood pressure or heart rate. This is, of course, the exact opposite of what would be expected of a beta-agonist like ephedrine, which is a potent stimulant. Side effects are still always possible with this drug however, and can include increased heart rate, sweating, nervousness, tremor, irritability, headache, dizziness and flushing. But these effects do tend to be very dose-related, so it is important not to overuse this drug in an attempt to produce a more dramatic fat-loss effect. One of the great advantages to yohimbine is that it can be a relatively comfortable compound to use. If taken in too high a dosage, you will see that change very quickly.

Overall I have to say that, at least as an oral product, the effects of yohimbine are not extremely dramatic. Most users notice "something", but rarely rave about a dramatic and rapid shedding of fat. It is of note that yohimbine seems to work most effectively in the fasted state, and its lipolytic action may be blocked if it is taken with a meal[161]. This may account for some of the negative reports at least. Still, you are likely to notice much greater fat loss with clenbuterol or an E/C (ephedrine, caffeine) stack than you will this agent. But then again, you would have to endure the strong stimulant properties of these drugs as well. It is also important to point out that several topical yohimbine hcl products have been introduced to the market recently, and many consumers are reporting greater success with these formulations. Some are claiming a strong "spot loss" effect, even to the point of being successfully used to locally treat lipomastia (fat buildup under the nipple that resembles/precedes hard-tissue gynecomastia). Although this is a controversial idea, and it is premature to make sweeping judgments, I can say for certain that topical yohimbine hcl products like "Yohimburn" are gathering a small cult following of users. This is probably for good reason, as products like this are not being heavily marketed right now.

Zaditen (ketotifen)

Ketotifen is an antihistamine, which is, oddly enough, used for the treatment of asthma in addition to allergy symptoms (the main focus of antihistamine use). It is sold in a number of countries around the world, including Canada where it is available in both its brand name and generic forms. The drug is approved for sale in the U.S., but currently only as an ophthalmic anti-allergy solution (Zaditor), and not as an oral allergy/asthma medication. When used for asthma it is not effective in treating an immediate attack (it is not an immediate bronchodilator), but does seem to reduce the frequency and severity of problems overall when taken on a daily basis, as well as increase the efficacy of other asthma medications. This drug seems to have proven itself in the marketplace as a very safe, and effective, treatment option for persistent asthma or allergy symptoms.

Ketotifen works to alleviate allergy symptoms by blocking histamine H1 receptors. But it is through its second, extremely unique, mode of action that this agent helps with asthma: ketotifen is a potent upregulator of beta-adrenergic receptors, especially beta-2 receptors. This also makes it an extremely valuable compound when it comes to fat loss, at least in the bodybuilding world. Perhaps maybe not this drug directly, but when taken with a beta-2 agonist thermogenic like clenbuterol, the benefits are both obvious and dramatic. You see, clenbuterol has a limited scope of usefulness because beta-2-adrenergic receptors downregulate very quickly. Soon after you start using the drug, its benefits begin to diminish. Within several weeks, the drug is usually discontinued because it is no longer working very effectively as a fat loss agent. Zaditen changes all that. A dosage of 2-3mg per day (two to three 1mg tablets) seems more than sufficient to prevent the normal receptor downregulation with clenbuterol, allowing you to run long cycles instead of brief intermittent ones. Some are finding the combination of clen and ketotifen to be effective for 12-week cycles or longer, something nobody would have dreamed possible before Zaditen.

The ability of ketotifen to potentiate the effects of beta-adrenergic agents is not just theory. This fact has been demonstrated in a number of placebo-controlled human medical studies. For example, one study published back in 1990 demonstrated that when ketotifen and clenbuterol were taken together, there was a clear increase in beta-adrenergic receptor density compared to the use of clenbuterol alone[162]. Other studies with salbuterol show that the downregulation that had been caused by long-term use of this beta-adrenergic agent, was rapidly reversed with as little as 2mg of ketotifen per day[163]. All this just solidifies what almost everyone who uses the drug will tell you: it works, and it works well. There is little questioning how much of a breakthrough this agent is in the world of bodybuilding drugs. I suspect before long, you will not be able to mention the word clenbuterol without following up with Zaditen shortly after.

This drug does tend to produce some side effects that you should be aware of. This may include dry mouth, appetite stimulation, weight gain, or the drowsiness often associated with strong antihistamine compounds. But then again, this compound does seem to have a very good record when it comes to patient compliance and comfort, with users rarely reporting much trouble. Provided the drowsiness doesn't get to you (this side effect seems to be most noticeable with higher doses like 6-10mg per day), this drug can make a night and day difference on your next fat loss cycle, at least if you are planning to include a beta-agonist such as clenbuterol or ephedrine.

FAT LOSS AGENTS - THYROID

DRUG PROFILES

Cytomel (liothyronine sodium)

Cytomel® is the popularly recognized brand name for the drug liothyronine sodium. This is not an anabolic steroid but a thyroid hormone. It is used medically to treat cases of thyroid insufficiency, obesity, certain metabolic disorders and fatigue. Specifically this drug is a pharmaceutical preparation of the natural thyroid hormone triiodothyronine (T-3). When administered, Cytomel® increases the patient's metabolism. The result is an increased rate of cellular activity (noted by a more rapid utilization of carbohydrates, fats and proteins). Bodybuilders are particularly attracted to this drug for its ability to burn off body excess fat. Most often utilized during contest preparation, one can greatly decrease the amount of stored fat without being forced to severely restrict calories. To this end Cytomel® is commonly used in conjunction with clenbuterol and can produce extremely dramatic results. This combination has become very popular in recent years, no doubt responsible for many "ripped" on-stage physiques. It is also noted by many that when thyroid hormones are taken in conjunction with steroids, an increased anabolic effect can be seen (noticeably greater than if the steroids are used alone). This is likely due to faster utilization of proteins by the body, increasing the rate for new muscle accumulation.

One should take caution if considering using this drug. Cytomel® comes with an extensive list of warnings and precautions which are not to be ignored. Side effects include, but are not limited to, heart palpitations, agitation, shortness of breath, irregular heartbeat, sweating, nausea, headaches, and psychic/metabolic disorders. It is a powerful hormone, and one that could potentially alter the normal functioning of the body if misused. When administering Cytomel®, one must remember to increase the dosage slowly. Generally one 25mcg tablet is taken on the first day, and the dosage is thereafter increased by one tablet every three of four days for a maximum dosage of 100mcg. This will help the body adjust to the increased thyroid hormone, hopefully avoiding any sudden "shock" to the system. The daily dose is also to be split evenly throughout the day, in an effort to keep blood levels steadier. Women are more sensitive to the side effects of Cytomel® than men, and usually opt to take no more than 50mcg daily.

It is important to stress that a cycle should last no longer than 6 weeks and it should never be halted abruptly. As slowly as the dosage was built up it should also be lowered, one tablet every 3-4 days. Taking Cytomel® for too long and/or at too high a dosage can result in a permanent thyroid deficiency. After doing such, one might need to be treated with a drug like Cytomel® for life. It is also a good idea to first consult your physician and have your thyroid function tested. An undiagnosed hyperfunction would not mix well with the added hormone. An athlete should also be sure never to purchase an injectable form of the drug. It is generally an emergency room product, much too powerful for athletic use. Since T-3 is the most powerful thyroid hormone athletes are using, this is generally not the starting point for a beginner. Before using such a powerful item, it is a good idea to become familiar with a weaker substance. The highly popular Triacana is very mild, allowing the user much more latitude (from severe side effects) than Cytomel®. An in-between point is Synthroid (synthetic T-4), still weaker in action than Cytomel®. Once the user is ready however, the fat burning effect of this hormone can be extremely dramatic.

On the black market, Cytomel® is readily available. 100 tablets (50 mcg) will sell for approximately $50. This price is considerably reduced when purchasing this drug from a variety of mail-order sources. Even lower in price is the Cynomel brand in Mexico. The pharmacy price for 100 25mcg tablets is only a few U.S. dollars.

Synthroid (levothyroxine sodium)

Synthroid is a popularly referenced brand name (U.S.) for the drug levothyroxine sodium. Specifically this is a synthetically manufactured thyroid hormone, with the effect of the endogenous hormone thyroxine (T-4). Thyroid hormones are primarily responsible for regulating the body's metabolic rate, and play an important role in determining one's physical disposition. When thyroid preparations are administered, the metabolism is markedly stimulated. This is noted by the faster conversion of carbohydrates, proteins and fats, as the body utilizes more calories throughout the day. These hormones are used medically to treat cases of both thyroid dysfunction and obesity (due to a related deficiency).

The action of this drug is very similar to that of the popular thyroid preparation Cytomel®. Cytomel® is slightly different is structure however, being a synthetic triiodothyronine (T-3) hormone. A healthy individual with actually have sufficient levels of both T-3 and T-4 thyroid hormones present in the body. In comparison, T-3 has an effect roughly four times stronger than that of T-4 on a weight basis (most of T-4's action actually comes from converting to T-3). This is clear when we look at the average tablet strength of both items, Cytomel® produced in much smaller microgram amounts. Likewise the preparation Cytomel® is a much stronger product than Synthroid, and is usually the preference should both items be available. Since Synthroid is much weaker, an athlete will generally expect to take the drug for a longer duration than Cytomel® in order to achieve a similar result.

Thyroid hormones are among the most efficient cutting agents in the athlete's drug arsenal. Administration should noticeably increase the rate in which the body breaks down fat stores, allowing more muscle definition to become visible. And since the body is utilizing more calories during treatment, the need for drastic dieting is greatly reduced. This is an added benefit during contest time, as muscle mass is often sacrificed when nutrients are severely deprived. Thyroid use will generally allow the athlete to burn off body fat while still consuming a comfortable level of calories each day. Anabolic steroids are generally used in conjunction with these hormones, as the metabolism boosting effect may result in faster muscle gains (increased protein utilization). This leads some to use thyroids during off-season bulk cycles, looking to obtain a greater muscle mass gain while accumulating less body fat than typically expected.

The dosage of this drug, as with all thyroid medications, must be built up slowly and evenly. An athlete will generally start with a low dosage of 25-100mcg (1/4-1 100mcg tablet) and slowly increase the amount 25-50mcg each day or two. The final dosage should not exceed 200-400mcg (2-4 100mcg tablets). With thyroid medications you run the risk of permanently altering your metabolic functioning when administering too high a dose or continuing treating for too long a period. Cautious individuals will be sure not to use excessive amounts nor continue treatment for longer than 6 or 8 weeks. On the same note it is important to reduce your Synthroid dosage gradually at the end of your cycle, just as the dosage was built up in the beginning. Dropping the dosage by 25-50mcg every second or third day should be an acceptably gradual withdrawal. This will give your body a chance to become more adjusted to the changing hormone level and avoid the "shock" that is possible when the drug is suddenly discontinued.

There are a number of side effects associated with Synthroid that a potential user should be aware of. These include, but are not limited to, trembling, excessive sweating, diarrhea, insomnia, nausea, elevated heart rate, inner unrest and weight loss. Mild occurrences of such side effects are usually eliminated by temporarily lowering the daily dosage. If the side effects are becoming uncomfortably pronounced, the drug of course should be discontinued. Again, abruptly stopping the drug may produce more unwelcome side effects; so tapering at this point is still recommended if possible. In an effort to avoid any severe problems, many athletes opt to first visit a doctor and have thyroid functions screened before committing to use. A previously unnoticed thyroid hyperfunction can prove very troublesome to someone administering this drug.

Although L-thyroxine is a widely manufactured drug, it is not a regular item on the black market. This is likely due to that fact that the stronger Cytomel® or much weaker Triacana are usually preferred. If this item is found in circulation there should be little doubt about its legitimacy.

Triacana (tiratricol)

Triacana is a popular trade name for the thyroid preparation tiratricol. Specifically this compound is a naturally occurring metabolite of the endogenous thyroid hormone triiodothyronine (T-3). The thyroid gland in fact produces two primary hormones, identified as T-3 and T-4 (thyroxine, which converts to T-3 in the body). Together these structures are the main regulators of the body's metabolism. Both of these basic hormones are also being synthetically manufactured, and are sold under the brand names (among others) of Cytomel® (T-3) and Synthroid (T-4). Triacana is a rapidly metabolized form of the T-3 hormone, and its action is comparatively much weaker than both of these preparations. When administered, all of these substances should markedly increase the metabolic rate. This is noted by an increase in the conversion rate of carbohydrates, proteins and fats. This basically means that the body will utilize nutrients at a much faster speed, due to increased cellular activity.

The medical use for thyroid preparations is for the treatment of thyroid dysfunction and obesity. In addition, Triacana is particularly effective with cases of hyperthyroidism (a disorder in which the body overproduces thyroid hormones). The intake of tiratricol can markedly reduce the secretion of TSH (thyroid stimulating hormone), thus regulating hormone production in the body. Bodybuilders however, find the metabolic boosting effects of these substances exceptional for burning off excess body fat. Even without extreme dieting, Triacana (and related) can lower subcutaneous fat stores, bringing about a harder, more defined look as muscle features become more visible. Without the use of thyroid hormones, the athlete will no doubt be forced to diet much more extremely. This is often done at the expense of muscle tissue, as it is difficult to retain the mass while the proper nutrients are being restricted. Competitive bodybuilders therefore find these hormones invaluable, used to drastically improve the quality of a show physique.

When looking to a thyroid product, the user obviously will have to decide which hormone to utilize. Triacana is the most popular choice since it is considered much safer than the others. When manipulating thyroid levels, a gamut of side effects should be taken into consideration. These include, but are not limited to, trembling, excessive sweating, diarrhea, insomnia, nausea, elevated heart rate, inner unrest and weight loss. The most unwanted side effect being the possibility of permanent thyroid dysfunction. While the use of Cytomel® must be carefully planned and specifically carried out, Triacana allows the user much more latitude. For starters, it is much less likely that a mistake in dosage or duration will result in severe and/or permanent side effects with this drug. Serious disturbances in thyroid functioning just do not seem to be an issue with this compound. Triacana is also cleared from the body much more rapidly than other thyroid hormones, a very welcome trait should the user begin to notice discomfort during treatment. It is no doubt the thyroid hormone a beginner should select.

The administration of Triacana is similar to that of the other hormones. The maximum dosage should not be taken from the onset; instead it is to be built up slowly. Being such a mild product, the effective dosage is in the range of ten to fourteen .35mg tablets per day. Two tablets is the customary starting point, a dosage that is to be increased by two tablets every day (or two). Tiratricol has a half-life of approximately six hours, so the daily dosage should be divided evenly through the day to keep blood levels more uniform. Also, athletes usually use thyroid hormones in conjunction with steroids, noting an increased anabolic effect due to faster protein conversion. It can also be combined with other cutting agents like clenbuterol, providing an even more dramatic fat burning effect. Athletes will generally limit the duration Triacana is to be taken, fearful of running into health complications. Although this is not a huge risk, using this compound for no longer than three months, with longer break intervals, is a good way to be sure. Remember that the dosage must be lowered in the same manner it was built up; two tablets less each day or two. Sudden discontinuance of thyroid hormones is likely to bring about many unwanted problems.

On the U.S. black market 100 tablets of Triacana usually costs approximately $75-100 when located. The French version is found almost exclusively, produced by the Medgenix Company. This version is packaged in boxes of 100, packed in four strips of 25 tablets each. It is interesting to note that this item was introduced to the. Sports supplement market briefly a few years ago, making tiratricol available to U.S. bodybuilders over-the-counter at a very reasonable cost. However its status as a legitimate supplement quickly came into question by the FDA. Deeming it an unapproved new drug, and not a natural supplement as claimed by the manufacturer, the product was pulled. The FDA went so far as to show up at the warehouses of a few supplement companies to confiscate their inventories. To the best of my knowledge no charges were ever filed, but they did succeed in quickly making the product unavailable. The total life span of tiratricol as a supplement was only about 8 months, after which the black market once again became the only source for this drug.

FAT LOSS AGENTS - OTHER

DRUG PROFILES

Adipex-P (phentermine hydrochloride)

Phentermine is a very popular prescription weight-loss drug in the United States. You may recognize it as one of the constituents in the controversial and now illegal weight-loss stack Fen-Phen, which stood for fenfluramine and phentermine. Fenfluramine was withdrawn from the market not long ago due to side-effect potential, however phentermine is still being sold. It is specifically a sympathomimetic stimulant of the amphetamine family, and is categorized (as other amphetamine derivatives) as an anorectic agent. This is just a scientific term for describing an appetite suppressant. Phentermine is prescribed for short-term use (usually 3-4 weeks) by obese patients, as an adjunct to support an ongoing exercise and dieting regimen.

The main focus, obviously, is to curb the desire to eat and thereby reduce the total caloric intake. To accomplish this, the typical daily dosage used is a single 37.5mg tablet per day, which is taken in the morning before breakfast (for optimal effectiveness it should not be taken with food). In some cases only a half a tablet per day is required, while in other it is best to take the full 37.5mg dosage each day, but to divide it between two separate applications instead of one. When taken more than once per day, the second dose should never be taken within 4-6 hours of bed. Although the data seems to vary from trial to trial, much of it supports at least a modest additional loss of fat mass with the use of phentermine[164].

As an amphetamine derivative, this medication also has a tendency to be habit forming if overused. For this reason it has been added to the U.S. controlled substances list, specifically as a schedule IV medication. If you are looking at including this in your next diet, make sure to take caution only to use it for a limited duration. There are also a number of potential side effects with a stimulant drug like this, including overstimulation, restlessness, insomnia, dizziness, headache, increased blood pressure, hypertension, heart palpitations, dry mouth, constipation, diarrhea, libido changes and impotence. Obviously the dosage should never be increased for the sake of trying to obtain a euphoric effect from the drug.

Phentermine is commonly sold in strengths of 15mg, 30mg and 37.5mg per tablet/capsule. At a U.S. pharmacy, the higher dosed version will run you about a dollar or so per dose. Name brand Adipex-P will run you another 50 cents or so. If you don't have a regular doctor to prescribe this agent, it would not be advised to try ordering it from overseas. Being a schedule IV controlled substance, having it mailed to you would carry the same legal ramifications as ordering Valium or anabolic steroids. Should you decide you want to take it, your best bet (legally) would be to look for a U.S. doctor that specializes in weight loss medications. I, for one, get about a dozen unsolicited emails each week from clinics offering to prescribe me phentermine, so I don't think it will be too hard for you to find one if you look.

DNP (2,4-Dinitrophenol)

DNP is one of the most controversial drugs in use by bodybuilders today. This agent is not sold for human use anywhere in the world at this time, but is readily available as an industrial chemical. Among other things, it is used as an intermediary for the production of certain dyes, for photographic development, as a fungicide, in wood pressure-treatment to prevent rotting, and as an insecticide. Although quite incongruous with this list of strong industrial/chemical uses, it was also sold a long time ago as a diet drug for humans. In fact, it was the first synthetic drug that was ever used for weight reduction in this country. Popular brand names included Dinitriso, Nitromet, Dinitrenal and Alpha Dinitrophenol, and at the peak of DNP's popularity could be found in pharmacies all across the country.

As the story goes, the fat-loss properties of DNP were first noticed during World War I, when overweight men working with DNP in munitions plants started losing substantial amounts of weight. It did not take very long for this chemical to be packaged as a drug product, and by 1935 more than 100,000 Americans had used "patent medicine" remedies that included DNP. It was being widely advertised as a new, safe and effective way to get thin. But it didn't take long for reports of side effects to start pouring in. One such incident involved a dozen women in California, who were temporarily blinded by the drug. Numerous reports of DNP linked cataracts were coming in from all over, from countries like the U.S., France and Italy. It was said to be happening with doses as little as 100mg daily when taken for longer periods. With such highly unfavorable safety reports, the drug was soon pulled. By 1938, just three years later, it was off the market for good.

Dinitrophenol induces weight loss by uncoupling oxidative phosphorylation, thereby markedly increasing the metabolic rate and body temperature[165]. While this is an extremely effective way of producing rapid weight loss, there seems to be no ceiling to DNP's temperature increasing effect. Herein lies perhaps its most dangerous trait; it may allow body temperature to rise to level that can be damaging, even fatal. Writer Carl Malmberg made perhaps one of the earliest and most famous quotes about this back in the 1930's, when he reported about a physician who was "literally cooked to death" from using it. This was no isolated case either, and the dose used was probably not frighteningly high. A man recently died on Long Island, for example, after taking DNP for only four days. The dose used was reportedly 600mg per day, just three capsules of the now underground "standard" amount of 200mg. No doubt he thought the dose he was using was going to be safe – it wasn't.

The typical dose used by bodybuilders is reportedly 2mg per kg of bodyweight each day. This would mean a dose of 200mg if you weigh in at about 220 pounds. This seems to be the dose most underground sellers of DNP are putting in their capsules. At this level, admittedly, the fat loss can be scary it is so rapid. Some people are capable of losing ½ to one pound of fat weight, each and every day, with its use. This can mean a drop of 15 or 20 pounds in only a few weeks. Not many weight-loss drugs even come close to this. But then there are its many potential side effects, including increased heart rate, breathing rate, nausea, elevated body temperature, insomnia, profuse sweating, rash, decreased white blood cell count and death. The strong incidence of any side effect should immediately indicate a need to stop using the drug, unless of course you are dead, in which case this will work itself out.

I was hesitant to even include a profile on this drug in my book, for fear it might entice someone, who otherwise may not have known about it, to use it. But ultimately I decided it would be better to include it. The true story of DNP is a scary one, and now more than ever needs to be told. Bodybuilders need to understand that the reemergence of underground DNP in the 1990's is not a revolutionary new achievement in fat loss, but a scary reiteration of one of our biggest past mistakes. It is a drug from a time when an unregulated market was allowing dangerous chemicals like this to harm the public. The Food and Drug Administration (FDA) exists today because we need to protect ourselves form things like this. The lessons learned in the 1930's should not be forgotten. DNP is a dangerous drug, and should be avoided. There are much safer ways of losing fat!

Capoten (captopril)

Captopril is an angiotensin-converting enzyme (ACE) inhibitor, used medically for the treatment of high blood pressure. Although the exact underlying mechanisms behind the activity of captopril are not fully understood, it appears to lower blood pressure and have beneficial effects on blood circulation in patients with congestive heart failure mainly by suppressing the renin-angiotensin-aldosterone system. It is a particularly effective medication in fact, and considered both as the first course of therapy or after other less powerful agents have failed to produce a desired response. Athletes are usually not using this drug to lower blood pressure however, at least not as the primarily purpose. In this arena captopril is of interest for its potential anabolic, thermogenic and diuretic qualities. Before going any further it is important to state that it is not recommend for anyone to take captopril unless they are already hypertensive from using anabolic steroids, as a potential dangerous drop in blood pressure may result.

Most athletes using this drug are hoping it will help promote fat loss. This use of captopril was first brought to our attention in and article by the writer Dharkham in Dan Duchaine's Dirty Dieting newsletter[166]. The suggested mechanism of action was a reduction of alpha-2 adrenoceptors, receptors that work against lipolysis in fat cells. If captopril were able to effectively lower alpha-2 levels in fat cells, it would certainly have quite a bit of potential in this regard. And indeed many who have used it do attest to the fact that it is a good cutting drug, often claiming they have a higher calorie threshold for fat loss/gain when taking the substance. Others however vehemently disagree with this use for captopril, and say they found it sorely lacking as a fat-loss agent. I did notice one study of great interest, showing that with 2 weeks of chronic administration it caused no significant changes and alpha-2 or beta-2 adrenoceptors[167]. A second however, using the drug for 16 weeks, did note a reduction in alpha-2 receptors[168]. If it simply takes longer to notice strong receptor downregulation, then captopril would work with prolonged use. However this would also make it a definite delayed gratification drug, and no doubt less than popular with bodybuilders. More immediately however, this drug does lower aldosterone levels and water retention. Even if not highly thermogenic, many will still no doubt find a use for the mild diuretic action of this drug.

Another interesing thing about captopril is that it has been shown to increase insulin sensitivity. Despite being integral to the deposition of body fat, we must remember that insulin is also an extremely potent anabolic agent in the human body. It is a nutrient transport hormone, responsible for the uptake and utilization of proteins, carbohydrates and fats, and is even a strong promoter of protein synthesis in muscle tissues. Athletes have found that by manipulating insulin levels, and even insulin sensitivity, in the right window of time after training, they can produce dramatic anabolic effects. To this end studies with captopril look very promising. One for instance looked at the effect of captopril on insulin sensitivity in obese rats, noting it to increase this in both liver and muscle tissues[169]. Perhaps an even better study to look it is one conducted in Japan in 1994, investigating the underlying mechanisms involved in this action of captopril. Here researchers showed that the drug actually increased the expression of glucose transporter 4 (GLUT4) in skeletal muscle[170], a definite positive effect in terms of glucose transport and metabolism in muscles. One would likely take captopril in conjunction with insulin for maximum effects, however should be cautious with the dosage as the effects of insulin may be notably enhanced in the presence of this drug.

The suggested dosage schedule includes starting with only 25 mg, or 1/2 tablet per day. Due to its tendency to cause fatigue, the dosage is usually taken at night before bed so as to not interfere with the quality of ones day or training. This dosage can be increased over time, but no more than 50 or 100 mg is ever suggested per day. And due to the previously mentioned risk of low blood pressure, one should certainly not mistake this as a recommendation to take one or two tabs per day and not worry about it. Due to the already mentioned risk of low blood pressure, one should take extreme caution when fiddling with this drug. Symptoms of this include dizziness and weakness, which may indicate a need for immediate medical intervention, so take extreme caution. It is especially advisable to take care and follow your blood pressure. Aside from the primary worry of low blood pressure, other potential side effects of this drug are numerous and include the mentioned dizziness, headaches, diarrhea, constipation, loss of appetite, nausea, flushes and fatigue.

Parlodel (bromocriptine mesylate)

Bromocriptine is a dopaminomimetic ergot derivative with D2 dopamine receptor agonist and D1 dopamine receptor antagonist activities. It is used most commonly as a prolactin inhibitor in cases of hyperprolactinemia, a growth hormone suppressant in acromegaly (high doses are required), and as an adjunctive medication to levodopa in the management of Parkinson's disease.

The most vocal proponent of bromocriptine use for fat loss is probably Lyle McDonald, author of the online e-Book "*Bromocriptine: An Old Drug With New Uses".* In this McDonald describes how the drug can be used to normalize the metabolism, such that some of the normal physiological responses to dieting (which begin to slow the loss of body fat as the duration of dieting increases) are hindered. A lot of this focuses on leptin, a hormone looked at as sort of a fat thermostat, telling your brain how much adipose tissue you have on your body and how many calories you are regularly consuming (an "anti-starvation" hormone). Dieting tends to lower leptin levels significantly, which causes your body to respond in an appropriate way for survival (it tries to hold on to its nutrient stores as much as possible). Maintaining normal leptin stimulation could be key to keeping any diet productive, and bromocriptine may indeed allow us to do that.

The human medical data on this drug is very encouraging. In cases where it was given while dieting, bromocriptine was capable of increasing total fat loss by a measurable degree, and seemed to extend the duration in which the diet was most effective. In one case, both placebo and treatment groups were noticing a good level of fat loss during the first 6 weeks of calorie restriction, however only the bromocriptine group continued to lose noticeable amounts of weight for the remaining 12 weeks of intervention. Looking over the dosing regimens of several human studies like this, McDonald is recommending that dieting bodybuilders take between 2.5 and 5mg per day. This is given in a single morning dose, due to the relatively long half-life of the drug.

Bromocriptine can produce a number of unwanted side effects, the most notable being low blood pressure, dizziness, confusion and nausea. These side effects do tend to be dose related, with the low recommended doses used in bodybuilding probably not likely to be much trouble for many. Further, initial nausea sometimes goes away after a couple of applications, once the user becomes accustomed to the drug. Obviously the strong incidence of any unwelcome side effects should warrant discontinuing therapy, especially if your blood pressure is becoming negatively affected (too low a drop). Less common adverse reactions include anxiety, dry mouth, edema, seizures, fatigue, headache, lethargy, nasal congestion, rash or changes in urinary frequency.

Bromocriptine is produced in a number of countries, including the United States where it is sold under the Parlodel brand name. This product comes in the form of both 2.5mg tablets and 5mg capsules, with 100 doses of either strength being packaged per bottle. At the pharmacy, 100 5mg capsules will run close to $400, so this drug is not really that cheap. But then again, that would be 100 days worth of drug, so you are really only talking about four dollars per day. If purchasing this drug from on overseas pharmacy, the cost can be considerably reduced as well, to as little as .50 to $2 per daily dose.

Thiomucase (mucopolysaccharidase)

Thiomucase is a mucopolysaccharidase obtained from the tissues of sheep. A mucopolysaccharidase is an enzyme that breaks down mucopolysaccharide substances such as mucins, which are proteins produced in the mucous membranes. Thiomucase is usually found as a topical formulation, where it is used to facilitate the diffusion of local anesthetics and in the treatment of cellulites (inflammation of subcutaneous or connective tissue). It is also used as a general spreading agent, mixed with other topical drugs to help increase their speed/area of transport. Bodybuilders have additionally found an effective off-label use for Thiomucase, namely as a "spot reduction" agent. It is used in the days leading up to a show to pull water from fat cells and cellulite, and tighten up last minute troubled areas before a stage appearance.

There are some misconceptions surrounding the potential use of this product with injectable steroids. Thiomucase cream is used to aid in the dispersion and transport of topical or subcutaneously administered drug products. It will not have any effect on the release of a steroid deposit sitting deep inside the belly of a muscle. In the world of bodybuilding, this agent is not really used for drug transport. There is, likewise, a lot of science that could be discussed concerning the mechanisms in which Thiomucase works, but it would be of little relevance. In this arena, Thiomucase has only one primary purpose – spot reduction. It is administered in a manner not unlike how some models use preparation-H to remove puffiness from their eyes, or small traces of cellulite on their buttocks, before a photo shoot. To use Thiomucase, one simply rubs it directly into the targeted areas, once or twice daily for a period of 1-2 weeks.

Thiomucase is readily available throughout Europe and South America, where it is typically sold as a non-prescription product. Bodybuilders in the U.S. will routinely order it from international pharmacies, being that there are no legal restrictions on its importation. The going price for a 45g tube is around $10-20, which is probably about as much as shipping is going to cost to get it here. Many American companies have also imported this product over the years, mainly from France, and have sold it on the open market as a cosmetic or "gray area" supplement. However, such sources do not currently seem abundant, leaving international sellers as the primary source for this product in the U.S.

Growth Hormones & Related

Drug Profiles

Catapres (clonidine hydrochloride)

Catapres® is a widely used high blood pressure medication containing the drug clonidine hydrochloride. It is available in a number of different preparations worldwide, designed for injectable, oral or ocular administration. Athletes are interested in Clonidine for two reasons. The first being the prescribed purpose for the drug, namely lowering high blood pressure. Athletes often encounter this side effect when using strong androgens (usually with a high rate of estrogen conversion). High blood pressure can be not only uncomfortable, but also dangerous. The risk for serious cardiac (among others) disorders greatly increases as blood pressure rises. This worry is amplified by the fact that the steroids are likely interfering with cholesterol levels at the same time. In an effort to suppress this side effect, some users will addition an anti-hypertensive drug like Catapres instead of quitting the offending anabolics. In many cases the blood pressure can be lowered and the cycle safely continued. In other instances taking a break from steroids and visiting the doctor for a full exam would much better serve the person.

Catapres provides the athlete another interesting benefit. The technical literature regarding this drug shows that it can stimulate endogenous growth hormone secretion. This effect seems to occur soon after administration and lasts for several hours. It can apparently raise levels enough to elicit an anabolic and thermogenic effect. The general regimen among athletes is to take two doses per day, morning and night. A single 150mcg tablet is administered upon rising in an effort to elevate growth hormone levels throughout the day. An additional dose of 300mcg is administered right before sleep, hopefully resulting in a significantly raised GH level overnight. The higher dose, although more effective, is to be given at night and not when rising. This should minimize some of the more undesirable side effects from happening during the day. Such side effects include fatigue, lethargy, dry mouth, dizziness and sexual disturbances. It is also particularly important not to use this product if you already have low blood pressure. It is generally only used when blood pressure is rising, so as to warrant an action by the athlete and not solely as an anabolic. A healthy individual with a slow, athletic heartbeat and low-normal blood pressure runs the risk of severely compromising their health by lowering their blood pressure to an unsafe level. The consequences can be drastic, if not life threatening.

Although somewhat of an interesting compound, Catapres is not in high demand among athletes. The side effects and safety issues associated with it make it unattractive to most potential buyers. Should one come across this on the black market it can be considered a safe buy, as no counterfeit operation is likely to be interested in duplicating this.

GH-RH (sermorelin acetate)

GH-RH, or Growth Hormone Releasing Hormone, is an extremely new pharmaceutical compound that may be of future interest to the athlete/bodybuilder. GH-RH contains the active substance sermorelin acetate, which is a synthetically manufactured form of the endogenous growth hormone-releasing hormone (GHRH or GRF). The composition of sermorelin is actually just a portion of this polypeptide hormone, containing 29 of the 44 amino acids that make up its structure. It does however display the full activity of the parent, so the lack of entirety should not affect the potency of this drug. GH-RH, specifically the Geref brand name from Serono, was approved for sale in the U.S. in 1997 as a diagnostic tool to evaluate a possible pituitary deficiency. It is being further assessed as a substitute to injectable growth hormone in patients with an existing deficiency.

GH-RH increases the level of Growth Hormone in the blood by stimulating the pituitary gland to manufacture more of this hormone. This makes it a useful diagnostic tool, since a failed response to a Geref injection (no GH elevation) should indicate a problem with the pituitary gland (or related). The standard practice is to sample the blood growth hormone level, then administer a single intravenous injection of Geref. The blood GH level is then recorded every subsequent 15 minutes (4 samples taken during the first hour after the shot), and compared against the first reading. Many are confident this is just the beginning, and believe GH-RH will ultimately prove to be an efficient GH replacement drug. One can liken such a practice to the way HCG (human chorionic gonadotropin) is used to increase the production of testosterone in the body. Just as is the case with testosterone, the body is capable of producing much more GH than it typically does. It is quite possible that regular use can produce a level of elevation consistent with an HGH replacement regimen.

Athletes would of course be attracted to this drug for the same reasons they use HGH. Among other things, an elevated growth hormone level can elicit new muscle growth, increase fat loss, enhance energy levels and strengthen connective tissues. The thermogenic and anabolic properties of growth hormone are readily known among bodybuilders and competitive athletes, many of who rely heavily on this compound. If GH-RH is able to sustain a GH elevation great enough for a beneficial effect (it appears to be), then it may enjoy great popularity on the black market in the years to come. As with HGH, one should remember that the full anabolic effect would be achieved only with the addition of other compounds. Most importantly, the body will have a heightened requirement for thyroid hormones, insulin and androgens. It is typical to add a small dosage of Cytomel® (T-3 thyroid) and a long acting injectable androgen like testosterone enanthate. In addition, many find the periodic use of insulin to be particularly beneficial for enhancing new muscle growth.

Sermorelin acetate does not remain active in the body for very long, so injections of this drug are to be given daily. The athlete will inject the solution intramuscularly or subcutaneously (never IV), in order to extend its release time. The exact dosage that would be needed by a healthy athlete is currently unclear however. Early reports suggest that 1mg of GH-RH would have roughly the equivalent effect of 1mg HGH (approximately 3 IU's). This of course seems like a very promising figure. With this level of efficiency, one would assume that a daily dosage of .5 to 1mg would prove sufficient for performance enhancement. This drug is of course so new that a standard injection protocol has not yet been established with athletes. It may come to be that more or less GH-RH is actually needed in order to receive noteworthy results.

The physical appearance of GH-RH is very similar to Growth Hormone. It comes packaged in two separate ampules, one containing a lyophilized powder (the active constituent) and the other a sterile dilutant. Each ampule pair will typically contain .5mg or 1mg of sermorelin acetate, and will obviously need mixing before use. Just as with HGH, the patient must be very careful not to disturb the contents much during this process. As with HGH, the accompanying paperwork states that if a cloudy or discolored solution is produced, the drug should be discarded. Unlike HGH however, an unused potion of GH-RH cannot be refrigerated for later use. One obviously would not want to be stuck purchasing 1mg vials if they only needed .5mg per day. This would not seem very important if GH-RH was cheap, but this is not the case. Overseas sources are currently showing the price of this drug to be very comparable to HGH; at about $75 per a daily dosage of 1mg. Perhaps we will see a reduction in price as the manufacture and use of this compound become more widespread.

Human Growth Hormone (somatropin)

In the human body growth hormone is produced by the pituitary gland. It exists at especially high levels during adolescence when it promotes the growth of tissues, protein deposition and the breakdown of subcutaneous fat stores. Upon maturation endogenous levels of GH decrease, but remain present in the body at a substantially lower level. In the body the actual structure of growth hormone is a sequence of 191 amino acids. Once scientists isolated this hormone, many became convinced it would exhibit exceptional therapeutic properties. It would be especially effective in cases of pituitary deficient dwarfism, the drug perhaps restoring much linear growth if administered during adolescence.

The 1980's brought about the first prepared drugs containing human growth hormone. The content was taken from a biological origin, the hormone being extracted from the pituitary glands of human corpses then prepared as a medical injection. This production method was short lived however, since it was linked to the spread of a rare and fatal brain disease. Today virtually all forms of HGH are synthetically manufactured. The recombinant DNA process is very intricate; using transformed e-coli bacterial or mouse cell lines to genetically produce the hormone structure. It is highly unlikely you will ever cross the old biologically active item on the black market (such as Grorm), as all such products should now be discontinued.

The use of growth hormone has been increasing in popularity among athletes, due of course to the numerous benefits associated with use. To begin with, GH stimulates growth in most body tissues, primarily due to increases in cell number rather than size. This includes skeletal muscle tissue, and with the exception of eyes and brain all other body organs. The transport of amino acids is also increased, as is the rate of protein synthesis. All of these effect are actually mediated by IGF-1 (insulin-like growth factor), a highly anabolic hormone produced in the liver and other tissues in response to growth hormone (peak levels of IGF-1 are noted approximately 20 hours after HGH administration). Growth hormone itself also stimulated triglyceride hydrolysis in adipose tissue, usually producing notable fat loss during treatment. GH also increases glucose output in the liver, and induces insulin resistance by blocking the activity of this hormone in target cells. A shift is seen where fats become a more primary source of fuel, further enhancing body fat loss.

Its growth promoting effect also seems to strengthen connective tissues, cartilage and tendons. This effect should reduce the susceptibility to injury (due to heavy weight training), and increase lifting ability (strength). HGH is also a safe drug for the "piss-test". Although athletic committees ban its use, there is no reliable detection method. This makes clear its attraction to (among others) professional bodybuilders, strength athletes and Olympic competitors, who are able to use this drug straight through a competition. There is talk however that a reliable test for the exogenous administration of growth hormone has been developed, and is close to being implemented. Until this happens, growth hormone will remain a highly sought after drug for the tested athlete.

But the degree in which HGH actually works for an athlete has been the topic of a long running debate. Some claim it to be the holy grail of anabolics, capable of amazing things. Able to provide incredible muscle growth and unbelievable fat loss in a very short period of time. Since it is used primarily by serious competitors who can afford such an expensive drug, a great body of myth further surrounds HGH discussion (among those personally unfamiliar). Many will state with the utmost confidence that the incredible mass of the Olympian competitors each year is 100% due to the use of HGH. Others have crossed bodybuilding materials claiming it to be a complete waste of money, an ineffective anabolic and barely worthwhile for fat loss. With its high price tag, certainly an incredibly poor buy in the face of steroids. So we have a very wide variety of opinions regarding this drug, whom should we believe?

It is first important to understand why there the results obtained from this drug seem to vary so much. A logical factor in this regard would seem to be the price of this drug. Due to the elaborate manufacturing techniques used to produce it, it is extremely costly. Even a moderately dosed cycle could cost an athlete between $75-$150 per daily dosage. Most are unable or unwilling to spend so much, and instead tinker around with low dosages of the drug. Most who have used this item extensively claim it will only be effective at higher doses. Poor results would then be expected if low amounts were used, or the drug not administered daily. If you cannot commit to the full expense of an HGH cycle, you should really not be trying to use the drug.

The average male athlete will usually need a dosage in the range of 4 to 6 I.U. per day to elicit the best results. On the low end perhaps 1 to 2 I.U. can be used daily, but this is still a considerable expense. Daily dosing is important, as HGH has a very short life span in the body. Peak blood concentrations are noted quickly (2 to 6 hours) after injection, and the hormone is cleared from the body with a half-life of only 20-30 minutes. Clearly it does not stick around very long, making stable blood levels difficult to maintain. The effects of this drug are also most pronounced when it is used for longer periods of time, often many months long. Some do use it for shorter periods, but generally only when looking for fat loss. For this purpose a cycle of at least four weeks would be used. This compound can be administered in both an intramuscular and subcutaneous injection. "Sub-Q" injections are particularly noted for producing a localized loss of fat, requiring the user to change injection points regularly to even out the effect. A general loss of fat seems to be the one characteristic most people agree on. It appears that the fat burning properties of this drug are more quickly apparent, and less dependent on high doses.

Other drugs also need to be used in conjunction with HGH in order to elicit the best results. Your body seems to require an increased amount of thyroid hormones, insulin and androgens while HGH levels are elevated (HGH therapy in fact is shown to lower thyroid and insulin levels). To begin with, the addition of thyroid hormones will greatly increase the thermogenic effectiveness of a cycle. Taking either Cytomel® or Synthroid® (prescription versions of T-3 and T-4) would seem to make the most sense (the more powerful Cytomel® is usually preferred). Insulin as well is very welcome during a cycle, used most commonly in an anabolic routine as described in this book under the insulin heading. Aside from replacing lowered insulin levels, use of this hormone is important as it can increase receptor sensitivity to IGF-1, and reduce levels of IGF binding protein-1 allowing for more free circulating IGF-1[171] (growth hormone itself also lowers IGF binding protein levels[172]). Steroids as well prove very necessary for the full anabolic effect of GH to become evident. Particularly something with a notable androgenic component such as testosterone or trenbolone (if worried about estrogen) should be used. The added androgen is quite useful, as it promotes anabolism by enhancing muscle cell size (remember GH primarily effects cell number). Steroid use may also increase free IGF-1 via a lowering of IGF binding proteins[173]. The combination of all of these (HGH, anabolics, insulin and T-3) proves to be the most synergistic combination, providing clearly amplified results. It is of course important to note that thyroid and insulin are particularly powerful drugs that involve a number of additional risks.

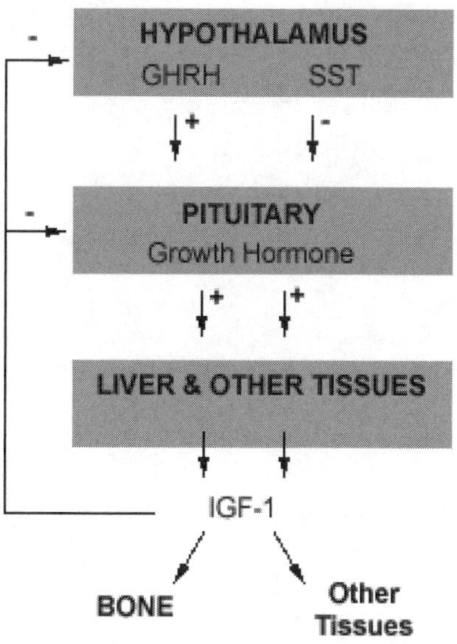

Release and action of GH and IGF-1: GHRH (growth hormone releasing hormone) and SST (somatostatin) are released by the hypothalamus to stimulate or inhibit the output of GH by the pituitary. GH has direct effects on many tissues, as well as indirect effects via the production of IGF-1. IGF-1 also causes negative feedback inhibition at the pituitary and hypothalamus. Heightened release of somatostatin affects not only the release of GH, but insulin and thyroid hormones as well.

HGH itself does carry with it some of its own risks. The most predominantly discussed side effect would be acromegaly, or a noticeable thickening of the bones (notably the feet, forehead, hands, jaw and elbows). The drug can also enlarge vital organs such as the heart and kidney, and has been linked to hypoglycemia and diabetes (presumably due to its ability to induce insulin resistance). Theoretically, overuse of this hormone can bring about a number of conditions, some life threatening. Such problems however are extremely rare. Among the many athletes using growth hormone, we have very few documented cases of a serious problem developing. When used periodically at a moderate dosage, the athlete should have little cause for worry. Of course if there are any noticeable changes in bone structure, skin texture or normal health and well being during use, HGH therapy should be completely halted.

In summary, the biggest mistake we can make with this drug is to get confused by the price tag. Even a relatively short cycle of this drug (and ancillaries) will cost in the thousand(s), not hundreds of dollars. We cannot jump to the conclusion that GH is therefore the most unbelievable anabolic. This hormone is simply very complex, and costly to manufacture (though it should be getting cheaper). If you were looking to achieve just a great mass gain the $1,000 would be better spent on steroids. Growth Hormone will not turn you into an overnight "freaky" monster and it is certainly not "the answer". Yes, it is a very effective performance enhancement tool. But it is more a tool for the competitive athlete looking for more than steroids alone can provide. There is little doubt that GH contributes considerably to the physiques and performance of many top bodybuilders and athletes. In this arena, the money spent on it is well justified, the drug obviously necessary. But outside of competitive sports it is usually not.

The high price of human growth hormone has provided a very strong motivation for the creation of counterfeit product so one must be cautious when purchasing it. A large percentage of the GH found on the black market will in actuality be re-labeled HCG, which bears a very close resemblance. Fear not, a trip to the corner drug store provides us with a cheap and effective way to test our product. A home pregnancy test works by detecting HCG in the urine, which will be present during pregnancy. In this case we want to use it to determine if there is HCG in our growth hormone vials. A few days into your GH cycle, take a full 1ml injection prior to bed. This would ensure a high level of HCG in the urine (if that's what your actually taking). Upon rising, take the pregnancy test. A positive will let you know that you have been swindled.

Both HCG and HGH are packaged in 2 separate vials, which are mixed before use (except for the new Nutropin aqueous product). One vial contains a sterile solution, the other a powder. With both the powder will not be loose but in a solid disc (lyophilized). The few fakes which are not re-labeled HCG vials will likely contain some form of loose powder, avoid.

IGF-1 (Insulin-Like Growth Factor 1)

Insulin-Like Growth Factor-1 is a peptide hormone found naturally in the human body, belonging to the same family of hormones as insulin. As peptide hormones go, IGF-1 is relatively small, containing only 70 amino acids. That, however, bears no relevance to how important this hormone is biologically. IGF-1 is the mediator of all of the anabolic activity of growth hormone, which, in of itself, is not anabolic at all. It is the ability of growth hormone to stimulate the release of IGF-1 that makes this drug an effective muscle-building agent. The IGF-1 hormone was discovered back in 1957. At first it was believed to exert its main functions of the growth of cartilage. It was not until the late 1970's that the name IGF-1 was finally adopted, and a more detailed understanding of its full properties began to develop. The recent introduction of recombinant human IGF-1 for clinical study (and its potential as an actual therapeutic drug) has opened new doors into the exploration of this powerful anabolic hormone.

IGF-1 stimulates the growth of nearly all tissues. This includes not just skeletal muscle, but almost all organs in the body barring the brain and eyes. Being that muscle tissue is meant to respond to external stress stimulus with rapid changes in size and strength, it is much more responsive to IGF-1 therapy than other internal organs. Even though IGF-1 exerts a "whole body" anabolic effect, it is not so pronounced that the drug cannot be used safely to support skeletal muscle growth (one must never ignore the possibility of organ enlargement, however). Early drug trials with both animals and humans have been promising thus far. We can be optimistic that the next decade will bring a number of new clinical investigations, perhaps looking at many potential uses of IGF-1 including: a lean mass preservative for patients suffering from HIV and AIDS, an anabolic for patients suffering from cancer or other debilitating conditions, and even as a general recovery aid for burn victims.

The anabolic effect of IGF-1 toward skeletal muscle tissue is characterized by increases in satellite cell activity, muscle DNA content, and muscle protein content. It is believed to enhance the incorporation of new satellite cells into muscle fibers mainly through a reduction in the output of the growth inhibitor "p27Kip1"[174]. We further understand that both GH and IGF-1 therapy coincide with suppressed levels of myostatin[175 176], a powerful growth-regulating (limiting) hormone. GH and IGF-1 are both powerful anabolic drugs, which exert their actions on muscle tissue in ways different from classic anabolic steroids. They are looked upon more so as drugs that stimulate hyperplasia, or increases in cell number (although admittedly these drugs trigger both hyperplasia and hypertrophy). There is no question that IGF-1 increases muscle size via a valid growth effect, not the increases in cell volume due to swelling that were suggested in earlier liver studies[177]. The main question now is, how strong is this effect? As this drug leaves the medical books and enters real world application, this question is being answered fairly quickly.

There were initially some issues with potentially using IGF-1 as a therapeutic drug that needed to be overcome. The main problem is its rate of metabolic clearance, which is far too rapid for effective blood levels to be sustained with plain recombinant IGF-1. It is the same early issue scientists noticed with testosterone, except magnified many times over, as free testosterone actually lasts far longer in the blood than IGF-1. Scientists were forced to search out ways to maximize the half-life of the drug before it could be used therapeutically. By the late 1990's, much progress had been made. One way discovered, was to complex IGF-1 with one of its primary binding proteins, IGFBP-3. This IGF-1/IGFBP-3 binary complex is readily distributed through the body, protecting IGF-1 from immediate metabolic breakdown. It is normal for IGF-1 to disassociate from its binding protein, which allows IGF-1/IGFBP-3 to be somewhat of a sustained acting drug. This formulation is currently available in limited quantities for research. Other methods were discovered that involved synthetically modifying the hormone. One extremely popular variant in the research has an arginine at residue 3 and an N-terminal extension, and has been named LR3-IGF-I or "IGF-1 Long R3". It has a longer half-life than insulin, and is resistant to binding proteins, such that the drug is highly active next to endogenous IGF-1. Another IGF-1 analog is a truncated form of the hormone, called des(1-3)IGF-I. Both of these variants were, in fact, shown in studies to be 2.5-3 times more potent than regular IGF-I in restoring growth[178].

IGF-1 Long R3 is currently being manufactured by GroPep in Australia, which hold patent on this unique synthetic form of IGF-1. As a potential therapeutic drug, it is officially in the experimental stages of development. Some bodybuilders have been able to obtain it "for research projects" through international distributors who sell to Universities and biotechnology companies. It usually costs around $175-400 per milligram, for a standard "media" grade form of the drug. This is said to be >85% purity, and has been working fine for bodybuilding purposes. It is also sold as a "receptor grade" material, which exceeds 99% purity. This material is used for the most sensitive studies, and has come to be looked at as the “choice” form of IGF-1 for the discriminating bodybuilder. It can be located at a reasonable price (somewhat close to media grade) when purchased in bulk; otherwise it can be exceedingly expensive (over $700 per milligram). Both grades of research material usually come as plain lyophilized powder, or suspended in a solvent like benzyl alcohol. If you have the former, it is typically mixed with benzyl alcohol for storage, and diluted with sterile saline or bacteriostatic water for use. When obtained in benzyl alcohol, the user would typically draw a tiny amount (the immediate dosage) into an insulin syringe, and dilute it before injection by drawing in extra bacteriostatic water. All unused portions of the drug should be refrigerated.

IGF-1 Long R3 is also sold under the brand name IGtropin, produced by the Chinese manufacturer GenSci (the makers of JinTropin rHGH). This is supposed to be the same exact compound supplied by GroPep, however, it is uncertain at this time if they obtain the material through any agreements with the company. Feedback on the product has been very good thus far, suggesting that whatever the source, they are indeed supplying real IGF-1 Long R3. The GenSci product is a little bit more expensive than raw research powers, selling for over $500 per 1-milligram kit when purchased directly from an overseas pharmacy. This price will usually increase to nearly $700 when the kit is found on the U.S. black market. The higher price of the GenSci product is balanced by greater convenience and trust, as it is packaged in a similar “ready to use” manner as prescription growth hormone. In each box you will find 10 vials with 100mcg hormone in each, and the necessary 10 ampules of sterile diluent to mix them with. Once reconstituted, any unused portion should be refrigerated to preserve the stability of the protein.

Unlike HGH, which is given subcutaneously, IGF-1 is usually given as an intramuscular injection. Although SubQ injections are possible, they tend to involve a little more discomfort than regular IM injections. The bodybuilder will typically inject it into the muscle that they are training that day, in an effort to stimulate spot growth and a greater overall anabolic response. The dose given is usually in the range of 20-80mcg, and given every day. The daily dosage can be further divided into two applications (spaced 10-12 hours apart) to allow for better stability in blood hormone levels. Some bodybuilders do venture above the 100mcg daily mark, and some “top pros” are even rumored to take as much as 200mcg per day during bulking cycles. With the astronomical costs that would be associated with such high-dosage use, it is likely that these amounts are more the product of speculation than real common practice in the professional ranks. 30mcg per day is probably the most commonly used dosage for the recreational bodybuilder, which allows a 1mg vial to last for about a month. At $35 or so per day, this would seem to be a fairly reasonable investment in one’s physique by most accounts. $100 per day is a crack habit, and probably not warranted for most users.

Typical results from IGF-1 administration (with a delayed acting form of the drug such as IGF-1 Long R3) include intensified pumps, increased appetite, increases in lean muscle mass & strength, and the stimulation of thermogenesis (fat loss). A 30-day cycle usually imparts at least several pounds of new muscle tissue gain, and by most accounts its local spot-growth effect works very well. Some bodybuilders claim to have gained as much as 12-15 pounds off of a single 4-week cycle of just IGF-1. When taken alone, IGF-1 is not quite as good as anabolic steroids for most of its users, but it is certainly not shabby for a non-steroidal anabolic either. By all accounts, muscle retention is also very high post-cycle, which can’t be said for steroids. This is due to a couple factors, including the lack of hormonal crash when the drug is discontinued, and a tendency to produce lasting (permanent) gains in satellite cell proliferation instead of mainly supporting increases in protein synthesis.

When it comes to cutting, IGF-1 is definitely not as potent as classic human growth hormone. This is quite understandable, as we know that this is an activity that is inherent in the human growth hormone molecule itself. Increased lipolysis is, likewise, not dependent on the stimulation of IGF-1 release the same way the anabolic attributes of GH are. However, that is not to say IGF-1 is entirely without benefit here. Users do still seem to comment that the drug has some noticeable effect as a fat loss agent. It seems to allow them to keep fat mass at bay, even when they are on a high-calorie (bulking) diet. Often they can even lose fat mass and tighten up their physiques while taking the drug during building phases of training, but individual metabolism seems to play a strong role in how noticeable this effect is. We can therefore say that IGF-1 is not going to be your number one drug choice for cutting up, but it will still make an excellent addition to any stack focused on lean muscle mass gains.

There are concerns that natural antibody reactions will start to work against the effectiveness of synthetic IGF-1 analogs as the usage duration becomes prolonged. You will recall that this has been investigated with somatrem, the synthetic 192 amino acid analog of human growth hormone (see Drug Profiles: Somatrem). For this reason, cycle length is usually limited to somewhere between 4 and 8 weeks. After this point a break of at least 4 weeks is usually taken, to ensure maximum responsiveness when drug therapy is again initiated. It is uncertain how crucial this is, however at this time it seems like good advice given how little we currently know about the use of IGF-1.

But ensuring maximum effectiveness is not the only reason for limiting drug duration and dosage. There are other potentially serious side effects to IGF-1 therapy that need to be considered. These mimic the risks associated with GH therapy very closely, and include pronounced internal organ growth, thickening of the bones and skin (GH jaw), insulin resistance, water retention and edema, and even gynecomasita in very sensitive users. Some people also report carpel tunnel syndrome from the overuse of GH or IGF-1, which may be preceded by numbness or discomfort in the hands and wrists. GH is known to be a strong drug, and IGF-1 is its powerful big brother in almost all regards. This agent should be respected, not abused.

The fact that IGF-1 is not yet an approved prescription drug in any country has definitely not stopped athletes from taking advantage of this agent. The potential benefit of this drug was simply too enticing to be ignored. As soon as the word was out about IGF-1, the wheels started turning about how to get it onto the black market. Although not in abundant supply, enough channels for this drug have been established to ensure that a steady stream of athletes are able to use it. At least one drug manufacturing company has taken notice, and since started marketing it in a prepared form for human use. Several other companies are likely to follow suit in the next year or two. Many that have used IGF-1 (as IGF-1 Long R3) are calling it "Super GH", which in many regards is a fair perspective. IGF-1 drugs like this allow us the full anabolic benefit of this hormone, without being forced to rely on our own body's ability to produce it in response to the administration of HGH. The difference can be likened to taking HCG to stimulate increased testosterone levels, or injecting an actual drug form of the hormone like testosterone cypionate. We can see why IGF-1 has earned the nickname "I Grow Faster", and become the cult drug of interest the past few years. Its popularity is only sure to grow as more athletes are given the opportunity to use it.

Nutropin AQ (somatropin aqueous suspension)

Nutropin AQ is a new injectable growth hormone preparation from the U.S. biotechnologies firm Genentech. Like their Nutropin Depot product, Nutropin AQ stands out as being extremely unique and innovative in design. In this case, Genentech has been able to develop the world's first liquid-stable GH product. As such, it comes in one vial, which does not require reconstitution (mixing) with a liquid solvent before use. Genentech is, of course, also the same company that manufacturers and sells Protropin (somatrem), which is a GH product that uses a 192 amino acid variant of the endogenous growth hormone molecule instead of the correct 191 amino acid sequence found in somatropin. For this product, however, Genentech has decided to use somatropin instead of somatrem, even though they still manufacture and sell Protropin. Growth hormone itself is a powerful lipolytic (fat loss) and anabolic agent, making it a common appearance on the underground bodybuilding drug market (for a more comprehensive discussion, please refer to the somatropin drug profile).

The advantages to be found in Nutropin AQ are ultimately not great. Essentially this is just a preconstituted form of the drug, saving you only the couple of minutes required to mix the vials in a standard GH product. For this slight timesaving benefit you meet with one main drawback, namely that the product needs to be refrigerated at all times. This makes dealing with it on the black market very difficult, as you never know if your product was correctly handled before it reached you. What if it was shipped across the country in the back of a hot UPS truck without refrigeration, or sat in some guy's dresser drawer for weeks? GH is not a cheap product to purchase to begin with, making inherent risks like this an extremely unwelcome fact. Serostim and Saizen are both also sold in the U.S., but the unused vials do not require refrigeration before they are mixed. This makes them safer to buy in comparison, and probably recommended if you are not buying the drug from a pharmacy.

Unlike Nutropin Depot, which is still being investigated in regards to other therapeutic claims, Nutropin AQ has already been approved by the FDA for the treatment of growth hormone deficiency in adults. This assures that bodybuilders have much greater access to the drug; as such applications are vast, and manufacturing volume need to meet them great, compared to the small number of patients each year given the drug to treat childhood GH-related growth deficiencies. Likewise, I expect it to start becoming a popular item with many of the longevity clinics that operate in the U.S., who cater to men and women (typically over 30) who are looking for the health and vitality restoring benefits of growth hormone replacement therapy.

Nutropin AQ is manufactured in 2ml vials and pre-loaded 2ml injectable "pen-cartridges". Both forms contain 5mg/mL (10mg total), or about 30IU units of human growth hormone each. At the pharmacy, each 2ml box of Nutropin AQ runs about $500. For a daily dose of 1-4 IU, this equates to anywhere from 7 to 30 days worth of the drug ($2000 a month at the full 4IU dose). Oddly enough, we should probably expect the black market price to be considerably cheaper than if you purchased this drug directly from a pharmacy with a prescription. Serostim, for example, runs about $1,400 in the pharmacy, yet the kits are commonly found on the black market for $500-600, sometimes even $450, each. Hopefully the same thing will happen with Nutropin AQ.

Nutropin Depot (somatropin)

Nutropin Depot is a brand new long-acting injectable growth hormone product, produced by the U.S. biotechnologies firm Genentech. In this product the growth hormone molecule is encased in biodegradable microspheres, which slowly break down in the body releasing the GH contained inside. Genentech is the same company that manufactures Protropin (somatrem), which is a 192 amino acid variant of the human growth hormone molecule. Although somatrem essentially has all of the physiological activities of the correct 191 amino acid growth hormone molecule (somatropin), Genentech has decided to use somatropin in this and most of its other growth hormone products (they still do manufacture Protropin). Human growth hormone can be a powerful lipolytic and anabolic hormone, making it somewhat of a “standard-issue” drug in the world of bodybuilding (for a more comprehensive discussion, please refer to the somatropin profile).

This product is designed to form a long acting hormone deposit at the site of injection, which takes weeks to be fully absorbed and utilized by the body. As such, the recommended administration schedule of Nutropin Depot is only a single application once or twice per month. This represents a great step forward in the technology of growth hormone medications, finally freeing patients from the uncomfortable repetitive daily injections they have had to endure for decades with preceding medications. But as we learned with injectable steroid hormones, long-acting depot drugs rarely work in an even manner. In this case, levels of growth hormone fluctuate a great deal between applications. In fact, studies show that as much as 50% of the dosage is dispersed in the body, in a strong supraphysiological rush, within the first two days following injection (see the included graph). In a second, long acting, phase, the remaining 50% of the miscrosphere-encased hormone slowly breaks down and enters circulation over a period of 2 to 4 weeks. This variability does also seem to come at a price. Genentech makes note in their packaging insert that in one of their long-term studies, 19% of the patients who switched to Nutropin Depot from daily growth hormone injections experienced decreased growth rates, and discontinued therapy.

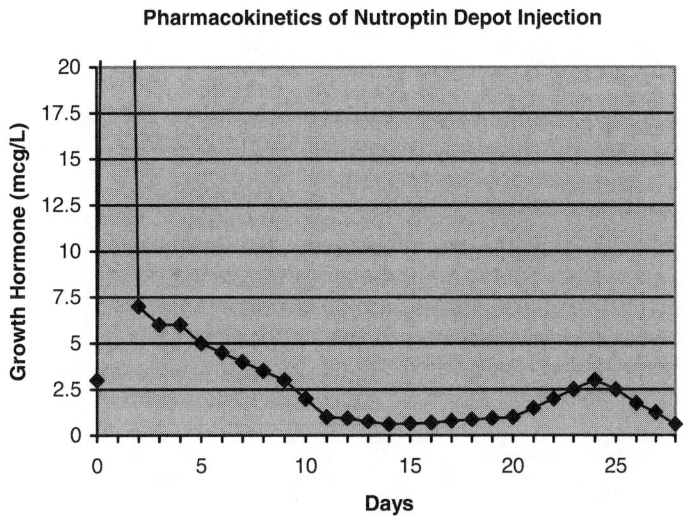

Figure 1. Mean serum GH concentrations (mcg/L) measured after single-dose application of Nutropin Depot. Data shows an extremely strong supraphysiological rush on day 1, peaking around 90 mcg/L. Source: Nutropin Depot® prescribing information. Genentech, Inc.

Nutropin Depot comes in single use vials (you cannot store unused portions for later use), of 13.5, 18 and 22.5mg. Even before reconstitution, the vials of Nutropin Depot must remain refrigerated at all times in order for the drug to keep its full potency. This is a major disadvantage next to products like Saizen and Serostim, which are fully stable at room temperature for a couple of years after the date of manufacture. Dealing with Nutropin Depot on the black market is likewise going to be very difficult. Even if you are able to find it, you are always going to wonder if it your vials were properly handled at all times before they reached your hands. Were they properly refrigerated, or did they sit in the hot trunk of some guy's car for two days? Unless you are getting the product directly from a pharmacy, this will always be a risk you will have to take when purchasing this drug.

Nutropin Depot is approved in the United States at this time for the long-term treatment of growth failure due to a lack of endogenous GH secretion (dwarfism). It has not yet been officially approved for treatment of somatopause (declining GH secretion in adults) or weight gain with HIV+ patients like Humatrope and Serostim (respectively). This greatly limits the access bodybuilders have to this drug, as only a small number of prescriptions are written each year to treat dwarfism; a vastly lower number than are written for HIV+ wasting and somatopause treatment. The illicit market for domestic GH products only seemed to explode once these new uses for Serostim and Humatrope were given the green light by the FDA. We might alternately come to find a good source for the drug in another country, should Genentech decide to aggressively market it internationally. Whatever the case, if anything ultimately opens up supply lines to this drug, there is little question it will quickly become *the* growth hormone product of choice amongst bodybuilders.

Protropin (somatrem)

Here in the United States two distinctly structured versions of growth hormone are being manufactured for the pharmaceutical market. Most items, such as Humatrope, Serostim, Saizen and Nutropin have the correct 191 amino acid sequence somatropin molecule. Genentech's Protropin uses somatrem, which is a 192 amino acid variant of the growth hormone molecule. Both products are roughly biologically equivalent, and can be used to treat cases of GH deficient dwarfism in children.

This unnatural structure of somatrem has been documented to increase the chance for developing an antibody reaction to the growth hormone treatment. The antibodies work by binding with the growth hormone molecule, interfering with its ability to exert activity in the body. In one clinical investigation, as much as two thirds of the 54 children treated wound up developed antibodies to growth hormone after one year of use[179]. This is quite a profound figure compared to what was noted in a similarly configured investigation, involving the administration of somatropin to 21 GH deficient children for one year. With the correct 191 amino acid hormone, only one in seven patients produced serum antibodies to GH[180]. It is important to note that in both studies the antibody reactions were not strong, and never diminished the ability of the drugs to be therapeutically effective. Still, there is a difference between the two forms of GH here, and obviously the correct 191 amino acid configuration of somatropin is considered the more reliable drug to use.

Protropin is still considered an effective product and is prescribed regularly in the U.S. Outside of the U.S., the vast majority of HGH in circulation will be the correct 191 amino acid sequence, so this distinction is not as great a concern. The only notable product to hit the market as of late is Fitropin, which is a popular somatrem product from China.

HYPOGLYCEMICS

DRUG PROFILES

Glucophage (metformin Hcl)

Glucophage is a trade name for the oral anti-hyperglycemic agent metformin HCL. This type of drug is generally used in the management of mature onset (Type-II) diabetes. It is utilized when dietary management and exercise alone have not been able to control the disease, yet injectable insulin is not appropriate since this hormone is still present in the body. While the main activity of metformin HCL is the increased utilization of glucose, it does not directly mimic the action of insulin. The precise mode of action is actually unknown, but it is believed to increase insulin sensitivity through some peripheral process. Use of this agent will certainly lower the patient's blood sugar, but its activity makes it unlikely to cause a state of hypoglycemia if the dosage is accidentally misjudged (a major concern with injectable insulin).

The concept of harnessing insulin for performance enhancement has been catching on in recent years. As you may know, insulin is considered a "storage hormone". It transports amino acids, fatty acids and carbohydrates (glucose) into various cells of your body. This process includes the storage of protein in skeletal muscle cells, equating to a possible anabolic effect. But insulin is a little tricky because it can also direct storage to fat cells, obviously an unwanted result. It is however possible to "guide" insulin in the right direction. Athletes have found that during periods of intense weight training, and a diet without excess caloric intake, insulin can show a much greater affinity for protein and carbohydrate storage in muscle cells. By manipulating insulin levels (or insulin sensitivity) under these conditions, we can see notable growth. Implemented correctly, the result should be a fuller, more defined look to the muscles. Injectable insulin can be extremely risky however, an incorrect dosage or insufficient carbohydrate intake having grave consequences to the user's health. In extreme cases, hypoglycemia (low blood sugar) can lead to coma or even death. Since this effect is rare with Glucophage, it is considered by many athletes to be an introduction to insulin manipulation.

When administered, the absorption rate of metformin HCL is very slow. The drug will make its way to circulation slowly, over a period of about six hours. The general intake schedule among bodybuilders is to take 850mg (one tablet) twice per day. The user will be sure to additionally supplement with a carbohydrate replacement (such as Ultra Fuel) and with creatine monohydrate, particularly after periods of training. The result of this treatment will probably not be as dramatic as when using insulin, but a notable anabolic effect can be achieved nonetheless. Most athletes opt to use this drug for a limited duration, cycles of Glucophage usually lasting only a couple of months. This would be followed by an equally long break (at a minimum).

While Glucophage is considered much safer than insulin, it is not without its own unique risks. The most serious complication is the possible development of lactic acidosis. This is an often-fatal metabolic disorder involving (among other factors) an increase in lactate levels (lactic) and a pronounced decrease in blood pH (acidosis). The package insert displays the additional warning: the administration of oral hypoglycemics may be associated with increased cardiovascular mortality as compared to treatment with diet alone or diet with insulin. The risk for severe side effects is increased in people suffering from liver dysfunction or who drink excessive alcohol. Or those with renal dysfunction, noting impaired creatine clearance (a serum concentration above 1,2 mg per 100 ml is considered the cut-off point for treatment). A number of other "minor" side effects may include, but are not limited to, anorexia, nausea, vomiting, diarrhea, metallic taste, fatigue, weakness and malabsorbtion of vitamin B12. Quite often these effects will subside if the dosage is lowered, stubborn cases requiring the drug to be discontinued. If vomiting occurs, the athlete will usually discontinue the drug immediately for fear this may be an early symptom of lacticacidosis.

Glucophage belongs to the same family of antidiabetic agents (biguanide derivatives) as Debeone (Phenformin HCL). Debeone was removed from the U.S. market (and others) in the late 70's, exhibiting a high tendency for lacticacidosis. While this compound is still available in Mexico, it is really too risky to justify using for performance enhancement. Since Glucophage has a much more reliable safety record, it is the preferred agent of the two (and usually never substituted). The reports on this drug have actually been mixed, with many bodybuilders being very disappointed with the results. Those looking for a more pronounced effect than this drug can provide will generally avoid stronger oral agents, and instead advance to injectable insulin. Others might first wish to give Rezulin® a try, which is another recently developed oral agent. This drug appears to have a more intense effect (through a different mechanism) than Glucophage, but does present a number of unique risks to the user as well (see: Rezulin®).

Insulin

Insulin is a powerful hormone in the human body, responsible for regulating glucose levels in the blood. This is a function that your life constantly depends on. Before going any further I must stress that **insulin use by those who do not medically require it can be a very risky endeavor.** It is important not only to research and understand the risks involved, but to really give some thought to just how important a little extra boost is to you. Misusing insulin can have tragic results. Immediate death, coma or the possible development of insulin dependent diabetes in a previously healthy athlete are all possible, be extremely careful.

In the human body insulin is secreted by the pancreas. The release of this hormone is most closely tied to glucose, although a number of other factors including pancreatic & gastrointestinal hormones, amino acids, fatty acids and ketone bodies are also involved. Its role in the body is to control the uptake, utilization and storage of amino acids, carbohydrates and fatty acids by various cells of your body. The activity of insulin is both anabolic and anti-catabolic, the hormone stimulating the use and retention cellular nutrients while inhibiting their breakdown. Skeletal muscle cells are among the many targets of this hormone's action, and the reason pharmaceutical insulin has made its way into the realm of athletics. But this is a little tricky because insulin can also promote nutrient storage in fat cells, obviously an unwanted result. Athletes have found however, that a strict regimen of intense weight training and a diet without excess caloric intake can result in insulin showing a much higher affinity for protein and carbohydrate storage in muscle cells. This could produce rapid and noticeable growth, the muscles beginning to look fuller (and sometimes more defined) almost immediately after starting insulin therapy.

The fact that insulin use cannot be detected by urinalysis has ensured it a place in the drug regimens of many professional bodybuilders. Insulin is often used in combination with other "contest safe" drugs like human growth hormone, thyroid medications and low dose testosterone injections, and together can have a dramatic effect on the users physique without fear of a positive urinalysis result. Those who do not have to worry about drug testing however, find insulin and anabolic/androgenic steroids a very synergistic combination. This is because the two actively support an anabolic state through different mechanisms, insulin enhancing the transport of nutrients into muscle cells and steroids (among other things) increasing the rate of cellular protein synthesis.

The actual medical purpose for insulin is to treat different forms of diabetes. Specifically the human body may not be producing insulin (Type-I diabetes) or may not recognize insulin well at the cell site although some level is present in the blood (Type-II diabetes). Type-I diabetics are therefore required to inject insulin on a regular basis, as they are left without a sufficient level of this hormone. Along with medication, the individual will need to constantly monitor blood glucose levels and regulate their sugar intake. Together with lifestyle modifications such as regular exercise and developing a balanced diet, insulin dependent individuals can live a healthy and full life. Untreated, diabetes can be a fatal disease.

Insulin is available from pharmacies in the United States without a prescription. This is so that an insulin-dependent diabetic will have easy access to medication when traveling about. Arguing over forms or having to call a doctor for verification is all the delay needed to cost someone who needs this medication their life. Pharmaceutical insulin comes from one of two basic origins, animal or synthetic. With Animal source insulin, the hormone is extracted from the pancreas of either pigs or cows (or both) and prepared for medical use. These preparations are further divided into the categories "standard" and "purified", dependent on the level of purity and non-insulin content of the solution. With such products there is always the slight possibility of pancreatic contaminants making their way into the prepared drug. On the other hand there is "synthetic" insulin. Specifically "biosynthetic", it is produced by a recombinant DNA procedure similar to the process used to manufacture human growth hormone. The result is a polypeptide hormone, consisting of one 21-amino acid "A-chain" coupled by two disulfide bonds with one 30-amino acid "B-chain". The biosynthetic process will produce a drug free of the pancreatic protein contaminants possible with animal insulin, and is biologically equivalent in all important ways to human pancreatic insulin. With the innate (remote) risk involved with animal insulin, coupled with the fact that the structure is (very slightly) different from human insulin, most opt for the synthetic product. Biosynthetic human insulin, hereon referred to as Humulin, is the standard insulin among athletes, and the subject of this section.

There are a number of different insulin preparations, separated by variable factors such as speed of onset, peak and the duration of activity. Regular synthetic insulin is generally faster acting that animal source insulin, with a shorter duration of activity in the body. But scientists have found that by adding substances such as protamine or zinc, they can produce a drug with a much slower release and a prolonged duration of effect. Following we will show you the distinctions between the various forms of Humulin.

Humalog® (Insulin Lispro Inj): Humalog® is a newer, rapid acting form of insulin. It reaches peak effect in less than two hours, and by the four hour mark is almost out of the body completely. It was designed to mimic the body's natural insulin response to meals, and allow a diabetic patient to take their medication before or immediately after eating. Medically this type does not replace other insulin products, but is used in conjunction with them. For athletes the fact that it works in such a short window of time makes it an extremely interesting product. It may in fact be the most ideal type of insulin to use, as it would work almost exclusively in the post-training nutrient uptake window.

Humulin®-R or "regular" insulin: This product has a short duration of effect, approximately 6 to 8 hours. This is the insulin of choice among athletes, as it is fast acting and easier to control than most other forms (except Humalog®). Should one encounter problems with glucose levels in the blood, the shorter the drug will remain active in the body the better. Occasionally athletes do experiment with the longer acting forms described below, but this is generally unadvised. While all other forms of insulin will be cloudy due to their mixture, regular insulin should be a clear solution. One should not use regular insulin if the solution is cloudy or has floating particles.

Humulin®-N, NPH (insulin isophane): Intermediate length insulin, lasts up to 24 hours.

Humulin®-L, Lente (medium zinc suspension): Intermediate length insulin, lasts up to 24 hours

Humulin®-U, Utalente (prolonged zinc suspension): Long acting insulin. Can remain active for over 24 hours.

Humulin® Mixtures: These are mixtures of regular insulin for fast onset and a longer acting insulin for prolonged effect. These are labeled by the mixture percentage, commonly 10/90, 20/80, 30/70, 40/60 and 50/50.

As we have discussed earlier, regular insulin is the most popular choice and will be the subject of our intake discussion. Before one even considers using insulin, they should become very familiar with using a glucometer. This device gives you a quick number reading of your blood glucose level and can be indispensable in helping you manage your insulin/carbohydrate intake.

Insulin is used in a wide variety of ways. The dosages can vary significantly among athletes, and are often dependent upon factors like insulin sensitivity and the use of other drugs. Most users choose to administer insulin immediately after a workout, which is likely the most "anabolic" time of the day to use this drug. Insulin is always injected subcutaneously, or below the surface of the skin but without entering muscle tissue. This is given by pinching a fold of skin, commonly in the arm or abdominal area. A small "insulin needle" is used, approximately ½" long, 27-29 gauge thickness and holding one third to one full cc. These are available over-the-counter in many states. A full cc (or ml) equates to 100 international units (I.U.), a scale that is clearly labeled on an insulin syringe. It is important that the injection site be left alone after insulin has been injected and not rubbed. This is to prevent the drug from releasing into circulation too quickly. It is also a good idea to rotate injection sites regularly; otherwise a localized buildup of subcutaneous fat may develop due to the lipogenic properties of this hormone.

Among bodybuilders, dosages used are usually in the range of 1IU per 15-20 pounds of lean bodyweight. First-time users should at first ignore body weight guidelines however, and instead start at a low dosage with the intention of gradually working up to this point. For example, on the first day of insulin therapy you could begin with a dose as low as only 2 IU. Each consecutive post-workout application this dosage can be increased by 1IU, until the user determines a comfortable range. This is safer and much more tailored to the individual than simply calculating and injecting a dose, as many find they tolerate much more or less insulin than weight guidelines would dictate. Athletes using growth hormone in particular often have higher insulin requirements, as HGH therapy is shown to both lower secretion of, and induce cellular resistance to, this hormone.

One also must remember that it is very important to consume carbohydrates for several hours following insulin use. One will generally follow the rule-of-thumb, of ingesting at least 10 grams of simple carbohydrates per IU of insulin injected (with a minimum immediate intake of 100 grams regardless of dose). This is timed approximately 20 to 30 minutes after the drug has been administered. The use of a carbohydrate replacement drink such as Ultra Fuel® by Twin Labs would probably be a good idea, as this is a fast and reliable carbohydrate source. It is best to always have something like this on-hand should you begin to notice too low a drop in glucose levels. Many athletes will also take creatine monohydrate with their carbohydrate drink, since the insulin may help force the creatine into the muscles. An hour or so after injecting insulin, one will eat a good meal or consume a protein shake. The carbohydrate drink and meal/protein shake are absolutely necessary. Without them, blood sugar levels can drop dangerously low, and the athlete will most likely enter a state of hypoglycemia.

Hypoglycemia is the primary worry of insulin users. This is a dangerous condition that occurs when blood glucose levels fall too low. It is a common and potentially fatal reaction experienced at some time or another by most insulin users. It is therefore critical to understand the warning signs of hypoglycemia. The following is a list of symptoms which may indicate a mild to moderate hypoglycemia: hunger, drowsiness, blurred vision, depressive mood, dizziness, sweating, palpitation, tremor, restlessness, tingling in the hands, feet, lips, or tongue, lightheadedness, inability to concentrate, headache, sleep disturbances, anxiety, slurred speech, irritability, abnormal behavior, unsteady movement and personality changes. If any of these warning signs should occur, one should immediately consume a food or drink containing simple sugars such as a candy bar or carbohydrate drink. This will hopefully raise blood glucose levels sufficiently enough to ward off mild to moderate hypoglycemia. There is always a possibility of severe hypoglycemia, which is very serious and requires immediate emergency medical attention. Symptoms of this include disorientation, seizure, unconsciousness, and death.

Many taking insulin will also notice a tendency to get sleepy some time after injecting the drug. This is an early symptom of hypoglycemia, and a clear sign the user should be consuming more carbohydrates. One should absolutely avoid the temptation to go to sleep at this point, as the insulin may take its peak effect during rest and blood glucose levels could be left to drop significantly. Unaware of this condition during sleep, the athlete may be at a high risk for going into a state of severe hypoglycemia. We have of course already discussed the serious dangers of such a state, and unfortunately here simply consuming more carbohydrates will not be an option. Those experimenting with insulin would therefore be wise to always stay awake for the duration of the drug's effect, and also avoid using insulin in the early evening to ensure the drug will not be inadvertently active when retiring for the night.

Many athletes prefer to bring their insulin with them to the gym, injecting in the locker room (or car) immediately after a workout. Although insulin should be refrigerated, it is fine to keep it in a gym bag or car so long as it is not left out for too long and it is kept away from heat/direct sunlight. Rather than waiting to the end of a workout, some actually prefer to inject their insulin dosage during training, 30 minutes prior to the end of a session. Immediately following the workout the user will consume a carbohydrate drink in this case. Such timing may make the insulin more efficient at bringing glycogen to the muscles, but also increases the danger of hypoglycemia as carbohydrate consumption may be inadvertently delayed. Some will go so far as to inject a few units before lifting to improve their pump. This practice is risky and best left to those very experienced with insulin. Finally, some bodybuilders opt to inject insulin upon waking in the morning. After the injection they will consume a carbohydrate drink. Later, perhaps one hour after the injection, a full breakfast will be consumed. Some athletes find this application of insulin very beneficial for putting on extra mass while others will tend to store excess fat. If using more than one application of insulin per day it would also be a good idea to restrict the total daily intake to no more than 20-40 IU.

In America, regular human insulin is available by the name of Humulin R by Eli Lilly and Company. It costs about $20 for a 10 ml vial with a strength of 100 IU per ml. Remember to be very careful, **one mistake in dosage or diet can be potentially fatal**.

Rezulin (troglitazone)

Rezulin® is a very interesting new oral antihyperglycemic medication, approved for U.S. sale in 1997. Specifically we are speaking of the active compound troglitazone, which is classified as a thiazolidinedione antidiabetic agent. This drug was designed for use on patients with Type-II (noninsulin-dependent diabetes mellitus (NIDDM) also known as adult-onset diabetes). Rezulin® is useful in this situation because it acts by increasing the body's sensitivity to insulin, therefore requiring some amount of endogenous insulin to be present in order to have an effect (Type-I diabetics produce no appreciable amount of insulin). The action of this drug is quite advanced from the oral agents we are familiar with like Glucophage (metformin HCL). Rezulin® works by increasing the number of active insulin receptor sites, allowing the hormone to have a more pronounced effect. This enables Rezulin® to be a much more potent compound, and therefore more useful than Glucophage (which acts via a less direct mechanism). The one worry is that a state of hypoglycemia (low blood sugar) may be easier to produce with Rezulin®. Since insulin is needed for the drug to work however, this problem is usually only seen when injectable insulin is used at the same time. Glucophage is perhaps less dangerous if the dosage is misjudged, although most feel it is still a much cruder product and less worth consideration at this time.

In the short time this drug has been available, safety concerns have generated it quite a bit of attention as well. This began in the end of 1997, about the time that Glaxo-Wellcome voluntarily halted production of the Romozin brand (UK) due to the death of five patients receiving treatment. These deaths were due to serious liver complications, brought about by a somewhat toxic nature of this substance. Soon after investigating, Parke-Davis decided not to discontinue their U.S. product, believing the benefits of Rezulin® to greatly outweigh any risks. And the risks were certainly made clear in our country as well. By November of 1997 35 people taking it had developed serious liver complications, resulting in two deaths. Parke-Davis promptly issued a warning to medical professionals, urging them to monitor their patients' liver enzymes during the first year of therapy. Subsequent to the warning, an additional 150 cases of liver difficulty were reported. The manufacturer quickly pointed out that statistically such occurrences we consistent with those found acceptable in clinical trials, noting that only about 2 percent of patients will show elevated liver enzymes and fewer will develop an actual problem.

The use of insulin and insulin enhancing medications for athletic purposes has been increasingly popular in recent years. This is due to the fact that the main action of insulin is to transport carbohydrates (glucose), fatty acids and amino acids into various body cells. This is how blood sugar is lowered, as insulin deposits glucose into the target cells, removing this nutrient from circulation. The negative to this hormone is that fat cells are possible targets for this effect, potentially increasing the athlete's body fat percentage. But insulin will also store carbohydrates and protein into the body's muscle tissue cells. During intense periods of weight training (and a diet without excess fat and calories) it has been shown that insulin can display a much greater tendency for storage in muscle cells than fat cells. The result could be a notable anabolic effect, producing a fuller and harder look to the physique. Since injectable insulin carries with it a number of considerable risks, many athletes first choose to experiment with oral diabetes medications.

But Glucophage has received very mixed reviews. Many athletes claimed to have received little or no benefit when taking this drug. Others have reported an anabolic effect, but usually only when higher dosages or longer cycles were utilized. Since Rezulin® appears to be much more active in the body than Glucophage, it may prove to be a more potent anabolic for athletes. But this drug is not without its own unique risks. For starters, one cannot ignore the risks for liver damage with this drug. This is especially true with athletes, as most of the individuals who would use Rezulin® are probably regular steroid users. Since most would of course be periodically taking c17-alpha alkylated (liver toxic) orals, this risk for liver damage may be amplified with such a combination. The fact that much shorter periods of intake are going to be used by athletes may not provide the most comfort, being that the medical cases in question involved both long and short-term treatment with this compound. Nausea, vomiting, abdominal pain, fatigue, anorexia, jaundice and dark urine are all symptoms that liver trouble may be developing, at which point the drug should be quickly discontinued. Also common with Rezulin® is an increase of total, HDL and LDL cholesterol values. Since these values typically rise evenly, leaving the actual HDL/LDL ratio generally unchanged, trouble with cardiac functioning does not commonly result from this effect.

Since Rezulin® is so new, it will probably take some time before a standard intake regimen becomes popular. It would seem like the best advice to begin taking the drug with a low dosage, perhaps 100-200mg. Being that this drug has a very long half life, it is taken only once per day. Food also increases the absorption of Rezulin®, so it is always taken with a meal so that the optimal blood level is achieved. The athlete will presumably take the dose one to two hours before a training session, as the drug will take two to three hours to achieve its peak blood level. Afterwards (and throughout the day) a carbohydrate replacement drink like Ultra Fuel® may be indispensable when managing the blood sugar level. Creatine monohydrate is also a common adjunct to insulin manipulation therapies, as the hormone will enhance the storing effect of the creatine supplementation by helping to shuttle it into muscle cells. Also, the user will probably have no need to exceed the standard medical dosage of 400mg-600mg. Perhaps he/she may even find it most comfortable to stay below this point, as the healthy athlete will not be suffering the same insulin related dysfunction's as the target patient.

Liver Detoxification

DRUG PROFILES

LIV-52

Liv-52 is an herbal product that has its roots in ayurvedic medicine, an ages old form of Hindu science and medicine that centers on the use of natural remedies. Liv-52 is manufactured by the Himalaya Drug Co. in Bombay, India, and was first introduced to the global market in 1955. This product is not a synthesized drug but an herbal blend, with a number of natural constituents including Capparis spinosa, Terminalia arjuna, Cichorium intybus, Achillea millefolium, Solanum nigrum, Tamarix gallica, Cassia occidentalis, and Mandur bhasma. It is primarily used to aid digestion, improve appetite, increase metabolism and protect and regenerate the liver. As the first three letters of its name would hint at, overall liver health is the primary focus of this product.

Numerous medical studies have been conducted on Liv-52 in recent years, many of which involve its ability to protect the liver from damage by alcohol or other toxins[181 182 183 184]. One investigation in particular looked at how the herbal medication affected the breakdown of alcohol in the body, showing it to notably increase its excretion, even to the point of being able to reduce next day hangover symptoms after binge drinking[185]. Another wanted to investigate what underlying mechanism might be involved in Liv-52's ability to protect the liver against alcohol toxicity. It was able to demonstrate that one avenue involved a specific ability to slow the rate of glutathione depletion[186]. This may be very important to the steroid-using athlete, as glutathione depletion is looked at as a direct marker of liver stress with c-17 alpha alkylated orals.

Many bodybuilders feel it is good to take this product during all steroid cycles that include c-17 alpha alkylated compounds. They will typically take a dosage of 1-2 tablets per application, which is repeated anywhere from once to four times daily. Many swear by it, even claiming they noticed it kept their liver enzymes down during routine visits with the doctor. Others have even insisted that for them, Liv-52 has made the difference between being able to use oral steroids (safely) or not. That might be a little strong, and this is by no means meant to suggest that this is some magic pill that can make otherwise toxic steroids 100% safe. There are always going to be risks when oral steroids are involved, and there is nothing available that can remove them completely. The trick is mitigating them as much as possible, and Liv-52 may indeed by one way to help do that.

Liv-52 is readily available in the United States, where 100 tablets will run you somewhere around $20-40 at your local supplement store. You would be well advised to be sure the Himalaya Drug Company produced your product, as many copycat versions of unknown quality are circulating the health supplement market right now, probably owing to the widespread recognition of the Liv-52 brand name. Thankfully, the real thing is not at all difficult to find. With the large body of evidence surrounding this product and its ability to support liver health, it is good advice that if you are considering oral steroids, you should consider looking into this.

Silymarin (Milk Thistle extract)

Silymarin is an herbal medicine made from the seeds of the Silybummarianum plant (also known as "milk thistle"). It has been used for more than 2,000 years as a folk remedy for liver disorders, and is still used widely today for the same purpose. More specifically, it is most commonly used as a natural treatment for cirrhosis of the liver, hepatitis or liver damage or poisoning with mushrooms, acetaminophen or other toxins. It is also used by many people as a general antioxidant and digestive aid, taken as part of a wellness regimen of natural herbs and vitamins. The active ingredients in milk thistle extract are the flavonoids silybin, silydianin, and silychristin, collectively referred to as Silymarin. Silymarin is widely sold in the United States, where it is considered a natural dietary supplement and not subject to prescription requirements.

Literally hundreds of medical studies have been conducted on Silymarin in recent times, and nearly all of them support strong liver protective and regenerative properties inherent in this natural remedy. Just one paper published in 1980, for example, concerns a double-blind investigation on Silymarin and its effect in treating cirrhosis of the liver. This study made note of a significantly higher survival rate in seriously ill patients when they were treated with this herbal medicine[187]. Another, looking into its underlying hepatoprotective properties, suggests that one if its most important activities may be to increase levels of stored glutathione in the liver[188]. Glutathione is an antioxidant amino acid peptide that is vital to the liver's ability to remove toxins from the body. Depletion of this vital nutrient is also an important marker of liver stress with the use of c-17 alpha alkylated compounds, suggesting that Silymarin may indeed be directly beneficial to the steroid-using athlete.

The typical dosage used is in the range of 300mg to 600mg daily. A standardized milk thistle extract contains about 80% active Silymarin, which would equate to about 240 mg to 480mg of total Silymarin flavonoids. Bodybuilders will typically use this product daily during a cycle with liver toxic steroids, and continue to use it for 4 to 6 weeks after the cycle is discontinued in hopes that it will help normalize liver enzyme values, and repair damage that may have been done during the cycle. Studies do suggest, however, that Silymarin also has notable anti-inflammatory properties (inhibiting prostaglandin biosynthesis)[189], which we know through recent studies is a trait that interferes with the protein synthesis response to resistance exercise (for a more detailed discussion, please refer to the NSAIDs drug profile). This may indicate the need to take somewhat of a "use if necessary" position, at least if absolute maximum muscle growth is the primary focus of your cycle.

Tationil (reduced glutathione)

Tationil is an injectable medication produced by Roche in Italy. It provides L-Glutathione in a form (called reduced glutathione) that may be given by intravenous infusion. Although this amino acid derivative is also readily obtained as a natural over-the-counter supplement, oral ingestion is an extremely ineffective route of administration. For example, studies have demonstrated that it is not possible to increase circulating glutathione levels with oral doses as high as three grams[190]. Injection, thus far, seems the only truly effective way to increase plasma and tissue concentrations of this important nutrient. Supplements containing L-Glutathione are, likewise, far from equivalents to this prescription medication.

L-Glutathione is an antioxidant that is made up of a tripeptide of three amino acids, L-Cysteine, L-Glutamic Acid and Glycine. Most glutathione in the body resides in the liver, where it is used in the breakdown and biliary excretion of many harmful compounds. It also plays an important role in the functioning of red and white blood cells, lungs, and intestinal tract. Although glutathione is an important antioxidant itself, it also is a vital building block for other antioxidant enzyme systems including glutathione-peroxidase, glutathione-reductase, and glutathione-transferase. Glutamine deficiency may manifest itself as coordination problems, cell damage, mental and nervous system disorders or tremors. Red and white blood cells may begin to stop functioning properly, and nerve tissues may even start to degenerate if ample levels of this antioxidant are not present in the body. Glutathione deficiency has been associated with a variety of health conditions including HIV infection, liver disease and some forms of cancer.

Normal glutathione levels are essential to the proper functioning of the liver, and glutathione depletion is a known marker of hepatic stress. Some studies, in fact, directly measure glutathione depletion as an indicator of how much strain a particular anabolic steroid compound may be placing on the liver. Oral (c-17alpha alkylated) steroid administration, of course, always places some strain on the liver due to the difficult-to-metabolize nature of these drugs. Replacing levels of glutathione that were lost because of them seems like an excellent way to minimize some of this stress. It is difficult to say just how much of a difference Tationil makes without a lot of blood work, but at the very least anecdotal evidence does seem to support that it makes a difference. The medical data certainly supports the hepatoprotective nature of this drug[191]. It is also being looked at as a treatment for Parkinson's disease, with one study reporting a notable improvement in neuromuscular functioning with IV use[192]. If your next cycle is to include a lot of oral steroids, or, perhaps more importantly, if you use them for prolonged durations and/or in regular intervals, Tationil may be something you want to look at.

Tationil comes in vials containing 300mg or 600mg of reduced glutathione. It is packaged in two separate containers, the same way recombinant human growth hormone is made. One vial contains a disc of lyophilized powder, and the other ampule contains a water solution. The two are mixed before use. In a medical setting, the typical recommended dose is 500mg daily, given patients via IV hookup. Bodybuilders are probably not going to use this much drug, and will typically experiment with 2-3 injections per week of either the 300mg or 600mg dose. Although IV is probably a much better way of using this drug, most athletes using this outside of a hospital setting are probably going to opt to use it as an intramuscular injection. We have no data on exactly how much of a difference this makes to the total bioavailability of glutathione. For this reason, proper IV infusion (with fluids), for those who can find a way to do this, would be the preferred method of use.

Masking Agents

DRUG PROFILES

Epitestosterone

Epitestosterone is an epimer of testosterone that is naturally produced in the body parallel with our primary androgen. It is identical to testosterone except for the lack of a 17-beta hydroxyl group, a trait necessary for androgen receptor binding. Although scientists long thought that epitestosterone was inert and served no biological function, we have since come to understand that it does play a role in regulating hormone activity. It weakly antagonizes the androgen receptor, inhibits testosterone biosynthesis, and prevents the reduction of testosterone to DHT[193]. Through these actions, it is believed to play a counter role in regulating such things as prostate growth and body hair distribution. If you think these facts make epitestosterone completely worthless as a performance-enhancing drug, think again. "Epitest" holds tremendous value as a masking agent, capable of skewing the results of a urinalysis screen so the illicit use of exogenous testosterone can be hidden. It may not improve performance itself, but it definitely is used in the realm of performance enhancement.

To understand how epitestosterone works as a masking agent, you need to first understand how testosterone is detected in the dreaded "piss test". Because testosterone is a material found in your body naturally, it hasn't been easy for scientists to come up with a method for detecting it. Early analytical methods, which are still largely applied today, can't tell the difference between testosterone that was injected and testosterone that your body manufactured itself. It all just appears as testosterone. To plug a hole in testing that is comparable to the size of the Holland Tunnel, a detection method was devised that relies on comparing levels of testosterone to those of epitestosterone, which your body manufactures at the same time. Normally these two compounds are produced in a 1:1 ratio; however, there are some variances in the natural chemistry of people that would allow for this figure to be different. Therefore, the IOC adopted a 6:1 ratio threshold that would allow for the natural differences in people without wrongly failing anyone. This means that if your urine screen shows your level of testosterone to be more than 6 times your level of epitestosterone, it is assumed you are using testosterone drugs.

Because the majority of people fall well below the 6:1 ratio threshold, the average athlete can get away with using a couple hundred milligrams of testosterone per week without failing a drug test. It is often thought of as a welcome loophole that allows for "a little something" to be used. But epitestosterone changes things considerably. It allows the athlete to break out of the constraints of testosterone/epitestosterone ratio testing, and use as much exogenous testosterone as they deem necessary to aid their performance. You simply need to take epitestosterone in similar doses to the testosterone drugs you are using, and your ratio will continue to read normal on a urine test. It can also be used in a single high dose shortly before testing, to correct an imbalanced ratio quickly. This way the athlete only needs to obtain a small amount of epitestosterone, which they can hold for the day it will be needed. Even if your testosterone to epitestosterone ratio becomes abnormally low from this practice, it will likely be perceived as a testing error instead of a failure for epitestosterone use.

Epitestosterone is not considered an anabolic steroid, nor is it a controlled drug in the United States at this time. Even though it is technically not an illegal substance, it is not an easy one to obtain. It is not sold as a commercial steroid, and is only scarcely available as a research chemical. Don't expect to pick some up with a couple of phone calls. However, for many in the upper echelons of competitive sports, it does seem to make itself available. Sources are likely diverting research material, or having it synthesized in private labs inside and outside the country. The existence of manufactured epitestosterone, and its ability to defeat a urine screen, has been known to testing officials for a long time. This has driven scientists to search for detection methods that do not rely on hormone profiling for a long time. After decades of work, a test was finally developed, and it might just close the ratio loophole for good. It relies on isotope ratio mass spectrometry (GC/C/IRMS) to determine if the testosterone in your body was actually of endogenous origin. Until this detection method becomes adopted in all drug-tested tested sports, epitestosterone will remain a compound of unique and profound value to those athletes who can use it.

Probenecid

Probenecid is a competitive inhibitor of organic acid transport in the kidneys and other organs. It was first developed in 1951 by Bayer as an adjunct to penicillin therapy, at a time when this antibiotic was in clinically short supply. Probenecid was the result of a long drug development program at Bayer, who saw an urgent need for a pharmaceutical that would inhibit the tubular secretion of penicillin. Probenecid would increase the levels of antibiotic in the blood (sometimes by several hundred percent), as well as its overall active lifespan, so that a therapeutic effect could be achieved at a much lower dosage. Although this technically remains an approved use of probenecid today, the drug is now more often prescribed as a uricosuric agent. It promotes the excretion of uric acid (the only endogenous compound it is known to increase the excretion of), which makes it important in the treatment of gout and gouty arthritis.

This drug is of no interest to athletes as a uricosuric agent. They have discovered a very unique "off label" use for probenecid, namely that it can be taken to mask the detection of anabolic steroids and other banned medications during urine testing at athletic competitions. This is accomplished by the drug's very strong ability to inhibit renal glucuronidation, a chemical reaction that attaches a water-soluble molecule (glucose) to a compound it wants to clear from the body. This shift in solubility allows the kidneys to remove byproducts from the blood, transferring them into the urine and bladder. Glucuronidation is a primary pathway for the disposal of anabolic steroids. While probenecid is being taken, the level of steroid byproducts in the urine will be dramatically lowered[194]. Combined this with a large volume of water intake and the pre-event secession of drug use, the metabolite density in the athlete's urine can suppressed to a low enough level to bypass detection. Detection is more difficult with probenecid, but not impossible.

Probenecid is a relatively old drug by today's standards, and has seen extensive clinical use. It is considered safe and reliable, however, like any medication, it is not without its potential risks and side effects. For one, great care should be taken when using it with other medications. It will alter the blood concentrations, half-lives, and excretion patterns of many medicines, sometimes with dangerous consequences. Other potential side effects include headache, upset stomach, vomiting, loss of appetite, dizziness, skin rash, difficulty breathing or swallowing, or unusual bleeding or bruising. The latter side effects are most serious, and warrant immediate medical attention. Although a case could be made that this could the anabolic effect of anabolic steroids by preventing their excretion, there seems to be little interest in taking probenecid for this purpose. Most athletes feel there are too many unanswered questions with extended use, as such, have instead adopted it as a last minute (short-term) masking agent, and not an "anabolic enhancer".

The fact that Probenecid can block the renal excretion of steroid metabolites is not news to athletic organizations. Its value as a masking agent has long been uncovered and eliminated. Banning the use of this drug in competitive sports and developing a detection method for this compound itself[195] have successfully accomplished this, feats that were undertaken and actualized over a decade ago. To this day, the International Olympic Committee and related governing athletic organizations continue to test for the prohibited use of Probenecid, and consider its use as serious an offense as any drug that it might be potentially masking. Therefore, there is currently no practical application for this drug unless you have somehow found a sport that has decided not (or doesn't know) to test for it.

Probenecid is sold by prescription in most countries, and found in numerous generic and "brand name" forms. U.S. brands include Benemid and Probalan, while Benuryl is most popular in Canada. Most formulations contain either 250 or 500mg, the latter being more popular. The typical therapeutic dose is in the range of 250-500mg (1 tablet) twice daily, amounts that would be common for use with athletes as well as patients. Sometimes, clinical requirements will call for as much as 2,000mg per day, which is considered the upper threshold of the safe dosage range for all purposes. There is a potential for death with severe overdose, so a "more is better" attitude should definitely not be taken with this agent. Also, you need to remember that this drug is being tested for practically every sport that tests their athletes for steroid use. It has become the official "masking agent of abuse" on all of the banned drug lists, and offers no value as such today.

REDUCTASE INHIBITORS

DRUG PROFILES

Avodart (dutasteride)

Avodart® (dutasteride) is one of the latest drugs in the treatment of benign prostate enlargement (BPH), gaining FDA approval as a prescription drug in 2002. Specifically, this agent is a 5-alpha reductase inhibitor, similar in action to Propecia (finasteride). Reductase inhibitors prevent the conversion of testosterone to its more androgenic counterpart, DHT (dihydrotestosterone). With androgens being implicated in numerous disorders in men including male pattern hair loss and benign prostate enlargement, DHT inhibition is an important treatment focus. Avodart® differs from the first generation reductase inhibitor, finasteride, in its tissue selectivity. Finasteride inhibits the type-2 isozyme of the 5-alpha reductase enzyme, which is found prominently in the scalp and prostate. Dutasteride, on the other hand, is non-specific for isotype (it inhibits both type-1 and type-2 reductase), and inhibits DHT conversion in all active tissues including the scalp, liver, prostate, and skin. It lowers systemic (whole body) levels of DHT much more effectively than finasteride, and represents a more effective "next generation" anti-DHT drug.

For bodybuilders concerned with the androgenic component of testosterone-based steroids, the release of Avodart® is big news. This drug is a substantial achievement in the minimization of androgenic side effects produced by DHT conversion, and is capable of changing the profile of testosterone measurably. When used with dutasteride, this potent androgen starts to become more like nandrolone in terms of its side effect profile. Maybe it will not be quite as weak in its level of androgenic activity as Deca (one of the least androgenic drugs known), but dutasteride will definitely allow testosterone to be a lot more "friendly" than it is normally. Occurrences of oily skin and acne should be considerably dampened, and the impact a steroid cycle will have on the hairline (for those genetically prone to baldness) somewhat reduced. Avodart® essentially finishes off what was started with finasteride. As a selective type-2 inhibitor, finasteride is effective at lowering DHT levels in the scalp, but it does not work as well for reducing oily skin and acne. Avodart® is an all around anti-DHT drug, effective at reducing androgenic side effects across the board.

It is important to remember a few things about dutasteride before running out to buy it. For starters, this drug does not stop all chances of noticing hair loss and acne. It works to minimize their occurrence by reducing, *not eliminating*, the level of androgenic activity in the body. This happens by preventing a moderately potent steroid (testosterone) from converting into a significantly stronger one (dihydrotestosterone). Testosterone is still a steroid. It mediates its effects through the same receptor that DHT does. This means that even if DHT conversion is blocked, testosterone is still capable of doing its job. There is a popular misconception that DHT is an unusual steroid in regard to hair loss, producing a side effect that other (non-DHT converting) steroids can't. Those who have this mindset might be tempted to take high doses of testosterone along with a reductase inhibitor, feeling they will not have any worries at all. They soon find that it is possible to take enough testosterone to compensate for the reduced levels of DHT conversion, making the cycle every bit as androgenic as a testosterone cycle.

You also need to remember that reductase inhibitors only effect testosterone, and its derivatives methyltestosterone and Halotestin. These three drugs are converted to stronger "dihydro" derivatives by the reductase enzyme. Nandrolone and most of its derivatives become weaker upon interaction with this enzyme, as their "dihydro" counterparts bind the androgen receptor very poorly. You definitely don't want to take Avodart® with Deca-Durabolin®, at least if side effects are your motivation. It will make them worse. Methandrostenolone and boldenone will undergo conversion to stronger 5-alpha reduced metabolites, but it occurs at such a slight extent in humans that it probably does not warrant the use of a drug like Avodart®. The rest of the synthetic anabolic agents are unaffected by reductase, making Avodart® inconsequential. Taking it during a cycle with anything like Winstrol, Primobolan, Dianabol, trenbolone, Anadrol, Anavar would be a waste of money. Avodart® is not a silver bullet anti-side effect drug, but is definitely worthy of consideration under the right circumstances.

Just as there are pluses to lowering 5-alpha reductase activity (less androgenic side effects), there are also minuses to the practice that should be taken into account. For one, the buildup of a strong androgen like DHT may be vital to the neuromuscular interaction, fostering strength, and even some muscle gain. Users of reductase inhibitors commonly report a drop in their maximum lifts soon after the drug is added, which is thought to be caused specifically by the drop in DHT levels. Libido may also decline as DHT concentrations are lowered, somewhat of a frequent complaint amongst users of the drug. A small percentage of men even find the need to keep Viagra on hand, as Avodart® renders them totally impotent. Dihydrotestosterone also serves as a potent endogenous anti-estrogen, as this non-aromatizable steroid competes with other substrates (like testosterone, which aromatizes) to bind with the aromatase enzyme. Gynecomastia or other estrogenic side effects may, therefore, start to occur when this competition is absent. Gyno is, in fact, listed in the warnings taking this product, although the frequency of this in testing was very low (1.1% of users).

In terms of exactly how effective this drug is as a reductase inhibitor compared to finasteride, we see a very substantial difference in how well these two agents work. This is demonstrated in a study published in the Journal of Clinical Endocrinology and Metabolism (May, 2004). It looks directly at dutasteride and finasteride and how these two drugs compare[196]. In this investigation 399 males suffering with benign prostatic hypertrophy (a large group of patients by most standards) was assembled. They were separated into three general groups, each receiving dutasteride (subdivided by doses of .01, .05, .5, 2.5 or 5.0 mg daily), finasteride (.5mg daily) or placebo, for a period of 24 weeks. Over the 24-week period, the dutasteride group noted by far the strongest level of DHT inhibition. The beneficial effects of this drug also occurred over a wide range of dosages. For example, 5mg daily amount caused 98.4% inhibition in DHT levels, while 1/10th of this amount (.5mg daily, the adopted therapeutic dose) lowered levels by an average of 94.7%. This was in great contrast to the 5mg finasteride group, which noticed only 70.8% inhibition. Researchers also noted that there was significantly more of a variation in the results of the finasteride group, with some patients noting DHT suppression in the range of only 50-55%. Clearly, dutasteride is much more effective.

Currently the price of Avodart® in your average U.S. discount pharmacy is about $2 per .5mg softgel capsule. This drug is also sold under the brand names Avolve and Duogen in Europe, which may offer slightly different pricing. One capsule per day is the given therapeutic dose, and since this drug is so effective at .5mg daily, there should be no need to exceed this amount. It is likely that even .25mg per day will provide strong inhibition in many users, however, being a softgel, you don't really have the option of breaking it in half to try this out. That means that on a per month basis, you are adding about $60 to your cycle, not a bad value if you want to use a testosterone product and acne and hair loss are strong concerns. Combine this with a new generation anti-estrogen like raloxifene ($3 per pill), and your monthly costs for keeping side effects down will be about $150. With such a hefty price tag, it is understandable why many athletes opt to ignore reductase inhibitors (or buy primarily anabolic drugs and avoid testosterone) and instead use the much cheaper Nolvadex to prevent gyno. But for those who would like optimal benefit and don't mind paying for it, a stack of Evista® and Avodart® is about the best you can get right now. They can't promise a side effect free cycle, but should make one based on testosterone, Halotestin, or methyltestosterone much more comfortable.

Proscar (finasteride)

Finasteride is a specific inhibitor of 5a-reductase, which is the enzyme responsible for converting testosterone into DHT (dihydrotestosterone). This drug can efficiently reduce the serum concentration of DHT, therefore minimizing the unwanted androgenic effects that result from its presence. The effect of this drug is quite rapid, suppressing serum DHT concentrations as much as 65% within 24 hours after taking a single 1mg tablet. Medically, this drug has been marketed to treat two specific conditions. The first release of finasteride in the U.S. was under the brand name of Proscar®, made for use by patients with benign prostate hyperplasia (prostate enlargement). More recently (December 1997), finasteride was approved for use as an anti-balding medication. We now have the additional brand name Propecia®, which is the same drug but the tablet contains only 1/5th of the Proscar® dosage. Scientists have long believed that DHT was the main culprit in many cases of male hair loss (along with genetic factors), so there was little doubt after the release of Proscar® that finasteride would eventually be used for this purpose. It has provided what many feel is a breakthrough for men with hair-loss problems.

Due to the very specific nature of finasteride, it has little effect on the other hormones in the body. It has no affinity for the androgen receptor, and does not exhibit any androgenic, antiandrogenic, estrogenic or antiestrogenic properties. It should have no impact on circulating levels of cortisol, thyroid-stimulating hormone, or thyroxine, nor should it alter HDL/LDL cholesterol levels. Changes in luteinizing hormone (LH) or follicle-stimulating hormone (FSH) are also not notable, and it is not shown to have an effect on the hypothalamic-pituitary-testicular axis. In a small percentage of cases the decreased DHT level did produce symptoms of sexual disinterest/dysfunction. Although this is not a common complaint, this problem can usually be resolved quickly by discontinuing the drug. It is also interesting that finasteride has been shown to increase the circulating levels of testosterone by roughly 15%, since a greater amount of the androgen is being left unaltered by the reductase enzyme.

Proscar®/Propecia® shows great potential for the steroid using athlete. And as you know, the dihydrotestosterone (DHT) metabolite is responsible for many of the unwanted androgenic side effects associated with testosterone use. The high levels of DHT that form in certain tissues produce oily skin, acne, facial/body hair growth and accelerated male pattern baldness. By minimizing the production of DHT, we should greatly reduce many of these harsh side effects and make our testosterone cycles more comfortable. In many instances, Proscar®/Propecia® can allow the athlete the use of steroid compounds (testosterone esters such as cypionate, enanthate, Sustanon etc.), Halotestin® and methyltestosterone with much less androgenic side activity. Of course we must not forget that all steroids activate the androgen receptor, so while this item offers help by means of reduced androgenic activity, not drug exists that can completely block androgenic side effects from appearing with steroid use.

One other thing to note is that finasteride specifically blocks the type II 5a reductase enzyme. There are actually two "isozymes" in the human body, labeled as type I and type II. Type I 5a-reductase is predominant in the sebaceous glands of most regions of skin. The Type II 5a-reductase isozyme is primarily found in prostate and hair follicles (among others). So although the type II enzyme is responsible for about two-thirds of the circulating DHT, a small amount of DHT may still be produced in the body by the type I enzyme. Finasteride may therefore have a more pronounced effect when preventing hair loss, and be somewhat of a lesser benefit when dealing with acne and body/facial hair growth (tissues where the type I enzyme is still active). Of course the drop in serum DHT will still have some beneficial effect on all related side effects. This is not a major concern in any event, as hair loss is really the primary worry amongst most male steroid users who would use this drug. A little oily skin or new hair growth on the back/shoulders can be dealt with by other means or simply endured. The user knows these problems will only be temporary. But the advancement of a balding condition can be very difficult, if not impossible to reverse. We must also remember that testosterone, Halotestin® and methyltestosterone are really the only hormones that converts to stronger steroids via 5-alpha reductase. Boldenone and methandrostenolone do also I guess, but to such a low degree that one would think Proscar would be of little significance. Perhaps we will come to find that some other steroids are broken down into stronger metabolites via 5a-reductase, but needless to say for now the uses of this drug are not great in number.

There is no research to site on exactly what dosage would be the most appropriate for a steroid user. Logic would dictate that the typically prescribed amount of Propecia®, a single 1mg tablet per day, would most likely be sufficient. In clinical trials the effect of just a single tablet is clearly dramatic. But if after a while the androgenic content of the cycle is still perceived as too high, increasing the number of tablets per day or perhaps switching to the stronger Proscar® (5mg tablet) may be necessary. Proscar®/Propecia® is also a relatively expensive compound, so it can become quite costly as the dosage increases. It is probably best to keep the dosage at the lowest effective amount. Cost may not be the only basis for such a decision, as DHT is believed to affect the nervous & reproductive system in many beneficial ways. By minimizing this conversion we not only face the possibility of interference with sexual functioning, but might also be inadvertently lessening the level of strength gained during testosterone therapy (this being tied to the actions of DHT on the neuromuscular system). A “use only when necessary” position should likewise be taken in regard to this drug.

It is also important to note that while Women may receive some small benefit from the drug (although testosterone is really not a steroid for females), they must be very careful with it. Those who are, or might become pregnant, should never take or even handle a finasteride tablet. The DHT blocking action can cause severe developmental problems to an unborn fetus, even in very small amounts. Since the drug can be absorbed through the skin, handling a broken tablet may be all that is needed for such an occurrence. Since women generally stay away from testosterone, and the design of Proscar®/Propecia® has been strictly for men, as of yet there is little to report on the effectiveness of this compound for combating virilization symptoms.

SITE ENHANCEMENT

DRUG PROFILES

Caverject (alprostadil)

Caverject is Pharmacia & Upjohn's brand name for the injectable impotence drug alprostadil. This product appeared on the U.S. drug market in 1995, and was the first real effective drug introduced to treat impotence. Alprostadil is specifically a synthetically manufactured form of the natural prostaglandin PGE1, which has the ability to almost immediately (5-20 minutes) produce an erection when injected directly into the penis (PGE1 stimulates nitric oxide release, which is vital to the erectogenic process). This will be sustained for about an hour (in certain cases it can last as long as 4-6 hours, which is considered a prolonged erection). Injecting Caverject is probably not a pleasant experience (never tried it myself), however many patients do seem to report this form of impotency treatment extremely effective and reliable. Caverject was most popular before the advent of Viagra, which essentially accomplishes the same thing without the need for uncomfortable and embarrassing injections. Viagra was introduced only a few years after Caverject, so it no doubt has been cut into the expected sales of this drug considerably.

But bodybuilders (at least those without impotency issues) are looking at Caverject with something very different in mind. They are hoping it can be used as an effective pre-contest "site-enhancing" agent. I guess someone looked at Caverject with the idea that if it can swell the penis tissues, maybe injections into small muscles like the biceps, triceps, deltoids and calves can produce swell in these tissues as well. Caverject is definitely being pushed hard by a number of overseas online steroid-selling pharmacies with this very effect in mind. But is this a valid use for the drug, or just an attempt by these pharmacies to find an alternative to offer customers requesting the now discontinued site-enhancing steroid Esiclene? Unfortunately, there is little real-world feedback on Caverject in this regard, but the few people who have experimented with the drug seem to have been disappointed with its results. It may offer some effect, but if there is a true replacement for Esiclene, it is probably not going to be found here. The non-opioid analgesic Nolotil seems to be much more promising in this regard, and is also comparatively much less expensive to use.

Side effects from this drug seem to be very limited, and usually concern pain or discomfort at the site of injection. With a sensitive area such as the penis, a misplaced shot can definitely be an uncomfortable experience. In some cases this has included painful erections, burning or soreness, blood in the urine, numbness, or irregular ejaculation. Obviously many of these potential pitfalls are avoided with the "extra-penile" administration of the drug, leaving only some typical injection site pain to deal with. Aside from this, it is a relatively side-effect-free compound. Many patients actually continue to use Caverject over Viagra as their chosen form of impotency treatment because it does not cause the same problems for them (such as blurred or irregular vision, flushing, headaches, stomach discomfort or indigestion). Even factoring in the injection procedure, these people find Caverject to be the more comfortable option.

Alprostadil is readily available in the United States, where it is sold as a prescription drug. The brand name Caverject from Pharmacia & Upjohn is found in vials containing 10, 20 or 40mcg of alprostadil, as well as single-use syringe kits that contain a total dose of 5, 10 or 20mcg. At the pharmacy, a single kit of 6 vials of the 20mcg product will run you around $175, while the 40mcg version will run you a little shy of $200. The price for a 20mcg dose, in a single vial kit, is about $50 from a popular overseas mail-order pharmacy. There is little chance you will find this drug for a remarkably low price at any of the mail-order pharmacies. The market for this drug is pretty small, and as a consequence is not widely manufactured (not many companies competing for market share). Caverject is not considered a controlled substance, making it easy to divert this drug to the black market should a large demand arise (I do not expect it to).

Nolotil (metamizol)

Nolotil is a current popular trade name for the non-opioid antipyretic (fever reducing) and analgesic (painkilling) drug metamizol. It is also sold under the generic name dipyrone in many countries. On a milligram for milligram basis this agent displays a level of analgesic potency very similar to that of mild opiate agonists/antagonists tramadol and pentacozine[197]. Like these opioid drugs, it possesses no additional anti-inflammatory properties. Being first used as a medicinal product in the early 1920's, metamizol has a long history in the medical world. But since drugs of its class (pyrazolone derivatives) were thought to have too much potential for side effects, and more effective analgesics (opiates) were being readily utilized, the uses for metamizol remained very limited for decades. Only toward the end of the 20th century did this drug become (somewhat) more accepted for use in certain areas of the world.

Metamizol is sought after in the bodybuilding arena not for its analgesic properties, but because it has the odd benefit of being a reliable "site-enhancement drug" when given by injection. By this, I mean it can cause a temporary swelling of the muscle in which it was administered, giving the appearance of a larger and fuller muscle. Within a short period of time it can help a bodybuilder bring up a lagging body part, or even enhance an already prominent muscle to a noticeable (eye-catching) degree. The typical procedure involves injecting 2.5-5ml of Nolotil (1/2 to 1 5ml ampule) deep into the belly of the muscle. A *very* light workout is then done focusing on that muscle part in order to get blood flowing and help disperse the drug. This may be repeated for a few days to optimize the overall effect of the drug. Reports are that as much as an inch increase can be made on the arms in a single day with the use of this compound. If used in larger muscle groups, it is likely to produce an uneven "bumpy" look however, so it is recommended only to inject this drug on smaller muscle groups such as the biceps, triceps, delts or calves. The site-enhancing effect of this drug is unfortunately temporary, and tends to subside within a few days after the last injection.

Metamizol is considered somewhat of a controversial medication. Its known and potentially dangerous side effects include shock, blood abnormalities, kidney failure, and agranulocytosis (a sudden high fever and drop in white blood cell count). In a number of cases these effects have been fatal. Unfavorable safety data has actually caused a number of countries to withdraw the drug from the market, including the United States and Canada where sales were discontinued in 1977 and 1997 respectively. The incidence of such severe side effects appears to be low (by one estimate one in 20,000 patients will develop agranulocytosis), however, the fact that they do occur is cause for many to rethink the use of this medication. Certainly the opiates, barring their risks for addiction, have a much better safety profile as pain killing drugs when used under medical guidance. If you plan on using this drug as a site-enhancing agent, you should at the very least be aware of why this drug is no longer being sold in the U.S.

Metamizol is available as an oral, suppository and injectable medication. The latter, of course, is the sole interest of the bodybuilding community, as it is the only form that is capable of imparting a site-enhancing effect. The correct use of site-enhancement compounds have no doubt meant the difference between winning and losing for many competitive bodybuilders. The now-discontinued steroid Esiclene was a highly sought-after drug for years for this reason, earning itself a reputation amongst bodybuilders as *the* agent of choice for pre-contest body sculpting. Nolotil only seems to be an improvement on Esiclene. Those experimenting with this drug in particular have been extremely satisfied with the rapid onset of its effect, the user not needing the weeks of continuous injections required with Synthol. With Nolotil, the same thing can be accomplished in a fraction of the time, with no concerns over where all that deposited slowly metabolized oil will end up (I don't love Synthol for this reason). Nolotil is not a long-term fix by any means, but is definitely a standout product in the market for effective pre-contest "site-enhancement" agents.

Synthol

Synthol is perhaps one of the most controversial tools in the bodybuilders' arsenal of performance-enhancing compounds. Chris Clark, a German inventor and bodybuilder, developed it several years ago. When it first hit the market it was immediately met with widespread skepticism and criticism. Much of the criticism centered on ethical grounds, as Synthol is an injectable spot-enhancing agent that can produce a rapid increase in the size of muscles; but the increase is totally artificial. What I mean is that the product is purely cosmetic. It offers no strength or performance enhancing benefit, and any increase you are going to see is not going to be actual muscle tissue. For lack of a better description, Synthol is the do-it-yourself answer to plastic surgery.

There is no active drug in Synthol, only an oily solution that is difficult for your body to metabolize. How it works is remarkably simple. You inject the solution into your smaller muscle groups, and it will sit in the tissues for a very long time because your body has trouble breaking it down. It will sit for so long actually, that the body will start to encapsulate it between the fascicles (muscle fiber bundles). With repeated injections, a bolus deposit of encapsulated solution will build in the muscle, expanding its total girth. It reportedly will take years for the body to fully break it down, giving the impression of a solid and permanent gain in overall muscle size. Gains of 1 inch or more are very typical with this product.

What was in the bottle was supposed to be a closely guarded secret. Early on, it was said to contain some synthetically developed oil that could not be disclosed or duplicated. That apparently was not really the case. Dan Duchaine reportedly had a vial analyzed, finding it to contain only a simple blend of C8-C12 fatty acids (medium-chain triglycerides). This was mixed with small amounts of lidocaine, a local anesthetic often included in irritating medications to reduce injection site pain. Benzyl alcohol was also added, which is a common antimicrobial (preservative) agent in injectable drugs. It looked like we had cheap bottles of injectable MCT oil, which were being marked up to a price of a few hundred dollars a piece. Not quite a good deal for the consumer. But then again, the ingenuity of the idea probably did deserve to be rewarded.

The original Synthol has been copied countless times now, no doubt owing to the fact that Duchaine was able to give the world access to the "secret" recipe. You can probably find a half a dozen or so different Synthol-type products advertised in the back of your favorite bodybuilding magazine right now, with a wide variety of different names and gimmicked add-on ingredients. Like the original Synthol, all of them are sold under the guise of being topically applied "posing oils". Sitting in vials with normal "multi-dose injectable" rubber-stoppers, the clear unspoken fact, however, is that these are anything but topical products. After all, if they were, you would be spending an awful lot of money just to get a bottle of MCT oil to rub on yourself.

Since injections of Synthol in larger muscle groups tend to produce a very unsightly bumpy and uneven look, bodybuilders typically only use this product in the biceps, triceps, shoulders or calves. The typical procedure involved starting with an injection of 1ML, placed deep into the belly of each muscle group targeted. This is repeated every day or two for about a week, maybe ten days. After this point, the amount administered is increased to 1.5-2ml per injection. This is continued for another week to ten days. If a desired increase is not produced after this, the user may increase the amount to 2.5-3ml per injection, given every day or two for another week or so. At this point the "loading" of Synthol is typically discontinued, and at best the bodybuilder will take a 1ml injection once or twice per week for a while (typically to around the time of a particular event) to help maintain the size increase. It might not actually be permanent, but the size gained with a cycle like this can stick around for quite some time, giving appearance it is.

I think if you told any doctor what the product was and how you intended to use it, he or she would tell you that you were fucking insane. The idea seems very risky, with a number of clear potential health concerns. We do not know if the product can cause long-term damage to your muscles for one, possibly leaving them with scarred tissues from the invasive injection solution. Such voluminous injections may also lead to infection and abscess. You might inject the fat into a vein or artery causing other serious problems. The bolus dose of oil could be transported into the lungs, causing a pulmonary embolism, or maybe even into the brain causing a stroke. There are just too many unanswered questions to ever recommend this product. But even with these risks known, many feel the rewards far outweigh them. Until people start dropping like flies from using this product, which does not appear to be happening, Synthol will likely remain a popular, but rarely talked about, part of bodybuilding

TANNING AGENTS

DRUG PROFILES

Trisoralen (trioxsalen)

Trisoralen® is a trade name (ICN) for the synthetic melanizing agent trioxsalen. As you may be familiar with, the normal pigmentation of the skin is due to melanin. This chemical is produced in the melanocytes, which are located in the base layers of the epidermis (skin). Melanin is formed by an enzyme reaction, involving the conversion of tyrosine to DOPA via the enzyme tyrosinase. Radiant energy in the form of ultraviolet light is needed to complete this process, hence the procedure of tanning. The exact mechanism in which Trisoralen takes its action is not clear however. Some investigators feel that this drug has a direct impact on the epidermis, or more specifically the melanocytes. Others feel its action is an inflammatory one, and that the process of increased melanogenesis is only a secondary effect. Whatever the exact path, Trisoralen can clearly increase the rate in which the skin is pigmented.

Medically this drug is used to treat a number of specific skin conditions. For starters, it is used effectively with various cases of vitiligo. This is a disorder that involves a marked loss of skin pigmentation. In many instances it will take on a very blotchy, uneven appearance. Depending on the intensity of this problem, Trisoralen may need to be used for a number of consecutive months in order to slowly and safely rebuild the skin's appearance. In many instances periodic treatment will be continued indefinitely so as to control any future progress of the disease. Trisoralen is also used when an increase in a patient's tolerance to sunlight is necessary. The extreme would be cases of albinism, in which the body is manufacturing no pigment. While Trisoralen will not stimulate new coloring, it can prevent severe sunburns by increasing the exposure time it will take for damage to occur. This protective action is accomplished by a greater retention of melanin in the skin, although the full melanagenic process cannot be completed. More basically, fair skinned individuals use Trisoralen in order to reduce the tendency to burn when tanning or out in direct sunlight. In many instances people will use this drug in order to prepare themselves for a tropical vacation. Regular use prior to the trip should greatly increase the amount of time one can spend in direct sunlight, and also increase the tendency to tan instead of burn.

Competitive bodybuilders find this drug extremely useful when readying for a stage appearance. It is no secret that a dark tan will make the physique look much more appealing. Muscle features seem to be markedly improved with tanning, resulting in a more "ripped" and impressive look on stage. Many bodybuilders, especially fair skinned individuals, have trouble developing a very dark skin base. Although the use of various skin dyes (sun-less tanning products) may be popular, a tanning agent like Trisoralen will produce a much more natural look. This drug has therefore proven to be invaluable to many top-level competitors, whom may otherwise have a frustrating time when developing their show physiques.

The typical routine is to take two 5mg tablets, 2 to 4 hours before sun exposure. When beginning therapy, it is important to gradually increase the sun (or tanning bed) exposure time, as this drug may cause severe burning if exposure is too great. It is also important not to increase the amount of tablets taken from this point, as the chance for burning (or blistering!) will notably increase with the dosage. Should the user accidentally take too high a dosage, or be noticing an uncomfortable burn after the drug is taken, he/she should remove themselves from light (as much as possible) for the next 8 hours. It is also of note that some users complain about stomach upset with this compound. Taking the drug with milk or after a meal will generally diminish this effect. Others may need to lower the dosage to 5mg, which in many instances is more tolerable. This amount is still enough to elicit a beneficial effect, but it will appear more slowly. This drug has also been shown to place some strain on the liver. Cautious individuals may therefore wish to limit the intake of Trisoralen to no more than two to four weeks. In fact two weeks is the typical cut-off point when the drug is prescribed to increase a patient's sun tolerance. Since bodybuilders are generally only taking this drug for short periods of time before a show, this is probably not a major concern.

Oxsoralen (methoxsalen)

Oxsoralen (methoxsalen) is a repigmenting agent that is being manufactured by the international pharmaceutical firm ICN. It is similar in structure and action to Trisoralen (trioxsalen), a drug that ICN used to market in the U.S. Both of these drugs belong to a class of medicines known as psoralens, which are used along with ultra violet light exposure to treat certain disorders of the skin such as Vitiligo (where skin pigment is lost) and psoriasis (a skin condition characterized by red and scaly blotches). Although the exact underlying mechanism behind these agents is unknown, they ultimately work to increase the output of melanin in response to stimulation by sunlight (or artificial UV exposure). This enhances the rate of pigmentation, which in many cases will allow the lighter areas of the skin to become more evenly colored.

Bodybuilders are attracted to psoralens because they may be used to help them develop that deep tan that is so favored in the world of competition and modeling. A good tan helps bring out muscle separation and definition tremendously, to the point it is just about considered a necessity (most bodybuilders who won't tan on their own will apply an artificial brush-on tan). A natural tan usually looks much better (at least in an immediate sense), especially when you are going to be seeing people face to face. This drives many fairer skinned people to look for drugs that can help them achieve a deep bronze look that is otherwise difficult or impossible to achieve on their own. In this regard, Oxsoralen most certainly seems to deliver, at least for most people who have carefully and correctly used the drug.

It is important to remember that this drug offers you no protection from the sun. It is most certainly nothing like using suntan lotion. In fact, since it increases the skin's sensitivity to sunlight, it can actually make one much more prone to skin damage. Medical professionals never prescribe it for the simple purpose of cosmetic enhancement of ones "tan" for this reason. If asked, your doctor will most likely point out that it has caused very serious sunburns when it was not properly used, even to the point of increasing a person's chance of suffering from skin cancer and cataracts. Like getting too much sunlight, it can also cause your skin to prematurely age. There are many serious concerns with the use of this drug, so do not let the fact that it is used for something as simple as tanning fool you into thinking it is benign. It most certainly is not. I assure you, if you use it incorrectly, you may wind up wishing you never heard of Oxsoralen.

The actual dose used is usually tailored to one's bodyweight and individual sensitivity to the drug. For this reason most bodybuilders will start by taking a single capsule or tablet per day, and increase the drug slowly, over time, to a point no more than the recommended medical dose for their bodyweight. According to the accompanying paperwork, this would be a maximum of 40mg for one weighing 146-176 pounds, 50mg for a weight of 179-198lbs, and 60mg for people less than 255lbs. Exposure to sunlight or ultraviolet light also must take place a certain number of hours after you take the medicine, or it will not work. For patients taking the normal capsules of methoxsalen, this will be 2 to 4 hours after administration. For patients taking the Oxsoralin Ultra softgels (which are digested much more rapidly), they will need to wait only 1½ to 2 hours. The amount of time one spends exposed to light will usually also be increased slowly, starting with very brief intervals as the user becomes accustomed to the drug. The sheer number of variables, with both natural and artificial sunlight (time of year, location, total UV exposure), makes it impossible to give exact recommendations as to how long, so it will be important to judge your own exposure time and dosage response very carefully.

At the pharmacy, 30 tablets of Oxsoralen Ultra (10mg per capsule) will cost you about $180-$200. If you are lucky enough to find a way to get a prescription for it, there is only a slight savings advantage to be found in buying it from a pharmacy in Canada. With such prices, Oxsoralen is much more costly than Trisoralen on a per dose basis, but then again Trisoralen has been discontinued in both the U.S. and Canada, so it may be the only thing available to you. It may be possible to find a generic version, offering a much larger savings, if you look hard enough.

Testosterone-Stimulating Drugs

DRUG PROFILES

HCG (Human chorionic gonadotropin)

Chorionic gonadotropin is a hormone found in the female body during the early months of pregnancy (it is produced in the placenta). It is in fact the pregnancy indicator looked at by the over the counter pregnancy test kits, as due to its origin it is not found in the body at any other time. Blood levels of this hormone will become noticeable as early as seven days after ovulation. The level will rise evenly, reaching a peak at approximately two to three months into gestation. After this point, the hormone level will drop gradually until the point of birth. As a prescription drug, HCG offers us some interesting benefits. In the United States, we have the two popular brands, Pregnyl, made by Organon, and Profasi, made by Serono. These are FDA approved for the treatment of undescended testicles in young boys, hypogonadism (underproduction of testosterone) and as a fertility drug used to aid in inducing ovulation in women. When prepared as a medical item, this hormone comes from a human origin. Although there is often a fear of biological origin products, there is little research to be found regarding pathogen or sterility problems with HCG. The problems seen with human origin growth hormone are certainly not to be repeated with HCG, as this compound is obtained in a much different way.

While HCG offers the female no performance enhancing ability, it does prove very useful to the male steroid user. The obvious use of course being to stimulate the production of endogenous testosterone. The activity of HCG in the male body is due to its ability to mimic LH (luteinizing hormone), a pituitary hormone that stimulates the Leydig's cells in the testes to manufacture testosterone. Restoring endogenous testosterone production is a special concern at the end of each steroid cycle, a time when a subnormal androgen level (due to steroid induced suppression) could be very costly. The main concern is the action of cortisol, which in many ways is balanced out by the effect of androgens. Cortisol sends the opposite message to the muscles than testosterone, or to breakdown protein in the cell. Left unchecked (by an extremely low testosterone level) in the body, cortisol can quickly strip much of your new muscle mass away.

The main focus with HCG is to restore the normal ability of the testes to respond to endogenous luteinizing hormone. After a long period of inactivity, this ability may have been seriously reduced. In such a state testosterone levels may not reach a normal point, even though the release of endogenous LH has been resumed. Many who have suffered severe testicular shrinkage may be able to relate, as it is often some time before normal testicle size and feelings of virility are restored if ancillary drugs had not been used. The excessive stimulation brought forth by administration of HCG can likewise cause the testicles to rapidly return to their normal size and level of activity. We are not simply looking for it to fix the problem however, as the resulting high testosterone level can itself trigger negative feedback inhibition at the hypothalamus. Estrogen production is also heightened with the use of HCG, due to its ability to increase aromatase activity in the Leydig's cells[198]. This is due to the main action of HCG, namely the increase of cyclicAMP (a secondary messenger that regulates cellular activity). When stimulated by HCG, the ability of the testes to aromatize androgens could potentially be heightened several times greater than normal. This also may inhibit testosterone production, so we therefore use HCG only as a quick shock to the testes.

The usual protocol is to inject 1500-3000 I.U. every 4th or 5th day, for a duration usually no longer than 2 or 3 weeks. If used for too long or at too high a dose, the drug may actually function to desensitize the Leydig's cells to luteinizing hormone, further hindering a return to homeostasis. Timing the initial dose is also very crucial. If your were coming off a cycle of Sustanon for example, testosterone levels in your blood will likely stay elevated for at least 3 to 4 weeks after your last injection. Taking HCG on the day of your last shot would therefore be useless. Instead one would want to calculate the last week in which androgen levels are likely to be above normal, and begin ancillary drug therapy at this point. In this case HCG would be started around the third or fourth week. Likewise, after ending a cycle of Dianabol (an oral) your blood levels will be sub normal after the third day. Here you may want to begin HCG therapy a few days before your last intake of tablets, giving it a few days to take effect. One would also want to give some thought to the level of suppression that the cycle might have brought about. After an 8 week cycle of Equipoise® for example, 1500-2500 I.U. would likely be a sufficient initial dosage. The lower amount of hormonal suppression one associates with this drug would probably not require much more. On the other hand, 750-1000mg of Sustanon per week might incline the user to inject a much larger HCG dose, perhaps as much as 5000 I.U. for the opening application. It may thereafter also be a good idea to reduce the dosage on subsequent shots, so as to step down the intake of HCG during the two or three weeks of intake.

As discussed above, HCG acts only to mimic the action of LH. It is likewise not the perfect hormone to combat testosterone suppression, and for this reason it is used most often in conjunction with estrogen antagonists such as Clomid®, Nolvadex® or cyclofenil. These drugs have a different effect on the regulating system, namely inhibiting estrogen-induced suppression at the hypothalamus. This of course also helps to restore the release of testosterone, although through a much different mechanism than HCG. A combination of both drugs appears to be very synergistic, HCG providing an immediate effect on the testes (shocking them out of inactivity) while the antiestrogen helps later to block inhibition on the hypothalamus and resume the normal release of gonadotropins from the pituitary. The typical procedure involves giving the Clomid®/Nolvadex® dose from the start with HCG, but continuing it alone for a few weeks once HCG has been discontinued. This practice should effectively raise testosterone levels, which will hopefully remain stable once Clomid®/Nolvadex® have been discontinued. While unfortunately there is no way to retain all of the muscle gains produced by anabolic steroids, using ancillaries to restore a balanced hormonal state is the best way to minimize the loss felt with ending a cycle.

Below is a sample ancillary drug schedule after ending a moderate cycle of Sustanon® 250

MON	TUE	WED	THU	FRI	SAT	SUN
*Sustanon 500mg						
HCG 5000IU Clomid100mg	Clomid100mg	Clomid100mg	**HCG 2500IU** Clomid100mg	Clomid100mg	Clomid100mg	Clomid100mg
HCG 2500IU Clomid100mg	Clomid100mg	Clomid100mg	Clomid100mg	**HCG 2500IU** Clomid100mg	Clomid100mg	Clomid100mg
Clomid100mg	**HCG 2500IU** Clomid100mg	Clomid100mg	Clomid100mg	Clomid100mg	**HCG 1250IU** Clomid100mg	Clomid100mg
Clomid50mg	Clomid50mg	Clomid50mg	Clomid50mg	Clomid50mg	Clomid50mg	Clomid50mg
Clomid50mg	Clomid50mg	Clomid50mg	Clomid50mg	Clomid50mg	Clomid50mg	Clomid50mg
Clomid50mg						

*Last shot of cycle

When we find HCG, we see it is always packaged in 2 different vials (one with a powder and the other with a sterile solvent). These vials need to be mixed before injecting, and are to be refrigerated should any be left over for later use. This product is widely manufactured and easily obtained on the black market. To date counterfeits have not been much of a concern, although a couple of oddities have popped up (all in multi-dose vials). The current popular fake matches the fake green/gold Steris boxes in circulation (see counterfeit photos). Since many other preparations are available, this item is easily avoided.

Bibliography

[1] Role of androgens in growth and development of the fetus, child, and adolescent. Rosenfield R.L. Adv Pediatr. 19 (1972) 172-213

[2] Metabolism of Anabolic Androgenic Steroids, Victor A. Rogozkin, CRC Press 1991

[3] Androgens and Erythropoeisis. J Clin Pharmacol. Feb-Mar 1974 p94-101

[4] Effects of various modes of androgen substitution therapy on erythropoiesis. Jockenhovel F, Vogel E, Reinhardt W, Reinwein D. *Eur J Med Res* 1997 Jul 28;2(7):293-8

[5] Testosterone increases lipolysis and the number of beta-adrenoceptors in male rat adipocytes. Xu XF, De Pergola G, Bjorntorp P. Endocrinology 1991 Jan;128(1):379-82

[6] The effects of androgens on the regulation of lipolysis in adipose precursor cells. Endocrinol 126 (1990) 1229-34

[7] Visceral fat accumulation in men is positively associated with insulin, glucose, and C-peptide levels, but negatively with testosterone levels. Seidell JC, Bjorntorp L, Sjostrom L, et al.Metabolism 39 (1990) 897-901

[8] Effects of testosterone and estrogens on deltoid and trochanter adipocytes in two cases of transsexualism. Vague J, Meignen J.M. and Negrin J.F. Horm. Metabol. Res. 16 (1984) 380-381

[9] Testosterone injection stimulates net protein synthesis but not tissue amino acid transport. Fernando A, Tipton K, Doyle D et al. Am J. Physiol (Endocrinology and Metabolism) 38:E864-71,1998.

[10] Glucorticoid antagonism by exercise and androgenic-anabolic steroids. Hickson RC, Czerwinski SM, Falduto MT, Young AP. Med Sci Sports Exerc 22 (1990) 331-40

[11] Binding of glucorticoid antagonists to androgen and glucorticoid hormone receptors in rat skeletal muscle. Danhaive PA, Rousseau GG. J Steroid Biochem Mol Biol 24 (1986) 481-71

[12] Evidence for a sex-dependent anabolic response to androgenic steroids mediated by muscle glucorticoid receptors in the rat. Danhaive PA, Rousseau GG. J. Steroid Biochem Mol Biol. 29 (1988) 575-81

[13] Glucorticoid antagonism by exercise and androgenic-anabolic steroids. Hickson RC, Czerwinski SM, Falduto MT, Young AP. Med Sci Sports Exerc 22 (1990) 331-40

[14] The source of excess creatine following methyl testosterone. Samuels L. T., Sellers D. M., McCaulay C. J. J. Clin.

Endocrinol. Metab. 6 (1946) 655-63

[15] Ontogeny of growth hormone, insulin-like growth factor, estradiol and cortisol in the growing lamb: effect of testosterone. Arnold AM, Peralta JM, Tonney MI. J Endocrinol 150 (1996) 391-9

[16] Testosterone administration to elderly men increases skeletal muscle strength and protein synthesis. Am J Physiol 269 (1995) E820-6

[17] Testosterone deficiency in young men: marked alterations in whole body protein kinetics, strength, and adiposity. Mausas N, Hayes V, Welch S et al. J Clin Endocrin Metab 83 (1998) 1886-92

[18] Endocrinology 114(6):2100-06 1984 June, "Relative Binding Affinity of Anabolic-Androgenic Steroids…", Saartok T; Dahlberg E; Gustafsson JA

[19] Endocrinology 114(6):2100-06 1984 June, "Relative Binding Affinity of Anabolic-Androgenic Steroids…", Saartok T; Dahlberg E; Gustafsson JA

[20] Sex Hormone-Binding Globulin Response to the Anabolic Steroid Stanozolol: Evidence for Its Suitability as a Biological Androgen Sensitivity Test. J Clin Endocrinol Metab 68:1195,1989

[21] Twenty two weeks of transdermal estradiol increases sex hormone-binding globulin in surgical menopausal women. Eur J Obstet Gynecol Reprod Biol 73: 149-52,1997

[22] Aromatization of androgens by muscle and adipose tissue in vivo. Longcope C, Pratt JH, Schneider SH, Fineberg SE. J Clin Endocrinol Metab 1978 Jan;46(1):146-52

[23] The aromatization of androstenedione by human adipose and liver tissue. J Steroid Biochem. 1980 Dec;13(12):1427-31.

[24] Aromatase expression in the human male. Brodie A, Inkster S, Yue W. Mol Cell Endocrinol 2001 Jun 10;178(1-2):23-8

[25] A review of brain aromatase cytochrome P450. Lephart ED. Brain Res Brain Res Rev 1996 Jun;22(1):1-26

[26] Aromatization by skeletal muscle. Matsumine H, Hirato K, Yanaihara T, Tamada T, Yoshida M. J Clin Endocrinol Metab 1986 Sep;63(3):717-20

[27] Pentose Cycle Activity in Muscle from Fetal, Neonatal and Infant Rhesus Monkeys. Arch Biochem Biophys 117:275-81 1966

[28] The pentose phosphate pathway in regenerating skeletal muscle. Biochem J 170: 17 1978

[29] Aromatization of androgens to estrogens mediates increased activity of glucose 6-phosphate dehydrogenase in rat levator ani muscle. Endocrinol 106(2):440-43 1980

[30] Influence of tamoxifen, aminoglutethimide and goserelin on human plasma IGF-1 levels in breast cancer patients. J steroid Biochem Mol Bio 41:541-3,1992

[31] Activation of the somatotropic axis by testosterone in adult males: Evidence for the role of aromatization. J Clin. Endocrinol Metab 76:1407-12 1993

[32] Testosterone administration increases insulin-like growth factor-I levels in normal men. J Clin Endocrinol Metab 77(3):776-9 1993

[33] Androgen-stimulated pubertal growth:the effects of testosterone and dihydrotestosterone on growth hormone and insulin-like growth factor-I in the treatment of short stature and delayed puberty. J Clin Endocrinol Metab 76(4)996-1001 1993

[34] Modulation of the cytosolic androgen receptor in striated muscle by sex steroids. Endocrinology. 1984 Sep;115(3):862-6.

[35] Neural androgen receptor regulation: effects of androgen and antiandrogen. Lu S, Simon NG, Wang Y, Hu S. J Neurobiol 1999 Dec;41(4):505-12

[36] A comparative study of the metabolic fate of testosterone, 17alpha-methyltestosterone, 19-nor-testosterone, 17alpha-methyl-19-nor-testosterone and 17alpha-methyl-estr-5(10)-ene-17beta-ol-3-one in normal males. Dimick D, Heron M, et al. Clin Chim Acta 6(1961) 63-71.

[37] Unique steroid congeners for receptor studies. Ojasoo T, Raynaud J. Cancer Research 38 (1978) 4186-98

[38] Cytosolic androgen receptor in regenerating rat levator ani muscle. Max S.R. Mufti S, Carlson B.M. J Biochem 200 (1981) 77

[39] In vitro binding and metabolism of androgens in various organs: a comparative study. Kreig M., Voigt K.D. J Steroid Biochem 7 (1976) 1005

[40] Androgen concentrations in sexual and non-sexual skin as well as striated muscle in man. Deslypere J.P., Sayed A., Verdonck L., Vermeulen A. J Steroid Biochem 13 (1980) 1455-8

[41] Contrasting effects of testosterone and stanozolol on serum lipoprotein levels. JAMA 261:1165-8,1989

[42] High-Density Lipoprotein Cholesterol Is Not Decreased if an Aromatizable Androgen Is Administered. Metabolism, 39:69-74,1990

[43] Testosterone dose-response relationships in healthy yo0ung men. Shalender, Woodhouse et al. Am J Physiol Endocrinol Metab 281: e1172-81 2001

[44] Metabolic effects of nandrolone decanoate and resistance training in men with HIV. Sattler et al. Am J Physiol Endocrinol Metab 283: e1214-22

[45] Effects of an oral androgen on muscle and metabolism in older, community-dwelling men. Schroeder et al. Am J Physiol Endocrinol Metab 284: E120-28

[46] Detection of nandrolone metabolites in urine after a football game in professional and amateur players: a Bayesian comparison. Robinson N, Taroni F, Saugy M, Ayotte C, Mangin P, Dvorak J. Forensic Sci Int 2001 Nov 1;122(2-3):130-5

[47] Detection of norbolethone, an anabolic steroid never marketed, in athletes' urine. Catlin D, Ahrens B, Kucherova Y. Rapid Commun. Mass Spectrom. 2002; 16: 1273-75

[48] Schanzer W, Donike M. Anal Chim. Acta. 1993; 275: 23

[49] Androgens and Anabolic Agents: Chemistry and Pharmacology, Julius A. Vida, Academic Press 1969

[50] Les hormones anabolisantes du point de vue experimental. P.A. Desaulles. Helv. Med. Acta 1960 479-503

[51] Studies on anabolic steroids-8. GC/MS characterization of unusual seco acidic metabolites of oxymetholone in human urine. J Steroid Biochem Mol Bio 42:229-42,1992

[52] Methyltestosterone, related steroids, and liver function. DeLorimier, Gordan G, Lowe R. et al. Arch Int. Med 116 (1965) 289-94

[53] Short-term oxandrolone administration stimulated net protein synthesis in young men. Sheffield-Moore et al. J Clin Endocrinol Metab 84(8) 2705-11 (1999)

[54] Effects of Oxandrolone on Plasma Lipoproteins and the Intravenous Fat tolerance in Man. Atherosclerosis 19:337-46, 1974

[55] Oxandrolone and Plasma Triglyceride Reduction: Effect of Triglyceride-Rich Diet and High Density Lipoproteins. Artery 9:328-41,1981

[56] Plasma and Lipoprotein Lipid Responses to Four Hypolipid Drugs. Lipids 19:73-79, 1984

[57] Studies on the treatment of idiopathic gynaecomastia with percutaneous dihydrotestosterone. Clin Endocrinol (Oxf). 1983 Oct;19(4):513-20.

[58] Gynecomastia: effect of prolonged treatment with dihydrotestosterone by the percutaneous route] Presse Med. 1983 Jan 8;12(1):21-5.

[59] Comparative pharmacokinetics of three doses of percutaneous dihydrotestosterone gel in healthy elderly men--a clinical research center study. Wang C, Iranmanesh A, Berman N et al. J Clin Endocrinol Metab 1998 Aug;83(8):2749-57

[60] Transdermal dihydrotestosterone treatment of 'andropause'. Ann Med. 1993 Jun;25(3):235-41.

[61] Which testosterone replacement therapy? Cantrill JA, Dewis P, Large DM et al. Clin Endocrinol (oxf) 21 (1984) 97-107

[62] Contribution of Lymphatically Transported Testosterone Undecanoate to the Systemic Exposure of Testosterone after Oral Administration of Two Andriol Formulations in Conscious Lymph Duct-Cannulated Dogs. D. Shackleford, W. A.Faassen et al. J of Pharm and Exper Ther. 306:925–933, 2003

[63] The biological activity of 7 alpha-methyl-19-nortestosterone is not amplified in male reproductive tract as is that of testosterone. Endocrinology. 1992 Jun;130(6):3677-83

[64] Different Pattern of Metabolism Determine the Relative Anabolic Activity of 19-Norandrogens. J Steroid Biochem Mol Bio 53:255-7,1995

[65] Relative binding affinities of testosterone, 19-nortestosterone and their 5-alpha reduced derivatives to the androgen receptor and to other androgen-bidning proteins: A suggested role of 5alpha-reductive steroid metabolism in the dissociation of "myotropic" and "androgenic" activities of 19-nortestosterone. Toth M, Zakar T. J Steroid Biochem 17 (1982) 653-60

[66] Biosynthesis of Estrogens, Gual C, Morato T, Hayano M, Gut M and Dorfman R. Endocrinology 71 (1962) 920-25

[67] Aromatization of androstenedione and 19-nortestosterone in human placental, liver and adipose tissues (abstract). Nippon Naibunpi Gakkai Zasshi 62:18-25,1986

[68] Competitive progesterone antagonists: receptor binding and biologic activity of testosterone and 19-nortestosterone derivatives. Reel JR, Humphrey RR, Shih YH, Windsor BL, Sakowski R, Creger PL, Edgren RA. Fertil Steril 1979 May;31(5):552-61

[69] Studies of the biological activity of certain 19-nor steroids in female animals. Pincus G., Chang M., Zarrow M., Hafez E., Merrill A. December 1956.

[70] Influence of nandrolonedecanoate on the pituitary-gonadal axis in males. Bijlsma J., Duursma S, Thijssen J, Huber O. Acta Endocrinol 101 (1982) 108-12

[71] Norandrostenolone and noretiocholanolone: metabolite markers. Acta Clin Belg (suppl) 1:68-73,1999

[72] Biological half-lives of [4-14C]testosterone and some of its esters after injection into the rat. K.C. James, P.J. Nicholls and M. Roberts. J. Pharm. Pharmacol 1969 v21 p24-27

[73] Relative imporance of 5alpha reduction for the androgenic and LH-inhibiting activities of delta-4-3-ketosteroids. Steroids 29: 331-48,1997

[74] Estrogen receptor binding radiopharmaceuticals: II. Tissue distribution of 17 alpha-methylestradiol in normal and tumor-

bearing rats. J Nucl Med. 1983 Jun:24(6):522-8.

[75] Biosynthesis of Estrogens, Gual C, Morato T, Hayano M, Gut M and Dorfman R. Endocrinology 71 (1962) 920-25

[76] Metabolism of Boldenone in Man: gas Chromatographic/Mass Spectrometric Identification of Urinary Excreted Metabolites and Determination of Excretion Rates. Schanzer, Donike. Bol Mass Spec. 21 (1992) 3-16

[77] Nutritional and metabolic effects of some newer steroids. V. Norbolethone. Albanese, Lorenze, Orto, Wein et al. New York State Journal of Medicine (1968), 68(18), 2392-406.

[78] Testing for fluoxymesterone (Halotestin®) administration to man: Identification of urinary metabolites by gas chromatography-mass spectrometry. Kammerer R., Mardink J., Jangels M et al. J Steroid Biochem 36 (1990) 659-66

[79] Liver toxicity of a new anabolic agent: methyltrienolone (17-alpha-methyl-4,9,11-estratriene-17 beta-ol-3-one). Kruskemper, Noell. Steroids. 1966 Jul;8(1):13-24.

[80] T. Feyel-Cabanes, Compt. Rend. Soc. Biol. 157, 1428 (1963)

[81] Liver toxicity of a new anabolic agent: methyltrienolone (17-alpha-methyl-4,9,11-estratriene-17 beta-ol-3-one). Kruskemper, Noell. Steroids. 1966 Jul;8(1):13-24.

[82] Aromatization of 7 alpha-methyl-19-nortestosterone by human placental microsomes in vitro. LaMorte A, Kumar N, Bardin CW, Sundaram K. J Steroid Biochem Mol Biol 1994 Feb;48(2-3):297-304

[83] Clin Pharmacol Ther. 1963 Nov-Dec;30:734-9.

[84] Metabolism of anabolic steroid drugs in man and the marmoset monkey (callithrix jacchus)-I. Nilevar and Orabolin. Ward R., Lawson A.M., Shackleton C.L.H. J Steroid Biochem 8 (1977) 1057-63

[85] U.S. Patent # 3,060,201. 4-hydroxy-17alpha-methyl-3-keto-delta4-steroids of androstane and 19-nor-androstane series and esters therof. Camerino, Patelli, Sala. Oct 23, 1962.

[86] Anabolic steroid abuse and cardiac death. Kennedy MC, Lawrence C. Med J Aust. 1993 Mar 1;158(5):346-8.

[87] Comparative studies about the influence of metenoloneacetate and mesterolone on hypophysis and male gonads. Trenkner R, Senge T, Hienz H et al. Arzneimittelforschung. 1970 20(4) 545-7.

[88] Contraceptive efficacy and adverse effects of testosterone enanthate in Thai men. Sukcharoen N, Aribarg A, Kriangsinyos R, Chanprasit Y, Ngeamvijawat J. J Med Assoc Thai 1996 Dec;79(12):767-73

[89] Hormonal therapy of endometriosis. Metzger DA, Luciano AA. Obstet Gynecol Clin North Am. 1989 Mar;16(1):105-22.

[90] Edgren, Peterson, Jones, et al. Recent Progr. Hormone Res. 22, 305 (1966)

[91] Tetrahydrogestrinone Is a Potent Androgen and Progestin. Alison Death, Kristine McGrath et al. J Clin Endocrinol and Metab. 89: 2498-2500, 2004.

[92] Disposition of 17 beta-trenbolone in humans. Spranger, Metzler. J Chromatogr 564 (1991) 485-92

[93] Unique steroid congeners for receptor studies. Ojasoo, Raynaud. Cancer Research 38 (1978) 4186-98

[94] Characterisation of the affinity of different anabolics and synthetic hormones to the human androgen receptor, human sex hormone binding globulin and to the bovine progestin receptor. Bauer, Meyer et al. Acta Pathol Microbiol Imunol Scand Suppl 108 (2000) 838-46

[95] Unique steroid congeners for receptor studies. Ojasoo, Raynaud. Cancer Research 38 (1978) 4186-98

[96] Progesterone is not essential to the differentiative potential of mammary epithelium in the male mouse. Freeman, Topper. Endocrinology. 1978 Jul;103(1):186-92

[97] Protein synthesis in isolated forelimb muscles. The possible role of metabolites of arachidonic acid in the response to intermittent stretching. Smith, Palmer et al. Biochem J. 1983 214,153-61

[98] The influence of changes in tension on protein synthesis and prostaglandin release in isolated rabbit muscles. Palemr, Reeds et al. Biochem J. 1983 214,1011-14

[99] Protein synthesis and degradation in isolated muscle. Effect of n3 and n6 fatty acids. Palmer, Wahle. Biochem J. 1987 242, 615-18

[100] Dietary effects of arachidonate-rich fungal oil and fish oil on murine hepatic and hippocampal gene expression. Alvin Berger, David M. Mutch, J Bruce German, Matthew A. Roberts. Lipids Health Dis. 2002; 1 (1): 2

[101] Regular exercise modulates muscle membrane phospholipid profile in rats. Helge et al. J. Nutr. 1999 129:1636-42

[102] Exercise training reduces skeletal muscle membrane arachidonate in obese (fa/fa) Zucker rat. Ayre et al. J. Appl. Physiol. 1998 85(5):1898-1902

[103] Effects of physical exercise on phospholipid fatty acid composition in skeletal muscle. Andersson et al. Am. J. Physiol. 274 (Endocrinol. Metab. 37):E432-38 1998

[104] A human dietary arachidonic acid supplementation study conducted in a metabolic research unit: rationale and design. Lipids 32:415-20

[105] Effects of dietary arachidonic acid on human immune response. Nelson et al. Lipids 32:449-56

[106] Effects of dietary arachidonic acid on metabolism of deuterated linoleic acid by adult male subjects. Nelson et al. Lipids 33:471-80

[107] Influence of dietary arachidonic acid on metabolism in-vivo of 8cis,11cis,14-eicosatrienoic acid in humans. Nelson et al. Lipids 32:441-48

[108] A human dietary arachidonic acid supplementation study conducted in a metabolic research unit: rationale and design. Lipids 32:415-20

[109] Action of heptaminol hydrochloride on contractile properties in frog isolated twitch muscle fibre. Allard B, Jacquemond V, Lemtiri-Chlieh F, Pourrias B, Rougier O. Br J Pharmacol. 1991 Nov;104(3):714-8.

[110] Heptaminol chlorhydrate: new data. Pourrias B. Ann Pharm Fr. 1991;49(3):127-38.

[111] On the mode of action of heptaminol (author's transl)] Grobecker H, Grobecker H. Arzneimittelforschung. 1976;26(12):2167-71.

[112] Prostaglandins and the control of muscle protein synthesis and degradation. Prostaglandins Leukot Essent Fatty Acids. 1990 Feb;39(2):95-104

[113] Prostaglandins promote and block adipogenesis through opposing effects on peroxisome proliferator-activated receptor gamma. Reginato MJ, Krakow SL, Bailey ST, Lazar MA. J Biol Chem 1998 Jan 23;273(4):1855-8

[114] Effect of ibuprofen and acetaminophen on postexercise muscle protein synthesis. Trappe, White et al. Am J Physiol Endocrinol Metab. 2002 Mar;282(3):E551-6.

[115] Skeletal muscle PGF(2)(alpha) and PGE(2) in response to eccentric resistance exercise: influence of ibuprofen acetaminophen. Trappe, White et al. J Clin Endocrinol Metab. 2001 Oct;86(10):5067-70.

[116] Preclinical pharmacology of "Arimidex" (anastrozole; ZD1033)--a potent, selective aromatase inhibitor. J Steroid Biochem Mol Biol 1996 Jul;58(4):439-45

[117] High activity and tolerability demonstrated for exemestane in postmenopausal women with metastatic breast cancer who had previously failed on tamoxifen treatment. Kvinnsland S, Anker G et al. Eur J Cancer 2000 May;36(8):976-82

[118] The minimal effective exemestane dose for endocrine activity in advanced breast cancer. Bajetta E, Zilembo N et al. Eur J Cancer 1997 Apr;33(4):587-91

[119] Inhibition of adrenal corticosteroid synthesis by aminoglutethimide: Studies on the mechanism of action. Dexter RN, FishmanLM, Ney RC et al. J Clin Endocrinol 27 (1967) 473-80

[120] First generation aromatase inhibitors –aminoglutethimide and testololactone. Cocconi G. Breast Cancer Res Treat 1994;30(1):57-80

[121] Stereoselective inhibition of aromatase by enantiomers of aminoglutethimide. Graves PE, Salhanick HA. Endocrinol 105 (1979) 52-57

1.Beneficial effects of raloxifene and tamoxifen in the treatment of pubertal gynecomastia. Lawrence SE, Faught et al. J. Pediatr. 2004 Jul;145(1):71-6

2.Effects of raloxifene on gonadotropins, sex hormones, bone turnover and lipids in healthy elderly men. Eur J Endocrinol. 2004 Apr;150(4):539-46

3.Raloxifene decreases serum IGF-1 in male patients with active acromegaly. Dimaraki EV, Symons KV, Barkan AL. Eur J Endocrinol. 2004 Apr;150(4):481-7

[122] Antiatherogenic effects of adjuvant antiestrogens: a randomized trial comparing the effects of tamoxifen and toremifene on plasma lipid levels in postmenopausal women with node-positive breast cancer. Saarto T, Blomqvist C, Ehnholm C, Taskinen MR, Elomaa I. J Clin Oncol 1996 Feb;14(2):429-33

[123] Fulvestrant, Formerly ICI 182,780, Is as Effective as Anastrozole in Postmenopausal Women With Advanced Breast Cancer Progressing After Prior Endocrine Treatment. Howell A, Robertson JFR, Quaresma Albano J, Aschermannova A, et al. *J Clin Oncol.* 2002; 1:57.

[124] Fulvestrant, an estrogen receptor downregulator, reduces cell turnover index more effectively than tamoxifen. Anticancer Res. 2002 Jul-Aug;22(4):2317-9.

[125] Fulvestrant. Cheung KL, Robertson JF. Expert Opin Investig Drugs 2002 Feb;11(2):303-308

[126] Treatment of advanced breast cancer with formestane. Murray R, Pitt P. Ann Oncol 1994;5 Suppl 7:S11-3

[127] Pilot study of formestane in postmenopausal women with breast cancer. Joseph JK, Lim AK. Med J Malaysia 1998 Mar;53(1):37-41

[128] Formestane is feasible and effective in elderly breast cancer patients with comorbidity and disability. Venturino A, Comandini D. Breast Cancer Res Treat 2000 Aug;62(3):217-22

[129] Formestane versus megestrol acetate in postmenopausal breast cancer patients after failure of tamoxifen: a phase III prospective randomised cross over trial of second-line hormonal treatment (SAKK 20/90). Swiss Group for Clinical Cancer Research (SAKK). Thurlimann B, Castiglione M. Eur J Cancer 1997 Jun;33(7):1017-24

[130] Formestane in the treatment of advanced postmenopausal breast cancer. Possinger K, Jonat W, Hoffken K. Ann Oncol 1994;5 Suppl 7:S7-10

[131] Comparison of the selective aromatase inhibitor formestane with tamoxifen as first-line hormonal therapy in postmenopausal women with advanced breast cancer. Perez Carrion R, Alberola Candel V. Ann Oncol 1994;5 Suppl 7:S19-24

[132] An endocrine and pharmacokinetic study of four oral doses of formestane in postmenopausal breast cancer patients. Dowsett M, Mehta A. et al. Eur J Cancer 1992;28(2-3):415-20

[133] Formestane is feasible and effective in elderly breast cancer patients with comorbidity and disability. Venturino A, Comandini D. et al. Breast Cancer Res Treat 2000 Aug;62(3):217-22

[134] Formestane. A review of its pharmacological properties and clinical efficacy in the treatment of postmenopausal breast cancer. Wiseman LR, Goa KL. Drugs Aging 1996 Oct;9(4):292-306

[135] An endocrine and pharmacokinetic study of four oral doses of formestane in postmenopausal breast cancer patients. Dowsett M, Mehta A, King N, Smith IE, Powles TJ, Stein RC, Coombes RC. Eur J Cancer 1992;28(2-3):415-20

[136] A randomized, open, parallel-group trial to compare the endocrine effects of oral anastrozole (Arimidex) with intramuscular formestane in postmenopausal women with advanced breast cancer. Vorobiof DA, Kleeberg et al. Ann Oncol 1999 Oct;10(10):1219-25

[137] Hormonal effects of an antiestrogen, tamoxifen, in normal and oligospermic men. Vermuelen A, Comhaire F. Fertil Ster 29 (1978) 320-27

[138] Tamoxifen, serum lipoproteins and cardiovascular risk. Bruning P.F., Bonfrer J.M.G., Hart A.A.M., Jong-Bakker M. Br J Cancer 1988 Oct;58(4):497-9

[139] The antiandrogenic effects of delta 1-testolactone (Teslac) in vivo in rats and in vitro in human cultured fibroblasts, rat mammary carcinoma cells, and rat prostate cytosol. Vigersky RA, Mozingo D, Eil C, Purohit V, Bruton J. Endocrinology 1982 Jan;110(1):214-9

[140] Aromatase inhibition by delta 1-testolactone does not relieve the gonadotropin-induced late steroidogenic block in normal men. Smals AG, Dony JM, Smals AE et al. J Clin Endocrinol Metab 1985 Jun;60(6):1127-31

[141] Rapid endocrine effects of tamoxifen and testolactone in prostatic carcinoma patients. Leinonen P, Bolton NJ, Kontturi M, Vihko R. Prostate 1982;3(6):589-97 Related Articles, Links

[142] Enhancement of linear growth and weight gain by cyproheptadine in children with hypopituitarism receiving growth hormone therapy. Kaplowitz PB, Jennings S. Pediatr. 1987 Jan;110(1):140-3.

[143] Megestrol acetate vs cyproheptadine in the treatment of weight loss associated with HIV infection. Summerbell CD, Youle M, McDonald V, Catalan J, Gazzard BG. Int J STD AIDS. 1992 Jul-Aug;3(4):278-80.

[144] Effects of modafinil ingestion on exercise time to exhaustion. Jacobs I, Bell DG. Med Sci Sports Exerc. 2004 Jun;36(6):1078-82.

[145] Spiropent (clenbuterol): another choice for patients with chronic reversible airways obstruction. Su WJ, Perng RP..Chung Hua I Hsueh Tsa Chih (Taipei) 1991 Jan;47(1):13-7

[146] Oral tocolytic therapy with clenbuterol--clinical facts. Meinen K, Rahn M, Hermer M, Rominger KL, Kanitz T. Z Geburtshilfe Perinatol 1988 Jul-Aug;192(4):163-8

[147] Oral tocolytic therapy with clenbuterol--determination of the plasma level. Meinen K, Rominger KL, Hermer M, Rahn M, Kanitz T. Z Geburtshilfe Perinatol 1988 Jul-Aug;192(4):158-62

[148] Effects of beta(2)-agonist clenbuterol on biochemical and contractile properties of unloaded soleus fibers of rat. Ricart-

Firinga C, Stevens L, Canu MH, Nemirovskaya TL, Mounier Y. Am J Physiol Cell Physiol 2000 Mar;278(3):C582-8

[149] Long-term clenbuterol administration alters the isometric contractile properties of skeletal muscle from normal and dystrophin-deficient mdx mice. Hayes A, Williams DA. Clin Exp Pharmacol Physiol 1994 Oct;21(10):757-65

[150] The effect of the anabolic agent, clenbuterol, on overloaded rat skeletal muscle. Maltin CA, Delday MI, Hay SM, Smith FG, Lobley GE, Reeds PJ. Biosci Rep 1987 Feb;7(2):143-9

[151] Human fat cell beta-adrenergic receptors: beta-agonist-dependent lipolytic responses and characterization of beta-adrenergic binding sites on human fat cell membranes with highly selective beta 1-antagonists. J Lipid Res 1988 May;29(5):587-601

[152] Clenbuterol: a substitute for anabolic steroids? Prather ID, Brown DE, North P, Wilson JR. Med Sci Sports Exerc 1995 Aug;27(8):1118-21

[153] Clenbuterol and Spot Reduction. Dharkam. Muscle Monthly May 15,2001.

[154] Modalities of the food intake-reducing effect of sibutramine in humans. Chapelot D, Marmonier C, Thomas F, Hanotin C. Physiol Behav. 2000 Jan;68(3):299-308.

[155]Thermogenic effects of sibutramine and its metabolites. Connoley IP, Liu YL, Frost I, Reckless IP, Heal DJ, Stock MJ. Br J Pharmacol. 1999 Mar;126(6):1487-95.

[156]A randomized, double-blind, placebo-controlled, multicenter study on sibutramine in over-weighted and obese subjects. Zhao Y, Wang X, Yan Z. Zhonghua Yu Fang Yi Xue Za Zhi. 2001 Sep;35(5):329-32.

[157] Alpha-2 adrenoceptors in lipolysis: A2 antagonists and lipid-mobilizing strategies. Lafontan, Berlan et al. Am J Clin Nutr (1992) 22:219s-27s

[158] Adrenergic receptor function in fat cells. Arner P. Am J Clin Nutr 1992;55:228S-36S

[159] Alpha2-Antagonist compounds and lipid mobilization: evidence for a lipid mobilizing effect of oral yohimbine in healthy male volunteers. Galitzky, Taouis et al. Eur J Clin Invest (1998) 18, 587-94

[160] Plasma catecholamine levels and lipid mobilization induced induced by yohimbine in obese and non-obese women. Berlan, Galitzky et al. Int J Obesity (1991), 15, 305-15

[161] Effects of Yohimbine on Autonomic Measures are Determined by Individual Values for Area Under the Concentration-Time Curve. Grasing, Sturgill et al. J Clin Pharm (1996) 36:814-22

[162] Effects of ketotifen and clenbuterol on beta-adrenergic receptor functions of lymphocytes and on plasma TXB-2 levels of asthmatic patients. Huszar E, Herjavecz I et al. Z Erkr Atmungsorgane 1990;175(3):141-6

[163] Effect of prednisolone and ketotifen on beta 2-adrenoceptors in asthmatic patients receiving beta 2-bronchodilators. Brodde OE, Howe U et al. Eur J Clin Pharmacol 1988;34(2):145-50

[164] A double-blind clinical trial in weight control. Use of fenfluramine and phentermine alone and in combination. Weintraub M, Hasday JD, Mushlin AI, Lockwood DH.Arch Intern Med. 1984 Jun;144(6):1143-8

[165] Use and abuse of appetite- suppressant drugs in the treatment of obesity. Bray GA. Ann Intern Med 1993;119(7 pt 2):707-13.

[166] Alpha-2 Adrenoceptor Downregulation. Michalovich Dharkam Greutstein. Dirty Dieting Newsletter 1 (1997)

[167] The effect of chronic captopril therapy on adrenergic receptors, plasma noradrenaline and the vascular response to infused nopradrenaline. Kondowe GB, Copelad S, Passmore AP et al. Eur J Clin Pharmacol 32 (1987) 229-35

[168] Changes in plasma norepinephrine concentration and thrombocyte alpha 2-adrenoceptor density during long-term antihypertensive therapy with nitrendipine and captopril. Muller R, et al. J Cardiovasc Pharmacol. 1994 Sep;24(3):429-33

[169] Effect of captopril, losartan, and bradykinin on early steps of insulin action. Carvalho CR, Thirone AC, Gontijo JA, Velloso LA, Sand MJ. Diabetes 46 (1997) 1950-7

[170] Glucose intolerance in spontaneously hypertensive and Wistar-Kyoto rate: enhanced gene expression and synthesis of skeletal muscle glucose transporter 4. Katayama S, Inaba M, Maruno Y et al. Hypertens Res 20 (1997) 279-86

[171] Identification of an insulin-responsive element in the promoter of the human gene for insulin-like growth factor binding protein-1. J Biol Chem 268:17063-68,1995

[172] Evidence supporting a direct suppressive effect of growth hormone on serum IGFBP-1 levels. Experimental studies in normal, obese and GH-deficient adults. Growth Hormone and IGF Research 9:52-60,1999

[173] Growth hormone induced increase in serum IGFBP-3 level is reversed by anabolic steroids in substance abusing power athletes. Clin Endocrinol (Oxf) 49:459-63,1998

[174] The molecular responses of skeletal muscle satellite cells to continuous expression of IGF-1: implications for the rescue of induced muscular atrophy in aged rats. Chakravarthy MV, Booth FW, Spangenburg EE. Int J Sport Nutr Exerc Metab. 2001 Dec;11 Suppl:S44-8.

[175] Myostatin Is a Skeletal Muscle Target of Growth Hormone Anabolic Action. Wie Liu, Scott G. Thomas, et al. J Clin Endocrinol Metab 88:5490–5496, 2003

[176] Recombinant human growth hormone and recombinant human insulin-like growth factor I diminish the catabolic effects of hypogonadism in man: metabolic and molecular effects.
J Clin Endocrinol Metab. 2001 May;86(5):2211-9.

[177] The anabolic effects of IGF-1 in skeletal muscle after burn injury are not caused by increased cell volume. Fang CH, Li BG, James JH, Fischer JE, Hasselgren PO. JPEN J Parenter Enteral Nutr. 1998 May-Jun;22(3):115-9.

[178] Insulin-like growth factor-I and more potent variants restore growth of diabetic rats without inducing all characteristic insulin effects. Tomas FM, Knowles SE, Owens PC, Chandler CS, Francis GL, Ballard FJ. Biochem. J. (1993) 291 (781–786)

[179] United Kingdom multicentre clinical trial of somatrem. Milner RD, Barnes ND, Buckler JM, Carson DJ, Hadden DR, Hughes IA, Johnston DI, Parkin JM, Price DA, Rayner PH, et al. Arch Dis Child 1987 Aug;62(8):776-9

[180] Antigenicity and efficacy of authentic sequence recombinant human growth hormone (somatropin): first-year experience in the United Kingdom. Buzi F, Buchanan CR, Morrell DJ, Preece MA. Clin Endocrinol (Oxf) 1989 May;30(5):531-8

[181] Hepatoprotective effects of Liv-52 on ethanol induced liver damage in rats. Indian J Exp Biol. 1999 Aug;37(8):762-6.

[182] The effect of the heptoprotective agent LIV 52 on liver damage. Cas Lek Cesk. 1997 Dec 17;136(24):758-60.

[183] Hepatoprotective effect of Liv-52 and kumaryasava on carbon tetrachloride induced hepatic damage in rats. Indian J Exp Biol. 1997 Jun;35(6):655-7.

[184] Role of Liv-52 in protection against beryllium intoxication. Biol Trace Elem Res. 1994 Jun;41(3):201-15.

[185] Alcohol hangover and Liv.52. Chauhan BL, Kulkarni RD. Eur J Clin Pharmacol. 1991;40(2):187-8.

[186] Hepatoprotective effects of Liv-52 on ethanol induced liver damage in rats. Sandhir R, Gill KD. Indian J Exp Biol. 1999 Aug;37(8):762-6.

[187] [The influence of therapy with silymarin on the survival rate of patients with liver cirrhosis (author's transl)] Wien Klin Wochenschr. 1980 Oct 10;92(19):678-83.

[188] Selectivity of silymarin on the increase of the glutathione content in different tissues of the rat. Valenzuela A, Aspillaga M, Vial S, Guerra R. Planta Med. 1989 Oct;55(5):420-2.

[189] Silymarin, an inhibitor of prostaglandin synthetase. Experientia. 1979 Dec 15;35(12):1550-2.

[190] Johnston CS, et al. Am J Clin Nutr. 1993 Jul;58(1):103-105; Witschi A, et al. Eur J Clin Pharmacol. 1992;43(6):667-669

[191] Reduced glutathione protection against rat liver microsomal injury by carbon tetrachloride. Dependence on O2. Biochem J. 1983 Dec 1;215(3):441-5.

[192] Reduced intravenous glutathione in the treatment of early Parkinson's disease. Prog Neuropsychopharmacol Biol Psychiatry. 1996 Oct;20(7):1159-70.

[193] Epitestosterone. Starka L. J Steroid Biochem Mol Biol. 2003 Oct;87(1):27-34.

[194] Effects of drugs which influence renal transport systems on the urinary excretion of the beta 2-adrenoceptor agonist clenbuterol and the anabolic steroids ethinylestradiol and methyltestosterone. Gleixner A, Sauerwein H, Meyer HH. Food Addit Contam. 1997 Feb-Mar;14(2):143-50.

[195] Approach to the analysis of diuretics and masking agents by high-performance liquid chromatography-mass spectrometry in doping control. Ventura R, Fraisse D, Becchi M, Paisse O, Segura J. J Chromatogr. 1991 Jan 2;562(1-2):723-36.

[196] Marked suppression of dihydrotestosterone in men with benign prostatic hyperplasia by dutasteride, a dual 5-alpha reductase inhibitor. Clark RV, Hermann DJ, Cunningham GR et al. J Clin Endocrinol Metab 2004 May;89(5):2179-84

[197] Metamizol--a new effective analgesic with a long history. Overview of its pharmacology and clinical use. Fendrich Z. Cas Lek Cesk 2000 Jul 19;139(14):440-4

[198] Acute stimulation of aromatization in Leydig cells by human chorionic gonadotropin in vitro. Proc Natl Acad Sci USA 76:4460-3,1979

Appendix A: Drug Availability Tables - Listings by Generic Name

Generic Name	Trade Name	Dose	Packaging	Company	Country	Status	Vet
boldenone (blend)	Equilon 100	100 mg/ml	6 ml vial	WDV	Myanmar/Burma		VET
boldenone undecylenate	Ana-Bolde	50 mg/ml	10 ml vial	Forti	Argentina		VET
boldenone undecylenate	Anabolic BD	50 mg/ml	10 ml vial	SYD Group	Australia		VET
boldenone undecylenate	Anabolic BD	100, 200 mg/ml	10 ml vial	SYD Group	Mexico		VET
boldenone undecylenate	Anabolic-BD	100 mg/ml	10 ml vial	Grupo Tarasco	Mexico	[NLM]	VET
boldenone undecylenate	Bold 200	200 mg/ml	10 ml vial	Animal Power	Mexico		VET
boldenone undecylenate	Bold QV 200	200 mg/ml	10 ml vial	Quality Vet	Mexico		VET
boldenone undecylenate	Boldabol	200 mg/ml	10 ml vial	British Dragon	Thailand		
boldenone undecylenate	Boldebal-H	50 mg/ml	10 ml vial	Ilium/Troy	Australia		VET
boldenone undecylenate	Boldenol 25	25 mg/ml	10, 50, 100, 250ml vial	Comandina	Colombia		VET
boldenone undecylenate	Boldenol R	50 mg/ml	10, 50, 100, 250ml vial	Comandina	Colombia		VET
boldenone undecylenate	Boldenon	200 mg/ml	10 ml vial	Ttokkyo	Mexico		VET
boldenone undecylenate	Boldenona	50 mg/ml	10, 20, 100 ml vial	Biogen	Colombia		VET
boldenone undecylenate	Boldenona	50 mg/ml	10, 50, 100, 250ml vial	Vecol	Colombia		VET
boldenone undecylenate	Boldenona 200	200 mg/ml	10 ml vial	Pet's Pharma	Mexico		VET
boldenone undecylenate	Boldenona 50	50 mg/ml	10, 50, 100, 250ml vial	Servinsumos	Colombia		VET
boldenone undecylenate	Boldenona 50 Gen-Far	50 mg/ml	10, 50, 100, 250ml vial	Gen-Far	Bolivia		VET
boldenone undecylenate	Boldenona 50 Gen-Far	50 mg/ml	10, 50, 100, 250ml vial	Gen-Far	Colombia		VET
boldenone undecylenate	Boldenona 50 Gen-Far	50 mg/ml	10, 50, 100, 250ml vial	Gen-Far	Costa Rica		VET
boldenone undecylenate	Boldenona 50 Gen-Far	50 mg/ml	10, 50, 100, 250ml vial	Gen-Far	Dom. Rep.		VET
boldenone undecylenate	Boldenona 50 Gen-Far	50 mg/ml	10, 50, 100, 250ml vial	Gen-Far	Ecuador		VET
boldenone undecylenate	Boldenona 50 Gen-Far	50 mg/ml	10, 50, 100, 250ml vial	Gen-Far	El Salvador		VET
boldenone undecylenate	Boldenona 50 Gen-Far	50 mg/ml	10, 50, 100, 250ml vial	Gen-Far	Guatemala		VET
boldenone undecylenate	Boldenona 50 Gen-Far	50 mg/ml	10, 50, 100, 250ml vial	Gen-Far	Honduras		VET
boldenone undecylenate	Boldenona 50 Gen-Far	50 mg/ml	10, 50, 100, 250ml vial	Gen-Far	Nicaragua		VET
boldenone undecylenate	Boldenona 50 Gen-Far	50 mg/ml	10, 50, 100, 250ml vial	Gen-Far	Panama		VET
boldenone undecylenate	Boldenona 50 Gen-Far	50 mg/ml	10, 50, 100, 250ml vial	Gen-Far	Peru		VET
boldenone undecylenate	Boldenone-50	50 mg/ml	10 ml vial	Jurox	Australia	[NLM]	VET
boldenone undecylenate	Cebulin 50	50 mg/ml	10, 50, 250 ml vial	Provet	Colombia		VET
boldenone undecylenate	Crecibol	25 mg/ml	10, 30 ml vial	Unimed	Mexico		VET
boldenone undecylenate	Dynabolin 50	50 mg/ml	10, 50, 100, 250ml vial	Kryovet	Colombia		VET
boldenone undecylenate	Equifort	50 mg/ml	10, 50 ml vial	Purina	Brazil		VET
boldenone undecylenate	Equi-gan	50 mg/ml	10, 50, 100, 250 ml vial	Tornel	Mexico		VET
boldenone undecylenate	Equipoise®	50 mg/ml	10, 50 ml vial	Fort Dodge	Mexico		VET
boldenone undecylenate	Equipoise®	50 mg/ml	50 ml vial	Fort Dodge	U.S.		VET
boldenone undecylenate	Equipoise®	25, 50 mg/ml	50 ml vial	Ciba-Geigy	Canada	[NLM]	VET
boldenone undecylenate	Equipoise®	25, 50 mg/ml	50 ml vial	Solvay	Mexico	[NLM]	VET
boldenone undecylenate	Equipoise®	25, 50 mg/ml	50 ml vial	Squibb	Canada	[NLM]	VET
boldenone undecylenate	Equipoise®	25, 50 mg/ml	50 ml vial	Squibb	Mexico	[NLM]	VET
boldenone undecylenate	Equipoise®	25, 50 mg/ml	50 ml vial	Squibb	U.S.	[NLM]	VET
boldenone undecylenate	Equipoise®	50 mg/ml	50 ml vial	Wyeth	Canada		VET

Appendix A: Drug Availability Tables - Listings by Generic Name

Generic Name	Trade Name	Dose	Packaging	Company	Country	Status	Vet
boldenone undecylenate	Ex-Pois	50 mg/ml	10 ml vial	Agofarma	Argentina		VET
boldenone undecylenate	Ganabol	50 mg/ml	500 ml vial	Laboratorios VM	Bolivia		VET
boldenone undecylenate	Ganabol	25, 50 mg/ml	10, 50, 100, 250ml vial	Laboratorios VM	Bolivia		VET
boldenone undecylenate	Ganabol	50 mg/ml	500 ml vial	Laboratorios VM	Chile		VET
boldenone undecylenate	Ganabol	25, 50 mg/ml	10, 50, 100, 250ml vial	Laboratorios VM	Chile		VET
boldenone undecylenate	Ganabol	50 mg/ml	500 ml vial	Laboratorios VM	Colombia		VET
boldenone undecylenate	Ganabol	25, 50 mg/ml	10, 50, 100, 250ml vial	Laboratorios VM	Colombia		VET
boldenone undecylenate	Ganabol	50 mg/ml	500 ml vial	Laboratorios VM	Dom. Rep.		VET
boldenone undecylenate	Ganabol	25, 50 mg/ml	10, 50, 100, 250ml vial	Laboratorios VM	Dom. Rep.		VET
boldenone undecylenate	Ganabol	50 mg/ml	500 ml vial	Laboratorios VM	Ecuador		VET
boldenone undecylenate	Ganabol	25, 50 mg/ml	10, 50, 100, 250ml vial	Laboratorios VM	Ecuador		VET
boldenone undecylenate	Ganabol	50 mg/ml	500 ml vial	Laboratorios VM	El Salvador		VET
boldenone undecylenate	Ganabol	25, 50 mg/ml	10, 50, 100, 250ml vial	Laboratorios VM	El Salvador		VET
boldenone undecylenate	Ganabol	50 mg/ml	500 ml vial	Laboratorios VM	Guatemala		VET
boldenone undecylenate	Ganabol	25, 50 mg/ml	10, 50, 100, 250ml vial	Laboratorios VM	Guatemala		VET
boldenone undecylenate	Ganabol	50 mg/ml	500 ml vial	Laboratorios VM	Honduras		VET
boldenone undecylenate	Ganabol	25, 50 mg/ml	10, 50, 100, 250ml vial	Laboratorios VM	Honduras		VET
boldenone undecylenate	Ganabol	50 mg/ml	500 ml vial	Laboratorios VM	Panama		VET
boldenone undecylenate	Ganabol	25, 50 mg/ml	10, 50, 100, 250ml vial	Laboratorios VM	Panama		VET
boldenone undecylenate	Ganabol	50 mg/ml	500 ml vial	Laboratorios VM	Paraguay		VET
boldenone undecylenate	Ganabol	25, 50 mg/ml	10, 50, 100, 250ml vial	Laboratorios VM	Paraguay		VET
boldenone undecylenate	Ganabol	50 mg/ml	500 ml vial	Laboratorios VM	Peru		VET
boldenone undecylenate	Ganabol	25, 50 mg/ml	10, 50, 100, 250ml vial	Laboratorios VM	Peru		VET
boldenone undecylenate	Ganabol	50 mg/ml	500 ml vial	Laboratorios VM	Venezuela		VET
boldenone undecylenate	Ganabol	25, 50 mg/ml	10, 50, 100, 250ml vial	Laboratorios VM	Venezuela		VET
boldenone undecylenate	Legacy	50 mg/ml	50 ml vial	Technoquimicas	Colombia		VET
boldenone undecylenate	Maxigan	50 mg/ml	10, 50 ml vial	Inpel/Denkall	Mexico	[NLM]	VET
boldenone undecylenate	Mitgan 50	50 mg/ml	50 ml vial	California	Colombia		VET
boldenone undecylenate	Porkybol 1%	10 mg/ml	10, 50, 100 ml vial	Compania California	Colombia		VET
boldenone undecylenate	Sybolin	25 mg/ml	10 ml vial	Ranvet	Australia		VET
boldenone undecylenate	Ultragan	100 mg/ml	10 ml vial	Denkall	Mexico		VET
boldenone undecylenate	Ultragan	50 mg/ml	50 ml vial	Denkall	Mexico		VET
boldenone undecylenate	Vebonol	25 mg/ml	10 ml vial	Ciba-Geigy	Australia	[NLM]	VET
boldenone undecylenate	Vebonol	25 mg/ml	10 ml vial	Ciba-Geigy	Germany		VET
boldenone undecylenate	Vebonol	25 mg/ml	10 ml vial	Ciba-Geigy	Switzerland	[NLM]	VET
chlorodehydromethyltestosterone	Turanabol	10 mg tablet	500 tablet pouch	British Dragon	Thailand		
clostebol acetate	Alfa-Trofodermin	.5% gel	n/a	Farmitalia	Italy	[NLM]	
clostebol acetate	Alfa-Trofodermin	.5% gel	n/a	Pharmacia & Upjohn	Italy		
clostebol acetate	Megagrisevit-Mono	15 mg dragee	30 dragee box	Pharmacia	Germany	[NLM]	
clostebol acetate	Megagrisevit-Mono	10 mg/1.5ml	1.5 ml vial	Pharmacia	Germany	[NLM]	
clostebol acetate	Steranabol	20 mg/ml	2 ml ampule	Farmitalia	Italy	[NLM]	

Appendix A: Drug Availability Tables - Listings by Generic Name

Generic Name	Trade Name	Dose	Packaging	Company	Country	Status	Vet
clostebol acetate	Trofodermin Crema	cream	30 gram tube	Carlo Erba OTC	Italy		
clostebol acetate	Trofodermin Spray	n/a	30 ml spray	Carlo Erba OTC	Italy		
dihydrotestosterone	Andractim	25 mg/g	100 gram gel	Besins-Iscovesco	France		
dihydrotestosterone	Andractim	25 mg/g	100 gram gel	Chemec	India		
dihydrotestosterone	Andractim	25 mg/g	80 gram gel	n/a	Korea		
dihydrotestosterone	Andractim	25 mg/g	80 gram gel	Piette	Belgium		
dihydrotestosterone	Andractim	25 mg/g	80 gram gel	Servimedic	Uruguay		
drostanolone	Dromostan	50 mg/ml	5 ml vial	Xelox (export)	Philippines		
drostanolone propionate	Drolban	50 mg/1ml	1 ml vial	Lilly	U.S.	[NLM]	
drostanolone propionate	Mastabol	50 mg/ml	10 ml vial	British Dragon	Thailand	[NLM]	
drostanolone propionate	Mastabol	100 mg/ml	10 ml vial	British Dragon	Thailand		
drostanolone propionate	Masterid	100 mg/2ml	2 ml amp	Gruenthal	Germany	[NLM]	
drostanolone propionate	Masteril	100 mg/2ml	2 ml ampule	Syntex	Bulgaria	[NLM]	
drostanolone propionate	Masteril	100 mg/2ml	2 ml amp	Syntex	United Kingdom	[NLM]	
drostanolone propionate	Masteron	100 mg/2ml	2 ml amp	Cilag	Portugal	[NLM]	
drostanolone propionate	Masteron	100 mg/2ml	2 ml amp	Sarva-Syntex	Belgium	[NLM]	
drostanolone propionate	Mastisol	5% injection sol.	n/a	Shionogi	Japan	[NLM]	
drostanolone propionate	Metormon	100 mg/2ml	2 ml amp	Syntex	Spain	[NLM]	
drostanolone propionate	Permastril	100 mg/2ml	2 ml ampule	Cassenne	France	[NLM]	
ethylestrenol	Maxibolin	2 mg tablet	n/a	Organon	U.S.	[NLM]	
ethylestrenol	Maxibolin Elixir	2 mg/5ml	n/a	Organon	U.S.	[NLM]	
ethylestrenol	Nandoral	.5 mg tablet	100, 500 tablet bottle	Intervet	Australia		VET
ethylestrenol	Nitrotain	15 mg/4gram	60, 250, 1000 gram tube	Nature-Vet	Australia		VET
ethylestrenol	Orabol-H	100 mg/5g paste	30 ml plastic tube	Vetsearch	Australia	[NLM]	VET
ethylestrenol	Orabolin®	2 mg tablet	n/a	Donmed/Organon	South Africa	[NLM]	
ethylestrenol	Orabolin®	2 mg tablet	10 tablet box	Infar	India		
ethylestrenol	Orabolin®	2 mg tablet	n/a	Organon	Belgium	[NLM]	
ethylestrenol	Orabolin®	2 mg tablet	100 tablet box	Organon	Pakistan		
ethylestrenol	Orabolin®	2 mg tablet	n/a	Organon	United Kingdom	[NLM]	
ethylestrenol	Orgabolin	2 mg tablet	n/a	Organon	Indonesia		
ethylestrenol	Orgabolin	2 mg tablet	n/a	Organon	Netherlands	[NLM]	
ethylestrenol	Orgabolin	2 mg tablet	n/a	Santa	Turkey	[NLM]	
ethylestrenol	Orgabolin Drops	2 mg	n/a	Santa	Turkey	[NLM]	
ethylestrenol	Silabolin	25, 50 mg/ml	1 ml ampule	Farmadon	Russia	[NLM]	
fluoxymesterone	Android-F	10 mg tablet	100 tablet bottle	Brown	U.S.	[NLM]	
fluoxymesterone	Baojen	5 mg capsule	n/a	Ta Fong	Taiwan		
fluoxymesterone	Chinglicosan	5 mg capsule	n/a	Ciiphar	Taiwan		
fluoxymesterone	Ferona	1 mg tablet	30 tablet box	Sidus	Argentina		
fluoxymesterone	Flouoxymesterone cap	5 mg capsule	n/a	Yuan Chou	Taiwan		
fluoxymesterone	Floxymesterone	5 mg capsule	n/a	Chen Ho	Taiwan		
fluoxymesterone	Fluoxymesterone	10 mg tablet	100 tablet bottle	Rosemont	U.S.		

Appendix A: Drug Availability Tables - Listings by Generic Name

Generic Name	Trade Name	Dose	Packaging	Company	Country	Status	Vet
fluoxymesterone	Fosteron	5 mg capsule	n/a	Health Chemical	Taiwan		
fluoxymesterone	Fu Lao Shu	10 mg capsule	n/a	Ming Ta	Taiwan		
fluoxymesterone	Fuloan	10 mg capsule	n/a	New Chem & Pharm	Taiwan		
fluoxymesterone	Halotestin®	5 mg tablet	n/a	Galenika	YugoslaviaFRMR	[NLM]	
fluoxymesterone	Halotestin®	2, 5 mg tablet	n/a	n/a	Japan		
fluoxymesterone	Halotestin®	5 mg tablet	50 tablet bottle	Pharmacia	Canada		
fluoxymesterone	Halotestin®	5 mg tablet	100 tablet bottle	Pharmacia	Thailand		
fluoxymesterone	Halotestin®	5 mg tablet	n/a	Pharmacia & Upjohn	Philippines		
fluoxymesterone	Halotestin®	2, 5, 10 mg tablet	100 tablet bottle	Pharmacia & Upjohn	U.S.		
fluoxymesterone	Halotestin®	5 mg tablet	n/a	Pharmacia-Upjohn	France	[NLM]	
fluoxymesterone	Halotestin®	5 mg tablet	n/a	Upjohn	Denmark	[NLM]	
fluoxymesterone	Halotestin®	5 mg tablet	n/a	Upjohn	Finland		
fluoxymesterone	Halotestin®	5 mg tablet	20 tablet box	Upjohn	Greece		
fluoxymesterone	Halotestin®	5 mg tablet	20 tablet box	Upjohn	Italy	[NLM]	
fluoxymesterone	Halotestin®	5 mg tablet	n/a	Upjohn	Netherlands	[NLM]	
fluoxymesterone	Halotestin®	5 mg tablet	n/a	Upjohn	Norway	[NLM]	
fluoxymesterone	Halotestin®	5 mg tablet	n/a	Upjohn	Sweden	[NLM]	
fluoxymesterone	Halotestin®	10 mg tablet	100 tablet bottle	Warner-Chilcott	U.S.	[NLM]	
fluoxymesterone	Hysterone	20 mg tablet	100 tablet bottle	Major	U.S.	[NLM]	
fluoxymesterone	Lipaw	10 mg capsule	n/a	Long Der	Taiwan		
fluoxymesterone	Long	10 mg capsule	n/a	Century	Taiwan		
fluoxymesterone	ODK	5 mg capsule	n/a	Winston	Taiwan		
fluoxymesterone	Oralsterone	5 mg capsule	n/a	Long Der	Taiwan		
fluoxymesterone	Ora-Testryl	5 mg tablet	100 tablet bottle	Squibb Mark	U.S.	[NLM]	
fluoxymesterone	Sidomon	5 mg capsule	n/a	n/a	Taiwan		
fluoxymesterone	Stenox	2.5 mg tablet	20 tablet box	Atlantis	Mexico		
fluoxymesterone	Tealigen	5 mg capsule	n/a	Ming ta	Taiwan		
fluoxymesterone	Ton Lin	10 mg capsule	n/a	Chin Teng	Taiwan		
fluoxymesterone	Ultandren	1,5 mg tablet	n/a	Ciba	United Kingdom	[NLM]	
fluoxymesterone	Vewon	5 mg tablet	n/a	Yung Shin	Taiwan		
fluoxymesterone	Vi Jane	10 mg capsule	n/a	Shyh Sar	Taiwan		
fluoxymesterone	Waromom	5 mg tablet	n/a	Washington	Taiwan		
formebolone	Esiclene	1 mg drops	n/a	Biofarma	Portugal	[NLM]	
formebolone	Esiclene	5 mg tablet	n/a	Biofarma	Portugal	[NLM]	
formebolone	Esiclene	1 mg drops	n/a	LPB	Italy	[NLM]	
formebolone	Esiclene	2 mg/ml	2 ml ampule	LPB	Italy	[NLM]	
formebolone	Esiclene	5 mg tablet	n/a	LPB	Italy	[NLM]	
formebolone	Hubernol	5 mg dragee	n/a	ICN Hubber	Spain	[NLM]	
formebolone	Hubernol	1 mg drops	n/a	ICN Hubber	Spain	[NLM]	
furazabol	Miotolan	1 mg tablet	n/a	Daiichi Seiyaku	Japan	[NLM]	
mesterolone	Mesterolon	25 mg tablet	n/a	Brown & Burk	Philippines		

Appendix A: Drug Availability Tables - Listings by Generic Name

Generic Name	Trade Name	Dose	Packaging	Company	Country	Status	Vet
mesterolone	Mesterolon	25 mg tablet	n/a	Schering	Sweden	[NLM]	
mesterolone	Mestoranum	25 mg tablet	n/a	Schering	Denmark		
mesterolone	Mestoranum	25 mg tablet	n/a	Schering	Norway	[NLM]	
mesterolone	Pluriviron	25 mg dragee	30 dragee box	Asche	Germany	[NLM]	
mesterolone	Proviron	25 mg tablet	20 tablet box	Schering	Algeria		
mesterolone	Proviron	25 mg tablet	50 tablet box	Schering	Taiwan		
mesterolone	Proviron	25 mg tablet	20 tablet box	Schering	Turkey		
mesterolone	Proviron®	25 mg tablet	n/a	Alkoid	YugoslaviaFRMR		
mesterolone	Proviron®	25 mg tablet	n/a	Leiras	Finland		
mesterolone	Proviron®	25 mg tablet	20 tablet box	Scherimed	Spain		
mesterolone	Proviron®	25 mg tablet	n/a	Schering	Argentina		
mesterolone	Proviron®	25, 50 mg tablet	n/a	Schering	Australia		
mesterolone	Proviron®	25 mg tablet	50 tablet bottle	Schering	Austria		
mesterolone	Proviron®	25 mg tablet	50 tablet bottle	Schering	Belgium		
mesterolone	Proviron®	25 mg tablet	20 tablet box	Schering	Brazil		
mesterolone	Proviron®	25 mg tablet	20, 50 tablet box	Schering	Bulgaria		
mesterolone	Proviron®	25 mg tablet	20 tablet box	Schering	Colombia		
mesterolone	Proviron®	25 mg tablet	n/a	Schering	Costa Rica		
mesterolone	Proviron®	25 mg tablet	20 tablet box	Schering	Croatia		
mesterolone	Proviron®	25 mg tablet	20, 50 tablet box	Schering	Czech. Rep.		
mesterolone	Proviron®	25 mg tablet	20 tablet bottle	Schering	Dom. Rep.		
mesterolone	Proviron®	25 mg tablet	n/a	Schering	El Salvador		
mesterolone	Proviron®	25 mg tablet	20 tablet box	Schering	Estonia	[NLM]	
mesterolone	Proviron®	25 mg tablet	n/a	Schering	France	[NLM]	
mesterolone	Proviron®	25 mg tablet	50 tablet bottle	Schering	Germany	[NLM]	
mesterolone	Proviron®	25 mg tablet	20 tablet bottle	Schering	Greece		
mesterolone	Proviron®	25 mg tablet	n/a	Schering	Guatemala		
mesterolone	Proviron®	25 mg tablet	n/a	Schering	Honduras		
mesterolone	Proviron®	25 mg tablet	10, 15, 20, 50, 100, 150 tab btl	Schering	Hungary		
mesterolone	Proviron®	25 mg tablet	30 tablet box	Schering	India		
mesterolone	Proviron®	25 mg tablet	n/a	Schering	Indonesia		
mesterolone	Proviron®	25 mg tablet	20, 50 tablet box	Schering	Israel		
mesterolone	Proviron®	50 mg tablet	20 tablet box	Schering	Italy		
mesterolone	Proviron®	25 mg tablet	20 tablet box	Schering	Latvia	[NLM]	
mesterolone	Proviron®	25 mg tablet	20 tablet box	Schering	Lithuania	[NLM]	
mesterolone	Proviron®	25 mg tablet	10 tablet box	Schering	Mexico		
mesterolone	Proviron®	25 mg tablet	50 tablet bottle	Schering	Netherlands		
mesterolone	Proviron®	25 mg tablet	n/a	Schering	Nicaragua		
mesterolone	Proviron®	25 mg tablet	n/a	Schering	Panama		
mesterolone	Proviron®	25 mg tablet	20 tablet box	Schering	Paraguay		
mesterolone	Proviron®	25 mg tablet	20 tablet box	Schering	Poland		

Appendix A: Drug Availability Tables - Listings by Generic Name

Generic Name	Trade Name	Dose	Packaging	Company	Country	Status	Vet
mesterolone	Proviron®	25 mg tablet	20 tablet box	Schering	Portugal		
mesterolone	Proviron®	25 mg tablet	20 tablet bottle	Schering	Russia		
mesterolone	Proviron®	25 mg tablet	20, 50 tablet bottle	Schering	Slovakia		
mesterolone	Proviron®	25 mg tablet	20 tablet box	Schering	Spain	[NLM]	
mesterolone	Proviron®	25 mg tablet	n/a	Schering	Switzerland	[NLM]	
mesterolone	Proviron®	25 mg tablet	20 tablet box	Schering	Ukraine		
mesterolone	Proviron®	25 mg tablet	30 tablet box	Schering	United Kingdom		
mesterolone	Proviron®	25 mg tablet	n/a	Schering	Uruguay		
mesterolone	Proviron®	25 mg tablet	15 tablet box	Schering	Venezuela		
mesterolone	Proviron®	25 mg tablet	20, 100 tablet bottle	Schering/Berlimed	South Africa		
mesterolone	Proviron®	25 mg tablet	20 tablet box	Schering/CID	Egypt	[NLM]	
mesterolone	Provironum	25 mg tablet	50 tablet box	Organon	Singapore		
mesterolone	Provironum	25 mg tablet	150 tablet box	Schering	Thailand		
mesterolone	Restore	25 mg tablet	20 tablet box	Brown & Burk	India		
mesterolone	Vistimon	25 mg tablet	30 tablet box	Jenapharm	Taiwan		
mesterolone	Vistimon	25 mg tablet	20 tablet box	Jenapharm	Germany	[NLM]	
mesterolone	Vistimon	25 mg tablet	n/a	n/a	Korea		
methandrostenolone	Ammipire	5 mg tablet	1000 tablet bottle	Ammipire	Thailand		
methandrostenolone	Anabol	50 mg tablet	n/a	British Dragon	Thailand	[NLM]	
methandrostenolone	Anabol Tablets	5 mg tablet	1000 tablet bottle	British Dispensary	Thailand		
methandrostenolone	Anabol Tablets	5 mg tablet	1000 tablet bottle	L.P Standard	Thailand	[NLM]	
methandrostenolone	Anabolex	3 mg tablet	100 tablet box	Ethical	Dom. Rep.		
methandrostenolone	Anabolikum 2.5%	25 mg/ml	50 ml vial	Meca G	Germany	[NLM]	VET
methandrostenolone	Anabolin	5 mg tablet	n/a	Leiras	Finland	[NLM]	
methandrostenolone	Anabolin	0.5% cream	n/a	Leiras	Finland	[NLM]	
methandrostenolone	Anabol-Jet	25 mg/ml	30, 100, 250 ml vial	Norvet	Mexico		VET
methandrostenolone	Anabol-Jet ADE	30 mg/ml	100, 250 ml vial	Norvet	Mexico		VET
methandrostenolone	Anabol-Pet's	10, 25 mg tablet	200 tablet bottle	Norvet	Mexico		VET
methandrostenolone	Andoredan	5 mg tablet	n/a	Takeshima-Kodama	Japan	[NLM]	
methandrostenolone	Averbol 25	25 mg/ml	20 ml vial	British Dragon	Thailand		
methandrostenolone	Bionabol	2, 5 mg tab	40 tablet box	Balkanpharma	Bulgaria		
methandrostenolone	Bionabol	2 mg tablet	40 tablet bottle	Pharmacia	Bulgaria	[NLM]	
methandrostenolone	Bionabol	5 mg tab	40 tablet bottle	Pharmacia	Bulgaria	[NLM]	
methandrostenolone	Chinlipan Tab	2 mg tablet	n/a	Chin Tien	Taiwan		
methandrostenolone	Danabol DS	10 mg tablet	500 tablet bottle	Body Research	Thailand		
methandrostenolone	D-Bol	10 mg tablet	100 tablet bottle	Denkall	Mexico		VET
methandrostenolone	D-Bol	10 mg capsule	96 capsule box	Denkall	Mexico		VET
methandrostenolone	D-Bol	10 mg capsule	300 capsule bottle	Denkall	Mexico		VET
methandrostenolone	D-Bol	25 mg/ml	10 ml vial	Denkall	Mexico		VET
methandrostenolone	Dialone	5 mg tablet	100 tablet bottle	Major	U.S.	[NLM]	
methandrostenolone	Dianabol	10 mg tablet	100 tablet bottle	Salud	Mexico		VET

Appendix A: Drug Availability Tables - Listings by Generic Name

Generic Name	Trade Name	Dose	Packaging	Company	Country	Status	Vet
methandrostenolone	Dianabol	25 mg/ml	10, 50, 100 ml vial	Salud	Mexico		VET
methandrostenolone	Dianabol	5 mg tablet	100 tablet bottle	Ciba	Germany	[NLM]	
methandrostenolone	Dianabol	5 mg tablet	100 tablet bottle	Ciba	U.S.	[NLM]	
methandrostenolone	Dianabol	5 mg tablet	100 tablet bottle	Ciba	United Kingdom	[NLM]	
methandrostenolone	Dianabol	25 mg tablet	30 tablet bottle	Planet Pharmacy	Belize		
methandrostenolone	Encephan	5 mg tablet	n/a	Sato	Japan	[NLM]	
methandrostenolone	Ganabol	25 mg/ml	50 ml vial	Salud	Mexico	[NLM]	VET
methandrostenolone	Melic	5 mg tablet	1000 tablet box, bottle	Pharmasant	Thailand		
methandrostenolone	Metaboline	2 mg tablet	60, 500 tablet bottle	Desbergers	Canada	[NLM]	
methandrostenolone	Metanabol	5 mg tablet	20 tablet box	Jelfa	Poland		
methandrostenolone	Metanabol	5 mg tablet	20 tablet box	Polfa	Poland	[NLM]	
methandrostenolone	Metanabol	I mg tablet	20 tablet box	Polfa	Poland	[NLM]	
methandrostenolone	Metanabol	0.5% cream	n/a	Polfa	Poland	[NLM]	
methandrostenolone	Metandiabol	25 mg/ml	50 ml vial	Quimper	Mexico		VET
methandrostenolone	Metandienon	5 mg tablet	100 tablet box	Bioreaktor	Russia		
methandrostenolone	Metandiol 60	60 mg/ml	10 ml vial	Pet's Pharma	Mexico		VET
methandrostenolone	Metandiol Tab	10 mg tablet	100 tablet bottle	Pet's Pharma	Mexico		VET
methandrostenolone	Metandrol 10	10 mg tablet	500 tablet bottle	Bratis Labs	Mexico		VET
methandrostenolone	Metandrostenolon	5 mg tablet	100 tablet box	Akrihin	Russia	[NLM]	
methandrostenolone	Metandrostenolon	5 mg tablet	100 tablet box	Akrikhin	Russia		
methandrostenolone	Metandrostenolon	5 mg tablet	100 tablet box	Bioreaktor	Russia	[NLM]	
methandrostenolone	Methan Tabs	10 mg tablet	100 tablet bottle	Animal Power	Mexico		VET
methandrostenolone	Methanabol	5 mg tablet	500 tablet pouch	British Dragon	Thailand	[NLM]	
methandrostenolone	Methanabol	10 mg tablet	500 tablet pouch	British Dragon	Thailand		
methandrostenolone	Methanabol	50 mg tablet	100 tablet pouch	British Dragon	Thailand		
methandrostenolone	Methandienone	5, 10 mg tablet	100, 1000 tablet bottle	Ttokkyo	Mexico		VET
methandrostenolone	Methandon	5 mg tablet	1000 tablet bottle	Acdhon Co.	Thailand		
methandrostenolone	Naposim	5 mg tablet	20 tablet box	Terapia	Rumania		
methandrostenolone	Neo-Anabolene	5 mg tablet	10 tablet strip	Haurus	Indonesia		
methandrostenolone	Nerobol	5 mg tablet	20 tablet box	Galenika	YugoslaviaFRMR	[NLM]	
methandrostenolone	Nerobol	5 mg tablet	20 tablet box	Gedeon Richter	Bulgaria	[NLM]	
methandrostenolone	Nerobol	5 mg tablet	20 tablet box	Gedeon Richter	Hungary	[NLM]	
methandrostenolone	Pronabol-5	5 mg tablet	100 tablet box	P&B Labs	India	[NLM]	
methandrostenolone	Reforvit Simple	5, 10, 25 mg tab	100, 500, 1000 tablet bottle	Loeffler	Mexico		VET
methandrostenolone	Reforvit-B	25 mg/ml	10, 50 ml	Loeffler	Mexico		VET
methandrostenolone	Restauvit	2 mg tablet	n/a	Ciba, Rugby	Mexico	[NLM]	
methandrostenolone	Stenolon	5 mg tablet	20 tablet box	Leciva	Czech. Rep.	[NLM]	
methandrostenolone	Stenolon	1 mg tablet	20 tablet box	Leciva	Czech. Rep.	[NLM]	
methandrostenolone	Trinergic	5 mg capsule	n/a	Unimed	India	[NLM]	
methandrostenolone/stanozolol	Diosterol	50 mg tablet	30 tablet bottle	Planet Pharmacy	Belize		
methenolone acetate	Metabolon 25	25 mg tablet	100 tablet bottle	Bratis Labs	Mexico		VET

Appendix A: Drug Availability Tables - Listings by Generic Name

Generic Name	Trade Name	Dose	Packaging	Company	Country	Status	Vet
methenolone acetate	Metenol QV	50 mg tablet	50 tablet bottle	Quality Vet	Mexico		VET
methenolone acetate	Primobolan®	5 mg tablet	n/a	Schering	Austria	[NLM]	
methenolone acetate	Primobolan®	5 mg tablet	n/a	Schering	Belgium	[NLM]	
methenolone acetate	Primobolan®	5 mg tablet	n/a	Schering	Bolivia	[NLM]	
methenolone acetate	Primobolan®	5 mg tablet	n/a	Schering	Costa Rica	[NLM]	
methenolone acetate	Primobolan®	5 mg tablet	n/a	Schering	Dom. Rep.	[NLM]	
methenolone acetate	Primobolan®	5 mg tablet	n/a	Schering	Ecuador	[NLM]	
methenolone acetate	Primobolan®	5 mg tablet	n/a	Schering	El Salvador	[NLM]	
methenolone acetate	Primobolan®	5 mg tablet	n/a	Schering	Germany	[NLM]	
methenolone acetate	Primobolan®	5 mg tablet	n/a	Schering	Guatemala	[NLM]	
methenolone acetate	Primobolan®	5 mg tablet	n/a	Schering	Honduras	[NLM]	
methenolone acetate	Primobolan®	5 mg tablet	100, 1000 tablet box	Schering	Japan		
methenolone acetate	Primobolan®	5 mg tablet	n/a	Schering	Mexico	[NLM]	
methenolone acetate	Primobolan®	5 mg tablet	n/a	Schering	Nicaragua	[NLM]	
methenolone acetate	Primobolan®	5 mg tablet	n/a	Schering	Panama	[NLM]	
methenolone acetate	Primobolan®	50 mg tablet	n/a	Schering	France	[NLM]	
methenolone acetate	Primobolan®	5 mg tablet	n/a	Schering/Berlimed	South Africa	[NLM]	
methenolone acetate	Primobolan® Acetate	25 mg/ml	1 ml ampule	Schering	Germany	[NLM]	
methenolone acetate	Primobolan® S	25 mg tablet	n/a	Leiras	Finland	[NLM]	
methenolone acetate	Primobolan® S	25 mg tablet	n/a	Schering	Germany	[NLM]	
methenolone acetate	Primobolan® S	25 mg tablet	n/a	Schering	Netherlands	[NLM]	
methenolone acetate	Primobolan® S	25 mg tablet	n/a	Schering	Thailand	[NLM]	
methenolone acetate	Primobolan® S	25 mg tablet	50 tablet bottle	Schering/Berlimed	South Africa		
methenolone acetate	Primo-Plus 50	50 mg tablet	100 tablet bottle	Ttokkyo	Mexico		VET
methenolone enanthate	Primobol	100 mg/ml	10 ml vial	British Dragon	Thailand		
methenolone enanthate	Primobolan Depot	100 mg/ml	1 ml ampule	Schering/CID	Egypt	[NLM]	
methenolone enanthate	Primobolan® Depot	100 mg/ml	1 ml ampule	Scherimed	Spain		
methenolone enanthate	Primobolan® Depot	100 mg/ml	1 ml ampule	Schering	Ecuador		
methenolone enanthate	Primobolan® Depot	100 mg/ml	1 ml ampule	Schering	France	[NLM]	
methenolone enanthate	Primobolan® Depot	100 mg/ml	1 ml ampule	Schering	Guatemala		
methenolone enanthate	Primobolan® Depot	50 mg/ml	1 ml ampule	Schering	Japan	[NLM]	
methenolone enanthate	Primobolan® Depot	100 mg/ml	1 ml ampule	Schering	Japan		
methenolone enanthate	Primobolan® Depot	50 mg/ml	1 ml ampule	Schering	Mexico		
methenolone enanthate	Primobolan® Depot	100 mg/ml	1 ml ampule	Schering	Paraguay		
methenolone enanthate	Primobolan® Depot	100 mg/ml	1 ml ampule	Schering	Austria	[NLM]	
methenolone enanthate	Primobolan® Depot	100 mg/ml	1 ml ampule	Schering	Belgium	[NLM]	
methenolone enanthate	Primobolan® Depot	100 mg/ml	1 ml ampule	Schering	Czech. Rep.	[NLM]	
methenolone enanthate	Primobolan® Depot	100 mg/ml	1 ml ampule	Schering	Germany	[NLM]	
methenolone enanthate	Primobolan® Depot	100 mg/ml	1 ml ampule	Schering	Greece	[NLM]	
methenolone enanthate	Primobolan® Depot	100 mg/ml	1 ml ampule	Schering	Italy	[NLM]	
methenolone enanthate	Primobolan® Depot	100 mg/ml	1 ml ampule	Schering	Portugal	[NLM]	

Appendix A: Drug Availability Tables - Listings by Generic Name

Generic Name	Trade Name	Dose	Packaging	Company	Country	Status	Vet
methenolone enanthate	Primobolan® Depot	100 mg/ml	1 ml ampule	Schering	Spain	[NLM]	
methenolone enanthate	Primobolan® Depot	100 mg/ml	1 ml ampule	Schering	Switzerland	[NLM]	
methenolone enanthate	Primobolan® Depot	100 mg/ml	1 ml ampule	Schering	Turkey		
methenolone enanthate	Primobolan® Depot	100 mg/ml	1 ml ampule	Schering/Berlimed	South Africa	[NLM]	
methenolone enanthate	Primobolan® Depot mite	50 mg/ml	1 ml ampule	Schering	Germany	[NLM]	
methenolone enanthate	Primo-Plus 100	100 mg/ml	1 ml ampule	Ttokkyo	Mexico		VET
methenolone enanthate	Suprimo 100	100 mg/ml	10 ml vial	SYD Group	Mexico		VET
methylandrostenediol	Andris	10 mg tablet	n/a	Chifar	Greece	[NLM]	
methylandrostenediol	Methyldiol	2 mg tablet	n/a	Vortech	U.S.	[NLM]	
methylandrostenediol	Methyldiol Aqueous	50 mg/ml	n/a	Vortech	U.S.	[NLM]	
methylandrostenediol	Metylandrostendiol	10, 25 mg tablet	n/a	Jelfa	Poland	[NLM]	
methylandrostenediol	Novandrol	10, 25 mg dragee	n/a	Galenika	YugoslaviaFRMR	[NLM]	
methylandrostenediol (blend)	Anabolic NA	75 mg/ml	10 ml vial	SYD Group	Australia		VET
methylandrostenediol (blend)	Anabolic NA	75 mg/ml	10 ml vial	SYD Group	Mexico		VET
methylandrostenediol (blend)	Anabolic-NA	75 mg/ml	10 ml vial	Grupo Tarasco	Mexico	[NLM]	VET
methylandrostenediol (blend)	Drive	55 mg/ml	10 ml vial	RWR	Australia		VET
methylandrostenediol (blend)	Filybol	70 mg/ml	10, 20 ml vial	Ranvet	Australia		VET
methylandrostenediol (blend)	Libriol	75 mg/ml	10, 20 ml vial	RWR	Australia		VET
methylandrostenediol (blend)	Spectriol	65 mg/ml	10 ml vial	RWR	Australia		VET
methylandrostenediol (blend)	Tribolin	75 mg/ml	10, 20 ml vial	Ranvet	Australia		VET
methylandrostenediol dipropionate	Anadiol	5 mg tab	10, 100 tablet bottle	Ilium/Troy	Australia		VET
methylandrostenediol dipropionate	Anadiol Depot	75 mg/ml	10 ml vial	Ilium/Troy	Australia		VET
methylandrostenediol dipropionate	Arbolic	50 mg/ml	n/a	Burgin Arden	U.S.	[NLM]	
methylandrostenediol dipropionate	Crestabolic	50 mg/ml	n/a	Nutrition	U.S.	[NLM]	
methylandrostenediol dipropionate	Denkadiol	75 mg/ml	10 ml vial	Denkall	Mexico	[NLM]	VET
methylandrostenediol dipropionate	Durandrol	50 mg/ml	n/a	Pharmex	U.S.	[NLM]	
methylandrostenediol dipropionate	Hybolin	50 mg/ml	n/a	Hyrex	U.S.	[NLM]	
methylandrostenediol dipropionate	Methandriol	75 mg/ml	10 ml vial	Ilium/Troy	Australia	[NLM]	VET
methylandrostenediol dipropionate	Methasus 50	50 mg/ml	20 ml vial	Jurox	Australia	[NLM]	VET
methylandrostenediol dipropionate	Protabol	75 mg/ml	10 ml vial	Protabol	Australia		VET
methylandrostenediol dipropionate	Superbolin	75 mg/ml	10 ml vial	Vetsearch	Australia		VET
methyltestosterone	Afro	25 mg tablet	40 tablet box	Casel	Turkey		
methyltestosterone	Agovirin	10 mg dragee	100 dragee bottle	Leciva	Czech. Rep.	[NLM]	
methyltestosterone	Android	5, 10, 25 mg tablet	60 tablet bottle	ICN Pharm	U.S.		
methyltestosterone	Android	5, 10, 25 mg tablet	n/a	Brown	U.S.	[NLM]	
methyltestosterone	Androral	10 mg tablet	n/a	Gedeon Richter	Hungary		
methyltestosterone	Arcosterone	10 mg sub.	n/a	Acrum	U.S.	[NLM]	
methyltestosterone	Arcosterone	10, 25 mg tablet	n/a	Acrum	U.S.	[NLM]	
methyltestosterone	Debosteron	n/a	n/a	n/a	Korea		
methyltestosterone	Geri Tabs	2 mg tablet	50, 200 tablet bottle	Vetcom	Canada		VET
methyltestosterone	Glando Stridox	10 mg tablet	20 tablet box	Ion	Uruguay		

Appendix A: Drug Availability Tables - Listings by Generic Name

Generic Name	Trade Name	Dose	Packaging	Company	Country	Status	Vet
methyltestosterone	Hormobin	5 mg tablet	40 tablet box	Munrin Sahin	Turkey		
methyltestosterone	KangJungBing	n/a	n/a	n/a	Korea		
methyltestosterone	Longivol (plus estrogen)	1 mg tablet	n/a	Medical S.A.	Spain		
methyltestosterone	Mediatric	10 mg tablet	n/a	Wyeth-Ayerst	U.S.	[NLM]	
methyltestosterone	Mesteron	10 mg tablet	n/a	Jelfa	Poland	[NLM]	
methyltestosterone	Metandren	5 mg sub. dragee	n/a	Ciba	U.S.	[NLM]	
methyltestosterone	Metandren	10, 25 mg tablet	n/a	Ciba	U.S.	[NLM]	
methyltestosterone	Metandren	10, 25 mg tablet	100 tablet bottle	Novartis	U.S.	[NLM]	
methyltestosterone	Metesto	25 mg tablet	100 tablet bottle	Acdhon	Thailand		
methyltestosterone	Methyltestosterone	10 mg tablet	n/a	Global	U.S.		
methyltestosterone	Methyltestosterone	10 mg tablet	n/a	Goldline	U.S.	[NLM]	
methyltestosterone	Metil Testosteron	10 mg tablet	50 tablet box	Terapia	Rumania		
methyltestosterone	Metil Thomsina S	10 mg tablet	20 tablet box	Celsius	Uruguay		
methyltestosterone	Metil-Test	50 mg tablet	100 tablet bottle	Brovel	Mexico		VET
methyltestosterone	Metiltestosterona	n/a	n/a	Botica	Paraguay		
methyltestosterone	Neo Aphro	5 mg tablet	30 tablet	Misr	Egypt		
methyltestosterone	Oreton	n/a	n/a	n/a	Venezuela		
methyltestosterone	Oreton Methyl	10 mg tablet	n/a	Schering	U.S.	[NLM]	
methyltestosterone	Oreton Methyl	10 mg sub. tablet	n/a	Schering	U.S.	[NLM]	
methyltestosterone	T. Lingvalete	5 mg sub. dragee	n/a	Galenika	YugoslaviaFRMR	[NLM]	
methyltestosterone	Testo Tab	25 mg tablet	n/a	Samil	Korea		
methyltestosterone	Teston	25 mg tablet	30 tablet box	Remek	Greece		
methyltestosterone	Testopropon	25 mg tablet	n/a	Scanpharm	Malaysia		
methyltestosterone	Testormon	10 mg tablet	n/a	Unitas	Portugal		
methyltestosterone	Testosteron	5 mg tablet	n/a	Berco	Germany	[NLM]	
methyltestosterone	Testosure	n/a	n/a	Europharm	Hong Kong		
methyltestosterone	Testovis	10 mg tablet	n/a	SIT	Italy		
methyltestosterone	Testoyohim	25 mg dragee	30 dragee box	Paul Mehner	Germany	[NLM]	
methyltestosterone	Testred	10 mg capsule	100 capsule bottle	ICN	U.S.		
methyltestosterone	TP Men Hormone	10 mg dragee	24 tablets	TP Drugs	Thailand		
methyltestosterone	Virilon (time released)	10 mg capsule	100,1000 capsule bottle	Star	U.S.		
mibolerone	Cheque Drops	100 mcg/ml	55 mg bottle	Upjohn	U.S.	[NLM]	VET
mibolerone	mibolerone drops	100 mcg/ml	55 mg bottle	Wedgewood	U.S.		VET
nandrolone (blend)	Dinandrol	100 mg/ml	2 ml vial	Xelox (export)	Philippines		
nandrolone cyclohexylpropionate	Sanabolicum	25, 50 mg/ml	1 ml ampule	Biochemie/Nile	Egypt		
nandrolone cyclohexylpropionate	Sanabolicum-Vet	50 mg/ml	10 ml vial	Werfft-Chemie	Austria		VET
nandrolone cypionate	Anabolic DN	50 mg/ml	10 ml vial	SYD Group	Australia		VET
nandrolone cypionate	Anabolic DN	50, 300 mg/ml	10 ml vial	SYD Group	Mexico		VET
nandrolone cypionate	Anabolic-DN	50 mg/ml	10 ml vial	Grupo Tarasco	Mexico	[NLM]	VET
nandrolone cypionate	Dynabol	50 mg/ml	10 ml vial	Jurox	Australia	[NLM]	VET
nandrolone decanoate	Anabolicum	25 mg/ml	10, 50 ml vial	Bela-Pharm	Germany		VET

Appendix A: Drug Availability Tables - Listings by Generic Name

Generic Name	Trade Name	Dose	Packaging	Company	Country	Status	Vet
nandrolone decanoate	Anabolin Forte	50 mg/ml	10 ml vial	Alfasan	Netherlands		VET
nandrolone decanoate	Anabolin Forte	50 mg/ml	10 ml vial	Alfasan	Rumania		VET
nandrolone decanoate	Anabolin Forte	50 mg/ml	10, 50 ml vial	Alfasan	Spain		VET
nandrolone decanoate	Anaboline Depot	50 mg/ml	1 ml	Adelco	Greece		
nandrolone decanoate	Anaprolina	25, 50 mg/ml	1 ml ampule	Silesia	Chile		
nandrolone decanoate	Androlone-D 200	200 mg/ml	1 ml	Keene	U.S.	[NLM]	
nandrolone decanoate	Canoate Inj	25, 50 mg/ml	n/a	n/a	Korea		
nandrolone decanoate	Deca 300	300 mg/ml	10 ml vial	Animal Power	Mexico		VET
nandrolone decanoate	Deca QV 200	200 mg/ml	10, 50 ml vial	Quality Vet	Mexico		VET
nandrolone decanoate	Deca QV 300	300 mg/ml	10 ml vial	Quality Vet	Mexico		VET
nandrolone decanoate	Decabol	250 mg/ml	10 ml vial	British Dragon	Thailand		
nandrolone decanoate	Deca-Dubol-100	100 mg/ml	2 ml vial	BM Pharmaceuticals	India		
nandrolone decanoate	Deca-Durabolin®	25, 50 mg/ml	1 ml ampule	Donmed/Organon	South Africa		
nandrolone decanoate	Deca-Durabolin®	25, 50, 100 mg/ml	1 ml ampule	Infar	India		
nandrolone decanoate	Deca-Durabolin®	25, 50 mg/ml	1 ml ampule	Organon	Bulgaria		
nandrolone decanoate	Deca-Durabolin®	25, 50, 100 mg/ml	1 ml ampule	Organon	Chile		
nandrolone decanoate	Deca-Durabolin®	25, 50 mg/ml	1 ml ampule	Organon	Colombia		
nandrolone decanoate	Deca-Durabolin®	25, 50 mg/ml	1 ml	Organon	Denmark	[NLM]	
nandrolone decanoate	Deca-Durabolin®	n/a	n/a	Organon	Ireland		
nandrolone decanoate	Deca-Durabolin®	25, 50 mg/ml	1 ml ampule	Organon	Korea		
nandrolone decanoate	Deca-Durabolin®	25 mg/ml	1 ml ampule	Organon	Malaysia		
nandrolone decanoate	Deca-Durabolin®	50 mg/ml	1 ml ampule	Organon	New Zealand		
nandrolone decanoate	Deca-Durabolin®	50 mg/ml	1 ml ampule	Organon	Norway		
nandrolone decanoate	Deca-Durabolin®	50 mg/ml	1 ml ampule	Organon	Peru		
nandrolone decanoate	Deca-Durabolin®	25 mg/ml	1 ml ampule	Organon	Poland	[NLM]	
nandrolone decanoate	Deca-Durabolin®	50 mg/ml	1 ml ampule	Organon	Poland		
nandrolone decanoate	Deca-Durabolin®	25 mg/ml	1 ml ampule	Organon	Singapore		
nandrolone decanoate	Deca-Durabolin®	50 mg/ml	1 ml ampule	Organon	Taiwan		
nandrolone decanoate	Deca-Durabolin®	25, 50 mg/ml	1 ml ampule	Organon	Thailand		
nandrolone decanoate	Deca-Durabolin®	25, 50 mg/ml	1 ml	Organon	Argentina		
nandrolone decanoate	Deca-Durabolin®	50 mg/ml	2 ml	Organon	Argentina		
nandrolone decanoate	Deca-Durabolin®	25 mg/ml	1 ml	Organon	Austria	[NLM]	
nandrolone decanoate	Deca-Durabolin®	25, 50 mg/ml	1 ml ampule, syringe	Organon	Belgium		
nandrolone decanoate	Deca-Durabolin®	25, 50 mg/ml	1 ml ampule	Organon	Brazil		
nandrolone decanoate	Deca-Durabolin®	50 mg/ml	2 ml	Organon	Canada	[NLM]	
nandrolone decanoate	Deca-Durabolin®	100 mg/ml	2 ml	Organon	Canada		
nandrolone decanoate	Deca-Durabolin®	25, 50 mg/ml	1 ml	Organon	Finland		
nandrolone decanoate	Deca-Durabolin®	100 mg/ml	1,2 ml	Organon	Finland		
nandrolone decanoate	Deca-Durabolin®	50 mg/ml	1 ml	Organon	France	[NLM]	
nandrolone decanoate	Deca-Durabolin®	25, 50 mg/ml	1 ml	Organon	Germany	[NLM]	
nandrolone decanoate	Deca-Durabolin®	50 mg/ml	1 ml vial	Organon	Greece		

Appendix A: Drug Availability Tables - Listings by Generic Name

Generic Name	Trade Name	Dose	Packaging	Company	Country	Status	Vet
nandrolone decanoate	Deca-Durabolin®	100 mg/ml	2 ml vial	Organon	Greece		
nandrolone decanoate	Deca-Durabolin®	100 mg/ml	2 ml vial	Organon	Greece		
nandrolone decanoate	Deca-Durabolin®	25, 50 mg/ml	1 ml ampule	Organon	Indonesia		
nandrolone decanoate	Deca-Durabolin®	25, 50 mg/ml	1 ml ampule	Organon	Italy		
nandrolone decanoate	Deca-Durabolin®	25, 50 mg/ml	1 ml ampule	Organon	Netherlands		
nandrolone decanoate	Deca-Durabolin®	50 mg/ml	1 ml ampule	Organon	Rumania		
nandrolone decanoate	Deca-Durabolin®	25, 50 mg/ml	1 ml ampule	Organon	Spain		
nandrolone decanoate	Deca-Durabolin®	50 mg/ml	1 ml ampule	Organon	Sweden		
nandrolone decanoate	Deca-Durabolin®	25, 100 mg/ml	1, 2 ml	Organon	Sweden	[NLM]	
nandrolone decanoate	Deca-Durabolin®	25 mg/ml	1 ml ampule	Organon	Switzerland	[NLM]	
nandrolone decanoate	Deca-Durabolin®	50 mg/ml	1 ml ampule	Organon	Switzerland		
nandrolone decanoate	Deca-Durabolin®	100 mg/ml	1, 2 ml vial	Organon	U.S.	[NLM]	
nandrolone decanoate	Deca-Durabolin®	200 mg/ml	1 ml vial	Organon	U.S.	[NLM]	
nandrolone decanoate	Deca-Durabolin®	50 mg/ml	1 ml ampule	Organon	United Kingdom		
nandrolone decanoate	Deca-Durabolin®	100 mg/ml	1, 2 ml ampule	Organon	United Kingdom	[NLM]	
nandrolone decanoate	Deca-Durabolin®	25 mg/ml	1 ml ampule	Organon	Venezuela		
nandrolone decanoate	Deca-Durabolin®	50 mg/ml	1 ml syringe	Organon	Venezuela		
nandrolone decanoate	Deca-Durabolin®	25, 50 mg/ml	1 ml ampule	Organon/Nile	Egypt		
nandrolone decanoate	Deca-Durabolin®	100 mg/ml	2 ml vial	Organon	Netherlands		
nandrolone decanoate	Deca-Evabolin	25 mg/ml	1 ml ampule	Concept	India		
nandrolone decanoate	Decagic	100 mg/ml	10 ml vial	Unichem	India	[NLM]	
nandrolone decanoate	Decanandrolen	200mg/ml	10 ml vial	Denkall	Mexico		VET
nandrolone decanoate	Decandrol 300	300 mg/ml	10 ml vial	Pet's Pharma	Mexico		VET
nandrolone decanoate	Decaneurabol	25, 50 mg/ml	1 ml ampule	Cadila	India		
nandrolone decanoate	Decaneurophen	25, 50 mg/ml	1 ml ampule	Ind-Swift	India		
nandrolone decanoate	Decanoato de Nandrolona	200 mg/ml	10 ml vial	Tornel	Mexico		VET
nandrolone decanoate	Decanoato Nandrolona	25, 50 mg/ml	1 ml ampule	Astorga	Chile		
nandrolone decanoate	Decanoato Nandrolona	50 mg/ml	1 ml ampule	Biosano	Chile		
nandrolone decanoate	Decanofort	25 mg/ml	1 ml ampule	Terapia	Rumania		
nandrolone decanoate	Deca-Pronabol	100 mg/ml	2 ml ampule	P & B Labs	India	[NLM]	
nandrolone decanoate	Decatron 250	250 mg/ml	10 ml vial	Brovel	Mexico		VET
nandrolone decanoate	Dimetabol	50 mg/ml	50 ml vial	Bremer Pharma	Dom. Rep.	[NLM]	VET
nandrolone decanoate	Dimetabol ADE	25 mg/ml	50, 100 ml vial	Lapisa	Mexico		VET
nandrolone decanoate	Dynabolon Inj	40 mg/.5 ml	1 ml ampule	n/a	Korea		
nandrolone decanoate	Elpihormo	50 mg/ml	1 ml	Chemica	Greece	[NLM]	
nandrolone decanoate	Extraboline	50 mg/ml	2 ml vial	Genepharm	Greece		
nandrolone decanoate	Gerabolin	25 mg/ml	1 ml ampule	Nile	Egypt		
nandrolone decanoate	Hybolin Decanoate	50, 100 mg/ml	1, 2 ml vial	Hyrex	U.S.		
nandrolone decanoate	Jebolan	50 mg/ml	1 ml ampule	Etem	Turkey	[NLM]	
nandrolone decanoate	Metadec	25, 50 mg/ml	1 ml ampule	Jagsonpal	India		
nandrolone decanoate	Myobolin	25 mg/ml	1 ml ampule	Troikaa	India		

Generic Name	Trade Name	Dose	Packaging	Company	Country	Status	Vet
nandrolone decanoate	Nandrobolic L.A.	100 mg/ml	1, 2 ml vial	Forest	U.S.	[NLM]	
nandrolone decanoate	Nandrolona 300 L.A.	300mg/ml	10 ml vial	Ttokkyo	Mexico		VET
nandrolone decanoate	nandrolona decanoato	50 mg/ml	1 ml ampule	Chile	Chile		
nandrolone decanoate	nandrolone decanoate	100 mg/ml	1, 2 ml vial	Lyphomed	U.S.	[NLM]	
nandrolone decanoate	nandrolone decanoate	200 mg/2ml	2 ml vial	Norma Hellas	Greece		
nandrolone decanoate	nandrolone decanoate	100 mg/ml	1, 2 ml vial	Quad	U.S.	[NLM]	
nandrolone decanoate	nandrolone decanoate	50, 100, 200 mg/ml	1, 2 ml vial	Steris	U.S.	[NLM]	
nandrolone decanoate	Nandrolone Decanoate Inj	100 mg/ml	2 ml vial	Watson Pharma	U.S.		
nandrolone decanoate	Nandrolone Decanoate Inj	200 mg/ml	1 ml vial	Watson Pharma	U.S.		
nandrolone decanoate	Nandrosande	25, 50, 100 mg/ml	1 ml ampule	Sanderson	Chile		
nandrolone decanoate	Neo-Durabolic	100, 200 mg/ml	1, 2 ml vial	Hauck	U.S.	[NLM]	
nandrolone decanoate	Norandren	50, 200 mg/ml	10, 50 ml vial	Brovel	Mexico		VET
nandrolone decanoate	Nurezan	50 mg/ml	1 ml ampule	Rafarm	Greece		
nandrolone decanoate	Retabolil	25, 50 mg/ml	1 ml ampule	Gedeon Richter	Bulgaria	[NLM]	
nandrolone decanoate	Retabolil	50 mg/ml	1 ml ampule	Gedeon Richter	Estonia		
nandrolone decanoate	Retabolil	25, 50 mg/ml	1 ml ampule	Gedeon Richter	Hungary		
nandrolone decanoate	Retabolil	25, 50 mg/ml	1 ml ampule	Gedeon Richter	Malaysia		
nandrolone decanoate	Retabolil	50 mg/ml	1 ml ampule	Medimpex/Alxndria	Egypt		
nandrolone decanoate	Retabolin	50 mg/ml	1 ml ampule	Medexport Russia	Russia	[NLM]	
nandrolone decanoate	RWR Deca 50	50 mg/ml	10 ml vial	RWR	Australia		VET
nandrolone decanoate	Sterobolin	50 mg/ml	1 ml ampule	Orion	Finland	[NLM]	
nandrolone decanoate	Turinabol Depot	50 mg/ml	1 ml ampule	Jenapharm	Bulgaria	[NLM]	
nandrolone decanoate	Turinabol Depot	50 mg/ml	1 ml ampule	Jenapharm	Czech. Rep.	[NLM]	
nandrolone decanoate	Turinabol Depot	50 ma/ ml	1 ml ampule	Jenapharm	Germany	[NLM]	
nandrolone decanoate	Ziremilon	50 mg/ml	1 ml ampule	Demo	Greece		
nandrolone hexyloxyphenylpropionate	Anador	25 mg/ml	2 ml ampule	Pharmacia-Upjohn	France	[NLM]	
nandrolone hexyloxyphenylpropionate	Anadur	25 mg/ml	2 ml ampule	Eczacibasi	Turkey	[NLM]	
nandrolone hexyloxyphenylpropionate	Anadur	25, 50 mg/ml	1, 2 ml ampule	Kabi Pharmacia	Switzerland	[NLM]	
nandrolone hexyloxyphenylpropionate	Anadur	25, 50 mg/ml	1, 2 ml ampule	Kabi Pharmacia	Austria	[NLM]	
nandrolone hexyloxyphenylpropionate	Anadur	25, 50 mg/ml	1, 2 ml ampule	Kabi Pharmacia	Germany	[NLM]	
nandrolone hexyloxyphenylpropionate	Anadur	25, 50 mg/ml	1, 2 ml ampule	Kabi Pharmacia	Norway	[NLM]	
nandrolone hexyloxyphenylpropionate	Anadur	25 mg/ml	2 ml ampule	Leo	Spain	[NLM]	
nandrolone hexyloxyphenylpropionate	Anadur	25 mg/ml	2 ml ampule	Lundbeck	Denmark	[NLM]	
nandrolone hexyloxyphenylpropionate	Anadur	25, 50 mg/ml	1, 2 ml ampule	Pharmacia	Belgium	[NLM]	
nandrolone hexyloxyphenylpropionate	Anadur	25, 50 mg/ml	1, 2 ml ampule	Pharmacia	Czech. Rep.	[NLM]	
nandrolone hexyloxyphenylpropionate	Anadur	25, 50 mg/ml	1, 2 ml ampule	Pharmacia	Finland	[NLM]	
nandrolone hexyloxyphenylpropionate	Anadur	25, 50 mg/ml	1, 2 ml ampule	Pharmacia	Netherlands	[NLM]	
nandrolone hexyloxyphenylpropionate	Anadurin	50 mg/ml	1 ml ampule	Xponei	Greece	[NLM]	
nandrolone laurate	Fortabol	20 mg/ml	10, 50 ml vial	Parfam	Mexico		VET
nandrolone laurate	Fortadex	25, 50 mg/ml	n/a	Hydro	Germany		VET
nandrolone laurate	Laudrol LA	250 mg/ml	10 ml vial	Loeffler	Mexico		VET

Appendix A: Drug Availability Tables - Listings by Generic Name

Generic Name	Trade Name	Dose	Packaging	Company	Country	Status	Vet
nandrolone laurate	Laurabolin	25, 50 mg/ml	10 ml vial	Intervet	Australia		VET
nandrolone laurate	Laurabolin	50 mg/ml	10, 50 ml	Intervet	Colombia		VET
nandrolone laurate	Laurabolin	20, 50 mg/ml	10, 50 ml vial	Intervet	Mexico		VET
nandrolone laurate	Laurabolin	25, 50 mg/ml	5, 10, 50 ml	Vemie	Germany		VET
nandrolone laurate	Laurabolin	50 mg/ml	n/a	Werfft-Chemie	Austria		VET
nandrolone laurate	Laurabolin V	50 mg/ml	10, 50 ml	Intervet	Netherlands		VET
nandrolone phenylpropionate	Activin	10 mg/ml	n/a	Aristegvi	Spain	[NLM]	
nandrolone phenylpropionate	Anabolin	50 mg/ml	n/a	Alto	U.S.	[NLM]	
nandrolone phenylpropionate	Anabolin-IM	50 mg/ml	n/a	Alto	U.S.	[NLM]	
nandrolone phenylpropionate	Anabolin-LA	100 mg/ml	n/a	Alto	U.S.	[NLM]	
nandrolone phenylpropionate	Androlone	50 mg/ml	n/a	Keene	U.S.	[NLM]	
nandrolone phenylpropionate	Daily Reborn Inj	25 mg/ml	n/a	Shiteh	Taiwan		
nandrolone phenylpropionate	Dubol-100	100 mg/ml	2 ml vial	BM Pharmaceuticals	India		
nandrolone phenylpropionate	Dubol-50	50 mg/ml	1 ml ampule	BM Pharmaceuticals	India		
nandrolone phenylpropionate	Durabol	200 mg/ml	10 ml vial	British Dragon	Thailand		
nandrolone phenylpropionate	Durabol	100 mg/ml	10 ml vial	British Dragon	Thailand	[NLM]	
nandrolone phenylpropionate	Durabolin®	25 mg/ml	1 ml ampule	Infar	India		
nandrolone phenylpropionate	Durabolin®	25 mg/ml	n/a	Opopharma	Switzerland	[NLM]	
nandrolone phenylpropionate	Durabolin®	25 mg/ml	1 ml ampule	Organon	Malaysia		
nandrolone phenylpropionate	Durabolin®	25 mg/ml	2 ml vial	Organon	Taiwan		
nandrolone phenylpropionate	Durabolin®	25 mg/ml	n/a	Organon	Belgium	[NLM]	
nandrolone phenylpropionate	Durabolin®	25, 50 mg/ml	n/a	Organon	Canada	[NLM]	
nandrolone phenylpropionate	Durabolin®	25 mg/ml	n/a	Organon	Finland		
nandrolone phenylpropionate	Durabolin®	25 mg/ml	1 ml ampule	Organon	Greece	[NLM]	
nandrolone phenylpropionate	Durabolin®	12.5 mg/ml	2 ml ampule	Organon	Indonesia		
nandrolone phenylpropionate	Durabolin®	25 mg/ml	1 ml ampule	Organon	Netherlands		
nandrolone phenylpropionate	Durabolin®	50 mg/ml	n/a	Organon	Portugal		
nandrolone phenylpropionate	Durabolin®	25 mg/ml	1 ml ampule	Organon	Spain	[NLM]	
nandrolone phenylpropionate	Durabolin®	25, 50 mg/ml	n/a	Organon	U.S.	[NLM]	
nandrolone phenylpropionate	Durabolin®	50 mg/ml	1 ml ampule	Organon	United Kingdom	[NLM]	
nandrolone phenylpropionate	Durabolin®	50 mg/ml	n/a	Organon	YugoslaviaFRMR		
nandrolone phenylpropionate	Equibolin-50	50 mg/ml	n/a	Vortech	U.S.	[NLM]	
nandrolone phenylpropionate	Estigor	10 mg/ml	250 ml	Burnet	Argentina		VET
nandrolone phenylpropionate	Evabolin	25 mg/ml	1 ml ampule	Concept	India		
nandrolone phenylpropionate	Fenobolin	20 mg/ml	n/a	Medexport Russia	Russia	[NLM]	
nandrolone phenylpropionate	Fherbolico	50 mg/ml	n/a	Fher	Spain	[NLM]	
nandrolone phenylpropionate	Ganekyl	50 mg/ml	10, 100 ml vial	Over Labs	Argentina		VET
nandrolone phenylpropionate	Hybolin	25, 50 mg/ml	n/a	Hyrex	U.S.	[NLM]	
nandrolone phenylpropionate	Macrabone	25 mg/ml	n/a	Ta Fong	Taiwan		
nandrolone phenylpropionate	Menabolin	25 mg/ml	1 ml ampule	Theramex/Memphis	Egypt		
nandrolone phenylpropionate	Metabol	25 mg/ml	1 ml ampule	Jagsonpal	India		

Appendix A: Drug Availability Tables - Listings by Generic Name

Generic Name	Trade Name	Dose	Packaging	Company	Country	Status	Vet
nandrolone phenylpropionate	Metrobolin	25 mg/ml	n/a	Metro	Taiwan		
nandrolone phenylpropionate	Nandrobolic	25 mg/ml	n/a	Forest	U.S.	[NLM]	
nandrolone phenylpropionate	Nandrolin	50 mg/ml	25 ml vial	Intervet	Australia		VET
nandrolone phenylpropionate	Nandrolin	25 mg/ml	10 ml vial	Intervet	Australia		VET
nandrolone phenylpropionate	nandrolone phenylpropionate	50, 100mg/ml	2 ml vial	Hayrian Biologicals	India	[NLM]	
nandrolone phenylpropionate	nandrolone phenylpropionate	25 mg/ml	1 ml ampule	Iran Hormone	Iran		
nandrolone phenylpropionate	nandrolone phenylpropionate	50 mg/ml	n/a	Quad	U.S.	[NLM]	
nandrolone phenylpropionate	Nerobolil	25 mg/ml	1 ml ampule	Godeon Richter	Bulgaria	[NLM]	
nandrolone phenylpropionate	Nerobolil	25 mg/ml	n/a	Godeon Richter	Hungary	[NLM]	
nandrolone phenylpropionate	Neurabol Inj	25 mg/ml	1 ml ampule	Cadila	India		
nandrolone phenylpropionate	Neurophen	25 mg/ml	1 ml ampule	Ind-Swift	India		
nandrolone phenylpropionate	Norabon	25 mg/ml	1 ml ampule	Phihalab	Thailand		
nandrolone phenylpropionate	Nu-Bolic	25 mg/ml	n/a	Seatrace	U.S.	[NLM]	
nandrolone phenylpropionate	Protosin Inj	25 mg/ml	n/a	Astar	Taiwan		
nandrolone phenylpropionate	Rubolin	25 mg/ml	n/a	Ying Yuan	Taiwan		
nandrolone phenylpropionate	Sinbolin	25 mg/ml	n/a	Sinton	Taiwan		
nandrolone phenylpropionate	Superanabolon	25 mg/ml	1 ml ampule	Spofa	Czech. Rep.		
nandrolone phenylpropionate	Turinabol	25 mg/ml	n/a	Germed	Czech. Rep.	[NLM]	
nandrolone phenylpropionate	Turinabol	25 mg/ml	n/a	Jenapharm	Bulgaria	[NLM]	
nandrolone phenylpropionate	Turinabol	25 mg/ml	n/a	Jenapharm	Germany	[NLM]	
nandrolone undecanoate	Dynabolon	80.5 mg/ml	1 ml ampule	Farmasister	Italy	[NLM]	
nandrolone undecanoate	Dynabolon	80.5 mg/ml	1 ml ampule	Fournier	Italy		
nandrolone undecanoate	Dynabolon	80.5 mg/ml	1 ml ampule	Theramex	France	[NLM]	
nandrolone undecanoate	Psychobolan	80.5 mg/ml	1ml ampule	Theramex	Greece	[NLM]	
norethandrolone	Anaplex	5 mg tablet	100 tablet bottle	Jurox	Australia		VET
norethandrolone	Nilevar	10 mg tablet	30 tablet bottle	Searle	France		
norethandrolone	Nilevar	10 mg tablet	30 tablet bottle	Searle	Switzerland	[NLM]	
norethandrolone	Nilevar	10 mg tablet	100 tablet bottle	Searle	U.S.		
Omnadren (testosterone blend)	Omnadren	250 mg/ml	1ml ampule	Jelfa	Poland		
Omnadren (testosterone blend)	Omnadren	250 mg/ml	1ml ampule	Polfa	Poland	[NLM]	
Omnadren (testosterone blend)	Omnadren 250	250 mg/ml	1 ml ampule	Jelfa	Bulgaria		
oxabolone cypionate	Steranabol Ritardo	12.5 mg/ml	2 ml ampule	Pharmacia & Upjohn	Italy	[NLM]	
oxandrolone	Anatrophill	2.5 mg tablet	n/a	Searle	France	[NLM]	
oxandrolone	Anavar	5 mg tablet	30 tablet strip	Hubei Huangshi	China		
oxandrolone	Anavar	2.5 mg tablet	100 tablet bottle	Searle	U.S.	[NLM]	
oxandrolone	Bonavar	2.5 mg tablet	10 tablet strip	Body Research	Thailand		
oxandrolone	Kicker Tab	2.5 mg tablet	n/a	n/a	Korea		
oxandrolone	Lipidex	2.5 mg tablet	n/a	Searle	Brazil	[NLM]	
oxandrolone	Lonavar	2.5 mg tablet	100 tablet bottle	BTG	Israel		
oxandrolone	Lonavar	2 mg tablet	n/a	Dainippon	Japan	[NLM]	
oxandrolone	Lonavar	2.5 mg tablet	n/a	Searle	Argentina	[NLM]	

Appendix A: Drug Availability Tables - Listings by Generic Name

Generic Name	Trade Name	Dose	Packaging	Company	Country	Status	Vet
oxandrolone	Oxafort	5 mg tablet	100 tablet bottle	Loeffler	Mexico		VET
oxandrolone	Oxanabol	5 mg tablet	100 tablet pouch	British Dragon	Thailand	[NLM]	
oxandrolone	Oxanabol	10 mg tablet	100 tablet pouch	British Dragon	Thailand		
oxandrolone	Oxandrin®	2.5, 10 mg tablet	100 tablet bottle	BTG	U.S.		
oxandrolone	Oxandro Tabs	5 mg tablet	100 tablet bottle	Animal Power	Mexico		VET
oxandrolone	Oxandrol 10	10 mg tablet	100 tablet bottle	Bratis Labs	Mexico		VET
oxandrolone	Oxandrolone	5 mg tablet	30 tablet bottle	Planet Pharmacy	Belize		
oxandrolone	Oxandrolone	2.5 tablet	100 tablet bottle	Ttokkyo	Mexico	[NLM]	VET
oxandrolone	Oxandrolone	5 mg tablet	100 tablet bottle	Ttokkyo	Mexico		VET
oxandrolone	Oxandrolone SPA	2.5 mg tablet	30 tablet box	SPA	Italy	[NLM]	
oxandrolone	Oxandrolone SPA (Export)	2.5 mg tablet	30 tablet box	SPA	Italy		
oxandrolone	Oxandrovet	5 mg tablet	100 tablet bottle	Denkall	Mexico		VET
oxandrolone	Oxavet QV	5 mg tablet	100 tablet bottle	Quality Vet	Mexico		VET
oxandrolone	Vasorome	0.5 mg tablet	n/a	Kowa	Japan	[NLM]	
oxandrolone	Vasorome	2 mg tablet	n/a	Kowa	Japan	[NLM]	
oxymetholone	Anabrol	50 mg tablet	100 tablet bottle	Brovel	Mexico		VET
oxymetholone	Anadrol	5 mg tablet	n/a	n/a	Japan		
oxymetholone	Anadrol 50®	50 mg tablet	100 tablet bottle	Unimed	U.S.		
oxymetholone	Anadrol 50®	50 mg tablet	100 tablet bottle	Syntex	Canada	[NLM]	
oxymetholone	Anadrol 50®	50 mg tablet	100 tablet bottle	Syntex	U.S.	[NLM]	
oxymetholone	Anapolon	50 mg tablet	20 tablet box	Ibrahim	Turkey		
oxymetholone	Anapolon	50 mg tablet	n/a	Syntex	Bulgaria	[NLM]	
oxymetholone	Anapolon	2.5, 5 mg tablet	20 tablet box	Ibrahim	Turkey	[NLM]	
oxymetholone	Anapolon 50	50 mg tablet	100 tablet bottle	Syntex	Malaysia	[NLM]	
oxymetholone	Anapolon 50	50 mg tablet	20 tablet strip	Syntex	Mexico	[NLM]	
oxymetholone	Anapolon 50	50 mg tablet	100 tablet bottle	Syntex	United Kingdom	[NLM]	
oxymetholone	Anapolon 50®	50 mg tablet	100 tablet bottle	Hoffman-La Rouche	Canada	[NLM]	
oxymetholone	Anasteron	25 mg tablet	60 tablet bottle	Farmaprod	Greece		
oxymetholone	Anasteron	50 mg tablet	n/a	Syntex	Greece	[NLM]	
oxymetholone	Anasteron	50 mg tablet	n/a	Syntex	Sweden	[NLM]	
oxymetholone	Androlic	50 mg tablet	100 tablet bottle	British Dispensary	Thailand		
oxymetholone	Androlic	50 mg tablet	100 tablet pouch	British Dispensary	Thailand	[NLM]	
oxymetholone	Androlic (Export)	50 mg tablet	20 tablet pouch	British Dragon	Thailand		
oxymetholone	Androyd	5 mg tablet	100 tablet	Parke Davis	India		
oxymetholone	Bonalone	50 mg tablet	100 tablet bottle	Body Research	Thailand		
oxymetholone	Dynasten	50 mg tablet	n/a	Cilag	Portugal	[NLM]	
oxymetholone	Hemogenin	50 mg tablet	10 tablet box	Syntex	Brazil	[NLM]	
oxymetholone	Hemogenin	50 mg tablet	n/a	Aventis	Brazil		
oxymetholone	Hemogenin	50 mg tablet	10 tablet box	Sarsa	Brazil	[NLM]	
oxymetholone	Kanestron	50 mg tablet	100 tablet bottle	Loeffler	Mexico		VET
oxymetholone	Metalon Tabs	75 mg tablet	100 tablet bottle	Animal Power	Mexico		VET

Appendix A: Drug Availability Tables - Listings by Generic Name

Generic Name	Trade Name	Dose	Packaging	Company	Country	Status	Vet
oxymetholone	Oximetalon	75 mg tablet	100 tablet bottle	Denkall	Mexico		VET
oxymetholone	Oxitosona 50	50 mg tablet	100 tablet box	Syntex	Spain	[NLM]	
oxymetholone	Oxitron 50	50 mg tablet	100 tablet bottle	Bratis Labs	Mexico		VET
oxymetholone	Oxivet QV	75 mg tablet	100 tablet bottle	Quality Vet	Mexico		VET
oxymetholone	Oxybolone	50 mg tablet	20 tablet box	Genapharm	Greece		
oxymetholone	Oxydrol	50 mg tablet	100 tablet pouch	British Dragon	Thailand		
oxymetholone	Oxydrol	100 mg tablet	50 tablet pouch	British Dragon	Thailand	[NLM]	
oxymetholone	Oxylone	50 mg tablet	100 tablet bottle	Duopharma	Malaysia		
oxymetholone	Oxymetholone	50 mg tablet	100 tablets	Alhavi	Israel		
oxymetholone	Oxymetholone	50 mg tablet	100 tablet pouch	British Dispensary	Thailand	[NLM]	
oxymetholone	Oxymetholone	50 mg tablet	30 tablet bottle	Planet Pharmacy	Belize		
oxymetholone	oxymetholone	50 mg tablet	n/a	Sime Darby	Malaysia		
oxymetholone	Oxymetholone DongIndang	n/a	n/a	Dongindang	Korea		
oxymetholone	Oxymetholone HanBul	50 mg tablet	n/a	HanBul	Korea		
oxymetholone	Oxymetholone HanSeo	50 mg tablet	100 tablet bottle	HanSeo	Korea		
oxymetholone	Oxymetholone Korea United	50 mg tablet	n/a	Korea United	Korea		
oxymetholone	Oxymetholone Miverva	50 mg tablet	100 tablet	Minerva	Greece	[NLM]	
oxymetholone	Oxymetolona 50	50 mg tablet	100 tablet bottle	Ttokkyo	Mexico		VET
oxymetholone	Oxytone 50	50 mg tablet	100 tablet bottle	SB Laboratories	Thailand		
oxymetholone	Plenastril	50 mg tablet	n/a	Grunenthal	Austria	[NLM]	
oxymetholone	Plenastril	50 mg tablet	n/a	Proto chemie	Switzerland	[NLM]	
oxymetholone	Roboral	50 mg tablet	100 tablets	Abic/Ramat-Gan	Israel	[NLM]	
oxymetholone	Synasteron	50 mg tablet	50 tablet bottle	Sarva	Belgium	[NLM]	
quinbolone	Anabolicum Vister	10 mg capsule	30 capsule bottle	Parke Davis	Italy	[NLM]	
quinbolone	Anabolicum Vister	oral drops	n/a	Parke Davis	Italy	[NLM]	
stanozolol	Stanozolol	10 mg tablet	100 tablet pouch	British Dispensary	Thailand		
stanozolol (inj)	Anabolic ST	50 mg/ml	20 ml vial	SYD Group	Australia		VET
stanozolol (inj)	Anabolic ST	50 mg/ml	20 ml vial	SYD Group	Mexico		VET
stanozolol (inj)	Anabolico Cimol	60 mg/ml	5 ml vial	Cimol	Argentina		VET
stanozolol (inj)	Anabolico Produvet	10 mg/ml	25 ml vial	Cimol	Argentina		VET
stanozolol (inj)	Anabolic-ST	50 mg/ml	20 ml vial	Grupo Tarasco	Mexico	[NLM]	VET
stanozolol (inj)	Estanozolol	50 mg/ml	30 ml vial	Industria Argentina	Argentina		VET
stanozolol (inj)	Estrombol	25 mg/ml	10 ml vial	Fundacion	Argentina		VET
stanozolol (inj)	Nabolic	2 mg/ml	50 ml vial	Chinfield Ind.	Argentina		VET
stanozolol (inj)	Nabolic Strong	50 mg/ml	30 ml vial	Chinfield Ind.	Argentina		VET
stanozolol (inj)	Stan 50	50 mg/ml	10 ml vial	Animal Power	Mexico		VET
stanozolol (inj)	Stan QV 100	100 mg/ml	20 ml vial	Quality Vet	Mexico		VET
stanozolol (inj)	Stan QV 50	50 mg/ml	20 ml vial	Quality Vet	Mexico		VET
stanozolol (inj)	Stanabolic	50 mg/ml	20 ml vial	Ilium/Troy	Australia		VET
stanozolol (inj)	Stanazol	50 mg/ml	20, 50 ml vial	RWR	Australia	[NLM]	VET
stanozolol (inj)	Stanazolic	50, 100 mg/ml	20 ml, 10ml vial	Denkall	Mexico		VET

Appendix A: Drug Availability Tables - Listings by Generic Name

Generic Name	Trade Name	Dose	Packaging	Company	Country	Status	Vet
stanozolol (inj)	Stanol 50	50 mg/ml	20 ml vial	Bratis Labs	Mexico		VET
stanozolol (inj)	Stanol-V	50, 100 mg/ml	20 ml vial	Ttokkyo	Mexico		VET
stanozolol (inj)	Stanosus	50 mg/ml	20 ml vial	Jurox	Australia	[NLM]	VET
stanozolol (inj)	Stromba	50 mg/ml	n/a	Sterling Research	United Kingdom	[NLM]	
stanozolol (inj)	Stromba	50 mg/ml	n/a	Sterling-Winthrop	Sweden	[NLM]	
stanozolol (inj)	Stromba	50 mg/ml	n/a	Winthrop	Sweden	[NLM]	
stanozolol (inj)	Strombaject	50 mg/ml	n/a	Winthrop	Belgium	[NLM]	
stanozolol (inj)	Strombaject	50 mg/ml	n/a	Winthrop	Germany	[NLM]	
stanozolol (inj)	Tanoxol	25 mg/ml	10 ml vial	Burnet	Argentina		VET
stanozolol (inj)	Vitabolic	20 mg/ml	10, 100 ml vial	Over Labs	Argentina		VET
stanozolol (inj)	Winstrol®	50 mg/ml	n/a	Winthrop	Greece	[NLM]	
stanozolol (inj)	Winstrol® Depot	50 mg/ml	1 ml vial	Zambon	Italy	[NLM]	
stanozolol (inj)	Winstrol® Depot	50 mg/ml	1 ml ampule	Zambon	Spain		
stanozolol (inj)	Winstrol® V	50 mg/ml	10, 30ml vial	Pharmacia	Canada		VET
stanozolol (inj)	Winstrol® V	50 mg/ml	10, 30ml vial	Pharmacia & Upjohn	U.S.		VET
stanozolol (inj)	Winstrol® V	50 mg/ml	10, 30ml vial	Winthrop	U.S.	[NLM]	VET
stanozolol (oral)	Anazol	2 mg tablet	100 tablet box	Xelox (export)	Philippines		
stanozolol (oral)	Anazol	2 mg tablet	100, 1000 tablet bottle	Xelox (export)	Philippines		
stanozolol (oral)	Apetil	4 mg/ml	10 ml dropper bottle	Holliday	Argentina		VET
stanozolol (oral)	Cetabon	2 mg tablet	10 tablet strip	Therapharma	Thailand		
stanozolol (oral)	Estano-Pet's	10, 25 mg tablet	100 tablet bottle	Norvet	Mexico		VET
stanozolol (oral)	Menabol	5 mg tablet	100 tablet box	n/a	India		
stanozolol (oral)	Neurabol	2 mg capsule	10 capsule box	Cadila	India		
stanozolol (oral)	Seidon	2 mg tablet	100 tablet box	Seoul Pharm	Korea		
stanozolol (oral)	Stabon	2 mg tablet	n/a	n/a	Korea		
stanozolol (oral)	Stan QV 10	10 mg tablet	100 tablet bottle	Quality Vet	Mexico		VET
stanozolol (oral)	Stan Tabs	10 mg tablet	100 tablet bottle	Animal Power	Mexico		VET
stanozolol (oral)	Stanabol	5 mg tablet	250 tablet pouch	British Dragon	Thailand	[NLM]	
stanozolol (oral)	Stanabol	5 mg tablet	200, 1000 tablet bottle	British Dragon	Thailand	[NLM]	
stanozolol (oral)	Stanabol	5 mg tablet	200 tablet pouch	British Dragon	Thailand	[NLM]	
stanozolol (oral)	Stanabol	10 mg tablet	100 tablet pouch	British Dragon	Thailand		
stanozolol (oral)	Stanabol	50 mg tablet	100 tablet pouch	British Dragon	Thailand		
stanozolol (oral)	Stanazolic	6 mg cap	300 capsule bottle	Denkall	Mexico		VET
stanozolol (oral)	Stanazolic	10 mg tablet	100 tablet bottle	Denkall	Mexico		VET
stanozolol (oral)	Stanol	5 mg tablet	200 tablet bottle	Body Research	Thailand		
stanozolol (oral)	Stanol	2 mg tablet	n/a	Hua Shin	Taiwan		
stanozolol (oral)	Stanol 10	10 mg tablet	250 tablet bottle	Bratis Labs	Mexico		VET
stanozolol (oral)	Stanol-V	10 mg tablet	100, 500 tablet bottle	Ttokkyo	Mexico		VET
stanozolol (oral)	Stanozodon	2 mg tablet	1000 tablet bottle	Acdhon Co.	Thailand		
stanozolol (oral)	stanozolol	5 mg tablet	30 tablet box	Genepharm	Greece		
stanozolol (oral)	stanozolol	25 mg tablet	30 tablet bottle	Planet Pharmacy	Belize		

Appendix A: Drug Availability Tables - Listings by Generic Name

Generic Name	Trade Name	Dose	Packaging	Company	Country	Status	Vet
stanozolol (oral)	Stanozolol Tab	2 mg tablet	n/a	Chen Ho	Taiwan		
stanozolol (oral)	Stanzol	5 mg tablet	200 tablet bottle	SB Laboratories	Thailand		
stanozolol (oral)	Stromba	5 mg tablet	56 tablet box	n/a	Greece		
stanozolol (oral)	Stromba	5 mg tablet	n/a	Sterling-Health	Hungary		
stanozolol (oral)	Stromba	5 mg tablet	10 tablet box	Winthrop	Belgium	[NLM]	
stanozolol (oral)	Stromba	5 mg tablet	n/a	Berger	Austria	[NLM]	
stanozolol (oral)	Stromba	5 mg tablet	100 tablet box	Sanofi	Netherlands		
stanozolol (oral)	Stromba	5 mg tablet	n/a	Sanofi	United Kingdom	[NLM]	
stanozolol (oral)	Stromba	5 mg tablet	n/a	Sterling	United Kingdom	[NLM]	
stanozolol (oral)	Stromba	5 mg tablet	n/a	Sterling-Health	Czech. Rep.	[NLM]	
stanozolol (oral)	Stromba	5 mg tablet	n/a	Winthrop	Denmark	[NLM]	
stanozolol (oral)	Stromba	5 mg tablet	n/a	Winthrop	Germany	[NLM]	
stanozolol (oral)	Stromba	5 mg tablet	n/a	Winthrop	Netherlands	[NLM]	
stanozolol (oral)	Stromba	5 mg tablet	n/a	Winthrop	Sweden	[NLM]	
stanozolol (oral)	Stromba	5 mg tablet	n/a	Winthrop	Switzerland	[NLM]	
stanozolol (oral)	Terabon	2 mg tablet	10 tablet strip	Jin Yang	Korea		
stanozolol (oral)	Winstrol	2 mg tablet	n/a	n/a	Japan		
stanozolol (oral)	Winstrol®	2 mg tablet	100 tablet bottle	Sanofi	U.S.		
stanozolol (oral)	Winstrol®	2 mg tablet	100 tablet bottle	Upjohn	U.S.	[NLM]	
stanozolol (oral)	Winstrol®	2 mg tablet	100 tablet bottle	Winthrop	U.S.	[NLM]	
stanozolol (oral)	Winstrol®	2 mg tablet	20 tablet box	Zambon	Italy	[NLM]	
stanozolol (oral)	Winstrol®	2 mg tablet	20 tablet box	Zambon	Spain		
stanozolol (oral)	Winstrol®	2 mg tablet	n/a	Winthrop	Portugal	[NLM]	
stanozolol (oral)	Winstrol®	2 mg tablet	n/a	Winthrop	Greece	[NLM]	
stanozolol (oral)	Winstrol-V®	2 mg tablet	100 tablet bottle	Pharmacia	Canada		VET
stanozolol (oral)	Winstrol-V®	2 mg tablet	100 tablet bottle	Pharmacia & Upjohn	U.S.		VET
stanozolol (oral)	Winstrol-V®	2 mg chewable tab	100 tablet bottle	Pharmacia & Upjohn	U.S.		VET
Sten (testosterone blend)	Sten	50 mg/ml	2 ml ampule	Atlantis	Mexico		
Sustanon 100 (testosterone blend)	Sustanon (Cyctahoh)	100 mg/ml	1 ml ampule	Infar	India		
Sustanon 100 (testosterone blend)	Sustanon 100	100 mg/ml	1 ml ampule	Organon	Germany	[NLM]	
Sustanon 100 (testosterone blend)	Sustanon '100'®	100 mg/ml	1 ml ampule	Organon	Netherlands		
Sustanon 100 (testosterone blend)	Sustanon '100'®	100 mg/ml	1 ml ampule	Organon	United Kingdom		
Sustanon 100 (testosterone blend)	Sustanon '100'®	100 mg/ml	1 ml ampule	Organon/Nile	Egypt		
Sustanon 100 (testosterone blend)	Testonon '100'®	100 mg/ml	1 ml ampule	Nile	Egypt		
Sustanon 250 (testosterone blend)	Andropen 275	275mg/ml	10 ml vial	British Dragon	Thailand		
Sustanon 250 (testosterone blend)	Durandron	250 mg/ml	1 ml ampule	Organon	Spain	[NLM]	
Sustanon 250 (testosterone blend)	Durateston	250 mg/ml	5 ml vial	Intervet	Australia		VET
Sustanon 250 (testosterone blend)	Durateston 250®	250 mg/ml	1 ml ampule	Organon	Bolivia		
Sustanon 250 (testosterone blend)	Durateston 250®	250 mg/ml	1 ml ampule	Organon	Brazil		
Sustanon 250 (testosterone blend)	Polysteron 250	250 mg/ml	1 ml ampule	Organon	Venezuela		
Sustanon 250 (testosterone blend)	Sostenon 250®	250 mg/ml	1 ml ampule	Organon	Mexico		

Appendix A: Drug Availability Tables - Listings by Generic Name

Generic Name	Trade Name	Dose	Packaging	Company	Country	Status	Vet
Sustanon 250 (testosterone blend)	Sostenon 250®	250 mg/ml	1 ml ampule	Organon	Spain	[NLM]	
Sustanon 250 (testosterone blend)	Super Test-250	250 mg/ml	5, 10 ml vial	Tornel	Mexico		VET
Sustanon 250 (testosterone blend)	Sustanon	250 mg/ml	1 ml ampule	Organon	Ireland		
Sustanon 250 (testosterone blend)	Sustanon	250 mg/ml	1 ml ampule	Organon	Israel		
Sustanon 250 (testosterone blend)	Sustanon	250 mg/ml	1 ml ampule	Organon	Slovakia		
Sustanon 250 (testosterone blend)	Sustanon "250"	250 mg/ml	1 ml ampule	Organon	Indonesia		
Sustanon 250 (testosterone blend)	Sustanon "250"	250 mg/ml	1 ml ampule	Organon	Singapore		
Sustanon 250 (testosterone blend)	Sustanon "250"	250 mg/ml	1 ml ampule	Organon	Argentina		
Sustanon 250 (testosterone blend)	Sustanon "250"	250 mg/ml	1ml ampule	Organon	Vietnam		
Sustanon 250 (testosterone blend)	Sustanon (Cyctahoh 250)	250 mg/ml	1 ml ampule	Organon	Russia		
Sustanon 250 (testosterone blend)	Sustanon 250	250 mg/ml	1 ml ampule	Organon	Germany	[NLM]	
Sustanon 250 (testosterone blend)	Sustanon 250	250 mg/ml	1 ml ampule	Organon	New Zealand		
Sustanon 250 (testosterone blend)	Sustanon 250	250 mg/ml	1 ml ampule	Organon	Taiwan		
Sustanon 250 (testosterone blend)	Sustanon 250	250 mg/ml	1 ml ampule	Organon	Czech. Rep.		
Sustanon 250 (testosterone blend)	Sustanon 250 (Cyctahon)	250 mg/ml	1 ml ampule	Infar	India		
Sustanon 250 (testosterone blend)	Sustanon 250®	250 mg/ml	1 ml ampule	Organon	Belgium		
Sustanon 250 (testosterone blend)	Sustanon 250®	250 mg/ml	1 ml ampule	Organon	Estonia		
Sustanon 250 (testosterone blend)	Sustanon 250®	250 mg/ml	1 ml ampule	Organon	Finland		
Sustanon 250 (testosterone blend)	Sustanon 250®	250 mg/ml	1 ml ampule	Organon	Netherlands		
Sustanon 250 (testosterone blend)	Sustanon 250®	250 mg/ml	1 ml ampule	Organon	Turkey		
Sustanon 250 (testosterone blend)	Sustanon '250'®	250 mg/ml	1 ml ampule	Donmed/Organon	South Africa		
Sustanon 250 (testosterone blend)	Sustanon '250'®	250 mg/ml	1 ml ampule	Organon	Malaysia		
Sustanon 250 (testosterone blend)	Sustanon '250'®	250 mg/ml	1ml ampule	Organon	Pakistan		
Sustanon 250 (testosterone blend)	Sustanon '250'®	250 mg/ml	1 ml ampule	Organon	Thailand		
Sustanon 250 (testosterone blend)	Sustanon '250'®	250 mg/ml	1 ml ampule	Organon	United Kingdom		
Sustanon 250 (testosterone blend)	Sustanon '250'®	250 mg/ml	1 ml ampule	Organon/Nile	Egypt		
Sustanon 250 (testosterone blend)	Sustanon®	250 mg/ml	1 ml ampule	Organon	Italy		
Sustanon 250 (testosterone blend)	Sustaretard 250	250 mg/ml	1 ml ampule	BM Pharmaceuticals	India		
Sustanon 250 (testosterone blend)	Sustenan 250	250 mg/ml	1 ml ampule	Organon	Chile		
Sustanon 250 (testosterone blend)	Sustenon 250®	250 mg/ml	1 ml ampule	Organon	Portugal		
Sustanon 250 (testosterone blend)	Testenon 250	250 mg/ml	5 ml vial	Ttokkyo	Mexico		VET
Sustanon 250 (testosterone blend)	Testo-Jet L.A.	250 mg/ml	10 ml vial	Norvet	Mexico		VET
Sustanon 250 (testosterone blend)	Testonon '250'®	250 mg/ml	1 ml ampule	Nile	Egypt		
Sustanon 250 (testosterone blend)	Testosteron 250	250 mg/ml	1 ml ampule	Rotex Medica	Germany	[NLM]	
Sustanon 250 (testosterone blend)	Testosterona 250	250 mg/ml	10 ml vial	Qualityvet	Costa Rica		VET
Sustanon 250 (testosterone blend)	Testosterona IV L/A	250 mg/ml	10 ml vial	Loeffler	Mexico		VET
Sustanon 250 (testosterone blend)	Testron 4 250	250 mg/ml	10 ml vial	Bratis Labs	Mexico		VET
Test 400 (testosterone blend)	Test 400	400 mg/ml	10 ml vial	Denkall	Mexico		VET
testosterone (gel)	Androgel	25, 50 mg	single dose packet	Besins	Netherlands		
testosterone (gel)	Androgel	25, 50 mg	single dose packet	Besins	Sweden		
testosterone (gel)	Androgel	25, 50 mg	single dose packet	Solvay	Canada		

Appendix A: Drug Availability Tables - Listings by Generic Name

Generic Name	Trade Name	Dose	Packaging	Company	Country	Status	Vet
testosterone (gel)	Androgel	50, 75, 100 mg	single dose packet	Unimed	U.S.		
testosterone (gel)	Androtop Gel	50 mg	single dose packet	Kade/Besins	Germany		
testosterone (gel)	Testogel	25, 50 mg	single dose packet	Besins	Netherlands		
testosterone (gel)	Testogel	25, 50 mg	single dose packet	Besins	Sweden		
testosterone (gel)	Testogel	25, 50 mg	single dose packet	Jenapharm	Germany		
testosterone (gel)	Testogel	25, 50 mg	single dose packet	Schering	Australia		
testosterone (gel)	Testogel	50 mg	single dose packet	Schering	Austria		
testosterone (implant)	Ropel Testosterone Pellets	23.5 mg pellet	450, 600 pellet bottle	Jurox	Australia		VET
testosterone (patch)	Androderm®	12.2 mg patch.	10, 30, 60 patches/box	AstraZenica	Germany		
testosterone (patch)	Androderm®	12.2 mg patch	n/a	Astrazenica	Switzerland		
testosterone (patch)	Androderm®	12.2 mg patch.	n/a	n/a	Korea		
testosterone (patch)	Androderm®	12.2 mg patch.	30 patches/box	Pharmascience	Canada		
testosterone (patch)	Androderm®	12.2 mg patch.	n/a	Schwarz Pharma	Italy		
testosterone (patch)	Androderm®	2.5 mg patch	30, 60 patch box	Schwarz Pharma	Spain		
testosterone (patch)	Androderm®	5 mg patch	30 patch box	Schwarz Pharma	Spain		
testosterone (patch)	Androderm®	12.2 mg patch	60 patches/box	SmithKline Beecham	U.S.	[NLM]	
testosterone (patch)	Androderm®	12.2, 24.3 mg patch	60 patches/box	Watson Pharma	U.S.		
testosterone (patch)	Andropatch	2.5 mg patch	60 patches/box	GSK	United Kingdom		
testosterone (patch)	Andropatch	5 mg patch	30 patches/box	GSK	United Kingdom		
testosterone (patch)	Andropatch	12.2 mg patch	30, 60 patch box	Schwarz Pharma	Netherlands		
testosterone (patch)	Atmos	5 mg patch	n/a	Astra	Sweden		
testosterone (patch)	Atmos	5 mg patch	30 patch box	Astra Zenica	Norway		
testosterone (patch)	Testoderm	15 mg patch	n/a	Alza	Malaysia		
testosterone (patch)	Testoderm	6 mg patch	10, 30 patch box	Esteve	Spain		
testosterone (patch)	Testoderm	4 mg patch	10 patch box	Esteve	Spain		
testosterone blend (misc)	Deposterona	60 mg/ml	10 ml vial	Fort Dodge	Mexico		VET
testosterone blend (misc)	Deposterona	60 mg/ml	10 ml vial	Syntex	Mexico	[NLM]	VET
testosterone blend (misc)	Equitest 200	200 mg/ml	6 ml vial	WDV	Myanmar/Burma		VET
testosterone blend (misc)	Triolandren	250 mg/ml	1 ml ampule	Novartis	Egypt		
testosterone blend (misc)	Triolandren	250 mg/ml	1 ml ampule	Novartis	Taiwan		
testosterone cyclohexylpropionate	Testosterone CHP Theramex	296, 148, 37 mg/ml	1 ml ampule	Theramex	France	[NLM]	
testosterone cypionate	Anabolic TL	100 mg/ml	10 ml vial	SYD Group	Australia		VET
testosterone cypionate	Anabolic TL	200 mg/ml	10 ml vial	SYD Group	Mexico		VET
testosterone cypionate	Andro-Cyp	100, 200 mg/ml	10 ml vial	Brown	U.S.	[NLM]	
testosterone cypionate	Andro-Cyp	100, 200 mg/ml	10 ml vial	Keene	U.S.	[NLM]	
testosterone cypionate	Andronaq LA	100, 200 mg/ml	10 ml vial	Central	U.S.	[NLM]	
testosterone cypionate	Andronate	100, 200 mg/ml	10 ml vial	Pasadena	U.S.	[NLM]	
testosterone cypionate	Banrot	75 mg/ml	200 ml bladder	Coopers	Australia	[NLM]	VET
testosterone cypionate	Biselmon Depot	50 mg/ml	n/a	Ta Fong	Taiwan		
testosterone cypionate	Cyclo-Testosterone Depot	130 mg/ml	n/a	Astar	Taiwan		
testosterone cypionate	Cypionax	100 mg/ml	2 ml ampule	Body Research	Thailand		

Appendix A: Drug Availability Tables - Listings by Generic Name

Generic Name	Trade Name	Dose	Packaging	Company	Country	Status	Vet
testosterone cypionate	Cypiotest 250	250 mg/ml	10 ml vial	Animal Power	Mexico		VET
testosterone cypionate	CypioTest 250	250 mg/ml	10 ml vial	Denkall	Mexico		VET
testosterone cypionate	Cypriotest L/A	250 mg/ml	10 ml vial	Loeffler	Mexico		VET
testosterone cypionate	Dep Andro-100-200	100, 200 mg/ml	10 ml vial	Forest	U.S.	[NLM]	
testosterone cypionate	Deposteron	100 mg/ml	2 ml ampule	Novaquimica/Sigma	Brazil		
testosterone cypionate	Depot-Bifuron	50 mg/ml	n/a	Gentle	Taiwan		
testosterone cypionate	Depo-TCP	200mg/ml	n/a	n/a	Korea		
testosterone cypionate	Depotest	100, 200 mg/ml	10 ml vial	Hyrex	U.S.	[NLM]	
testosterone cypionate	Depotest	100, 200 mg/ml	10 ml vial	Kay	U.S.	[NLM]	
testosterone cypionate	Depo-Testermon	200 mg/ml	n/a	CCPC	Taiwan		
testosterone cypionate	Depo-Testerone	200 mg/ml	n/a	Metro	Taiwan		
testosterone cypionate	Depo-Testomon	100 mg/ml	n/a	Li Ta	Taiwan		
testosterone cypionate	Depo-Testosterone	100 mg/ml	10 ml vial	Pharmacia & Upjohn	South Africa		
testosterone cypionate	Depo-Testosterone CPP	100 mg/ml	n/a	Metro	Taiwan		
testosterone cypionate	Depo-Testosterone®	100 mg/ml	n/a	Pharmacia	Malaysia		
testosterone cypionate	Depo-Testosterone®	100 mg/ml	10 ml vial	Pharmacia	Canada		
testosterone cypionate	Depo-Testosterone®	100 mg/ml	10 ml vial	Pharmacia & Upjohn	New Zealand		
testosterone cypionate	Depo-Testosterone®	100 mg/ml	10 ml vial	Pharmacia & Upjohn	Singapore		
testosterone cypionate	Depo-Testosterone®	100, 200 mg/ml	10 ml vial	Pharmacia & Upjohn	U.S.		
testosterone cypionate	Depo-Testosterone®	200 mg/ml	1 ml vial	Pharmacia & Upjohn	U.S.		
testosterone cypionate	Depot-Hormon MF	50 mg/ml	n/a	Sintong	Taiwan		
testosterone cypionate	Depotrone	100 mg/ml	2 ml ampule	Propan-Zurich	South Africa		
testosterone cypionate	Depovirin Inj	125 mg/ml	2 ml	n/a	Korea		
testosterone cypionate	Dep-Test	100 mg/ml	10 ml vial	Rocky Mountain	U.S.	[NLM]	
testosterone cypionate	D-Test 100/200	100, 200 mg/ml	10 ml vial	Sig	U.S.	[NLM]	
testosterone cypionate	Duratest-100-200	100, 200 mg/ml	10 ml vial	Roberts	U.S.	[NLM]	
testosterone cypionate	Duratest-100-200	100, 200 mg/ml	10 ml vial	Hauck	U.S.	[NLM]	
testosterone cypionate	Malogen Cyp	100, 200 mg/ml	10 ml vial	Forest	U.S.	[NLM]	
testosterone cypionate	Miro Depo	125 mg/ml	2 ml vial	Hanil Pharm	Korea		
testosterone cypionate	Nannismon Depot	50, 100 mg/ml	n/a	Chi Sheng	Taiwan		
testosterone cypionate	Ridrot Testosterone Inj.	75 mg/ml	250 ml vial	Troy	Australia		VET
testosterone cypionate	Scheinpharma Testone-Cyp	100 mg/ml	10 ml vial	Schein	Canada		
testosterone cypionate	Testabol Depot	200 mg/ml	10 ml vial	British Dragon	Thailand		
testosterone cypionate	Testa-C	200 mg/ml	10 ml vial	Vortech	U.S.	[NLM]	
testosterone cypionate	Testacyp	100 mg/ml	2 ml vial	BM Pharmaceuticals	India		
testosterone cypionate	Testadiate-Depo	200 mg/ml	10 ml vial	Kay	U.S.	[NLM]	
testosterone cypionate	Testex Leo prolongatum	50, 125 mg/ml	2 ml ampule	Altana Pharma	Spain		
testosterone cypionate	Testex Leo prolongatum	50, 125 mg/ml	2 ml ampule	Leo	Spain	[NLM]	
testosterone cypionate	Testo LA	100 mg/ml	10 ml vial	Jurox	Australia	[NLM]	VET
testosterone cypionate	Testoject	100 mg/ml	n/a	Mayrand	U.S.	[NLM]	
testosterone cypionate	Testoject 50	50 mg/ml	n/a	Mayrand	U.S.	[NLM]	

Appendix A: Drug Availability Tables - Listings by Generic Name

Generic Name	Trade Name	Dose	Packaging	Company	Country	Status	Vet
testosterone cypionate	Testoject-LA	200 mg/ml	n/a	Mayrand	U.S.	[NLM]	
testosterone cypionate	Teston QV 200	200 mg/ml	10 ml vial	Quality Vet	Mexico		VET
testosterone cypionate	Testorone Depot	100 mg/ml	n/a	Gentle	Taiwan		
testosterone cypionate	Testosterona Ultra Lenta	100 mg/ml	20 ml vial	Dispert Labs.	Uruguay		VET
testosterone cypionate	Testosterona Ultra Lenta Fuerte	200 mg/ml	5 ml ampule	Dispert Labs.	Uruguay		VET
testosterone cypionate	Testosterona Ultra Lenta Fuerte	200 mg/ml	20 ml vial	Dispert Labs.	Uruguay		VET
testosterone cypionate	testosterone cypionate	100 mg/ml	10 ml vial	Geneva Geriatrics	U.S.	[NLM]	
testosterone cypionate	testosterone cypionate	100, 200 mg/ml	10 ml vial	Goldline	U.S.	[NLM]	
testosterone cypionate	testosterone cypionate	50, 100, 200 mg/ml	10 ml vial	Huffman	U.S.	[NLM]	
testosterone cypionate	testosterone cypionate	200 mg/ml	10 ml vial	Legere	U.S.	[NLM]	
testosterone cypionate	testosterone cypionate	100, 200 mg/ml	10 ml vial	Schein	U.S.	[NLM]	
testosterone cypionate	testosterone cypionate	100, 200 mg/ml	10 ml vial	Steris	U.S.	[NLM]	
testosterone cypionate	Testosterone Cypionate 200	200 mg/ml	10 ml vial	Ttokkyo	Mexico		VET
testosterone cypionate	Testosterone Cypionate Inj	200 mg/ml	n/a	Charmaine	Hong Kong		
testosterone cypionate	Testosterone Cypionate Inj	200 mg/ml	n/a	Gwo Chyang	Taiwan		
testosterone cypionate	Testosterone Cypionate Inj	200 mg/ml	n/a	Tai Yu	Taiwan		
testosterone cypionate	Testosterone Cypionate Inj.	100 mg/ml	2 ml vial	Cytex	Canada		
testosterone cypionate	Testosterone Cypionate Inj.	200 mg/ml	10 ml vial	Sabex	Canada		
testosterone cypionate	Testosterone Cypionate L.A.	100 mg/ml	10 ml vial	Ttokkyo	Mexico	[NLM]	VET
testosterone cypionate	Testosterone Depositum	n/a	n/a	SPA	Italy		
testosterone cypionate	Testred Cypionate	200 mg/ml	10 ml vial	INC	U.S.	[NLM]	
testosterone cypionate	Vironate	200 mg/ml	5 ml vial	Xelox (export)	Philippines		
testosterone decanoate	Neotest 250	250 mg/ml	10 ml bottle	Loeffler	Mexico		
testosterone enanthate	Anderone 100/200	100, 200 mg/ml	10 ml vial	Burgin-Arden	U.S.	[NLM]	
testosterone enanthate	Andro 100	100 mg/ml	10 ml vial	Forest	U.S.	[NLM]	
testosterone enanthate	Andro L.A. 200	200 mg/ml	10 ml vial	Forest	U.S.	[NLM]	
testosterone enanthate	Andropository	200 mg/ml	10 ml vial	Rugby	U.S.	[NLM]	
testosterone enanthate	Androtardyl®	250 mg/ml	1 ml ampule	Schering	Algeria		
testosterone enanthate	Androtardyl®	250 mg/ml	1 ml ampule	Schering	France		
testosterone enanthate	Androtardyl®	250 mg/ml	1 ml ampule	Schering	Morocco		
testosterone enanthate	Androtardyl®	250 mg/ml	1 ml ampule	Schering	Tunisia		
testosterone enanthate	Andryl 200	200 mg/ml	10 ml vial	Keene	U.S.	[NLM]	
testosterone enanthate	Delatest	100/mg/ml	10 ml vial	Dunhall	U.S.	[NLM]	
testosterone enanthate	Delatestryl	200 mg/ml	10 ml vial	Brovel	Mexico	[NLM]	VET
testosterone enanthate	Delatestryl	200 mg/ml	1 ml syringe	BTG	U.S.		
testosterone enanthate	Delatestryl	200 mg/ml	5 ml vial	BTG	U.S.		
testosterone enanthate	Delatestryl	200 mg/ml	10 ml vial	Mead Johnson	U.S.	[NLM]	
testosterone enanthate	Delatestryl	200 mg/ml	5 ml vial	Theramed	Canada		
testosterone enanthate	DepoTestmon Inj	65 mg/ml	n/a	CCPC	Taiwan		
testosterone enanthate	Dura-Testosterone	200 mg/ml	10 ml vial	Pharmex	U.S.	[NLM]	
testosterone enanthate	Durathate-200 Injection	200 mg/ml	n/a	Hauck	U.S.	[NLM]	

Appendix A: Drug Availability Tables - Listings by Generic Name

Generic Name	Trade Name	Dose	Packaging	Company	Country	Status	Vet
testosterone enanthate	Durathate-200 Injection	200 mg/ml	n/a	Roberts	U.S.	[NLM]	
testosterone enanthate	Enantat QV 250	250 mg/ml	10, 50 ml vial	Quality Vet	Mexico		VET
testosterone enanthate	Enantato 350	350 mg/ml	10 ml vial	Pet's Pharma	Mexico		VET
testosterone enanthate	Enantest 250	250 mg/ml	10 ml vial	Animal Power	Mexico		VET
testosterone enanthate	Enarmon-Depot	125 mg/ml	n/a	Teskoku Hormone	Japan		
testosterone enanthate	Everone	100, 200 mg/ml	10 ml vial	Hyrex	U.S.	[NLM]	
testosterone enanthate	Jenasteron Inj	250 mg/ml	1 ml ampule	Jenahexal	Malaysia		
testosterone enanthate	Jenasteron Inj	250 mg/ml	n/a	n/a	Korea		
testosterone enanthate	Malogen 100/200 L.A.	100, 200 mg/ml	10 ml vial	Forest	U.S.	[NLM]	
testosterone enanthate	Malogex LA200	200 mg/ml	10 ml vial	Germiphene	Canada	[NLM]	
testosterone enanthate	PMS-Testosterone Enanthate	200 mg/ml	10 ml vial	Pharmascience	Canada		
testosterone enanthate	Primoniat®-Depot 250	250 mg/ml	1 ml ampule	Schering-Chile	Chile	[NLM]	
testosterone enanthate	Primoteston®-Depot	250 mg/ml	1 ml ampule	Leiras	Finland	[NLM]	
testosterone enanthate	Primoteston®-Depot	250 mg/ml	1 ml ampule	Schering	Norway		
testosterone enanthate	Primoteston®-Depot	250 mg/ml	1 ml ampule	Schering	United Kingdom	[NLM]	
testosterone enanthate	Primoteston®-Depot	250 mg/ml	1 ml ampule	Schering/CID	Egypt		
testosterone enanthate	Primoteston®-Depot	250 mg/ml	1 ml ampule	Schering	Australia		
testosterone enanthate	Primoteston®-Depot	250 mg/ml	1 ml ampule	Schering	Ecuador		
testosterone enanthate	Primoteston®-Depot	250 mg/ml	1 ml ampule	Schering	Guatemala		
testosterone enanthate	Primoteston®-Depot	250 mg/ml	1 ml ampule	Schering	Jordan		
testosterone enanthate	Primoteston®-Depot	250 mg/ml	1 ml ampule	Schering	Kuwait	[NLM]	
testosterone enanthate	Primoteston®-Depot	250 mg/ml	1 ml ampule	Schering	Mauritius		
testosterone enanthate	Primoteston®-Depot	250 mg/ml	1 ml ampule	Schering	Mexico		
testosterone enanthate	Primoteston®-Depot	250 mg/ml	1 ml syringe	Schering	New Zealand		
testosterone enanthate	Primoteston®-Depot	250 mg/ml	1 ml ampule	Schering	Sudan		
testosterone enanthate	Proviron®-Depot	250 mg/ml	1 ml ampule	Schering	Venezuela		
testosterone enanthate	Ropel Liquid Testosterone	75 mg/ml	200 ml vial	Jurox	Australia		VET
testosterone enanthate	Sunamon Depot Inj	130 mg/ml	n/a	Astar	Taiwan		
testosterone enanthate	Sunamon Inj	250 mg/ml	n/a	Astar	Taiwan		
testosterone enanthate	Tesone L.A.	200 mg/ml	10 ml vial	Sig	U.S.	[NLM]	
testosterone enanthate	Testanate No. 1	100 mg/ml	n/a	Kenyon	U.S.	[NLM]	
testosterone enanthate	Testaval	100, 200 mg/ml	10 ml vial	Legere	U.S.	[NLM]	
testosterone enanthate	Testen-250	250 mg/ml	2 ml vial	BM Pharmaceuticals	India		
testosterone enanthate	Testenan Depot	250 mg/ml	n/a	Sinton	Taiwan		
testosterone enanthate	Testenat 10%	100 mg/ml	1 ml ampule	Farmadon	Russia		
testosterone enanthate	Testermon	25 mg/ml	n/a	CCPC	Taiwan		
testosterone enanthate	Testinon-Depot	n/a	n/a	n/a	Japan		
testosterone enanthate	Testoenan L/A	250 mg/ml	10 ml vial	Loeffler	Mexico		VET
testosterone enanthate	Testo-Enant	125 mg/ml	2 ml ampule	Geymonat	Italy		
testosterone enanthate	Testo-Enant	250 mg/ml	1 ml ampule	Geymonat	Italy		
testosterone enanthate	Testosteron Depot	100 mg/ml	1 ml ampule	Rotex Medica	Germany	[NLM]	

Appendix A: Drug Availability Tables - Listings by Generic Name

Generic Name	Trade Name	Dose	Packaging	Company	Country	Status	Vet
testosterone enanthate	Testosteron Depot	250 mg/ml	1 ml ampule	Rotex Medica	Germany		
testosterone enanthate	Testosterona 200	200 mg/ml	10 ml vial	Brovel	Mexico		VET
testosterone enanthate	testosterona enantato	250 mg/ml	1 ml ampule	Biosano	Chile		
testosterone enanthate	testosterona enantato	100 mg/ml	1 ml ampule	Chile	Chile	[NLM]	
testosterone enanthate	testosterona enantato	250 mg/ml	1 ml ampule	Chile	Chile		
testosterone enanthate	Testosteron-Depo	100 mg/ml	1 ml ampule	Galenika	YugoslaviaFRMR	[NLM]	
testosterone enanthate	Testosteron-Depo	250 mg/ml	1 ml ampule	Galenika	YugoslaviaFRMR		
testosterone enanthate	Testosteron-Depo	100, 250 mg/ml	1 ml ampule	Hemofarm	YugoslaviaFRMR	[NLM]	
testosterone enanthate	Testosteron-Depot	250 mg/ml	1 ml ampule	Eifelfango	Germany		
testosterone enanthate	Testosteron-Depot	250 mg/ml	1 ml ampule	Jenapharm	Bulgaria		
testosterone enanthate	Testosteron-Depot	250 mg/ml	1 ml ampule	Jenapharm	Germany		
testosterone enanthate	Testosterone 200 Depot	200 mg/ml	10 ml vial	Tornel	Mexico		VET
testosterone enanthate	testosterone enanthate	100, 200 mg/ml	10 ml vial	Geneva Geriatrics	U.S.	[NLM]	
testosterone enanthate	testosterone enanthate	100, 200 mg/ml	10 ml vial	Goldline	U.S.	[NLM]	
testosterone enanthate	testosterone enanthate	250 mg/ml	1 ml ampule	Norma Hellas	Greece		
testosterone enanthate	testosterone enanthate	100, 200 mg/ml	10 ml vial	Quad	U.S.	[NLM]	
testosterone enanthate	testosterone enanthate	100, 200 mg/ml	10 ml vial	Schein	U.S.	[NLM]	
testosterone enanthate	testosterone enanthate	100, 200 mg/ml	10 ml vial	Steris	U.S.	[NLM]	
testosterone enanthate	Testosterone Enanthate 250	250 mg/ml	1 ml ampule	Aburaihan	Iran		
testosterone enanthate	Testosterone Enanthate Dalim	250 mg/ml	n/a	Dalim	Korea		
testosterone enanthate	Testosterone Enanthate Inj	200 mg/ml	10 ml vial	Taro	Canada	[NLM]	
testosterone enanthate	Testosterone Heptylate	50, 100, 250 mg/ml	1 ml ampule	Theramex	France		
testosterone enanthate	Testosteronum Prolongatum	100 mg/ml	1 ml ampule	Jelfa	Bulgaria	[NLM]	
testosterone enanthate	Testosteronum Prolongatum	100 mg/ml	1 ml ampule	Jelfa	Poland		
testosterone enanthate	Testosteronum Prolongatum	100 mg/ml	1 ml ampule	Polfa	Belgium	[NLM]	
testosterone enanthate	Testosteronum Prolongatum	100 mg/ml	1 ml ampule	Polfa	Poland	[NLM]	
testosterone enanthate	Testoviron Depot	250 mg/ml	1 ml ampule	Schering	Taiwan		
testosterone enanthate	Testoviron® Depot	250 mg/ml	1 ml ampule	Schering	Argentina		
testosterone enanthate	Testoviron® Depot	250 mg/ml	1 ml ampule	Schering	Hungary	[NLM]	
testosterone enanthate	Testoviron® Depot	250 mg/ml	1 ml ampule	Schering	Ireland	[NLM]	
testosterone enanthate	Testoviron® Depot	250 mg/ml	1 ml ampule	Schering	Peru		
testosterone enanthate	Testoviron®-Depot	250 mg/ml	1 ml ampule	Schering	Hong Kong		
testosterone enanthate	Testoviron®-Depot	250 mg/ml	1 ml ampule	Schering	Iceland		
testosterone enanthate	Testoviron®-Depot	250 mg/ml	1 ml ampule	Schering	Thailand		
testosterone enanthate	Testoviron®-Depot	250 mg/ml	1 ml ampule	Schering	Yemen		
testosterone enanthate	Testoviron®-Depot	250 mg/ml	1 ml ampule	Scherimed	Spain		
testosterone enanthate	Testoviron®-Depot	250 mg/ml	1 ml ampule	Schering	Austria		
testosterone enanthate	Testoviron®-Depot	250 mg/ml	1 ml ampule	Schering	Bahrain	[NLM]	
testosterone enanthate	Testoviron®-Depot	250 mg/ml	1 ml ampule	Schering	Colombia		
testosterone enanthate	Testoviron®-Depot	250 mg/ml	1 ml ampule	Schering	Czech. Rep.	[NLM]	
testosterone enanthate	Testoviron®-Depot	250 mg/ml	1 ml ampule	Schering	Denmark		

Appendix A: Drug Availability Tables - Listings by Generic Name

Generic Name	Trade Name	Dose	Packaging	Company	Country	Status	Vet
testosterone enanthate	Testoviron®-Depot	250 mg/ml	1 ml ampule	Schering	Dom. Rep.		
testosterone enanthate	Testoviron®-Depot	250 mg/ml	1 ml ampule	Schering	Ethiopia		
testosterone enanthate	Testoviron®-Depot	250 mg/ml	1 ml ampule	Schering	Germany		
testosterone enanthate	Testoviron®-Depot	250 mg/ml	1 ml ampule	Schering	Greece		
testosterone enanthate	Testoviron®-Depot	250 mg/ml	1 ml ampule	Schering	India		
testosterone enanthate	Testoviron®-Depot	250 mg/ml	1 ml ampule	Schering	Israel		
testosterone enanthate	Testoviron®-Depot	250 mg/ml	1 ml ampule	Schering	Italy		
testosterone enanthate	Testoviron®-Depot	250 mg/ml	1 ml ampule	Schering	Japan		
testosterone enanthate	Testoviron®-Depot	250 mg/ml	1 ml ampule	Schering	Lebanon	[NLM]	
testosterone enanthate	Testoviron®-Depot	250 mg/ml	1 ml ampule	Schering	Malaysia		
testosterone enanthate	Testoviron®-Depot	250 mg/ml	1 ml ampule	Schering	Malta		
testosterone enanthate	Testoviron®-Depot	250 mg/ml	1 ml ampule	Schering	Pakistan		
testosterone enanthate	Testoviron®-Depot	250 mg/ml	1 ml ampule	Schering	Paraguay		
testosterone enanthate	Testoviron®-Depot	250 mg/ml	1 ml ampule	Schering	Portugal		
testosterone enanthate	Testoviron®-Depot	250 mg/ml	1 ml ampule	Schering	Qatar	[NLM]	
testosterone enanthate	Testoviron®-Depot	250 mg/ml	1 ml ampule	Schering	Saudi Arabia		
testosterone enanthate	Testoviron®-Depot	250 mg/ml	1 ml ampule	Schering	Spain	[NLM]	
testosterone enanthate	Testoviron®-Depot	250 mg/ml	1 ml ampule	Schering	Sri Lanka		
testosterone enanthate	Testoviron®-Depot	250 mg/ml	1 ml ampule	Schering	Sweden		
testosterone enanthate	Testoviron®-Depot	250 mg/ml	1 ml ampule	Schering	Switzerland		
testosterone enanthate	Testoviron®-Depot	250 mg/ml	1 ml ampule	Schering	Uruguay		
testosterone enanthate	Testrin-P.A.	200 mg/ml	n/a	Pasadena Res.	U.S.	[NLM]	
testosterone enanthate	Testron Depot	125, 250 mg/ml	1 ml vial	n/a	Japan		
testosterone enanthate	Weratestone 250	250 mg/ml	1 ml ampule	Weimer Pharma	Algeria		
testosterone enanthate	Weratestone 250	250 mg/ml	1 ml ampule	Weimer Pharma	Mozambique		
testosterone enanthate	Weratestone 250	250 mg/ml	1 ml ampule	Weimer Pharma	Zimbabwe		
testosterone enanthate	Weratestone 250	250 mg/ml	1 ml ampule	Weimer Pharma	Zimbabwe		
testosterone phenylpropionate	Testolent	100 mg/ml	1 ml ampule	Sicomed	Rumania	[NLM]	
testosterone propionate	Agovirin injectable	25 mg/ml	n/a	Leciva	Czech. Rep.	[NLM]	
testosterone propionate	Anatest	100 mg/ml	10 ml vial	Rhone	Canada	[NLM]	VET
testosterone propionate	Anatest	100 mg/ml	10 ml vial	Sterivet	Canada	[NLM]	VET
testosterone propionate	Anatest	100 mg/ml	10 ml vial	Vetoquinol	Canada		VET
testosterone propionate	Androfort-Richter	10, 25 mg/ml	n/a	Gedeon Richter	Hungary		
testosterone propionate	Androlan	50, 100 mg/ml	n/a	Lannett	U.S.	[NLM]	
testosterone propionate	Ara-Test	25 mg/ml	10 ml vial	Aranda Laboratories	Mexico	[NLM]	VET
testosterone propionate	Astrapin	50 mg/ml	1 ml ampule	Astrapin	Malaysia		
testosterone propionate	AVP Supertest	50 mg/ml	10 ml vial	Vetsearch	Australia		VET
testosterone propionate	Dubol	25 mg/ml	1 ml ampule	n/a	China		
testosterone propionate	Facovit	1 mg/ml	10 ml vial	Teofarma	Italy		
testosterone propionate	Hybolin Imp.	25, 50 mg/ml	n/a	Hyrex	U.S.	[NLM]	
testosterone propionate	Malogen In Oil	100 mg/ml	10 ml vial	Germiphene	Canada	[NLM]	

Appendix A: Drug Availability Tables - Listings by Generic Name

Generic Name	Trade Name	Dose	Packaging	Company	Country	Status	Vet
testosterone propionate	Nansmon Depot	25 mg/ml	n/a	Chi Sheng	Taiwan		
testosterone propionate	Neo-Hombreol	50 mg/ml	n/a	Organon	Netherlands	[NLM]	
testosterone propionate	Oreton	25 mg/ml	n/a	Goldline	Mexico	[NLM]	
testosterone propionate	Propionat QV 100	100 mg/ml	10 ml vial	Quality Vet	Mexico		VET
testosterone propionate	Propionato de Testosterona	25 mg/ml	20 ml vial	Induvet	Argentina		VET
testosterone propionate	Propiotest 100	100 mg/ml	10 ml vial	Animal Power	Mexico		VET
testosterone propionate	Tepro Hormone	100 mg/ml	500 ml vial	Virbac	Australia		VET
testosterone propionate	Testabol Propionate	100 mg/ml	10 ml vial	British Dragon	Thailand		
testosterone propionate	Testex	50, 100 mg/ml	n/a	Pasadena	U.S.	[NLM]	
testosterone propionate	Testex Leo	25 mg/ml	1 ml ampule	Altana Pharma	Spain		
testosterone propionate	Testex Leo	25 mg/ml	1 ml ampule	Leo	Spain	[NLM]	
testosterone propionate	Testo	50 mg/ml	10 ml vial	Samil	Korea		
testosterone propionate	Testogan	25 mg/ml	50 ml vial	Laguinsa	Costa Rica		VET
testosterone propionate	Testogan	25 mg/ml	50 ml vial	Laguinsa	Dom. Rep.		VET
testosterone propionate	Testogan	25 mg/ml	50 ml vial	Laguinsa	Ecuador		VET
testosterone propionate	Testogan	25 mg/ml	50 ml vial	Laguinsa	El Salvador		VET
testosterone propionate	Testogan	25 mg/ml	50 ml vial	Laguinsa	Guatemala		VET
testosterone propionate	Testogan	25 mg/ml	50 ml vial	Laguinsa	Honduras		VET
testosterone propionate	Testogan	25 mg/ml	50 ml vial	Laguinsa	Nicaragua		VET
testosterone propionate	Testogan	25 mg/ml	50 ml vial	Laguinsa	Panama		VET
testosterone propionate	Testolic	50 mg/ml	2 ml ampule	Body Research	Thailand		
testosterone propionate	Testone-E	25 mg/ml	1 ml ampule	Misr	Egypt		
testosterone propionate	Testopin-100	100 mg/ml	2 ml vial	BM Pharmaceuticals	India		
testosterone propionate	Testopin-100	100 mg/ml	1 ml ampule	BM Pharmaceuticals	India		
testosterone propionate	Testopro L/A	250 mg/ml	10 ml vial	Loeffler	Mexico		VET
testosterone propionate	Testosteron	25 mg/ml	1 ml ampule	Sicomed	Rumania	[NLM]	
testosterone propionate	Testosteron	5, 10, 25, 50 mg/ml	1 ml ampule	Galenika	YugoslaviaFRMR	[NLM]	
testosterone propionate	Testosteron	5, 10, 25, 50 mg/ml	1 ml ampule	Hemofarm	Hungary	[NLM]	
testosterone propionate	Testosteron	50 mg/ml	1 ml ampule	Sopharma	Bulgaria		
testosterone propionate	Testosteron	50 mg/ml	1 ml ampule	Streuli & Co. AG	Switzerland	[NLM]	
testosterone propionate	Testosteron Depot	25 mg/ml	n/a	Gentle	Taiwan		
testosterone propionate	Testosterona	50, 100 mg/ml	10, 20 ml vial	Brovel	Mexico		VET
testosterone propionate	Testosterona Propionat	50, 100 mg/ml	1 ml ampule	Farmadon	Russia	[NLM]	
testosterone propionate	Testosterona Propionato	n/a	n/a	Botica	Paraguay		
testosterone propionate	Testosterone Berco Supp.	40 mg/suppository	18 supp. box	Funke	Germany	[NLM]	
testosterone propionate	Testosterone Jenapharm	25 mg/ml	1 ml ampule	Jenapharm	Germany	[NLM]	
testosterone propionate	testosterone propionate	50 mg/ml	n/a	Quad & Lilly	U.S.	[NLM]	
testosterone propionate	testosterone propionate	100 mg/ml	10, 30 ml vial	Rugby	U.S.	[NLM]	
testosterone propionate	testosterone propionate	100 mg/ml	10 ml vial	Steris	U.S.	[NLM]	
testosterone propionate	Testosterone Propionate Inj.	100 mg/ml	10 ml vial	Cytex	Canada		
testosterone propionate	Testosterone Propionate Inj.	100 mg/ml	10 ml vial	Dominion	Canada		VET

Appendix A: Drug Availability Tables - Listings by Generic Name

Generic Name	Trade Name	Dose	Packaging	Company	Country	Status	Vet
testosterone propionate	Testosterone Propionate Inj.	100 mg/ml	10 ml vial	Taro	Canada	[NLM]	
testosterone propionate	Testosterone Propionate Inj	25 mg/ml	n/a	Charmaine	Hong Kong		
testosterone propionate	Testosterone Propionate Inj	50 mg/ml	n/a	Hong Kong Med	Hong Kong		
testosterone propionate	Testosterone Propionate Inj	50 mg/ml	1 ml ampule	n/a	China		
testosterone propionate	Testosterone Propionate Inj	25 mg/ml	n/a	Tai Yu	Taiwan		
testosterone propionate	Testosterone Streuli	n/a	5, 10, 25, 50 mg/ml	Streuli & Co. AG	Austria	[NLM]	
testosterone propionate	Testosterone Vitis	n/a	10, 25 mg/ml	Neopharma	Germany	[NLM]	
testosterone propionate	Testosterone-Prop. Disp.	n/a	10, 20 mg/ml	Disperga	Austria	[NLM]	
testosterone propionate	testosteronpropionat	10, 25 mg/ml	1 ml ampule	Eifelfango	Germany	[NLM]	
testosterone propionate	testosteronpropionat	50 mg/ml	1 ml ampule	Eifelfango	Germany		
testosterone propionate	Testosteronum Propionicum	25 mg/ml	1 ml ampule	Jelfa	Poland		
testosterone propionate	Testoviron®	50 mg/ml	1 ml ampule	Schering	Greece		
testosterone propionate	Testoviron®	10, 25, 50 mg/ml	1 ml ampule	Schering	Italy	[NLM]	
testosterone propionate	Testoviron®	10, 25 mg/ml	1 ml ampule	Schering	Spain	[NLM]	
testosterone propionate	Testovis	50 mg/ml	2 ml ampule	SIT	Italy		
testosterone propionate	Triolandren	20 mg/ml	n/a	Ciba Geigy CH	Switzerland	[NLM]	
testosterone propionate	Uni-Test Inj	100 mg/ml	10 ml vial	Univet	Canada		VET
testosterone propionate	Virormone	50 mg/ml	2 ml ampule	Ferring	United Kingdom	[NLM]	
testosterone propionate	Virormone	50 mg/ml	2 ml ampule	Nordic	United Kingdom		
testosterone propionate	Virormone	50, 100 mg/ml	1 ml ampule	Paines	Thailand		
testosterone propionate	VR Testprop	50 mg/ml	10 ml vial	Jurox	Australia		VET
testosterone propionate (implant)	Implus-H	22 mg/pellet	n/a	Upjohn	U.S.		
testosterone propionate (implant)	Progro-H (plus estradiol)	20 mg/pellet	n/a	Pro Beef	Australia		VET
testosterone propionate (implant)	Synovex®-H (plus estradiol)	20 mg/pellet	n/a	Ayerst	Canada		
testosterone propionate (implant)	Synovex®-H (plus estrogen)	20 mg/pellet	n/a	Fort Dodge	Australia		VET
testosterone propionate (implant)	Synovex®-H (plus estrogen)	25 mg/pellet	80 pellet cartridge	Fort Dodge	Mexico		
testosterone propionate (implant)	Synovex®-H (plus estrogen)	20 mg/pellet	n/a	Fort Dodge	U.S.		VET
testosterone propionate (implant)	Synovex®-H (plus estrogen)	20 mg/pellet	n/a	Syntex	Mexico	[NLM]	
testosterone propionate (implant)	Synovex®-H (plus estrogen)	20 mg/pellet	n/a	Syntex	U.S.	[NLM]	VET
testosterone propionate (implant)	Virbac Tepro Pellets	23.5 mg pellet	450 pellets	Virbac	Australia		VET
testosterone suspension	Anabolic TS	100 mg/ml	20 ml vial	SYD Group	Australia		VET
testosterone suspension	Anabolic TS	100 mg/ml	20 ml vial	SYD Group	Mexico		VET
testosterone suspension	Anabolic-TS	100 mg/ml	20 ml vial	Grupo Tarasco	Mexico	[NLM]	VET
testosterone suspension	Androlan Aqueous	25, 50, 100 mg/ml	n/a	Lannet	U.S.	[NLM]	
testosterone suspension	Androlin	100 mg/ml	n/a	Lincoln	U.S.	[NLM]	
testosterone suspension	Andronaq-50	50 mg/ml	n/a	Central	U.S.	[NLM]	
testosterone suspension	AquaTest	100 mg/ml	10 ml vial	Denkall	Mexico		VET
testosterone suspension	Aquaviron	25 mg/ml	1 ml ampule	Nicholas	India		
testosterone suspension	Histerone Injection	100 mg/ml	n/a	Roberts	U.S.	[NLM]	
testosterone suspension	Histerone Injection	100 mg/ml	n/a	Hauck	U.S.	[NLM]	
testosterone suspension	Malogen	25, 50, 100, mg/ml	n/a	Forest	U.S.	[NLM]	

Appendix A: Drug Availability Tables - Listings by Generic Name

Generic Name	Trade Name	Dose	Packaging	Company	Country	Status	Vet
testosterone suspension	Malogen Aqueous	100 mg/ml	10 ml vial	Germiphene	Canada	[NLM]	
testosterone suspension	Malotrone	25, 50 mg/ml	n/a	Bluco	U.S.	[NLM]	
testosterone suspension	RWR Suspension	100 mg/ml	20 ml vial	RWR	Australia		VET
testosterone suspension	Tesamone	25, 50, 100, mg/ml	n/a	Dunhall	U.S.	[NLM]	
testosterone suspension	Testolin	25, 50, 100, mg/ml	n/a	Pasadena	U.S.	[NLM]	
testosterone suspension	Testos 100	100 mg/ml	10 ml vial	Vetcom	Canada		VET
testosterone suspension	testosterone suspension	100 mg/ml	n/a	Legere	U.S.	[NLM]	
testosterone suspension	testosterone suspension	50, 100 mg/ml	10, 30 ml vial	Schein	U.S.	[NLM]	
testosterone suspension	testosterone suspension	50, 100 mg/ml	10, 30 ml vial	Steris	U.S.	[NLM]	
testosterone suspension	Testosus 100	100 mg/ml	20 ml vial	Jurox	Australia	[NLM]	VET
testosterone suspension	Uni-Test Suspension	100 mg/ml	30 ml vial	Univet	Canada		VET
testosterone suspension	Veto-Test Sus	100 mg/ml	30 ml vial	Austin	Canada		VET
testosterone suspension (isobutyrate)	Agovirin-Depot	25 mg/ml	2 ml ampule	Biotika	Czech. Rep.		
testosterone undecanoate	Andriol	40 mg capsules	60 capsule bottle	Organon	Algeria		
testosterone undecanoate	Andriol	40 mg capsules	n/a	Organon	Aruba		
testosterone undecanoate	Andriol	40 mg capsules	60 capsule bottle	Organon	Australia		
testosterone undecanoate	Andriol	40 mg capsules	60 capsule bottle	Organon	Austria		
testosterone undecanoate	Andriol	40 mg capsules	n/a	Organon	Bahrain		
testosterone undecanoate	Andriol	40 mg capsules	n/a	Organon	Bangladesh		
testosterone undecanoate	Andriol	40 mg capsules	n/a	Organon	Belarus		
testosterone undecanoate	Andriol	40 mg capsules	60 capsule bottle	Organon	Canada		
testosterone undecanoate	Andriol	40 mg capsules	16 capsule box	Organon	China		
testosterone undecanoate	Andriol	40 mg capsules	n/a	Organon	Cyprus		
testosterone undecanoate	Andriol	40 mg capsules	n/a	Organon	Dutch Antilles		
testosterone undecanoate	Andriol	40 mg capsules	n/a	Organon	Ecuador		
testosterone undecanoate	Andriol	40 mg capsules	n/a	Organon	Georgia		
testosterone undecanoate	Andriol	40 mg capsules	30, 60 capsule bottle	Organon	Germany		
testosterone undecanoate	Andriol	40 mg capsules	n/a	Organon	Ghana		
testosterone undecanoate	Andriol	40 mg capsules	n/a	Organon	Hong-Kong		
testosterone undecanoate	Andriol	40 mg capsules	n/a	Organon	Hungary		
testosterone undecanoate	Andriol	40 mg capsules	n/a	Organon	Indonesia		
testosterone undecanoate	Andriol	40 mg capsules	60 capsule bottle	Organon	Italy		
testosterone undecanoate	Andriol	40 mg capsules	n/a	Organon	Jordan		
testosterone undecanoate	Andriol	40 mg capsules	n/a	Organon	Kenya		
testosterone undecanoate	Andriol	40 mg capsules	n/a	Organon	Korea		
testosterone undecanoate	Andriol	40 mg capsules	n/a	Organon	Kuwait		
testosterone undecanoate	Andriol	40 mg capsules	n/a	Organon	Lebanon		
testosterone undecanoate	Andriol	40 mg capsules	60 capsule bottle	Organon	Malaysia		
testosterone undecanoate	Andriol	40 mg capsules	n/a	Organon	Mauritius		
testosterone undecanoate	Andriol	40 mg capsules	n/a	Organon	Morocco		
testosterone undecanoate	Andriol	40 mg capsules	n/a	Organon	Myanmar/Burma		VET

Appendix A: Drug Availability Tables - Listings by Generic Name

Generic Name	Trade Name	Dose	Packaging	Company	Country	Status	Vet
testosterone undecanoate	Andriol	40 mg capsules	n/a	Organon	Netherlands		
testosterone undecanoate	Andriol	40 mg capsules	n/a	Organon	Nigeria		
testosterone undecanoate	Andriol	40 mg capsules	n/a	Organon	Oman		
testosterone undecanoate	Andriol	40 mg capsules	n/a	Organon	Philippines		
testosterone undecanoate	Andriol	40 mg capsules	n/a	Organon	Portugal		
testosterone undecanoate	Andriol	40 mg capsules	n/a	Organon	Qatar		
testosterone undecanoate	Andriol	40 mg capsules	n/a	Organon	Russia		
testosterone undecanoate	Andriol	40 mg capsules	n/a	Organon	Saudi Arabia		
testosterone undecanoate	Andriol	40 mg capsules	60 capsule bottle	Organon	Singapore		
testosterone undecanoate	Andriol	40 mg capsules	n/a	Organon	Sri Lanka		
testosterone undecanoate	Andriol	40 mg capsules	n/a	Organon	Switzerland		
testosterone undecanoate	Andriol	40 mg capsules	10 capsule strip	Organon	Thailand		
testosterone undecanoate	Andriol	40 mg capsules	n/a	Organon	Tunisia		
testosterone undecanoate	Andriol	40 mg capsules	n/a	Organon	Ukraine		
testosterone undecanoate	Andriol	40 mg capsules	n/a	Organon	United Arab E		
testosterone undecanoate	Andriol	40 mg capsules	n/a	Organon	Vietnam		
testosterone undecanoate	Andriol	40 mg capsules	n/a	Organon	Yemen		
testosterone undecanoate	Andriol	40 mg capsules	n/a	Organon	YugoslaviaFRMR		
testosterone undecanoate	Andriol	40 mg capsules	20 capsule box	Organon/Sedico	Egypt		
testosterone undecanoate	Andriol capsulas	40 mg capsules	30 capsule bottle	Organon	Mexico		
testosterone undecanoate	Andriol capsulas	40 mg capsules	n/a	Organon	Venezuela		
testosterone undecanoate	Androxon	40 mg capsules	60 capsule bottle	Donmed/Organon	South Africa		
testosterone undecanoate	Androxon	40 mg capsules	20 capsule box	Organon	Brazil		
testosterone undecanoate	Androxon	40 mg capsules	30 capsule bottle	Organon	Israel		
testosterone undecanoate	Androxon	40 mg capsules	60 capsule bottle	Organon	Norway		
testosterone undecanoate	Androxon	40 mg capsules	n/a	Organon	Pakistan		
testosterone undecanoate	Nuvir	40 mg capsules	30 capsule bottle	Organon	India		
testosterone undecanoate	Panteston	40 mg capsules	60 capsule bottle	Organon	Finland		
testosterone undecanoate	Panteston	40 mg capsules	n/a	Organon	Latvia		
testosterone undecanoate	Panteston	40 mg capsules	n/a	Organon	Lithuania		
testosterone undecanoate	Panteston	40 mg capsules	30, 60 capsule bottle	Organon	Peru		
testosterone undecanoate	Panteston capsules	40 mg capsules	n/a	Organon	New Zealand		
testosterone undecanoate	Pantestone	40 mg capsules	60 capsule bottle	Organon	Estonia		
testosterone undecanoate	Pantestone	40 mg capsules	60 capsule bottle	Organon	France		
testosterone undecanoate	Restandol	40 mg capsules	60 capsule bottle	Organon	Denmark		
testosterone undecanoate	Restandol	40 mg capsules	60 capsule bottle	Organon	Greece		
testosterone undecanoate	Restandol	40 mg capsules	n/a	Organon	Taiwan		
testosterone undecanoate	Restandol	40 mg capsules	28, 56 capsule box	Organon	United Kingdom		
testosterone undecanoate	Sustenan Oral	40 mg capsules	n/a	Organon	Chile		
testosterone undecanoate	Undestor	40 mg capsules	n/a	Organon	Argentina		
testosterone undecanoate	Undestor	40 mg capsules	60 capsule bottle	Organon	Belgium		

Appendix A: Drug Availability Tables - Listings by Generic Name

Generic Name	Trade Name	Dose	Packaging	Company	Country	Status	Vet
testosterone undecanoate	Undestor	40 mg capsules	60 capsule bottle	Organon	Bulgaria		
testosterone undecanoate	Undestor	40 mg capsules	60 capsule bottle	Organon	Czech. Rep.		
testosterone undecanoate	Undestor	40 mg capsules	n/a	Organon	Luxemburg		
testosterone undecanoate	Undestor	40 mg capsules	60 capsule bottle	Organon	Poland		
testosterone undecanoate	Undestor	40 mg capsules	60 capsule bottle	Organon	Rumania		
testosterone undecanoate	Undestor	40 mg capsules	n/a	Organon	Slovakia		
testosterone undecanoate	Undestor	40 mg capsules	n/a	Organon	Sweden		
testosterone undecanoate	Virigen	40 mg capsules	30 capsule bottle	Organon	Turkey		
Testoviron (testosterone blend)	Aratest 2500	250 mg/ml	10 ml vial	Aranda	Mexico		VET
Testoviron (testosterone blend)	Bi-Testo	60 mg/ml	10 ml vial	Cimol	Argentina		VET
Testoviron (testosterone blend)	Primoniat®-Depot 100	135 mg/ml	1 ml ampule	Schering-Chile	Chile	[NLM]	
Testoviron (testosterone blend)	Primoteston Depot 100	135 mg/ml	1 ml ampule	Schering	Australia	[NLM]	
Testoviron (testosterone blend)	Primoteston Depot 50	75 mg/ml	1 ml ampule	Schering	Australia	[NLM]	
Testoviron (testosterone blend)	Primoteston®-Depot 100	135 mg/ml	1 ml ampule	Schering/CID	Egypt		
Testoviron (testosterone blend)	Testenat	100 mg/ml	1 ml ampule	Farmadon	Russia	[NLM]	
Testoviron (testosterone blend)	Testenon	135 mg/ml	2 ml vial	BM Pharmaceuticals	India		
Testoviron (testosterone blend)	Testenon	135 mg/ml	1 ml ampule	BM Pharmaceuticals	India		
Testoviron (testosterone blend)	Testoprim-D	250 mg/ml	1 ml ampule	Labs. Tocogino	Mexico		
Testoviron (testosterone blend)	Testoviron® Depot	135 mg/ml	1 ml ampule	Schering	Argentina	[NLM]	
Testoviron (testosterone blend)	Testoviron® Depot	135 mg/ml	1 ml ampule	Schering	Hungary	[NLM]	
Testoviron (testosterone blend)	Testoviron® Depot 100	135 mg/ml	1 ml ampule	Schering	Austria	[NLM]	
Testoviron (testosterone blend)	Testoviron® Depot 100	135 mg/ml	1 ml ampule	Schering	Dom. Rep.		
Testoviron (testosterone blend)	Testoviron® Depot 100	135 mg/ml	1 ml ampule	Schering	Germany	[NLM]	
Testoviron (testosterone blend)	Testoviron® Depot 100	135 mg/ml	1 ml ampule	Schering	Greece	[NLM]	
Testoviron (testosterone blend)	Testoviron® Depot 100	135 mg/ml	1 ml ampule	Schering	Italy		
Testoviron (testosterone blend)	Testoviron® Depot 100	135 mg/ml	1 ml ampule	Schering	Netherlands	[NLM]	
Testoviron (testosterone blend)	Testoviron® Depot 100	135 mg/ml	1 ml ampule	Schering	Portugal	[NLM]	
Testoviron (testosterone blend)	Testoviron® Depot 100	135 mg/ml	1 ml ampule	Schering	Spain	[NLM]	
Testoviron (testosterone blend)	Testoviron® Depot 100	135 mg/ml	1 ml ampule	Schering	Switzerland	[NLM]	
Testoviron (testosterone blend)	Testoviron® Depot 135	135 mg/ml	1 ml ampule	Schering	Denmark		
Testoviron (testosterone blend)	Testoviron® Depot 135	135 mg/ml	1 ml ampule	Schering	Sweden	[NLM]	
Testoviron (testosterone blend)	Testoviron® Depot 50	75 mg/ml	1 ml ampule	Schering	Austria	[NLM]	
Testoviron (testosterone blend)	Testoviron® Depot 50	75 mg/ml	1 ml ampule	Schering	Germany	[NLM]	
Testoviron (testosterone blend)	Testoviron® Depot 50	75 mg/ml	1 ml ampule	Schering	Italy	[NLM]	
Testoviron (testosterone blend)	Testoviron® Depot 50	75 mg/ml	1 ml ampule	Schering	Spain	[NLM]	
trenbolone (blend)	Trinabol 150	150 mg/ml	10 ml vial	British Dragon	Thailand		
trenbolone acetate	Acetrenbo 50	50 mg tablet	20 tablet bottle	Loeffler	Mexico		VET
trenbolone acetate	ComponentTE-G® (+ estradiol)	20 mg pellet	40 pellet cartridge	VetLife	U.S.		VET
trenbolone acetate	ComponentTE-S® (+ estradiol)	20 mg pellet	120 pellet cartridge	VetLife	U.S.		VET
trenbolone acetate	ComponentT-H®	20 mg pellet	200 pellet cartridge	VetLife	U.S.		VET
trenbolone acetate	ComponentT-S®	20 mg pellet	140 pellet cartridge	VetLife	U.S.		VET

Appendix A: Drug Availability Tables - Listings by Generic Name

Generic Name	Trade Name	Dose	Packaging	Company	Country	Status	Vet
trenbolone acetate	Finaject	30 mg/ml	n/a	Roussel	France	[NLM]	VET
trenbolone acetate	Finajet	30 mg/ml	50 ml vial	Hoechst	U.S.	[NLM]	VET
trenbolone acetate	Finajet	30 mg/ml	50 ml vial	Hoechst	United Kingdom	[NLM]	VET
trenbolone acetate	Finaplix-H®	20 mg pellet	100 pellet cartridge	Hoechst-Roussel	U.S.	[NLM]	VET
trenbolone acetate	Finaplix-H®	20 mg pellet	100 pellet cartridge	Intervet	U.S.		VET
trenbolone acetate	Finaplix-H®	20 mg pellet	70, 100 pellet cartridge	Roussel	Mexico	[NLM]	VET
trenbolone acetate	Finaplix-S®	20 mg pellet	70 pellet cartridge	Hoechst-Roussel	U.S.	[NLM]	VET
trenbolone acetate	Parabolan Tabs (Export)	25 mg tablet	20 tablet pouch	British Dragon	Thailand		
trenbolone acetate	Revalor-200 (plus estradiol)	20 mg pellet	100 pellet cartridge	Intervet	U.S.		VET
trenbolone acetate	Revalor-G (plus estradiol)	20 mg pellet	20 pellet cartridge	Intervet	U.S.		VET
trenbolone acetate	Revalor-H (plus estradiol)	20 mg pellet	70 pellet cartridge	Hoechst-Roussel	U.S.	[NLM]	VET
trenbolone acetate	Revalor-H (plus estradiol)	20 mg pellet	70 pellet cartridge	Intervet	Canada		VET
trenbolone acetate	Revalor-H (plus estradiol)	20 mg pellet	70 pellet cartridge	Intervet	U.S.		VET
trenbolone acetate	Revalor-IH (plus estradiol)	20 mg pellet	40 pellet cartridge	Intervet	U.S.		VET
trenbolone acetate	Revalor-IS (plus estradiol)	20 mg pellet	40 pellet cartridge	Intervet	U.S.		VET
trenbolone acetate	Revalor-S (plus estradiol)	20 mg pellet	60 pellet cartridge	Hoechst-Roussel	U.S.	[NLM]	VET
trenbolone acetate	Revalor-S (plus estradiol)	20 mg pellet	60 pellet cartridge	Intervet	Canada		VET
trenbolone acetate	Revalor-S (plus estradiol)	20 mg pellet	60 pellet cartridge	Intervet	U.S.		VET
trenbolone acetate	Synovex plus (plus estradiol)	25 mg pellet	80 pellet cartridge	Fort Dodge	Mexico		VET
trenbolone acetate	Synovex plus (plus estradiol)	25 mg pellet	80 pellet cartridge	Fort Dodge	U.S.		VET
trenbolone acetate	Synovex plus (plus estradiol)	25 mg pellet	80 pellet cartridge	Syntex	U.S.	[NLM]	VET
trenbolone acetate	Synovex plus (plus estradiol)	25 mg pellet	80 pellet cartridge	Wyeth	Canada		VET
trenbolone acetate	Trembolone QV 75	75 mg/ml	10 ml vial	Quality Vet	Mexico		VET
trenbolone acetate	Trenabol	75 mg/ml	10 ml vial	British Dragon	Thailand		
trenbolone acetate	Trenbo 75	75 mg/ml	10 ml vial	Animal Power	Mexico		VET
trenbolone acetate	Trenbol 75	75 mg/ml	20 ml vial	Ttokkyo	Mexico		VET
trenbolone acetate	Trenbolon 75	75 mg/ml	10, 20 ml vial	Pet's Pharma	Mexico		VET
trenbolone acetate	Trenol 50	50 mg/ml	6 ml vial	WDV	Myanmar/Burma		VET
trenbolone hexahydrobenzylcarbonate	Danabolan	76 mg/ml	1.5 ml ampule	Body Research	Thailand		
trenbolone hexahydrobenzylcarbonate	Parabolan	76 mg/1.5 ml	1.5 ml ampule	Negma	France	[NLM]	
trenbolone hexahydrobenzylcarbonate	Trenabol Depot	100 mg/ml	10 ml vial	British Dragon	Thailand		

ABBREVIATIONS:

[NLM] = No Longer Manufactured
VET = Veterinary Drug

Appendix B: Drug Availability Tables - Listings by Trade Name

Trade Name	Generic Name	Dose	Packaging	Company	Country	Status	Vet
Acetrenbo 50	trenbolone acetate	50 mg tablet	20 tablet bottle	Loeffler	Mexico		VET
Activin	nandrolone phenylpropionate	10 mg/ml	n/a	Aristegvi	Spain	[NLM]	
Afro	methyltestosterone	25 mg tablet	40 tablet box	Casel	Turkey		
Agovirin	methyltestosterone	10 mg dragee	100 dragee bottle	Leciva	Czech. Rep.	[NLM]	
Agovirin injectable	testosterone propionate	25 mg/ml	n/a	Leciva	Czech. Rep.	[NLM]	
Agovirin-Depot	testosterone suspension (isobutyrate)	25 mg/ml	2 ml ampule	Biotika	Czech. Rep.		
Alfa-Trofodermin	clostebol acetate	.5% gel	n/a	Farmitalia	Italy	[NLM]	
Alfa-Trofodermin	clostebol acetate	.5% gel	n/a	Pharmacia & Upjohn	Italy		
Ammipire	methandrostenolone	5 mg tablet	1000 tablet bottle	Ammipire	Thailand		
Anabol	methandrostenolone	50 mg tablet	n/a	British Dragon	Thailand	[NLM]	
Anabol Tablets	methandrostenolone	5 mg tablet	1000 tablet bottle	British Dispensary	Thailand		
Anabol Tablets	methandrostenolone	5 mg tablet	1000 tablet bottle	L.P Standard	Thailand	[NLM]	
Ana-Bolde	boldenone undecylenate	50 mg/ml	10 ml vial	Forti	Argentina		VET
Anabolex	methandrostenolone	3 mg tablet	100 tablet box	Ethical	Dom. Rep.		
Anabolic BD	boldenone undecylenate	50 mg/ml	10 ml vial	SYD Group	Australia		VET
Anabolic BD	boldenone undecylenate	100, 200 mg/ml	10 ml vial	SYD Group	Mexico		VET
Anabolic DN	nandrolone cypionate	50 mg/ml	10 ml vial	SYD Group	Australia		VET
Anabolic DN	nandrolone cypionate	50, 300 mg/ml	10 ml vial	SYD Group	Mexico		VET
Anabolic NA	methylandrostenediol (blend)	75 mg/ml	10 ml vial	SYD Group	Australia		VET
Anabolic NA	methylandrostenediol (blend)	75 mg/ml	10 ml vial	SYD Group	Mexico		VET
Anabolic ST	stanozolol (inj)	50 mg/ml	20 ml vial	SYD Group	Australia		VET
Anabolic ST	stanozolol (inj)	50 mg/ml	20 ml vial	SYD Group	Mexico		VET
Anabolic TL	testosterone cypionate	100 mg/ml	10 ml vial	SYD Group	Australia		VET
Anabolic TL	testosterone cypionate	200 mg/ml	10 ml vial	SYD Group	Mexico		VET
Anabolic TS	testosterone suspension	100 mg/ml	20 ml vial	SYD Group	Australia		VET
Anabolic TS	testosterone suspension	100 mg/ml	20 ml vial	SYD Group	Mexico		VET
Anabolic-BD	boldenone undecylenate	100 mg/ml	10 ml vial	Grupo Tarasco	Mexico	[NLM]	VET
Anabolic-DN	nandrolone cypionate	50 mg/ml	10 ml vial	Grupo Tarasco	Mexico	[NLM]	VET
Anabolic-NA	methylandrostenediol (blend)	75 mg/ml	10 ml vial	Grupo Tarasco	Mexico	[NLM]	VET
Anabolico Cimol	stanozolol (inj)	60 mg/ml	5 ml vial	Cimol	Argentina		VET
Anabolico Produvet	stanozolol (inj)	10 mg/ml	25 ml vial	Cimol	Argentina		VET
Anabolic-ST	stanozolol (inj)	50 mg/ml	20 ml vial	Grupo Tarasco	Mexico	[NLM]	VET
Anabolic-TS	testosterone suspension	100 mg/ml	20 ml vial	Grupo Tarasco	Mexico	[NLM]	VET
Anabolicum	nandrolone decanoate	25 mg/ml	10, 50 ml vial	Bela-Pharm	Germany		VET
Anabolicum Vister	quinbolone	10 mg capsule	30 capsule bottle	Parke Davis	Italy	[NLM]	
Anabolicum Vister	quinbolone	oral drops	n/a	Parke Davis	Italy	[NLM]	
Anabolikum 2.5%	methandrostenolone	25 mg/ml	50 ml vial	Meca G	Germany	[NLM]	VET
Anabolin	nandrolone phenylpropionate	50 mg/ml	n/a	Alto	U.S.	[NLM]	
Anabolin	methandrostenolone	5 mg tablet	n/a	Leiras	Finland	[NLM]	
Anabolin	methandrostenolone	0.5% cream	n/a	Leiras	Finland	[NLM]	
Anabolin Forte	nandrolone decanoate	50 mg/ml	10 ml vial	Alfasan	Netherlands		VET

Appendix B: Drug Availability Tables - Listings by Trade Name

Trade Name	Generic Name	Dose	Packaging	Company	Country	Status	Vet
Anabolin Forte	nandrolone decanoate	50 mg/ml	10 ml vial	Alfasan	Rumania		VET
Anabolin Forte	nandrolone decanoate	50 mg/ml	10, 50 ml vial	Alfasan	Spain		VET
Anaboline Depot	nandrolone decanoate	50 mg/ml	1 ml	Adelco	Greece		
Anabolin-IM	nandrolone phenylpropionate	50 mg/ml	n/a	Alto	U.S.	[NLM]	
Anabolin-LA	nandrolone phenylpropionate	100 mg/ml	n/a	Alto	U.S.	[NLM]	
Anabol-Jet	methandrostenolone	25 mg/ml	30, 100, 250 ml vial	Norvet	Mexico		VET
Anabol-Jet ADE	methandrostenolone	30 mg/ml	100, 250 ml vial	Norvet	Mexico		VET
Anabol-Pet's	methandrostenolone	10, 25 mg tablet	200 tablet bottle	Norvet	Mexico		VET
Anabrol	oxymetholone	50 mg tablet	100 tablet bottle	Brovel	Mexico		VET
Anadiol	methylandrostenediol dipropionate	5 mg tab	10, 100 tablet bottle	Ilium/Troy	Australia		VET
Anadiol Depot	methylandrostenediol dipropionate	75 mg/ml	10 ml vial	Ilium/Troy	Australia		VET
Anador	nandrolone hexyloxyphenylpropionate	25 mg/ml	2 ml ampule	Pharmacia-Upjohn	France	[NLM]	
Anadrol	oxymetholone	5 mg tablet	n/a	n/a	Japan		
Anadrol 50®	oxymetholone	50 mg tablet	100 tablet bottle	Unimed	U.S.		
Anadrol 50®	oxymetholone	50 mg tablet	100 tablet bottle	Syntex	Canada	[NLM]	
Anadrol 50®	oxymetholone	50 mg tablet	100 tablet bottle	Syntex	U.S.	[NLM]	
Anadur	nandrolone hexyloxyphenylpropionate	25 mg/ml	2 ml ampule	Eczacibasi	Turkey	[NLM]	
Anadur	nandrolone hexyloxyphenylpropionate	25, 50 mg/ml	1, 2 ml ampule	Kabi Pharmacia	Switzerland	[NLM]	
Anadur	nandrolone hexyloxyphenylpropionate	25, 50 mg/ml	1, 2 ml ampule	Kabi Pharmacia	Austria	[NLM]	
Anadur	nandrolone hexyloxyphenylpropionate	25, 50 mg/ml	1, 2 ml ampule	Kabi Pharmacia	Germany	[NLM]	
Anadur	nandrolone hexyloxyphenylpropionate	25, 50 mg/ml	1, 2 ml ampule	Kabi Pharmacia	Norway	[NLM]	
Anadur	nandrolone hexyloxyphenylpropionate	25 mg/ml	2 ml ampule	Leo	Spain	[NLM]	
Anadur	nandrolone hexyloxyphenylpropionate	25 mg/ml	2 ml ampule	Lundbeck	Denmark	[NLM]	
Anadur	nandrolone hexyloxyphenylpropionate	25, 50 mg/ml	1, 2 ml ampule	Pharmacia	Belgium	[NLM]	
Anadur	nandrolone hexyloxyphenylpropionate	25, 50 mg/ml	1, 2 ml ampule	Pharmacia	Czech. Rep.	[NLM]	
Anadur	nandrolone hexyloxyphenylpropionate	25, 50 mg/ml	1, 2 ml ampule	Pharmacia	Finland	[NLM]	
Anadur	nandrolone hexyloxyphenylpropionate	25, 50 mg/ml	1, 2 ml ampule	Pharmacia	Netherlands	[NLM]	
Anadurin	nandrolone hexyloxyphenylpropionate	50 mg/ml	1 ml ampule	Xponei	Greece	[NLM]	
Anaplex	norethandrolone	5 mg tablet	100 tablet bottle	Jurox	Australia		VET
Anapolon	oxymetholone	50 mg tablet	20 tablet box	Ibrahim	Turkey		
Anapolon	oxymetholone	50 mg tablet	n/a	Syntex	Bulgaria	[NLM]	
Anapolon	oxymetholone	2.5, 5 mg tablet	20 tablet box	Ibrahim	Turkey	[NLM]	
Anapolon 50	oxymetholone	50 mg tablet	100 tablet bottle	Syntex	Malaysia	[NLM]	
Anapolon 50	oxymetholone	50 mg tablet	20 tablet strip	Syntex	Mexico	[NLM]	
Anapolon 50	oxymetholone	50 mg tablet	100 tablet bottle	Syntex	United Kingdom	[NLM]	
Anapolon 50®	oxymetholone	50 mg tablet	100 tablet bottle	Hoffman-La Rouche	Canada	[NLM]	
Anaprolina	nandrolone decanoate	25, 50 mg/ml	1 ml ampule	Silesia	Chile		
Anasteron	oxymetholone	25 mg tablet	60 tablet bottle	Farmaprod	Greece		
Anasteron	oxymetholone	50 mg tablet	n/a	Syntex	Greece	[NLM]	
Anasteron	oxymetholone	50 mg tablet	n/a	Syntex	Sweden	[NLM]	
Anatest	testosterone propionate	100 mg/ml	10 ml vial	Rhone	Canada	[NLM]	VET

Appendix B: Drug Availability Tables - Listings by Trade Name

Trade Name	Generic Name	Dose	Packaging	Company	Country	Status	Vet
Anatest	testosterone propionate	100 mg/ml	10 ml vial	Sterivet	Canada	[NLM]	VET
Anatest	testosterone propionate	100 mg/ml	10 ml vial	Vetoquinol	Canada		VET
Anatrophill	oxandrolone	2.5 mg tablet	n/a	Searle	France	[NLM]	
Anavar	oxandrolone	5 mg tablet	30 tablet strip	Hubei Huangshi	China		
Anavar	oxandrolone	2.5 mg tablet	100 tablet bottle	Searle	U.S.	[NLM]	
Anazol	stanozolol (oral)	2 mg tablet	100 tablet box	Xelox (export)	Philippines		
Anazol	stanozolol (oral)	2 mg tablet	100, 1000 tablet bottle	Xelox (export)	Philippines		
Anderone 100/200	testosterone enanthate	100, 200 mg/ml	10 ml vial	Burgin-Arden	U.S.	[NLM]	
Andoredan	methandrostenolone	5 mg tablet	n/a	Takeshima-Kodama	Japan	[NLM]	
Andractim	dihydrotestosterone	25 mg/g	100 gram gel	Besins-Iscovesco	France		
Andractim	dihydrotestosterone	25 mg/g	100 gram gel	Chemec	India		
Andractim	dihydrotestosterone	25 mg/g	80 gram gel	n/a	Korea		
Andractim	dihydrotestosterone	25 mg/g	80 gram gel	Piette	Belgium		
Andractim	dihydrotestosterone	25 mg/g	80 gram gel	Servimedic	Uruguay		
Andriol	testosterone undecanoate	40 mg capsules	60 capsule bottle	Organon	Algeria		
Andriol	testosterone undecanoate	40 mg capsules	n/a	Organon	Aruba		
Andriol	testosterone undecanoate	40 mg capsules	60 capsule bottle	Organon	Australia		
Andriol	testosterone undecanoate	40 mg capsules	60 capsule bottle	Organon	Austria		
Andriol	testosterone undecanoate	40 mg capsules	n/a	Organon	Bahrain		
Andriol	testosterone undecanoate	40 mg capsules	n/a	Organon	Bangladesh		
Andriol	testosterone undecanoate	40 mg capsules	n/a	Organon	Belarus		
Andriol	testosterone undecanoate	40 mg capsules	60 capsule bottle	Organon	Canada		
Andriol	testosterone undecanoate	40 mg capsules	16 capsule box	Organon	China		
Andriol	testosterone undecanoate	40 mg capsules	n/a	Organon	Cyprus		
Andriol	testosterone undecanoate	40 mg capsules	n/a	Organon	Dutch Antilles		
Andriol	testosterone undecanoate	40 mg capsules	n/a	Organon	Ecuador		
Andriol	testosterone undecanoate	40 mg capsules	n/a	Organon	Georgia		
Andriol	testosterone undecanoate	40 mg capsules	30, 60 capsule bottle	Organon	Germany		
Andriol	testosterone undecanoate	40 mg capsules	n/a	Organon	Ghana		
Andriol	testosterone undecanoate	40 mg capsules	n/a	Organon	Hong-Kong		
Andriol	testosterone undecanoate	40 mg capsules	n/a	Organon	Hungary		
Andriol	testosterone undecanoate	40 mg capsules	n/a	Organon	Indonesia		
Andriol	testosterone undecanoate	40 mg capsules	60 capsule bottle	Organon	Italy		
Andriol	testosterone undecanoate	40 mg capsules	n/a	Organon	Jordan		
Andriol	testosterone undecanoate	40 mg capsules	n/a	Organon	Kenya		
Andriol	testosterone undecanoate	40 mg capsules	n/a	Organon	Korea		
Andriol	testosterone undecanoate	40 mg capsules	n/a	Organon	Kuwait		
Andriol	testosterone undecanoate	40 mg capsules	n/a	Organon	Lebanon		
Andriol	testosterone undecanoate	40 mg capsules	60 capsule bottle	Organon	Malaysia		
Andriol	testosterone undecanoate	40 mg capsules	n/a	Organon	Mauritius		
Andriol	testosterone undecanoate	40 mg capsules	n/a	Organon	Morocco		

Appendix B: Drug Availability Tables - Listings by Trade Name

Trade Name	Generic Name	Dose	Packaging	Company	Country	Status	Vet
Andriol	testosterone undecanoate	40 mg capsules	n/a	Organon	Myanmar/Burma		VET
Andriol	testosterone undecanoate	40 mg capsules	n/a	Organon	Netherlands		
Andriol	testosterone undecanoate	40 mg capsules	n/a	Organon	Nigeria		
Andriol	testosterone undecanoate	40 mg capsules	n/a	Organon	Oman		
Andriol	testosterone undecanoate	40 mg capsules	n/a	Organon	Philippines		
Andriol	testosterone undecanoate	40 mg capsules	n/a	Organon	Portugal		
Andriol	testosterone undecanoate	40 mg capsules	n/a	Organon	Qatar		
Andriol	testosterone undecanoate	40 mg capsules	n/a	Organon	Russia		
Andriol	testosterone undecanoate	40 mg capsules	n/a	Organon	Saudi Arabia		
Andriol	testosterone undecanoate	40 mg capsules	60 capsule bottle	Organon	Singapore		
Andriol	testosterone undecanoate	40 mg capsules	n/a	Organon	Sri Lanka		
Andriol	testosterone undecanoate	40 mg capsules	n/a	Organon	Switzerland		
Andriol	testosterone undecanoate	40 mg capsules	10 capsule strip	Organon	Thailand		
Andriol	testosterone undecanoate	40 mg capsules	n/a	Organon	Tunisia		
Andriol	testosterone undecanoate	40 mg capsules	n/a	Organon	Ukraine		
Andriol	testosterone undecanoate	40 mg capsules	n/a	Organon	United Arab E		
Andriol	testosterone undecanoate	40 mg capsules	n/a	Organon	Vietnam		
Andriol	testosterone undecanoate	40 mg capsules	n/a	Organon	Yemen		
Andriol	testosterone undecanoate	40 mg capsules	n/a	Organon	YugoslaviaFRMR		
Andriol	testosterone undecanoate	40 mg capsules	20 capsule box	Organon/Sedico	Egypt		
Andriol capsulas	testosterone undecanoate	40 mg capsules	30 capsule bottle	Organon	Mexico		
Andriol capsulas	testosterone undecanoate	40 mg capsules	n/a	Organon	Venezuela		
Andris	methylandrostenediol	10 mg tablet	n/a	Chifar	Greece	[NLM]	
Andro 100	testosterone enanthate	100 mg/ml	10 ml vial	Forest	U.S.	[NLM]	
Andro L.A. 200	testosterone enanthate	200 mg/ml	10 ml vial	Forest	U.S.	[NLM]	
Andro-Cyp	testosterone cypionate	100, 200 mg/ml	10 ml vial	Brown	U.S.	[NLM]	
Andro-Cyp	testosterone cypionate	100, 200 mg/ml	10 ml vial	Keene	U.S.	[NLM]	
Androderm®	testosterone (patch)	12.2 mg patch.	10, 30, 60 patches/box	AstraZenica	Germany		
Androderm®	testosterone (patch)	12.2 mg patch	n/a	Astrazenica	Switzerland		
Androderm®	testosterone (patch)	12.2 mg patch.	n/a	n/a	Korea		
Androderm®	testosterone (patch)	12.2 mg patch.	30 patches/box	Pharmascience	Canada		
Androderm®	testosterone (patch)	12.2 mg patch.	n/a	Schwarz Pharma	Italy		
Androderm®	testosterone (patch)	2.5 mg patch	30, 60 patch box	Schwarz Pharma	Spain		
Androderm®	testosterone (patch)	5 mg patch	30 patch box	Schwarz Pharma	Spain		
Androderm®	testosterone (patch)	12.2 mg patch	60 patches/box	SmithKline Beecham	U.S.	[NLM]	
Androderm®	testosterone (patch)	12.2, 24.3 mg patch	60 patches/box	Watson Pharma	U.S.		
Androfort-Richter	testosterone propionate	10, 25 mg/ml	n/a	Gedeon Richter	Hungary		
Androgel	testosterone (gel)	25, 50 mg	single dose packet	Besins	Netherlands		
Androgel	testosterone (gel)	25, 50 mg	single dose packet	Besins	Sweden		
Androgel	testosterone (gel)	25, 50 mg	single dose packet	Solvay	Canada		
Androgel	testosterone (gel)	50, 75, 100 mg	single dose packet	Unimed	U.S.		

Appendix B: Drug Availability Tables - Listings by Trade Name

Trade Name	Generic Name	Dose	Packaging	Company	Country	Status	Vet
Android	methyltestosterone	5, 10, 25 mg tablet	60 tablet bottle	ICN Pharm	U.S.		
Android	methyltestosterone	5, 10, 25 mg tablet	n/a	Brown	U.S.	[NLM]	
Android-F	fluoxymesterone	10 mg tablet	100 tablet bottle	Brown	U.S.	[NLM]	
Androlan	testosterone propionate	50, 100 mg/ml	n/a	Lannett	U.S.	[NLM]	
Androlan Aqueous	testosterone suspension	25, 50, 100 mg/ml	n/a	Lannet	U.S.	[NLM]	
Androlic	oxymetholone	50 mg tablet	100 tablet bottle	British Dispensary	Thailand		
Androlic	oxymetholone	50 mg tablet	100 tablet pouch	British Dispensary	Thailand	[NLM]	
Androlic (Export)	oxymetholone	50 mg tablet	20 tablet pouch	British Dragon	Thailand		
Androlin	testosterone suspension	100 mg/ml	n/a	Lincoln	U.S.	[NLM]	
Androlone	nandrolone phenylpropionate	50 mg/ml	n/a	Keene	U.S.	[NLM]	
Androlone-D 200	nandrolone decanoate	200 mg/ml	1 ml	Keene	U.S.	[NLM]	
Andronaq LA	testosterone cypionate	100, 200 mg/ml	10 ml vial	Central	U.S.	[NLM]	
Andronaq-50	testosterone suspension	50 mg/ml	n/a	Central	U.S.	[NLM]	
Andronate	testosterone cypionate	100, 200 mg/ml	10 ml vial	Pasadena	U.S.	[NLM]	
Andropatch	testosterone (patch)	2.5 mg patch	60 patches/box	GSK	United Kingdom		
Andropatch	testosterone (patch)	5 mg patch	30 patches/box	GSK	United Kingdom		
Andropatch	testosterone (patch)	12.2 mg patch	30, 60 patch box	Schwarz Pharma	Netherlands		
Andropen 275	Sustanon 250 (testosterone blend)	275mg/ml	10 ml vial	British Dragon	Thailand		
Andropository	testosterone enanthate	200 mg/ml	10 ml vial	Rugby	U.S.	[NLM]	
Androral	methyltestosterone	10 mg tablet	n/a	Gedeon Richter	Hungary		
Androtardyl®	testosterone enanthate	250 mg/ml	1 ml ampule	Schering	Algeria		
Androtardyl®	testosterone enanthate	250 mg/ml	1 ml ampule	Schering	France		
Androtardyl®	testosterone enanthate	250 mg/ml	1 ml ampule	Schering	Morocco		
Androtardyl®	testosterone enanthate	250 mg/ml	1 ml ampule	Schering	Tunisia		
Androtop Gel	testosterone (gel)	50 mg	single dose packet	Kade/Besins	Germany		
Androxon	testosterone undecanoate	40 mg capsules	60 capsule bottle	Donmed/Organon	South Africa		
Androxon	testosterone undecanoate	40 mg capsules	20 capsule box	Organon	Brazil		
Androxon	testosterone undecanoate	40 mg capsules	30 capsule bottle	Organon	Israel		
Androxon	testosterone undecanoate	40 mg capsules	60 capsule bottle	Organon	Norway		
Androxon	testosterone undecanoate	40 mg capsules	n/a	Organon	Pakistan		
Androyd	oxymetholone	5 mg tablet	100 tablet	Parke Davis	India		
Andryl 200	testosterone enanthate	200 mg/ml	10 ml vial	Keene	U.S.	[NLM]	
Apetil	stanozolol (oral)	4 mg/ml	10 ml dropper bottle	Holliday	Argentina		VET
AquaTest	testosterone suspension	100 mg/ml	10 ml vial	Denkall	Mexico		VET
Aquaviron	testosterone suspension	25 mg/ml	1 ml ampule	Nicholas	India		
Ara-Test	testosterone propionate	25 mg/ml	10 ml vial	Aranda Laboratories	Mexico	[NLM]	VET
Aratest 2500	Testoviron (testosterone blend)	250 mg/ml	10 ml vial	Aranda	Mexico		VET
Arbolic	methylandrostenediol dipropionate	50 mg/ml	n/a	Burgin Arden	U.S.	[NLM]	
Arcosterone	methyltestosterone	10 mg sub.	n/a	Acrum	U.S.	[NLM]	
Arcosterone	methyltestosterone	10, 25 mg tablet	n/a	Acrum	U.S.	[NLM]	
Astrapin	testosterone propionate	50 mg/ml	1 ml ampule	Astrapin	Malaysia		

Appendix B: Drug Availability Tables - Listings by Trade Name

Trade Name	Generic Name	Dose	Packaging	Company	Country	Status	Vet
Atmos	testosterone (patch)	5 mg patch	n/a	Astra	Sweden		
Atmos	testosterone (patch)	5 mg patch	30 patch box	Astra Zenica	Norway		
Averbol 25	methandrostenolone	25 mg/ml	20 ml vial	British Dragon	Thailand		
AVP Supertest	testosterone propionate	50 mg/ml	10 ml vial	Vetsearch	Australia		VET
Banrot	testosterone cypionate	75 mg/ml	200 ml bladder	Coopers	Australia	[NLM]	VET
Baojen	fluoxymesterone	5 mg capsule	n/a	Ta Fong	Taiwan		
Bionabol	methandrostenolone	2, 5 mg tab	40 tablet box	Balkanpharma	Bulgaria		
Bionabol	methandrostenolone	2 mg tablet	40 tablet bottle	Pharmacia	Bulgaria	[NLM]	
Bionabol	methandrostenolone	5 mg tab	40 tablet bottle	Pharmacia	Bulgaria	[NLM]	
Biselmon Depot	testosterone cypionate	50 mg/ml	n/a	Ta Fong	Taiwan		
Bi-Testo	Testoviron (testosterone blend)	60 mg/ml	10 ml vial	Cimol	Argentina		VET
Bold 200	boldenone undecylenate	200 mg/ml	10 ml vial	Animal Power	Mexico		VET
Bold QV 200	boldenone undecylenate	200 mg/ml	10 ml vial	Quality Vet	Mexico		VET
Boldabol	boldenone undecylenate	200 mg/ml	10 ml vial	British Dragon	Thailand		
Boldebal-H	boldenone undecylenate	50 mg/ml	10 ml vial	Ilium/Troy	Australia		VET
Boldenol 25	boldenone undecylenate	25 mg/ml	10, 50, 100, 250ml vial	Comandina	Colombia		VET
Boldenol R	boldenone undecylenate	50 mg/ml	10, 50, 100, 250ml vial	Comandina	Colombia		VET
Boldenon	boldenone undecylenate	200 mg/ml	10 ml vial	Ttokkyo	Mexico		VET
Boldenona	boldenone undecylenate	50 mg/ml	10, 20, 100 ml vial	Biogen	Colombia		VET
Boldenona	boldenone undecylenate	50 mg/ml	10, 50, 100, 250ml vial	Vecol	Colombia		VET
Boldenona 200	boldenone undecylenate	200 mg/ml	10 ml vial	Pet's Pharma	Mexico		VET
Boldenona 50	boldenone undecylenate	50 mg/ml	10, 50, 100, 250ml vial	Servinsumos	Colombia		VET
Boldenona 50 Gen-Far	boldenone undecylenate	50 mg/ml	10, 50, 100, 250ml vial	Gen-Far	Bolivia		VET
Boldenona 50 Gen-Far	boldenone undecylenate	50 mg/ml	10, 50, 100, 250ml vial	Gen-Far	Colombia		VET
Boldenona 50 Gen-Far	boldenone undecylenate	50 mg/ml	10, 50, 100, 250ml vial	Gen-Far	Costa Rica		VET
Boldenona 50 Gen-Far	boldenone undecylenate	50 mg/ml	10, 50, 100, 250ml vial	Gen-Far	Dom. Rep.		VET
Boldenona 50 Gen-Far	boldenone undecylenate	50 mg/ml	10, 50, 100, 250ml vial	Gen-Far	Ecuador		VET
Boldenona 50 Gen-Far	boldenone undecylenate	50 mg/ml	10, 50, 100, 250ml vial	Gen-Far	El Salvador		VET
Boldenona 50 Gen-Far	boldenone undecylenate	50 mg/ml	10, 50, 100, 250ml vial	Gen-Far	Guatemala		VET
Boldenona 50 Gen-Far	boldenone undecylenate	50 mg/ml	10, 50, 100, 250ml vial	Gen-Far	Honduras		VET
Boldenona 50 Gen-Far	boldenone undecylenate	50 mg/ml	10, 50, 100, 250ml vial	Gen-Far	Nicaragua		VET
Boldenona 50 Gen-Far	boldenone undecylenate	50 mg/ml	10, 50, 100, 250ml vial	Gen-Far	Panama		VET
Boldenona 50 Gen-Far	boldenone undecylenate	50 mg/ml	10, 50, 100, 250ml vial	Gen-Far	Peru		VET
Boldenone-50	boldenone undecylenate	50 mg/ml	10 ml vial	Jurox	Australia	[NLM]	VET
Bonalone	oxymetholone	50 mg tablet	100 tablet bottle	Body Research	Thailand		
Bonavar	oxandrolone	2.5 mg tablet	10 tablet strip	Body Research	Thailand		
Canoate Inj	nandrolone decanoate	25, 50 mg/ml	n/a	n/a	Korea		
Cebulin 50	boldenone undecylenate	50 mg/ml	10, 50, 250 ml vial	Provet	Colombia		VET
Cetabon	stanozolol (oral)	2 mg tablet	10 tablet strip	Therapharma	Thailand		
Cheque Drops	mibolerone	100 mcg/ml	55 mg bottle	Upjohn	U.S.	[NLM]	VET
Chinglicosan	fluoxymesterone	5 mg capsule	n/a	Ciiphar	Taiwan		

Appendix B: Drug Availability Tables - Listings by Trade Name

Trade Name	Generic Name	Dose	Packaging	Company	Country	Status	Vet
Chinlipan Tab	methandrostenolone	2 mg tablet	n/a	Chin Tien	Taiwan		
ComponentTE-G® (+ estradiol)	trenbolone acetate	20 mg pellet	40 pellet cartridge	VetLife	U.S.		VET
ComponentTE-S® (+ estradiol)	trenbolone acetate	20 mg pellet	120 pellet cartridge	VetLife	U.S.		VET
ComponentT-H®	trenbolone acetate	20 mg pellet	200 pellet cartridge	VetLife	U.S.		VET
ComponentT-S®	trenbolone acetate	20 mg pellet	140 pellet cartridge	VetLife	U.S.		VET
Crecibol	boldenone undecylenate	25 mg/ml	10, 30 ml vial	Unimed	Mexico		VET
Crestabolic	methylandrostenediol dipropionate	50 mg/ml	n/a	Nutrition	U.S.	[NLM]	
Cyclo-Testosterone Depot	testosterone cypionate	130 mg/ml	n/a	Astar	Taiwan		
Cypionax	testosterone cypionate	100 mg/ml	2 ml ampule	Body Research	Thailand		
Cypiotest 250	testosterone cypionate	250 mg/ml	10 ml vial	Animal Power	Mexico		VET
CypioTest 250	testosterone cypionate	250 mg/ml	10 ml vial	Denkall	Mexico		VET
Cypriotest L/A	testosterone cypionate	250 mg/ml	10 ml vial	Loeffler	Mexico		VET
Daily Reborn Inj	nandrolone phenylpropionate	25 mg/ml	n/a	Shiteh	Taiwan		
Danabol DS	methandrostenolone	10 mg tablet	500 tablet bottle	Body Research	Thailand		
Danabolan	trenbolone hexahydrobenzylcarbonate	76 mg/ml	1.5 ml ampule	Body Research	Thailand		
D-Bol	methandrostenolone	10 mg tablet	100 tablet bottle	Denkall	Mexico		VET
D-Bol	methandrostenolone	10 mg capsule	96 capsule box	Denkall	Mexico		VET
D-Bol	methandrostenolone	10 mg capsule	300 capsule bottle	Denkall	Mexico		VET
D-Bol	methandrostenolone	25 mg/ml	10 ml vial	Denkall	Mexico		VET
Debosteron	methyltestosterone	n/a	n/a	n/a	Korea		
Deca 300	nandrolone decanoate	300 mg/ml	10 ml vial	Animal Power	Mexico		VET
Deca QV 200	nandrolone decanoate	200 mg/ml	10, 50 ml vial	Quality Vet	Mexico		VET
Deca QV 300	nandrolone decanoate	300 mg/ml	10 ml vial	Quality Vet	Mexico		VET
Decabol	nandrolone decanoate	250 mg/ml	10 ml vial	British Dragon	Thailand		
Deca-Dubol-100	nandrolone decanoate	100 mg/ml	2 ml vial	BM Pharmaceuticals	India		
Deca-Durabolin®	nandrolone decanoate	25, 50 mg/ml	1 ml ampule	Donmed/Organon	South Africa		
Deca-Durabolin®	nandrolone decanoate	25, 50, 100 mg/ml	1 ml ampule	Infar	India		
Deca-Durabolin®	nandrolone decanoate	25, 50 mg/ml	1 ml ampule	Organon	Bulgaria		
Deca-Durabolin®	nandrolone decanoate	25, 50, 100 mg/ml	1 ml ampule	Organon	Chile		
Deca-Durabolin®	nandrolone decanoate	25, 50 mg/ml	1 ml ampule	Organon	Colombia		
Deca-Durabolin®	nandrolone decanoate	25, 50 mg/ml	1 ml	Organon	Denmark	[NLM]	
Deca-Durabolin®	nandrolone decanoate	n/a	n/a	Organon	Ireland		
Deca-Durabolin®	nandrolone decanoate	25, 50 mg/ml	1 ml ampule	Organon	Korea		
Deca-Durabolin®	nandrolone decanoate	25 mg/ml	1 ml ampule	Organon	Malaysia		
Deca-Durabolin®	nandrolone decanoate	50 mg/ml	1 ml ampule	Organon	New Zealand		
Deca-Durabolin®	nandrolone decanoate	50 mg/ml	1 ml ampule	Organon	Norway		
Deca-Durabolin®	nandrolone decanoate	50 mg/ml	1 ml ampule	Organon	Peru		
Deca-Durabolin®	nandrolone decanoate	25 mg/ml	1 ml ampule	Organon	Poland	[NLM]	
Deca-Durabolin®	nandrolone decanoate	50 mg/ml	1 ml ampule	Organon	Poland		
Deca-Durabolin®	nandrolone decanoate	25 mg/ml	1 ml ampule	Organon	Singapore		
Deca-Durabolin®	nandrolone decanoate	50 mg/ml	1 ml ampule	Organon	Taiwan		

Appendix B: Drug Availability Tables - Listings by Trade Name

Trade Name	Generic Name	Dose	Packaging	Company	Country	Status	Vet
Deca-Durabolin®	nandrolone decanoate	25, 50 mg/ml	1 ml ampule	Organon	Thailand		
Deca-Durabolin®	nandrolone decanoate	25, 50 mg/ml	1 ml	Organon	Argentina		
Deca-Durabolin®	nandrolone decanoate	50 mg/ml	2 ml	Organon	Argentina		
Deca-Durabolin®	nandrolone decanoate	25 mg/ml	1 ml	Organon	Austria	[NLM]	
Deca-Durabolin®	nandrolone decanoate	25, 50 mg/ml	1 ml ampule, syringe	Organon	Belgium		
Deca-Durabolin®	nandrolone decanoate	25, 50 mg/ml	1 ml ampule	Organon	Brazil		
Deca-Durabolin®	nandrolone decanoate	50 mg/ml	2 ml	Organon	Canada	[NLM]	
Deca-Durabolin®	nandrolone decanoate	100 mg/ml	2 ml	Organon	Canada		
Deca-Durabolin®	nandrolone decanoate	25, 50 mg/ml	1 ml	Organon	Finland		
Deca-Durabolin®	nandrolone decanoate	100 mg/ml	1,2 ml	Organon	Finland		
Deca-Durabolin®	nandrolone decanoate	50 mg/ml	1 ml	Organon	France	[NLM]	
Deca-Durabolin®	nandrolone decanoate	25, 50 mg/ml	1 ml	Organon	Germany	[NLM]	
Deca-Durabolin®	nandrolone decanoate	50 mg/ml	1 ml vial	Organon	Greece		
Deca-Durabolin®	nandrolone decanoate	100 mg/ml	2 ml vial	Organon	Greece		
Deca-Durabolin®	nandrolone decanoate	100 mg/ml	2 ml vial	Organon	Greece		
Deca-Durabolin®	nandrolone decanoate	25, 50 mg/ml	1 ml ampule	Organon	Indonesia		
Deca-Durabolin®	nandrolone decanoate	25, 50 mg/ml	1 ml ampule	Organon	Italy		
Deca-Durabolin®	nandrolone decanoate	25, 50 mg/ml	1 ml ampule	Organon	Netherlands		
Deca-Durabolin®	nandrolone decanoate	50 mg/ml	1 ml ampule	Organon	Rumania		
Deca-Durabolin®	nandrolone decanoate	25, 50 mg/ml	1 ml ampule	Organon	Spain		
Deca-Durabolin®	nandrolone decanoate	50 mg/ml	1 ml ampule	Organon	Sweden		
Deca-Durabolin®	nandrolone decanoate	25, 100 mg/ml	1, 2 ml	Organon	Sweden	[NLM]	
Deca-Durabolin®	nandrolone decanoate	25 mg/ml	1 ml ampule	Organon	Switzerland	[NLM]	
Deca-Durabolin®	nandrolone decanoate	50 mg/ml	1 ml ampule	Organon	Switzerland		
Deca-Durabolin®	nandrolone decanoate	100 mg/ml	1, 2 ml vial	Organon	U.S.	[NLM]	
Deca-Durabolin®	nandrolone decanoate	200 mg/ml	1 ml vial	Organon	U.S.	[NLM]	
Deca-Durabolin®	nandrolone decanoate	50 mg/ml	1 ml ampule	Organon	United Kingdom		
Deca-Durabolin®	nandrolone decanoate	100 mg/ml	1, 2 ml ampule	Organon	United Kingdom	[NLM]	
Deca-Durabolin®	nandrolone decanoate	25 mg/ml	1 ml ampule	Organon	Venezuela		
Deca-Durabolin®	nandrolone decanoate	50 mg/ml	1 ml syringe	Organon	Venezuela		
Deca-Durabolin®	nandrolone decanoate	25, 50 mg/ml	1 ml ampule	Organon/Nile	Egypt		
Deca-Durabolin®	nandrolone decanoate	100 mg/ml	2 ml vial	Organon	Netherlands		
Deca-Evabolin	nandrolone decanoate	25 mg/ml	1 ml ampule	Concept	India		
Decagic	nandrolone decanoate	100 mg/ml	10 ml vial	Unichem	India	[NLM]	
Decanandrolen	nandrolone decanoate	200mg/ml	10 ml vial	Denkall	Mexico		VET
Decandrol 300	nandrolone decanoate	300 mg/ml	10 ml vial	Pet's Pharma	Mexico		VET
Decaneurabol	nandrolone decanoate	25, 50 mg/ml	1 ml ampule	Cadila	India		
Decaneurophen	nandrolone decanoate	25, 50 mg/ml	1 ml ampule	Ind-Swift	India		
Decanoato de Nandrolona	nandrolone decanoate	200 mg/ml	10 ml vial	Tornel	Mexico		VET
Decanoato Nandrolona	nandrolone decanoate	25, 50 mg/ml	1 ml ampule	Astorga	Chile		
Decanoato Nandrolona	nandrolone decanoate	50 mg/ml	1 ml ampule	Biosano	Chile		

Appendix B: Drug Availability Tables - Listings by Trade Name

Trade Name	Generic Name	Dose	Packaging	Company	Country	Status	Vet
Decanofort	nandrolone decanoate	25 mg/ml	1 ml ampule	Terapia	Rumania		
Deca-Pronabol	nandrolone decanoate	100 mg/ml	2 ml ampule	P & B Labs	India	[NLM]	
Decatron 250	nandrolone decanoate	250 mg/ml	10 ml vial	Brovel	Mexico		VET
Delatest	testosterone enanthate	100/mg/ml	10 ml vial	Dunhall	U.S.	[NLM]	
Delatestryl	testosterone enanthate	200 mg/ml	10 ml vial	Brovel	Mexico	[NLM]	VET
Delatestryl	testosterone enanthate	200 mg/ml	1 ml syringe	BTG	U.S.		
Delatestryl	testosterone enanthate	200 mg/ml	5 ml vial	BTG	U.S.		
Delatestryl	testosterone enanthate	200 mg/ml	10 ml vial	Mead Johnson	U.S.	[NLM]	
Delatestryl	testosterone enanthate	200 mg/ml	5 ml vial	Theramed	Canada		
Denkadiol	methylandrostenediol dipropionate	75 mg/ml	10 ml vial	Denkall	Mexico	[NLM]	VET
Dep Andro-100-200	testosterone cypionate	100, 200 mg/ml	10 ml vial	Forest	U.S.	[NLM]	
Deposteron	testosterone cypionate	100 mg/ml	2 ml ampule	Novaquimica/Sigma	Brazil		
Deposterona	testosterone blend (misc)	60 mg/ml	10 ml vial	Fort Dodge	Mexico		VET
Deposterona	testosterone blend (misc)	60 mg/ml	10 ml vial	Syntex	Mexico	[NLM]	VET
Depot-Bifuron	testosterone cypionate	50 mg/ml	n/a	Gentle	Taiwan		
Depo-TCP	testosterone cypionate	200mg/ml	n/a	n/a	Korea		
Depotest	testosterone cypionate	100, 200 mg/ml	10 ml vial	Hyrex	U.S.	[NLM]	
Depotest	testosterone cypionate	100, 200 mg/ml	10 ml vial	Kay	U.S.	[NLM]	
Depo-Testermon	testosterone cypionate	200 mg/ml	n/a	CCPC	Taiwan		
Depo-Testerone	testosterone cypionate	200 mg/ml	n/a	Metro	Taiwan		
DepoTestmon Inj	testosterone enanthate	65 mg/ml	n/a	CCPC	Taiwan		
Depo-Testomon	testosterone cypionate	100 mg/ml	n/a	Li Ta	Taiwan		
Depo-Testosterone	testosterone cypionate	100 mg/ml	10 ml vial	Pharmacia & Upjohn	South Africa		
Depo-Testosterone CPP	testosterone cypionate	100 mg/ml	n/a	Metro	Taiwan		
Depo-Testosterone®	testosterone cypionate	100 mg/ml	n/a	Pharmacia	Malaysia		
Depo-Testosterone®	testosterone cypionate	100 mg/ml	10 ml vial	Pharmacia	Canada		
Depo-Testosterone®	testosterone cypionate	100 mg/ml	10 ml vial	Pharmacia & Upjohn	New Zealand		
Depo-Testosterone®	testosterone cypionate	100 mg/ml	10 ml vial	Pharmacia & Upjohn	Singapore		
Depo-Testosterone®	testosterone cypionate	100, 200 mg/ml	10 ml vial	Pharmacia & Upjohn	U.S.		
Depo-Testosterone®	testosterone cypionate	200 mg/ml	1 ml vial	Pharmacia & Upjohn	U.S.		
Depot-Hormon MF	testosterone cypionate	50 mg/ml	n/a	Sintong	Taiwan		
Depotrone	testosterone cypionate	100 mg/ml	2 ml ampule	Propan-Zurich	South Africa		
Depovirin Inj	testosterone cypionate	125 mg/ml	2 ml	n/a	Korea		
Dep-Test	testosterone cypionate	100 mg/ml	10 ml vial	Rocky Mountain	U.S.	[NLM]	
Dialone	methandrostenolone	5 mg tablet	100 tablet bottle	Major	U.S.	[NLM]	
Dianabol	methandrostenolone	10 mg tablet	100 tablet bottle	Salud	Mexico		VET
Dianabol	methandrostenolone	25 mg/ml	10, 50, 100 ml vial	Salud	Mexico		VET
Dianabol	methandrostenolone	5 mg tablet	100 tablet bottle	Ciba	Germany	[NLM]	
Dianabol	methandrostenolone	5 mg tablet	100 tablet bottle	Ciba	U.S.	[NLM]	
Dianabol	methandrostenolone	5 mg tablet	100 tablet bottle	Ciba	United Kingdom	[NLM]	
Dianabol	methandrostenolone	25 mg tablet	30 tablet bottle	Planet Pharmacy	Belize		

Appendix B: Drug Availability Tables - Listings by Trade Name

Trade Name	Generic Name	Dose	Packaging	Company	Country	Status	Vet
Dimetabol	nandrolone decanoate	50 mg/ml	50 ml vial	Bremer Pharma	Dom. Rep.	[NLM]	VET
Dimetabol ADE	nandrolone decanoate	25 mg/ml	50, 100 ml vial	Lapisa	Mexico		VET
Dinandrol	nandrolone (blend)	100 mg/ml	2 ml vial	Xelox (export)	Philippines		
Diosterol	methandrostenolone/stanozolol	50 mg tablet	30 tablet bottle	Planet Pharmacy	Belize		
Drive	methylandrostenediol (blend)	55 mg/ml	10 ml vial	RWR	Australia		VET
Drolban	drostanolone propionate	50 mg/1ml	1 ml vial	Lilly	U.S.	[NLM]	
Dromostan	drostanolone	50 mg/ml	5 ml vial	Xelox (export)	Philippines		
D-Test 100/200	testosterone cypionate	100, 200 mg/ml	10 ml vial	Sig	U.S.	[NLM]	
Dubol	testosterone propionate	25 mg/ml	1 ml ampule	n/a	China		
Dubol-100	nandrolone phenylpropionate	100 mg/ml	2 ml vial	BM Pharmaceuticals	India		
Dubol-50	nandrolone phenylpropionate	50 mg/ml	1 ml ampule	BM Pharmaceuticals	India		
Durabol	nandrolone phenylpropionate	200 mg/ml	10 ml vial	British Dragon	Thailand		
Durabol	nandrolone phenylpropionate	100 mg/ml	10 ml vial	British Dragon	Thailand	[NLM]	
Durabolin®	nandrolone phenylpropionate	25 mg/ml	1 ml ampule	Infar	India		
Durabolin®	nandrolone phenylpropionate	25 mg/ml	n/a	Opopharma	Switzerland	[NLM]	
Durabolin®	nandrolone phenylpropionate	25 mg/ml	1 ml ampule	Organon	Malaysia		
Durabolin®	nandrolone phenylpropionate	25 mg/ml	2 ml vial	Organon	Taiwan		
Durabolin®	nandrolone phenylpropionate	25 mg/ml	n/a	Organon	Belgium	[NLM]	
Durabolin®	nandrolone phenylpropionate	25, 50 mg/ml	n/a	Organon	Canada	[NLM]	
Durabolin®	nandrolone phenylpropionate	25 mg/ml	n/a	Organon	Finland		
Durabolin®	nandrolone phenylpropionate	25 mg/ml	1 ml ampule	Organon	Greece	[NLM]	
Durabolin®	nandrolone phenylpropionate	12.5 mg/ml	2 ml ampule	Organon	Indonesia		
Durabolin®	nandrolone phenylpropionate	25 mg/ml	1 ml ampule	Organon	Netherlands		
Durabolin®	nandrolone phenylpropionate	50 mg/ml	n/a	Organon	Portugal		
Durabolin®	nandrolone phenylpropionate	25 mg/ml	1 ml ampule	Organon	Spain	[NLM]	
Durabolin®	nandrolone phenylpropionate	25, 50 mg/ml	n/a	Organon	U.S.	[NLM]	
Durabolin®	nandrolone phenylpropionate	50 mg/ml	1 ml ampule	Organon	United Kingdom	[NLM]	
Durabolin®	nandrolone phenylpropionate	50 mg/ml	n/a	Organon	YugoslaviaFRMR		
Durandrol	methylandrostenediol dipropionate	50 mg/ml	n/a	Pharmex	U.S.	[NLM]	
Durandron	Sustanon 250 (testosterone blend)	250 mg/ml	1 ml ampule	Organon	Spain	[NLM]	
Duratest-100-200	testosterone cypionate	100, 200 mg/ml	10 ml vial	Roberts	U.S.	[NLM]	
Duratest-100-200	testosterone cypionate	100, 200 mg/ml	10 ml vial	Hauck	U.S.	[NLM]	
Durateston	Sustanon 250 (testosterone blend)	250 mg/ml	5 ml vial	Intervet	Australia		VET
Durateston 250®	Sustanon 250 (testosterone blend)	250 mg/ml	1 ml ampule	Organon	Bolivia		
Durateston 250®	Sustanon 250 (testosterone blend)	250 mg/ml	1 ml ampule	Organon	Brazil		
Dura-Testosterone	testosterone enanthate	200 mg/ml	10 ml vial	Pharmex	U.S.	[NLM]	
Durathate-200 Injection	testosterone enanthate	200 mg/ml	n/a	Hauck	U.S.	[NLM]	
Durathate-200 Injection	testosterone enanthate	200 mg/ml	n/a	Roberts	U.S.	[NLM]	
Dynabol	nandrolone cypionate	50 mg/ml	10 ml vial	Jurox	Australia	[NLM]	VET
Dynabolin 50	boldenone undecylenate	50 mg/ml	10, 50, 100, 250ml vial	Kryovet	Colombia		VET
Dynabolon	nandrolone undecanoate	80.5 mg/ml	1 ml ampule	Farmasister	Italy	[NLM]	

Appendix B: Drug Availability Tables - Listings by Trade Name

Trade Name	Generic Name	Dose	Packaging	Company	Country	Status	Vet
Dynabolon	nandrolone undecanoate	80.5 mg/ml	1 ml ampule	Fournier	Italy		
Dynabolon	nandrolone undecanoate	80.5 mg/ml	1 ml ampule	Theramex	France	[NLM]	
Dynabolon Inj	nandrolone decanoate	40 mg/.5 ml	1 ml ampule	n/a	Korea		
Dynasten	oxymetholone	50 mg tablet	n/a	Cilag	Portugal	[NLM]	
Elpihormo	nandrolone decanoate	50 mg/ml	1 ml	Chemica	Greece	[NLM]	
Enantat QV 250	testosterone enanthate	250 mg/ml	10, 50 ml vial	Quality Vet	Mexico		VET
Enantato 350	testosterone enanthate	350 mg/ml	10 ml vial	Pet's Pharma	Mexico		VET
Enantest 250	testosterone enanthate	250 mg/ml	10 ml vial	Animal Power	Mexico		VET
Enarmon-Depot	testosterone enanthate	125 mg/ml	n/a	Teskoku Hormone	Japan		
Encephan	methandrostenolone	5 mg tablet	n/a	Sato	Japan	[NLM]	
Equibolin-50	nandrolone phenylpropionate	50 mg/ml	n/a	Vortech	U.S.	[NLM]	
Equifort	boldenone undecylenate	50 mg/ml	10, 50 ml vial	Purina	Brazil		VET
Equi-gan	boldenone undecylenate	50 mg/ml	10, 50, 100, 250 ml vial	Tornel	Mexico		VET
Equilon 100	boldenone (blend)	100 mg/ml	6 ml vial	WDV	Myanmar/Burma		VET
Equipoise®	boldenone undecylenate	50 mg/ml	10, 50 ml vial	Fort Dodge	Mexico		VET
Equipoise®	boldenone undecylenate	50 mg/ml	50 ml vial	Fort Dodge	U.S.		VET
Equipoise®	boldenone undecylenate	25, 50 mg/ml	50 ml vial	Ciba-Geigy	Canada	[NLM]	VET
Equipoise®	boldenone undecylenate	25, 50 mg/ml	50 ml vial	Solvay	Mexico	[NLM]	VET
Equipoise®	boldenone undecylenate	25, 50 mg/ml	50 ml vial	Squibb	Canada	[NLM]	VET
Equipoise®	boldenone undecylenate	25, 50 mg/ml	50 ml vial	Squibb	Mexico	[NLM]	VET
Equipoise®	boldenone undecylenate	25, 50 mg/ml	50 ml vial	Squibb	U.S.	[NLM]	VET
Equipoise®	boldenone undecylenate	50 mg/ml	50 ml vial	Wyeth	Canada		VET
Equitest 200	testosterone blend (misc)	200 mg/ml	6 ml vial	WDV	Myanmar/Burma		VET
Esiclene	formebolone	1 mg drops	n/a	Biofarma	Portugal	[NLM]	
Esiclene	formebolone	5 mg tablet	n/a	Biofarma	Portugal	[NLM]	
Esiclene	formebolone	1 mg drops	n/a	LPB	Italy	[NLM]	
Esiclene	formebolone	2 mg/ml	2 ml ampule	LPB	Italy	[NLM]	
Esiclene	formebolone	5 mg tablet	n/a	LPB	Italy	[NLM]	
Estano-Pet's	stanozolol (oral)	10, 25 mg tablet	100 tablet bottle	Norvet	Mexico		VET
Estanozolol	stanozolol (inj)	50 mg/ml	30 ml vial	Industria Argentina	Argentina		VET
Estigor	nandrolone phenylpropionate	10 mg/ml	250 ml	Burnet	Argentina		VET
Estrombol	stanozolol (inj)	25 mg/ml	10 ml vial	Fundacion	Argentina		VET
Evabolin	nandrolone phenylpropionate	25 mg/ml	1 ml ampule	Concept	India		
Everone	testosterone enanthate	100, 200 mg/ml	10 ml vial	Hyrex	U.S.	[NLM]	
Ex-Pois	boldenone undecylenate	50 mg/ml	10 ml vial	Agofarma	Argentina		VET
Extraboline	nandrolone decanoate	50 mg/ml	2 ml vial	Genepharm	Greece		
Facovit	testosterone propionate	1 mg/ml	10 ml vial	Teofarma	Italy		
Fenobolin	nandrolone phenylpropionate	20 mg/ml	n/a	Medexport Russia	Russia	[NLM]	
Ferona	fluoxymesterone	1 mg tablet	30 tablet box	Sidus	Argentina		
Fherbolico	nandrolone phenylpropionate	50 mg/ml	n/a	Fher	Spain	[NLM]	
Filybol	methylandrostenediol (blend)	70 mg/ml	10, 20 ml vial	Ranvet	Australia		VET

Appendix B: Drug Availability Tables - Listings by Trade Name

Trade Name	Generic Name	Dose	Packaging	Company	Country	Status	Vet
Finaject	trenbolone acetate	30 mg/ml	n/a	Roussel	France	[NLM]	VET
Finajet	trenbolone acetate	30 mg/ml	50 ml vial	Hoechst	U.S.	[NLM]	VET
Finajet	trenbolone acetate	30 mg/ml	50 ml vial	Hoechst	United Kingdom	[NLM]	VET
Finaplix-H®	trenbolone acetate	20 mg pellet	100 pellet cartridge	Hoechst-Roussel	U.S.	[NLM]	VET
Finaplix-H®	trenbolone acetate	20 mg pellet	100 pellet cartridge	Intervet	U.S.		VET
Finaplix-H®	trenbolone acetate	20 mg pellet	70, 100 pellet cartridge	Roussel	Mexico	[NLM]	VET
Finaplix-S®	trenbolone acetate	20 mg pellet	70 pellet cartridge	Hoechst-Roussel	U.S.	[NLM]	VET
Flouoxymesterone cap	fluoxymesterone	5 mg capsule	n/a	Yuan Chou	Taiwan		
Floxymesterone	fluoxymesterone	5 mg capsule	n/a	Chen Ho	Taiwan		
Fluoxymesterone	fluoxymesterone	10 mg tablet	100 tablet bottle	Rosemont	U.S.		
Fortabol	nandrolone laurate	20 mg/ml	10, 50 ml vial	Parfam	Mexico		VET
Fortadex	nandrolone laurate	25, 50 mg/ml	n/a	Hydro	Germany		VET
Fosteron	fluoxymesterone	5 mg capsule	n/a	Health Chemical	Taiwan		
Fu Lao Shu	fluoxymesterone	10 mg capsule	n/a	Ming Ta	Taiwan		
Fuloan	fluoxymesterone	10 mg capsule	n/a	New Chem & Pharm	Taiwan		
Ganabol	boldenone undecylenate	50 mg/ml	500 ml vial	Laboratorios VM	Bolivia		VET
Ganabol	boldenone undecylenate	25, 50 mg/ml	10, 50, 100, 250ml vial	Laboratorios VM	Bolivia		VET
Ganabol	boldenone undecylenate	50 mg/ml	500 ml vial	Laboratorios VM	Chile		VET
Ganabol	boldenone undecylenate	25, 50 mg/ml	10, 50, 100, 250ml vial	Laboratorios VM	Chile		VET
Ganabol	boldenone undecylenate	50 mg/ml	500 ml vial	Laboratorios VM	Colombia		VET
Ganabol	boldenone undecylenate	25, 50 mg/ml	10, 50, 100, 250ml vial	Laboratorios VM	Colombia		VET
Ganabol	boldenone undecylenate	50 mg/ml	500 ml vial	Laboratorios VM	Dom. Rep.		VET
Ganabol	boldenone undecylenate	25, 50 mg/ml	10, 50, 100, 250ml vial	Laboratorios VM	Dom. Rep.		VET
Ganabol	boldenone undecylenate	50 mg/ml	500 ml vial	Laboratorios VM	Ecuador		VET
Ganabol	boldenone undecylenate	25, 50 mg/ml	10, 50, 100, 250ml vial	Laboratorios VM	Ecuador		VET
Ganabol	boldenone undecylenate	50 mg/ml	500 ml vial	Laboratorios VM	El Salvador		VET
Ganabol	boldenone undecylenate	25, 50 mg/ml	10, 50, 100, 250ml vial	Laboratorios VM	El Salvador		VET
Ganabol	boldenone undecylenate	50 mg/ml	500 ml vial	Laboratorios VM	Guatemala		VET
Ganabol	boldenone undecylenate	25, 50 mg/ml	10, 50, 100, 250ml vial	Laboratorios VM	Guatemala		VET
Ganabol	boldenone undecylenate	50 mg/ml	500 ml vial	Laboratorios VM	Honduras		VET
Ganabol	boldenone undecylenate	25, 50 mg/ml	10, 50, 100, 250ml vial	Laboratorios VM	Honduras		VET
Ganabol	boldenone undecylenate	50 mg/ml	500 ml vial	Laboratorios VM	Panama		VET
Ganabol	boldenone undecylenate	25, 50 mg/ml	10, 50, 100, 250ml vial	Laboratorios VM	Panama		VET
Ganabol	boldenone undecylenate	50 mg/ml	500 ml vial	Laboratorios VM	Paraguay		VET
Ganabol	boldenone undecylenate	25, 50 mg/ml	10, 50, 100, 250ml vial	Laboratorios VM	Paraguay		VET
Ganabol	boldenone undecylenate	50 mg/ml	500 ml vial	Laboratorios VM	Peru		VET
Ganabol	boldenone undecylenate	25, 50 mg/ml	10, 50, 100, 250ml vial	Laboratorios VM	Peru		VET
Ganabol	boldenone undecylenate	50 mg/ml	500 ml vial	Laboratorios VM	Venezuela		VET
Ganabol	boldenone undecylenate	25, 50 mg/ml	10, 50, 100, 250ml vial	Laboratorios VM	Venezuela		VET
Ganabol	methandrostenolone	25 mg/ml	50 ml vial	Salud	Mexico	[NLM]	VET
Ganekyl	nandrolone phenylpropionate	50 mg/ml	10, 100 ml vial	Over Labs	Argentina		VET

Appendix B: Drug Availability Tables - Listings by Trade Name

Trade Name	Generic Name	Dose	Packaging	Company	Country	Status	Vet
Gerabolin	nandrolone decanoate	25 mg/ml	1 ml ampule	Nile	Egypt		
Geri Tabs	methyltestosterone	2 mg tablet	50, 200 tablet bottle	Vetcom	Canada		VET
Glando Stridox	methyltestosterone	10 mg tablet	20 tablet box	Ion	Uruguay		
Halotestin®	fluoxymesterone	5 mg tablet	n/a	Galenika	YugoslaviaFRMR	[NLM]	
Halotestin®	fluoxymesterone	2, 5 mg tablet	n/a	n/a	Japan		
Halotestin®	fluoxymesterone	5 mg tablet	50 tablet bottle	Pharmacia	Canada		
Halotestin®	fluoxymesterone	5 mg tablet	100 tablet bottle	Pharmacia	Thailand		
Halotestin®	fluoxymesterone	5 mg tablet	n/a	Pharmacia & Upjohn	Philippines		
Halotestin®	fluoxymesterone	2, 5, 10 mg tablet	100 tablet bottle	Pharmacia & Upjohn	U.S.		
Halotestin®	fluoxymesterone	5 mg tablet	n/a	Pharmacia-Upjohn	France	[NLM]	
Halotestin®	fluoxymesterone	5 mg tablet	n/a	Upjohn	Denmark	[NLM]	
Halotestin®	fluoxymesterone	5 mg tablet	n/a	Upjohn	Finland		
Halotestin®	fluoxymesterone	5 mg tablet	20 tablet box	Upjohn	Greece		
Halotestin®	fluoxymesterone	5 mg tablet	20 tablet box	Upjohn	Italy	[NLM]	
Halotestin®	fluoxymesterone	5 mg tablet	n/a	Upjohn	Netherlands	[NLM]	
Halotestin®	fluoxymesterone	5 mg tablet	n/a	Upjohn	Norway	[NLM]	
Halotestin®	fluoxymesterone	5 mg tablet	n/a	Upjohn	Sweden	[NLM]	
Halotestin®	fluoxymesterone	10 mg tablet	100 tablet bottle	Warner-Chilcott	U.S.	[NLM]	
Hemogenin	oxymetholone	50 mg tablet	10 tablet box	Syntex	Brazil	[NLM]	
Hemogenin	oxymetholone	50 mg tablet	n/a	Aventis	Brazil		
Hemogenin	oxymetholone	50 mg tablet	10 tablet box	Sarsa	Brazil	[NLM]	
Histerone Injection	testosterone suspension	100 mg/ml	n/a	Roberts	U.S.	[NLM]	
Histerone Injection	testosterone suspension	100 mg/ml	n/a	Hauck	U.S.	[NLM]	
Hormobin	methyltestosterone	5 mg tablet	40 tablet box	Munrin Sahin	Turkey		
Hubernol	formebolone	5 mg dragee	n/a	ICN Hubber	Spain	[NLM]	
Hubernol	formebolone	1 mg drops	n/a	ICN Hubber	Spain	[NLM]	
Hybolin	methylandrostenediol dipropionate	50 mg/ml	n/a	Hyrex	U.S.	[NLM]	
Hybolin	nandrolone phenylpropionate	25, 50 mg/ml	n/a	Hyrex	U.S.	[NLM]	
Hybolin Decanoate	nandrolone decanoate	50, 100 mg/ml	1, 2 ml vial	Hyrex	U.S.		
Hybolin Imp.	testosterone propionate	25, 50 mg/ml	n/a	Hyrex	U.S.	[NLM]	
Hysterone	fluoxymesterone	20 mg tablet	100 tablet bottle	Major	U.S.	[NLM]	
Implus-H	testosterone propionate (implant)	22 mg/pellet	n/a	Upjohn	U.S.		
Jebolan	nandrolone decanoate	50 mg/ml	1 ml ampule	Etem	Turkey	[NLM]	
Jenasteron Inj	testosterone enanthate	250 mg/ml	1 ml ampule	Jenahexal	Malaysia		
Jenasteron Inj	testosterone enanthate	250 mg/ml	n/a	n/a	Korea		
Kanestron	oxymetholone	50 mg tablet	100 tablet bottle	Loeffler	Mexico		VET
KangJungBing	methyltestosterone	n/a	n/a	n/a	Korea		
Kicker Tab	oxandrolone	2.5 mg tablet	n/a	n/a	Korea		
Laudrol LA	nandrolone laurate	250 mg/ml	10 ml vial	Loeffler	Mexico		VET
Laurabolin	nandrolone laurate	25, 50 mg/ml	10 ml vial	Intervet	Australia		VET
Laurabolin	nandrolone laurate	50 mg/ml	10, 50 ml	Intervet	Colombia		VET

Appendix B: Drug Availability Tables - Listings by Trade Name

Trade Name	Generic Name	Dose	Packaging	Company	Country	Status	Vet
Laurabolin	nandrolone laurate	20, 50 mg/ml	10, 50 ml vial	Intervet	Mexico		VET
Laurabolin	nandrolone laurate	25, 50 mg/ml	5, 10, 50 ml	Vemie	Germany		VET
Laurabolin	nandrolone laurate	50 mg/ml	n/a	Werfft-Chemie	Austria		VET
Laurabolin V	nandrolone laurate	50 mg/ml	10, 50 ml	Intervet	Netherlands		VET
Legacy	boldenone undecylenate	50 mg/ml	50 ml vial	Technoquimicas	Colombia		VET
Libriol	methylandrostenediol (blend)	75 mg/ml	10, 20 ml vial	RWR	Australia		VET
Lipaw	fluoxymesterone	10 mg capsule	n/a	Long Der	Taiwan		
Lipidex	oxandrolone	2.5 mg tablet	n/a	Searle	Brazil	[NLM]	
Lonavar	oxandrolone	2.5 mg tablet	100 tablet bottle	BTG	Israel		
Lonavar	oxandrolone	2 mg tablet	n/a	Dainippon	Japan	[NLM]	
Lonavar	oxandrolone	2.5 mg tablet	n/a	Searle	Argentina	[NLM]	
Long	fluoxymesterone	10 mg capsule	n/a	Century	Taiwan		
Longivol (plus estrogen)	methyltestosterone	1 mg tablet	n/a	Medical S.A.	Spain		
Macrabone	nandrolone phenylpropionate	25 mg/ml	n/a	Ta Fong	Taiwan		
Malogen	testosterone suspension	25, 50, 100, mg/ml	n/a	Forest	U.S.	[NLM]	
Malogen 100/200 L.A.	testosterone enanthate	100, 200 mg/ml	10 ml vial	Forest	U.S.	[NLM]	
Malogen Aqueous	testosterone suspension	100 mg/ml	10 ml vial	Germiphene	Canada	[NLM]	
Malogen Cyp	testosterone cypionate	100, 200 mg/ml	10 ml vial	Forest	U.S.	[NLM]	
Malogen In Oil	testosterone propionate	100 mg/ml	10 ml vial	Germiphene	Canada	[NLM]	
Malogex LA200	testosterone enanthate	200 mg/ml	10 ml vial	Germiphene	Canada	[NLM]	
Malotrone	testosterone suspension	25, 50 mg/ml	n/a	Bluco	U.S.	[NLM]	
Mastabol	drostanolone propionate	50 mg/ml	10 ml vial	British Dragon	Thailand	[NLM]	
Mastabol	drostanolone propionate	100 mg/ml	10 ml vial	British Dragon	Thailand		
Masterid	drostanolone propionate	100 mg/2ml	2 ml amp	Gruenthal	Germany	[NLM]	
Masteril	drostanolone propionate	100 mg/2ml	2 ml ampule	Syntex	Bulgaria	[NLM]	
Masteril	drostanolone propionate	100 mg/2ml	2 ml amp	Syntex	United Kingdom	[NLM]	
Masteron	drostanolone propionate	100 mg/2ml	2 ml amp	Cilag	Portugal	[NLM]	
Masteron	drostanolone propionate	100 mg/2ml	2 ml amp	Sarva-Syntex	Belgium	[NLM]	
Mastisol	drostanolone propionate	5% injection sol.	n/a	Shionogi	Japan	[NLM]	
Maxibolin	ethylestrenol	2 mg tablet	n/a	Organon	U.S.	[NLM]	
Maxibolin Elixir	ethylestrenol	2 mg/5ml	n/a	Organon	U.S.	[NLM]	
Maxigan	boldenone undecylenate	50 mg/ml	10, 50 ml vial	Inpel/Denkall	Mexico	[NLM]	VET
Mediatric	methyltestosterone	10 mg tablet	n/a	Wyeth-Ayerst	U.S.	[NLM]	
Megagrisevit-Mono	clostebol acetate	15 mg dragee	30 dragee box	Pharmacia	Germany	[NLM]	
Megagrisevit-Mono	clostebol acetate	10 mg/1.5ml	1.5 ml vial	Pharmacia	Germany	[NLM]	
Melic	methandrostenolone	5 mg tablet	1000 tablet box, bottle	Pharmasant	Thailand		
Menabol	stanozolol (oral)	5 mg tablet	100 tablet box	n/a	India		
Menabolin	nandrolone phenylpropionate	25 mg/ml	1 ml ampule	Theramex/Memphis	Egypt		
Mesterolon	mesterolone	25 mg tablet	n/a	Brown & Burk	Philippines		
Mesterolon	mesterolone	25 mg tablet	n/a	Schering	Sweden	[NLM]	
Mesteron	methyltestosterone	10 mg tablet	n/a	Jelfa	Poland	[NLM]	

Appendix B: Drug Availability Tables - Listings by Trade Name

Trade Name	Generic Name	Dose	Packaging	Company	Country	Status	Vet
Mestoranum	mesterolone	25 mg tablet	n/a	Schering	Denmark		
Mestoranum	mesterolone	25 mg tablet	n/a	Schering	Norway	[NLM]	
Metabol	nandrolone phenylpropionate	25 mg/ml	1 ml ampule	Jagsonpal	India		
Metaboline	methandrostenolone	2 mg tablet	60, 500 tablet bottle	Desbergers	Canada	[NLM]	
Metabolon 25	methenolone acetate	25 mg tablet	100 tablet bottle	Bratis Labs	Mexico		VET
Metadec	nandrolone decanoate	25, 50 mg/ml	1 ml ampule	Jagsonpal	India		
Metalon Tabs	oxymetholone	75 mg tablet	100 tablet bottle	Animal Power	Mexico		VET
Metanabol	methandrostenolone	5 mg tablet	20 tablet box	Jelfa	Poland		
Metanabol	methandrostenolone	5 mg tablet	20 tablet box	Polfa	Poland	[NLM]	
Metanabol	methandrostenolone	I mg tablet	20 tablet box	Polfa	Poland	[NLM]	
Metanabol	methandrostenolone	0.5% cream	n/a	Polfa	Poland	[NLM]	
Metandiabol	methandrostenolone	25 mg/ml	50 ml vial	Quimper	Mexico		VET
Metandienon	methandrostenolone	5 mg tablet	100 tablet box	Bioreaktor	Russia		
Metandiol 60	methandrostenolone	60 mg/ml	10 ml vial	Pet's Pharma	Mexico		VET
Metandiol Tab	methandrostenolone	10 mg tablet	100 tablet bottle	Pet's Pharma	Mexico		VET
Metandren	methyltestosterone	5 mg sub. dragee	n/a	Ciba	U.S.	[NLM]	
Metandren	methyltestosterone	10, 25 mg tablet	n/a	Ciba	U.S.	[NLM]	
Metandren	methyltestosterone	10, 25 mg tablet	100 tablet bottle	Novartis	U.S.	[NLM]	
Metandrol 10	methandrostenolone	10 mg tablet	500 tablet bottle	Bratis Labs	Mexico		VET
Metandrostenolon	methandrostenolone	5 mg tablet	100 tablet box	Akrihin	Russia	[NLM]	
Metandrostenolon	methandrostenolone	5 mg tablet	100 tablet box	Akrikhin	Russia		
Metandrostenolon	methandrostenolone	5 mg tablet	100 tablet box	Bioreaktor	Russia	[NLM]	
Metenol QV	methenolone acetate	50 mg tablet	50 tablet bottle	Quality Vet	Mexico		VET
Metesto	methyltestosterone	25 mg tablet	100 tablet bottle	Acdhon	Thailand		
Methan Tabs	methandrostenolone	10 mg tablet	100 tablet bottle	Animal Power	Mexico		VET
Methanabol	methandrostenolone	5 mg tablet	500 tablet pouch	British Dragon	Thailand	[NLM]	
Methanabol	methandrostenolone	10 mg tablet	500 tablet pouch	British Dragon	Thailand		
Methanabol	methandrostenolone	50 mg tablet	100 tablet pouch	British Dragon	Thailand		
Methandienone	methandrostenolone	5, 10 mg tablet	100, 1000 tablet bottle	Ttokkyo	Mexico		VET
Methandon	methandrostenolone	5 mg tablet	1000 tablet bottle	Acdhon Co.	Thailand		
Methandriol	methylandrostenediol dipropionate	75 mg/ml	10 ml vial	Ilium/Troy	Australia	[NLM]	VET
Methasus 50	methylandrostenediol dipropionate	50 mg/ml	20 ml vial	Jurox	Australia	[NLM]	VET
Methyldiol	methylandrostenediol	2 mg tablet	n/a	Vortech	U.S.	[NLM]	
Methyldiol Aqueous	methylandrostenediol	50 mg/ml	n/a	Vortech	U.S.	[NLM]	
Methyltestosterone	methyltestosterone	10 mg tablet	n/a	Global	U.S.		
Methyltestosterone	methyltestosterone	10 mg tablet	n/a	Goldline	U.S.	[NLM]	
Metil Testosteron	methyltestosterone	10 mg tablet	50 tablet box	Terapia	Rumania		
Metil Thomsina S	methyltestosterone	10 mg tablet	20 tablet box	Celsius	Uruguay		
Metil-Test	methyltestosterone	50 mg tablet	100 tablet bottle	Brovel	Mexico		VET
Metiltestosterona	methyltestosterone	n/a	n/a	Botica	Paraguay		
Metormon	drostanolone propionate	100 mg/2ml	2 ml amp	Syntex	Spain	[NLM]	

Appendix B: Drug Availability Tables - Listings by Trade Name

Trade Name	Generic Name	Dose	Packaging	Company	Country	Status	Vet
Metrobolin	nandrolone phenylpropionate	25 mg/ml	n/a	Metro	Taiwan		
Metylandrostendiol	methylandrostenediol	10, 25 mg tablet	n/a	Jelfa	Poland	[NLM]	
mibolerone drops	mibolerone	100 mcg/ml	55 mg bottle	Wedgewood	U.S.		VET
Miotolan	furazabol	1 mg tablet	n/a	Daiichi Seiyaku	Japan	[NLM]	
Miro Depo	testosterone cypionate	125 mg/ml	2 ml vial	Hanil Pharm	Korea		
Mitgan 50	boldenone undecylenate	50 mg/ml	50 ml vial	California	Colombia		VET
Myobolin	nandrolone decanoate	25 mg/ml	1 ml ampule	Troikaa	India		
Nabolic	stanozolol (inj)	2 mg/ml	50 ml vial	Chinfield Ind.	Argentina		VET
Nabolic Strong	stanozolol (inj)	50 mg/ml	30 ml vial	Chinfield Ind.	Argentina		VET
Nandoral	ethylestrenol	.5 mg tablet	100, 500 tablet bottle	Intervet	Australia		VET
Nandrobolic	nandrolone phenylpropionate	25 mg/ml	n/a	Forest	U.S.	[NLM]	
Nandrobolic L.A.	nandrolone decanoate	100 mg/ml	1, 2 ml vial	Forest	U.S.	[NLM]	
Nandrolin	nandrolone phenylpropionate	50 mg/ml	25 ml vial	Intervet	Australia		VET
Nandrolin	nandrolone phenylpropionate	25 mg/ml	10 ml vial	Intervet	Australia		VET
Nandrolona 300 L.A.	nandrolone decanoate	300mg/ml	10 ml vial	Ttokkyo	Mexico		VET
nandrolona decanoato	nandrolone decanoate	50 mg/ml	1 ml ampule	Chile	Chile		
nandrolone decanoate	nandrolone decanoate	100 mg/ml	1, 2 ml vial	Lyphomed	U.S.	[NLM]	
nandrolone decanoate	nandrolone decanoate	200 mg/2ml	2 ml vial	Norma Hellas	Greece		
nandrolone decanoate	nandrolone decanoate	100 mg/ml	1, 2 ml vial	Quad	U.S.	[NLM]	
nandrolone decanoate	nandrolone decanoate	50, 100, 200 mg/ml	1, 2 ml vial	Steris	U.S.	[NLM]	
Nandrolone Decanoate Inj	nandrolone decanoate	100 mg/ml	2 ml vial	Watson Pharma	U.S.		
Nandrolone Decanoate Inj	nandrolone decanoate	200 mg/ml	1 ml vial	Watson Pharma	U.S.		
nandrolone phenylpropionate	nandrolone phenylpropionate	50, 100mg/ml	2 ml vial	Hayrian Biologicals	India	[NLM]	
nandrolone phenylpropionate	nandrolone phenylpropionate	25 mg/ml	1 ml ampule	Iran Hormone	Iran		
nandrolone phenylpropionate	nandrolone phenylpropionate	50 mg/ml	n/a	Quad	U.S.	[NLM]	
Nandrosande	nandrolone decanoate	25, 50, 100 mg/ml	1 ml ampule	Sanderson	Chile		
Nannismon Depot	testosterone cypionate	50, 100 mg/ml	n/a	Chi Sheng	Taiwan		
Nansmon Depot	testosterone propionate	25 mg/ml	n/a	Chi Sheng	Taiwan		
Naposim	methandrostenolone	5 mg tablet	20 tablet box	Terapia	Rumania		
Neo Aphro	methyltestosterone	5 mg tablet	30 tablet	Misr	Egypt		
Neo-Anabolene	methandrostenolone	5 mg tablet	10 tablet strip	Haurus	Indonesia		
Neo-Durabolic	nandrolone decanoate	100, 200 mg/ml	1, 2 ml vial	Hauck	U.S.	[NLM]	
Neo-Hombreol	testosterone propionate	50 mg/ml	n/a	Organon	Netherlands	[NLM]	
Neotest 250	testosterone decanoate	250 mg/ml	10 ml bottle	Loeffler	Mexico		
Nerobol	methandrostenolone	5 mg tablet	20 tablet box	Galenika	YugoslaviaFRMR	[NLM]	
Nerobol	methandrostenolone	5 mg tablet	20 tablet box	Gedeon Richter	Bulgaria	[NLM]	
Nerobol	methandrostenolone	5 mg tablet	20 tablet box	Gedeon Richter	Hungary	[NLM]	
Nerobolil	nandrolone phenylpropionate	25 mg/ml	1 ml ampule	Godeon Richter	Bulgaria	[NLM]	
Nerobolil	nandrolone phenylpropionate	25 mg/ml	n/a	Godeon Richter	Hungary	[NLM]	
Neurabol	stanozolol (oral)	2 mg capsule	10 capsule box	Cadila	India		
Neurabol Inj	nandrolone phenylpropionate	25 mg/ml	1 ml ampule	Cadila	India		

Appendix B: Drug Availability Tables - Listings by Trade Name

Trade Name	Generic Name	Dose	Packaging	Company	Country	Status	Vet
Neurophen	nandrolone phenylpropionate	25 mg/ml	1 ml ampule	Ind-Swift	India		
Nilevar	norethandrolone	10 mg tablet	30 tablet bottle	Searle	France		
Nilevar	norethandrolone	10 mg tablet	30 tablet bottle	Searle	Switzerland	[NLM]	
Nilevar	norethandrolone	10 mg tablet	100 tablet bottle	Searle	U.S.		
Nitrotain	ethylestrenol	15 mg/4gram	60, 250, 1000 gram tube	Nature-Vet	Australia		VET
Norabon	nandrolone phenylpropionate	25 mg/ml	1 ml ampule	Phihalab	Thailand		
Norandren	nandrolone decanoate	50, 200 mg/ml	10, 50 ml vial	Brovel	Mexico		VET
Novandrol	methylandrostenediol	10, 25 mg dragee	n/a	Galenika	YugoslaviaFRMR	[NLM]	
Nu-Bolic	nandrolone phenylpropionate	25 mg/ml	n/a	Seatrace	U.S.	[NLM]	
Nurezan	nandrolone decanoate	50 mg/ml	1 ml ampule	Rafarm	Greece		
Nuvir	testosterone undecanoate	40 mg capsules	30 capsule bottle	Organon	India		
ODK	fluoxymesterone	5 mg capsule	n/a	Winston	Taiwan		
Omnadren	Omnadren (testosterone blend)	250 mg/ml	1ml ampule	Jelfa	Poland		
Omnadren	Omnadren (testosterone blend)	250 mg/ml	1ml ampule	Polfa	Poland	[NLM]	
Omnadren 250	Omnadren (testosterone blend)	250 mg/ml	1 ml ampule	Jelfa	Bulgaria		
Orabol-H	ethylestrenol	100 mg/5g paste	30 ml plastic tube	Vetsearch	Australia	[NLM]	VET
Orabolin®	ethylestrenol	2 mg tablet	n/a	Donmed/Organon	South Africa	[NLM]	
Orabolin®	ethylestrenol	2 mg tablet	10 tablet box	Infar	India		
Orabolin®	ethylestrenol	2 mg tablet	n/a	Organon	Belgium	[NLM]	
Orabolin®	ethylestrenol	2 mg tablet	100 tablet box	Organon	Pakistan		
Orabolin®	ethylestrenol	2 mg tablet	n/a	Organon	United Kingdom	[NLM]	
Oralsterone	fluoxymesterone	5 mg capsule	n/a	Long Der	Taiwan		
Ora-Testryl	fluoxymesterone	5 mg tablet	100 tablet bottle	Squibb Mark	U.S.	[NLM]	
Oreton	methyltestosterone	n/a	n/a	n/a	Venezuela		
Oreton	testosterone propionate	25 mg/ml	n/a	Goldline	Mexico	[NLM]	
Oreton Methyl	methyltestosterone	10 mg tablet	n/a	Schering	U.S.	[NLM]	
Oreton Methyl	methyltestosterone	10 mg sub. tablet	n/a	Schering	U.S.	[NLM]	
Orgabolin	ethylestrenol	2 mg tablet	n/a	Organon	Indonesia		
Orgabolin	ethylestrenol	2 mg tablet	n/a	Organon	Netherlands	[NLM]	
Orgabolin	ethylestrenol	2 mg tablet	n/a	Santa	Turkey	[NLM]	
Orgabolin Drops	ethylestrenol	2 mg	n/a	Santa	Turkey	[NLM]	
Oxafort	oxandrolone	5 mg tablet	100 tablet bottle	Loeffler	Mexico		VET
Oxanabol	oxandrolone	5 mg tablet	100 tablet pouch	British Dragon	Thailand	[NLM]	
Oxanabol	oxandrolone	10 mg tablet	100 tablet pouch	British Dragon	Thailand		
Oxandrin®	oxandrolone	2.5, 10 mg tablet	100 tablet bottle	BTG	U.S.		
Oxandro Tabs	oxandrolone	5 mg tablet	100 tablet bottle	Animal Power	Mexico		VET
Oxandrol 10	oxandrolone	10 mg tablet	100 tablet bottle	Bratis Labs	Mexico		VET
Oxandrolone	oxandrolone	5 mg tablet	30 tablet bottle	Planet Pharmacy	Belize		
Oxandrolone	oxandrolone	2.5 tablet	100 tablet bottle	Ttokkyo	Mexico	[NLM]	VET
Oxandrolone	oxandrolone	5 mg tablet	100 tablet bottle	Ttokkyo	Mexico		VET
Oxandrolone SPA	oxandrolone	2.5 mg tablet	30 tablet box	SPA	Italy	[NLM]	

Appendix B: Drug Availability Tables - Listings by Trade Name

Trade Name	Generic Name	Dose	Packaging	Company	Country	Status	Vet
Oxandrolone SPA (Export)	oxandrolone	2.5 mg tablet	30 tablet box	SPA	Italy		
Oxandrovet	oxandrolone	5 mg tablet	100 tablet bottle	Denkall	Mexico		VET
Oxavet QV	oxandrolone	5 mg tablet	100 tablet bottle	Quality Vet	Mexico		VET
Oximetalon	oxymetholone	75 mg tablet	100 tablet bottle	Denkall	Mexico		VET
Oxitosona 50	oxymetholone	50 mg tablet	100 tablet box	Syntex	Spain	[NLM]	
Oxitron 50	oxymetholone	50 mg tablet	100 tablet bottle	Bratis Labs	Mexico		VET
Oxivet QV	oxymetholone	75 mg tablet	100 tablet bottle	Quality Vet	Mexico		VET
Oxybolone	oxymetholone	50 mg tablet	20 tablet box	Genapharm	Greece		
Oxydrol	oxymetholone	50 mg tablet	100 tablet pouch	British Dragon	Thailand		
Oxydrol	oxymetholone	100 mg tablet	50 tablet pouch	British Dragon	Thailand	[NLM]	
Oxylone	oxymetholone	50 mg tablet	100 tablet bottle	Duopharma	Malaysia		
Oxymetholone	oxymetholone	50 mg tablet	100 tablets	Alhavi	Israel		
Oxymetholone	oxymetholone	50 mg tablet	100 tablet pouch	British Dispensary	Thailand	[NLM]	
Oxymetholone	oxymetholone	50 mg tablet	30 tablet bottle	Planet Pharmacy	Belize		
oxymetholone	oxymetholone	50 mg tablet	n/a	Sime Darby	Malaysia		
Oxymetholone DongIndang	oxymetholone	n/a	n/a	Dongindang	Korea		
Oxymetholone HanBul	oxymetholone	50 mg tablet	n/a	HanBul	Korea		
Oxymetholone HanSeo	oxymetholone	50 mg tablet	100 tablet bottle	HanSeo	Korea		
Oxymetholone Korea United	oxymetholone	50 mg tablet	n/a	Korea United	Korea		
Oxymetholone Miverva	oxymetholone	50 mg tablet	100 tablet	Minerva	Greece	[NLM]	
Oxymetolona 50	oxymetholone	50 mg tablet	100 tablet bottle	Ttokkyo	Mexico		VET
Oxytone 50	oxymetholone	50 mg tablet	100 tablet bottle	SB Laboratories	Thailand		
Panteston	testosterone undecanoate	40 mg capsules	60 capsule bottle	Organon	Finland		
Panteston	testosterone undecanoate	40 mg capsules	n/a	Organon	Latvia		
Panteston	testosterone undecanoate	40 mg capsules	n/a	Organon	Lithuania		
Panteston	testosterone undecanoate	40 mg capsules	30, 60 capsule bottle	Organon	Peru		
Panteston capsules	testosterone undecanoate	40 mg capsules	n/a	Organon	New Zealand		
Pantestone	testosterone undecanoate	40 mg capsules	60 capsule bottle	Organon	Estonia		
Pantestone	testosterone undecanoate	40 mg capsules	60 capsule bottle	Organon	France		
Parabolan	trenbolone hexahydrobenzylcarbonate	76 mg/1.5 ml	1.5 ml ampule	Negma	France	[NLM]	
Parabolan Tabs (Export)	trenbolone acetate	25 mg tablet	20 tablet pouch	British Dragon	Thailand		
Permastril	drostanolone propionate	100 mg/2ml	2 ml ampule	Cassenne	France	[NLM]	
Plenastril	oxymetholone	50 mg tablet	n/a	Grunenthal	Austria	[NLM]	
Plenastril	oxymetholone	50 mg tablet	n/a	Proto chemie	Switzerland	[NLM]	
Pluriviron	mesterolone	25 mg dragee	30 dragee box	Asche	Germany	[NLM]	
PMS-Testosterone Enanthate	testosterone enanthate	200 mg/ml	10 ml vial	Pharmascience	Canada		
Polysteron 250	Sustanon 250 (testosterone blend)	250 mg/ml	1 ml ampule	Organon	Venezuela		
Porkybol 1%	boldenone undecylenate	10 mg/ml	10, 50, 100 ml vial	Compania California	Colombia		VET
Primobol	methenolone enanthate	100 mg/ml	10 ml vial	British Dragon	Thailand		
Primobolan Depot	methenolone enanthate	100 mg/ml	1 ml ampule	Schering/CID	Egypt	[NLM]	
Primobolan®	methenolone acetate	5 mg tablet	n/a	Schering	Austria	[NLM]	

Appendix B: Drug Availability Tables - Listings by Trade Name

Trade Name	Generic Name	Dose	Packaging	Company	Country	Status	Vet
Primobolan®	methenolone acetate	5 mg tablet	n/a	Schering	Belgium	[NLM]	
Primobolan®	methenolone acetate	5 mg tablet	n/a	Schering	Bolivia	[NLM]	
Primobolan®	methenolone acetate	5 mg tablet	n/a	Schering	Costa Rica	[NLM]	
Primobolan®	methenolone acetate	5 mg tablet	n/a	Schering	Dom. Rep.	[NLM]	
Primobolan®	methenolone acetate	5 mg tablet	n/a	Schering	Ecuador	[NLM]	
Primobolan®	methenolone acetate	5 mg tablet	n/a	Schering	El Salvador	[NLM]	
Primobolan®	methenolone acetate	5 mg tablet	n/a	Schering	Germany	[NLM]	
Primobolan®	methenolone acetate	5 mg tablet	n/a	Schering	Guatemala	[NLM]	
Primobolan®	methenolone acetate	5 mg tablet	n/a	Schering	Honduras	[NLM]	
Primobolan®	methenolone acetate	5 mg tablet	100, 1000 tablet box	Schering	Japan		
Primobolan®	methenolone acetate	5 mg tablet	n/a	Schering	Mexico	[NLM]	
Primobolan®	methenolone acetate	5 mg tablet	n/a	Schering	Nicaragua	[NLM]	
Primobolan®	methenolone acetate	5 mg tablet	n/a	Schering	Panama	[NLM]	
Primobolan®	methenolone acetate	50 mg tablet	n/a	Schering	France	[NLM]	
Primobolan®	methenolone acetate	5 mg tablet	n/a	Schering/Berlimed	South Africa	[NLM]	
Primobolan® Acetate	methenolone acetate	25 mg/ml	1 ml ampule	Schering	Germany	[NLM]	
Primobolan® Depot	methenolone enanthate	100 mg/ml	1 ml ampule	Scherimed	Spain		
Primobolan® Depot	methenolone enanthate	100 mg/ml	1 ml ampule	Schering	Ecuador		
Primobolan® Depot	methenolone enanthate	100 mg/ml	1 ml ampule	Schering	France	[NLM]	
Primobolan® Depot	methenolone enanthate	100 mg/ml	1 ml ampule	Schering	Guatemala		
Primobolan® Depot	methenolone enanthate	50 mg/ml	1 ml ampule	Schering	Japan	[NLM]	
Primobolan® Depot	methenolone enanthate	100 mg/ml	1 ml ampule	Schering	Japan		
Primobolan® Depot	methenolone enanthate	50 mg/ml	1 ml ampule	Schering	Mexico		
Primobolan® Depot	methenolone enanthate	100 mg/ml	1 ml ampule	Schering	Paraguay		
Primobolan® Depot	methenolone enanthate	100 mg/ml	1 ml ampule	Schering	Austria	[NLM]	
Primobolan® Depot	methenolone enanthate	100 mg/ml	1 ml ampule	Schering	Belgium	[NLM]	
Primobolan® Depot	methenolone enanthate	100 mg/ml	1 ml ampule	Schering	Czech. Rep.	[NLM]	
Primobolan® Depot	methenolone enanthate	100 mg/ml	1 ml ampule	Schering	Germany	[NLM]	
Primobolan® Depot	methenolone enanthate	100 mg/ml	1 ml ampule	Schering	Greece	[NLM]	
Primobolan® Depot	methenolone enanthate	100 mg/ml	1 ml ampule	Schering	Italy	[NLM]	
Primobolan® Depot	methenolone enanthate	100 mg/ml	1 ml ampule	Schering	Portugal	[NLM]	
Primobolan® Depot	methenolone enanthate	100 mg/ml	1 ml ampule	Schering	Spain	[NLM]	
Primobolan® Depot	methenolone enanthate	100 mg/ml	1 ml ampule	Schering	Switzerland	[NLM]	
Primobolan® Depot	methenolone enanthate	100 mg/ml	1 ml ampule	Schering	Turkey		
Primobolan® Depot	methenolone enanthate	100 mg/ml	1 ml ampule	Schering/Berlimed	South Africa	[NLM]	
Primobolan® Depot mite	methenolone enanthate	50 mg/ml	1 ml ampule	Schering	Germany	[NLM]	
Primobolan® S	methenolone acetate	25 mg tablet	n/a	Leiras	Finland	[NLM]	
Primobolan® S	methenolone acetate	25 mg tablet	n/a	Schering	Germany	[NLM]	
Primobolan® S	methenolone acetate	25 mg tablet	n/a	Schering	Netherlands	[NLM]	
Primobolan® S	methenolone acetate	25 mg tablet	n/a	Schering	Thailand	[NLM]	
Primobolan® S	methenolone acetate	25 mg tablet	50 tablet bottle	Schering/Berlimed	South Africa		

Appendix B: Drug Availability Tables - Listings by Trade Name

Trade Name	Generic Name	Dose	Packaging	Company	Country	Status	Vet
Primoniat®-Depot 100	Testoviron (testosterone blend)	135 mg/ml	1 ml ampule	Schering-Chile	Chile	[NLM]	
Primoniat®-Depot 250	testosterone enanthate	250 mg/ml	1 ml ampule	Schering-Chile	Chile	[NLM]	
Primo-Plus 100	methenolone enanthate	100 mg/ml	1 ml ampule	Ttokkyo	Mexico		VET
Primo-Plus 50	methenolone acetate	50 mg tablet	100 tablet bottle	Ttokkyo	Mexico		VET
Primoteston Depot 100	Testoviron (testosterone blend)	135 mg/ml	1 ml ampule	Schering	Australia	[NLM]	
Primoteston Depot 50	Testoviron (testosterone blend)	75 mg/ml	1 ml ampule	Schering	Australia	[NLM]	
Primoteston®-Depot	testosterone enanthate	250 mg/ml	1 ml ampule	Leiras	Finland	[NLM]	
Primoteston®-Depot	testosterone enanthate	250 mg/ml	1 ml ampule	Schering	Norway		
Primoteston®-Depot	testosterone enanthate	250 mg/ml	1 ml ampule	Schering	United Kingdom	[NLM]	
Primoteston®-Depot	testosterone enanthate	250 mg/ml	1 ml ampule	Schering/CID	Egypt		
Primoteston®-Depot	testosterone enanthate	250 mg/ml	1 ml ampule	Schering	Australia		
Primoteston®-Depot	testosterone enanthate	250 mg/ml	1 ml ampule	Schering	Ecuador		
Primoteston®-Depot	testosterone enanthate	250 mg/ml	1 ml ampule	Schering	Guatemala		
Primoteston®-Depot	testosterone enanthate	250 mg/ml	1 ml ampule	Schering	Jordan		
Primoteston®-Depot	testosterone enanthate	250 mg/ml	1 ml ampule	Schering	Kuwait	[NLM]	
Primoteston®-Depot	testosterone enanthate	250 mg/ml	1 ml ampule	Schering	Mauritius		
Primoteston®-Depot	testosterone enanthate	250 mg/ml	1 ml ampule	Schering	Mexico		
Primoteston®-Depot	testosterone enanthate	250 mg/ml	1 ml syringe	Schering	New Zealand		
Primoteston®-Depot	testosterone enanthate	250 mg/ml	1 ml ampule	Schering	Sudan		
Primoteston®-Depot 100	Testoviron (testosterone blend)	135 mg/ml	1 ml ampule	Schering/CID	Egypt		
Progro-H (plus estradiol)	testosterone propionate (implant)	20 mg/pellet	n/a	Pro Beef	Australia		VET
Pronabol-5	methandrostenolone	5 mg tablet	100 tablet box	P&B Labs	India	[NLM]	
Propionat QV 100	testosterone propionate	100 mg/ml	10 ml vial	Quality Vet	Mexico		VET
Propionato de Testosterona	testosterone propionate	25 mg/ml	20 ml vial	Induvet	Argentina		VET
Propiotest 100	testosterone propionate	100 mg/ml	10 ml vial	Animal Power	Mexico		VET
Protabol	methylandrostenediol dipropionate	75 mg/ml	10 ml vial	Protabol	Australia		VET
Protosin Inj	nandrolone phenylpropionate	25 mg/ml	n/a	Astar	Taiwan		
Proviron	mesterolone	25 mg tablet	20 tablet box	Schering	Algeria		
Proviron	mesterolone	25 mg tablet	50 tablet box	Schering	Taiwan		
Proviron	mesterolone	25 mg tablet	20 tablet box	Schering	Turkey		
Proviron®	mesterolone	25 mg tablet	n/a	Alkoid	YugoslaviaFRMR		
Proviron®	mesterolone	25 mg tablet	n/a	Leiras	Finland		
Proviron®	mesterolone	25 mg tablet	20 tablet box	Scherimed	Spain		
Proviron®	mesterolone	25 mg tablet	n/a	Schering	Argentina		
Proviron®	mesterolone	25, 50 mg tablet	n/a	Schering	Australia		
Proviron®	mesterolone	25 mg tablet	50 tablet bottle	Schering	Austria		
Proviron®	mesterolone	25 mg tablet	50 tablet bottle	Schering	Belgium		
Proviron®	mesterolone	25 mg tablet	20 tablet box	Schering	Brazil		
Proviron®	mesterolone	25 mg tablet	20, 50 tablet box	Schering	Bulgaria		
Proviron®	mesterolone	25 mg tablet	20 tablet box	Schering	Colombia		
Proviron®	mesterolone	25 mg tablet	n/a	Schering	Costa Rica		

Appendix B: Drug Availability Tables - Listings by Trade Name

Trade Name	Generic Name	Dose	Packaging	Company	Country	Status	Vet
Proviron®	mesterolone	25 mg tablet	20 tablet box	Schering	Croatia		
Proviron®	mesterolone	25 mg tablet	20, 50 tablet box	Schering	Czech. Rep.		
Proviron®	mesterolone	25 mg tablet	20 tablet bottle	Schering	Dom. Rep.		
Proviron®	mesterolone	25 mg tablet	n/a	Schering	El Salvador		
Proviron®	mesterolone	25 mg tablet	20 tablet box	Schering	Estonia	[NLM]	
Proviron®	mesterolone	25 mg tablet	n/a	Schering	France	[NLM]	
Proviron®	mesterolone	25 mg tablet	50 tablet bottle	Schering	Germany	[NLM]	
Proviron®	mesterolone	25 mg tablet	20 tablet bottle	Schering	Greece		
Proviron®	mesterolone	25 mg tablet	n/a	Schering	Guatemala		
Proviron®	mesterolone	25 mg tablet	n/a	Schering	Honduras		
Proviron®	mesterolone	25 mg tablet	10, 15, 20, 50, 100, 150 tab btl	Schering	Hungary		
Proviron®	mesterolone	25 mg tablet	30 tablet box	Schering	India		
Proviron®	mesterolone	25 mg tablet	n/a	Schering	Indonesia		
Proviron®	mesterolone	25 mg tablet	20, 50 tablet box	Schering	Israel		
Proviron®	mesterolone	50 mg tablet	20 tablet box	Schering	Italy		
Proviron®	mesterolone	25 mg tablet	20 tablet box	Schering	Latvia	[NLM]	
Proviron®	mesterolone	25 mg tablet	20 tablet box	Schering	Lithuania	[NLM]	
Proviron®	mesterolone	25 mg tablet	10 tablet box	Schering	Mexico		
Proviron®	mesterolone	25 mg tablet	50 tablet bottle	Schering	Netherlands		
Proviron®	mesterolone	25 mg tablet	n/a	Schering	Nicaragua		
Proviron®	mesterolone	25 mg tablet	n/a	Schering	Panama		
Proviron®	mesterolone	25 mg tablet	20 tablet box	Schering	Paraguay		
Proviron®	mesterolone	25 mg tablet	20 tablet box	Schering	Poland		
Proviron®	mesterolone	25 mg tablet	20 tablet box	Schering	Portugal		
Proviron®	mesterolone	25 mg tablet	20 tablet bottle	Schering	Russia		
Proviron®	mesterolone	25 mg tablet	20, 50 tablet bottle	Schering	Slovakia		
Proviron®	mesterolone	25 mg tablet	20 tablet box	Schering	Spain	[NLM]	
Proviron®	mesterolone	25 mg tablet	n/a	Schering	Switzerland	[NLM]	
Proviron®	mesterolone	25 mg tablet	20 tablet box	Schering	Ukraine		
Proviron®	mesterolone	25 mg tablet	30 tablet box	Schering	United Kingdom		
Proviron®	mesterolone	25 mg tablet	n/a	Schering	Uruguay		
Proviron®	mesterolone	25 mg tablet	15 tablet box	Schering	Venezuela		
Proviron®	mesterolone	25 mg tablet	20, 100 tablet bottle	Schering/Berlimed	South Africa		
Proviron®	mesterolone	25 mg tablet	20 tablet box	Schering/CID	Egypt	[NLM]	
Proviron®-Depot	testosterone enanthate	250 mg/ml	1 ml ampule	Schering	Venezuela		
Provironum	mesterolone	25 mg tablet	50 tablet box	Organon	Singapore		
Provironum	mesterolone	25 mg tablet	150 tablet box	Schering	Thailand		
Psychobolan	nandrolone undecanoate	80.5 mg/ml	1ml ampule	Theramex	Greece	[NLM]	
Reforvit Simple	methandrostenolone	5, 10, 25 mg tab	100, 500, 1000 tablet bottle	Loeffler	Mexico		VET
Reforvit-B	methandrostenolone	25 mg/ml	10, 50 ml	Loeffler	Mexico		VET
Restandol	testosterone undecanoate	40 mg capsules	60 capsule bottle	Organon	Denmark		

Appendix B: Drug Availability Tables - Listings by Trade Name

Trade Name	Generic Name	Dose	Packaging	Company	Country	Status	Vet
Restandol	testosterone undecanoate	40 mg capsules	60 capsule bottle	Organon	Greece		
Restandol	testosterone undecanoate	40 mg capsules	n/a	Organon	Taiwan		
Restandol	testosterone undecanoate	40 mg capsules	28, 56 capsule box	Organon	United Kingdom		
Restauvit	methandrostenolone	2 mg tablet	n/a	Ciba, Rugby	Mexico	[NLM]	
Restore	mesterolone	25 mg tablet	20 tablet box	Brown & Burk	India		
Retabolil	nandrolone decanoate	25, 50 mg/ml	1 ml ampule	Gedeon Richter	Bulgaria	[NLM]	
Retabolil	nandrolone decanoate	50 mg/ml	1 ml ampule	Gedeon Richter	Estonia		
Retabolil	nandrolone decanoate	25, 50 mg/ml	1 ml ampule	Gedeon Richter	Hungary		
Retabolil	nandrolone decanoate	25, 50 mg/ml	1 ml ampule	Gedeon Richter	Malaysia		
Retabolil	nandrolone decanoate	50 mg/ml	1 ml ampule	Medimpex/Alxndria	Egypt		
Retabolin	nandrolone decanoate	50 mg/ml	1 ml ampule	Medexport Russia	Russia	[NLM]	
Revalor-200 (plus estradiol)	trenbolone acetate	20 mg pellet	100 pellet cartridge	Intervet	U.S.		VET
Revalor-G (plus estradiol)	trenbolone acetate	20 mg pellet	20 pellet cartridge	Intervet	U.S.		VET
Revalor-H (plus estradiol)	trenbolone acetate	20 mg pellet	70 pellet cartridge	Hoechst-Roussel	U.S.	[NLM]	VET
Revalor-H (plus estradiol)	trenbolone acetate	20 mg pellet	70 pellet cartridge	Intervet	Canada		VET
Revalor-H (plus estradiol)	trenbolone acetate	20 mg pellet	70 pellet cartridge	Intervet	U.S.		VET
Revalor-IH (plus estradiol)	trenbolone acetate	20 mg pellet	40 pellet cartridge	Intervet	U.S.		VET
Revalor-IS (plus estradiol)	trenbolone acetate	20 mg pellet	40 pellet cartridge	Intervet	U.S.		VET
Revalor-S (plus estradiol)	trenbolone acetate	20 mg pellet	60 pellet cartridge	Hoechst-Roussel	U.S.	[NLM]	VET
Revalor-S (plus estradiol)	trenbolone acetate	20 mg pellet	60 pellet cartridge	Intervet	Canada		VET
Revalor-S (plus estradiol)	trenbolone acetate	20 mg pellet	60 pellet cartridge	Intervet	U.S.		VET
Ridrot Testosterone Inj.	testosterone cypionate	75 mg/ml	250 ml vial	Troy	Australia		VET
Roboral	oxymetholone	50 mg tablet	100 tablets	Abic/Ramat-Gan	Israel	[NLM]	
Ropel Liquid Testosterone	testosterone enanthate	75 mg/ml	200 ml vial	Jurox	Australia		VET
Ropel Testosterone Pellets	testosterone (implant)	23.5 mg pellet	450, 600 pellet bottle	Jurox	Australia		VET
Rubolin	nandrolone phenylpropionate	25 mg/ml	n/a	Ying Yuan	Taiwan		
RWR Deca 50	nandrolone decanoate	50 mg/ml	10 ml vial	RWR	Australia		VET
RWR Suspension	testosterone suspension	100 mg/ml	20 ml vial	RWR	Australia		VET
Sanabolicum	nandrolone cyclohexylpropionate	25, 50 mg/ml	1 ml ampule	Biochemie/Nile	Egypt		
Sanabolicum-Vet	nandrolone cyclohexylpropionate	50 mg/ml	10 ml vial	Werfft-Chemie	Austria		VET
Scheinpharma Testone-Cyp	testosterone cypionate	100 mg/ml	10 ml vial	Schein	Canada		
Seidon	stanozolol (oral)	2 mg tablet	100 tablet box	Seoul Pharm	Korea		
Sidomon	fluoxymesterone	5 mg capsule	n/a	n/a	Taiwan		
Silabolin	ethylestrenol	25, 50 mg/ml	1 ml ampule	Farmadon	Russia	[NLM]	
Sinbolin	nandrolone phenylpropionate	25 mg/ml	n/a	Sinton	Taiwan		
Sostenon 250®	Sustanon 250 (testosterone blend)	250 mg/ml	1 ml ampule	Organon	Mexico		
Sostenon 250®	Sustanon 250 (testosterone blend)	250 mg/ml	1 ml ampule	Organon	Spain	[NLM]	
Spectriol	methylandrostenediol (blend)	65 mg/ml	10 ml vial	RWR	Australia		VET
Stabon	stanozolol (oral)	2 mg tablet	n/a	n/a	Korea		
Stan 50	stanozolol (inj)	50 mg/ml	10 ml vial	Animal Power	Mexico		VET
Stan QV 10	stanozolol (oral)	10 mg tablet	100 tablet bottle	Quality Vet	Mexico		VET

Appendix B: Drug Availability Tables - Listings by Trade Name

Trade Name	Generic Name	Dose	Packaging	Company	Country	Status	Vet
Stan QV 100	stanozolol (inj)	100 mg/ml	20 ml vial	Quality Vet	Mexico		VET
Stan QV 50	stanozolol (inj)	50 mg/ml	20 ml vial	Quality Vet	Mexico		VET
Stan Tabs	stanozolol (oral)	10 mg tablet	100 tablet bottle	Animal Power	Mexico		VET
Stanabol	stanozolol (oral)	5 mg tablet	250 tablet pouch	British Dragon	Thailand	[NLM]	
Stanabol	stanozolol (oral)	5 mg tablet	200, 1000 tablet bottle	British Dragon	Thailand	[NLM]	
Stanabol	stanozolol (oral)	5 mg tablet	200 tablet pouch	British Dragon	Thailand	[NLM]	
Stanabol	stanozolol (oral)	10 mg tablet	100 tablet pouch	British Dragon	Thailand		
Stanabol	stanozolol (oral)	50 mg tablet	100 tablet pouch	British Dragon	Thailand		
Stanabolic	stanozolol (inj)	50 mg/ml	20 ml vial	Ilium/Troy	Australia		VET
Stanazol	stanozolol (inj)	50 mg/ml	20, 50 ml vial	RWR	Australia	[NLM]	VET
Stanazolic	stanozolol (inj)	50, 100 mg/ml	20 ml, 10ml vial	Denkall	Mexico		VET
Stanazolic	stanozolol (oral)	6 mg cap	300 capsule bottle	Denkall	Mexico		VET
Stanazolic	stanozolol (oral)	10 mg tablet	100 tablet bottle	Denkall	Mexico		VET
Stanol	stanozolol (oral)	5 mg tablet	200 tablet bottle	Body Research	Thailand		
Stanol	stanozolol (oral)	2 mg tablet	n/a	Hua Shin	Taiwan		
Stanol 10	stanozolol (oral)	10 mg tablet	250 tablet bottle	Bratis Labs	Mexico		VET
Stanol 50	stanozolol (inj)	50 mg/ml	20 ml vial	Bratis Labs	Mexico		VET
Stanol-V	stanozolol (inj)	50, 100 mg/ml	20 ml vial	Ttokkyo	Mexico		VET
Stanol-V	stanozolol (oral)	10 mg tablet	100, 500 tablet bottle	Ttokkyo	Mexico		VET
Stanosus	stanozolol (inj)	50 mg/ml	20 ml vial	Jurox	Australia	[NLM]	VET
Stanozodon	stanozolol (oral)	2 mg tablet	1000 tablet bottle	Acdhon Co.	Thailand		
stanozolol	stanozolol (oral)	5 mg tablet	30 tablet box	Genepharm	Greece		
stanozolol	stanozolol (oral)	25 mg tablet	30 tablet bottle	Planet Pharmacy	Belize		
Stanozolol	stanozolol	10 mg tablet	100 tablet pouch	British Dispensary	Thailand		
Stanozolol Tab	stanozolol (oral)	2 mg tablet	n/a	Chen Ho	Taiwan		
Stanzol	stanozolol (oral)	5 mg tablet	200 tablet bottle	SB Laboratories	Thailand		
Sten	Sten (testosterone blend)	50 mg/ml	2 ml ampule	Atlantis	Mexico		
Stenolon	methandrostenolone	5 mg tablet	20 tablet box	Leciva	Czech. Rep.	[NLM]	
Stenolon	methandrostenolone	1 mg tablet	20 tablet box	Leciva	Czech. Rep.	[NLM]	
Stenox	fluoxymesterone	2.5 mg tablet	20 tablet box	Atlantis	Mexico		
Steranabol	clostebol acetate	20 mg/ml	2 ml ampule	Farmitalia	Italy	[NLM]	
Steranabol Ritardo	oxabolone cypionate	12.5 mg/ml	2 ml ampule	Pharmacia & Upjohn	Italy	[NLM]	
Sterobolin	nandrolone decanoate	50 mg/ml	1 ml ampule	Orion	Finland	[NLM]	
Stromba	stanozolol (oral)	5 mg tablet	56 tablet box	n/a	Greece		
Stromba	stanozolol (inj)	50 mg/ml	n/a	Sterling Research	United Kingdom	[NLM]	
Stromba	stanozolol (oral)	5 mg tablet	n/a	Sterling-Health	Hungary		
Stromba	stanozolol (oral)	5 mg tablet	10 tablet box	Winthrop	Belgium	[NLM]	
Stromba	stanozolol (oral)	5 mg tablet	n/a	Berger	Austria	[NLM]	
Stromba	stanozolol (oral)	5 mg tablet	100 tablet box	Sanofi	Netherlands		
Stromba	stanozolol (oral)	5 mg tablet	n/a	Sanofi	United Kingdom	[NLM]	
Stromba	stanozolol (oral)	5 mg tablet	n/a	Sterling	United Kingdom	[NLM]	

Appendix B: Drug Availability Tables - Listings by Trade Name

Trade Name	Generic Name	Dose	Packaging	Company	Country	Status	Vet
Stromba	stanozolol (oral)	5 mg tablet	n/a	Sterling-Health	Czech. Rep.	[NLM]	
Stromba	stanozolol (inj)	50 mg/ml	n/a	Sterling-Winthrop	Sweden	[NLM]	
Stromba	stanozolol (oral)	5 mg tablet	n/a	Winthrop	Denmark	[NLM]	
Stromba	stanozolol (oral)	5 mg tablet	n/a	Winthrop	Germany	[NLM]	
Stromba	stanozolol (oral)	5 mg tablet	n/a	Winthrop	Netherlands	[NLM]	
Stromba	stanozolol (inj)	50 mg/ml	n/a	Winthrop	Sweden	[NLM]	
Stromba	stanozolol (oral)	5 mg tablet	n/a	Winthrop	Sweden	[NLM]	
Stromba	stanozolol (oral)	5 mg tablet	n/a	Winthrop	Switzerland	[NLM]	
Strombaject	stanozolol (inj)	50 mg/ml	n/a	Winthrop	Belgium	[NLM]	
Strombaject	stanozolol (inj)	50 mg/ml	n/a	Winthrop	Germany	[NLM]	
Sunamon Depot Inj	testosterone enanthate	130 mg/ml	n/a	Astar	Taiwan		
Sunamon Inj	testosterone enanthate	250 mg/ml	n/a	Astar	Taiwan		
Super Test-250	Sustanon 250 (testosterone blend)	250 mg/ml	5, 10 ml vial	Tornel	Mexico		VET
Superanabolon	nandrolone phenylpropionate	25 mg/ml	1 ml ampule	Spofa	Czech. Rep.		
Superbolin	methylandrostenediol dipropionate	75 mg/ml	10 ml vial	Vetsearch	Australia		VET
Suprimo 100	methenolone enanthate	100 mg/ml	10 ml vial	SYD Group	Mexico		VET
Sustanon	Sustanon 250 (testosterone blend)	250 mg/ml	1 ml ampule	Organon	Ireland		
Sustanon	Sustanon 250 (testosterone blend)	250 mg/ml	1 ml ampule	Organon	Israel		
Sustanon	Sustanon 250 (testosterone blend)	250 mg/ml	1 ml ampule	Organon	Slovakia		
Sustanon "250"	Sustanon 250 (testosterone blend)	250 mg/ml	1 ml ampule	Organon	Indonesia		
Sustanon "250"	Sustanon 250 (testosterone blend)	250 mg/ml	1 ml ampule	Organon	Singapore		
Sustanon "250"	Sustanon 250 (testosterone blend)	250 mg/ml	1 ml ampule	Organon	Argentina		
Sustanon "250"	Sustanon 250 (testosterone blend)	250 mg/ml	1ml ampule	Organon	Vietnam		
Sustanon (Cyctahoh 250)	Sustanon 250 (testosterone blend)	250 mg/ml	1 ml ampule	Organon	Russia		
Sustanon (Cyctahoh)	Sustanon 100 (testosterone blend)	100 mg/ml	1 ml ampule	Infar	India		
Sustanon 100	Sustanon 100 (testosterone blend)	100 mg/ml	1 ml ampule	Organon	Germany	[NLM]	
Sustanon '100'®	Sustanon 100 (testosterone blend)	100 mg/ml	1 ml ampule	Organon	Netherlands		
Sustanon '100'®	Sustanon 100 (testosterone blend)	100 mg/ml	1 ml ampule	Organon	United Kingdom		
Sustanon '100'®	Sustanon 100 (testosterone blend)	100 mg/ml	1 ml ampule	Organon/Nile	Egypt		
Sustanon 250	Sustanon 250 (testosterone blend)	250 mg/ml	1 ml ampule	Organon	Germany	[NLM]	
Sustanon 250	Sustanon 250 (testosterone blend)	250 mg/ml	1 ml ampule	Organon	New Zealand		
Sustanon 250	Sustanon 250 (testosterone blend)	250 mg/ml	1 ml ampule	Organon	Taiwan		
Sustanon 250	Sustanon 250 (testosterone blend)	250 mg/ml	1 ml ampule	Organon	Czech. Rep.		
Sustanon 250 (Cyctahon)	Sustanon 250 (testosterone blend)	250 mg/ml	1 ml ampule	Infar	India		
Sustanon 250®	Sustanon 250 (testosterone blend)	250 mg/ml	1 ml ampule	Organon	Belgium		
Sustanon 250®	Sustanon 250 (testosterone blend)	250 mg/ml	1 ml ampule	Organon	Estonia		
Sustanon 250®	Sustanon 250 (testosterone blend)	250 mg/ml	1 ml ampule	Organon	Finland		
Sustanon 250®	Sustanon 250 (testosterone blend)	250 mg/ml	1 ml ampule	Organon	Netherlands		
Sustanon 250®	Sustanon 250 (testosterone blend)	250 mg/ml	1 ml ampule	Organon	Turkey		
Sustanon '250'®	Sustanon 250 (testosterone blend)	250 mg/ml	1 ml ampule	Donmed/Organon	South Africa		
Sustanon '250'®	Sustanon 250 (testosterone blend)	250 mg/ml	1 ml ampule	Organon	Malaysia		

Appendix B: Drug Availability Tables - Listings by Trade Name

Trade Name	Generic Name	Dose	Packaging	Company	Country	Status	Vet
Sustanon '250'®	Sustanon 250 (testosterone blend)	250 mg/ml	1ml ampule	Organon	Pakistan		
Sustanon '250'®	Sustanon 250 (testosterone blend)	250 mg/ml	1 ml ampule	Organon	Thailand		
Sustanon '250'®	Sustanon 250 (testosterone blend)	250 mg/ml	1 ml ampule	Organon	United Kingdom		
Sustanon '250'®	Sustanon 250 (testosterone blend)	250 mg/ml	1 ml ampule	Organon/Nile	Egypt		
Sustanon®	Sustanon 250 (testosterone blend)	250 mg/ml	1 ml ampule	Organon	Italy		
Sustaretard 250	Sustanon 250 (testosterone blend)	250 mg/ml	1 ml ampule	BM Pharmaceuticals	India		
Sustenan 250	Sustanon 250 (testosterone blend)	250 mg/ml	1 ml ampule	Organon	Chile		
Sustenan Oral	testosterone undecanoate	40 mg capsules	n/a	Organon	Chile		
Sustenon 250®	Sustanon 250 (testosterone blend)	250 mg/ml	1 ml ampule	Organon	Portugal		
Sybolin	boldenone undecylenate	25 mg/ml	10 ml vial	Ranvet	Australia		VET
Synasteron	oxymetholone	50 mg tablet	50 tablet bottle	Sarva	Belgium	[NLM]	
Synovex plus (plus estradiol)	trenbolone acetate	25 mg pellet	80 pellet cartridge	Fort Dodge	Mexico		VET
Synovex plus (plus estradiol)	trenbolone acetate	25 mg pellet	80 pellet cartridge	Fort Dodge	U.S.		VET
Synovex plus (plus estradiol)	trenbolone acetate	25 mg pellet	80 pellet cartridge	Syntex	U.S.	[NLM]	VET
Synovex plus (plus estradiol)	trenbolone acetate	25 mg pellet	80 pellet cartridge	Wyeth	Canada		VET
Synovex®-H (plus estradiol)	testosterone propionate (implant)	20 mg/pellet	n/a	Ayerst	Canada		
Synovex®-H (plus estrogen)	testosterone propionate (implant)	20 mg/pellet	n/a	Fort Dodge	Australia		VET
Synovex®-H (plus estrogen)	testosterone propionate (implant)	25 mg/pellet	80 pellet cartridge	Fort Dodge	Mexico		
Synovex®-H (plus estrogen)	testosterone propionate (implant)	20 mg/pellet	n/a	Fort Dodge	U.S.		VET
Synovex®-H (plus estrogen)	testosterone propionate (implant)	20 mg/pellet	n/a	Syntex	Mexico	[NLM]	
Synovex®-H (plus estrogen)	testosterone propionate (implant)	20 mg/pellet	n/a	Syntex	U.S.	[NLM]	VET
T. Lingvalete	methyltestosterone	5 mg sub. dragee	n/a	Galenika	YugoslaviaFRMR	[NLM]	
Tanoxol	stanozolol (inj)	25 mg/ml	10 ml vial	Burnet	Argentina		VET
Tealigen	fluoxymesterone	5 mg capsule	n/a	Ming ta	Taiwan		
Tepro Hormone	testosterone propionate	100 mg/ml	500 ml vial	Virbac	Australia		VET
Terabon	stanozolol (oral)	2 mg tablet	10 tablet strip	Jin Yang	Korea		
Tesamone	testosterone suspension	25, 50, 100, mg/ml	n/a	Dunhall	U.S.	[NLM]	
Tesone L.A.	testosterone enanthate	200 mg/ml	10 ml vial	Sig	U.S.	[NLM]	
Test 400	Test 400 (testosterone blend)	400 mg/ml	10 ml vial	Denkall	Mexico		VET
Testabol Depot	testosterone cypionate	200 mg/ml	10 ml vial	British Dragon	Thailand		
Testabol Propionate	testosterone propionate	100 mg/ml	10 ml vial	British Dragon	Thailand		
Testa-C	testosterone cypionate	200 mg/ml	10 ml vial	Vortech	U.S.	[NLM]	
Testacyp	testosterone cypionate	100 mg/ml	2 ml vial	BM Pharmaceuticals	India		
Testadiate-Depo	testosterone cypionate	200 mg/ml	10 ml vial	Kay	U.S.	[NLM]	
Testanate No. 1	testosterone enanthate	100 mg/ml	n/a	Kenyon	U.S.	[NLM]	
Testaval	testosterone enanthate	100, 200 mg/ml	10 ml vial	Legere	U.S	[NLM]	
Testen-250	testosterone enanthate	250 mg/ml	2 ml vial	BM Pharmaceuticals	India		
Testenan Depot	testosterone enanthate	250 mg/ml	n/a	Sinton	Taiwan		
Testenat	Testoviron (testosterone blend)	100 mg/ml	1 ml ampule	Farmadon	Russia	[NLM]	
Testenat 10%	testosterone enanthate	100 mg/ml	1 ml ampule	Farmadon	Russia		
Testenon	Testoviron (testosterone blend)	135 mg/ml	2 ml vial	BM Pharmaceuticals	India		

Appendix B: Drug Availability Tables - Listings by Trade Name

Trade Name	Generic Name	Dose	Packaging	Company	Country	Status	Vet
Testenon	Testoviron (testosterone blend)	135 mg/ml	1 ml ampule	BM Pharmaceuticals	India		
Testenon 250	Sustanon 250 (testosterone blend)	250 mg/ml	5 ml vial	Ttokkyo	Mexico		VET
Testermon	testosterone enanthate	25 mg/ml	n/a	CCPC	Taiwan		
Testex	testosterone propionate	50, 100 mg/ml	n/a	Pasadena	U.S.	[NLM]	
Testex Leo	testosterone propionate	25 mg/ml	1 ml ampule	Altana Pharma	Spain		
Testex Leo	testosterone propionate	25 mg/ml	1 ml ampule	Leo	Spain	[NLM]	
Testex Leo prolongatum	testosterone cypionate	50, 125 mg/ml	2 ml ampule	Altana Pharma	Spain		
Testex Leo prolongatum	testosterone cypionate	50, 125 mg/ml	2 ml ampule	Leo	Spain	[NLM]	
Testinon-Depot	testosterone enanthate	n/a	n/a	n/a	Japan		
Testo	testosterone propionate	50 mg/ml	10 ml vial	Samil	Korea		
Testo LA	testosterone cypionate	100 mg/ml	10 ml vial	Jurox	Australia	[NLM]	VET
Testo Tab	methyltestosterone	25 mg tablet	n/a	Samil	Korea		
Testoderm	testosterone (patch)	15 mg patch	n/a	Alza	Malaysia		
Testoderm	testosterone (patch)	6 mg patch	10, 30 patch box	Esteve	Spain		
Testoderm	testosterone (patch)	4 mg patch	10 patch box	Esteve	Spain		
Testoenan L/A	testosterone enanthate	250 mg/ml	10 ml vial	Loeffler	Mexico		VET
Testo-Enant	testosterone enanthate	125 mg/ml	2 ml ampule	Geymonat	Italy		
Testo-Enant	testosterone enanthate	250 mg/ml	1 ml ampule	Geymonat	Italy		
Testogan	testosterone propionate	25 mg/ml	50 ml vial	Laguinsa	Costa Rica		VET
Testogan	testosterone propionate	25 mg/ml	50 ml vial	Laguinsa	Dom. Rep.		VET
Testogan	testosterone propionate	25 mg/ml	50 ml vial	Laguinsa	Ecuador		VET
Testogan	testosterone propionate	25 mg/ml	50 ml vial	Laguinsa	El Salvador		VET
Testogan	testosterone propionate	25 mg/ml	50 ml vial	Laguinsa	Guatemala		VET
Testogan	testosterone propionate	25 mg/ml	50 ml vial	Laguinsa	Honduras		VET
Testogan	testosterone propionate	25 mg/ml	50 ml vial	Laguinsa	Nicaragua		VET
Testogan	testosterone propionate	25 mg/ml	50 ml vial	Laguinsa	Panama		VET
Testogel	testosterone (gel)	25, 50 mg	single dose packet	Besins	Netherlands		
Testogel	testosterone (gel)	25, 50 mg	single dose packet	Besins	Sweden		
Testogel	testosterone (gel)	25, 50 mg	single dose packet	Jenapharm	Germany		
Testogel	testosterone (gel)	25, 50 mg	single dose packet	Schering	Australia		
Testogel	testosterone (gel)	50 mg	single dose packet	Schering	Austria		
Testoject	testosterone cypionate	100 mg/ml	n/a	Mayrand	U.S.	[NLM]	
Testoject 50	testosterone cypionate	50 mg/ml	n/a	Mayrand	U.S.	[NLM]	
Testoject-LA	testosterone cypionate	200 mg/ml	n/a	Mayrand	U.S.	[NLM]	
Testo-Jet L.A.	Sustanon 250 (testosterone blend)	250 mg/ml	10 ml vial	Norvet	Mexico		VET
Testolent	testosterone phenylpropionate	100 mg/ml	1 ml ampule	Sicomed	Rumania	[NLM]	
Testolic	testosterone propionate	50 mg/ml	2 ml ampule	Body Research	Thailand		
Testolin	testosterone suspension	25, 50, 100, mg/ml	n/a	Pasadena	U.S.	[NLM]	
Teston	methyltestosterone	25 mg tablet	30 tablet box	Remek	Greece		
Teston QV 200	testosterone cypionate	200 mg/ml	10 ml vial	Quality Vet	Mexico		VET
Testone-E	testosterone propionate	25 mg/ml	1 ml ampule	Misr	Egypt		

Appendix B: Drug Availability Tables - Listings by Trade Name

Trade Name	Generic Name	Dose	Packaging	Company	Country	Status	Vet
Testonon '100'®	Sustanon 100 (testosterone blend)	100 mg/ml	1 ml ampule	Nile	Egypt		
Testonon '250'®	Sustanon 250 (testosterone blend)	250 mg/ml	1 ml ampule	Nile	Egypt		
Testopin-100	testosterone propionate	100 mg/ml	2 ml vial	BM Pharmaceuticals	India		
Testopin-100	testosterone propionate	100 mg/ml	1 ml ampule	BM Pharmaceuticals	India		
Testoprim-D	Testoviron (testosterone blend)	250 mg/ml	1 ml ampule	Labs. Tocogino	Mexico		
Testopro L/A	testosterone propionate	250 mg/ml	10 ml vial	Loeffler	Mexico		VET
Testopropon	methyltestosterone	25 mg tablet	n/a	Scanpharm	Malaysia		
Testormon	methyltestosterone	10 mg tablet	n/a	Unitas	Portugal		
Testorone Depot	testosterone cypionate	100 mg/ml	n/a	Gentle	Taiwan		
Testos 100	testosterone suspension	100 mg/ml	10 ml vial	Vetcom	Canada		VET
Testosteron	methyltestosterone	5 mg tablet	n/a	Berco	Germany	[NLM]	
Testosteron	testosterone propionate	25 mg/ml	1 ml ampule	Sicomed	Rumania	[NLM]	
Testosteron	testosterone propionate	5, 10, 25, 50 mg/ml	1 ml ampule	Galenika	YugoslaviaFRMR	[NLM]	
Testosteron	testosterone propionate	5, 10, 25, 50 mg/ml	1 ml ampule	Hemofarm	Hungary	[NLM]	
Testosteron	testosterone propionate	50 mg/ml	1 ml ampule	Sopharma	Bulgaria		
Testosteron	testosterone propionate	50 mg/ml	1 ml ampule	Streuli & Co. AG	Switzerland	[NLM]	
Testosteron 250	Sustanon 250 (testosterone blend)	250 mg/ml	1 ml ampule	Rotex Medica	Germany	[NLM]	
Testosteron Depot	testosterone propionate	25 mg/ml	n/a	Gentle	Taiwan		
Testosteron Depot	testosterone enanthate	100 mg/ml	1 ml ampule	Rotex Medica	Germany	[NLM]	
Testosteron Depot	testosterone enanthate	250 mg/ml	1 ml ampule	Rotex Medica	Germany		
Testosterona	testosterone propionate	50, 100 mg/ml	10, 20 ml vial	Brovel	Mexico		VET
Testosterona 200	testosterone enanthate	200 mg/ml	10 ml vial	Brovel	Mexico		VET
Testosterona 250	Sustanon 250 (testosterone blend)	250 mg/ml	10 ml vial	Qualityvet	Costa Rica		VET
testosterona enantato	testosterone enanthate	250 mg/ml	1 ml ampule	Biosano	Chile		
testosterona enantato	testosterone enanthate	100 mg/ml	1 ml ampule	Chile	Chile	[NLM]	
testosterona enantato	testosterone enanthate	250 mg/ml	1 ml ampule	Chile	Chile		
Testosterona IV L/A	Sustanon 250 (testosterone blend)	250 mg/ml	10 ml vial	Loeffler	Mexico		VET
Testosterona Propionat	testosterone propionate	50, 100 mg/ml	1 ml ampule	Farmadon	Russia	[NLM]	
Testosterona Propionato	testosterone propionate	n/a	n/a	Botica	Paraguay		
Testosterona Ultra Lenta	testosterone cypionate	100 mg/ml	20 ml vial	Dispert Labs.	Uruguay		VET
Testosterona Ultra Lenta Fuerte	testosterone cypionate	200 mg/ml	5 ml ampule	Dispert Labs.	Uruguay		VET
Testosterona Ultra Lenta Fuerte	testosterone cypionate	200 mg/ml	20 ml vial	Dispert Labs.	Uruguay		VET
Testosteron-Depo	testosterone enanthate	100 mg/ml	1 ml ampule	Galenika	YugoslaviaFRMR	[NLM]	
Testosteron-Depo	testosterone enanthate	250 mg/ml	1 ml ampule	Galenika	YugoslaviaFRMR		
Testosteron-Depo	testosterone enanthate	100, 250 mg/ml	1 ml ampule	Hemofarm	YugoslaviaFRMR	[NLM]	
Testosteron-Depot	testosterone enanthate	250 mg/ml	1 ml ampule	Eifelfango	Germany		
Testosteron-Depot	testosterone enanthate	250 mg/ml	1 ml ampule	Jenapharm	Bulgaria		
Testosteron-Depot	testosterone enanthate	250 mg/ml	1 ml ampule	Jenapharm	Germany		
Testosterone 200 Depot	testosterone enanthate	200 mg/ml	10 ml vial	Tornel	Mexico		VET
Testosterone Berco Supp.	testosterone propionate	40 mg/suppository	18 supp. box	Funke	Germany	[NLM]	
Testosterone CHP Theramex	testosterone cyclohexylpropionate	296, 148, 37 mg/ml	1 ml ampule	Theramex	France	[NLM]	

Trade Name	Generic Name	Dose	Packaging	Company	Country	Status	Vet
testosterone cypionate	testosterone cypionate	100 mg/ml	10 ml vial	Geneva Geriatrics	U.S.	[NLM]	
testosterone cypionate	testosterone cypionate	100, 200 mg/ml	10 ml vial	Goldline	U.S.	[NLM]	
testosterone cypionate	testosterone cypionate	50, 100, 200 mg/ml	10 ml vial	Huffman	U.S.	[NLM]	
testosterone cypionate	testosterone cypionate	200 mg/ml	10 ml vial	Legere	U.S.	[NLM]	
testosterone cypionate	testosterone cypionate	100, 200 mg/ml	10 ml vial	Schein	U.S.	[NLM]	
testosterone cypionate	testosterone cypionate	100, 200 mg/ml	10 ml vial	Steris	U.S.	[NLM]	
Testosterone Cypionate 200	testosterone cypionate	200 mg/ml	10 ml vial	Ttokkyo	Mexico		VET
Testosterone Cypionate Inj	testosterone cypionate	200 mg/ml	n/a	Charmaine	Hong Kong		
Testosterone Cypionate Inj	testosterone cypionate	200 mg/ml	n/a	Gwo Chyang	Taiwan		
Testosterone Cypionate Inj	testosterone cypionate	200 mg/ml	n/a	Tai Yu	Taiwan		
Testosterone Cypionate Inj.	testosterone cypionate	100 mg/ml	2 ml vial	Cytex	Canada		
Testosterone Cypionate Inj.	testosterone cypionate	200 mg/ml	10 ml vial	Sabex	Canada		
Testosterone Cypionate L.A.	testosterone cypionate	100 mg/ml	10 ml vial	Ttokkyo	Mexico	[NLM]	VET
Testosterone Depositum	testosterone cypionate	n/a	n/a	SPA	Italy		
testosterone enanthate	testosterone enanthate	100, 200 mg/ml	10 ml vial	Geneva Geriatrics	U.S.	[NLM]	
testosterone enanthate	testosterone enanthate	100, 200 mg/ml	10 ml vial	Goldline	U.S.	[NLM]	
testosterone enanthate	testosterone enanthate	250 mg/ml	1 ml ampule	Norma Hellas	Greece		
testosterone enanthate	testosterone enanthate	100, 200 mg/ml	10 ml vial	Quad	U.S.	[NLM]	
testosterone enanthate	testosterone enanthate	100, 200 mg/ml	10 ml vial	Schein	U.S.	[NLM]	
testosterone enanthate	testosterone enanthate	100, 200 mg/ml	10 ml vial	Steris	U.S.	[NLM]	
Testosterone Enanthate 250	testosterone enanthate	250 mg/ml	1 ml ampule	Aburaihan	Iran		
Testosterone Enanthate Dalim	testosterone enanthate	250 mg/ml	n/a	Dalim	Korea		
Testosterone Enanthate Inj	testosterone enanthate	200 mg/ml	10 ml vial	Taro	Canada	[NLM]	
Testosterone Heptylate	testosterone enanthate	50, 100, 250 mg/ml	1 ml ampule	Theramex	France		
Testosterone Jenapharm	testosterone propionate	25 mg/ml	1 ml ampule	Jenapharm	Germany	[NLM]	
testosterone propionate	testosterone propionate	50 mg/ml	n/a	Quad & Lilly	U.S.	[NLM]	
testosterone propionate	testosterone propionate	100 mg/ml	10, 30 ml vial	Rugby	U.S.	[NLM]	
testosterone propionate	testosterone propionate	100 mg/ml	10 ml vial	Steris	U.S.	[NLM]	
Testosterone Propionate Inj.	testosterone propionate	100 mg/ml	10 ml vial	Cytex	Canada		
Testosterone Propionate Inj.	testosterone propionate	100 mg/ml	10 ml vial	Dominion	Canada		VET
Testosterone Propionate Inj.	testosterone propionate	100 mg/ml	10 ml vial	Taro	Canada	[NLM]	
Testosterone Propionate Inj	testosterone propionate	25 mg/ml	n/a	Charmaine	Hong Kong		
Testosterone Propionate Inj	testosterone propionate	50 mg/ml	n/a	Hong Kong Med	Hong Kong		
Testosterone Propionate Inj	testosterone propionate	50 mg/ml	1 ml ampule	n/a	China		
Testosterone Propionate Inj	testosterone propionate	25 mg/ml	n/a	Tai Yu	Taiwan		
Testosterone Streuli	testosterone propionate	n/a	5, 10, 25, 50 mg/ml	Streuli & Co. AG	Austria	[NLM]	
testosterone suspension	testosterone suspension	100 mg/ml	n/a	Legere	U.S.	[NLM]	
testosterone suspension	testosterone suspension	50, 100 mg/ml	10, 30 ml vial	Schein	U.S.	[NLM]	
testosterone suspension	testosterone suspension	50, 100 mg/ml	10, 30 ml vial	Steris	U.S.	[NLM]	
Testosterone Vitis	testosterone propionate	n/a	10, 25 mg/ml	Neopharma	Germany	[NLM]	
Testosterone-Prop. Disp.	testosterone propionate	n/a	10, 20 mg/ml	Disperga	Austria	[NLM]	

Appendix B: Drug Availability Tables - Listings by Trade Name

Trade Name	Generic Name	Dose	Packaging	Company	Country	Status	Vet
testosteronpropionat	testosterone propionate	10, 25 mg/ml	1 ml ampule	Eifelfango	Germany	[NLM]	
testosteronpropionat	testosterone propionate	50 mg/ml	1 ml ampule	Eifelfango	Germany		
Testosteronum Prolongatum	testosterone enanthate	100 mg/ml	1 ml ampule	Jelfa	Bulgaria	[NLM]	
Testosteronum Prolongatum	testosterone enanthate	100 mg/ml	1 ml ampule	Jelfa	Poland		
Testosteronum Prolongatum	testosterone enanthate	100 mg/ml	1 ml ampule	Polfa	Belgium	[NLM]	
Testosteronum Prolongatum	testosterone enanthate	100 mg/ml	1 ml ampule	Polfa	Poland	[NLM]	
Testosteronum Propionicum	testosterone propionate	25 mg/ml	1 ml ampule	Jelfa	Poland		
Testosure	methyltestosterone	n/a	n/a	Europharm	Hong Kong		
Testosus 100	testosterone suspension	100 mg/ml	20 ml vial	Jurox	Australia	[NLM]	VET
Testoviron Depot	testosterone enanthate	250 mg/ml	1 ml ampule	Schering	Taiwan		
Testoviron®	testosterone propionate	50 mg/ml	1 ml ampule	Schering	Greece		
Testoviron®	testosterone propionate	10, 25, 50 mg/ml	1 ml ampule	Schering	Italy	[NLM]	
Testoviron®	testosterone propionate	10, 25 mg/ml	1 ml ampule	Schering	Spain	[NLM]	
Testoviron® Depot	testosterone enanthate	250 mg/ml	1 ml ampule	Schering	Argentina		
Testoviron® Depot	Testoviron (testosterone blend)	135 mg/ml	1 ml ampule	Schering	Argentina	[NLM]	
Testoviron® Depot	testosterone enanthate	250 mg/ml	1 ml ampule	Schering	Hungary	[NLM]	
Testoviron® Depot	Testoviron (testosterone blend)	135 mg/ml	1 ml ampule	Schering	Hungary	[NLM]	
Testoviron® Depot	testosterone enanthate	250 mg/ml	1 ml ampule	Schering	Ireland	[NLM]	
Testoviron® Depot	testosterone enanthate	250 mg/ml	1 ml ampule	Schering	Peru		
Testoviron® Depot 100	Testoviron (testosterone blend)	135 mg/ml	1 ml ampule	Schering	Austria	[NLM]	
Testoviron® Depot 100	Testoviron (testosterone blend)	135 mg/ml	1 ml ampule	Schering	Dom. Rep.		
Testoviron® Depot 100	Testoviron (testosterone blend)	135 mg/ml	1 ml ampule	Schering	Germany	[NLM]	
Testoviron® Depot 100	Testoviron (testosterone blend)	135 mg/ml	1 ml ampule	Schering	Greece	[NLM]	
Testoviron® Depot 100	Testoviron (testosterone blend)	135 mg/ml	1 ml ampule	Schering	Italy		
Testoviron® Depot 100	Testoviron (testosterone blend)	135 mg/ml	1 ml ampule	Schering	Netherlands	[NLM]	
Testoviron® Depot 100	Testoviron (testosterone blend)	135 mg/ml	1 ml ampule	Schering	Portugal	[NLM]	
Testoviron® Depot 100	Testoviron (testosterone blend)	135 mg/ml	1 ml ampule	Schering	Spain	[NLM]	
Testoviron® Depot 100	Testoviron (testosterone blend)	135 mg/ml	1 ml ampule	Schering	Switzerland	[NLM]	
Testoviron® Depot 135	Testoviron (testosterone blend)	135 mg/ml	1 ml ampule	Schering	Denmark		
Testoviron® Depot 135	Testoviron (testosterone blend)	135 mg/ml	1 ml ampule	Schering	Sweden	[NLM]	
Testoviron® Depot 50	Testoviron (testosterone blend)	75 mg/ml	1 ml ampule	Schering	Austria	[NLM]	
Testoviron® Depot 50	Testoviron (testosterone blend)	75 mg/ml	1 ml ampule	Schering	Germany	[NLM]	
Testoviron® Depot 50	Testoviron (testosterone blend)	75 mg/ml	1 ml ampule	Schering	Italy	[NLM]	
Testoviron® Depot 50	Testoviron (testosterone blend)	75 mg/ml	1 ml ampule	Schering	Spain	[NLM]	
Testoviron®-Depot	testosterone enanthate	250 mg/ml	1 ml ampule	Schering	Hong Kong		
Testoviron®-Depot	testosterone enanthate	250 mg/ml	1 ml ampule	Schering	Iceland		
Testoviron®-Depot	testosterone enanthate	250 mg/ml	1 ml ampule	Schering	Thailand		
Testoviron®-Depot	testosterone enanthate	250 mg/ml	1 ml ampule	Schering	Yemen		
Testoviron®-Depot	testosterone enanthate	250 mg/ml	1 ml ampule	Scherimed	Spain		
Testoviron®-Depot	testosterone enanthate	250 mg/ml	1 ml ampule	Schering	Austria		
Testoviron®-Depot	testosterone enanthate	250 mg/ml	1 ml ampule	Schering	Bahrain	[NLM]	

Appendix B: Drug Availability Tables - Listings by Trade Name

Trade Name	Generic Name	Dose	Packaging	Company	Country	Status	Vet
Testoviron®-Depot	testosterone enanthate	250 mg/ml	1 ml ampule	Schering	Colombia		
Testoviron®-Depot	testosterone enanthate	250 mg/ml	1 ml ampule	Schering	Czech. Rep.	[NLM]	
Testoviron®-Depot	testosterone enanthate	250 mg/ml	1 ml ampule	Schering	Denmark		
Testoviron®-Depot	testosterone enanthate	250 mg/ml	1 ml ampule	Schering	Dom. Rep.		
Testoviron®-Depot	testosterone enanthate	250 mg/ml	1 ml ampule	Schering	Ethiopia		
Testoviron®-Depot	testosterone enanthate	250 mg/ml	1 ml ampule	Schering	Germany		
Testoviron®-Depot	testosterone enanthate	250 mg/ml	1 ml ampule	Schering	Greece		
Testoviron®-Depot	testosterone enanthate	250 mg/ml	1 ml ampule	Schering	India		
Testoviron®-Depot	testosterone enanthate	250 mg/ml	1 ml ampule	Schering	Israel		
Testoviron®-Depot	testosterone enanthate	250 mg/ml	1 ml ampule	Schering	Italy		
Testoviron®-Depot	testosterone enanthate	250 mg/ml	1 ml ampule	Schering	Japan		
Testoviron®-Depot	testosterone enanthate	250 mg/ml	1 ml ampule	Schering	Lebanon	[NLM]	
Testoviron®-Depot	testosterone enanthate	250 mg/ml	1 ml ampule	Schering	Malaysia		
Testoviron®-Depot	testosterone enanthate	250 mg/ml	1 ml ampule	Schering	Malta		
Testoviron®-Depot	testosterone enanthate	250 mg/ml	1 ml ampule	Schering	Pakistan		
Testoviron®-Depot	testosterone enanthate	250 mg/ml	1 ml ampule	Schering	Paraguay		
Testoviron®-Depot	testosterone enanthate	250 mg/ml	1 ml ampule	Schering	Portugal		
Testoviron®-Depot	testosterone enanthate	250 mg/ml	1 ml ampule	Schering	Qatar	[NLM]	
Testoviron®-Depot	testosterone enanthate	250 mg/ml	1 ml ampule	Schering	Saudi Arabia		
Testoviron®-Depot	testosterone enanthate	250 mg/ml	1 ml ampule	Schering	Spain	[NLM]	
Testoviron®-Depot	testosterone enanthate	250 mg/ml	1 ml ampule	Schering	Sri Lanka		
Testoviron®-Depot	testosterone enanthate	250 mg/ml	1 ml ampule	Schering	Sweden		
Testoviron®-Depot	testosterone enanthate	250 mg/ml	1 ml ampule	Schering	Switzerland		
Testoviron®-Depot	testosterone enanthate	250 mg/ml	1 ml ampule	Schering	Uruguay		
Testovis	methyltestosterone	10 mg tablet	n/a	SIT	Italy		
Testovis	testosterone propionate	50 mg/ml	2 ml ampule	SIT	Italy		
Testoyohim	methyltestosterone	25 mg dragee	30 dragee box	Paul Mehner	Germany	[NLM]	
Testred	methyltestosterone	10 mg capsule	100 capsule bottle	ICN	U.S.		
Testred Cypionate	testosterone cypionate	200 mg/ml	10 ml vial	INC	U.S.	[NLM]	
Testrin-P.A.	testosterone enanthate	200 mg/ml	n/a	Pasadena Res.	U.S.	[NLM]	
Testron 4 250	Sustanon 250 (testosterone blend)	250 mg/ml	10 ml vial	Bratis Labs	Mexico		VET
Testron Depot	testosterone enanthate	125, 250 mg/ml	1 ml vial	n/a	Japan		
Ton Lin	fluoxymesterone	10 mg capsule	n/a	Chin Teng	Taiwan		
TP Men Hormone	methyltestosterone	10 mg dragee	24 tablets	TP Drugs	Thailand		
Trembolone QV 75	trenbolone acetate	75 mg/ml	10 ml vial	Quality Vet	Mexico		VET
Trenabol	trenbolone acetate	75 mg/ml	10 ml vial	British Dragon	Thailand		
Trenabol Depot	trenbolone hexahydrobenzylcarbonate	100 mg/ml	10 ml vial	British Dragon	Thailand		
Trenbo 75	trenbolone acetate	75 mg/ml	10 ml vial	Animal Power	Mexico		VET
Trenbol 75	trenbolone acetate	75 mg/ml	20 ml vial	Ttokkyo	Mexico		VET
Trenbolon 75	trenbolone acetate	75 mg/ml	10, 20 ml vial	Pet's Pharma	Mexico		VET
Trenol 50	trenbolone acetate	50 mg/ml	6 ml vial	WDV	Myanmar/Burma		VET

Appendix B: Drug Availability Tables - Listings by Trade Name

Trade Name	Generic Name	Dose	Packaging	Company	Country	Status	Vet
Tribolin	methylandrostenediol (blend)	75 mg/ml	10, 20 ml vial	Ranvet	Australia		VET
Trinabol 150	trenbolone (blend)	150 mg/ml	10 ml vial	British Dragon	Thailand		
Trinergic	methandrostenolone	5 mg capsule	n/a	Unimed	India	[NLM]	
Triolandren	testosterone propionate	20 mg/ml	n/a	Ciba Geigy CH	Switzerland	[NLM]	
Triolandren	testosterone blend (misc)	250 mg/ml	1 ml ampule	Novartis	Egypt		
Triolandren	testosterone blend (misc)	250 mg/ml	1 ml ampule	Novartis	Taiwan		
Trofodermin Crema	clostebol acetate	cream	30 gram tube	Carlo Erba OTC	Italy		
Trofodermin Spray	clostebol acetate	n/a	30 ml spray	Carlo Erba OTC	Italy		
Turanabol	chlorodehydromethyltestosterone	10 mg tablet	500 tablet pouch	British Dragon	Thailand		
Turinabol	nandrolone phenylpropionate	25 mg/ml	n/a	Germed	Czech. Rep.	[NLM]	
Turinabol	nandrolone phenylpropionate	25 mg/ml	n/a	Jenapharm	Bulgaria	[NLM]	
Turinabol	nandrolone phenylpropionate	25 mg/ml	n/a	Jenapharm	Germany	[NLM]	
Turinabol Depot	nandrolone decanoate	50 mg/ml	1 ml ampule	Jenapharm	Bulgaria	[NLM]	
Turinabol Depot	nandrolone decanoate	50 mg/ml	1 ml ampule	Jenapharm	Czech. Rep.	[NLM]	
Turinabol Depot	nandrolone decanoate	50 ma/ ml	1 ml ampule	Jenapharm	Germany	[NLM]	
Ultandren	fluoxymesterone	1,5 mg tablet	n/a	Ciba	United Kingdom	[NLM]	
Ultragan	boldenone undecylenate	100 mg/ml	10 ml vial	Denkall	Mexico		VET
Ultragan	boldenone undecylenate	50 mg/ml	50 ml vial	Denkall	Mexico		VET
Undestor	testosterone undecanoate	40 mg capsules	n/a	Organon	Argentina		
Undestor	testosterone undecanoate	40 mg capsules	60 capsule bottle	Organon	Belgium		
Undestor	testosterone undecanoate	40 mg capsules	60 capsule bottle	Organon	Bulgaria		
Undestor	testosterone undecanoate	40 mg capsules	60 capsule bottle	Organon	Czech. Rep.		
Undestor	testosterone undecanoate	40 mg capsules	n/a	Organon	Luxemburg		
Undestor	testosterone undecanoate	40 mg capsules	60 capsule bottle	Organon	Poland		
Undestor	testosterone undecanoate	40 mg capsules	60 capsule bottle	Organon	Rumania		
Undestor	testosterone undecanoate	40 mg capsules	n/a	Organon	Slovakia		
Undestor	testosterone undecanoate	40 mg capsules	n/a	Organon	Sweden		
Uni-Test Inj	testosterone propionate	100 mg/ml	10 ml vial	Univet	Canada		VET
Uni-Test Suspension	testosterone suspension	100 mg/ml	30 ml vial	Univet	Canada		VET
Vasorome	oxandrolone	0.5 mg tablet	n/a	Kowa	Japan	[NLM]	
Vasorome	oxandrolone	2 mg tablet	n/a	Kowa	Japan	[NLM]	
Vebonol	boldenone undecylenate	25 mg/ml	10 ml vial	Ciba-Geigy	Australia	[NLM]	VET
Vebonol	boldenone undecylenate	25 mg/ml	10 ml vial	Ciba-Geigy	Germany		VET
Vebonol	boldenone undecylenate	25 mg/ml	10 ml vial	Ciba-Geigy	Switzerland	[NLM]	VET
Veto-Test Sus	testosterone suspension	100 mg/ml	30 ml vial	Austin	Canada		VET
Vewon	fluoxymesterone	5 mg tablet	n/a	Yung Shin	Taiwan		
Vi Jane	fluoxymesterone	10 mg capsule	n/a	Shyh Sar	Taiwan		
Virbac Tepro Pellets	testosterone propionate (implant)	23.5 mg pellet	450 pellets	Virbac	Australia		VET
Virigen	testosterone undecanoate	40 mg capsules	30 capsule bottle	Organon	Turkey		
Virilon (time released)	methyltestosterone	10 mg capsule	100,1000 capsule bottle	Star	U.S.		
Vironate	testosterone cypionate	200 mg/ml	5 ml vial	Xelox (export)	Philippines		

Appendix B: Drug Availability Tables - Listings by Trade Name

Trade Name	Generic Name	Dose	Packaging	Company	Country	Status	Vet
Virormone	testosterone propionate	50 mg/ml	2 ml ampule	Ferring	United Kingdom	[NLM]	
Virormone	testosterone propionate	50 mg/ml	2 ml ampule	Nordic	United Kingdom		
Virormone	testosterone propionate	50, 100 mg/ml	1 ml ampule	Paines	Thailand		
Vistimon	mesterolone	25 mg tablet	30 tablet box	Jenapharm	Taiwan		
Vistimon	mesterolone	25 mg tablet	20 tablet box	Jenapharm	Germany	[NLM]	
Vistimon	mesterolone	25 mg tablet	n/a	n/a	Korea		
Vitabolic	stanozolol (inj)	20 mg/ml	10, 100 ml vial	Over Labs	Argentina		VET
VR Testprop	testosterone propionate	50 mg/ml	10 ml vial	Jurox	Australia		VET
Waromom	fluoxymesterone	5 mg tablet	n/a	Washington	Taiwan		
Weratestone 250	testosterone enanthate	250 mg/ml	1 ml ampule	Weimer Pharma	Algeria		
Weratestone 250	testosterone enanthate	250 mg/ml	1 ml ampule	Weimer Pharma	Mozambique		
Weratestone 250	testosterone enanthate	250 mg/ml	1 ml ampule	Weimer Pharma	Zimbabwe		
Weratestone 250	testosterone enanthate	250 mg/ml	1 ml ampule	Weimer Pharma	Zimbabwe		
Winstrol	stanozolol (oral)	2 mg tablet	n/a	n/a	Japan		
Winstrol®	stanozolol (oral)	2 mg tablet	100 tablet bottle	Sanofi	U.S.		
Winstrol®	stanozolol (oral)	2 mg tablet	100 tablet bottle	Upjohn	U.S.	[NLM]	
Winstrol®	stanozolol (oral)	2 mg tablet	100 tablet bottle	Winthrop	U.S.	[NLM]	
Winstrol®	stanozolol (oral)	2 mg tablet	20 tablet box	Zambon	Italy	[NLM]	
Winstrol®	stanozolol (oral)	2 mg tablet	20 tablet box	Zambon	Spain		
Winstrol®	stanozolol (oral)	2 mg tablet	n/a	Winthrop	Portugal	[NLM]	
Winstrol®	stanozolol (inj)	50 mg/ml	n/a	Winthrop	Greece	[NLM]	
Winstrol®	stanozolol (oral)	2 mg tablet	n/a	Winthrop	Greece	[NLM]	
Winstrol® Depot	stanozolol (inj)	50 mg/ml	1 ml vial	Zambon	Italy	[NLM]	
Winstrol® Depot	stanozolol (inj)	50 mg/ml	1 ml ampule	Zambon	Spain		
Winstrol® V	stanozolol (inj)	50 mg/ml	10, 30ml vial	Pharmacia	Canada		VET
Winstrol® V	stanozolol (inj)	50 mg/ml	10, 30ml vial	Pharmacia & Upjohn	U.S.		VET
Winstrol® V	stanozolol (inj)	50 mg/ml	10, 30ml vial	Winthrop	U.S.	[NLM]	VET
Winstrol-V®	stanozolol (oral)	2 mg tablet	100 tablet bottle	Pharmacia	Canada		VET
Winstrol-V®	stanozolol (oral)	2 mg tablet	100 tablet bottle	Pharmacia & Upjohn	U.S.		VET
Winstrol-V®	stanozolol (oral)	2 mg chewable tab	100 tablet bottle	Pharmacia & Upjohn	U.S.		VET
Ziremilon	nandrolone decanoate	50 mg/ml	1 ml ampule	Demo	Greece		

ABBREVIATIONS: [NLM] = No Longer Manufactured

VET = Veterinary Drug

Appendix C: Drug Availability Tables - Listings by Country

Country	Generic Name	Trade Name	Dose	Packaging	Company	Status	Vet
Algeria	mesterolone	Proviron	25 mg tablet	20 tablet box	Schering		
Algeria	testosterone enanthate	Androtardyl®	250 mg/ml	1 ml ampule	Schering		
Algeria	testosterone enanthate	Weratestone 250	250 mg/ml	1 ml ampule	Weimer Pharma		
Algeria	testosterone undecanoate	Andriol	40 mg capsules	60 capsule bottle	Organon		
Argentina	boldenone undecylenate	Ana-Bolde	50 mg/ml	10 ml vial	Forti		VET
Argentina	boldenone undecylenate	Ex-Pois	50 mg/ml	10 ml vial	Agofarma		VET
Argentina	fluoxymesterone	Ferona	1 mg tablet	30 tablet box	Sidus		
Argentina	mesterolone	Proviron®	25 mg tablet	n/a	Schering		
Argentina	nandrolone decanoate	Deca-Durabolin®	25, 50 mg/ml	1 ml	Organon		
Argentina	nandrolone decanoate	Deca-Durabolin®	50 mg/ml	2 ml	Organon		
Argentina	nandrolone phenylpropionate	Estigor	10 mg/ml	250 ml	Burnet		VET
Argentina	nandrolone phenylpropionate	Ganekyl	50 mg/ml	10, 100 ml vial	Over Labs		VET
Argentina	oxandrolone	Lonavar	2.5 mg tablet	n/a	Searle	[NLM]	
Argentina	stanozolol (inj)	Anabolico Cimol	60 mg/ml	5 ml vial	Cimol		VET
Argentina	stanozolol (inj)	Anabolico Produvet	10 mg/ml	25 ml vial	Cimol		VET
Argentina	stanozolol (inj)	Estanozolol	50 mg/ml	30 ml vial	Industria Argentina		VET
Argentina	stanozolol (inj)	Estrombol	25 mg/ml	10 ml vial	Fundacion		VET
Argentina	stanozolol (inj)	Nabolic	2 mg/ml	50 ml vial	Chinfield Ind.		VET
Argentina	stanozolol (inj)	Nabolic Strong	50 mg/ml	30 ml vial	Chinfield Ind.		VET
Argentina	stanozolol (inj)	Tanoxol	25 mg/ml	10 ml vial	Burnet		VET
Argentina	stanozolol (inj)	Vitabolic	20 mg/ml	10, 100 ml vial	Over Labs		VET
Argentina	stanozolol (oral)	Apetil	4 mg/ml	10 ml dropper bottle	Holliday		VET
Argentina	Sustanon 250 (testosterone blend)	Sustanon "250"	250 mg/ml	1 ml ampule	Organon		
Argentina	testosterone enanthate	Testoviron® Depot	250 mg/ml	1 ml ampule	Schering		
Argentina	testosterone propionate	Propionato de Testosterona	25 mg/ml	20 ml vial	Induvet		VET
Argentina	testosterone undecanoate	Undestor	40 mg capsules	n/a	Organon		
Argentina	Testoviron (testosterone blend)	Bi-Testo	60 mg/ml	10 ml vial	Cimol		VET
Argentina	Testoviron (testosterone blend)	Testoviron® Depot	135 mg/ml	1 ml ampule	Schering	[NLM]	
Aruba	testosterone undecanoate	Andriol	40 mg capsules	n/a	Organon		
Australia	boldenone undecylenate	Anabolic BD	50 mg/ml	10 ml vial	SYD Group		VET
Australia	boldenone undecylenate	Boldebal-H	50 mg/ml	10 ml vial	Ilium/Troy		VET
Australia	boldenone undecylenate	Boldenone-50	50 mg/ml	10 ml vial	Jurox	[NLM]	VET
Australia	boldenone undecylenate	Sybolin	25 mg/ml	10 ml vial	Ranvet		VET
Australia	boldenone undecylenate	Vebonol	25 mg/ml	10 ml vial	Ciba-Geigy	[NLM]	VET
Australia	ethylestrenol	Nandoral	.5 mg tablet	100, 500 tablet bottle	Intervet		VET
Australia	ethylestrenol	Nitrotain	15 mg/4gram	60, 250, 1000 gram tube	Nature-Vet		VET
Australia	ethylestrenol	Orabol-H	100 mg/5g paste	30 ml plastic tube	Vetsearch	[NLM]	VET
Australia	mesterolone	Proviron®	25, 50 mg tablet	n/a	Schering		
Australia	methylandrostenediol (blend)	Anabolic NA	75 mg/ml	10 ml vial	SYD Group		VET
Australia	methylandrostenediol (blend)	Drive	55 mg/ml	10 ml vial	RWR		VET
Australia	methylandrostenediol (blend)	Filybol	70 mg/ml	10, 20 ml vial	Ranvet		VET

Appendix C: Drug Availability Tables - Listings by Country

Country	Generic Name	Trade Name	Dose	Packaging	Company	Status	Vet
Australia	methylandrostenediol (blend)	Libriol	75 mg/ml	10, 20 ml vial	RWR		VET
Australia	methylandrostenediol (blend)	Spectriol	65 mg/ml	10 ml vial	RWR		VET
Australia	methylandrostenediol (blend)	Tribolin	75 mg/ml	10, 20 ml vial	Ranvet		VET
Australia	methylandrostenediol dipropionate	Anadiol	5 mg tab	10, 100 tablet bottle	Ilium/Troy		VET
Australia	methylandrostenediol dipropionate	Anadiol Depot	75 mg/ml	10 ml vial	Ilium/Troy		VET
Australia	methylandrostenediol dipropionate	Methandriol	75 mg/ml	10 ml vial	Ilium/Troy	[NLM]	VET
Australia	methylandrostenediol dipropionate	Methasus 50	50 mg/ml	20 ml vial	Jurox	[NLM]	VET
Australia	methylandrostenediol dipropionate	Protabol	75 mg/ml	10 ml vial	Protabol		VET
Australia	methylandrostenediol dipropionate	Superbolin	75 mg/ml	10 ml vial	Vetsearch		VET
Australia	nandrolone cypionate	Anabolic DN	50 mg/ml	10 ml vial	SYD Group		VET
Australia	nandrolone cypionate	Dynabol	50 mg/ml	10 ml vial	Jurox	[NLM]	VET
Australia	nandrolone decanoate	RWR Deca 50	50 mg/ml	10 ml vial	RWR		VET
Australia	nandrolone laurate	Laurabolin	25, 50 mg/ml	10 ml vial	Intervet		VET
Australia	nandrolone phenylpropionate	Nandrolin	50 mg/ml	25 ml vial	Intervet		VET
Australia	nandrolone phenylpropionate	Nandrolin	25 mg/ml	10 ml vial	Intervet		VET
Australia	norethandrolone	Anaplex	5 mg tablet	100 tablet bottle	Jurox		VET
Australia	stanozolol (inj)	Anabolic ST	50 mg/ml	20 ml vial	SYD Group		VET
Australia	stanozolol (inj)	Stanabolic	50 mg/ml	20 ml vial	Ilium/Troy		VET
Australia	stanozolol (inj)	Stanazol	50 mg/ml	20, 50 ml vial	RWR	[NLM]	VET
Australia	stanozolol (inj)	Stanosus	50 mg/ml	20 ml vial	Jurox	[NLM]	VET
Australia	Sustanon 250 (testosterone blend)	Durateston	250 mg/ml	5 ml vial	Intervet		VET
Australia	testosterone (gel)	Testogel	25, 50 mg	single dose packet	Schering		
Australia	testosterone (implant)	Ropel Testosterone Pellets	23.5 mg pellet	450, 600 pellet bottle	Jurox		VET
Australia	testosterone cypionate	Anabolic TL	100 mg/ml	10 ml vial	SYD Group		VET
Australia	testosterone cypionate	Banrot	75 mg/ml	200 ml bladder	Coopers	[NLM]	VET
Australia	testosterone cypionate	Ridrot Testosterone Inj.	75 mg/ml	250 ml vial	Troy		VET
Australia	testosterone cypionate	Testo LA	100 mg/ml	10 ml vial	Jurox	[NLM]	VET
Australia	testosterone enanthate	Primoteston®-Depot	250 mg/ml	1 ml ampule	Schering		
Australia	testosterone enanthate	Ropel Liquid Testosterone	75 mg/ml	200 ml vial	Jurox		VET
Australia	testosterone propionate	AVP Supertest	50 mg/ml	10 ml vial	Vetsearch		VET
Australia	testosterone propionate	Tepro Hormone	100 mg/ml	500 ml vial	Virbac		VET
Australia	testosterone propionate	VR Testprop	50 mg/ml	10 ml vial	Jurox		VET
Australia	testosterone propionate (implant)	Progro-H (plus estradiol)	20 mg/pellet	n/a	Pro Beef		VET
Australia	testosterone propionate (implant)	Synovex®-H (plus estrogen)	20 mg/pellet	n/a	Fort Dodge		VET
Australia	testosterone propionate (implant)	Virbac Tepro Pellets	23.5 mg pellet	450 pellets	Virbac		VET
Australia	testosterone suspension	Anabolic TS	100 mg/ml	20 ml vial	SYD Group		VET
Australia	testosterone suspension	RWR Suspension	100 mg/ml	20 ml vial	RWR		VET
Australia	testosterone suspension	Testosus 100	100 mg/ml	20 ml vial	Jurox	[NLM]	VET
Australia	testosterone undecanoate	Andriol	40 mg capsules	60 capsule bottle	Organon		
Australia	Testoviron (testosterone blend)	Primoteston Depot 100	135 mg/ml	1 ml ampule	Schering	[NLM]	
Australia	Testoviron (testosterone blend)	Primoteston Depot 50	75 mg/ml	1 ml ampule	Schering	[NLM]	

Appendix C: Drug Availability Tables - Listings by Country

Country	Generic Name	Trade Name	Dose	Packaging	Company	Status	Vet
Austria	mesterolone	Proviron®	25 mg tablet	50 tablet bottle	Schering		
Austria	methenolone acetate	Primobolan®	5 mg tablet	n/a	Schering	[NLM]	
Austria	methenolone enanthate	Primobolan® Depot	100 mg/ml	1 ml ampule	Schering	[NLM]	
Austria	nandrolone cyclohexylpropionate	Sanabolicum-Vet	50 mg/ml	10 ml vial	Werfft-Chemie		VET
Austria	nandrolone decanoate	Deca-Durabolin®	25 mg/ml	1 ml	Organon	[NLM]	
Austria	nandrolone hexyloxyphenylpropionate	Anadur	25, 50 mg/ml	1, 2 ml ampule	Kabi Pharmacia	[NLM]	
Austria	nandrolone laurate	Laurabolin	50 mg/ml	n/a	Werfft-Chemie		VET
Austria	oxymetholone	Plenastril	50 mg tablet	n/a	Grunenthal	[NLM]	
Austria	stanozolol (oral)	Stromba	5 mg tablet	n/a	Berger	[NLM]	
Austria	testosterone (gel)	Testogel	50 mg	single dose packet	Schering		
Austria	testosterone enanthate	Testoviron®-Depot	250 mg/ml	1 ml ampule	Schering		
Austria	testosterone propionate	Testosterone Streuli	n/a	5, 10, 25, 50 mg/ml	Streuli & Co. AG	[NLM]	
Austria	testosterone propionate	Testosterone-Prop. Disp.	n/a	10, 20 mg/ml	Disperga	[NLM]	
Austria	testosterone undecanoate	Andriol	40 mg capsules	60 capsule bottle	Organon		
Austria	Testoviron (testosterone blend)	Testoviron® Depot 100	135 mg/ml	1 ml ampule	Schering	[NLM]	
Austria	Testoviron (testosterone blend)	Testoviron® Depot 50	75 mg/ml	1 ml ampule	Schering	[NLM]	
Bahrain	testosterone undecanoate	Andriol	40 mg capsules	n/a	Organon		
Bahrain	testosterone enanthate	Testoviron®-Depot	250 mg/ml	1 ml ampule	Schering	[NLM]	
Bangladesh	testosterone undecanoate	Andriol	40 mg capsules	n/a	Organon		
Belarus	testosterone undecanoate	Andriol	40 mg capsules	n/a	Organon		
Belgium	dihydrotestosterone	Andractim	25 mg/g	80 gram gel	Piette		
Belgium	drostanolone propionate	Masteron	100 mg/2ml	2 ml amp	Sarva-Syntex	[NLM]	
Belgium	ethylestrenol	Orabolin®	2 mg tablet	n/a	Organon	[NLM]	
Belgium	mesterolone	Proviron®	25 mg tablet	50 tablet bottle	Schering		
Belgium	methenolone acetate	Primobolan®	5 mg tablet	n/a	Schering	[NLM]	
Belgium	methenolone enanthate	Primobolan® Depot	100 mg/ml	1 ml ampule	Schering	[NLM]	
Belgium	nandrolone decanoate	Deca-Durabolin®	25, 50 mg/ml	1 ml ampule, syringe	Organon		
Belgium	nandrolone hexyloxyphenylpropionate	Anadur	25, 50 mg/ml	1, 2 ml ampule	Pharmacia	[NLM]	
Belgium	nandrolone phenylpropionate	Durabolin®	25 mg/ml	n/a	Organon	[NLM]	
Belgium	oxymetholone	Synasteron	50 mg tablet	50 tablet bottle	Sarva	[NLM]	
Belgium	stanozolol (inj)	Strombaject	50 mg/ml	n/a	Winthrop	[NLM]	
Belgium	stanozolol (oral)	Stromba	5 mg tablet	10 tablet box	Winthrop	[NLM]	
Belgium	Sustanon 250 (testosterone blend)	Sustanon 250®	250 mg/ml	1 ml ampule	Organon		
Belgium	testosterone enanthate	Testosteronum Prolongatum	100 mg/ml	1 ml ampule	Polfa	[NLM]	
Belgium	testosterone undecanoate	Undestor	40 mg capsules	60 capsule bottle	Organon		
Belize	methandrostenolone	Dianabol	25 mg tablet	30 tablet bottle	Planet Pharmacy		
Belize	methandrostenolone/stanozolol	Diosterol	50 mg tablet	30 tablet bottle	Planet Pharmacy		
Belize	oxandrolone	Oxandrolone	5 mg tablet	30 tablet bottle	Planet Pharmacy		
Belize	oxymetholone	Oxymetholone	50 mg tablet	30 tablet bottle	Planet Pharmacy		
Belize	stanozolol (oral)	stanozolol	25 mg tablet	30 tablet bottle	Planet Pharmacy		
Bolivia	boldenone undecylenate	Boldenona 50 Gen-Far	50 mg/ml	10, 50, 100, 250ml vial	Gen-Far		VET

Appendix C: Drug Availability Tables - Listings by Country

Country	Generic Name	Trade Name	Dose	Packaging	Company	Status	Vet
Bolivia	boldenone undecylenate	Ganabol	50 mg/ml	500 ml vial	Laboratorios VM		VET
Bolivia	boldenone undecylenate	Ganabol	25, 50 mg/ml	10, 50, 100, 250ml vial	Laboratorios VM		VET
Bolivia	methenolone acetate	Primobolan®	5 mg tablet	n/a	Schering	[NLM]	
Bolivia	Sustanon 250 (testosterone blend)	Durateston 250®	250 mg/ml	1 ml ampule	Organon		
Brazil	boldenone undecylenate	Equifort	50 mg/ml	10, 50 ml vial	Purina		VET
Brazil	mesterolone	Proviron®	25 mg tablet	20 tablet box	Schering		
Brazil	nandrolone decanoate	Deca-Durabolin®	25, 50 mg/ml	1 ml ampule	Organon		
Brazil	oxandrolone	Lipidex	2.5 mg tablet	n/a	Searle	[NLM]	
Brazil	oxymetholone	Hemogenin	50 mg tablet	10 tablet box	Syntex	[NLM]	
Brazil	oxymetholone	Hemogenin	50 mg tablet	n/a	Aventis		
Brazil	oxymetholone	Hemogenin	50 mg tablet	10 tablet box	Sarsa	[NLM]	
Brazil	Sustanon 250 (testosterone blend)	Durateston 250®	250 mg/ml	1 ml ampule	Organon		
Brazil	testosterone cypionate	Deposteron	100 mg/ml	2 ml ampule	Novaquimica/Sigma		
Brazil	testosterone undecanoate	Androxon	40 mg capsules	20 capsule box	Organon		
Bulgaria	drostanolone propionate	Masteril	100 mg/2ml	2 ml ampule	Syntex	[NLM]	
Bulgaria	mesterolone	Proviron®	25 mg tablet	20, 50 tablet box	Schering		
Bulgaria	methandrostenolone	Bionabol	2, 5 mg tab	40 tablet box	Balkanpharma		
Bulgaria	methandrostenolone	Bionabol	2 mg tablet	40 tablet bottle	Pharmacia	[NLM]	
Bulgaria	methandrostenolone	Bionabol	5 mg tab	40 tablet bottle	Pharmacia	[NLM]	
Bulgaria	methandrostenolone	Nerobol	5 mg tablet	20 tablet box	Gedeon Richter	[NLM]	
Bulgaria	nandrolone decanoate	Deca-Durabolin®	25, 50 mg/ml	1 ml ampule	Organon		
Bulgaria	nandrolone decanoate	Retabolil	25, 50 mg/ml	1 ml ampule	Gedeon Richter	[NLM]	
Bulgaria	nandrolone decanoate	Turinabol Depot	50 mg/ml	1 ml ampule	Jenapharm	[NLM]	
Bulgaria	nandrolone phenylpropionate	Nerobolil	25 mg/ml	1 ml ampule	Godeon Richter	[NLM]	
Bulgaria	nandrolone phenylpropionate	Turinabol	25 mg/ml	n/a	Jenapharm	[NLM]	
Bulgaria	Omnadren (testosterone blend)	Omnadren 250	250 mg/ml	1 ml ampule	Jelfa		
Bulgaria	oxymetholone	Anapolon	50 mg tablet	n/a	Syntex	[NLM]	
Bulgaria	testosterone enanthate	Testosteron-Depot	250 mg/ml	1 ml ampule	Jenapharm		
Bulgaria	testosterone enanthate	Testosteronum Prolongatum	100 mg/ml	1 ml ampule	Jelfa	[NLM]	
Bulgaria	testosterone propionate	Testosteron	50 mg/ml	1 ml ampule	Sopharma		
Bulgaria	testosterone undecanoate	Undestor	40 mg capsules	60 capsule bottle	Organon		
Canada	boldenone undecylenate	Equipoise®	25, 50 mg/ml	50 ml vial	Ciba-Geigy	[NLM]	VET
Canada	boldenone undecylenate	Equipoise®	25, 50 mg/ml	50 ml vial	Squibb	[NLM]	VET
Canada	boldenone undecylenate	Equipoise®	50 mg/ml	50 ml vial	Wyeth		VET
Canada	fluoxymesterone	Halotestin®	5 mg tablet	50 tablet bottle	Pharmacia		
Canada	methandrostenolone	Metaboline	2 mg tablet	60, 500 tablet bottle	Desbergers	[NLM]	
Canada	methyltestosterone	Geri Tabs	2 mg tablet	50, 200 tablet bottle	Vetcom		VET
Canada	nandrolone decanoate	Deca-Durabolin®	50 mg/ml	2 ml	Organon	[NLM]	
Canada	nandrolone decanoate	Deca-Durabolin®	100 mg/ml	2 ml	Organon		
Canada	nandrolone phenylpropionate	Durabolin®	25, 50 mg/ml	n/a	Organon	[NLM]	
Canada	oxymetholone	Anadrol 50®	50 mg tablet	100 tablet bottle	Syntex	[NLM]	

Appendix C: Drug Availability Tables - Listings by Country

Country	Generic Name	Trade Name	Dose	Packaging	Company	Status	Vet
Canada	oxymetholone	Anapolon 50®	50 mg tablet	100 tablet bottle	Hoffman-La Rouche	[NLM]	
Canada	stanozolol (inj)	Winstrol® V	50 mg/ml	10, 30ml vial	Pharmacia		VET
Canada	stanozolol (oral)	Winstrol-V®	2 mg tablet	100 tablet bottle	Pharmacia		VET
Canada	testosterone (gel)	Androgel	25, 50 mg	single dose packet	Solvay		
Canada	testosterone (patch)	Androderm®	12.2 mg patch.	30 patches/box	Pharmascience		
Canada	testosterone cypionate	Depo-Testosterone®	100 mg/ml	10 ml vial	Pharmacia		
Canada	testosterone cypionate	Scheinpharma Testone-Cyp	100 mg/ml	10 ml vial	Schein		
Canada	testosterone cypionate	Testosterone Cypionate Inj.	100 mg/ml	2 ml vial	Cytex		
Canada	testosterone cypionate	Testosterone Cypionate Inj.	200 mg/ml	10 ml vial	Sabex		
Canada	testosterone enanthate	Delatestryl	200 mg/ml	5 ml vial	Theramed		
Canada	testosterone enanthate	Malogex LA200	200 mg/ml	10 ml vial	Germiphene	[NLM]	
Canada	testosterone enanthate	PMS-Testosterone Enanthate	200 mg/ml	10 ml vial	Pharmascience		
Canada	testosterone enanthate	Testosterone Enanthate Inj	200 mg/ml	10 ml vial	Taro	[NLM]	
Canada	testosterone propionate	Anatest	100 mg/ml	10 ml vial	Rhone	[NLM]	VET
Canada	testosterone propionate	Anatest	100 mg/ml	10 ml vial	Sterivet	[NLM]	VET
Canada	testosterone propionate	Anatest	100 mg/ml	10 ml vial	Vetoquinol		VET
Canada	testosterone propionate	Malogen In Oil	100 mg/ml	10 ml vial	Germiphene	[NLM]	
Canada	testosterone propionate	Testosterone Propionate Inj.	100 mg/ml	10 ml vial	Cytex		
Canada	testosterone propionate	Testosterone Propionate Inj.	100 mg/ml	10 ml vial	Dominion		VET
Canada	testosterone propionate	Testosterone Propionate Inj.	100 mg/ml	10 ml vial	Taro	[NLM]	
Canada	testosterone propionate	Uni-Test Inj	100 mg/ml	10 ml vial	Univet		VET
Canada	testosterone propionate (implant)	Synovex®-H (plus estradiol)	20 mg/pellet	n/a	Ayerst		
Canada	testosterone suspension	Malogen Aqueous	100 mg/ml	10 ml vial	Germiphene	[NLM]	
Canada	testosterone suspension	Testos 100	100 mg/ml	10 ml vial	Vetcom		VET
Canada	testosterone suspension	Uni-Test Suspension	100 mg/ml	30 ml vial	Univet		VET
Canada	testosterone suspension	Veto-Test Sus	100 mg/ml	30 ml vial	Austin		VET
Canada	testosterone undecanoate	Andriol	40 mg capsules	60 capsule bottle	Organon		
Canada	trenbolone acetate	Revalor-H (plus estradiol)	20 mg pellet	70 pellet cartridge	Intervet		VET
Canada	trenbolone acetate	Revalor-S (plus estradiol)	20 mg pellet	60 pellet cartridge	Intervet		VET
Canada	trenbolone acetate	Synovex plus (plus estradiol)	25 mg pellet	80 pellet cartridge	Wyeth		VET
Chile	boldenone undecylenate	Ganabol	50 mg/ml	500 ml vial	Laboratorios VM		VET
Chile	boldenone undecylenate	Ganabol	25, 50 mg/ml	10, 50, 100, 250ml vial	Laboratorios VM		VET
Chile	nandrolone decanoate	Anaprolina	25, 50 mg/ml	1 ml ampule	Silesia		
Chile	nandrolone decanoate	Deca-Durabolin®	25, 50, 100 mg/ml	1 ml ampule	Organon		
Chile	nandrolone decanoate	Decanoato Nandrolona	25, 50 mg/ml	1 ml ampule	Astorga		
Chile	nandrolone decanoate	Decanoato Nandrolona	50 mg/ml	1 ml ampule	Biosano		
Chile	nandrolone decanoate	nandrolona decanoato	50 mg/ml	1 ml ampule	Chile		
Chile	nandrolone decanoate	Nandrosande	25, 50, 100 mg/ml	1 ml ampule	Sanderson		
Chile	Sustanon 250 (testosterone blend)	Sustenan 250	250 mg/ml	1 ml ampule	Organon		
Chile	testosterone enanthate	Primoniat®-Depot 250	250 mg/ml	1 ml ampule	Schering-Chile	[NLM]	
Chile	testosterone enanthate	testosterona enantato	250 mg/ml	1 ml ampule	Biosano		

Appendix C: Drug Availability Tables - Listings by Country

Country	Generic Name	Trade Name	Dose	Packaging	Company	Status	Vet
Chile	testosterone enanthate	testosterona enantato	100 mg/ml	1 ml ampule	Chile	[NLM]	
Chile	testosterone enanthate	testosterona enantato	250 mg/ml	1 ml ampule	Chile		
Chile	testosterone undecanoate	Sustenan Oral	40 mg capsules	n/a	Organon		
Chile	Testoviron (testosterone blend)	Primoniat®-Depot 100	135 mg/ml	1 ml ampule	Schering-Chile	[NLM]	
China	oxandrolone	Anavar	5 mg tablet	30 tablet strip	Hubei Huangshi		
China	testosterone propionate	Dubol	25 mg/ml	1 ml ampule	n/a		
China	testosterone propionate	Testosterone Propionate Inj	50 mg/ml	1 ml ampule	n/a		
China	testosterone undecanoate	Andriol	40 mg capsules	16 capsule box	Organon		
Colombia	boldenone undecylenate	Boldenol 25	25 mg/ml	10, 50, 100, 250ml vial	Comandina		VET
Colombia	boldenone undecylenate	Boldenol R	50 mg/ml	10, 50, 100, 250ml vial	Comandina		VET
Colombia	boldenone undecylenate	Boldenona	50 mg/ml	10, 20, 100 ml vial	Biogen		VET
Colombia	boldenone undecylenate	Boldenona	50 mg/ml	10, 50, 100, 250ml vial	Vecol		VET
Colombia	boldenone undecylenate	Boldenona 50	50 mg/ml	10, 50, 100, 250ml vial	Servinsumos		VET
Colombia	boldenone undecylenate	Boldenona 50 Gen-Far	50 mg/ml	10, 50, 100, 250ml vial	Gen-Far		VET
Colombia	boldenone undecylenate	Cebulin 50	50 mg/ml	10, 50, 250 ml vial	Provet		VET
Colombia	boldenone undecylenate	Dynabolin 50	50 mg/ml	10, 50, 100, 250ml vial	Kryovet		VET
Colombia	boldenone undecylenate	Ganabol	50 mg/ml	500 ml vial	Laboratorios VM		VET
Colombia	boldenone undecylenate	Ganabol	25, 50 mg/ml	10, 50, 100, 250ml vial	Laboratorios VM		VET
Colombia	boldenone undecylenate	Legacy	50 mg/ml	50 ml vial	Technoquimicas		VET
Colombia	boldenone undecylenate	Mitgan 50	50 mg/ml	50 ml vial	California		VET
Colombia	boldenone undecylenate	Porkybol 1%	10 mg/ml	10, 50, 100 ml vial	Compania California		VET
Colombia	mesterolone	Proviron®	25 mg tablet	20 tablet box	Schering		
Colombia	nandrolone decanoate	Deca-Durabolin®	25, 50 mg/ml	1 ml ampule	Organon		
Colombia	nandrolone laurate	Laurabolin	50 mg/ml	10, 50 ml	Intervet		VET
Colombia	testosterone enanthate	Testoviron®-Depot	250 mg/ml	1 ml ampule	Schering		
Costa Rica	boldenone undecylenate	Boldenona 50 Gen-Far	50 mg/ml	10, 50, 100, 250ml vial	Gen-Far		VET
Costa Rica	mesterolone	Proviron®	25 mg tablet	n/a	Schering		
Costa Rica	methenolone acetate	Primobolan®	5 mg tablet	n/a	Schering	[NLM]	
Costa Rica	Sustanon 250 (testosterone blend)	Testosterona 250	250 mg/ml	10 ml vial	Qualityvet		VET
Costa Rica	testosterone propionate	Testogan	25 mg/ml	50 ml vial	Laguinsa		VET
Croatia	mesterolone	Proviron®	25 mg tablet	20 tablet box	Schering		
Cyprus	testosterone undecanoate	Andriol	40 mg capsules	n/a	Organon		
Czech. Rep.	mesterolone	Proviron®	25 mg tablet	20, 50 tablet box	Schering		
Czech. Rep.	methandrostenolone	Stenolon	5 mg tablet	20 tablet box	Leciva	[NLM]	
Czech. Rep.	methandrostenolone	Stenolon	1 mg tablet	20 tablet box	Leciva	[NLM]	
Czech. Rep.	methenolone enanthate	Primobolan® Depot	100 mg/ml	1 ml ampule	Schering	[NLM]	
Czech. Rep.	methyltestosterone	Agovirin	10 mg dragee	100 dragee bottle	Leciva	[NLM]	
Czech. Rep.	nandrolone decanoate	Turinabol Depot	50 mg/ml	1 ml ampule	Jenapharm	[NLM]	
Czech. Rep.	nandrolone hexyloxyphenylpropionate	Anadur	25, 50 mg/ml	1, 2 ml ampule	Pharmacia	[NLM]	
Czech. Rep.	nandrolone phenylpropionate	Superanabolon	25 mg/ml	1 ml ampule	Spofa		
Czech. Rep.	nandrolone phenylpropionate	Turinabol	25 mg/ml	n/a	Germed	[NLM]	

Appendix C: Drug Availability Tables - Listings by Country

Country	Generic Name	Trade Name	Dose	Packaging	Company	Status	Vet
Czech. Rep.	stanozolol (oral)	Stromba	5 mg tablet	n/a	Sterling-Health	[NLM]	
Czech. Rep.	Sustanon 250 (testosterone blend)	Sustanon 250	250 mg/ml	1 ml ampule	Organon		
Czech. Rep.	testosterone enanthate	Testoviron®-Depot	250 mg/ml	1 ml ampule	Schering	[NLM]	
Czech. Rep.	testosterone propionate	Agovirin injectable	25 mg/ml	n/a	Leciva	[NLM]	
Czech. Rep.	testosterone suspension (isobutyrate)	Agovirin-Depot	25 mg/ml	2 ml ampule	Biotika		
Czech. Rep.	testosterone undecanoate	Undestor	40 mg capsules	60 capsule bottle	Organon		
Denmark	fluoxymesterone	Halotestin®	5 mg tablet	n/a	Upjohn	[NLM]	
Denmark	mesterolone	Mestoranum	25 mg tablet	n/a	Schering		
Denmark	nandrolone decanoate	Deca-Durabolin®	25, 50 mg/ml	1 ml	Organon	[NLM]	
Denmark	nandrolone hexyloxyphenylpropionate	Anadur	25 mg/ml	2 ml ampule	Lundbeck	[NLM]	
Denmark	stanozolol (oral)	Stromba	5 mg tablet	n/a	Winthrop	[NLM]	
Denmark	testosterone enanthate	Testoviron®-Depot	250 mg/ml	1 ml ampule	Schering		
Denmark	testosterone undecanoate	Restandol	40 mg capsules	60 capsule bottle	Organon		
Denmark	Testoviron (testosterone blend)	Testoviron® Depot 135	135 mg/ml	1 ml ampule	Schering		
Dom. Rep.	boldenone undecylenate	Boldenona 50 Gen-Far	50 mg/ml	10, 50, 100, 250ml vial	Gen-Far		VET
Dom. Rep.	boldenone undecylenate	Ganabol	50 mg/ml	500 ml vial	Laboratorios VM		VET
Dom. Rep.	boldenone undecylenate	Ganabol	25, 50 mg/ml	10, 50, 100, 250ml vial	Laboratorios VM		VET
Dom. Rep.	mesterolone	Proviron®	25 mg tablet	20 tablet bottle	Schering		
Dom. Rep.	methandrostenolone	Anabolex	3 mg tablet	100 tablet box	Ethical		
Dom. Rep.	methenolone acetate	Primobolan®	5 mg tablet	n/a	Schering	[NLM]	
Dom. Rep.	nandrolone decanoate	Dimetabol	50 mg/ml	50 ml vial	Bremer Pharma	[NLM]	VET
Dom. Rep.	testosterone enanthate	Testoviron®-Depot	250 mg/ml	1 ml ampule	Schering		
Dom. Rep.	testosterone propionate	Testogan	25 mg/ml	50 ml vial	Laguinsa		VET
Dom. Rep.	Testoviron (testosterone blend)	Testoviron® Depot 100	135 mg/ml	1 ml ampule	Schering		
Dutch Antilles	testosterone undecanoate	Andriol	40 mg capsules	n/a	Organon		
Ecuador	boldenone undecylenate	Boldenona 50 Gen-Far	50 mg/ml	10, 50, 100, 250ml vial	Gen-Far		VET
Ecuador	boldenone undecylenate	Ganabol	50 mg/ml	500 ml vial	Laboratorios VM		VET
Ecuador	boldenone undecylenate	Ganabol	25, 50 mg/ml	10, 50, 100, 250ml vial	Laboratorios VM		VET
Ecuador	methenolone acetate	Primobolan®	5 mg tablet	n/a	Schering	[NLM]	
Ecuador	methenolone enanthate	Primobolan® Depot	100 mg/ml	1 ml ampule	Schering		
Ecuador	testosterone enanthate	Primoteston®-Depot	250 mg/ml	1 ml ampule	Schering		
Ecuador	testosterone propionate	Testogan	25 mg/ml	50 ml vial	Laguinsa		VET
Ecuador	testosterone undecanoate	Andriol	40 mg capsules	n/a	Organon		
Egypt	mesterolone	Proviron®	25 mg tablet	20 tablet box	Schering/CID	[NLM]	
Egypt	methenolone enanthate	Primobolan Depot	100 mg/ml	1 ml ampule	Schering/CID	[NLM]	
Egypt	methyltestosterone	Neo Aphro	5 mg tablet	30 tablet	Misr		
Egypt	nandrolone cyclohexylpropionate	Sanabolicum	25, 50 mg/ml	1 ml ampule	Biochemie/Nile		
Egypt	nandrolone decanoate	Deca-Durabolin®	25, 50 mg/ml	1 ml ampule	Organon/Nile		
Egypt	nandrolone decanoate	Gerabolin	25 mg/ml	1 ml ampule	Nile		
Egypt	nandrolone decanoate	Retabolil	50 mg/ml	1 ml ampule	Medimpex/Alxndria		
Egypt	nandrolone phenylpropionate	Menabolin	25 mg/ml	1 ml ampule	Theramex/Memphis		

Appendix C: Drug Availability Tables - Listings by Country

Country	Generic Name	Trade Name	Dose	Packaging	Company	Status	Vet
Egypt	Sustanon 100 (testosterone blend)	Sustanon '100'®	100 mg/ml	1 ml ampule	Organon/Nile		
Egypt	Sustanon 100 (testosterone blend)	Testonon '100'®	100 mg/ml	1 ml ampule	Nile		
Egypt	Sustanon 250 (testosterone blend)	Sustanon '250'®	250 mg/ml	1 ml ampule	Organon/Nile		
Egypt	Sustanon 250 (testosterone blend)	Testonon '250'®	250 mg/ml	1 ml ampule	Nile		
Egypt	testosterone blend (misc)	Triolandren	250 mg/ml	1 ml ampule	Novartis		
Egypt	testosterone enanthate	Primoteston®-Depot	250 mg/ml	1 ml ampule	Schering/CID		
Egypt	testosterone propionate	Testone-E	25 mg/ml	1 ml ampule	Misr		
Egypt	testosterone undecanoate	Andriol	40 mg capsules	20 capsule box	Organon/Sedico		
Egypt	Testoviron (testosterone blend)	Primoteston®-Depot 100	135 mg/ml	1 ml ampule	Schering/CID		
El Salvador	boldenone undecylenate	Boldenona 50 Gen-Far	50 mg/ml	10, 50, 100, 250ml vial	Gen-Far		VET
El Salvador	boldenone undecylenate	Ganabol	50 mg/ml	500 ml vial	Laboratorios VM		VET
El Salvador	boldenone undecylenate	Ganabol	25, 50 mg/ml	10, 50, 100, 250ml vial	Laboratorios VM		VET
El Salvador	mesterolone	Proviron®	25 mg tablet	n/a	Schering		
El Salvador	methenolone acetate	Primobolan®	5 mg tablet	n/a	Schering	[NLM]	
El Salvador	testosterone propionate	Testogan	25 mg/ml	50 ml vial	Laguinsa		VET
Estonia	mesterolone	Proviron®	25 mg tablet	20 tablet box	Schering	[NLM]	
Estonia	nandrolone decanoate	Retabolil	50 mg/ml	1 ml ampule	Gedeon Richter		
Estonia	Sustanon 250 (testosterone blend)	Sustanon 250®	250 mg/ml	1 ml ampule	Organon		
Estonia	testosterone undecanoate	Pantestone	40 mg capsules	60 capsule bottle	Organon		
Ethiopia	testosterone enanthate	Testoviron®-Depot	250 mg/ml	1 ml ampule	Schering		
Finland	fluoxymesterone	Halotestin®	5 mg tablet	n/a	Upjohn		
Finland	mesterolone	Proviron®	25 mg tablet	n/a	Leiras		
Finland	methandrostenolone	Anabolin	5 mg tablet	n/a	Leiras	[NLM]	
Finland	methandrostenolone	Anabolin	0.5% cream	n/a	Leiras	[NLM]	
Finland	methenolone acetate	Primobolan® S	25 mg tablet	n/a	Leiras	[NLM]	
Finland	nandrolone decanoate	Deca-Durabolin®	25, 50 mg/ml	1 ml	Organon		
Finland	nandrolone decanoate	Deca-Durabolin®	100 mg/ml	1,2 ml	Organon		
Finland	nandrolone decanoate	Sterobolin	50 mg/ml	1 ml ampule	Orion	[NLM]	
Finland	nandrolone hexyloxyphenylpropionate	Anadur	25, 50 mg/ml	1, 2 ml ampule	Pharmacia	[NLM]	
Finland	nandrolone phenylpropionate	Durabolin®	25 mg/ml	n/a	Organon		
Finland	Sustanon 250 (testosterone blend)	Sustanon 250®	250 mg/ml	1 ml ampule	Organon		
Finland	testosterone enanthate	Primoteston®-Depot	250 mg/ml	1 ml ampule	Leiras	[NLM]	
Finland	testosterone undecanoate	Panteston	40 mg capsules	60 capsule bottle	Organon		
France	dihydrotestosterone	Andractim	25 mg/g	100 gram gel	Besins-Iscovesco		
France	drostanolone propionate	Permastril	100 mg/2ml	2 ml ampule	Cassenne	[NLM]	
France	fluoxymesterone	Halotestin®	5 mg tablet	n/a	Pharmacia-Upjohn	[NLM]	
France	mesterolone	Proviron®	25 mg tablet	n/a	Schering	[NLM]	
France	methenolone acetate	Primobolan®	50 mg tablet	n/a	Schering	[NLM]	
France	methenolone enanthate	Primobolan® Depot	100 mg/ml	1 ml ampule	Schering	[NLM]	
France	nandrolone decanoate	Deca-Durabolin®	50 mg/ml	1 ml	Organon	[NLM]	
France	nandrolone hexyloxyphenylpropionate	Anador	25 mg/ml	2 ml ampule	Pharmacia-Upjohn	[NLM]	

Appendix C: Drug Availability Tables - Listings by Country

Country	Generic Name	Trade Name	Dose	Packaging	Company	Status	Vet
France	nandrolone undecanoate	Dynabolon	80.5 mg/ml	1 ml ampule	Theramex	[NLM]	
France	norethandrolone	Nilevar	10 mg tablet	30 tablet bottle	Searle		
France	oxandrolone	Anatrophill	2.5 mg tablet	n/a	Searle	[NLM]	
France	testosterone cyclohexylpropionate	Testosterone CHP Theramex	296, 148, 37 mg/ml	1 ml ampule	Theramex	[NLM]	
France	testosterone enanthate	Androtardyl®	250 mg/ml	1 ml ampule	Schering		
France	testosterone enanthate	Testosterone Heptylate	50, 100, 250 mg/ml	1 ml ampule	Theramex		
France	testosterone undecanoate	Pantestone	40 mg capsules	60 capsule bottle	Organon		
France	trenbolone acetate	Finaject	30 mg/ml	n/a	Roussel	[NLM]	VET
France	trenbolone hexahydrobenzylcarbonate	Parabolan	76 mg/1.5 ml	1.5 ml ampule	Negma	[NLM]	
Georgia	testosterone undecanoate	Andriol	40 mg capsules	n/a	Organon		
Germany	boldenone undecylenate	Vebonol	25 mg/ml	10 ml vial	Ciba-Geigy		VET
Germany	clostebol acetate	Megagrisevit-Mono	15 mg dragee	30 dragee box	Pharmacia	[NLM]	
Germany	clostebol acetate	Megagrisevit-Mono	10 mg/1.5ml	1.5 ml vial	Pharmacia	[NLM]	
Germany	drostanolone propionate	Masterid	100 mg/2ml	2 ml amp	Gruenthal	[NLM]	
Germany	mesterolone	Pluriviron	25 mg dragee	30 dragee box	Asche	[NLM]	
Germany	mesterolone	Proviron®	25 mg tablet	50 tablet bottle	Schering	[NLM]	
Germany	mesterolone	Vistimon	25 mg tablet	20 tablet box	Jenapharm	[NLM]	
Germany	methandrostenolone	Anabolikum 2.5%	25 mg/ml	50 ml vial	Meca G	[NLM]	VET
Germany	methandrostenolone	Dianabol	5 mg tablet	100 tablet bottle	Ciba	[NLM]	
Germany	methenolone acetate	Primobolan®	5 mg tablet	n/a	Schering	[NLM]	
Germany	methenolone acetate	Primobolan® Acetate	25 mg/ml	1 ml ampule	Schering	[NLM]	
Germany	methenolone acetate	Primobolan® S	25 mg tablet	n/a	Schering	[NLM]	
Germany	methenolone enanthate	Primobolan® Depot	100 mg/ml	1 ml ampule	Schering	[NLM]	
Germany	methenolone enanthate	Primobolan® Depot mite	50 mg/ml	1 ml ampule	Schering	[NLM]	
Germany	methyltestosterone	Testosteron	5 mg tablet	n/a	Berco	[NLM]	
Germany	methyltestosterone	Testoyohim	25 mg dragee	30 dragee box	Paul Mehner	[NLM]	
Germany	nandrolone decanoate	Anabolicum	25 mg/ml	10, 50 ml vial	Bela-Pharm		VET
Germany	nandrolone decanoate	Deca-Durabolin®	25, 50 mg/ml	1 ml	Organon	[NLM]	
Germany	nandrolone decanoate	Turinabol Depot	50 ma/ ml	1 ml ampule	Jenapharm	[NLM]	
Germany	nandrolone hexyloxyphenylpropionate	Anadur	25, 50 mg/ml	1, 2 ml ampule	Kabi Pharmacia	[NLM]	
Germany	nandrolone laurate	Fortadex	25, 50 mg/ml	n/a	Hydro		VET
Germany	nandrolone laurate	Laurabolin	25, 50 mg/ml	5, 10, 50 ml	Vemie		VET
Germany	nandrolone phenylpropionate	Turinabol	25 mg/ml	n/a	Jenapharm	[NLM]	
Germany	stanozolol (inj)	Strombaject	50 mg/ml	n/a	Winthrop	[NLM]	
Germany	stanozolol (oral)	Stromba	5 mg tablet	n/a	Winthrop	[NLM]	
Germany	Sustanon 100 (testosterone blend)	Sustanon 100	100 mg/ml	1 ml ampule	Organon	[NLM]	
Germany	Sustanon 250 (testosterone blend)	Sustanon 250	250 mg/ml	1 ml ampule	Organon	[NLM]	
Germany	Sustanon 250 (testosterone blend)	Testosteron 250	250 mg/ml	1 ml ampule	Rotex Medica	[NLM]	
Germany	testosterone (gel)	Androtop Gel	50 mg	single dose packet	Kade/Besins		
Germany	testosterone (gel)	Testogel	25, 50 mg	single dose packet	Jenapharm		
Germany	testosterone (patch)	Androderm®	12.2 mg patch.	10, 30, 60 patches/box	AstraZenica		

Appendix C: Drug Availability Tables - Listings by Country

Country	Generic Name	Trade Name	Dose	Packaging	Company	Status	Vet
Germany	testosterone enanthate	Testosteron Depot	100 mg/ml	1 ml ampule	Rotex Medica	[NLM]	
Germany	testosterone enanthate	Testosteron Depot	250 mg/ml	1 ml ampule	Rotex Medica		
Germany	testosterone enanthate	Testosteron-Depot	250 mg/ml	1 ml ampule	Eifelfango		
Germany	testosterone enanthate	Testosteron-Depot	250 mg/ml	1 ml ampule	Jenapharm		
Germany	testosterone enanthate	Testoviron®-Depot	250 mg/ml	1 ml ampule	Schering		
Germany	testosterone propionate	Testosterone Berco Supp.	40 mg/suppository	18 supp. box	Funke	[NLM]	
Germany	testosterone propionate	Testosterone Jenapharm	25 mg/ml	1 ml ampule	Jenapharm	[NLM]	
Germany	testosterone propionate	Testosterone Vitis	n/a	10, 25 mg/ml	Neopharma	[NLM]	
Germany	testosterone propionate	testosteronpropionat	10, 25 mg/ml	1 ml ampule	Eifelfango	[NLM]	
Germany	testosterone propionate	testosteronpropionat	50 mg/ml	1 ml ampule	Eifelfango		
Germany	testosterone undecanoate	Andriol	40 mg capsules	30, 60 capsule bottle	Organon		
Germany	Testoviron (testosterone blend)	Testoviron® Depot 100	135 mg/ml	1 ml ampule	Schering	[NLM]	
Germany	Testoviron (testosterone blend)	Testoviron® Depot 50	75 mg/ml	1 ml ampule	Schering	[NLM]	
Ghana	testosterone undecanoate	Andriol	40 mg capsules	n/a	Organon		
Greece	fluoxymesterone	Halotestin®	5 mg tablet	20 tablet box	Upjohn		
Greece	mesterolone	Proviron®	25 mg tablet	20 tablet bottle	Schering		
Greece	methenolone enanthate	Primobolan® Depot	100 mg/ml	1 ml ampule	Schering	[NLM]	
Greece	methylandrostenediol	Andris	10 mg tablet	n/a	Chifar	[NLM]	
Greece	methyltestosterone	Teston	25 mg tablet	30 tablet box	Remek		
Greece	nandrolone decanoate	Anaboline Depot	50 mg/ml	1 ml	Adelco		
Greece	nandrolone decanoate	Deca-Durabolin®	50 mg/ml	1 ml vial	Organon		
Greece	nandrolone decanoate	Deca-Durabolin®	100 mg/ml	2 ml vial	Organon		
Greece	nandrolone decanoate	Deca-Durabolin®	100 mg/ml	2 ml vial	Organon		
Greece	nandrolone decanoate	Elpihormo	50 mg/ml	1 ml	Chemica	[NLM]	
Greece	nandrolone decanoate	Extraboline	50 mg/ml	2 ml vial	Genepharm		
Greece	nandrolone decanoate	nandrolone decanoate	200 mg/2ml	2 ml vial	Norma Hellas		
Greece	nandrolone decanoate	Nurezan	50 mg/ml	1 ml ampule	Rafarm		
Greece	nandrolone decanoate	Ziremilon	50 mg/ml	1 ml ampule	Demo		
Greece	nandrolone hexyloxyphenylpropionate	Anadurin	50 mg/ml	1 ml ampule	Xponei	[NLM]	
Greece	nandrolone phenylpropionate	Durabolin®	25 mg/ml	1 ml ampule	Organon	[NLM]	
Greece	nandrolone undecanoate	Psychobolan	80.5 mg/ml	1ml ampule	Theramex	[NLM]	
Greece	oxymetholone	Anasteron	25 mg tablet	60 tablet bottle	Farmaprod		
Greece	oxymetholone	Anasteron	50 mg tablet	n/a	Syntex	[NLM]	
Greece	oxymetholone	Oxybolone	50 mg tablet	20 tablet box	Genapharm		
Greece	oxymetholone	Oxymetholone Miverva	50 mg tablet	100 tablet	Minerva	[NLM]	
Greece	stanozolol (inj)	Winstrol®	50 mg/ml	n/a	Winthrop	[NLM]	
Greece	stanozolol (oral)	stanozolol	5 mg tablet	30 tablet box	Genepharm		
Greece	stanozolol (oral)	Stromba	5 mg tablet	56 tablet box	n/a		
Greece	stanozolol (oral)	Winstrol®	2 mg tablet	n/a	Winthrop	[NLM]	
Greece	testosterone enanthate	testosterone enanthate	250 mg/ml	1 ml ampule	Norma Hellas		
Greece	testosterone enanthate	Testoviron®-Depot	250 mg/ml	1 ml ampule	Schering		

Appendix C: Drug Availability Tables - Listings by Country

Country	Generic Name	Trade Name	Dose	Packaging	Company	Status	Vet
Greece	testosterone propionate	Testoviron®	50 mg/ml	1 ml ampule	Schering		
Greece	testosterone undecanoate	Restandol	40 mg capsules	60 capsule bottle	Organon		
Greece	Testoviron (testosterone blend)	Testoviron® Depot 100	135 mg/ml	1 ml ampule	Schering	[NLM]	
Guatemala	boldenone undecylenate	Boldenona 50 Gen-Far	50 mg/ml	10, 50, 100, 250ml vial	Gen-Far		VET
Guatemala	boldenone undecylenate	Ganabol	50 mg/ml	500 ml vial	Laboratorios VM		VET
Guatemala	boldenone undecylenate	Ganabol	25, 50 mg/ml	10, 50, 100, 250ml vial	Laboratorios VM		VET
Guatemala	mesterolone	Proviron®	25 mg tablet	n/a	Schering		
Guatemala	methenolone acetate	Primobolan®	5 mg tablet	n/a	Schering	[NLM]	
Guatemala	methenolone enanthate	Primobolan® Depot	100 mg/ml	1 ml ampule	Schering		
Guatemala	testosterone enanthate	Primoteston®-Depot	250 mg/ml	1 ml ampule	Schering		
Guatemala	testosterone propionate	Testogan	25 mg/ml	50 ml vial	Laguinsa		VET
Honduras	boldenone undecylenate	Boldenona 50 Gen-Far	50 mg/ml	10, 50, 100, 250ml vial	Gen-Far		VET
Honduras	boldenone undecylenate	Ganabol	50 mg/ml	500 ml vial	Laboratorios VM		VET
Honduras	boldenone undecylenate	Ganabol	25, 50 mg/ml	10, 50, 100, 250ml vial	Laboratorios VM		VET
Honduras	mesterolone	Proviron®	25 mg tablet	n/a	Schering		
Honduras	methenolone acetate	Primobolan®	5 mg tablet	n/a	Schering	[NLM]	
Honduras	testosterone propionate	Testogan	25 mg/ml	50 ml vial	Laguinsa		VET
Hong Kong	methyltestosterone	Testosure	n/a	n/a	Europharm		
Hong Kong	testosterone cypionate	Testosterone Cypionate Inj	200 mg/ml	n/a	Charmaine		
Hong Kong	testosterone enanthate	Testoviron®-Depot	250 mg/ml	1 ml ampule	Schering		
Hong Kong	testosterone propionate	Testosterone Propionate Inj	25 mg/ml	n/a	Charmaine		
Hong Kong	testosterone propionate	Testosterone Propionate Inj	50 mg/ml	n/a	Hong Kong Med		
Hong-Kong	testosterone undecanoate	Andriol	40 mg capsules	n/a	Organon		
Hungary	mesterolone	Proviron®	25 mg tablet	10, 15, 20, 50, 100, 150 tab btl	Schering		
Hungary	methandrostenolone	Nerobol	5 mg tablet	20 tablet box	Gedeon Richter	[NLM]	
Hungary	methyltestosterone	Androral	10 mg tablet	n/a	Gedeon Richter		
Hungary	nandrolone decanoate	Retabolil	25, 50 mg/ml	1 ml ampule	Gedeon Richter		
Hungary	nandrolone phenylpropionate	Nerobolil	25 mg/ml	n/a	Godeon Richter	[NLM]	
Hungary	stanozolol (oral)	Stromba	5 mg tablet	n/a	Sterling-Health		
Hungary	testosterone enanthate	Testoviron® Depot	250 mg/ml	1 ml ampule	Schering	[NLM]	
Hungary	testosterone propionate	Androfort-Richter	10, 25 mg/ml	n/a	Gedeon Richter		
Hungary	testosterone propionate	Testosteron	5, 10, 25, 50 mg/ml	1 ml ampule	Hemofarm	[NLM]	
Hungary	testosterone undecanoate	Andriol	40 mg capsules	n/a	Organon		
Hungary	Testoviron (testosterone blend)	Testoviron® Depot	135 mg/ml	1 ml ampule	Schering	[NLM]	
Iceland	testosterone enanthate	Testoviron®-Depot	250 mg/ml	1 ml ampule	Schering		
India	dihydrotestosterone	Andractim	25 mg/g	100 gram gel	Chemec		
India	ethylestrenol	Orabolin®	2 mg tablet	10 tablet box	Infar		
India	mesterolone	Proviron®	25 mg tablet	30 tablet box	Schering		
India	mesterolone	Restore	25 mg tablet	20 tablet box	Brown & Burk		
India	methandrostenolone	Pronabol-5	5 mg tablet	100 tablet box	P&B Labs	[NLM]	
India	methandrostenolone	Trinergic	5 mg capsule	n/a	Unimed	[NLM]	

Appendix C: Drug Availability Tables - Listings by Country

Country	Generic Name	Trade Name	Dose	Packaging	Company	Status	Vet
India	nandrolone decanoate	Deca-Dubol-100	100 mg/ml	2 ml vial	BM Pharmaceuticals		
India	nandrolone decanoate	Deca-Durabolin®	25, 50, 100 mg/ml	1 ml ampule	Infar		
India	nandrolone decanoate	Deca-Evabolin	25 mg/ml	1 ml ampule	Concept		
India	nandrolone decanoate	Decagic	100 mg/ml	10 ml vial	Unichem	[NLM]	
India	nandrolone decanoate	Decaneurabol	25, 50 mg/ml	1 ml ampule	Cadila		
India	nandrolone decanoate	Decaneurophen	25, 50 mg/ml	1 ml ampule	Ind-Swift		
India	nandrolone decanoate	Deca-Pronabol	100 mg/ml	2 ml ampule	P & B Labs	[NLM]	
India	nandrolone decanoate	Metadec	25, 50 mg/ml	1 ml ampule	Jagsonpal		
India	nandrolone decanoate	Myobolin	25 mg/ml	1 ml ampule	Troikaa		
India	nandrolone phenylpropionate	Dubol-100	100 mg/ml	2 ml vial	BM Pharmaceuticals		
India	nandrolone phenylpropionate	Dubol-50	50 mg/ml	1 ml ampule	BM Pharmaceuticals		
India	nandrolone phenylpropionate	Durabolin®	25 mg/ml	1 ml ampule	Infar		
India	nandrolone phenylpropionate	Evabolin	25 mg/ml	1 ml ampule	Concept		
India	nandrolone phenylpropionate	Metabol	25 mg/ml	1 ml ampule	Jagsonpal		
India	nandrolone phenylpropionate	nandrolone phenylpropionate	50, 100mg/ml	2 ml vial	Hayrian Biologicals	[NLM]	
India	nandrolone phenylpropionate	Neurabol Inj	25 mg/ml	1 ml ampule	Cadila		
India	nandrolone phenylpropionate	Neurophen	25 mg/ml	1 ml ampule	Ind-Swift		
India	oxymetholone	Androyd	5 mg tablet	100 tablet	Parke Davis		
India	stanozolol (oral)	Menabol	5 mg tablet	100 tablet box	n/a		
India	stanozolol (oral)	Neurabol	2 mg capsule	10 capsule box	Cadila		
India	Sustanon 100 (testosterone blend)	Sustanon (Cyctahoh)	100 mg/ml	1 ml ampule	Infar		
India	Sustanon 250 (testosterone blend)	Sustanon 250 (Cyctahon)	250 mg/ml	1 ml ampule	Infar		
India	Sustanon 250 (testosterone blend)	Sustaretard 250	250 mg/ml	1 ml ampule	BM Pharmaceuticals		
India	testosterone cypionate	Testacyp	100 mg/ml	2 ml vial	BM Pharmaceuticals		
India	testosterone enanthate	Testen-250	250 mg/ml	2 ml vial	BM Pharmaceuticals		
India	testosterone enanthate	Testoviron®-Depot	250 mg/ml	1 ml ampule	Schering		
India	testosterone propionate	Testopin-100	100 mg/ml	2 ml vial	BM Pharmaceuticals		
India	testosterone propionate	Testopin-100	100 mg/ml	1 ml ampule	BM Pharmaceuticals		
India	testosterone suspension	Aquaviron	25 mg/ml	1 ml ampule	Nicholas		
India	testosterone undecanoate	Nuvir	40 mg capsules	30 capsule bottle	Organon		
India	Testoviron (testosterone blend)	Testenon	135 mg/ml	2 ml vial	BM Pharmaceuticals		
India	Testoviron (testosterone blend)	Testenon	135 mg/ml	1 ml ampule	BM Pharmaceuticals		
Indonesia	ethylestrenol	Orgabolin	2 mg tablet	n/a	Organon		
Indonesia	mesterolone	Proviron®	25 mg tablet	n/a	Schering		
Indonesia	methandrostenolone	Neo-Anabolene	5 mg tablet	10 tablet strip	Haurus		
Indonesia	nandrolone decanoate	Deca-Durabolin®	25, 50 mg/ml	1 ml ampule	Organon		
Indonesia	nandrolone phenylpropionate	Durabolin®	12.5 mg/ml	2 ml ampule	Organon		
Indonesia	Sustanon 250 (testosterone blend)	Sustanon "250"	250 mg/ml	1 ml ampule	Organon		
Indonesia	testosterone undecanoate	Andriol	40 mg capsules	n/a	Organon		
Iran	nandrolone phenylpropionate	nandrolone phenylpropionate	25 mg/ml	1 ml ampule	Iran Hormone		
Iran	testosterone enanthate	Testosterone Enanthate 250	250 mg/ml	1 ml ampule	Aburaihan		

Appendix C: Drug Availability Tables - Listings by Country

Country	Generic Name	Trade Name	Dose	Packaging	Company	Status	Vet
Ireland	nandrolone decanoate	Deca-Durabolin®	n/a	n/a	Organon		
Ireland	Sustanon 250 (testosterone blend)	Sustanon	250 mg/ml	1 ml ampule	Organon		
Ireland	testosterone enanthate	Testoviron® Depot	250 mg/ml	1 ml ampule	Schering	[NLM]	
Israel	mesterolone	Proviron®	25 mg tablet	20, 50 tablet box	Schering		
Israel	oxandrolone	Lonavar	2.5 mg tablet	100 tablet bottle	BTG		
Israel	oxymetholone	Oxymetholone	50 mg tablet	100 tablets	Alhavi		
Israel	oxymetholone	Roboral	50 mg tablet	100 tablets	Abic/Ramat-Gan	[NLM]	
Israel	Sustanon 250 (testosterone blend)	Sustanon	250 mg/ml	1 ml ampule	Organon		
Israel	testosterone enanthate	Testoviron®-Depot	250 mg/ml	1 ml ampule	Schering		
Israel	testosterone undecanoate	Androxon	40 mg capsules	30 capsule bottle	Organon		
Italy	clostebol acetate	Alfa-Trofodermin	.5% gel	n/a	Farmitalia	[NLM]	
Italy	clostebol acetate	Alfa-Trofodermin	.5% gel	n/a	Pharmacia & Upjohn		
Italy	clostebol acetate	Steranabol	20 mg/ml	2 ml ampule	Farmitalia	[NLM]	
Italy	clostebol acetate	Trofodermin Crema	cream	30 gram tube	Carlo Erba OTC		
Italy	clostebol acetate	Trofodermin Spray	n/a	30 ml spray	Carlo Erba OTC		
Italy	fluoxymesterone	Halotestin®	5 mg tablet	20 tablet box	Upjohn	[NLM]	
Italy	formebolone	Esiclene	1 mg drops	n/a	LPB	[NLM]	
Italy	formebolone	Esiclene	2 mg/ml	2 ml ampule	LPB	[NLM]	
Italy	formebolone	Esiclene	5 mg tablet	n/a	LPB	[NLM]	
Italy	mesterolone	Proviron®	50 mg tablet	20 tablet box	Schering		
Italy	methenolone enanthate	Primobolan® Depot	100 mg/ml	1 ml ampule	Schering	[NLM]	
Italy	methyltestosterone	Testovis	10 mg tablet	n/a	SIT		
Italy	nandrolone decanoate	Deca-Durabolin®	25, 50 mg/ml	1 ml ampule	Organon		
Italy	nandrolone undecanoate	Dynabolon	80.5 mg/ml	1 ml ampule	Farmasister	[NLM]	
Italy	nandrolone undecanoate	Dynabolon	80.5 mg/ml	1 ml ampule	Fournier		
Italy	oxabolone cypionate	Steranabol Ritardo	12.5 mg/ml	2 ml ampule	Pharmacia & Upjohn	[NLM]	
Italy	oxandrolone	Oxandrolone SPA	2.5 mg tablet	30 tablet box	SPA	[NLM]	
Italy	oxandrolone	Oxandrolone SPA (Export)	2.5 mg tablet	30 tablet box	SPA		
Italy	quinbolone	Anabolicum Vister	10 mg capsule	30 capsule bottle	Parke Davis	[NLM]	
Italy	quinbolone	Anabolicum Vister	oral drops	n/a	Parke Davis	[NLM]	
Italy	stanozolol (inj)	Winstrol® Depot	50 mg/ml	1 ml vial	Zambon	[NLM]	
Italy	stanozolol (oral)	Winstrol®	2 mg tablet	20 tablet box	Zambon	[NLM]	
Italy	Sustanon 250 (testosterone blend)	Sustanon®	250 mg/ml	1 ml ampule	Organon		
Italy	testosterone (patch)	Androderm®	12.2 mg patch.	n/a	Schwarz Pharma		
Italy	testosterone cypionate	Testosterone Depositum	n/a	n/a	SPA		
Italy	testosterone enanthate	Testo-Enant	125 mg/ml	2 ml ampule	Geymonat		
Italy	testosterone enanthate	Testo-Enant	250 mg/ml	1 ml ampule	Geymonat		
Italy	testosterone enanthate	Testoviron®-Depot	250 mg/ml	1 ml ampule	Schering		
Italy	testosterone propionate	Facovit	1 mg/ml	10 ml vial	Teofarma		
Italy	testosterone propionate	Testoviron®	10, 25, 50 mg/ml	1 ml ampule	Schering	[NLM]	
Italy	testosterone propionate	Testovis	50 mg/ml	2 ml ampule	SIT		

Appendix C: Drug Availability Tables - Listings by Country

Country	Generic Name	Trade Name	Dose	Packaging	Company	Status	Vet
Italy	testosterone undecanoate	Andriol	40 mg capsules	60 capsule bottle	Organon		
Italy	Testoviron (testosterone blend)	Testoviron® Depot 100	135 mg/ml	1 ml ampule	Schering		
Italy	Testoviron (testosterone blend)	Testoviron® Depot 50	75 mg/ml	1 ml ampule	Schering	[NLM]	
Japan	drostanolone propionate	Mastisol	5% injection sol.	n/a	Shionogi	[NLM]	
Japan	fluoxymesterone	Halotestin®	2, 5 mg tablet	n/a	n/a		
Japan	furazabol	Miotolan	1 mg tablet	n/a	Daiichi Seiyaku	[NLM]	
Japan	methandrostenolone	Andoredan	5 mg tablet	n/a	Takeshima-Kodama	[NLM]	
Japan	methandrostenolone	Encephan	5 mg tablet	n/a	Sato	[NLM]	
Japan	methenolone acetate	Primobolan®	5 mg tablet	100, 1000 tablet box	Schering		
Japan	methenolone enanthate	Primobolan® Depot	50 mg/ml	1 ml ampule	Schering	[NLM]	
Japan	methenolone enanthate	Primobolan® Depot	100 mg/ml	1 ml ampule	Schering		
Japan	oxandrolone	Lonavar	2 mg tablet	n/a	Dainippon	[NLM]	
Japan	oxandrolone	Vasorome	0.5 mg tablet	n/a	Kowa	[NLM]	
Japan	oxandrolone	Vasorome	2 mg tablet	n/a	Kowa	[NLM]	
Japan	oxymetholone	Anadrol	5 mg tablet	n/a	n/a		
Japan	stanozolol (oral)	Winstrol	2 mg tablet	n/a	n/a		
Japan	testosterone enanthate	Enarmon-Depot	125 mg/ml	n/a	Teskoku Hormone		
Japan	testosterone enanthate	Testinon-Depot	n/a	n/a	n/a		
Japan	testosterone enanthate	Testoviron®-Depot	250 mg/ml	1 ml ampule	Schering		
Japan	testosterone enanthate	Testron Depot	125, 250 mg/ml	1 ml vial	n/a		
Jordan	testosterone enanthate	Primoteston®-Depot	250 mg/ml	1 ml ampule	Schering		
Jordan	testosterone undecanoate	Andriol	40 mg capsules	n/a	Organon		
Kenya	testosterone undecanoate	Andriol	40 mg capsules	n/a	Organon		
Korea	dihydrotestosterone	Andractim	25 mg/g	80 gram gel	n/a		
Korea	mesterolone	Vistimon	25 mg tablet	n/a	n/a		
Korea	methyltestosterone	Debosteron	n/a	n/a	n/a		
Korea	methyltestosterone	KangJungBing	n/a	n/a	n/a		
Korea	methyltestosterone	Testo Tab	25 mg tablet	n/a	Samil		
Korea	nandrolone decanoate	Canoate Inj	25, 50 mg/ml	n/a	n/a		
Korea	nandrolone decanoate	Deca-Durabolin®	25, 50 mg/ml	1 ml ampule	Organon		
Korea	nandrolone decanoate	Dynabolon Inj	40 mg/.5 ml	1 ml ampule	n/a		
Korea	oxandrolone	Kicker Tab	2.5 mg tablet	n/a	n/a		
Korea	oxymetholone	Oxymetholone DongIndang	n/a	n/a	Dongindang		
Korea	oxymetholone	Oxymetholone HanBul	50 mg tablet	n/a	HanBul		
Korea	oxymetholone	Oxymetholone HanSeo	50 mg tablet	100 tablet bottle	HanSeo		
Korea	oxymetholone	Oxymetholone Korea United	50 mg tablet	n/a	Korea United		
Korea	stanozolol (oral)	Seidon	2 mg tablet	100 tablet box	Seoul Pharm		
Korea	stanozolol (oral)	Stabon	2 mg tablet	n/a	n/a		
Korea	stanozolol (oral)	Terabon	2 mg tablet	10 tablet strip	Jin Yang		
Korea	testosterone (patch)	Androderm®	12.2 mg patch.	n/a	n/a		
Korea	testosterone cypionate	Depo-TCP	200mg/ml	n/a	n/a		

Appendix C: Drug Availability Tables - Listings by Country

Country	Generic Name	Trade Name	Dose	Packaging	Company	Status	Vet
Korea	testosterone cypionate	Depovirin Inj	125 mg/ml	2 ml	n/a		
Korea	testosterone cypionate	Miro Depo	125 mg/ml	2 ml vial	Hanil Pharm		
Korea	testosterone enanthate	Jenasteron Inj	250 mg/ml	n/a	n/a		
Korea	testosterone enanthate	Testosterone Enanthate Dalim	250 mg/ml	n/a	Dalim		
Korea	testosterone propionate	Testo	50 mg/ml	10 ml vial	Samil		
Korea	testosterone undecanoate	Andriol	40 mg capsules	n/a	Organon		
Kuwait	testosterone enanthate	Primoteston®-Depot	250 mg/ml	1 ml ampule	Schering	[NLM]	
Kuwait	testosterone undecanoate	Andriol	40 mg capsules	n/a	Organon		
Latvia	mesterolone	Proviron®	25 mg tablet	20 tablet box	Schering	[NLM]	
Latvia	testosterone undecanoate	Panteston	40 mg capsules	n/a	Organon		
Lebanon	testosterone enanthate	Testoviron®-Depot	250 mg/ml	1 ml ampule	Schering	[NLM]	
Lebanon	testosterone undecanoate	Andriol	40 mg capsules	n/a	Organon		
Lithuania	mesterolone	Proviron®	25 mg tablet	20 tablet box	Schering	[NLM]	
Lithuania	testosterone undecanoate	Panteston	40 mg capsules	n/a	Organon		
Luxemburg	testosterone undecanoate	Undestor	40 mg capsules	n/a	Organon		
Malaysia	methyltestosterone	Testopropon	25 mg tablet	n/a	Scanpharm		
Malaysia	nandrolone decanoate	Deca-Durabolin®	25 mg/ml	1 ml ampule	Organon		
Malaysia	nandrolone decanoate	Retabolil	25, 50 mg/ml	1 ml ampule	Gedeon Richter		
Malaysia	nandrolone phenylpropionate	Durabolin®	25 mg/ml	1 ml ampule	Organon		
Malaysia	oxymetholone	Anapolon 50	50 mg tablet	100 tablet bottle	Syntex	[NLM]	
Malaysia	oxymetholone	Oxylone	50 mg tablet	100 tablet bottle	Duopharma		
Malaysia	oxymetholone	oxymetholone	50 mg tablet	n/a	Sime Darby		
Malaysia	Sustanon 250 (testosterone blend)	Sustanon '250'®	250 mg/ml	1 ml ampule	Organon		
Malaysia	testosterone (patch)	Testoderm	15 mg patch	n/a	Alza		
Malaysia	testosterone cypionate	Depo-Testosterone®	100 mg/ml	n/a	Pharmacia		
Malaysia	testosterone enanthate	Jenasteron Inj	250 mg/ml	1 ml ampule	Jenahexal		
Malaysia	testosterone enanthate	Testoviron®-Depot	250 mg/ml	1 ml ampule	Schering		
Malaysia	testosterone propionate	Astrapin	50 mg/ml	1 ml ampule	Astrapin		
Malaysia	testosterone undecanoate	Andriol	40 mg capsules	60 capsule bottle	Organon		
Malta	testosterone enanthate	Testoviron®-Depot	250 mg/ml	1 ml ampule	Schering		
Mauritius	testosterone enanthate	Primoteston®-Depot	250 mg/ml	1 ml ampule	Schering		
Mauritius	testosterone undecanoate	Andriol	40 mg capsules	n/a	Organon		
Mexico	boldenone undecylenate	Anabolic BD	100, 200 mg/ml	10 ml vial	SYD Group		VET
Mexico	boldenone undecylenate	Anabolic-BD	100 mg/ml	10 ml vial	Grupo Tarasco	[NLM]	VET
Mexico	boldenone undecylenate	Bold 200	200 mg/ml	10 ml vial	Animal Power		VET
Mexico	boldenone undecylenate	Bold QV 200	200 mg/ml	10 ml vial	Quality Vet		VET
Mexico	boldenone undecylenate	Boldenon	200 mg/ml	10 ml vial	Ttokkyo	[NLM]	VET
Mexico	boldenone undecylenate	Boldenona 200	200 mg/ml	10 ml vial	Pet's Pharma		VET
Mexico	boldenone undecylenate	Crecibol	25 mg/ml	10, 30 ml vial	Unimed		VET
Mexico	boldenone undecylenate	Equi-gan	50 mg/ml	10, 50, 100, 250 ml vial	Tornel		VET
Mexico	boldenone undecylenate	Equipoise®	50 mg/ml	10, 50 ml vial	Fort Dodge		VET

Appendix C: Drug Availability Tables - Listings by Country

Country	Generic Name	Trade Name	Dose	Packaging	Company	Status	Vet
Mexico	boldenone undecylenate	Equipoise®	25, 50 mg/ml	50 ml vial	Solvay	[NLM]	VET
Mexico	boldenone undecylenate	Equipoise®	25, 50 mg/ml	50 ml vial	Squibb	[NLM]	VET
Mexico	boldenone undecylenate	Maxigan	50 mg/ml	10, 50 ml vial	Inpel/Denkall	[NLM]	VET
Mexico	boldenone undecylenate	Ultragan	100 mg/ml	10 ml vial	Denkall		VET
Mexico	boldenone undecylenate	Ultragan	50 mg/ml	50 ml vial	Denkall		VET
Mexico	fluoxymesterone	Stenox	2.5 mg tablet	20 tablet box	Atlantis		
Mexico	mesterolone	Proviron®	25 mg tablet	10 tablet box	Schering		
Mexico	methandrostenolone	Anabol-Jet	25 mg/ml	30, 100, 250 ml vial	Norvet		VET
Mexico	methandrostenolone	Anabol-Jet ADE	30 mg/ml	100, 250 ml vial	Norvet		VET
Mexico	methandrostenolone	Anabol-Pet's	10, 25 mg tablet	200 tablet bottle	Norvet		VET
Mexico	methandrostenolone	D-Bol	10 mg tablet	100 tablet bottle	Denkall		VET
Mexico	methandrostenolone	D-Bol	10 mg capsule	96 capsule box	Denkall		VET
Mexico	methandrostenolone	D-Bol	10 mg capsule	300 capsule bottle	Denkall		VET
Mexico	methandrostenolone	D-Bol	25 mg/ml	10 ml vial	Denkall		VET
Mexico	methandrostenolone	Dianabol	10 mg tablet	100 tablet bottle	Salud		VET
Mexico	methandrostenolone	Dianabol	25 mg/ml	10, 50, 100 ml vial	Salud		VET
Mexico	methandrostenolone	Ganabol	25 mg/ml	50 ml vial	Salud	[NLM]	VET
Mexico	methandrostenolone	Metandiabol	25 mg/ml	50 ml vial	Quimper		VET
Mexico	methandrostenolone	Metandiol 60	60 mg/ml	10 ml vial	Pet's Pharma		VET
Mexico	methandrostenolone	Metandiol Tab	10 mg tablet	100 tablet bottle	Pet's Pharma		VET
Mexico	methandrostenolone	Metandrol 10	10 mg tablet	500 tablet bottle	Bratis Labs		VET
Mexico	methandrostenolone	Methan Tabs	10 mg tablet	100 tablet bottle	Animal Power		VET
Mexico	methandrostenolone	Methandienone	5, 10 mg tablet	100, 1000 tablet bottle	Ttokkyo	[NLM]	VET
Mexico	methandrostenolone	Reforvit Simple	5, 10, 25 mg tab	100, 500, 1000 tablet bottle	Loeffler		VET
Mexico	methandrostenolone	Reforvit-B	25 mg/ml	10, 50 ml	Loeffler		VET
Mexico	methandrostenolone	Restauvit	2 mg tablet	n/a	Ciba, Rugby	[NLM]	
Mexico	methenolone acetate	Metabolon 25	25 mg tablet	100 tablet bottle	Bratis Labs		VET
Mexico	methenolone acetate	Metenol QV	50 mg tablet	50 tablet bottle	Quality Vet		VET
Mexico	methenolone acetate	Primobolan®	5 mg tablet	n/a	Schering	[NLM]	
Mexico	methenolone acetate	Primo-Plus 50	50 mg tablet	100 tablet bottle	Ttokkyo	[NLM]	VET
Mexico	methenolone enanthate	Primobolan® Depot	50 mg/ml	1 ml ampule	Schering		
Mexico	methenolone enanthate	Primo-Plus 100	100 mg/ml	1 ml ampule	Ttokkyo	[NLM]	VET
Mexico	methenolone enanthate	Suprimo 100	100 mg/ml	10 ml vial	SYD Group		VET
Mexico	methylandrostenediol (blend)	Anabolic NA	75 mg/ml	10 ml vial	SYD Group		VET
Mexico	methylandrostenediol (blend)	Anabolic-NA	75 mg/ml	10 ml vial	Grupo Tarasco	[NLM]	VET
Mexico	methylandrostenediol dipropionate	Denkadiol	75 mg/ml	10 ml vial	Denkall	[NLM]	VET
Mexico	methyltestosterone	Metil-Test	50 mg tablet	100 tablet bottle	Brovel		VET
Mexico	nandrolone cypionate	Anabolic DN	50, 300 mg/ml	10 ml vial	SYD Group		VET
Mexico	nandrolone cypionate	Anabolic-DN	50 mg/ml	10 ml vial	Grupo Tarasco	[NLM]	VET
Mexico	nandrolone decanoate	Deca 300	300 mg/ml	10 ml vial	Animal Power		VET
Mexico	nandrolone decanoate	Deca QV 200	200 mg/ml	10, 50 ml vial	Quality Vet		VET

Appendix C: Drug Availability Tables - Listings by Country

Country	Generic Name	Trade Name	Dose	Packaging	Company	Status	Vet
Mexico	nandrolone decanoate	Deca QV 300	300 mg/ml	10 ml vial	Quality Vet		VET
Mexico	nandrolone decanoate	Decanandrolen	200mg/ml	10 ml vial	Denkall		VET
Mexico	nandrolone decanoate	Decandrol 300	300 mg/ml	10 ml vial	Pet's Pharma		VET
Mexico	nandrolone decanoate	Decanoato de Nandrolona	200 mg/ml	10 ml vial	Tornel		VET
Mexico	nandrolone decanoate	Decatron 250	250 mg/ml	10 ml vial	Brovel		VET
Mexico	nandrolone decanoate	Dimetabol ADE	25 mg/ml	50, 100 ml vial	Lapisa		VET
Mexico	nandrolone decanoate	Nandrolona 300 L.A.	300mg/ml	10 ml vial	Ttokkyo	[NLM]	VET
Mexico	nandrolone decanoate	Norandren	50, 200 mg/ml	10, 50 ml vial	Brovel		VET
Mexico	nandrolone laurate	Fortabol	20 mg/ml	10, 50 ml vial	Parfam		VET
Mexico	nandrolone laurate	Laudrol LA	250 mg/ml	10 ml vial	Loeffler		VET
Mexico	nandrolone laurate	Laurabolin	20, 50 mg/ml	10, 50 ml vial	Intervet		VET
Mexico	oxandrolone	Oxafort	5 mg tablet	100 tablet bottle	Loeffler		VET
Mexico	oxandrolone	Oxandro Tabs	5 mg tablet	100 tablet bottle	Animal Power		VET
Mexico	oxandrolone	Oxandrol 10	10 mg tablet	100 tablet bottle	Bratis Labs		VET
Mexico	oxandrolone	Oxandrolone	2.5 tablet	100 tablet bottle	Ttokkyo	[NLM]	VET
Mexico	oxandrolone	Oxandrolone	5 mg tablet	100 tablet bottle	Ttokkyo	[NLM]	VET
Mexico	oxandrolone	Oxandrovet	5 mg tablet	100 tablet bottle	Denkall		VET
Mexico	oxandrolone	Oxavet QV	5 mg tablet	100 tablet bottle	Quality Vet		VET
Mexico	oxymetholone	Anabrol	50 mg tablet	100 tablet bottle	Brovel		VET
Mexico	oxymetholone	Anapolon 50	50 mg tablet	20 tablet strip	Syntex	[NLM]	
Mexico	oxymetholone	Kanestron	50 mg tablet	100 tablet bottle	Loeffler		VET
Mexico	oxymetholone	Metalon Tabs	75 mg tablet	100 tablet bottle	Animal Power		VET
Mexico	oxymetholone	Oximetalon	75 mg tablet	100 tablet bottle	Denkall		VET
Mexico	oxymetholone	Oxitron 50	50 mg tablet	100 tablet bottle	Bratis Labs		VET
Mexico	oxymetholone	Oxivet QV	75 mg tablet	100 tablet bottle	Quality Vet		VET
Mexico	oxymetholone	Oxymetolona 50	50 mg tablet	100 tablet bottle	Ttokkyo	[NLM]	VET
Mexico	stanozolol (inj)	Anabolic ST	50 mg/ml	20 ml vial	SYD Group		VET
Mexico	stanozolol (inj)	Anabolic-ST	50 mg/ml	20 ml vial	Grupo Tarasco	[NLM]	VET
Mexico	stanozolol (inj)	Stan 50	50 mg/ml	10 ml vial	Animal Power		VET
Mexico	stanozolol (inj)	Stan QV 100	100 mg/ml	20 ml vial	Quality Vet		VET
Mexico	stanozolol (inj)	Stan QV 50	50 mg/ml	20 ml vial	Quality Vet		VET
Mexico	stanozolol (inj)	Stanazolic	50, 100 mg/ml	20 ml, 10ml vial	Denkall		VET
Mexico	stanozolol (inj)	Stanol 50	50 mg/ml	20 ml vial	Bratis Labs		VET
Mexico	stanozolol (inj)	Stanol-V	50, 100 mg/ml	20 ml vial	Ttokkyo	[NLM]	VET
Mexico	stanozolol (oral)	Estano-Pet's	10, 25 mg tablet	100 tablet bottle	Norvet		VET
Mexico	stanozolol (oral)	Stan QV 10	10 mg tablet	100 tablet bottle	Quality Vet		VET
Mexico	stanozolol (oral)	Stan Tabs	10 mg tablet	100 tablet bottle	Animal Power		VET
Mexico	stanozolol (oral)	Stanazolic	6 mg cap	300 capsule bottle	Denkall		VET
Mexico	stanozolol (oral)	Stanazolic	10 mg tablet	100 tablet bottle	Denkall		VET
Mexico	stanozolol (oral)	Stanol 10	10 mg tablet	250 tablet bottle	Bratis Labs		VET
Mexico	stanozolol (oral)	Stanol-V	10 mg tablet	100, 500 tablet bottle	Ttokkyo	[NLM]	VET

Appendix C: Drug Availability Tables - Listings by Country

Country	Generic Name	Trade Name	Dose	Packaging	Company	Status	Vet
Mexico	Sten (testosterone blend)	Sten	50 mg/ml	2 ml ampule	Atlantis		
Mexico	Sustanon 250 (testosterone blend)	Sostenon 250®	250 mg/ml	1 ml ampule	Organon		
Mexico	Sustanon 250 (testosterone blend)	Super Test-250	250 mg/ml	5, 10 ml vial	Tornel		VET
Mexico	Sustanon 250 (testosterone blend)	Testenon 250	250 mg/ml	5 ml vial	Ttokkyo	[NLM]	VET
Mexico	Sustanon 250 (testosterone blend)	Testo-Jet L.A.	250 mg/ml	10 ml vial	Norvet		VET
Mexico	Sustanon 250 (testosterone blend)	Testosterona IV L/A	250 mg/ml	10 ml vial	Loeffler		VET
Mexico	Sustanon 250 (testosterone blend)	Testron 4 250	250 mg/ml	10 ml vial	Bratis Labs		VET
Mexico	Test 400 (testosterone blend)	Test 400	400 mg/ml	10 ml vial	Denkall		VET
Mexico	testosterone blend (misc)	Deposterona	60 mg/ml	10 ml vial	Fort Dodge		VET
Mexico	testosterone blend (misc)	Deposterona	60 mg/ml	10 ml vial	Syntex	[NLM]	VET
Mexico	testosterone cypionate	Anabolic TL	200 mg/ml	10 ml vial	SYD Group		VET
Mexico	testosterone cypionate	Cypiotest 250	250 mg/ml	10 ml vial	Animal Power		VET
Mexico	testosterone cypionate	CypioTest 250	250 mg/ml	10 ml vial	Denkall		VET
Mexico	testosterone cypionate	Cypriotest L/A	250 mg/ml	10 ml vial	Loeffler		VET
Mexico	testosterone cypionate	Teston QV 200	200 mg/ml	10 ml vial	Quality Vet		VET
Mexico	testosterone cypionate	Testosterone Cypionate 200	200 mg/ml	10 ml vial	Ttokkyo	[NLM]	VET
Mexico	testosterone cypionate	Testosterone Cypionate L.A.	100 mg/ml	10 ml vial	Ttokkyo	[NLM]	VET
Mexico	testosterone decanoate	Neotest 250	250 mg/ml	10 ml bottle	Loeffler		
Mexico	testosterone enanthate	Delatestryl	200 mg/ml	10 ml vial	Brovel	[NLM]	VET
Mexico	testosterone enanthate	Enantat QV 250	250 mg/ml	10, 50 ml vial	Quality Vet		VET
Mexico	testosterone enanthate	Enantato 350	350 mg/ml	10 ml vial	Pet's Pharma		VET
Mexico	testosterone enanthate	Enantest 250	250 mg/ml	10 ml vial	Animal Power		VET
Mexico	testosterone enanthate	Primoteston®-Depot	250 mg/ml	1 ml ampule	Schering		
Mexico	testosterone enanthate	Testoenan L/A	250 mg/ml	10 ml vial	Loeffler		VET
Mexico	testosterone enanthate	Testosterona 200	200 mg/ml	10 ml vial	Brovel		VET
Mexico	testosterone enanthate	Testosterone 200 Depot	200 mg/ml	10 ml vial	Tornel		VET
Mexico	testosterone propionate	Ara-Test	25 mg/ml	10 ml vial	Aranda Laboratories	[NLM]	VET
Mexico	testosterone propionate	Oreton	25 mg/ml	n/a	Goldline	[NLM]	
Mexico	testosterone propionate	Propionat QV 100	100 mg/ml	10 ml vial	Quality Vet		VET
Mexico	testosterone propionate	Propiotest 100	100 mg/ml	10 ml vial	Animal Power		VET
Mexico	testosterone propionate	Testopro L/A	250 mg/ml	10 ml vial	Loeffler		VET
Mexico	testosterone propionate	Testosterona	50, 100 mg/ml	10, 20 ml vial	Brovel		VET
Mexico	testosterone propionate (implant)	Synovex®-H (plus estrogen)	25 mg/pellet	80 pellet cartridge	Fort Dodge		
Mexico	testosterone propionate (implant)	Synovex®-H (plus estrogen)	20 mg/pellet	n/a	Syntex	[NLM]	
Mexico	testosterone suspension	Anabolic TS	100 mg/ml	20 ml vial	SYD Group		VET
Mexico	testosterone suspension	Anabolic-TS	100 mg/ml	20 ml vial	Grupo Tarasco	[NLM]	VET
Mexico	testosterone suspension	AquaTest	100 mg/ml	10 ml vial	Denkall		VET
Mexico	testosterone undecanoate	Andriol capsulas	40 mg capsules	30 capsule bottle	Organon		
Mexico	Testoviron (testosterone blend)	Aratest 2500	250 mg/ml	10 ml vial	Aranda		VET
Mexico	Testoviron (testosterone blend)	Testoprim-D	250 mg/ml	1 ml ampule	Labs. Tocogino		
Mexico	trenbolone acetate	Acetrenbo 50	50 mg tablet	20 tablet bottle	Loeffler		VET

Appendix C: Drug Availability Tables - Listings by Country

Country	Generic Name	Trade Name	Dose	Packaging	Company	Status	Vet
Mexico	trenbolone acetate	Finaplix-H®	20 mg pellet	70, 100 pellet cartridge	Roussel	[NLM]	VET
Mexico	trenbolone acetate	Synovex plus (plus estradiol)	25 mg pellet	80 pellet cartridge	Fort Dodge		VET
Mexico	trenbolone acetate	Trembolone QV 75	75 mg/ml	10 ml vial	Quality Vet		VET
Mexico	trenbolone acetate	Trenbo 75	75 mg/ml	10 ml vial	Animal Power		VET
Mexico	trenbolone acetate	Trenbol 75	75 mg/ml	20 ml vial	Ttokkyo	[NLM]	VET
Mexico	trenbolone acetate	Trenbolon 75	75 mg/ml	10, 20 ml vial	Pet's Pharma		VET
Morocco	testosterone enanthate	Androtardyl®	250 mg/ml	1 ml ampule	Schering		
Morocco	testosterone undecanoate	Andriol	40 mg capsules	n/a	Organon		
Mozambique	testosterone enanthate	Weratestone 250	250 mg/ml	1 ml ampule	Weimer Pharma		
Myanmar/Burma	boldenone (blend)	Equilon 100	100 mg/ml	6 ml vial	WDV		VET
Myanmar/Burma	testosterone blend (misc)	Equitest 200	200 mg/ml	6 ml vial	WDV		VET
Myanmar/Burma	testosterone undecanoate	Andriol	40 mg capsules	n/a	Organon		VET
Myanmar/Burma	trenbolone acetate	Trenol 50	50 mg/ml	6 ml vial	WDV		VET
Netherlands	ethylestrenol	Orgabolin	2 mg tablet	n/a	Organon	[NLM]	
Netherlands	fluoxymesterone	Halotestin®	5 mg tablet	n/a	Upjohn	[NLM]	
Netherlands	mesterolone	Proviron®	25 mg tablet	50 tablet bottle	Schering		
Netherlands	methenolone acetate	Primobolan® S	25 mg tablet	n/a	Schering	[NLM]	
Netherlands	nandrolone decanoate	Anabolin Forte	50 mg/ml	10 ml vial	Alfasan		VET
Netherlands	nandrolone decanoate	Deca-Durabolin®	25, 50 mg/ml	1 ml ampule	Organon		
Netherlands	nandrolone decanoate	Deca-Durabolin®	100 mg/ml	2 ml vial	Organon		
Netherlands	nandrolone hexyloxyphenylpropionate	Anadur	25, 50 mg/ml	1, 2 ml ampule	Pharmacia	[NLM]	
Netherlands	nandrolone laurate	Laurabolin V	50 mg/ml	10, 50 ml	Intervet		VET
Netherlands	nandrolone phenylpropionate	Durabolin®	25 mg/ml	1 ml ampule	Organon		
Netherlands	stanozolol (oral)	Stromba	5 mg tablet	100 tablet box	Sanofi		
Netherlands	stanozolol (oral)	Stromba	5 mg tablet	n/a	Winthrop	[NLM]	
Netherlands	Sustanon 100 (testosterone blend)	Sustanon '100'®	100 mg/ml	1 ml ampule	Organon		
Netherlands	Sustanon 250 (testosterone blend)	Sustanon 250®	250 mg/ml	1 ml ampule	Organon		
Netherlands	testosterone (gel)	Androgel	25, 50 mg	single dose packet	Besins		
Netherlands	testosterone (gel)	Testogel	25, 50 mg	single dose packet	Besins		
Netherlands	testosterone (patch)	Andropatch	12.2 mg patch	30, 60 patch box	Schwarz Pharma		
Netherlands	testosterone propionate	Neo-Hombreol	50 mg/ml	n/a	Organon	[NLM]	
Netherlands	testosterone undecanoate	Andriol	40 mg capsules	n/a	Organon		
Netherlands	Testoviron (testosterone blend)	Testoviron® Depot 100	135 mg/ml	1 ml ampule	Schering	[NLM]	
New Zealand	nandrolone decanoate	Deca-Durabolin®	50 mg/ml	1 ml ampule	Organon		
New Zealand	Sustanon 250 (testosterone blend)	Sustanon 250	250 mg/ml	1 ml ampule	Organon		
New Zealand	testosterone cypionate	Depo-Testosterone®	100 mg/ml	10 ml vial	Pharmacia & Upjohn		
New Zealand	testosterone enanthate	Primoteston®-Depot	250 mg/ml	1 ml syringe	Schering		
New Zealand	testosterone undecanoate	Panteston capsules	40 mg capsules	n/a	Organon		
Nicaragua	boldenone undecylenate	Boldenona 50 Gen-Far	50 mg/ml	10, 50, 100, 250ml vial	Gen-Far		VET
Nicaragua	mesterolone	Proviron®	25 mg tablet	n/a	Schering		
Nicaragua	methenolone acetate	Primobolan®	5 mg tablet	n/a	Schering	[NLM]	

Appendix C: Drug Availability Tables - Listings by Country

Country	Generic Name	Trade Name	Dose	Packaging	Company	Status	Vet
Nicaragua	testosterone propionate	Testogan	25 mg/ml	50 ml vial	Laguinsa		VET
Nigeria	testosterone undecanoate	Andriol	40 mg capsules	n/a	Organon		
Norway	fluoxymesterone	Halotestin®	5 mg tablet	n/a	Upjohn	[NLM]	
Norway	mesterolone	Mestoranum	25 mg tablet	n/a	Schering	[NLM]	
Norway	nandrolone decanoate	Deca-Durabolin®	50 mg/ml	1 ml ampule	Organon		
Norway	nandrolone hexyloxyphenylpropionate	Anadur	25, 50 mg/ml	1, 2 ml ampule	Kabi Pharmacia	[NLM]	
Norway	testosterone (patch)	Atmos	5 mg patch	30 patch box	Astra Zenica		
Norway	testosterone enanthate	Primoteston®-Depot	250 mg/ml	1 ml ampule	Schering		
Norway	testosterone undecanoate	Androxon	40 mg capsules	60 capsule bottle	Organon		
Oman	testosterone undecanoate	Andriol	40 mg capsules	n/a	Organon		
Pakistan	ethylestrenol	Orabolin®	2 mg tablet	100 tablet box	Organon		
Pakistan	Sustanon 250 (testosterone blend)	Sustanon '250'®	250 mg/ml	1ml ampule	Organon		
Pakistan	testosterone enanthate	Testoviron®-Depot	250 mg/ml	1 ml ampule	Schering		
Pakistan	testosterone undecanoate	Androxon	40 mg capsules	n/a	Organon		
Panama	boldenone undecylenate	Boldenona 50 Gen-Far	50 mg/ml	10, 50, 100, 250ml vial	Gen-Far		VET
Panama	boldenone undecylenate	Ganabol	50 mg/ml	500 ml vial	Laboratorios VM		VET
Panama	boldenone undecylenate	Ganabol	25, 50 mg/ml	10, 50, 100, 250ml vial	Laboratorios VM		VET
Panama	mesterolone	Proviron®	25 mg tablet	n/a	Schering		
Panama	methenolone acetate	Primobolan®	5 mg tablet	n/a	Schering	[NLM]	
Panama	testosterone propionate	Testogan	25 mg/ml	50 ml vial	Laguinsa		VET
Paraguay	boldenone undecylenate	Ganabol	50 mg/ml	500 ml vial	Laboratorios VM		VET
Paraguay	boldenone undecylenate	Ganabol	25, 50 mg/ml	10, 50, 100, 250ml vial	Laboratorios VM		VET
Paraguay	mesterolone	Proviron®	25 mg tablet	20 tablet box	Schering		
Paraguay	methenolone enanthate	Primobolan® Depot	100 mg/ml	1 ml ampule	Schering		
Paraguay	methyltestosterone	Metiltestosterona	n/a	n/a	Botica		
Paraguay	testosterone enanthate	Testoviron®-Depot	250 mg/ml	1 ml ampule	Schering		
Paraguay	testosterone propionate	Testosterona Propionato	n/a	n/a	Botica		
Peru	boldenone undecylenate	Boldenona 50 Gen-Far	50 mg/ml	10, 50, 100, 250ml vial	Gen-Far		VET
Peru	boldenone undecylenate	Ganabol	50 mg/ml	500 ml vial	Laboratorios VM		VET
Peru	boldenone undecylenate	Ganabol	25, 50 mg/ml	10, 50, 100, 250ml vial	Laboratorios VM		VET
Peru	nandrolone decanoate	Deca-Durabolin®	50 mg/ml	1 ml ampule	Organon		
Peru	testosterone enanthate	Testoviron® Depot	250 mg/ml	1 ml ampule	Schering		
Peru	testosterone undecanoate	Panteston	40 mg capsules	30, 60 capsule bottle	Organon		
Philippines	drostanolone	Dromostan	50 mg/ml	5 ml vial	Xelox (export)		
Philippines	fluoxymesterone	Halotestin®	5 mg tablet	n/a	Pharmacia & Upjohn		
Philippines	mesterolone	Mesterolon	25 mg tablet	n/a	Brown & Burk		
Philippines	nandrolone (blend)	Dinandrol	100 mg/ml	2 ml vial	Xelox (export)		
Philippines	stanozolol (oral)	Anazol	2 mg tablet	100 tablet box	Xelox (export)		
Philippines	stanozolol (oral)	Anazol	2 mg tablet	100, 1000 tablet bottle	Xelox (export)		
Philippines	testosterone cypionate	Vironate	200 mg/ml	5 ml vial	Xelox (export)		
Philippines	testosterone undecanoate	Andriol	40 mg capsules	n/a	Organon		

Appendix C: Drug Availability Tables - Listings by Country

Country	Generic Name	Trade Name	Dose	Packaging	Company	Status	Vet
Poland	mesterolone	Proviron®	25 mg tablet	20 tablet box	Schering		
Poland	methandrostenolone	Metanabol	5 mg tablet	20 tablet box	Jelfa		
Poland	methandrostenolone	Metanabol	5 mg tablet	20 tablet box	Polfa	[NLM]	
Poland	methandrostenolone	Metanabol	l mg tablet	20 tablet box	Polfa	[NLM]	
Poland	methandrostenolone	Metanabol	0.5% cream	n/a	Polfa	[NLM]	
Poland	methylandrostenediol	Metylandrostendiol	10, 25 mg tablet	n/a	Jelfa	[NLM]	
Poland	methyltestosterone	Mesteron	10 mg tablet	n/a	Jelfa	[NLM]	
Poland	nandrolone decanoate	Deca-Durabolin®	25 mg/ml	1 ml ampule	Organon	[NLM]	
Poland	nandrolone decanoate	Deca-Durabolin®	50 mg/ml	1 ml ampule	Organon		
Poland	Omnadren (testosterone blend)	Omnadren	250 mg/ml	1ml ampule	Jelfa		
Poland	Omnadren (testosterone blend)	Omnadren	250 mg/ml	1ml ampule	Polfa	[NLM]	
Poland	testosterone enanthate	Testosteronum Prolongatum	100 mg/ml	1 ml ampule	Jelfa		
Poland	testosterone enanthate	Testosteronum Prolongatum	100 mg/ml	1 ml ampule	Polfa	[NLM]	
Poland	testosterone propionate	Testosteronum Propionicum	25 mg/ml	1 ml ampule	Jelfa		
Poland	testosterone undecanoate	Undestor	40 mg capsules	60 capsule bottle	Organon		
Portugal	drostanolone propionate	Masteron	100 mg/2ml	2 ml amp	Cilag	[NLM]	
Portugal	formebolone	Esiclene	1 mg drops	n/a	Biofarma	[NLM]	
Portugal	formebolone	Esiclene	5 mg tablet	n/a	Biofarma	[NLM]	
Portugal	mesterolone	Proviron®	25 mg tablet	20 tablet box	Schering		
Portugal	methenolone enanthate	Primobolan® Depot	100 mg/ml	1 ml ampule	Schering	[NLM]	
Portugal	methyltestosterone	Testormon	10 mg tablet	n/a	Unitas		
Portugal	nandrolone phenylpropionate	Durabolin®	50 mg/ml	n/a	Organon		
Portugal	oxymetholone	Dynasten	50 mg tablet	n/a	Cilag	[NLM]	
Portugal	stanozolol (oral)	Winstrol®	2 mg tablet	n/a	Winthrop	[NLM]	
Portugal	Sustanon 250 (testosterone blend)	Sustenon 250®	250 mg/ml	1 ml ampule	Organon		
Portugal	testosterone enanthate	Testoviron®-Depot	250 mg/ml	1 ml ampule	Schering		
Portugal	testosterone undecanoate	Andriol	40 mg capsules	n/a	Organon		
Portugal	Testoviron (testosterone blend)	Testoviron® Depot 100	135 mg/ml	1 ml ampule	Schering	[NLM]	
Qatar	testosterone enanthate	Testoviron®-Depot	250 mg/ml	1 ml ampule	Schering	[NLM]	
Qatar	testosterone undecanoate	Andriol	40 mg capsules	n/a	Organon		
Rumania	methandrostenolone	Naposim	5 mg tablet	20 tablet box	Terapia		
Rumania	methyltestosterone	Metil Testosteron	10 mg tablet	50 tablet box	Terapia		
Rumania	nandrolone decanoate	Anabolin Forte	50 mg/ml	10 ml vial	Alfasan		VET
Rumania	nandrolone decanoate	Deca-Durabolin®	50 mg/ml	1 ml ampule	Organon		
Rumania	nandrolone decanoate	Decanofort	25 mg/ml	1 ml ampule	Terapia		
Rumania	testosterone phenylpropionate	Testolent	100 mg/ml	1 ml ampule	Sicomed	[NLM]	
Rumania	testosterone propionate	Testosteron	25 mg/ml	1 ml ampule	Sicomed	[NLM]	
Rumania	testosterone undecanoate	Undestor	40 mg capsules	60 capsule bottle	Organon		
Russia	ethylestrenol	Silabolin	25, 50 mg/ml	1 ml ampule	Farmadon	[NLM]	
Russia	mesterolone	Proviron®	25 mg tablet	20 tablet bottle	Schering		
Russia	methandrostenolone	Metandienon	5 mg tablet	100 tablet box	Bioreaktor		

Appendix C: Drug Availability Tables - Listings by Country

Country	Generic Name	Trade Name	Dose	Packaging	Company	Status	Vet
Russia	methandrostenolone	Metandrostenolon	5 mg tablet	100 tablet box	Akrihin	[NLM]	
Russia	methandrostenolone	Metandrostenolon	5 mg tablet	100 tablet box	Akrikhin		
Russia	methandrostenolone	Metandrostenolon	5 mg tablet	100 tablet box	Bioreaktor	[NLM]	
Russia	nandrolone decanoate	Retabolin	50 mg/ml	1 ml ampule	Medexport Russia	[NLM]	
Russia	nandrolone phenylpropionate	Fenobolin	20 mg/ml	n/a	Medexport Russia	[NLM]	
Russia	Sustanon 250 (testosterone blend)	Sustanon (Cyctahoh 250)	250 mg/ml	1 ml ampule	Organon		
Russia	testosterone enanthate	Testenat 10%	100 mg/ml	1 ml ampule	Farmadon		
Russia	testosterone propionate	Testosterona Propionat	50, 100 mg/ml	1 ml ampule	Farmadon	[NLM]	
Russia	testosterone undecanoate	Andriol	40 mg capsules	n/a	Organon		
Russia	Testoviron (testosterone blend)	Testenat	100 mg/ml	1 ml ampule	Farmadon	[NLM]	
Saudi Arabia	testosterone enanthate	Testoviron®-Depot	250 mg/ml	1 ml ampule	Schering		
Saudi Arabia	testosterone undecanoate	Andriol	40 mg capsules	n/a	Organon		
Singapore	mesterolone	Provironum	25 mg tablet	50 tablet box	Organon		
Singapore	nandrolone decanoate	Deca-Durabolin®	25 mg/ml	1 ml ampule	Organon		
Singapore	Sustanon 250 (testosterone blend)	Sustanon "250"	250 mg/ml	1 ml ampule	Organon		
Singapore	testosterone cypionate	Depo-Testosterone®	100 mg/ml	10 ml vial	Pharmacia & Upjohn		
Singapore	testosterone undecanoate	Andriol	40 mg capsules	60 capsule bottle	Organon		
Slovakia	mesterolone	Proviron®	25 mg tablet	20, 50 tablet bottle	Schering		
Slovakia	Sustanon 250 (testosterone blend)	Sustanon	250 mg/ml	1 ml ampule	Organon		
Slovakia	testosterone undecanoate	Undestor	40 mg capsules	n/a	Organon		
South Africa	ethylestrenol	Orabolin®	2 mg tablet	n/a	Donmed/Organon	[NLM]	
South Africa	mesterolone	Proviron®	25 mg tablet	20, 100 tablet bottle	Schering/Berlimed		
South Africa	methenolone acetate	Primobolan®	5 mg tablet	n/a	Schering/Berlimed	[NLM]	
South Africa	methenolone acetate	Primobolan® S	25 mg tablet	50 tablet bottle	Schering/Berlimed		
South Africa	methenolone enanthate	Primobolan® Depot	100 mg/ml	1 ml ampule	Schering/Berlimed	[NLM]	
South Africa	nandrolone decanoate	Deca-Durabolin®	25, 50 mg/ml	1 ml ampule	Donmed/Organon		
South Africa	Sustanon 250 (testosterone blend)	Sustanon '250'®	250 mg/ml	1 ml ampule	Donmed/Organon		
South Africa	testosterone cypionate	Depo-Testosterone	100 mg/ml	10 ml vial	Pharmacia & Upjohn		
South Africa	testosterone cypionate	Depotrone	100 mg/ml	2 ml ampule	Propan-Zurich		
South Africa	testosterone undecanoate	Androxon	40 mg capsules	60 capsule bottle	Donmed/Organon		
Spain	drostanolone propionate	Metormon	100 mg/2ml	2 ml amp	Syntex	[NLM]	
Spain	formebolone	Hubernol	5 mg dragee	n/a	ICN Hubber	[NLM]	
Spain	formebolone	Hubernol	1 mg drops	n/a	ICN Hubber	[NLM]	
Spain	mesterolone	Proviron®	25 mg tablet	20 tablet box	Schering	[NLM]	
Spain	mesterolone	Proviron®	25 mg tablet	20 tablet box	Scherimed		
Spain	methenolone enanthate	Primobolan® Depot	100 mg/ml	1 ml ampule	Schering	[NLM]	
Spain	methenolone enanthate	Primobolan® Depot	100 mg/ml	1 ml ampule	Scherimed		
Spain	methyltestosterone	Longivol (plus estrogen)	1 mg tablet	n/a	Medical S.A.		
Spain	nandrolone decanoate	Anabolin Forte	50 mg/ml	10, 50 ml vial	Alfasan		VET
Spain	nandrolone decanoate	Deca-Durabolin®	25, 50 mg/ml	1 ml ampule	Organon		
Spain	nandrolone hexyloxyphenylpropionate	Anadur	25 mg/ml	2 ml ampule	Leo	[NLM]	

Appendix C: Drug Availability Tables - Listings by Country

Country	Generic Name	Trade Name	Dose	Packaging	Company	Status	Vet
Spain	nandrolone phenylpropionate	Activin	10 mg/ml	n/a	Aristegvi	[NLM]	
Spain	nandrolone phenylpropionate	Durabolin®	25 mg/ml	1 ml ampule	Organon	[NLM]	
Spain	nandrolone phenylpropionate	Fherbolico	50 mg/ml	n/a	Fher	[NLM]	
Spain	oxymetholone	Oxitosona 50	50 mg tablet	100 tablet box	Syntex	[NLM]	
Spain	stanozolol (inj)	Winstrol® Depot	50 mg/ml	1 ml ampule	Zambon		
Spain	stanozolol (oral)	Winstrol®	2 mg tablet	20 tablet box	Zambon		
Spain	Sustanon 250 (testosterone blend)	Durandron	250 mg/ml	1 ml ampule	Organon	[NLM]	
Spain	Sustanon 250 (testosterone blend)	Sostenon 250®	250 mg/ml	1 ml ampule	Organon	[NLM]	
Spain	testosterone (patch)	Androderm®	2.5 mg patch	30, 60 patch box	Schwarz Pharma		
Spain	testosterone (patch)	Androderm®	5 mg patch	30 patch box	Schwarz Pharma		
Spain	testosterone (patch)	Testoderm	6 mg patch	10, 30 patch box	Esteve		
Spain	testosterone (patch)	Testoderm	4 mg patch	10 patch box	Esteve		
Spain	testosterone cypionate	Testex Leo prolongatum	50, 125 mg/ml	2 ml ampule	Altana Pharma		
Spain	testosterone cypionate	Testex Leo prolongatum	50, 125 mg/ml	2 ml ampule	Leo	[NLM]	
Spain	testosterone enanthate	Testoviron®-Depot	250 mg/ml	1 ml ampule	Schering	[NLM]	
Spain	testosterone enanthate	Testoviron®-Depot	250 mg/ml	1 ml ampule	Scherimed		
Spain	testosterone propionate	Testex Leo	25 mg/ml	1 ml ampule	Altana Pharma		
Spain	testosterone propionate	Testex Leo	25 mg/ml	1 ml ampule	Leo	[NLM]	
Spain	testosterone propionate	Testoviron®	10, 25 mg/ml	1 ml ampule	Schering	[NLM]	
Spain	Testoviron (testosterone blend)	Testoviron® Depot 100	135 mg/ml	1 ml ampule	Schering	[NLM]	
Spain	Testoviron (testosterone blend)	Testoviron® Depot 50	75 mg/ml	1 ml ampule	Schering	[NLM]	
Sri Lanka	testosterone enanthate	Testoviron®-Depot	250 mg/ml	1 ml ampule	Schering		
Sri Lanka	testosterone undecanoate	Andriol	40 mg capsules	n/a	Organon		
Sudan	testosterone enanthate	Primoteston®-Depot	250 mg/ml	1 ml ampule	Schering		
Sweden	fluoxymesterone	Halotestin®	5 mg tablet	n/a	Upjohn	[NLM]	
Sweden	mesterolone	Mesterolon	25 mg tablet	n/a	Schering	[NLM]	
Sweden	nandrolone decanoate	Deca-Durabolin®	50 mg/ml	1 ml ampule	Organon		
Sweden	nandrolone decanoate	Deca-Durabolin®	25, 100 mg/ml	1, 2 ml	Organon	[NLM]	
Sweden	oxymetholone	Anasteron	50 mg tablet	n/a	Syntex	[NLM]	
Sweden	stanozolol (inj)	Stromba	50 mg/ml	n/a	Sterling-Winthrop	[NLM]	
Sweden	stanozolol (inj)	Stromba	50 mg/ml	n/a	Winthrop	[NLM]	
Sweden	stanozolol (oral)	Stromba	5 mg tablet	n/a	Winthrop	[NLM]	
Sweden	testosterone (gel)	Androgel	25, 50 mg	single dose packet	Besins		
Sweden	testosterone (gel)	Testogel	25, 50 mg	single dose packet	Besins		
Sweden	testosterone (patch)	Atmos	5 mg patch	n/a	Astra		
Sweden	testosterone enanthate	Testoviron®-Depot	250 mg/ml	1 ml ampule	Schering		
Sweden	testosterone undecanoate	Undestor	40 mg capsules	n/a	Organon		
Sweden	Testoviron (testosterone blend)	Testoviron® Depot 135	135 mg/ml	1 ml ampule	Schering	[NLM]	
Switzerland	boldenone undecylenate	Vebonol	25 mg/ml	10 ml vial	Ciba-Geigy	[NLM]	VET
Switzerland	mesterolone	Proviron®	25 mg tablet	n/a	Schering	[NLM]	
Switzerland	methenolone enanthate	Primobolan® Depot	100 mg/ml	1 ml ampule	Schering	[NLM]	

Appendix C: Drug Availability Tables - Listings by Country

Country	Generic Name	Trade Name	Dose	Packaging	Company	Status	Vet
Switzerland	nandrolone decanoate	Deca-Durabolin®	25 mg/ml	1 ml ampule	Organon	[NLM]	
Switzerland	nandrolone decanoate	Deca-Durabolin®	50 mg/ml	1 ml ampule	Organon		
Switzerland	nandrolone hexyloxyphenylpropionate	Anadur	25, 50 mg/ml	1, 2 ml ampule	Kabi Pharmacia	[NLM]	
Switzerland	nandrolone phenylpropionate	Durabolin®	25 mg/ml	n/a	Opopharma	[NLM]	
Switzerland	norethandrolone	Nilevar	10 mg tablet	30 tablet bottle	Searle	[NLM]	
Switzerland	oxymetholone	Plenastril	50 mg tablet	n/a	Proto chemie	[NLM]	
Switzerland	stanozolol (oral)	Stromba	5 mg tablet	n/a	Winthrop	[NLM]	
Switzerland	testosterone (patch)	Androderm®	12.2 mg patch	n/a	Astrazenica		
Switzerland	testosterone enanthate	Testoviron®-Depot	250 mg/ml	1 ml ampule	Schering		
Switzerland	testosterone propionate	Testosteron	50 mg/ml	1 ml ampule	Streuli & Co. AG	[NLM]	
Switzerland	testosterone propionate	Triolandren	20 mg/ml	n/a	Ciba Geigy CH	[NLM]	
Switzerland	testosterone undecanoate	Andriol	40 mg capsules	n/a	Organon		
Switzerland	Testoviron (testosterone blend)	Testoviron® Depot 100	135 mg/ml	1 ml ampule	Schering	[NLM]	
Taiwan	fluoxymesterone	Baojen	5 mg capsule	n/a	Ta Fong		
Taiwan	fluoxymesterone	Chinglicosan	5 mg capsule	n/a	Ciiphar		
Taiwan	fluoxymesterone	Flouoxymesterone cap	5 mg capsule	n/a	Yuan Chou		
Taiwan	fluoxymesterone	Floxymesterone	5 mg capsule	n/a	Chen Ho		
Taiwan	fluoxymesterone	Fosteron	5 mg capsule	n/a	Health Chemical		
Taiwan	fluoxymesterone	Fu Lao Shu	10 mg capsule	n/a	Ming Ta		
Taiwan	fluoxymesterone	Fuloan	10 mg capsule	n/a	New Chem & Pharm		
Taiwan	fluoxymesterone	Lipaw	10 mg capsule	n/a	Long Der		
Taiwan	fluoxymesterone	Long	10 mg capsule	n/a	Century		
Taiwan	fluoxymesterone	ODK	5 mg capsule	n/a	Winston		
Taiwan	fluoxymesterone	Oralsterone	5 mg capsule	n/a	Long Der		
Taiwan	fluoxymesterone	Sidomon	5 mg capsule	n/a	n/a		
Taiwan	fluoxymesterone	Tealigen	5 mg capsule	n/a	Ming ta		
Taiwan	fluoxymesterone	Ton Lin	10 mg capsule	n/a	Chin Teng		
Taiwan	fluoxymesterone	Vewon	5 mg tablet	n/a	Yung Shin		
Taiwan	fluoxymesterone	Vi Jane	10 mg capsule	n/a	Shyh Sar		
Taiwan	fluoxymesterone	Waromom	5 mg tablet	n/a	Washington		
Taiwan	mesterolone	Proviron	25 mg tablet	50 tablet box	Schering		
Taiwan	mesterolone	Vistimon	25 mg tablet	30 tablet box	Jenapharm		
Taiwan	methandrostenolone	Chinlipan Tab	2 mg tablet	n/a	Chin Tien		
Taiwan	nandrolone decanoate	Deca-Durabolin®	50 mg/ml	1 ml ampule	Organon		
Taiwan	nandrolone phenylpropionate	Daily Reborn Inj	25 mg/ml	n/a	Shiteh		
Taiwan	nandrolone phenylpropionate	Durabolin®	25 mg/ml	2 ml vial	Organon		
Taiwan	nandrolone phenylpropionate	Macrabone	25 mg/ml	n/a	Ta Fong		
Taiwan	nandrolone phenylpropionate	Metrobolin	25 mg/ml	n/a	Metro		
Taiwan	nandrolone phenylpropionate	Protosin Inj	25 mg/ml	n/a	Astar		
Taiwan	nandrolone phenylpropionate	Rubolin	25 mg/ml	n/a	Ying Yuan		
Taiwan	nandrolone phenylpropionate	Sinbolin	25 mg/ml	n/a	Sinton		

Appendix C: Drug Availability Tables - Listings by Country

Country	Generic Name	Trade Name	Dose	Packaging	Company	Status	Vet
Taiwan	stanozolol (oral)	Stanol	2 mg tablet	n/a	Hua Shin		
Taiwan	stanozolol (oral)	Stanozolol Tab	2 mg tablet	n/a	Chen Ho		
Taiwan	Sustanon 250 (testosterone blend)	Sustanon 250	250 mg/ml	1 ml ampule	Organon		
Taiwan	testosterone blend (misc)	Triolandren	250 mg/ml	1 ml ampule	Novartis		
Taiwan	testosterone cypionate	Biselmon Depot	50 mg/ml	n/a	Ta Fong		
Taiwan	testosterone cypionate	Cyclo-Testosterone Depot	130 mg/ml	n/a	Astar		
Taiwan	testosterone cypionate	Depot-Bifuron	50 mg/ml	n/a	Gentle		
Taiwan	testosterone cypionate	Depo-Testermon	200 mg/ml	n/a	CCPC		
Taiwan	testosterone cypionate	Depo-Testerone	200 mg/ml	n/a	Metro		
Taiwan	testosterone cypionate	Depo-Testomon	100 mg/ml	n/a	Li Ta		
Taiwan	testosterone cypionate	Depo-Testosterone CPP	100 mg/ml	n/a	Metro		
Taiwan	testosterone cypionate	Depot-Hormon MF	50 mg/ml	n/a	Sintong		
Taiwan	testosterone cypionate	Nannismon Depot	50, 100 mg/ml	n/a	Chi Sheng		
Taiwan	testosterone cypionate	Testorone Depot	100 mg/ml	n/a	Gentle		
Taiwan	testosterone cypionate	Testosterone Cypionate Inj	200 mg/ml	n/a	Gwo Chyang		
Taiwan	testosterone cypionate	Testosterone Cypionate Inj	200 mg/ml	n/a	Tai Yu		
Taiwan	testosterone enanthate	DepoTestmon Inj	65 mg/ml	n/a	CCPC		
Taiwan	testosterone enanthate	Sunamon Depot Inj	130 mg/ml	n/a	Astar		
Taiwan	testosterone enanthate	Sunamon Inj	250 mg/ml	n/a	Astar		
Taiwan	testosterone enanthate	Testenan Depot	250 mg/ml	n/a	Sinton		
Taiwan	testosterone enanthate	Testermon	25 mg/ml	n/a	CCPC		
Taiwan	testosterone enanthate	Testoviron Depot	250 mg/ml	1 ml ampule	Schering		
Taiwan	testosterone propionate	Nansmon Depot	25 mg/ml	n/a	Chi Sheng		
Taiwan	testosterone propionate	Testosteron Depot	25 mg/ml	n/a	Gentle		
Taiwan	testosterone propionate	Testosterone Propionate Inj	25 mg/ml	n/a	Tai Yu		
Taiwan	testosterone undecanoate	Restandol	40 mg capsules	n/a	Organon		
Thailand	boldenone undecylenate	Boldabol	200 mg/ml	10 ml vial	British Dragon		
Thailand	chlorodehydromethyltestosterone	Turanabol	10 mg tablet	500 tablet pouch	British Dragon		
Thailand	drostanolone propionate	Mastabol	50 mg/ml	10 ml vial	British Dragon	[NLM]	
Thailand	drostanolone propionate	Mastabol	100 mg/ml	10 ml vial	British Dragon		
Thailand	fluoxymesterone	Halotestin®	5 mg tablet	100 tablet bottle	Pharmacia		
Thailand	mesterolone	Provironum	25 mg tablet	150 tablet box	Schering		
Thailand	methandrostenolone	Ammipire	5 mg tablet	1000 tablet bottle	Ammipire		
Thailand	methandrostenolone	Anabol	50 mg tablet	n/a	British Dragon	[NLM]	
Thailand	methandrostenolone	Anabol Tablets	5 mg tablet	1000 tablet bottle	British Dispensary		
Thailand	methandrostenolone	Anabol Tablets	5 mg tablet	1000 tablet bottle	L.P Standard	[NLM]	
Thailand	methandrostenolone	Averbol 25	25 mg/ml	20 ml vial	British Dragon		
Thailand	methandrostenolone	Danabol DS	10 mg tablet	500 tablet bottle	Body Research		
Thailand	methandrostenolone	Melic	5 mg tablet	1000 tablet box, bottle	Pharmasant		
Thailand	methandrostenolone	Methanabol	5 mg tablet	500 tablet pouch	British Dragon	[NLM]	
Thailand	methandrostenolone	Methanabol	10 mg tablet	500 tablet pouch	British Dragon		

Appendix C: Drug Availability Tables - Listings by Country

Country	Generic Name	Trade Name	Dose	Packaging	Company	Status	Vet
Thailand	methandrostenolone	Methanabol	50 mg tablet	100 tablet pouch	British Dragon		
Thailand	methandrostenolone	Methandon	5 mg tablet	1000 tablet bottle	Acdhon Co.		
Thailand	methenolone acetate	Primobolan® S	25 mg tablet	n/a	Schering	[NLM]	
Thailand	methenolone enanthate	Primobol	100 mg/ml	10 ml vial	British Dragon		
Thailand	methyltestosterone	Metesto	25 mg tablet	100 tablet bottle	Acdhon		
Thailand	methyltestosterone	TP Men Hormone	10 mg dragee	24 tablets	TP Drugs		
Thailand	nandrolone decanoate	Decabol	250 mg/ml	10 ml vial	British Dragon		
Thailand	nandrolone decanoate	Deca-Durabolin®	25, 50 mg/ml	1 ml ampule	Organon		
Thailand	nandrolone phenylpropionate	Durabol	200 mg/ml	10 ml vial	British Dragon		
Thailand	nandrolone phenylpropionate	Durabol	100 mg/ml	10 ml vial	British Dragon	[NLM]	
Thailand	nandrolone phenylpropionate	Norabon	25 mg/ml	1 ml ampule	Phihalab		
Thailand	oxandrolone	Bonavar	2.5 mg tablet	10 tablet strip	Body Research		
Thailand	oxandrolone	Oxanabol	5 mg tablet	100 tablet pouch	British Dragon	[NLM]	
Thailand	oxandrolone	Oxanabol	10 mg tablet	100 tablet pouch	British Dragon		
Thailand	oxymetholone	Androlic	50 mg tablet	100 tablet bottle	British Dispensary		
Thailand	oxymetholone	Androlic	50 mg tablet	100 tablet pouch	British Dispensary	[NLM]	
Thailand	oxymetholone	Androlic (Export)	50 mg tablet	20 tablet pouch	British Dragon		
Thailand	oxymetholone	Bonalone	50 mg tablet	100 tablet bottle	Body Research		
Thailand	oxymetholone	Oxydrol	50 mg tablet	100 tablet pouch	British Dragon		
Thailand	oxymetholone	Oxydrol	100 mg tablet	50 tablet pouch	British Dragon	[NLM]	
Thailand	oxymetholone	Oxymetholone	50 mg tablet	100 tablet pouch	British Dispensary	[NLM]	
Thailand	oxymetholone	Oxytone 50	50 mg tablet	100 tablet bottle	SB Laboratories		
Thailand	stanozolol	Stanozolol	10 mg tablet	100 tablet pouch	British Dispensary		
Thailand	stanozolol (oral)	Cetabon	2 mg tablet	10 tablet strip	Therapharma		
Thailand	stanozolol (oral)	Stanabol	5 mg tablet	250 tablet pouch	British Dragon	[NLM]	
Thailand	stanozolol (oral)	Stanabol	5 mg tablet	200, 1000 tablet bottle	British Dragon	[NLM]	
Thailand	stanozolol (oral)	Stanabol	5 mg tablet	200 tablet pouch	British Dragon	[NLM]	
Thailand	stanozolol (oral)	Stanabol	10 mg tablet	100 tablet pouch	British Dragon		
Thailand	stanozolol (oral)	Stanabol	50 mg tablet	100 tablet pouch	British Dragon		
Thailand	stanozolol (oral)	Stanol	5 mg tablet	200 tablet bottle	Body Research		
Thailand	stanozolol (oral)	Stanozodon	2 mg tablet	1000 tablet bottle	Acdhon Co.		
Thailand	stanozolol (oral)	Stanzol	5 mg tablet	200 tablet bottle	SB Laboratories		
Thailand	Sustanon 250 (testosterone blend)	Andropen 275	275mg/ml	10 ml vial	British Dragon		
Thailand	Sustanon 250 (testosterone blend)	Sustanon '250'®	250 mg/ml	1 ml ampule	Organon		
Thailand	testosterone cypionate	Cypionax	100 mg/ml	2 ml ampule	Body Research		
Thailand	testosterone cypionate	Testabol Depot	200 mg/ml	10 ml vial	British Dragon		
Thailand	testosterone enanthate	Testoviron®-Depot	250 mg/ml	1 ml ampule	Schering		
Thailand	testosterone propionate	Testabol Propionate	100 mg/ml	10 ml vial	British Dragon		
Thailand	testosterone propionate	Testolic	50 mg/ml	2 ml ampule	Body Research		
Thailand	testosterone propionate	Virormone	50, 100 mg/ml	1 ml ampule	Paines		
Thailand	testosterone undecanoate	Andriol	40 mg capsules	10 capsule strip	Organon		

Appendix C: Drug Availability Tables - Listings by Country

Country	Generic Name	Trade Name	Dose	Packaging	Company	Status	Vet
Thailand	trenbolone (blend)	Trinabol 150	150 mg/ml	10 ml vial	British Dragon		
Thailand	trenbolone acetate	Parabolan Tabs (Export)	25 mg tablet	20 tablet pouch	British Dragon		
Thailand	trenbolone acetate	Trenabol	75 mg/ml	10 ml vial	British Dragon		
Thailand	trenbolone hexahydrobenzylcarbonate	Danabolan	76 mg/ml	1.5 ml ampule	Body Research		
Thailand	trenbolone hexahydrobenzylcarbonate	Trenabol Depot	100 mg/ml	10 ml vial	British Dragon		
Tunisia	testosterone enanthate	Androtardyl®	250 mg/ml	1 ml ampule	Schering		
Tunisia	testosterone undecanoate	Andriol	40 mg capsules	n/a	Organon		
Turkey	ethylestrenol	Orgabolin	2 mg tablet	n/a	Santa	[NLM]	
Turkey	ethylestrenol	Orgabolin Drops	2 mg	n/a	Santa	[NLM]	
Turkey	mesterolone	Proviron	25 mg tablet	20 tablet box	Schering		
Turkey	methenolone enanthate	Primobolan® Depot	100 mg/ml	1 ml ampule	Schering		
Turkey	methyltestosterone	Afro	25 mg tablet	40 tablet box	Casel		
Turkey	methyltestosterone	Hormobin	5 mg tablet	40 tablet box	Munrin Sahin		
Turkey	nandrolone decanoate	Jebolan	50 mg/ml	1 ml ampule	Etem	[NLM]	
Turkey	nandrolone hexyloxyphenylpropionate	Anadur	25 mg/ml	2 ml ampule	Eczacibasi	[NLM]	
Turkey	oxymetholone	Anapolon	50 mg tablet	20 tablet box	Ibrahim		
Turkey	oxymetholone	Anapolon	2.5, 5 mg tablet	20 tablet box	Ibrahim	[NLM]	
Turkey	Sustanon 250 (testosterone blend)	Sustanon 250®	250 mg/ml	1 ml ampule	Organon		
Turkey	testosterone undecanoate	Virigen	40 mg capsules	30 capsule bottle	Organon		
U.S.	boldenone undecylenate	Equipoise®	50 mg/ml	50 ml vial	Fort Dodge		VET
U.S.	boldenone undecylenate	Equipoise®	25, 50 mg/ml	50 ml vial	Squibb	[NLM]	VET
U.S.	drostanolone propionate	Drolban	50 mg/1ml	1 ml vial	Lilly	[NLM]	
U.S.	ethylestrenol	Maxibolin	2 mg tablet	n/a	Organon	[NLM]	
U.S.	ethylestrenol	Maxibolin Elixir	2 mg/5ml	n/a	Organon	[NLM]	
U.S.	fluoxymesterone	Android-F	10 mg tablet	100 tablet bottle	Brown	[NLM]	
U.S.	fluoxymesterone	Fluoxymesterone	10 mg tablet	100 tablet bottle	Rosemont		
U.S.	fluoxymesterone	Halotestin®	2, 5, 10 mg tablet	100 tablet bottle	Pharmacia & Upjohn		
U.S.	fluoxymesterone	Halotestin®	10 mg tablet	100 tablet bottle	Warner-Chilcott	[NLM]	
U.S.	fluoxymesterone	Hysterone	20 mg tablet	100 tablet bottle	Major	[NLM]	
U.S.	fluoxymesterone	Ora-Testryl	5 mg tablet	100 tablet bottle	Squibb Mark	[NLM]	
U.S.	methandrostenolone	Dialone	5 mg tablet	100 tablet bottle	Major	[NLM]	
U.S.	methandrostenolone	Dianabol	5 mg tablet	100 tablet bottle	Ciba	[NLM]	
U.S.	methylandrostenediol	Methyldiol	2 mg tablet	n/a	Vortech	[NLM]	
U.S.	methylandrostenediol	Methyldiol Aqueous	50 mg/ml	n/a	Vortech	[NLM]	
U.S.	methylandrostenediol dipropionate	Arbolic	50 mg/ml	n/a	Burgin Arden	[NLM]	
U.S.	methylandrostenediol dipropionate	Crestabolic	50 mg/ml	n/a	Nutrition	[NLM]	
U.S.	methylandrostenediol dipropionate	Durandrol	50 mg/ml	n/a	Pharmex	[NLM]	
U.S.	methylandrostenediol dipropionate	Hybolin	50 mg/ml	n/a	Hyrex	[NLM]	
U.S.	methyltestosterone	Android	5, 10, 25 mg tablet	60 tablet bottle	ICN Pharm		
U.S.	methyltestosterone	Android	5, 10, 25 mg tablet	n/a	Brown	[NLM]	
U.S.	methyltestosterone	Arcosterone	10 mg sub.	n/a	Acrum	[NLM]	

Appendix C: Drug Availability Tables - Listings by Country

Country	Generic Name	Trade Name	Dose	Packaging	Company	Status	Vet
U.S.	methyltestosterone	Arcosterone	10, 25 mg tablet	n/a	Acrum	[NLM]	
U.S.	methyltestosterone	Mediatric	10 mg tablet	n/a	Wyeth-Ayerst	[NLM]	
U.S.	methyltestosterone	Metandren	5 mg sub. dragee	n/a	Ciba	[NLM]	
U.S.	methyltestosterone	Metandren	10, 25 mg tablet	n/a	Ciba	[NLM]	
U.S.	methyltestosterone	Metandren	10, 25 mg tablet	100 tablet bottle	Novartis	[NLM]	
U.S.	methyltestosterone	Methyltestosterone	10 mg tablet	n/a	Global		
U.S.	methyltestosterone	Methyltestosterone	10 mg tablet	n/a	Goldline	[NLM]	
U.S.	methyltestosterone	Oreton Methyl	10 mg tablet	n/a	Schering	[NLM]	
U.S.	methyltestosterone	Oreton Methyl	10 mg sub. tablet	n/a	Schering	[NLM]	
U.S.	methyltestosterone	Testred	10 mg capsule	100 capsule bottle	ICN		
U.S.	methyltestosterone	Virilon (time released)	10 mg capsule	100,1000 capsule bottle	Star		
U.S.	mibolerone	Cheque Drops	100 mcg/ml	55 mg bottle	Upjohn	[NLM]	VET
U.S.	mibolerone	mibolerone drops	100 mcg/ml	55 mg bottle	Wedgewood		VET
U.S.	nandrolone decanoate	Androlone-D 200	200 mg/ml	1 ml	Keene	[NLM]	
U.S.	nandrolone decanoate	Deca-Durabolin®	100 mg/ml	1, 2 ml vial	Organon	[NLM]	
U.S.	nandrolone decanoate	Deca-Durabolin®	200 mg/ml	1 ml vial	Organon	[NLM]	
U.S.	nandrolone decanoate	Hybolin Decanoate	50, 100 mg/ml	1, 2 ml vial	Hyrex		
U.S.	nandrolone decanoate	Nandrobolic L.A.	100 mg/ml	1, 2 ml vial	Forest	[NLM]	
U.S.	nandrolone decanoate	nandrolone decanoate	100 mg/ml	1, 2 ml vial	Lyphomed	[NLM]	
U.S.	nandrolone decanoate	nandrolone decanoate	100 mg/ml	1, 2 ml vial	Quad	[NLM]	
U.S.	nandrolone decanoate	nandrolone decanoate	50, 100, 200 mg/ml	1, 2 ml vial	Steris	[NLM]	
U.S.	nandrolone decanoate	Nandrolone Decanoate Inj	100 mg/ml	2 ml vial	Watson Pharma		
U.S.	nandrolone decanoate	Nandrolone Decanoate Inj	200 mg/ml	1 ml vial	Watson Pharma		
U.S.	nandrolone decanoate	Neo-Durabolic	100, 200 mg/ml	1, 2 ml vial	Hauck	[NLM]	
U.S.	nandrolone phenylpropionate	Anabolin	50 mg/ml	n/a	Alto	[NLM]	
U.S.	nandrolone phenylpropionate	Anabolin-IM	50 mg/ml	n/a	Alto	[NLM]	
U.S.	nandrolone phenylpropionate	Anabolin-LA	100 mg/ml	n/a	Alto	[NLM]	
U.S.	nandrolone phenylpropionate	Androlone	50 mg/ml	n/a	Keene	[NLM]	
U.S.	nandrolone phenylpropionate	Durabolin®	25, 50 mg/ml	n/a	Organon	[NLM]	
U.S.	nandrolone phenylpropionate	Equibolin-50	50 mg/ml	n/a	Vortech	[NLM]	
U.S.	nandrolone phenylpropionate	Hybolin	25, 50 mg/ml	n/a	Hyrex	[NLM]	
U.S.	nandrolone phenylpropionate	Nandrobolic	25 mg/ml	n/a	Forest	[NLM]	
U.S.	nandrolone phenylpropionate	nandrolone phenylpropionate	50 mg/ml	n/a	Quad	[NLM]	
U.S.	nandrolone phenylpropionate	Nu-Bolic	25 mg/ml	n/a	Seatrace	[NLM]	
U.S.	norethandrolone	Nilevar	10 mg tablet	100 tablet bottle	Searle		
U.S.	oxandrolone	Anavar	2.5 mg tablet	100 tablet bottle	Searle	[NLM]	
U.S.	oxandrolone	Oxandrin®	2.5, 10 mg tablet	100 tablet bottle	BTG		
U.S.	oxymetholone	Anadrol 50®	50 mg tablet	100 tablet bottle	Unimed		
U.S.	oxymetholone	Anadrol 50®	50 mg tablet	100 tablet bottle	Syntex	[NLM]	
U.S.	stanozolol (inj)	Winstrol® V	50 mg/ml	10, 30ml vial	Pharmacia & Upjohn		VET
U.S.	stanozolol (inj)	Winstrol® V	50 mg/ml	10, 30ml vial	Winthrop	[NLM]	VET

Appendix C: Drug Availability Tables - Listings by Country

Country	Generic Name	Trade Name	Dose	Packaging	Company	Status	Vet
U.S.	stanozolol (oral)	Winstrol®	2 mg tablet	100 tablet bottle	Sanofi		
U.S.	stanozolol (oral)	Winstrol®	2 mg tablet	100 tablet bottle	Upjohn	[NLM]	
U.S.	stanozolol (oral)	Winstrol®	2 mg tablet	100 tablet bottle	Winthrop	[NLM]	
U.S.	stanozolol (oral)	Winstrol-V®	2 mg tablet	100 tablet bottle	Pharmacia & Upjohn		VET
U.S.	stanozolol (oral)	Winstrol-V®	2 mg chewable tab	100 tablet bottle	Pharmacia & Upjohn		VET
U.S.	testosterone (gel)	Androgel	50, 75, 100 mg	single dose packet	Unimed		
U.S.	testosterone (patch)	Androderm®	12.2 mg patch	60 patches/box	SmithKline Beecham	[NLM]	
U.S.	testosterone (patch)	Androderm®	12.2, 24.3 mg patch	60 patches/box	Watson Pharma		
U.S.	testosterone cypionate	Andro-Cyp	100, 200 mg/ml	10 ml vial	Brown	[NLM]	
U.S.	testosterone cypionate	Andro-Cyp	100, 200 mg/ml	10 ml vial	Keene	[NLM]	
U.S.	testosterone cypionate	Andronaq LA	100, 200 mg/ml	10 ml vial	Central	[NLM]	
U.S.	testosterone cypionate	Andronate	100, 200 mg/ml	10 ml vial	Pasadena	[NLM]	
U.S.	testosterone cypionate	Dep Andro-100-200	100, 200 mg/ml	10 ml vial	Forest	[NLM]	
U.S.	testosterone cypionate	Depotest	100, 200 mg/ml	10 ml vial	Hyrex	[NLM]	
U.S.	testosterone cypionate	Depotest	100, 200 mg/ml	10 ml vial	Kay	[NLM]	
U.S.	testosterone cypionate	Depo-Testosterone®	100, 200 mg/ml	10 ml vial	Pharmacia & Upjohn		
U.S.	testosterone cypionate	Depo-Testosterone®	200 mg/ml	1 ml vial	Pharmacia & Upjohn		
U.S.	testosterone cypionate	Dep-Test	100 mg/ml	10 ml vial	Rocky Mountain	[NLM]	
U.S.	testosterone cypionate	D-Test 100/200	100, 200 mg/ml	10 ml vial	Sig	[NLM]	
U.S.	testosterone cypionate	Duratest-100-200	100, 200 mg/ml	10 ml vial	Roberts	[NLM]	
U.S.	testosterone cypionate	Duratest-100-200	100, 200 mg/ml	10 ml vial	Hauck	[NLM]	
U.S.	testosterone cypionate	Malogen Cyp	100, 200 mg/ml	10 ml vial	Forest	[NLM]	
U.S.	testosterone cypionate	Testa-C	200 mg/ml	10 ml vial	Vortech	[NLM]	
U.S.	testosterone cypionate	Testadiate-Depo	200 mg/ml	10 ml vial	Kay	[NLM]	
U.S.	testosterone cypionate	Testoject	100 mg/ml	n/a	Mayrand	[NLM]	
U.S.	testosterone cypionate	Testoject 50	50 mg/ml	n/a	Mayrand	[NLM]	
U.S.	testosterone cypionate	Testoject-LA	200 mg/ml	n/a	Mayrand	[NLM]	
U.S.	testosterone cypionate	testosterone cypionate	100 mg/ml	10 ml vial	Geneva Geriatrics	[NLM]	
U.S.	testosterone cypionate	testosterone cypionate	100, 200 mg/ml	10 ml vial	Goldline	[NLM]	
U.S.	testosterone cypionate	testosterone cypionate	50, 100, 200 mg/ml	10 ml vial	Huffman	[NLM]	
U.S.	testosterone cypionate	testosterone cypionate	200 mg/ml	10 ml vial	Legere	[NLM]	
U.S.	testosterone cypionate	testosterone cypionate	100, 200 mg/ml	10 ml vial	Schein	[NLM]	
U.S.	testosterone cypionate	testosterone cypionate	100, 200 mg/ml	10 ml vial	Steris	[NLM]	
U.S.	testosterone cypionate	Testred Cypionate	200 mg/ml	10 ml vial	INC	[NLM]	
U.S.	testosterone enanthate	Anderone 100/200	100, 200 mg/ml	10 ml vial	Burgin-Arden	[NLM]	
U.S.	testosterone enanthate	Andro 100	100 mg/ml	10 ml vial	Forest	[NLM]	
U.S.	testosterone enanthate	Andro L.A. 200	200 mg/ml	10 ml vial	Forest	[NLM]	
U.S.	testosterone enanthate	Andropository	200 mg/ml	10 ml vial	Rugby	[NLM]	
U.S.	testosterone enanthate	Andryl 200	200 mg/ml	10 ml vial	Keene	[NLM]	
U.S.	testosterone enanthate	Delatest	100/mg/ml	10 ml vial	Dunhall	[NLM]	
U.S.	testosterone enanthate	Delatestryl	200 mg/ml	1 ml syringe	BTG		

Appendix C: Drug Availability Tables - Listings by Country

Country	Generic Name	Trade Name	Dose	Packaging	Company	Status	Vet
U.S.	testosterone enanthate	Delatestryl	200 mg/ml	5 ml vial	BTG		
U.S.	testosterone enanthate	Delatestryl	200 mg/ml	10 ml vial	Mead Johnson	[NLM]	
U.S.	testosterone enanthate	Dura-Testosterone	200 mg/ml	10 ml vial	Pharmex	[NLM]	
U.S.	testosterone enanthate	Durathate-200 Injection	200 mg/ml	n/a	Hauck	[NLM]	
U.S.	testosterone enanthate	Durathate-200 Injection	200 mg/ml	n/a	Roberts	[NLM]	
U.S.	testosterone enanthate	Everone	100, 200 mg/ml	10 ml vial	Hyrex	[NLM]	
U.S.	testosterone enanthate	Malogen 100/200 L.A.	100, 200 mg/ml	10 ml vial	Forest	[NLM]	
U.S.	testosterone enanthate	Tesone L.A.	200 mg/ml	10 ml vial	Sig	[NLM]	
U.S.	testosterone enanthate	Testanate No. 1	100 mg/ml	n/a	Kenyon	[NLM]	
U.S.	testosterone enanthate	Testaval	100, 200 mg/ml	10 ml vial	Legere	[NLM]	
U.S.	testosterone enanthate	testosterone enanthate	100, 200 mg/ml	10 ml vial	Geneva Geriatrics	[NLM]	
U.S.	testosterone enanthate	testosterone enanthate	100, 200 mg/ml	10 ml vial	Goldline	[NLM]	
U.S.	testosterone enanthate	testosterone enanthate	100, 200 mg/ml	10 ml vial	Quad	[NLM]	
U.S.	testosterone enanthate	testosterone enanthate	100, 200 mg/ml	10 ml vial	Schein	[NLM]	
U.S.	testosterone enanthate	testosterone enanthate	100, 200 mg/ml	10 ml vial	Steris	[NLM]	
U.S.	testosterone enanthate	Testrin-P.A.	200 mg/ml	n/a	Pasadena Res.	[NLM]	
U.S.	testosterone propionate	Androlan	50, 100 mg/ml	n/a	Lannett	[NLM]	
U.S.	testosterone propionate	Hybolin Imp.	25, 50 mg/ml	n/a	Hyrex	[NLM]	
U.S.	testosterone propionate	Testex	50, 100 mg/ml	n/a	Pasadena	[NLM]	
U.S.	testosterone propionate	testosterone propionate	50 mg/ml	n/a	Quad & Lilly	[NLM]	
U.S.	testosterone propionate	testosterone propionate	100 mg/ml	10, 30 ml vial	Rugby	[NLM]	
U.S.	testosterone propionate	testosterone propionate	100 mg/ml	10 ml vial	Steris	[NLM]	
U.S.	testosterone propionate (implant)	Implus-H	22 mg/pellet	n/a	Upjohn		
U.S.	testosterone propionate (implant)	Synovex®-H (plus estrogen)	20 mg/pellet	n/a	Fort Dodge		VET
U.S.	testosterone propionate (implant)	Synovex®-H (plus estrogen)	20 mg/pellet	n/a	Syntex	[NLM]	VET
U.S.	testosterone suspension	Androlan Aqueous	25, 50, 100 mg/ml	n/a	Lannet	[NLM]	
U.S.	testosterone suspension	Androlin	100 mg/ml	n/a	Lincoln	[NLM]	
U.S.	testosterone suspension	Andronaq-50	50 mg/ml	n/a	Central	[NLM]	
U.S.	testosterone suspension	Histerone Injection	100 mg/ml	n/a	Roberts	[NLM]	
U.S.	testosterone suspension	Histerone Injection	100 mg/ml	n/a	Hauck	[NLM]	
U.S.	testosterone suspension	Malogen	25, 50, 100, mg/ml	n/a	Forest	[NLM]	
U.S.	testosterone suspension	Malotrone	25, 50 mg/ml	n/a	Bluco	[NLM]	
U.S.	testosterone suspension	Tesamone	25, 50, 100, mg/ml	n/a	Dunhall	[NLM]	
U.S.	testosterone suspension	Testolin	25, 50, 100, mg/ml	n/a	Pasadena	[NLM]	
U.S.	testosterone suspension	testosterone suspension	100 mg/ml	n/a	Legere	[NLM]	
U.S.	testosterone suspension	testosterone suspension	50, 100 mg/ml	10, 30 ml vial	Schein	[NLM]	
U.S.	testosterone suspension	testosterone suspension	50, 100 mg/ml	10, 30 ml vial	Steris	[NLM]	
U.S.	trenbolone acetate	ComponentTE-G® (+ estradiol)	20 mg pellet	40 pellet cartridge	VetLife		VET
U.S.	trenbolone acetate	ComponentTE-S® (+ estradiol)	20 mg pellet	120 pellet cartridge	VetLife		VET
U.S.	trenbolone acetate	ComponentT-H®	20 mg pellet	200 pellet cartridge	VetLife		VET
U.S.	trenbolone acetate	ComponentT-S®	20 mg pellet	140 pellet cartridge	VetLife		VET

Appendix C: Drug Availability Tables - Listings by Country

Country	Generic Name	Trade Name	Dose	Packaging	Company	Status	Vet
U.S.	trenbolone acetate	Finajet	30 mg/ml	50 ml vial	Hoechst	[NLM]	VET
U.S.	trenbolone acetate	Finaplix-H®	20 mg pellet	100 pellet cartridge	Hoechst-Roussel	[NLM]	VET
U.S.	trenbolone acetate	Finaplix-H®	20 mg pellet	100 pellet cartridge	Intervet		VET
U.S.	trenbolone acetate	Finaplix-S®	20 mg pellet	70 pellet cartridge	Hoechst-Roussel	[NLM]	VET
U.S.	trenbolone acetate	Revalor-200 (plus estradiol)	20 mg pellet	100 pellet cartridge	Intervet		VET
U.S.	trenbolone acetate	Revalor-G (plus estradiol)	20 mg pellet	20 pellet cartridge	Intervet		VET
U.S.	trenbolone acetate	Revalor-H (plus estradiol)	20 mg pellet	70 pellet cartridge	Hoechst-Roussel	[NLM]	VET
U.S.	trenbolone acetate	Revalor-H (plus estradiol)	20 mg pellet	70 pellet cartridge	Intervet		VET
U.S.	trenbolone acetate	Revalor-IH (plus estradiol)	20 mg pellet	40 pellet cartridge	Intervet		VET
U.S.	trenbolone acetate	Revalor-IS (plus estradiol)	20 mg pellet	40 pellet cartridge	Intervet		VET
U.S.	trenbolone acetate	Revalor-S (plus estradiol)	20 mg pellet	60 pellet cartridge	Hoechst-Roussel	[NLM]	VET
U.S.	trenbolone acetate	Revalor-S (plus estradiol)	20 mg pellet	60 pellet cartridge	Intervet		VET
U.S.	trenbolone acetate	Synovex plus (plus estradiol)	25 mg pellet	80 pellet cartridge	Fort Dodge		VET
U.S.	trenbolone acetate	Synovex plus (plus estradiol)	25 mg pellet	80 pellet cartridge	Syntex	[NLM]	VET
Ukraine	mesterolone	Proviron®	25 mg tablet	20 tablet box	Schering		
Ukraine	testosterone undecanoate	Andriol	40 mg capsules	n/a	Organon		
United Arab E	testosterone undecanoate	Andriol	40 mg capsules	n/a	Organon		
United Kingdom	drostanolone propionate	Masteril	100 mg/2ml	2 ml amp	Syntex	[NLM]	
United Kingdom	ethylestrenol	Orabolin®	2 mg tablet	n/a	Organon	[NLM]	
United Kingdom	fluoxymesterone	Ultandren	1,5 mg tablet	n/a	Ciba	[NLM]	
United Kingdom	mesterolone	Proviron®	25 mg tablet	30 tablet box	Schering		
United Kingdom	methandrostenolone	Dianabol	5 mg tablet	100 tablet bottle	Ciba	[NLM]	
United Kingdom	nandrolone decanoate	Deca-Durabolin®	50 mg/ml	1 ml ampule	Organon		
United Kingdom	nandrolone decanoate	Deca-Durabolin®	100 mg/ml	1, 2 ml ampule	Organon	[NLM]	
United Kingdom	nandrolone phenylpropionate	Durabolin®	50 mg/ml	1 ml ampule	Organon	[NLM]	
United Kingdom	oxymetholone	Anapolon 50	50 mg tablet	100 tablet bottle	Syntex	[NLM]	
United Kingdom	stanozolol (inj)	Stromba	50 mg/ml	n/a	Sterling Research	[NLM]	
United Kingdom	stanozolol (oral)	Stromba	5 mg tablet	n/a	Sanofi	[NLM]	
United Kingdom	stanozolol (oral)	Stromba	5 mg tablet	n/a	Sterling	[NLM]	
United Kingdom	Sustanon 100 (testosterone blend)	Sustanon '100'®	100 mg/ml	1 ml ampule	Organon		
United Kingdom	Sustanon 250 (testosterone blend)	Sustanon '250'®	250 mg/ml	1 ml ampule	Organon		
United Kingdom	testosterone (patch)	Andropatch	2.5 mg patch	60 patches/box	GSK		
United Kingdom	testosterone (patch)	Andropatch	5 mg patch	30 patches/box	GSK		
United Kingdom	testosterone enanthate	Primoteston®-Depot	250 mg/ml	1 ml ampule	Schering	[NLM]	
United Kingdom	testosterone propionate	Virormone	50 mg/ml	2 ml ampule	Ferring	[NLM]	
United Kingdom	testosterone propionate	Virormone	50 mg/ml	2 ml ampule	Nordic		
United Kingdom	testosterone undecanoate	Restandol	40 mg capsules	28, 56 capsule box	Organon		
United Kingdom	trenbolone acetate	Finajet	30 mg/ml	50 ml vial	Hoechst	[NLM]	VET
Uruguay	dihydrotestosterone	Andractim	25 mg/g	80 gram gel	Servimedic		
Uruguay	mesterolone	Proviron®	25 mg tablet	n/a	Schering		
Uruguay	methyltestosterone	Glando Stridox	10 mg tablet	20 tablet box	Ion		

Appendix C: Drug Availability Tables - Listings by Country

Country	Generic Name	Trade Name	Dose	Packaging	Company	Status	Vet
Uruguay	methyltestosterone	Metil Thomsina S	10 mg tablet	20 tablet box	Celsius		
Uruguay	testosterone cypionate	Testosterona Ultra Lenta	100 mg/ml	20 ml vial	Dispert Labs.		VET
Uruguay	testosterone cypionate	Testosterona Ultra Lenta Fuerte	200 mg/ml	5 ml ampule	Dispert Labs.		VET
Uruguay	testosterone cypionate	Testosterona Ultra Lenta Fuerte	200 mg/ml	20 ml vial	Dispert Labs.		VET
Uruguay	testosterone enanthate	Testoviron®-Depot	250 mg/ml	1 ml ampule	Schering		
Venezuela	boldenone undecylenate	Ganabol	50 mg/ml	500 ml vial	Laboratorios VM		VET
Venezuela	boldenone undecylenate	Ganabol	25, 50 mg/ml	10, 50, 100, 250ml vial	Laboratorios VM		VET
Venezuela	mesterolone	Proviron®	25 mg tablet	15 tablet box	Schering		
Venezuela	methyltestosterone	Oreton	n/a	n/a	n/a		
Venezuela	nandrolone decanoate	Deca-Durabolin®	25 mg/ml	1 ml ampule	Organon		
Venezuela	nandrolone decanoate	Deca-Durabolin®	50 mg/ml	1 ml syringe	Organon		
Venezuela	Sustanon 250 (testosterone blend)	Polysteron 250	250 mg/ml	1 ml ampule	Organon		
Venezuela	testosterone enanthate	Proviron®-Depot	250 mg/ml	1 ml ampule	Schering		
Venezuela	testosterone undecanoate	Andriol capsulas	40 mg capsules	n/a	Organon		
Vietnam	Sustanon 250 (testosterone blend)	Sustanon "250"	250 mg/ml	1ml ampule	Organon		
Vietnam	testosterone undecanoate	Andriol	40 mg capsules	n/a	Organon		
Yemen	testosterone enanthate	Testoviron®-Depot	250 mg/ml	1 ml ampule	Schering		
Yemen	testosterone undecanoate	Andriol	40 mg capsules	n/a	Organon		
YugoslaviaFRMR	fluoxymesterone	Halotestin®	5 mg tablet	n/a	Galenika	[NLM]	
YugoslaviaFRMR	mesterolone	Proviron®	25 mg tablet	n/a	Alkoid		
YugoslaviaFRMR	methandrostenolone	Nerobol	5 mg tablet	20 tablet box	Galenika	[NLM]	
YugoslaviaFRMR	methylandrostenediol	Novandrol	10, 25 mg dragee	n/a	Galenika	[NLM]	
YugoslaviaFRMR	methyltestosterone	T. Lingvalete	5 mg sub. dragee	n/a	Galenika	[NLM]	
YugoslaviaFRMR	nandrolone phenylpropionate	Durabolin®	50 mg/ml	n/a	Organon		
YugoslaviaFRMR	testosterone enanthate	Testosteron-Depo	100 mg/ml	1 ml ampule	Galenika	[NLM]	
YugoslaviaFRMR	testosterone enanthate	Testosteron-Depo	250 mg/ml	1 ml ampule	Galenika		
YugoslaviaFRMR	testosterone enanthate	Testosteron-Depo	100, 250 mg/ml	1 ml ampule	Hemofarm	[NLM]	
YugoslaviaFRMR	testosterone propionate	Testosteron	5, 10, 25, 50 mg/ml	1 ml ampule	Galenika	[NLM]	
YugoslaviaFRMR	testosterone undecanoate	Andriol	40 mg capsules	n/a	Organon		
Zimbabwe	testosterone enanthate	Weratestone 250	250 mg/ml	1 ml ampule	Weimer Pharma		
Zimbabwe	testosterone enanthate	Weratestone 250	250 mg/ml	1 ml ampule	Weimer Pharma		

ABBREVIATIONS: [NLM] = No Longer Manufactured
VET = Veterinary Drug

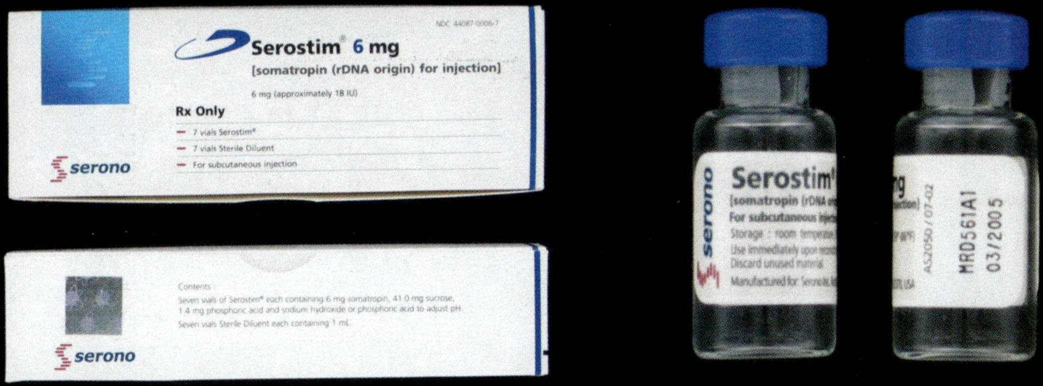

New U.S. Serostim box and vials

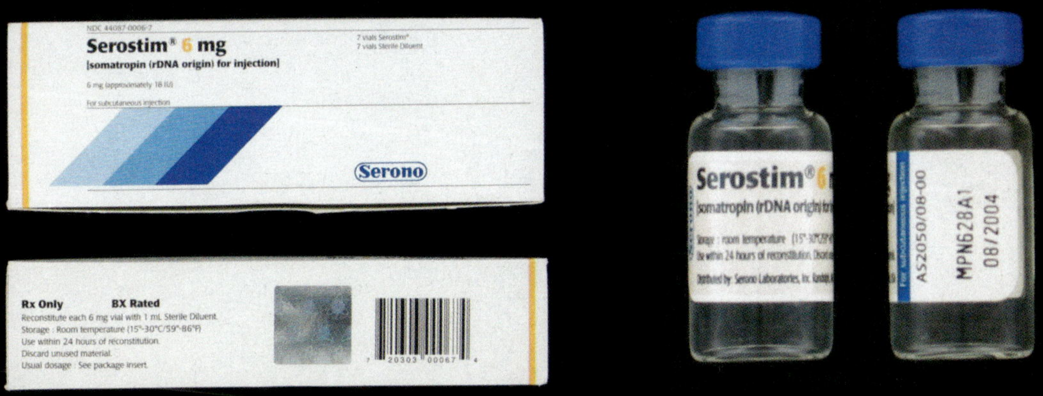

Older style packaging for U.S. Serostim

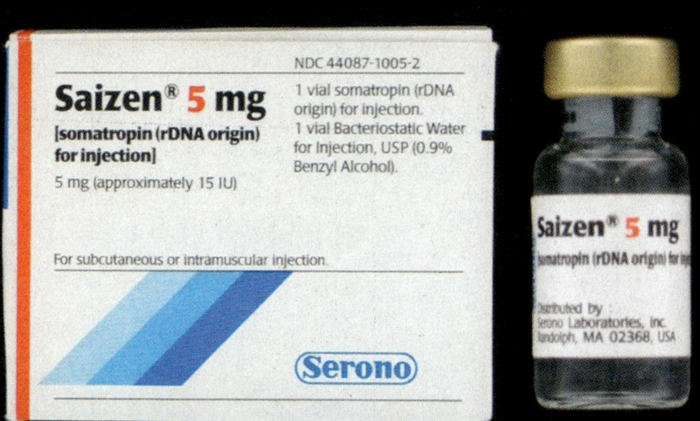

U.S. Saizen box and vial

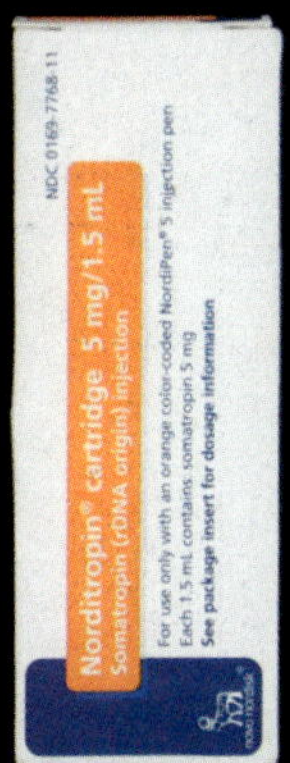

U.S. Norditropin

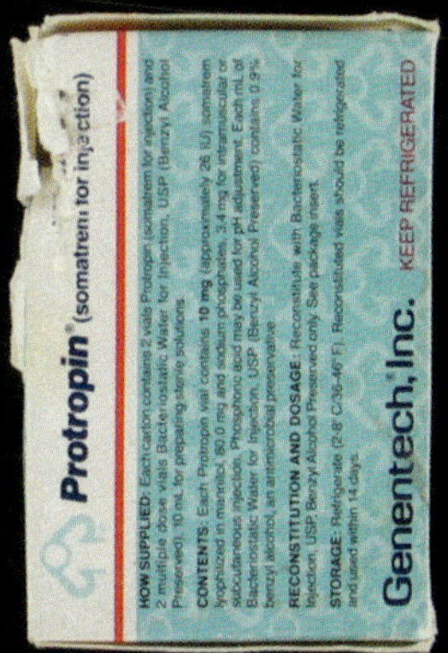

U.S. Protropin (somatrem)

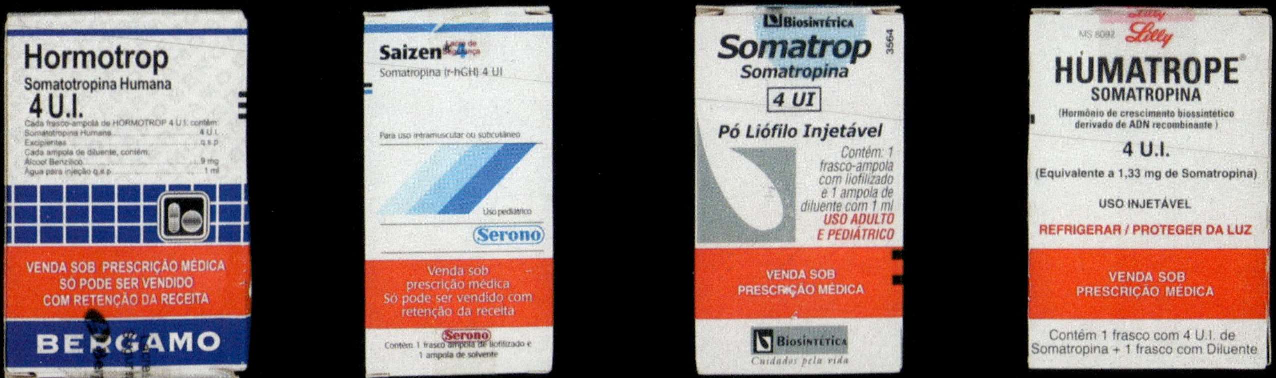

Four different brands from Brazil

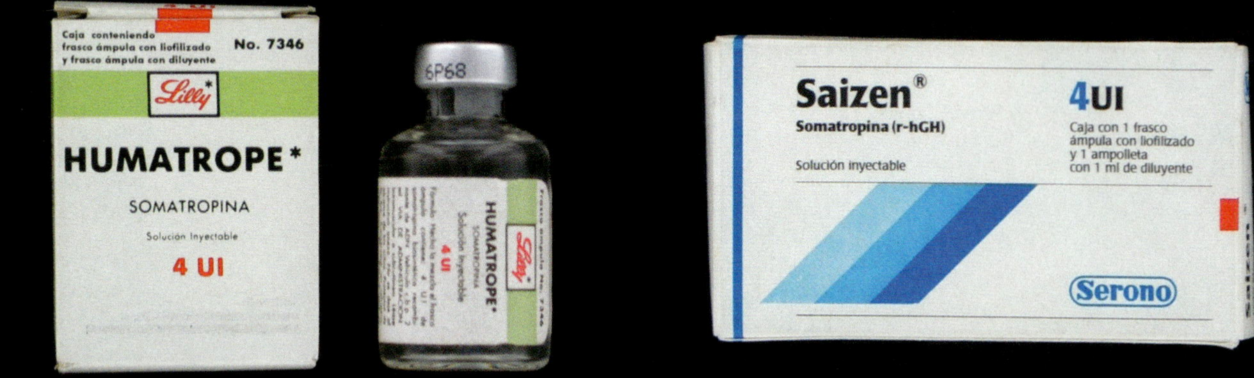

Lilly Humatrope and Serono Saizen (Mexico)

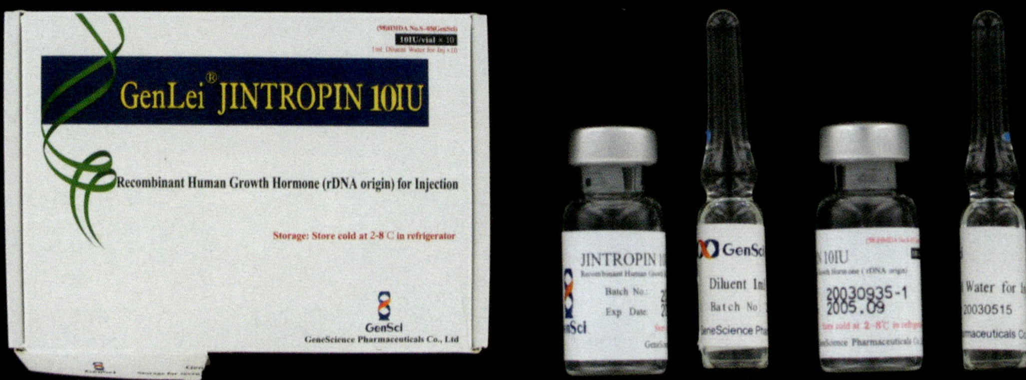

Jintropin from GenSci (China)

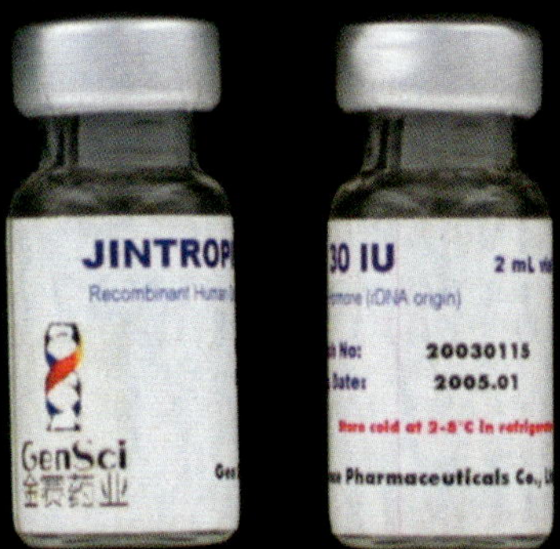

Counterfeit Jintropin

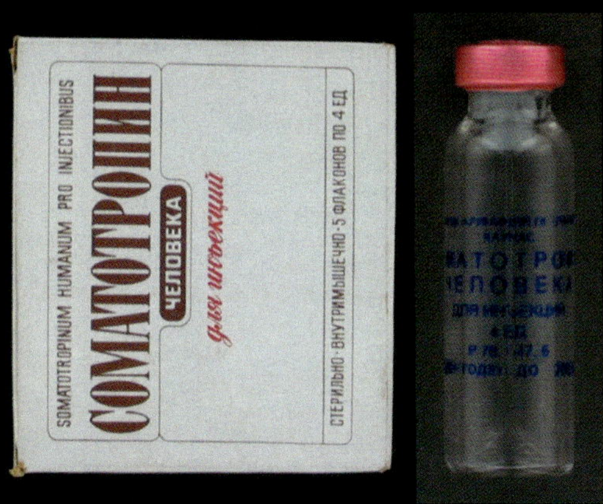

"Somatotropin" (Russia)

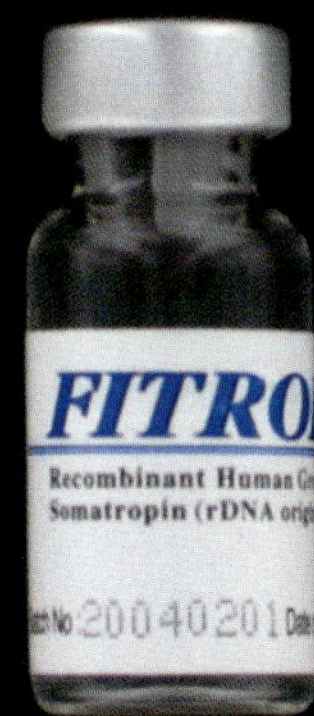

Chinese Fitropin (somatrem)

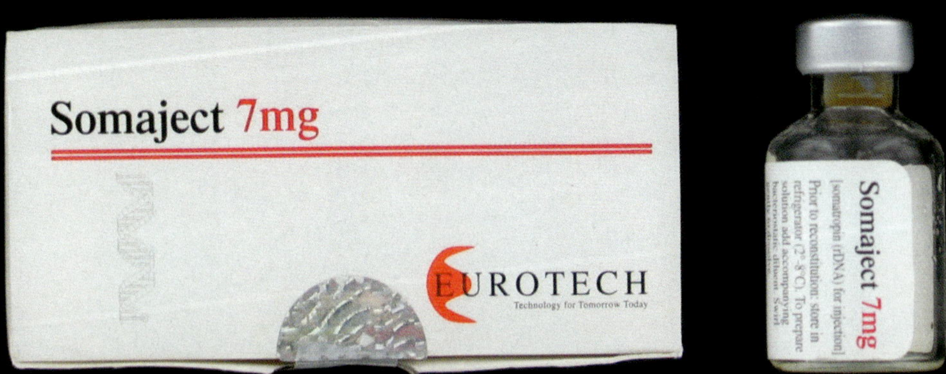

Somaject from Eurotech - Underground product (NLM)

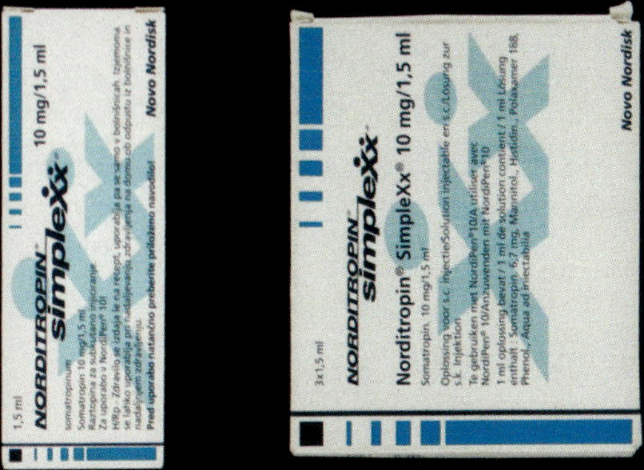

Norditropin Simplexx from Denmark and Belgium

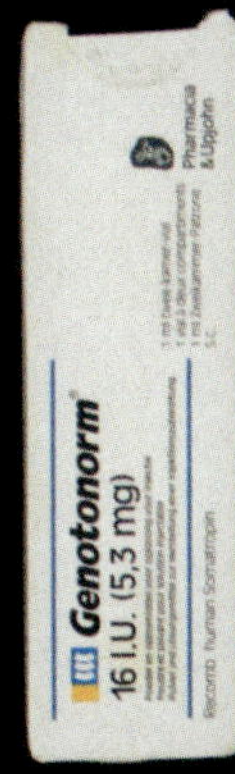

Genotonorm (Belgium)

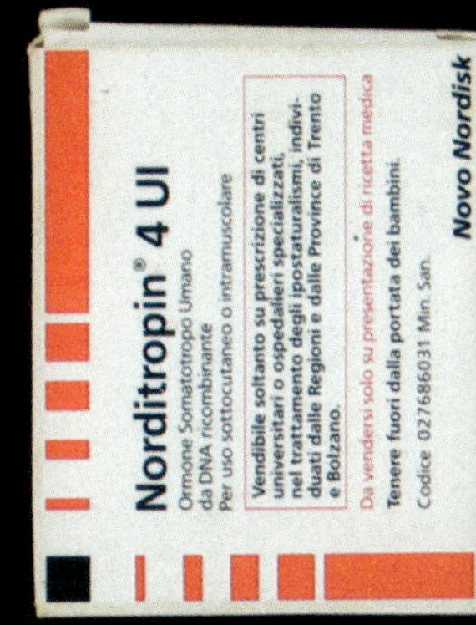

Italian Norditropin

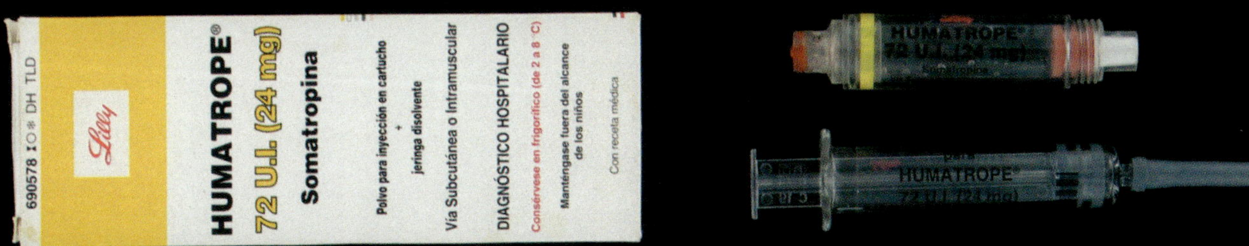

Humatrope from Spain

IGF-1

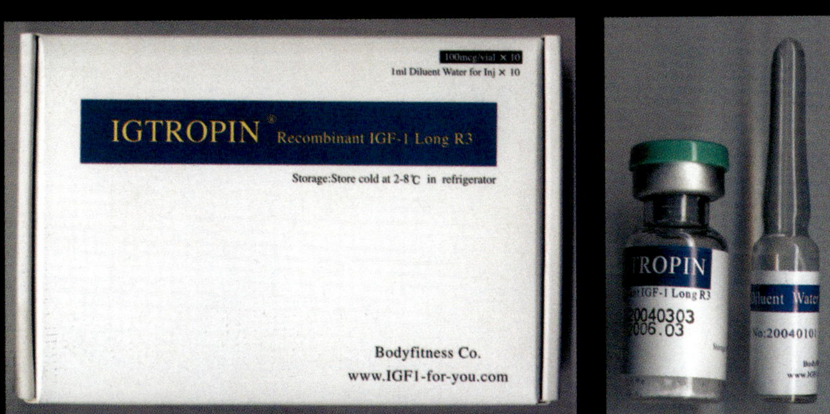

IGTropin from GenSci (China)

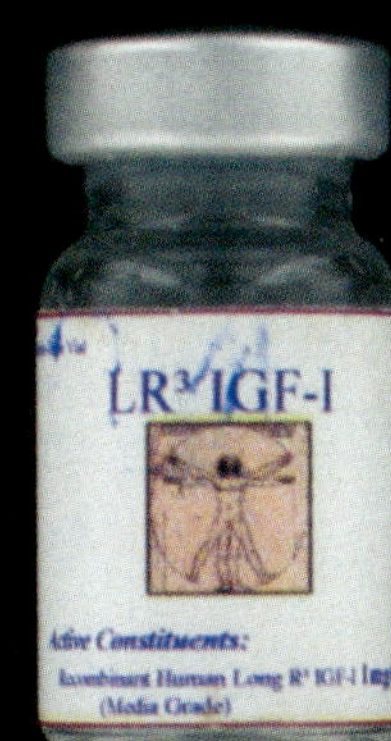

U.S. "Research" product

Adipex-P

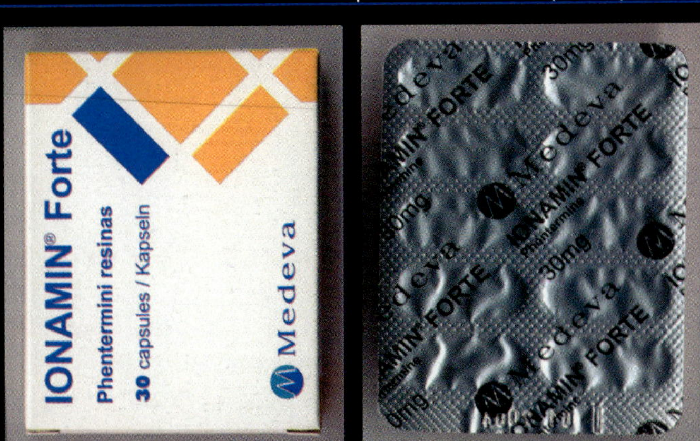

Ionamin (phentermine)

Aldactazide

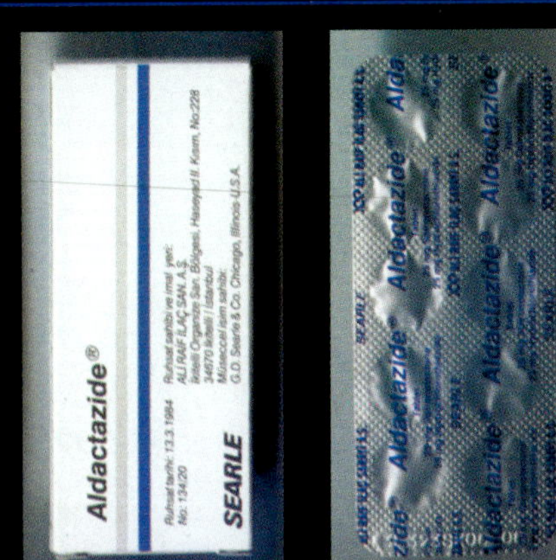

Aldactazide from Turkey (box/strip)

Aldactone

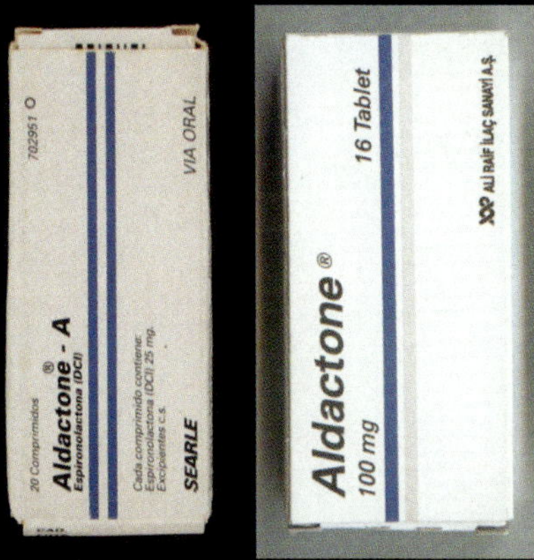

Aldactone from Spain and Turkey

Arimidex

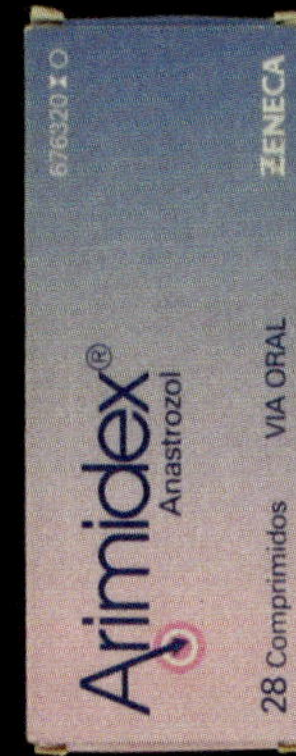

Spanish Arimidex

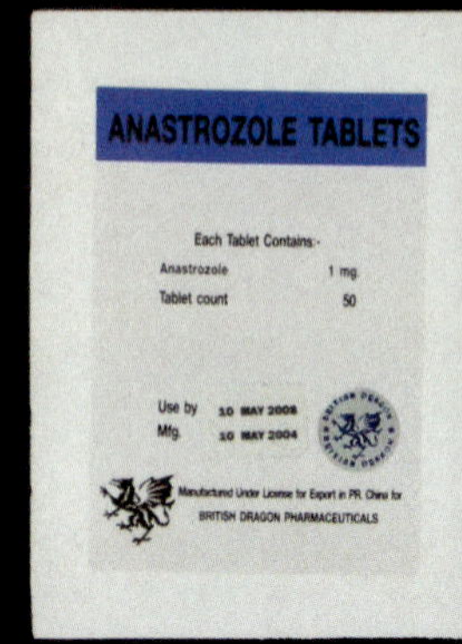

British Dragon (Thailand)

Avodart

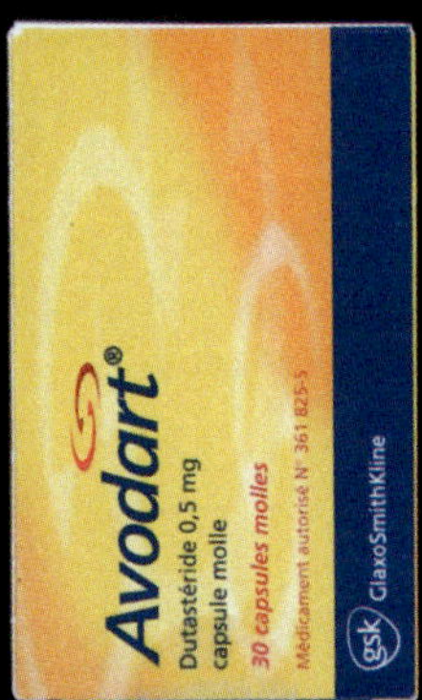

French Avodart

Capoten

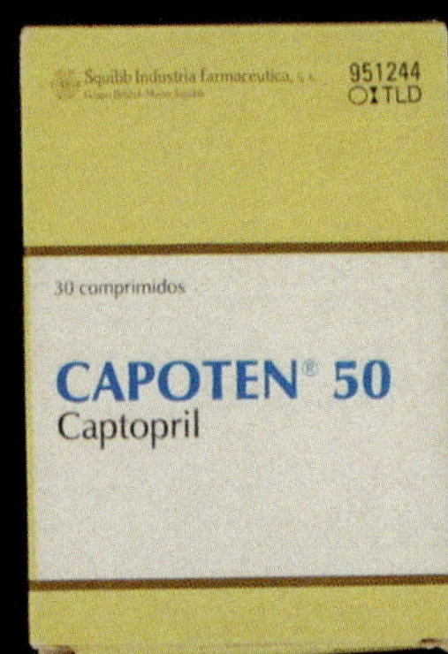

Spanish Capoten box

Catapres

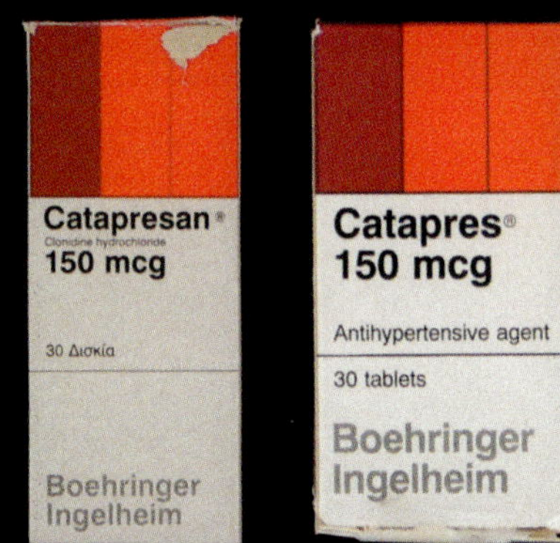

Greek and German Catapres

Clenbuterol

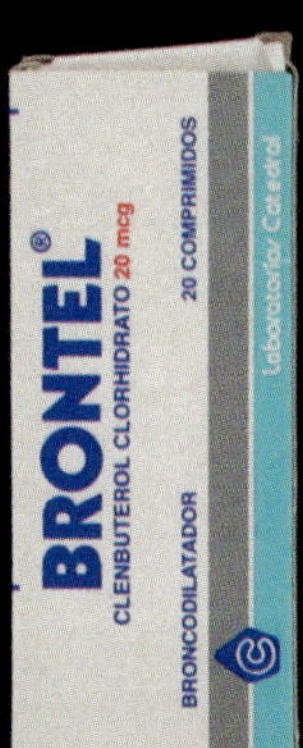

Brontel from Brazil

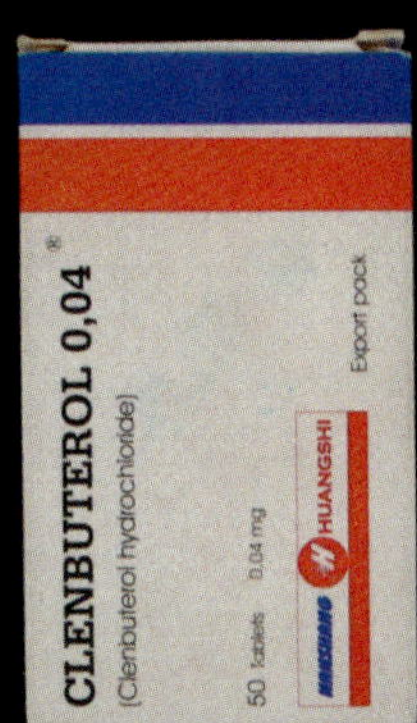

Chinese generic

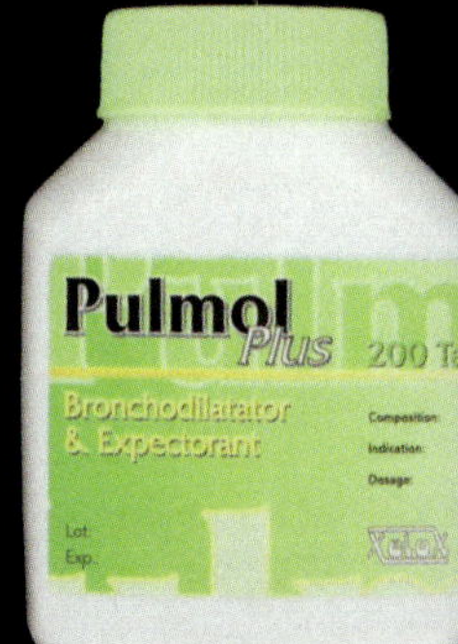

Pulmol from Xelox

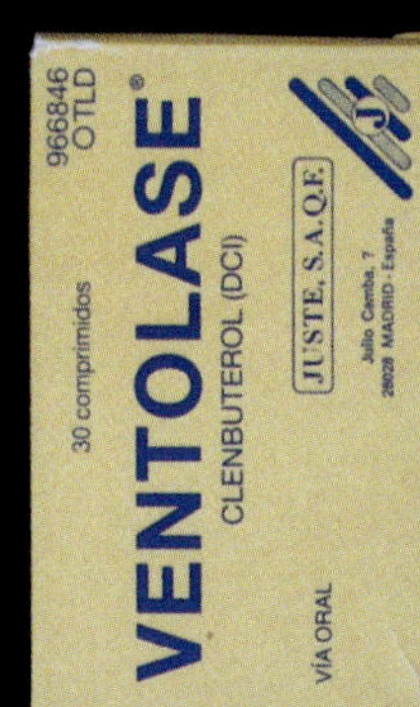

Ventolase from Spain

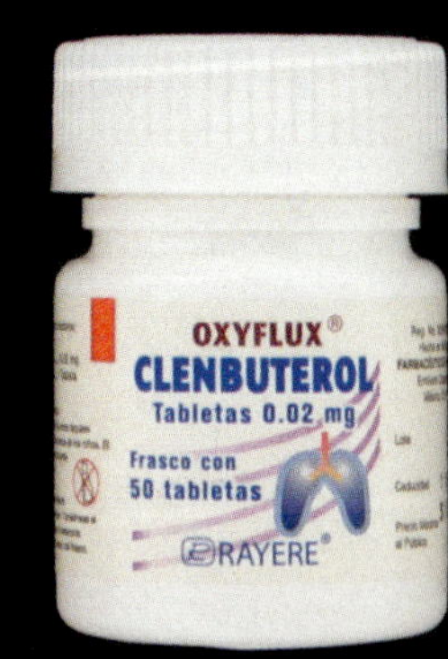

Oxyflux (Mexico)

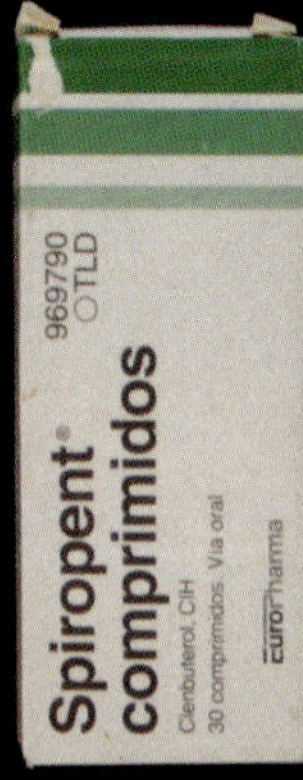

Spanish Spiropent

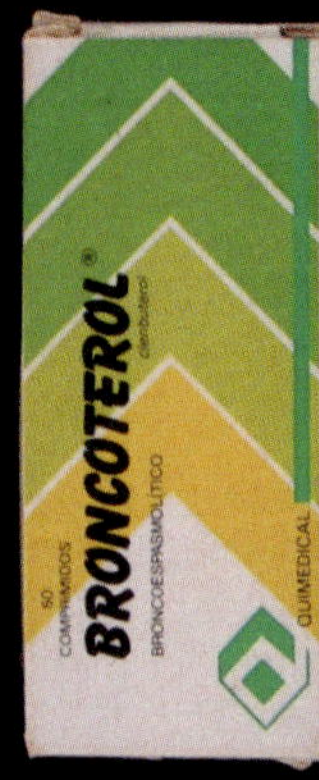

Broncoterol (Spain)

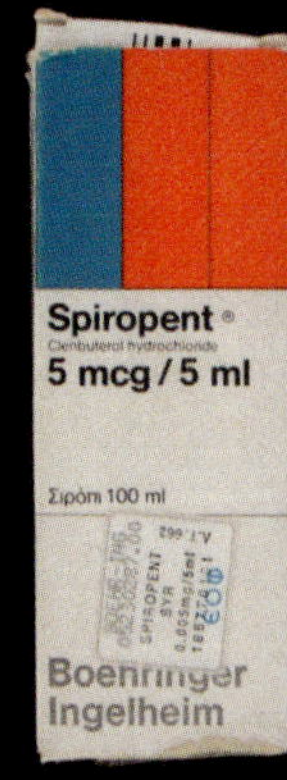

Greek clen

Clomid

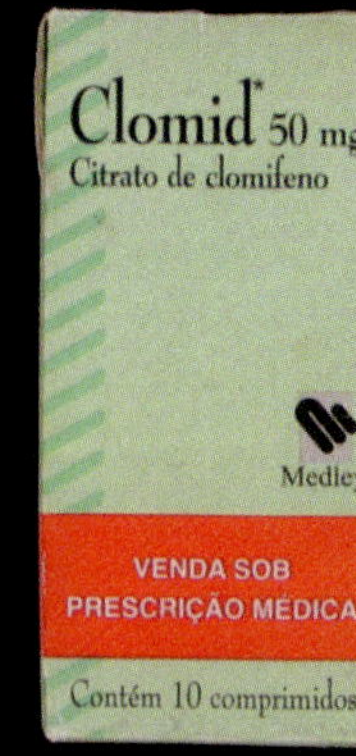

Clomid from Braz

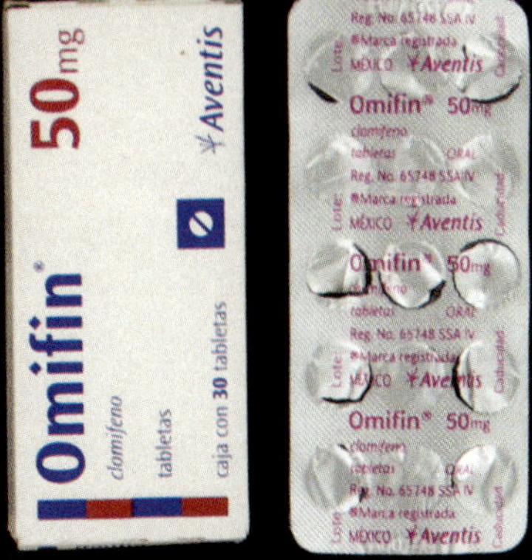

Omifin (Mexico)

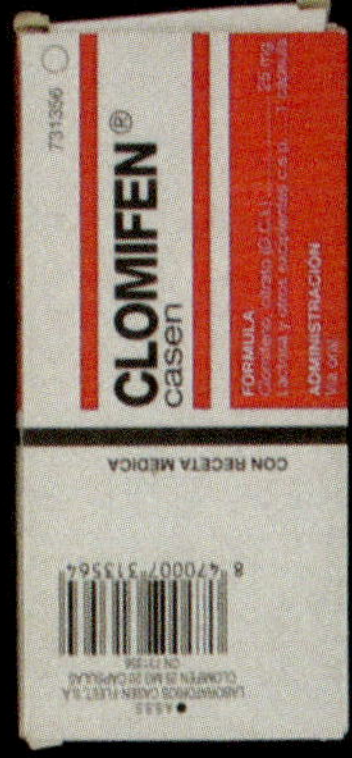

Spanish Clomifen

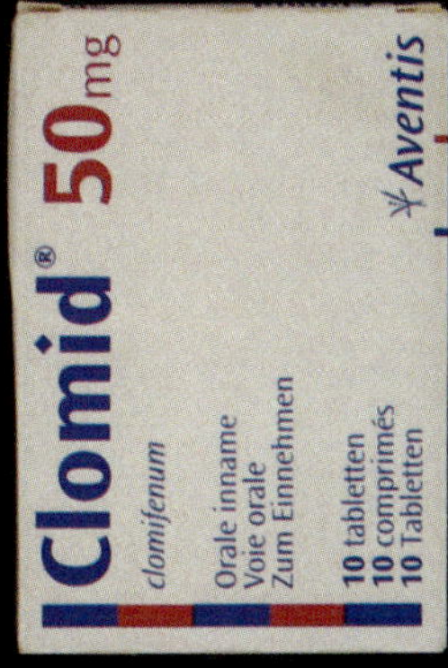

Clomid (Germany)

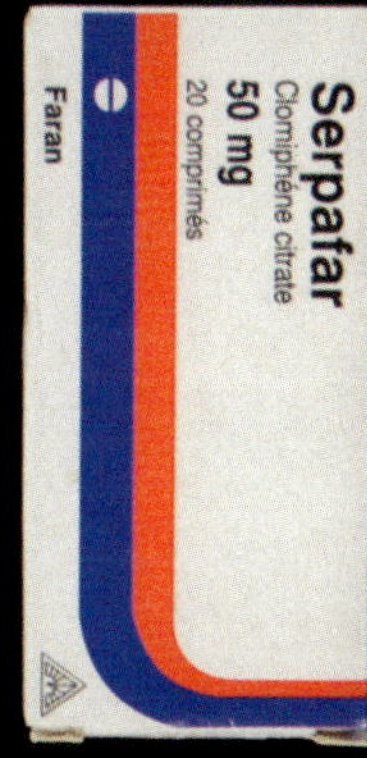

Serpafar (Greece)

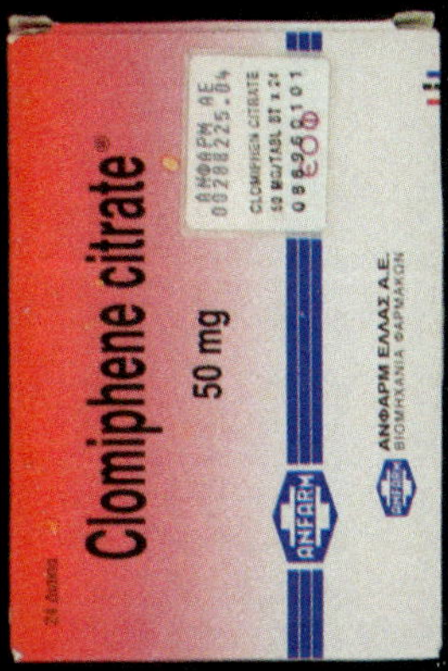

Anfarm generic (Greece)

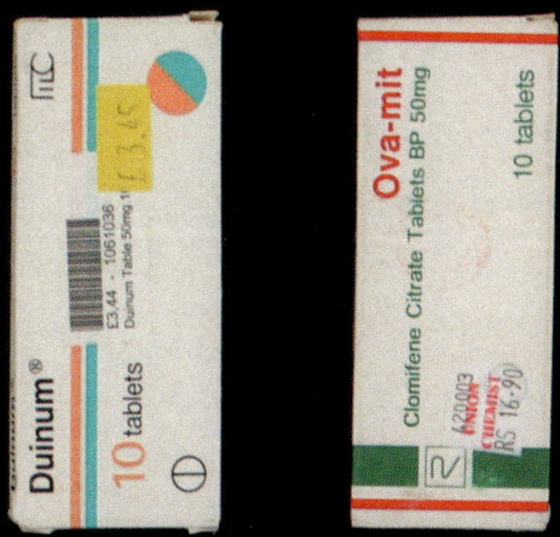

Duinum and Ova-mit (Cypress)

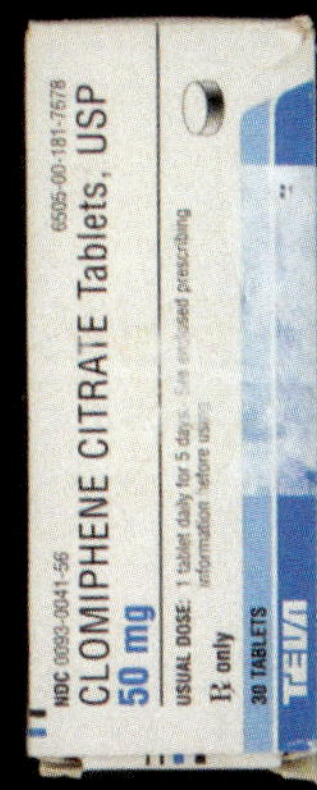

U.S. generic

Cyclofenil

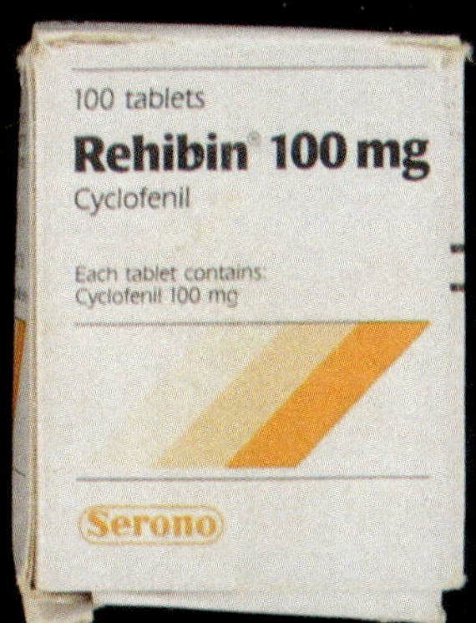

Rehibin (Sweden)

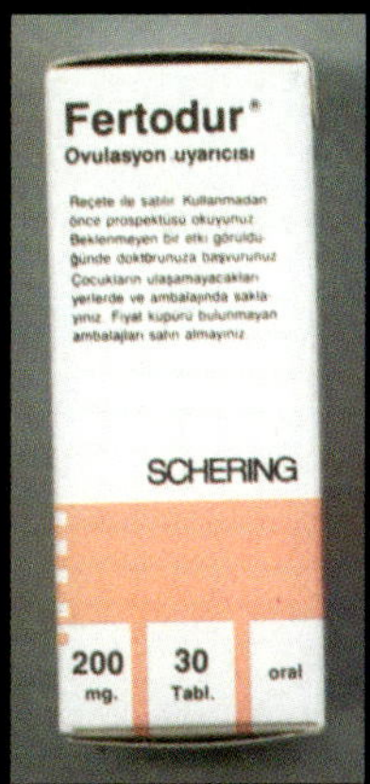

Fertodur (Turkey)

Cytadren

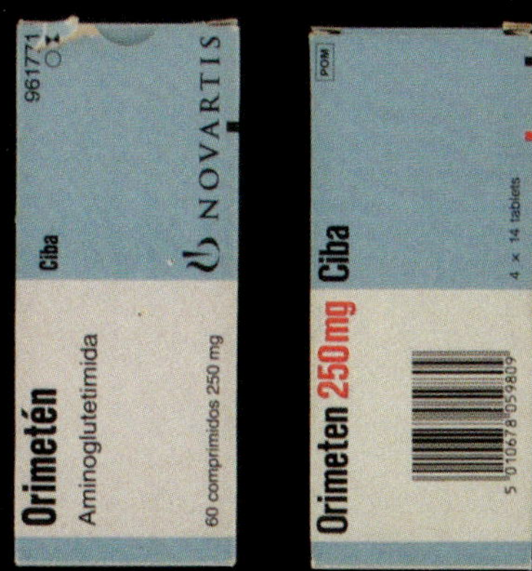

Orimiten from Spain and UK

Cytomel

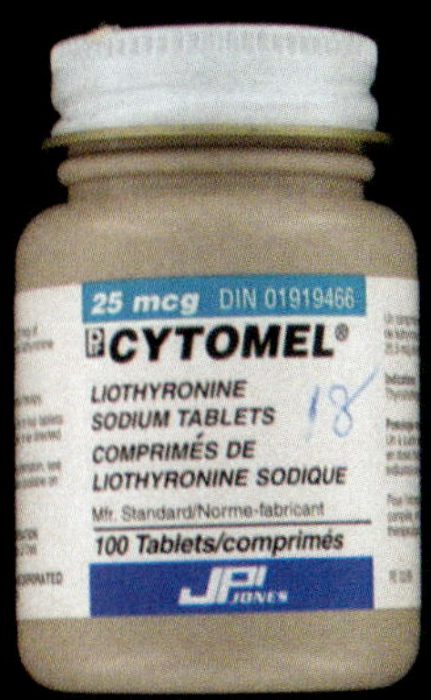

Cytomel (U.S.)

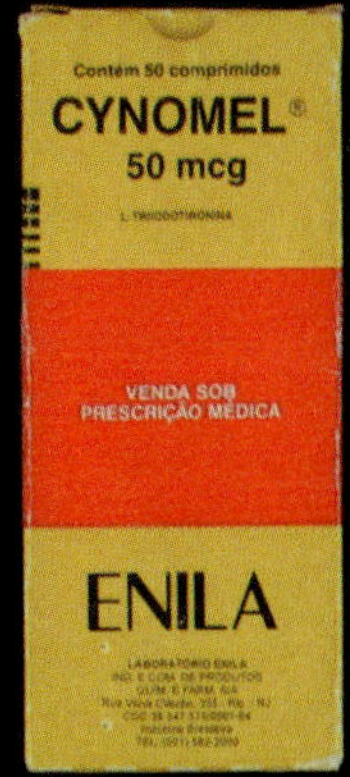

Cynomel (Mexico)

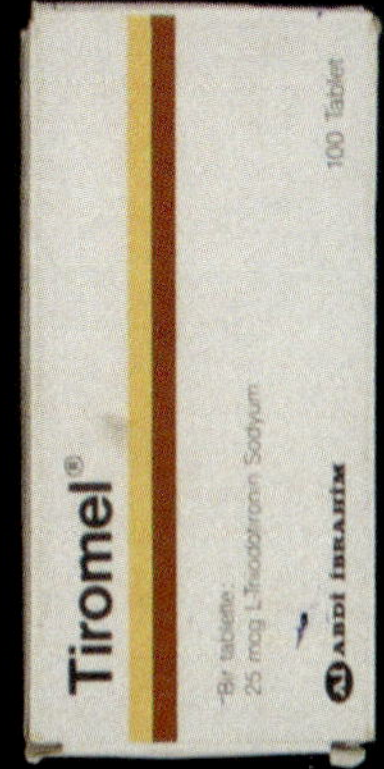

Tiromel (Turkey)

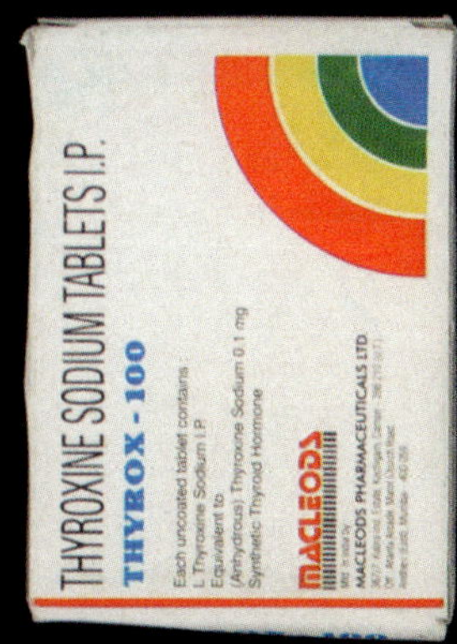

Thyrox-100 (India)

Ephedrine

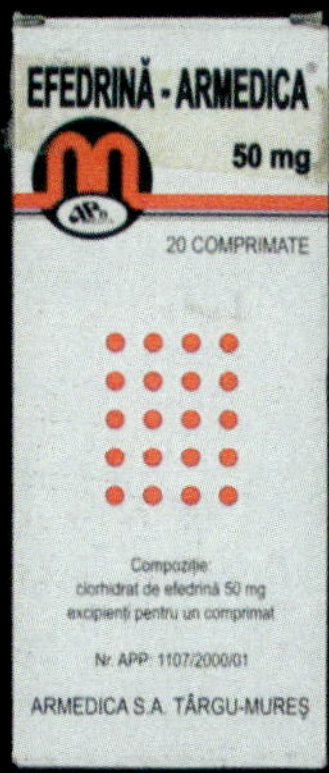

Epogen

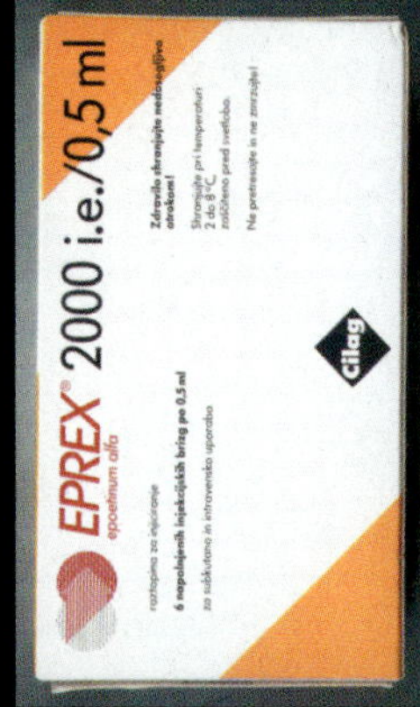

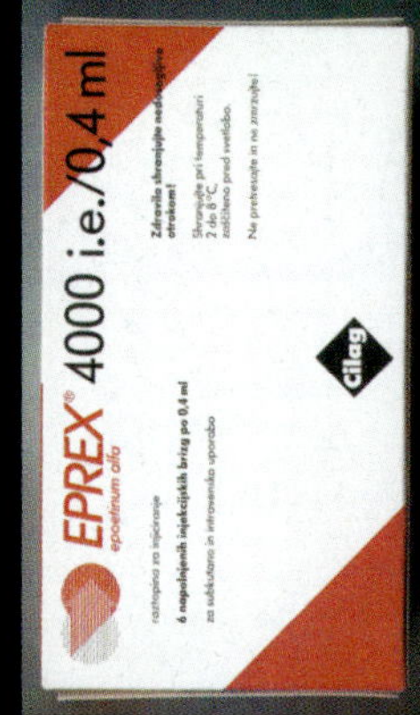

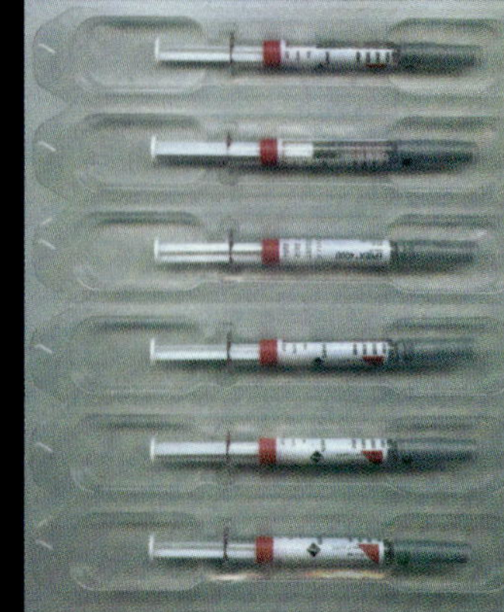

Armedica Ephedrine

Epogen from Cllag (boxes and preloaded syringes)

HCG

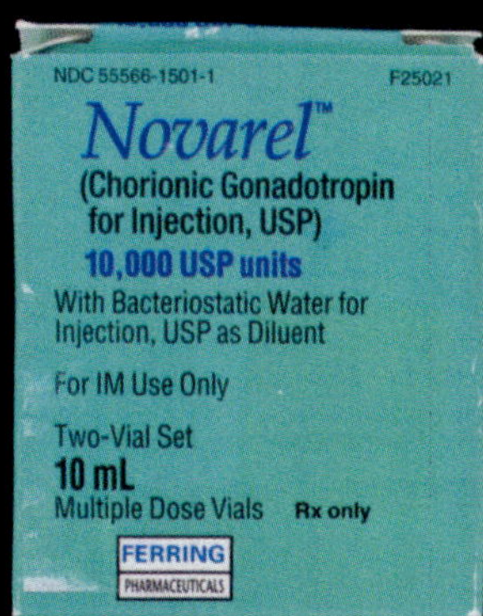

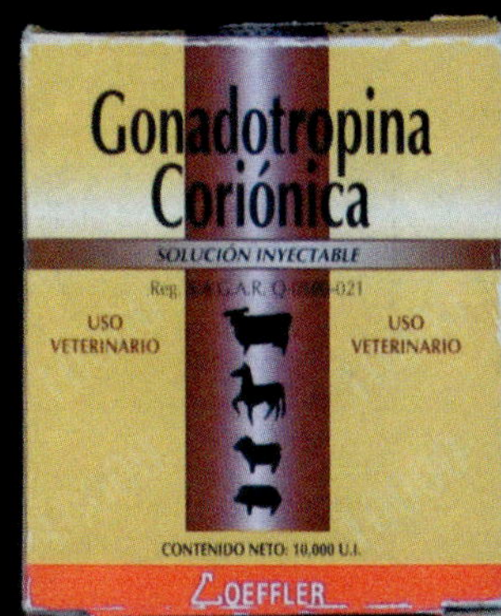

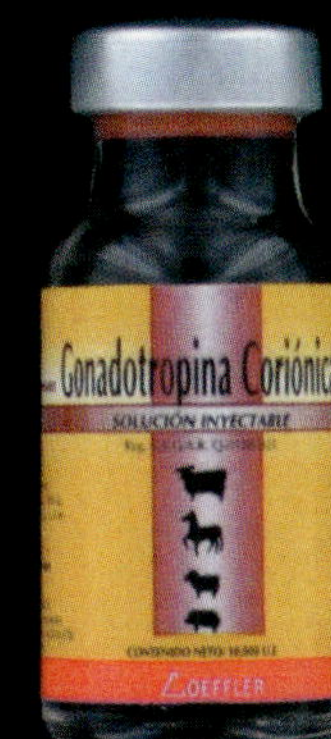

Novarel (U.S.)

Vet product from Loeffler (Mexico)

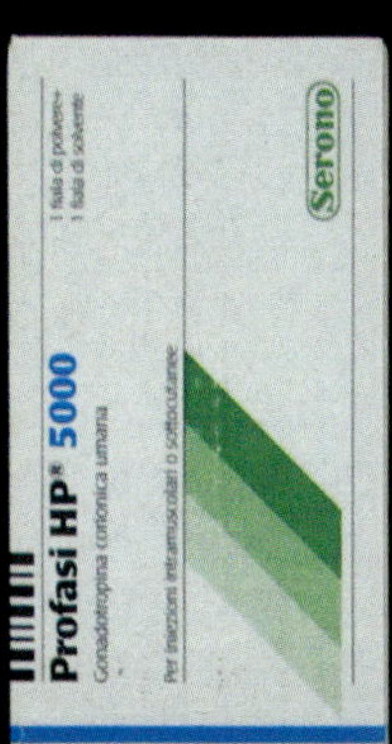

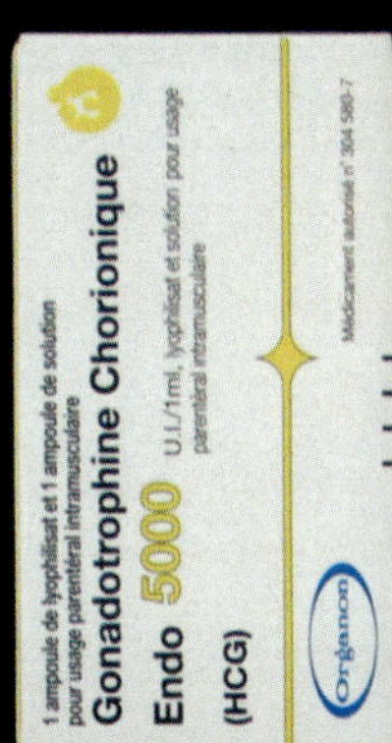

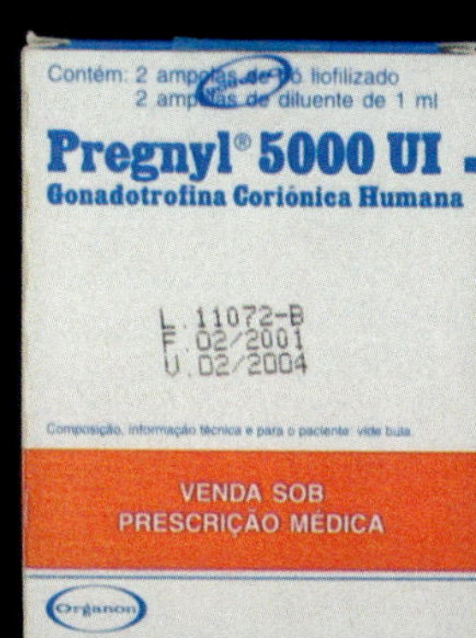

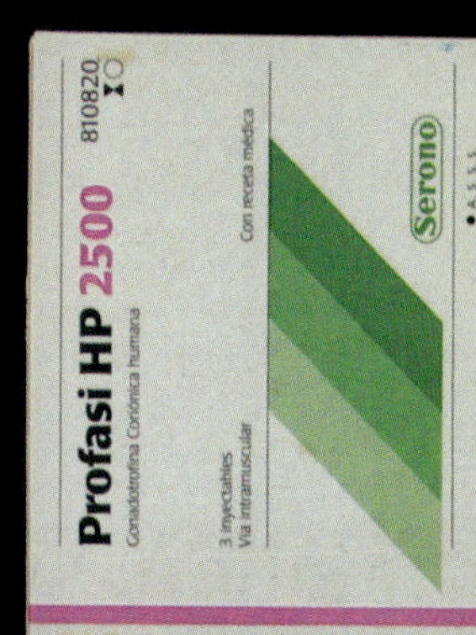

Profasi (Italy)

Endo (French)

Pregnyl (Brazil)

Profasi (Spain)

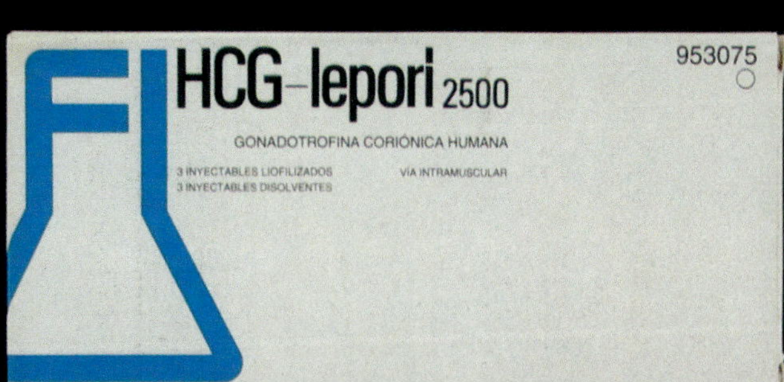

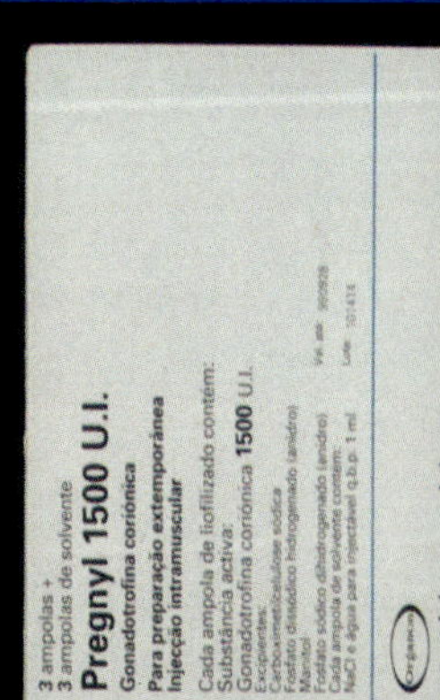

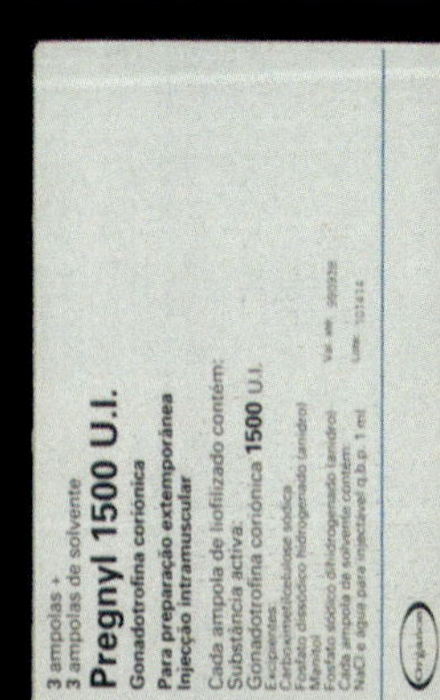

HCG-lepori (Spain)

Pregnyl from Greece and Portugal

HELIOS

Insulin

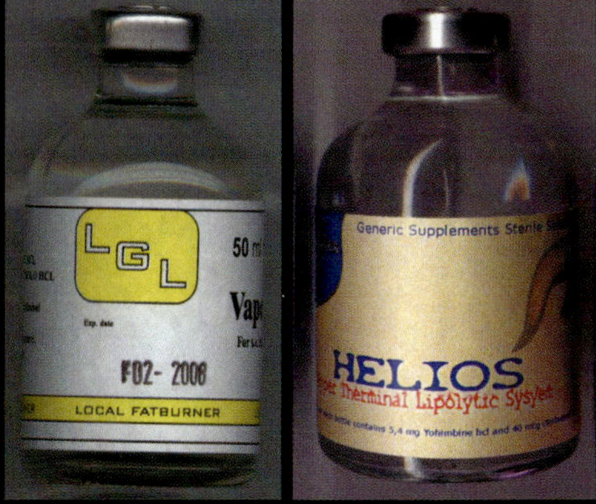

HELIOS from LGL and Generic Supplements

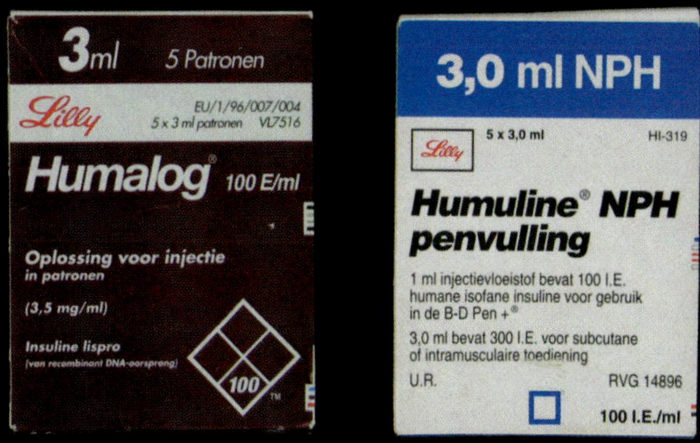

Lilly Humalog and Humuline

Lasix

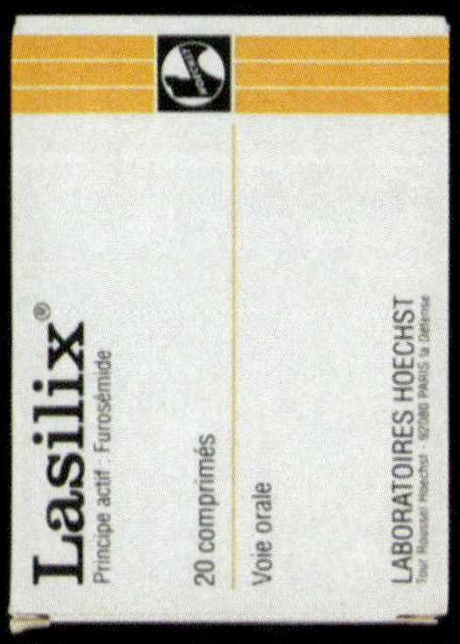

(France)

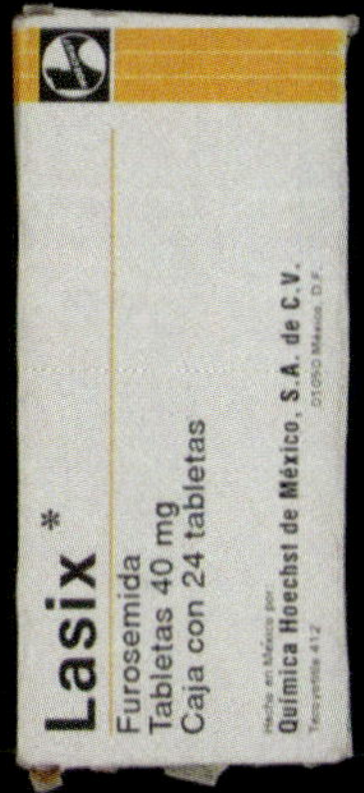

(Mexico)

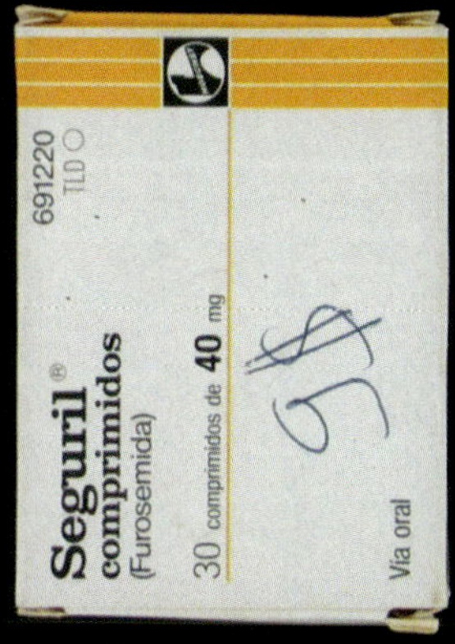

(Spain)

Kynoselen

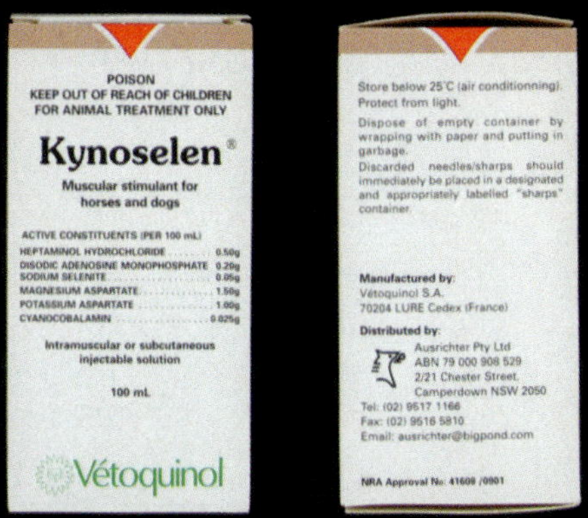

Kynoselen (U.K.)

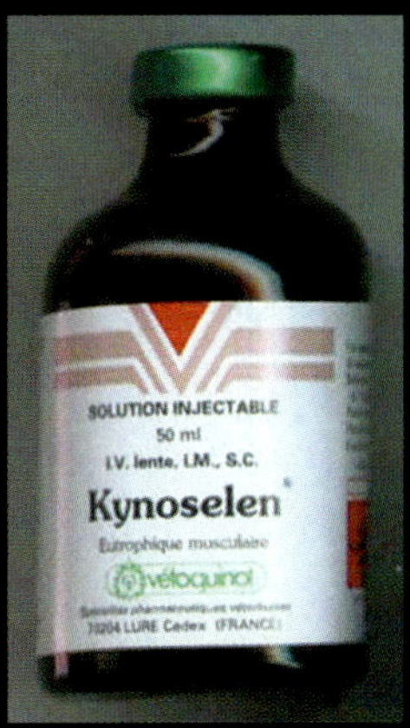

Kynoselen (France)

Lentaron

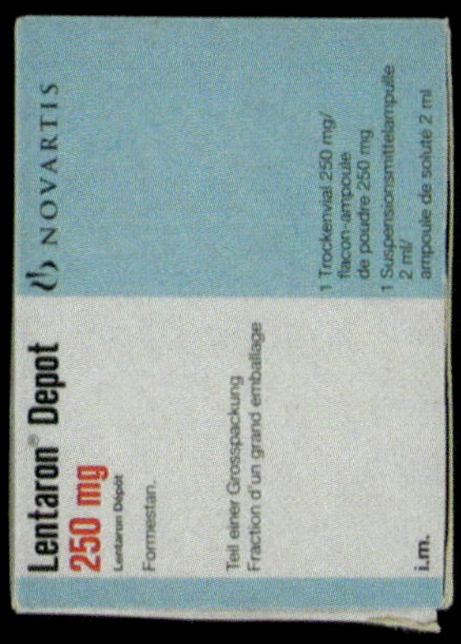

Lentaron (UK)

Lutalyse

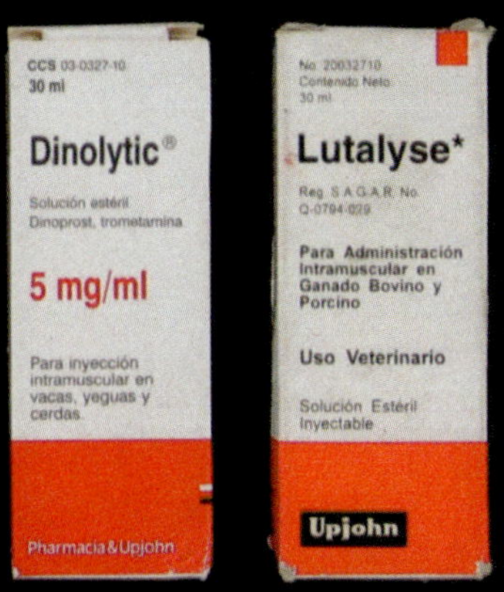

Spanish and American products

Nolvadex

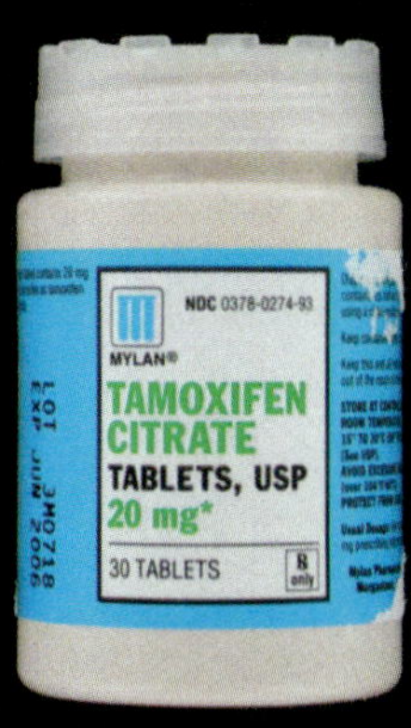

Mylan generic (U.S.)

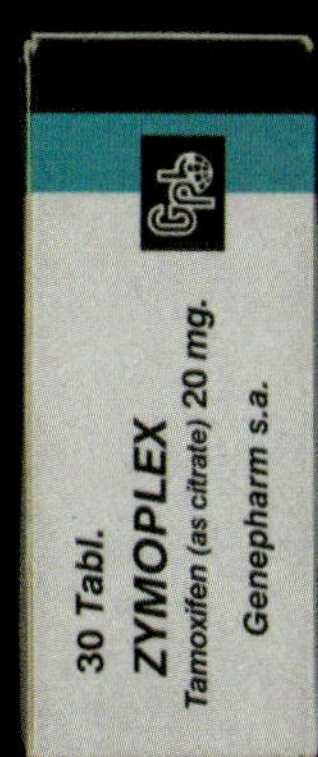

Zymoplex (Greece)

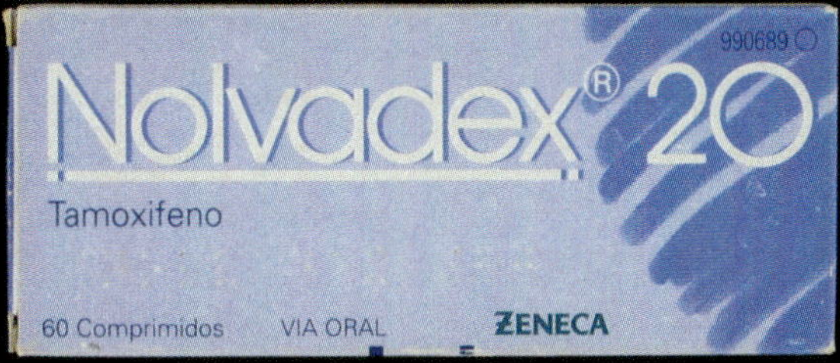

Nolvadex (Spain)

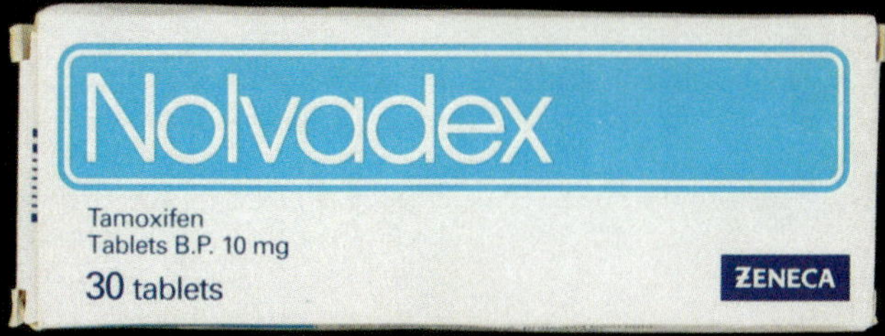

Nolvadex (Greece)

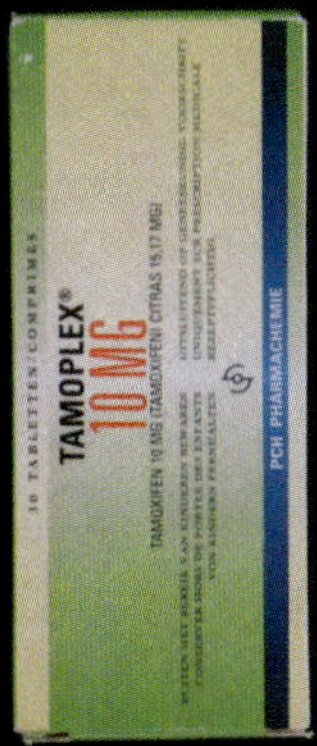

(Sri-Lanka)

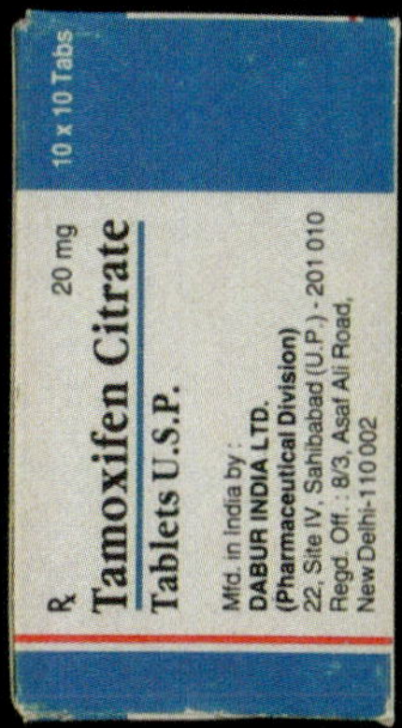

(India)

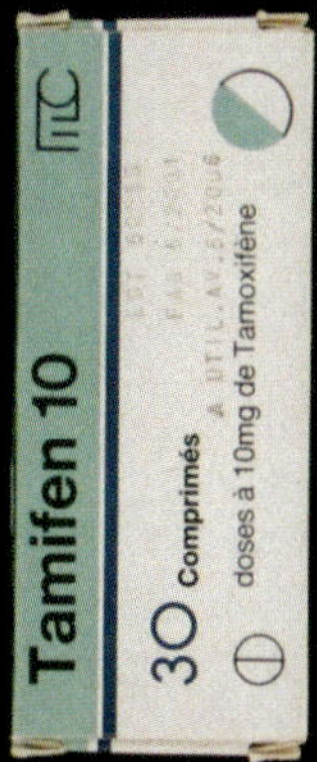

(Cypress)

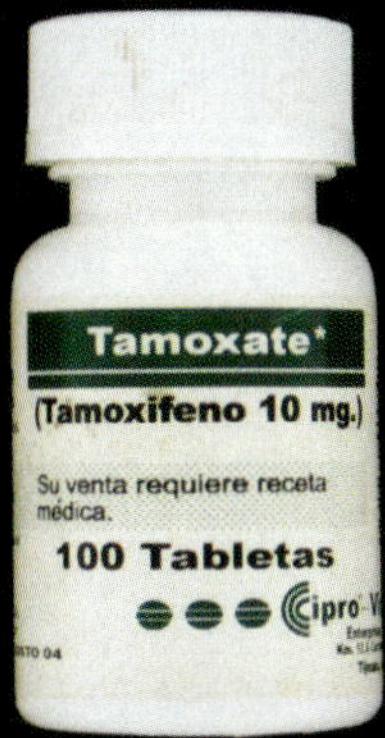

(Mexico)

Proscar

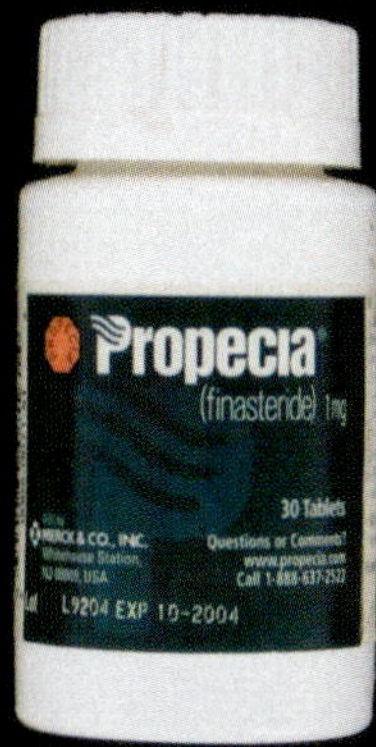

Propecia (U.S.)

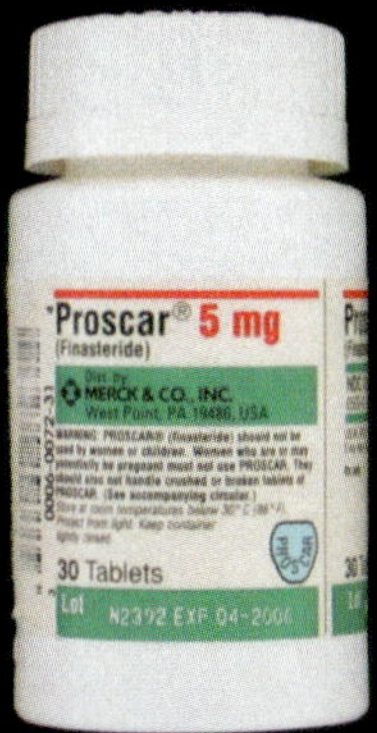

Proscar (U.S.)

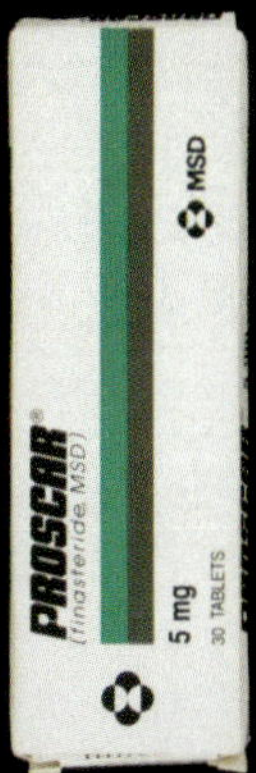

Thai Box

Parlodel

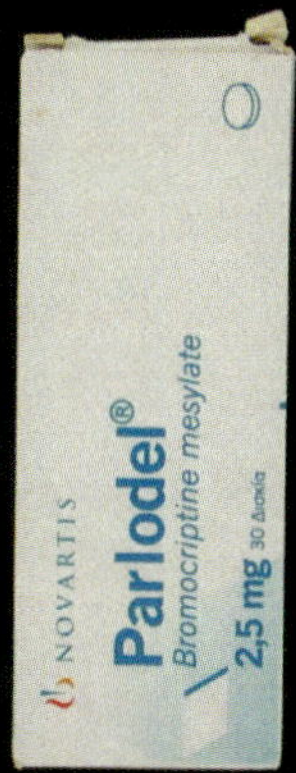

Greek Parlodel

Synthol

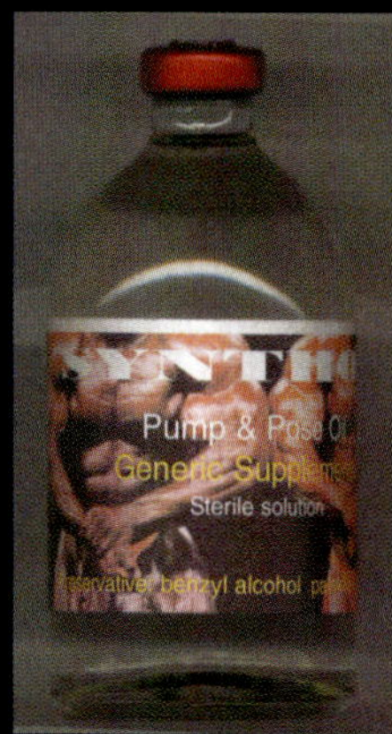

UG Synthol

Synthroid

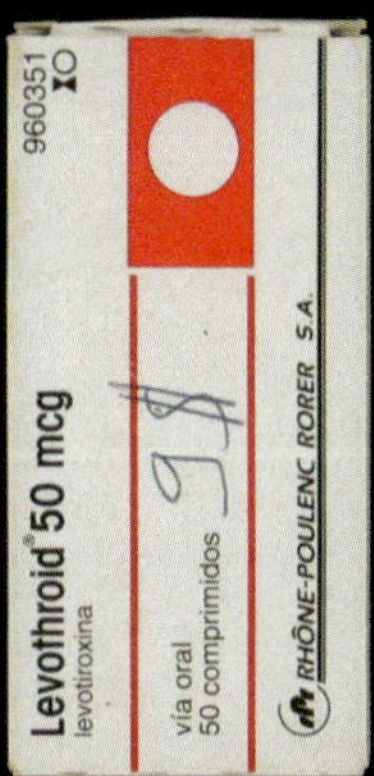

Levothroid (Spain)

Tationil

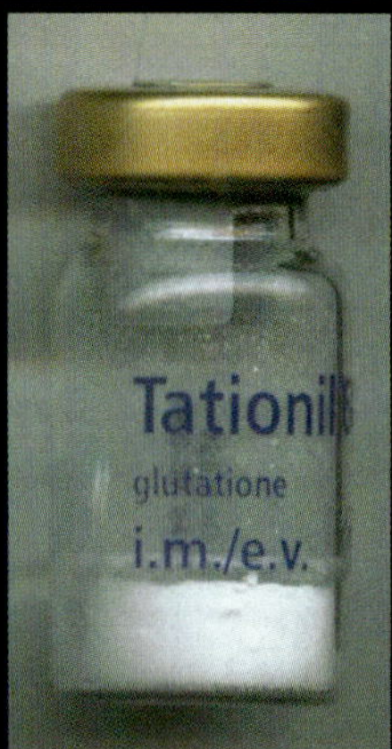

Tationil vial

Zaditen

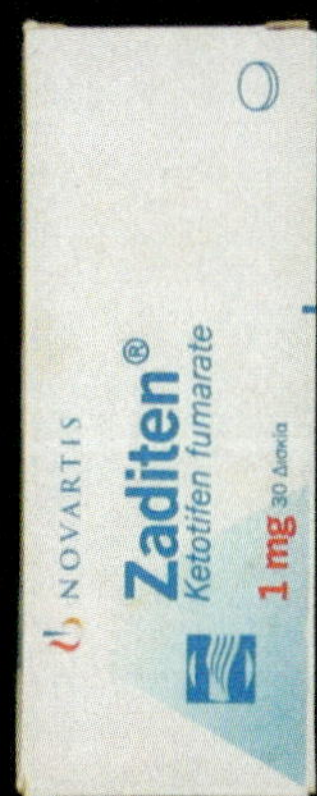

(Greece)

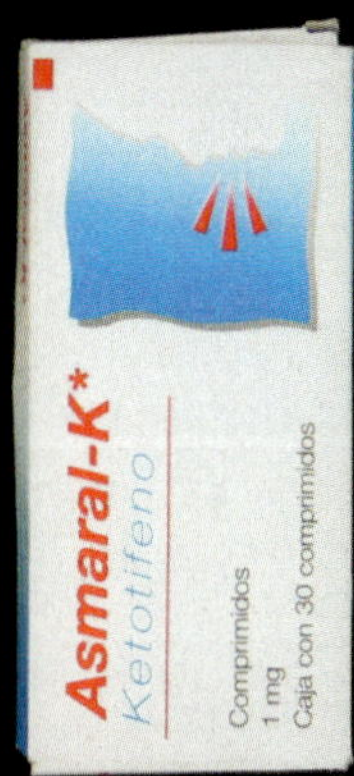

(Mexico)

Anabolic DN

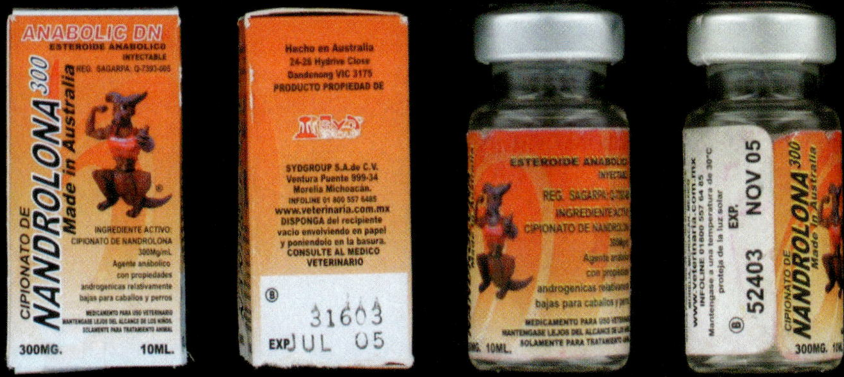

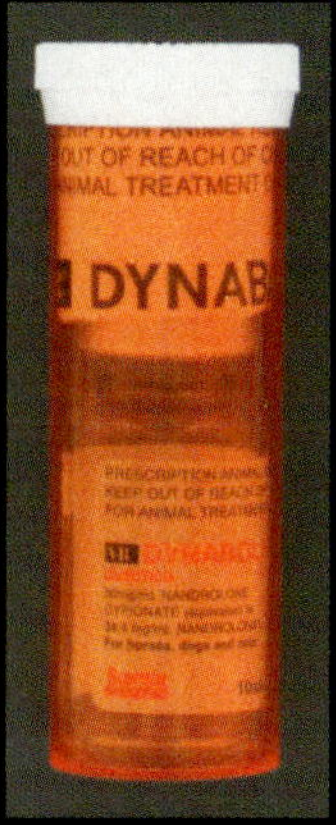

Anabolic DN from SYD Group (Mexico)

Jurox Dynabol (Australia)

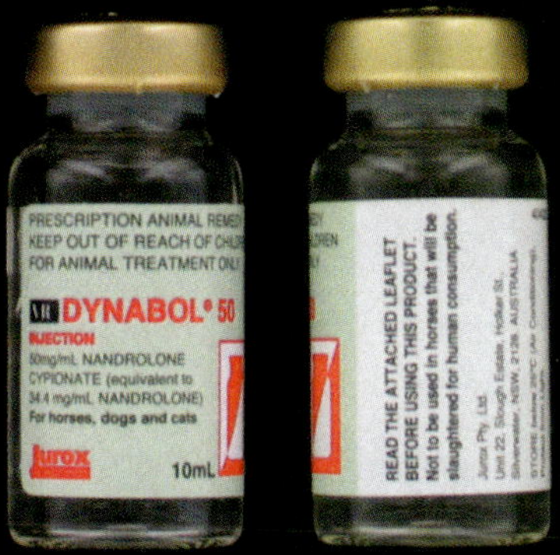

Anadrol

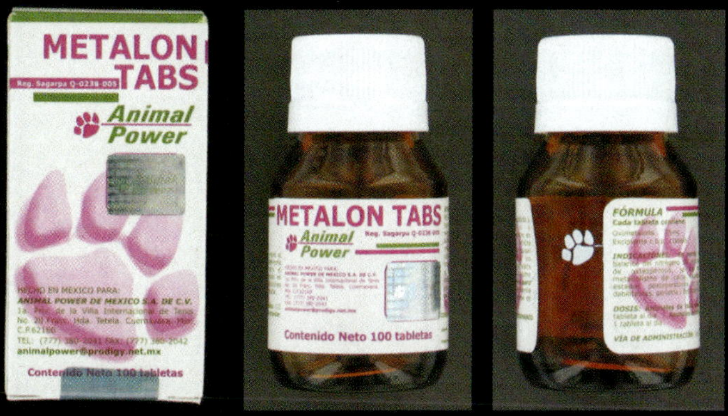

Jurox Dynabol 50 Vial

Metalon Tabs from Animal Power (Mexico)

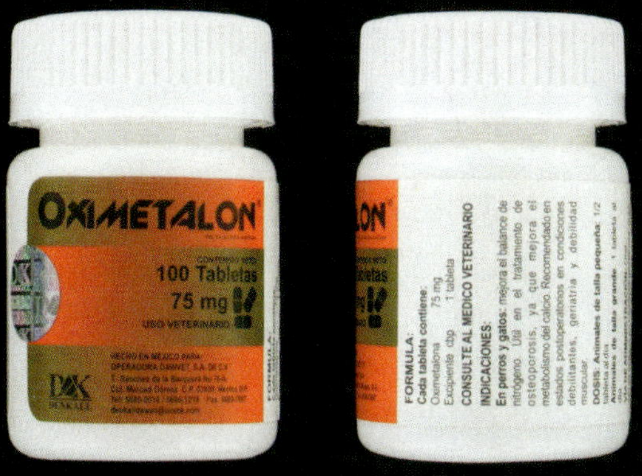

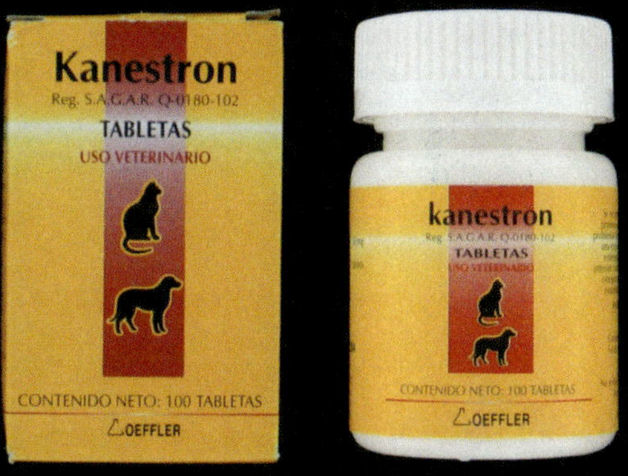

Oximetalon from Denkall (Mexico)

Kanestron from Loeffler (Mexico)

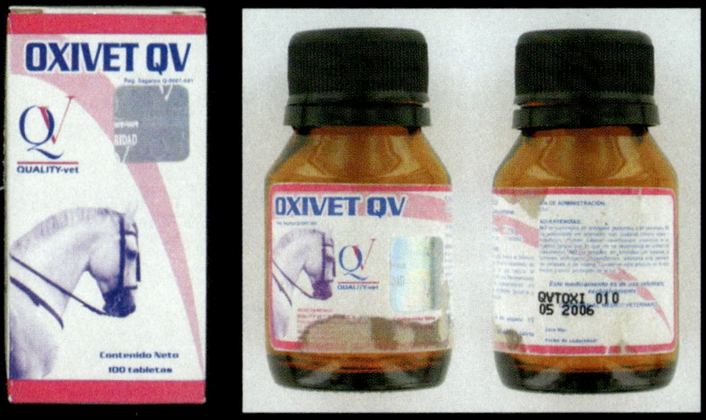

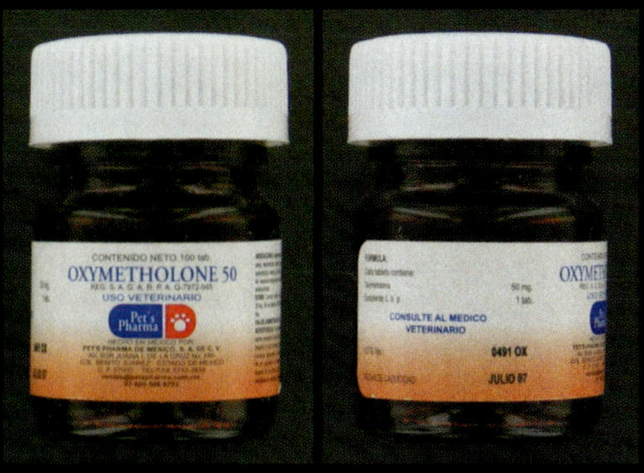

Oxivet box and vial from Quality Vet (Mexico)

Generic from Pet's Pharma (Mexico)

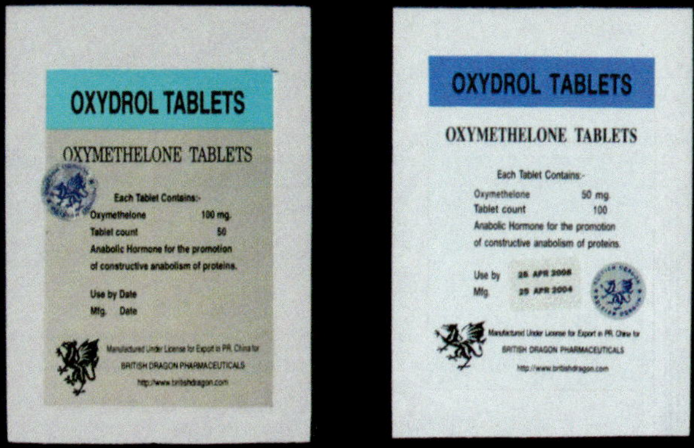

Oxydrol 100mg (NLM) and 50mg from British Dragon

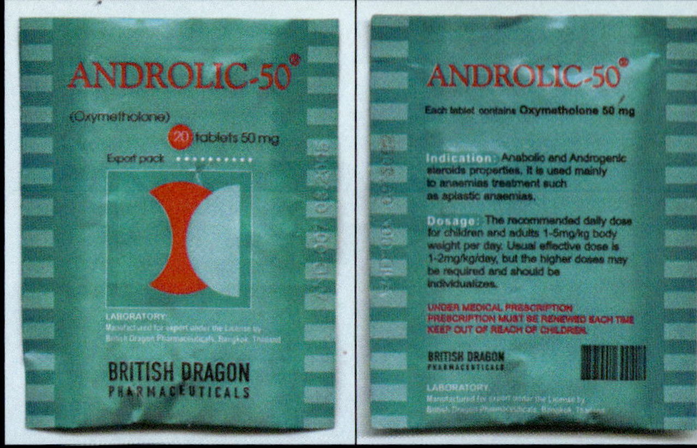

BD Eastern “Export” Pouch (NLM)

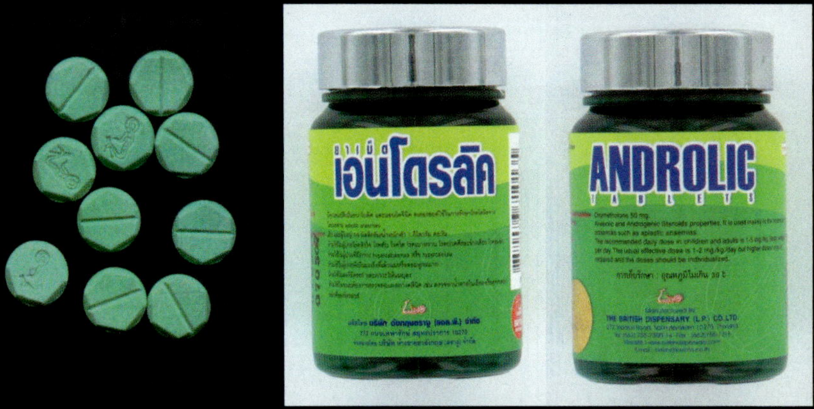

British Dispensary Androlic (Thailand)

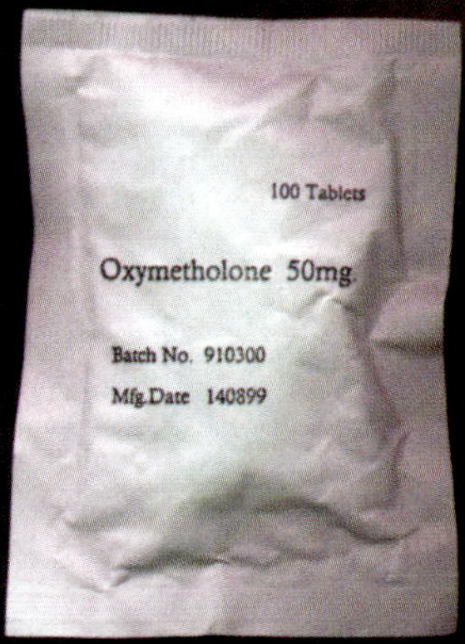

Old BD Pouch

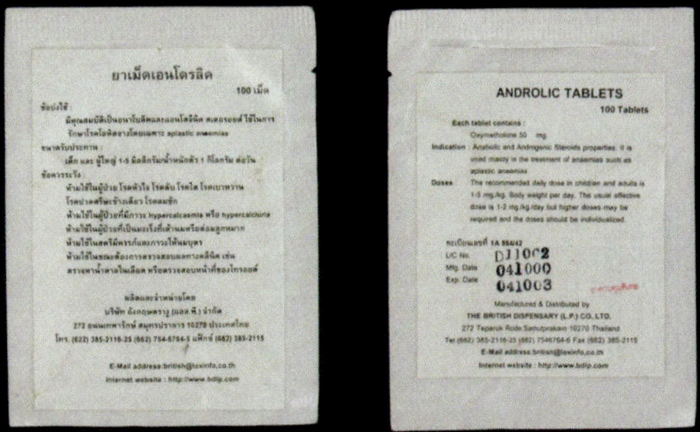

Another British Dispensary Pouch (NLM)

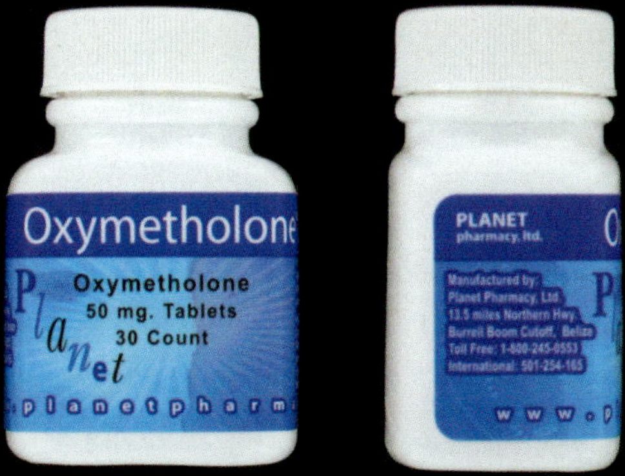

Generic from Planet Pharmacy (Belize)

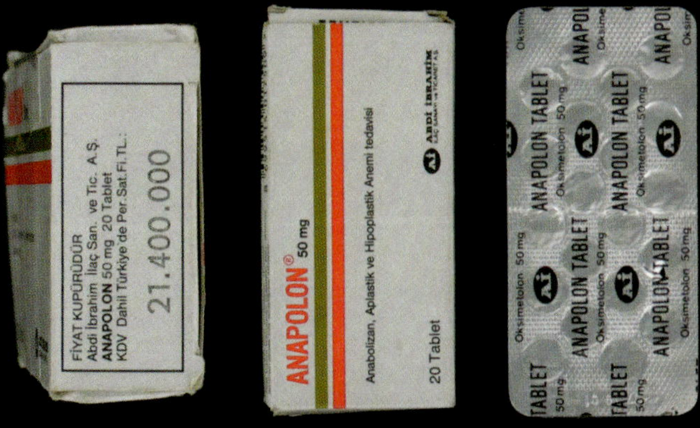

Anapolon from Turkey

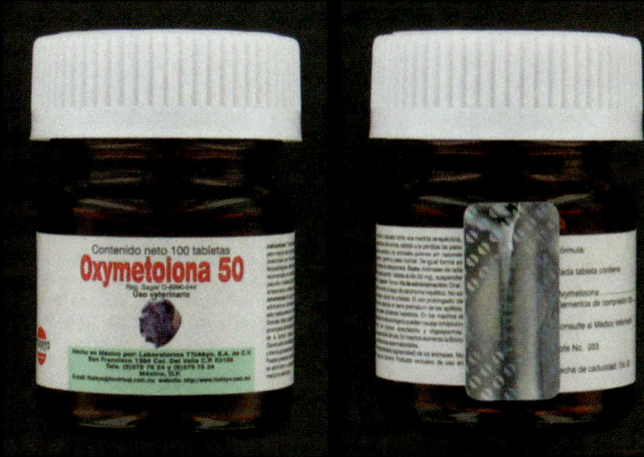

Ttokkyo generic from Mexico (NLM)

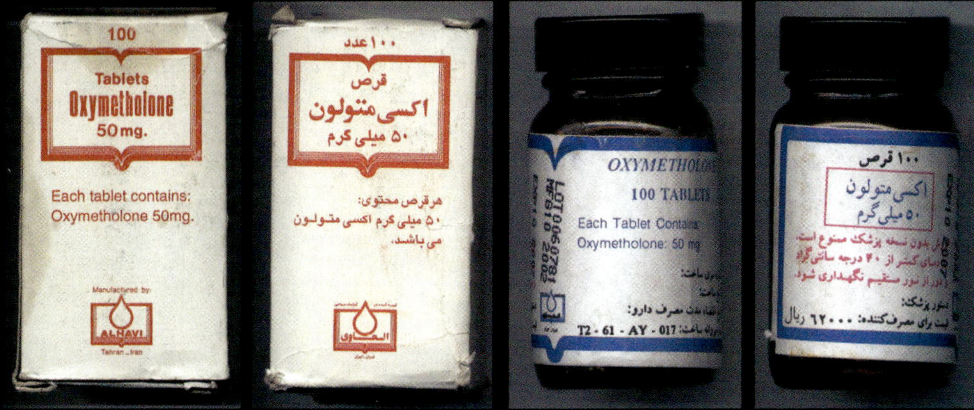

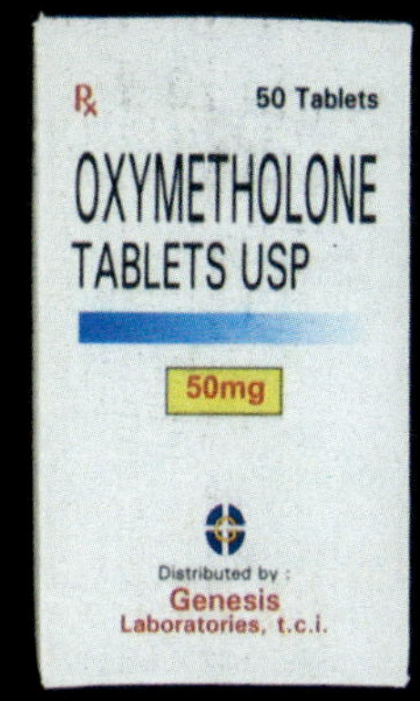

Generic from Alhavi (Israel) Genesis (Singapore)

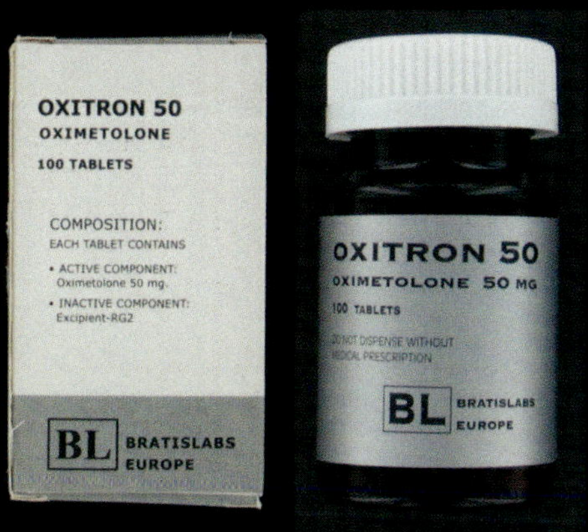

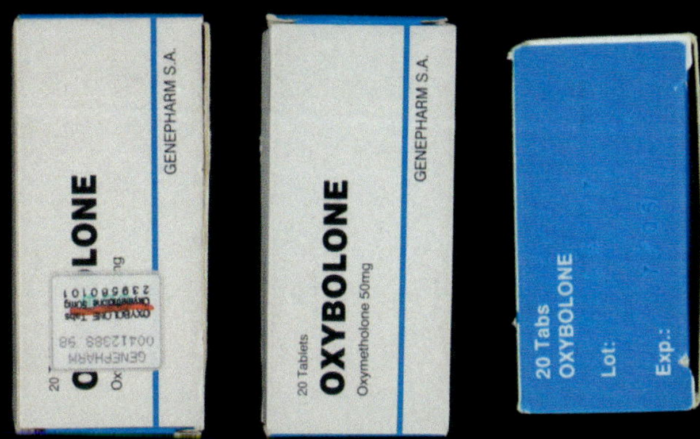

Bratis Oxitron (Mexico) Oxybolone from Greece

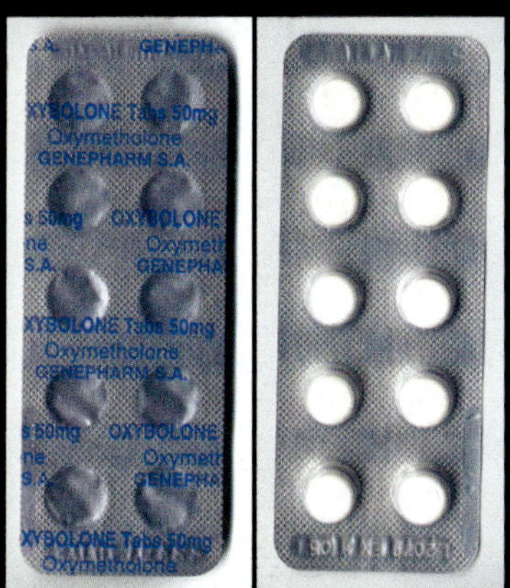

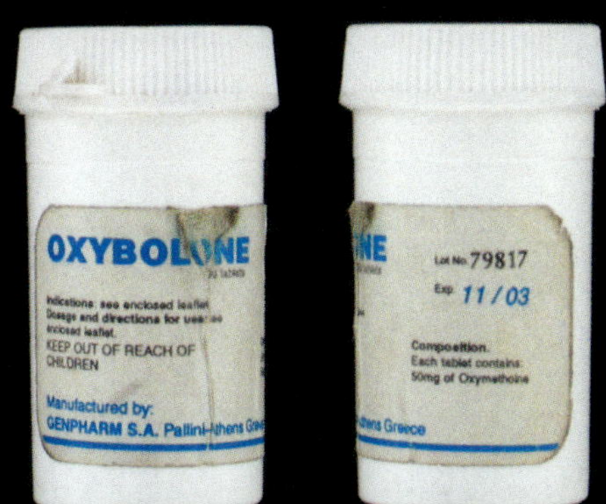

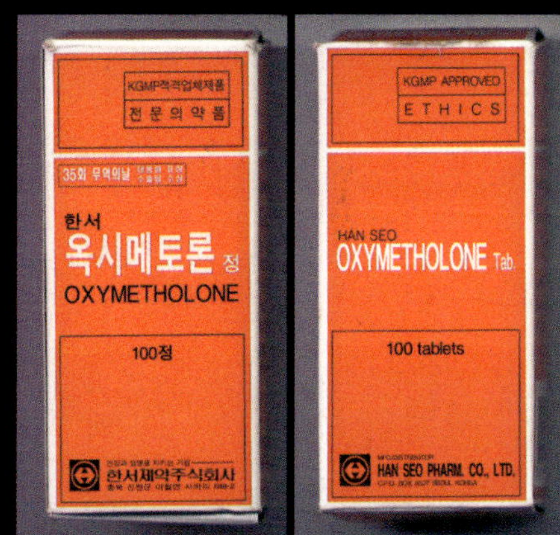

Oxybolone Strip (real) Oxybolone bottle (fake) Han Seo generic (Korea)

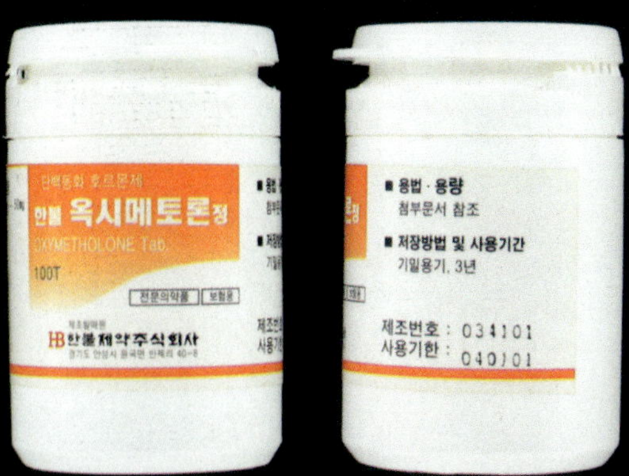

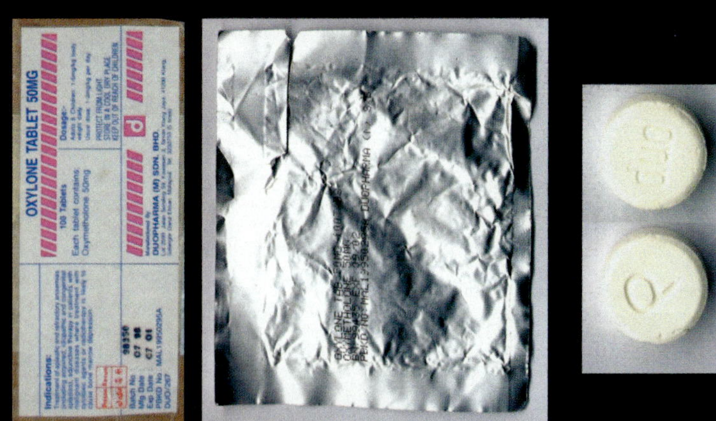

Han Bul generic (Korea) Oxylone from Duopharma (Malaysia)

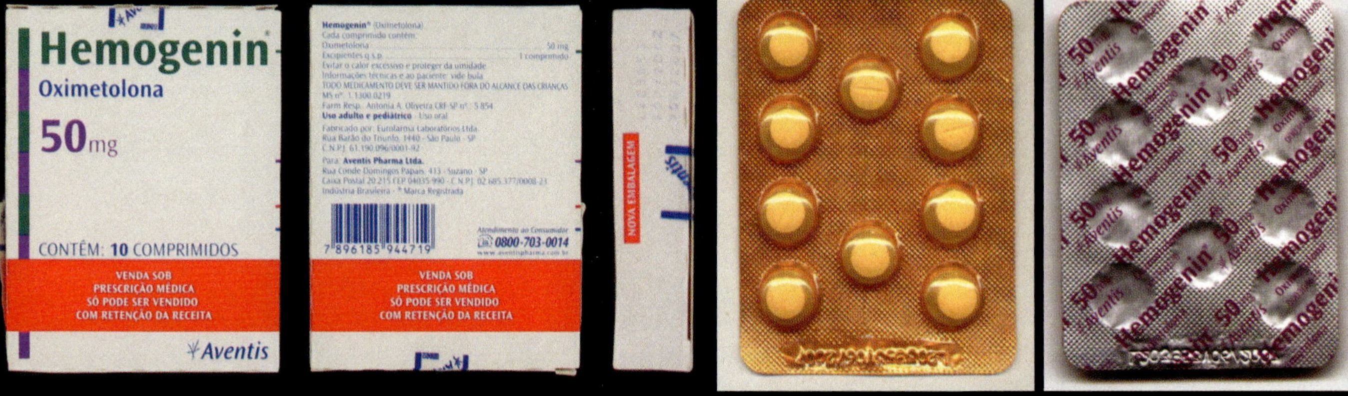

Hemogenin (50mg oxymetholone) from Aventis (Brazil) - Most recent version

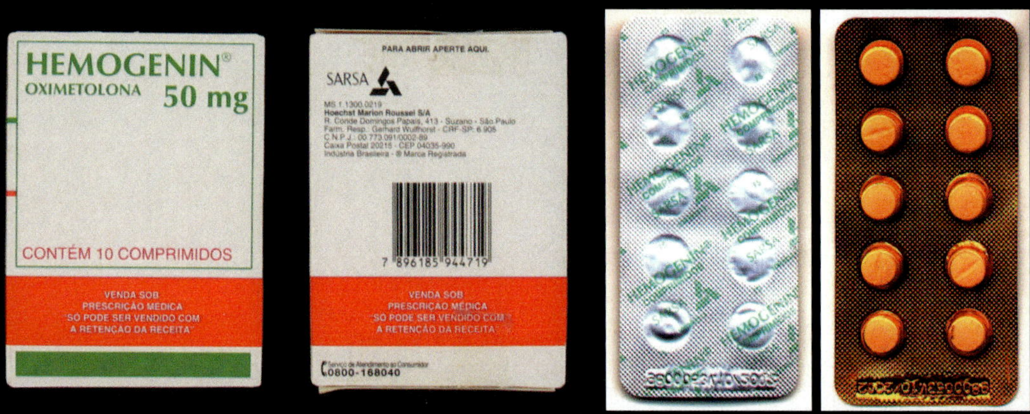

Older Hemogenin from Sarsa (Brazil)

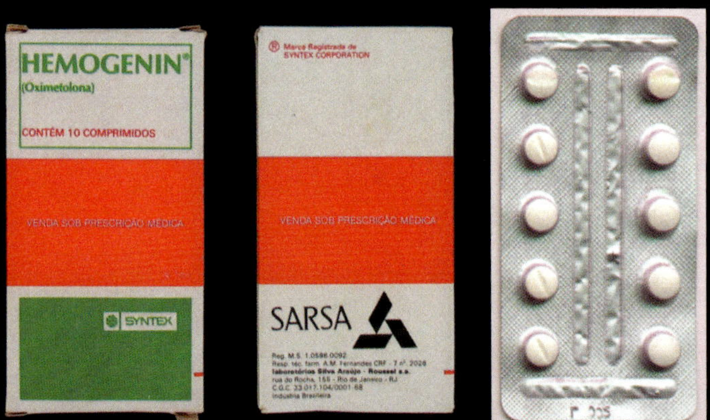

Oldest version of Hemogenin shown

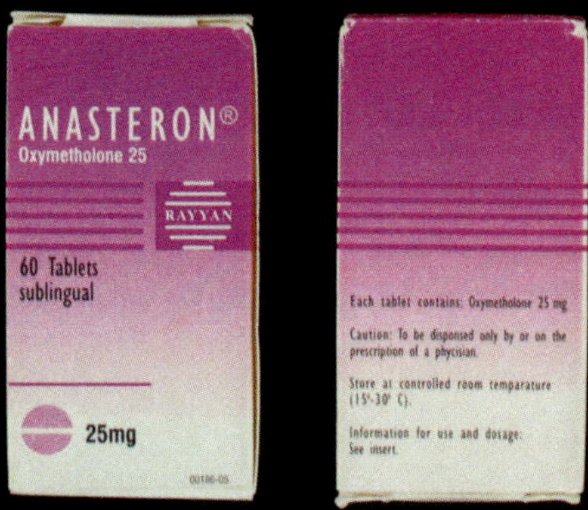

Anasteron - Old Greek Export (NLM)

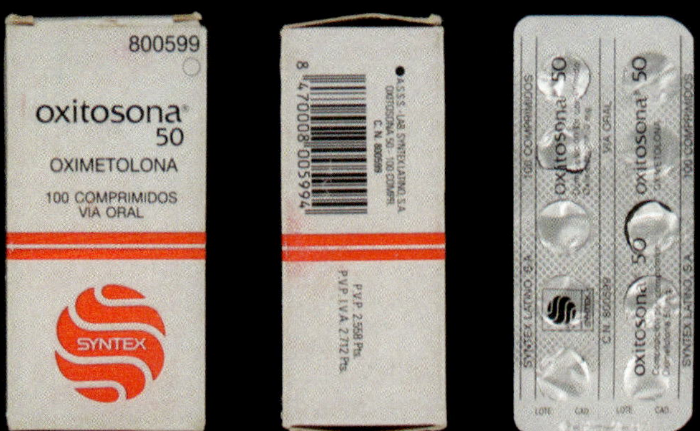

Real Oxitosona from Spain (NLM)

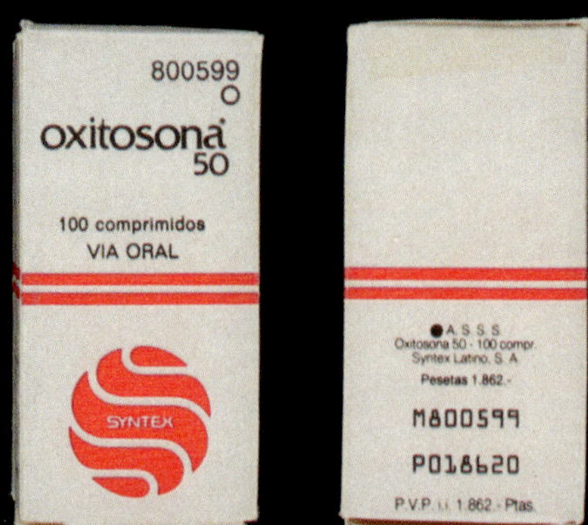

Counterfeit Oxitosona

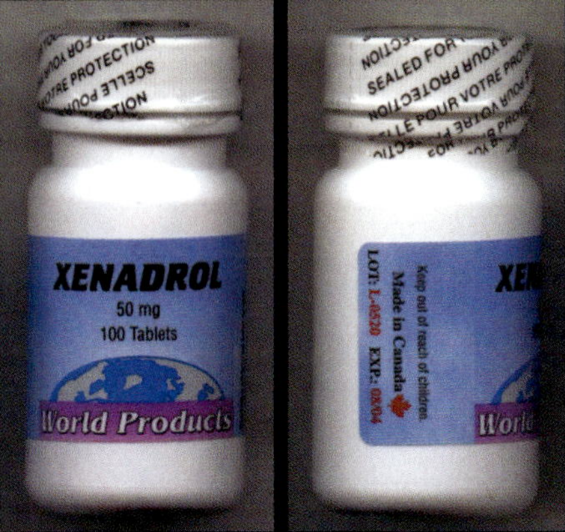

Underground product - World

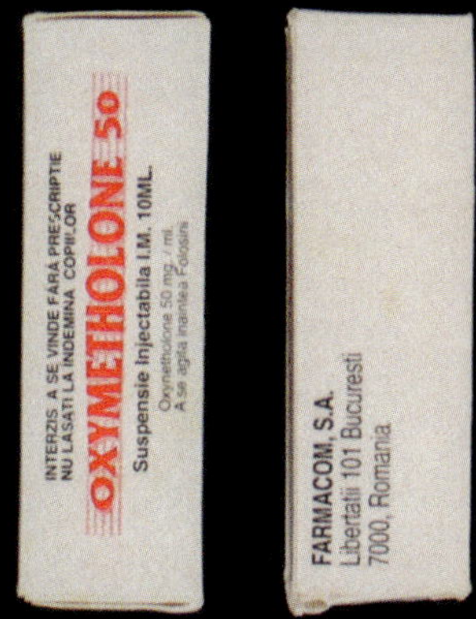

UG oxy injectable

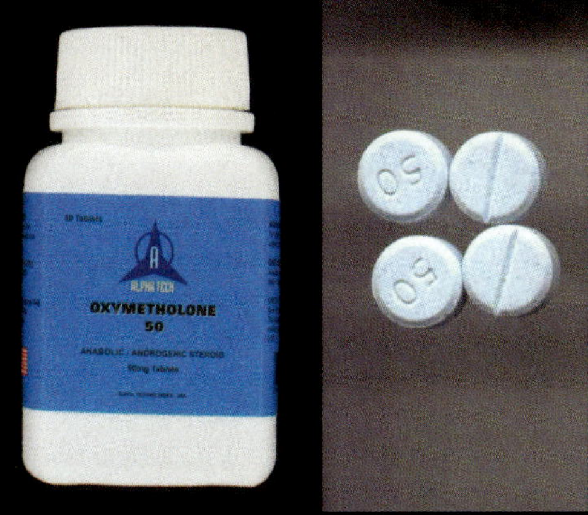

Alpha Tech (NLM) - UG Product

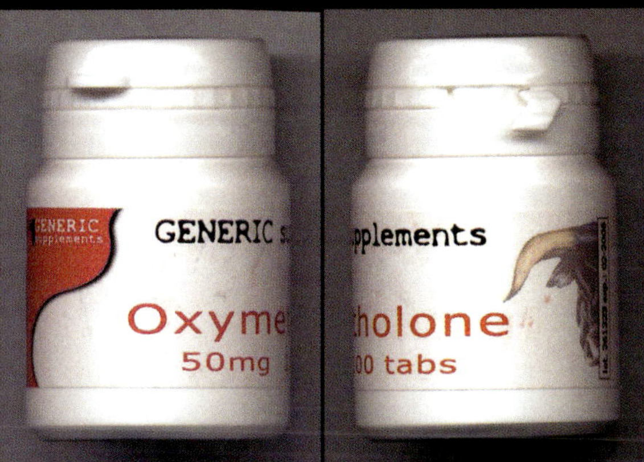

Generic Supplements oxymetholone (UG)

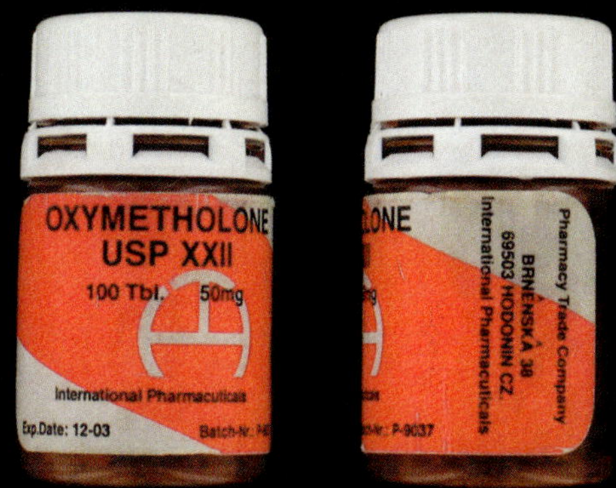

Underground IP generic

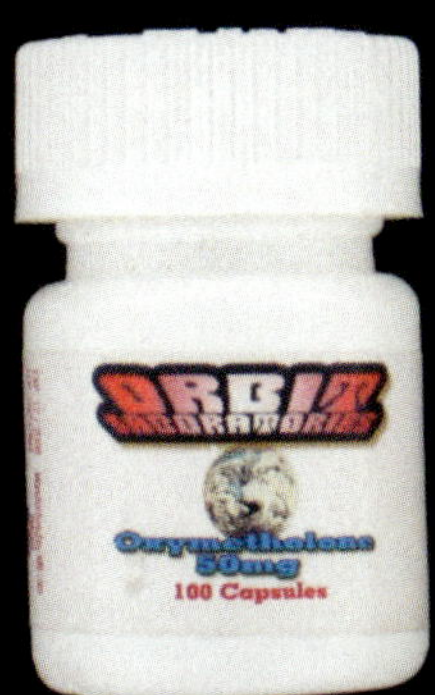

Orbit generic (UG)

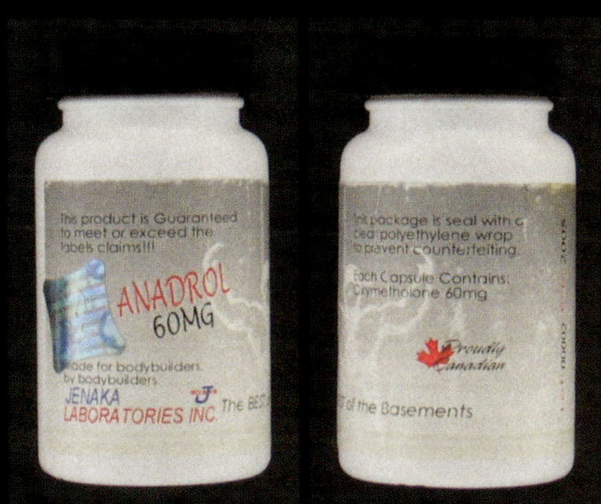

Jenaka UG oxy (NLM)

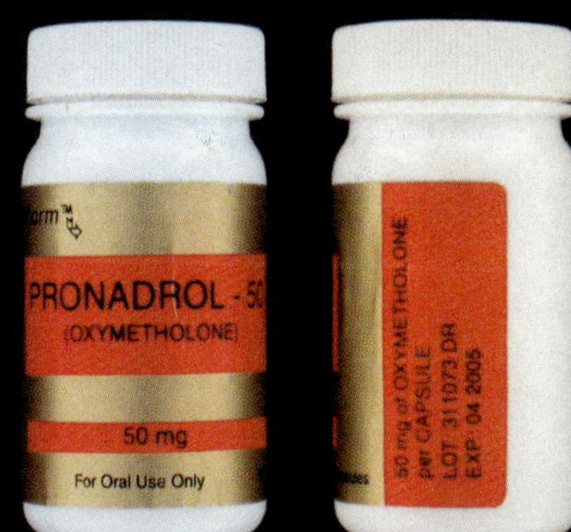

Valopharm UG product

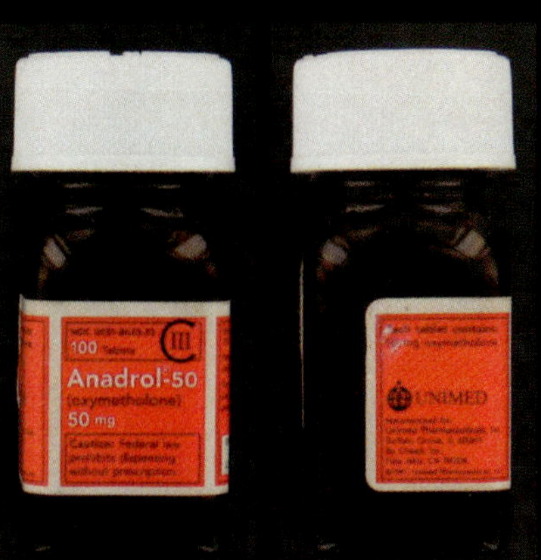

Counterfeit U.S. Unimed product

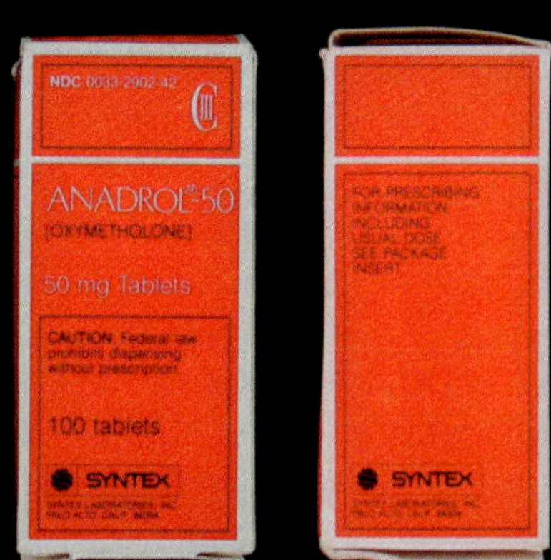

Counterfeit of the old Syntex brand

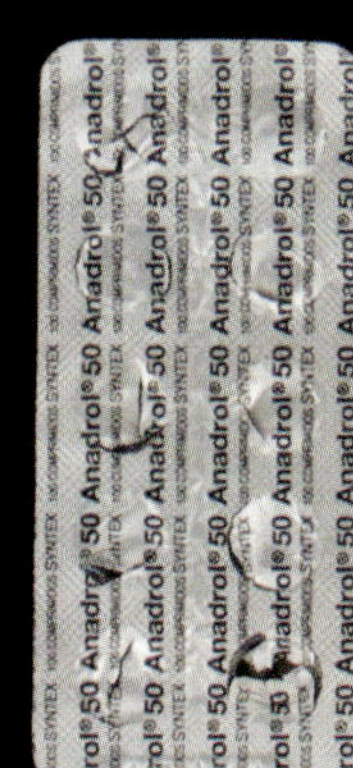

Bogus strip

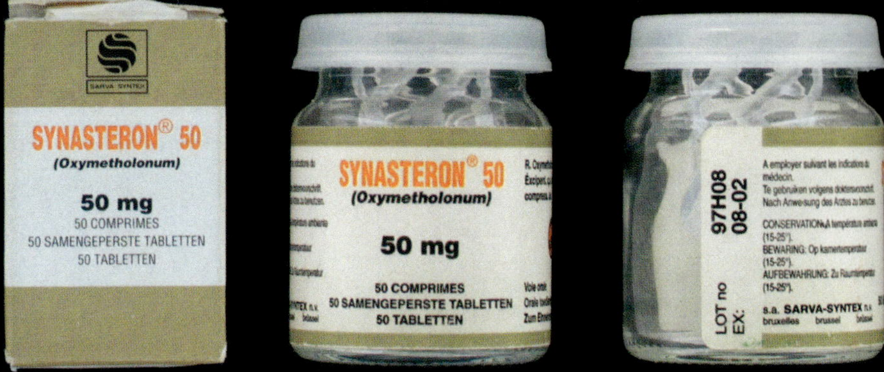

Counterfeit Belgian Synasteron

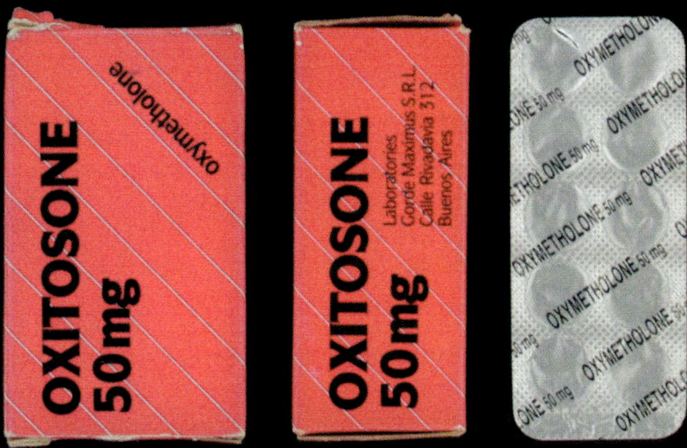

Bogus "Oxitosone" - No such brand is made

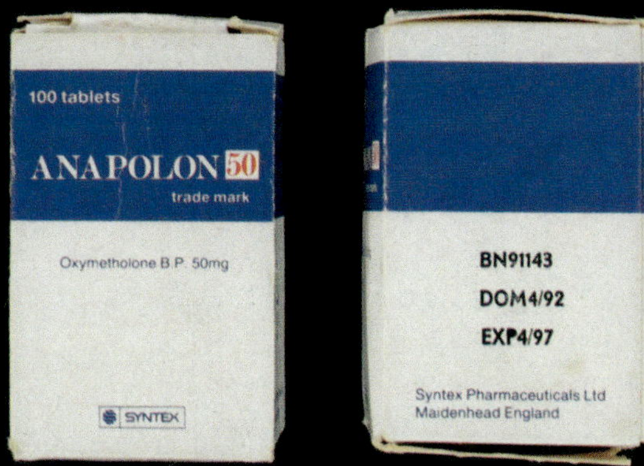

Counterfeit UK Anapolon

Anavar

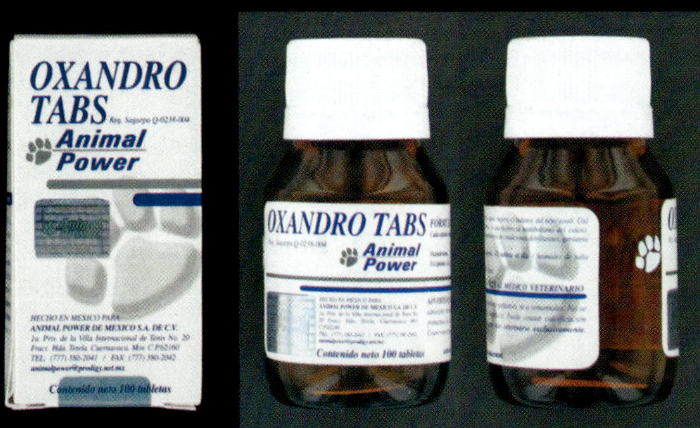

Oxandro Tabs from Animal Power (Mexico)

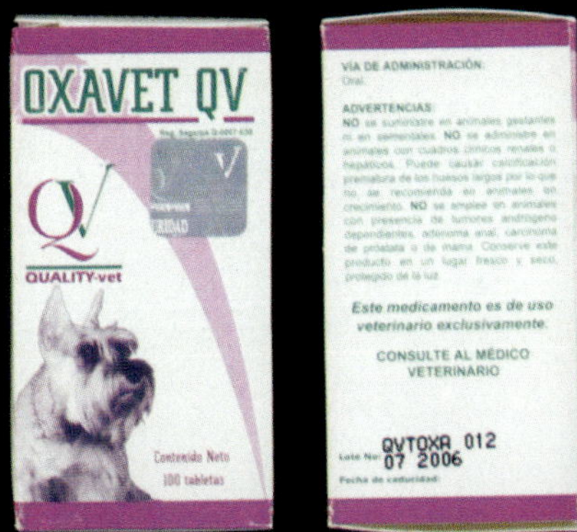

Oxavet from Quality Vet (Mexico)

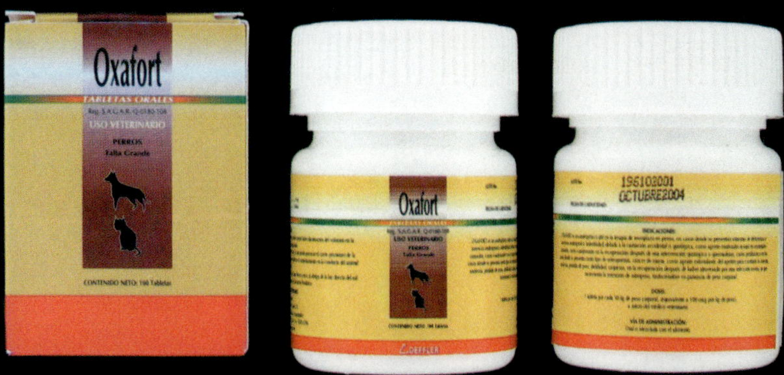

Oxafort from Loeffler (Mexico)

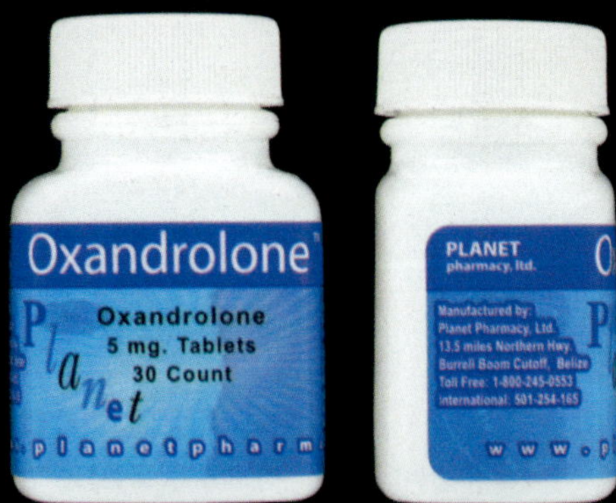

Generic from Planet Pharm (Belize)

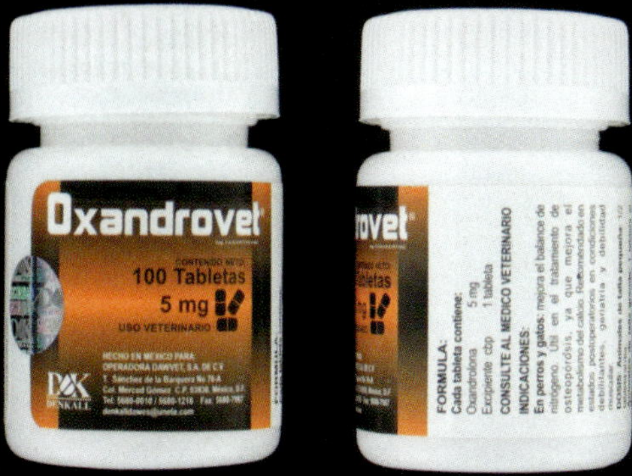

Oxandrovet from Denkall (Mexico)

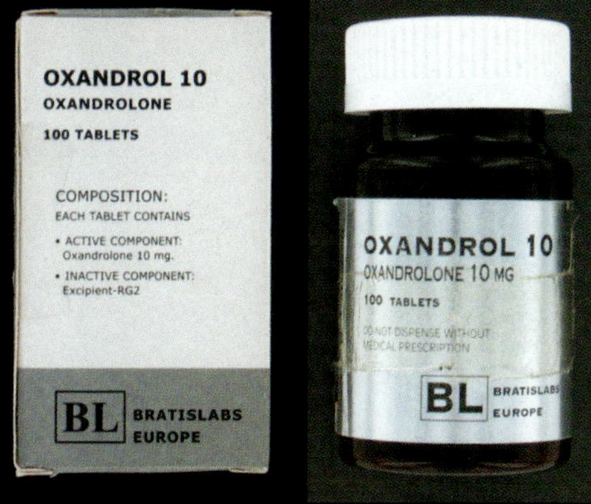

Old Oxandrol from Bratis (Mexico)

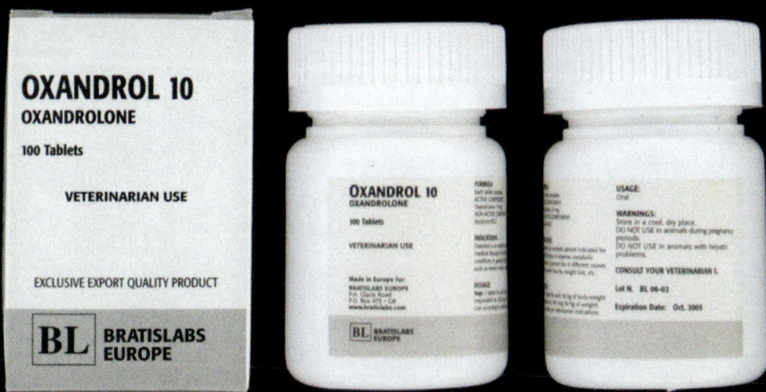

Newer style Bratis product

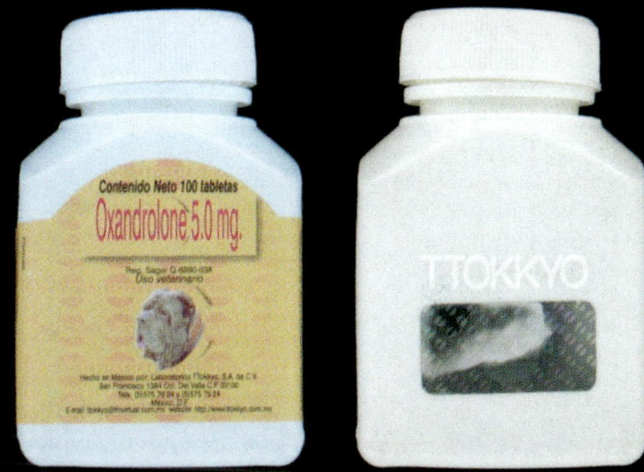

Ttokkyo 5mg generic from Mexico (NLM)

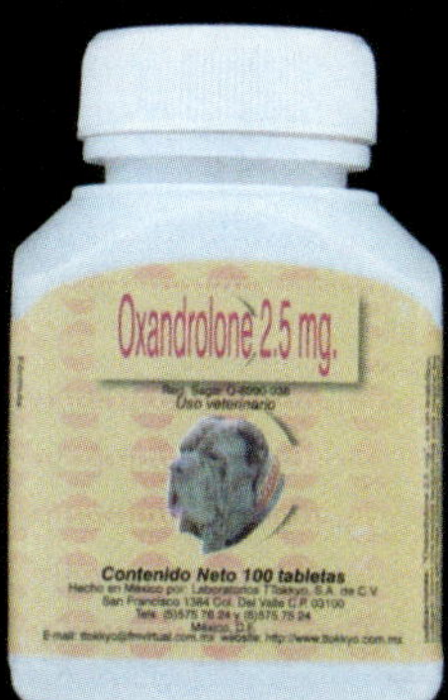

Ttokkyo 2.5mg (NLM)

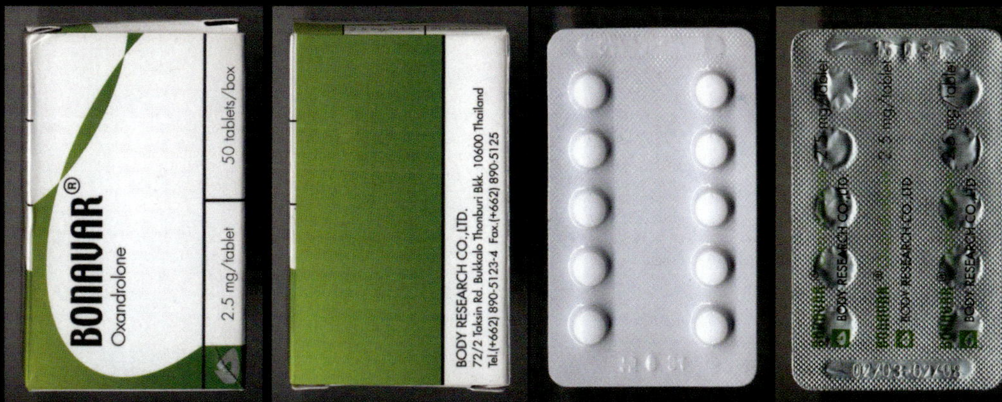

Bonavar from Body Research (Thailand)

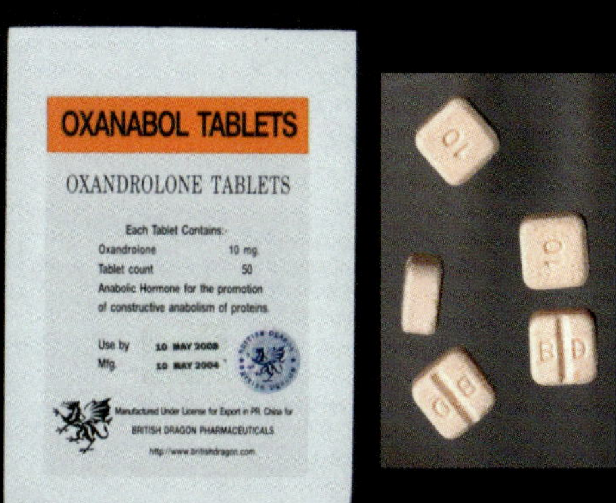

British Dragon Oxanabol (Thailand)

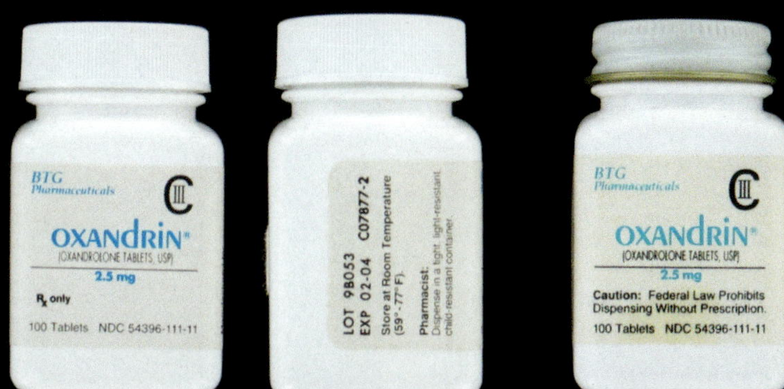

U.S. Oxandrin Newer and Older style bottles

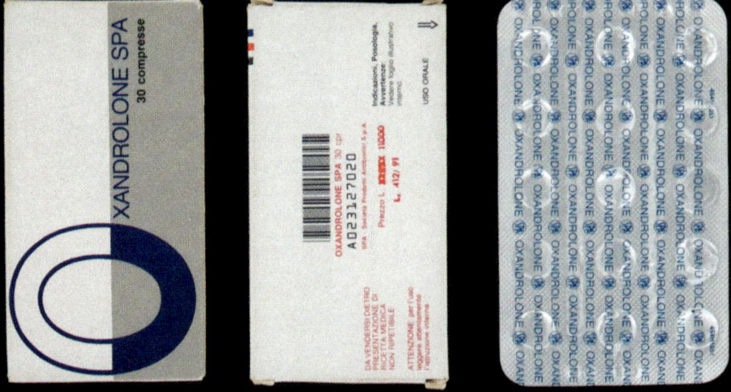

Italian domestic product from SPA (NLM)

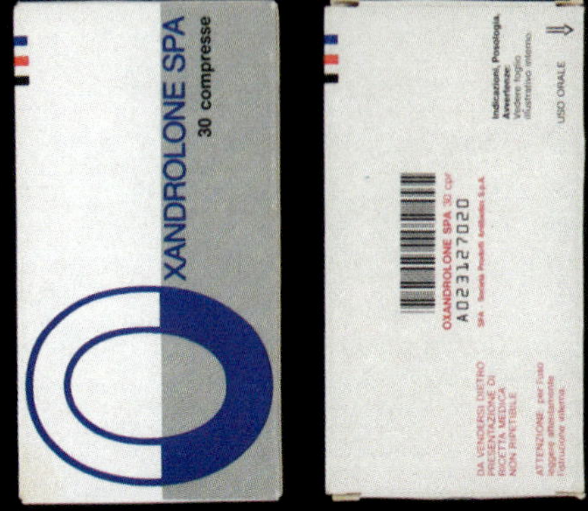

Counterfeit #1

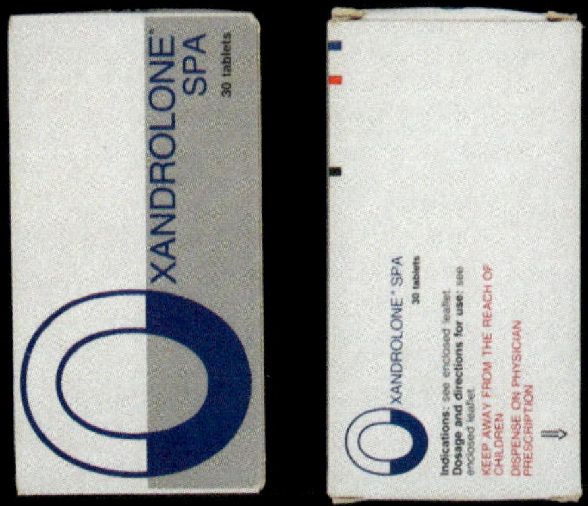

Counterfeit #2

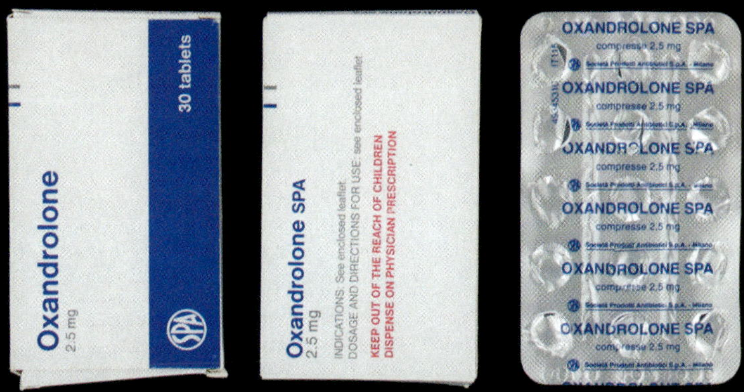

SPA Export item

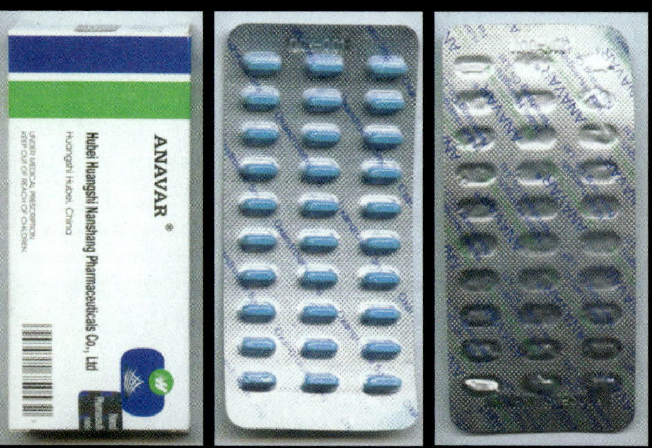

Anavar from China

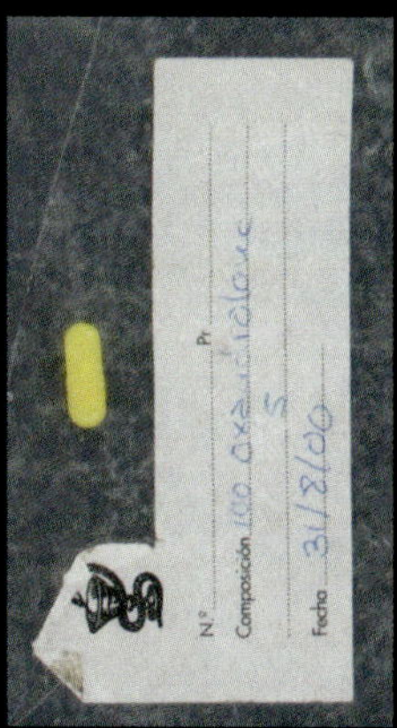

Spanish pharmacy prod

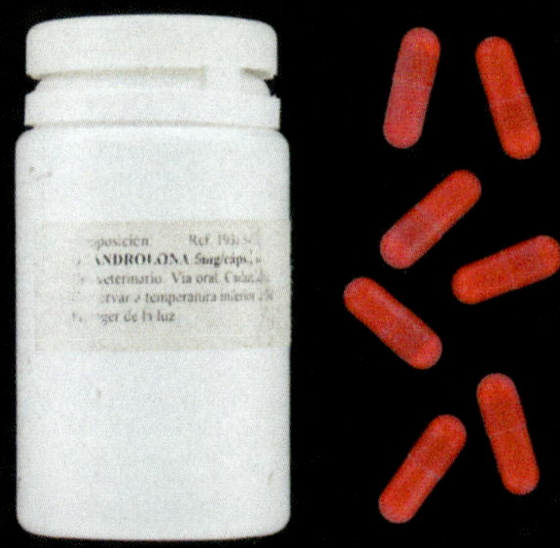

Spanish underground capsules

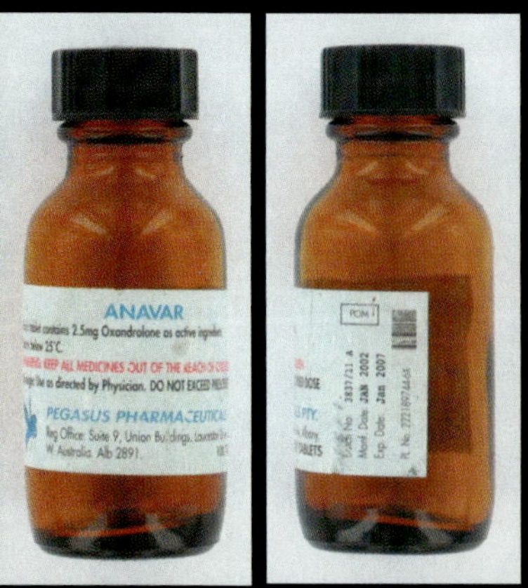

(UG) Pegasus product

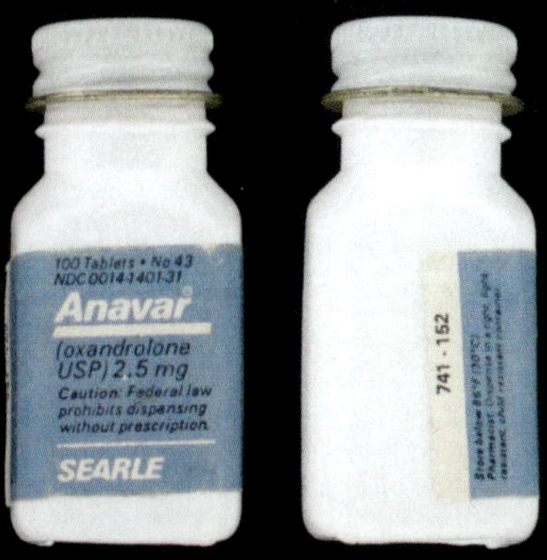

Counterfeit U.S. Anavar

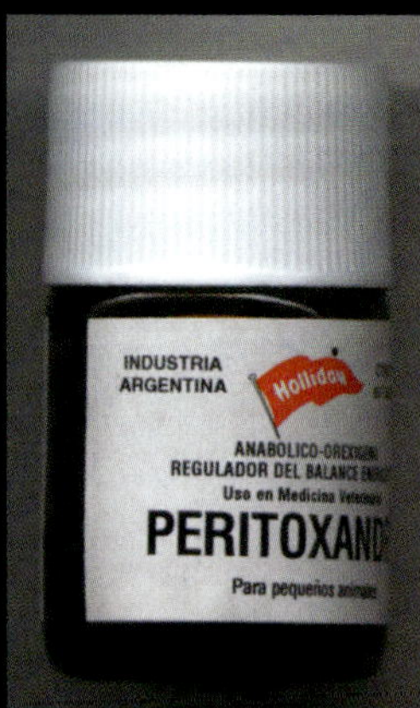

Counterfeit Holliday bottle

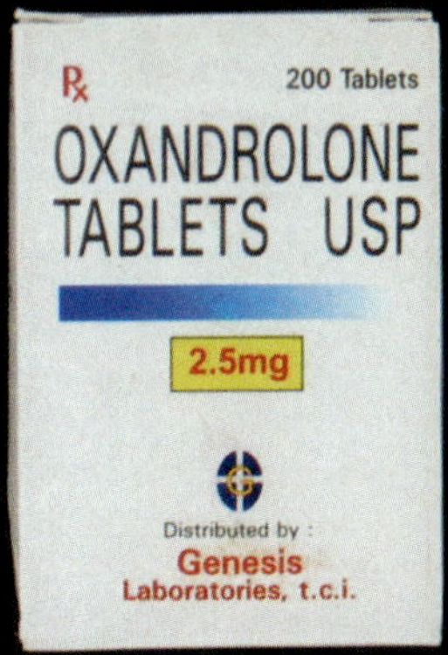

Genesis tabs (Singapore)

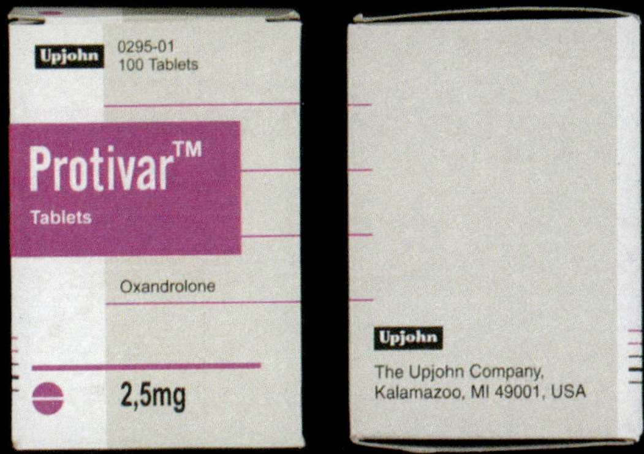

Bogus U.S. Protivar

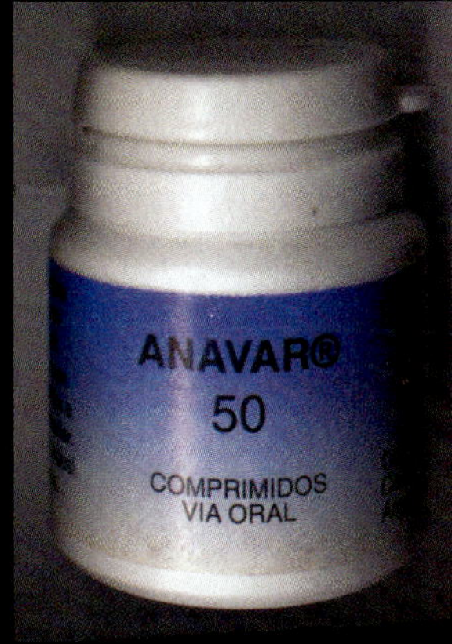

Counterfeit Anavar (Argentina)

Andriol

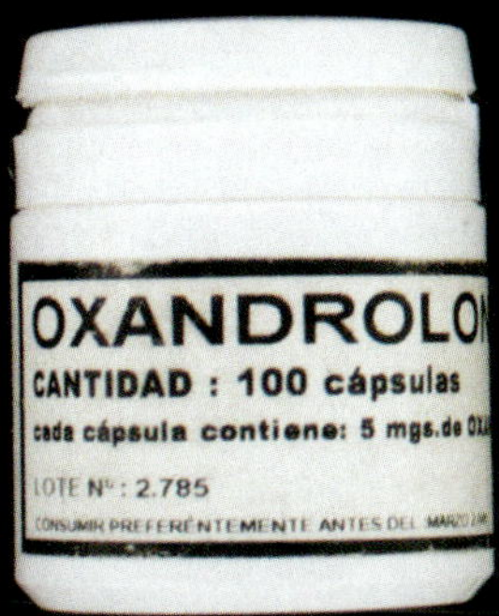

Fake generic bottle

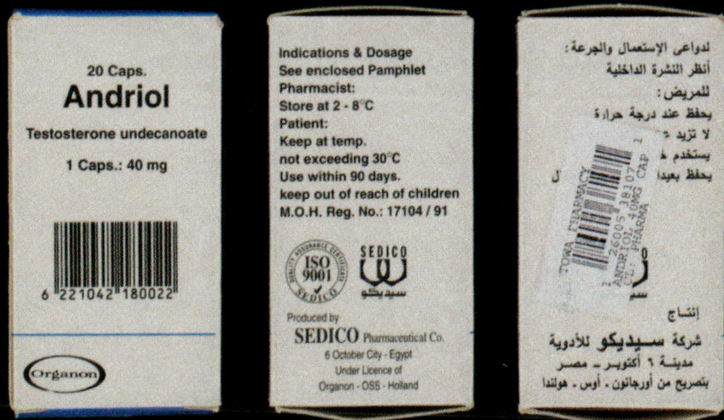

Andriol from Egypt

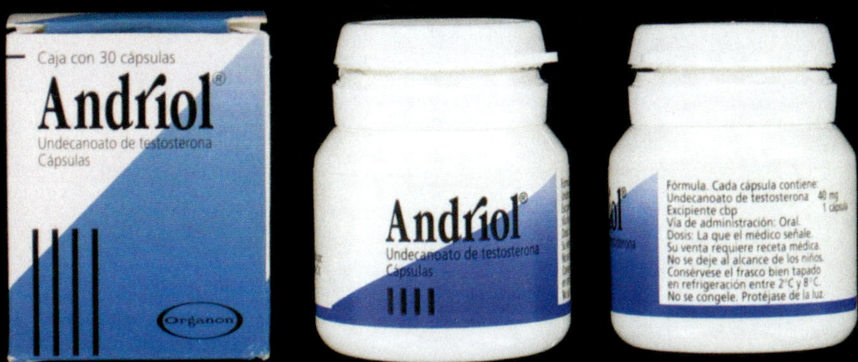

Andriol from Mexico

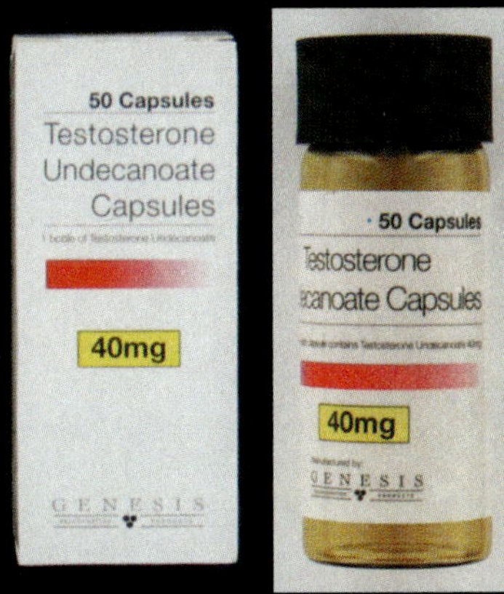

Genesis generic (Singapore)

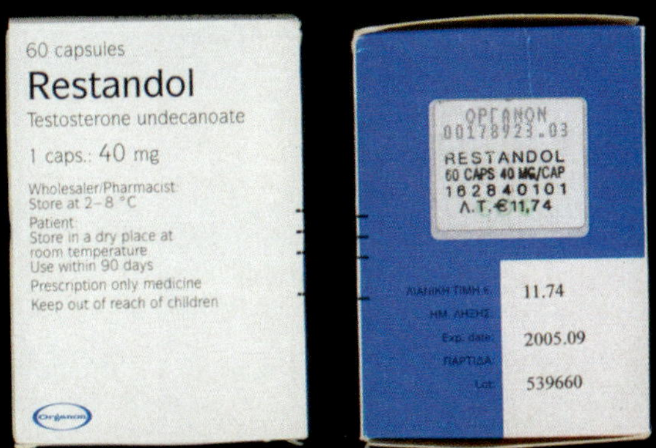

Greek Restandol

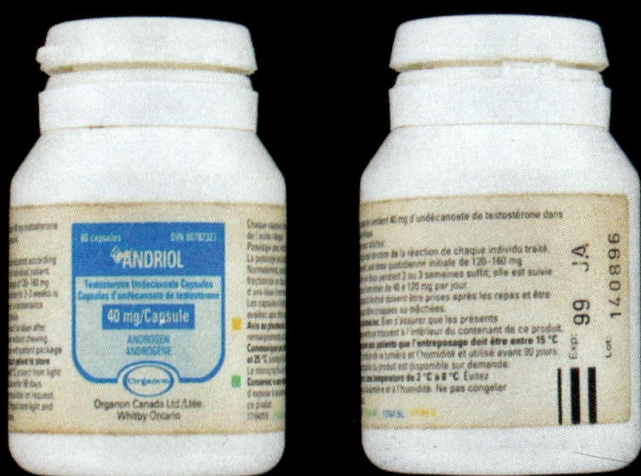

Canadian Andriol

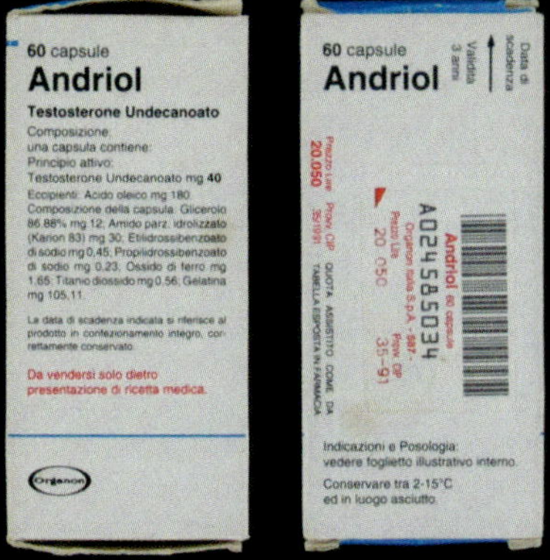

Italian Andriol

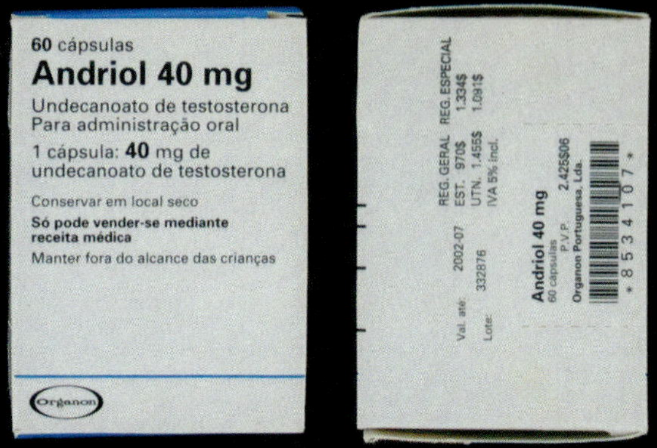

Andriol from Portugal

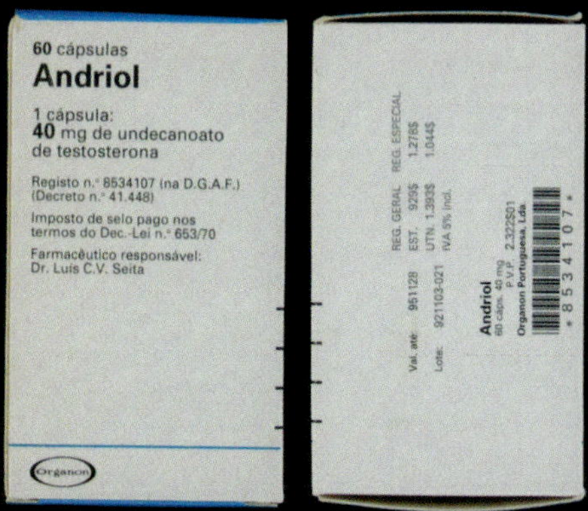

Old box from Portugal

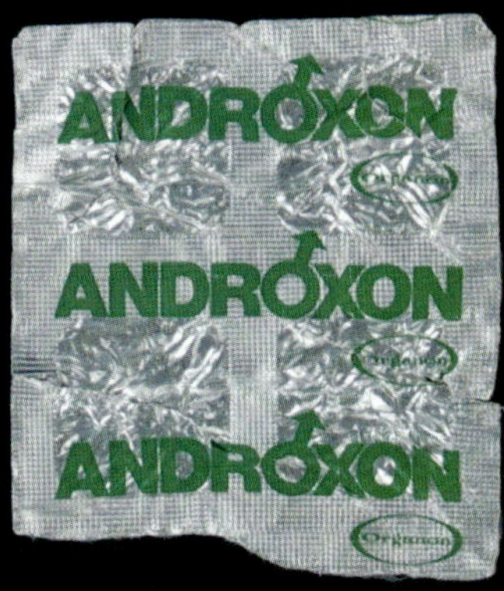

Androxon from Brazil

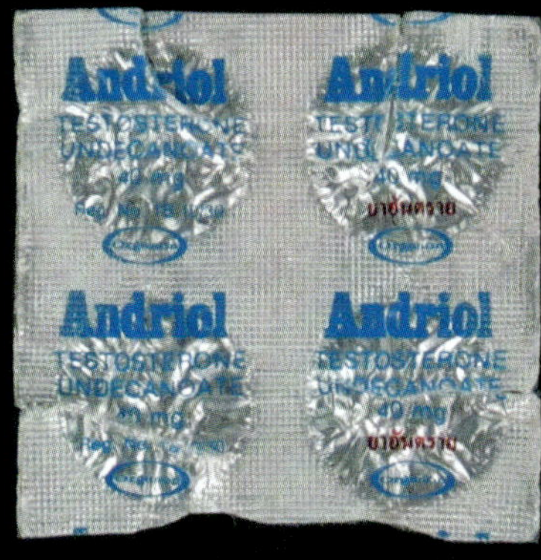

Thai Andriol

Androderm

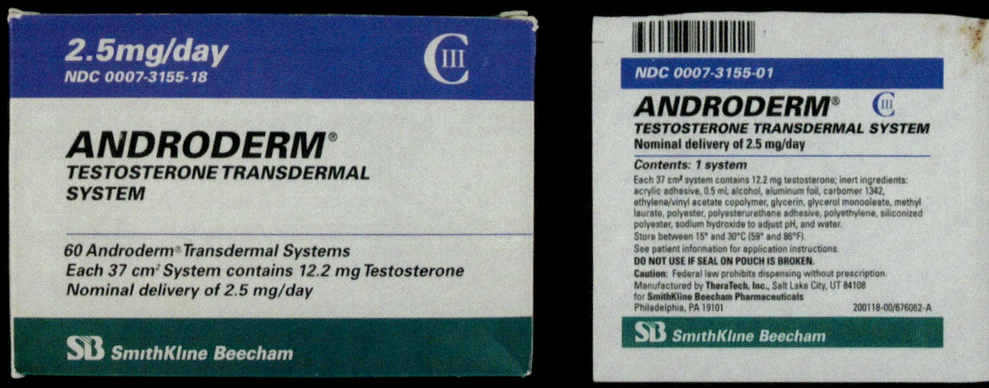

U.S. Androderm

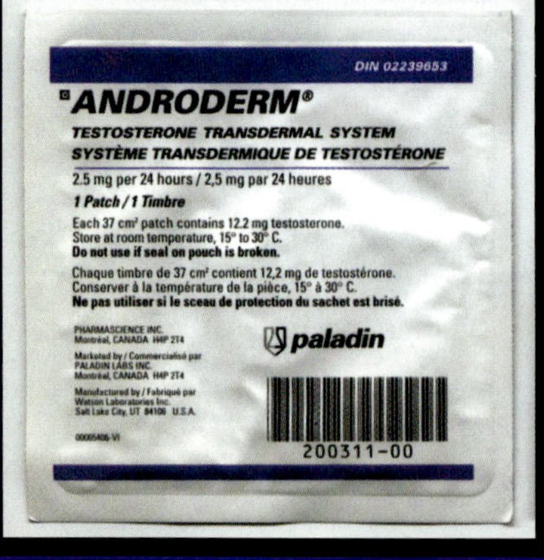

Canadian Patch

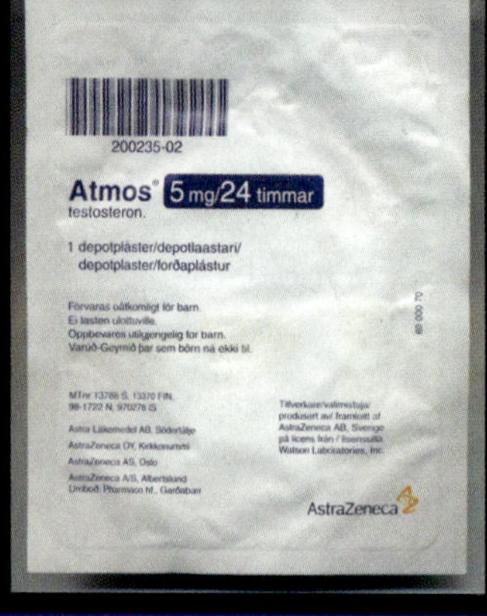

Atmos from Sweden

Androgel

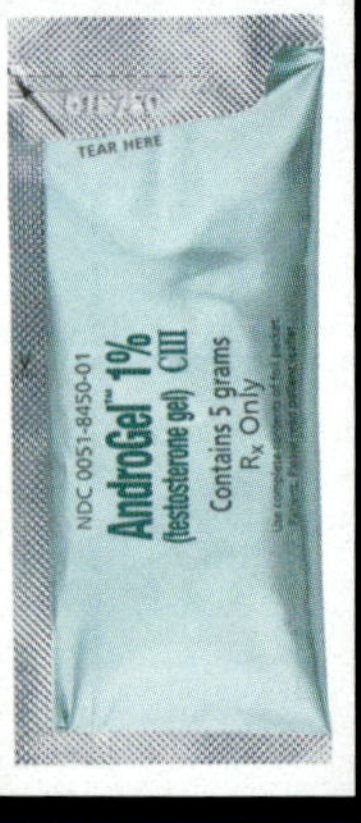

Androgel packet

Deca-Durabolin

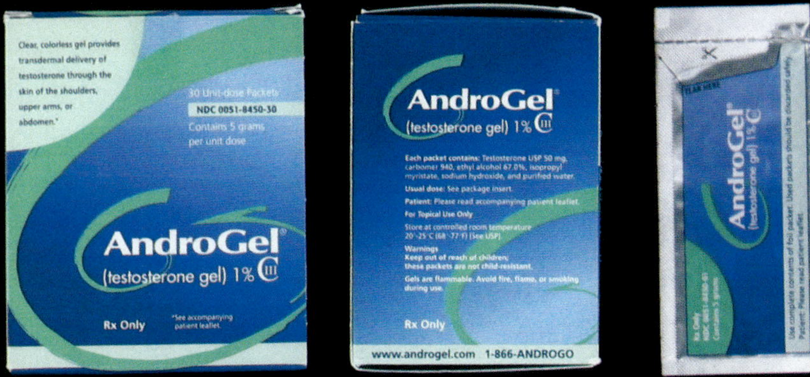

U.S. Androgel

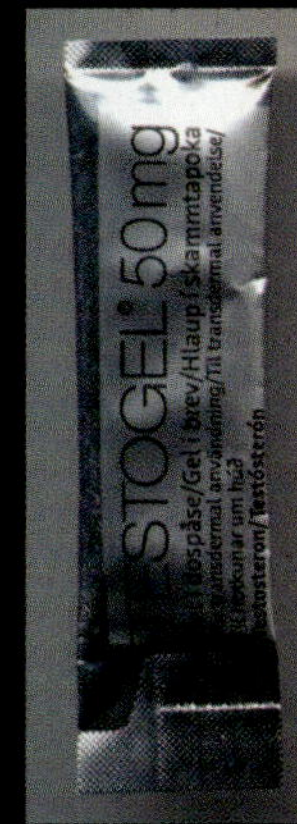

Testogel (Iceland)

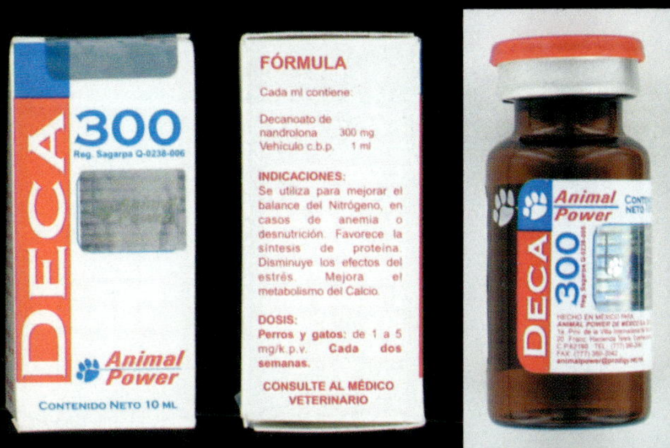

Deca 300 from Animal Power (Mexico)

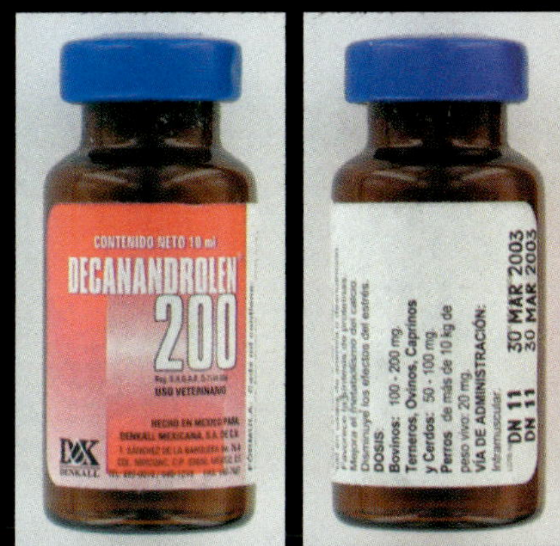

Denkall's Decanandrolen (Mexico)

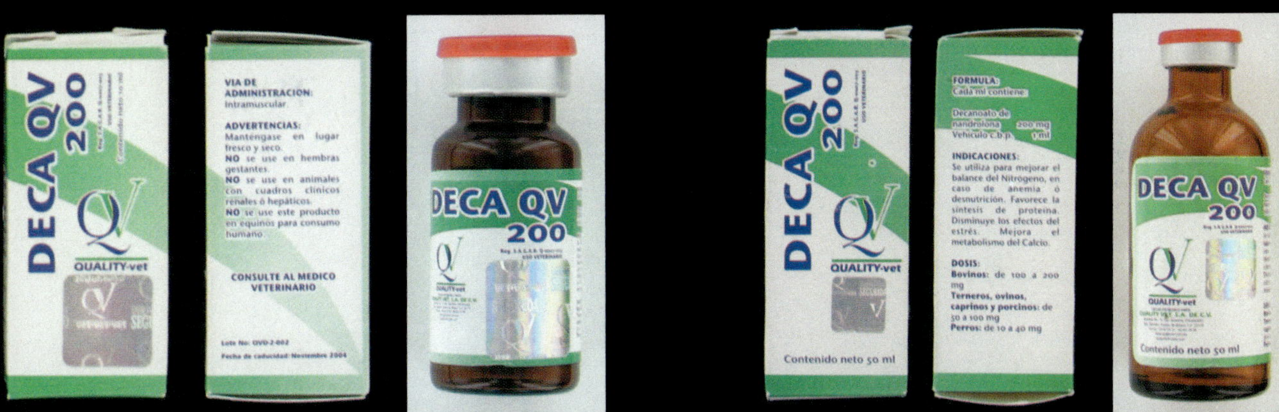

Quality Vet's Deca QV 200 - 10ml and 50ml versions (Mexico)

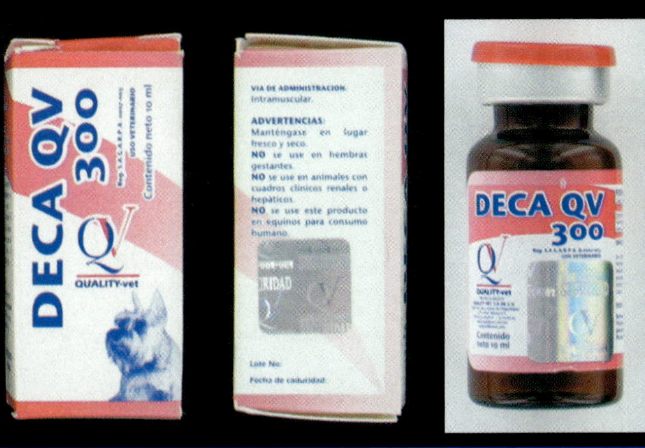

QV Deca 300 (new style)

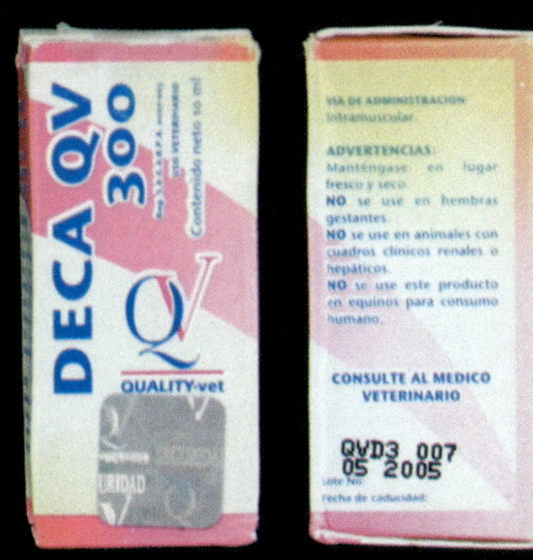

Older style box

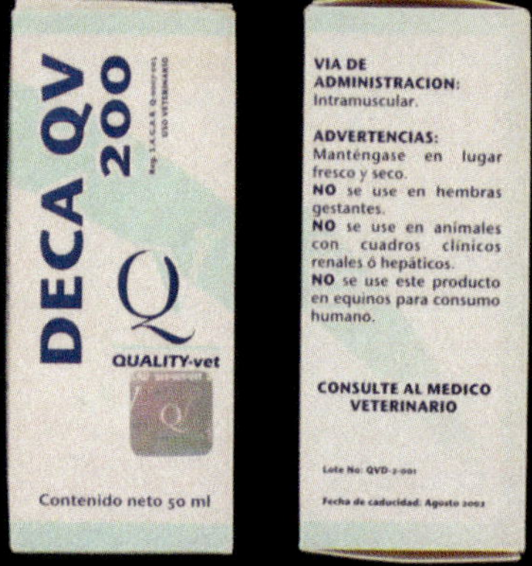

Old style QV Deca 200 box

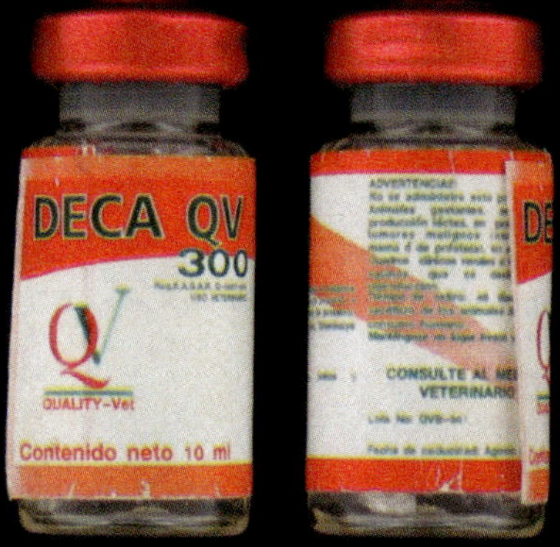

Counterfeit QV vial

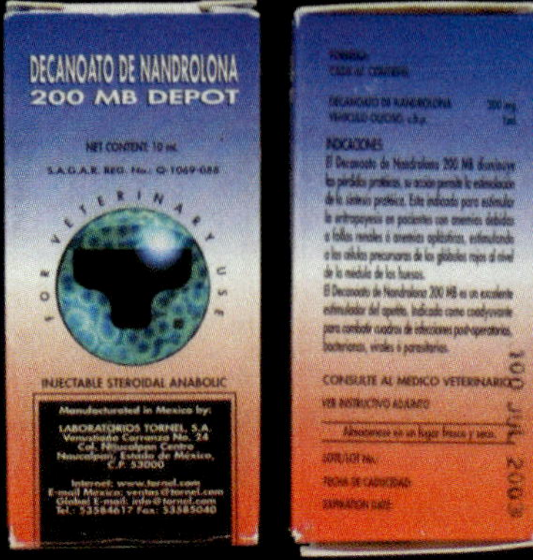

Generic from Tornel in Mexico

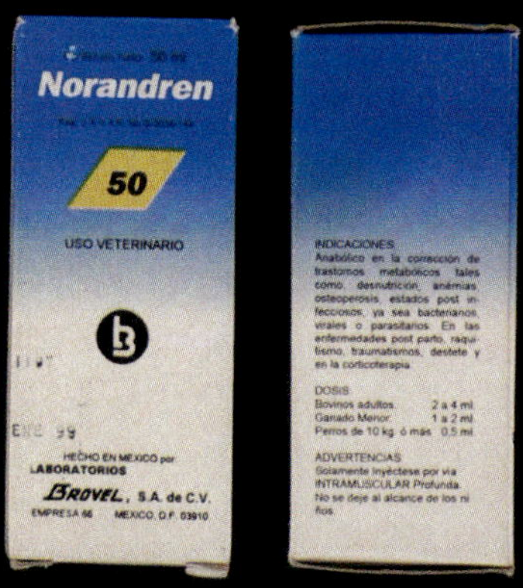

Brovel Norandren 50 (Mexico)

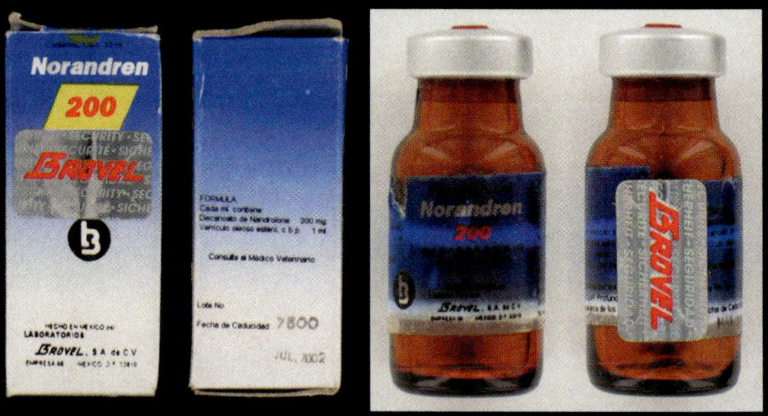

Brovel's 200mg/mL product (10ml)

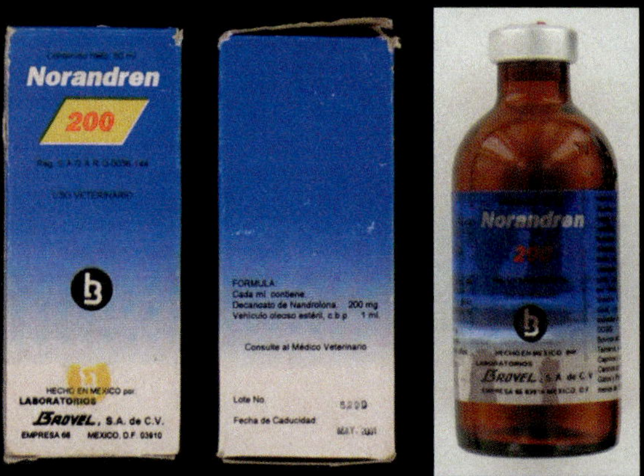

Norandren 200 - 50ml vial

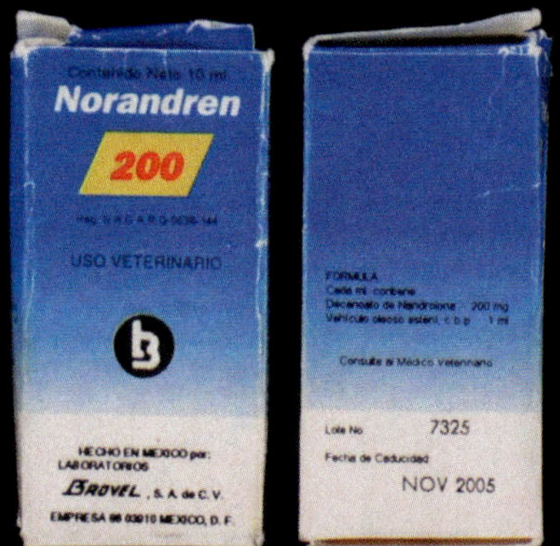

Counterfeit Norandren

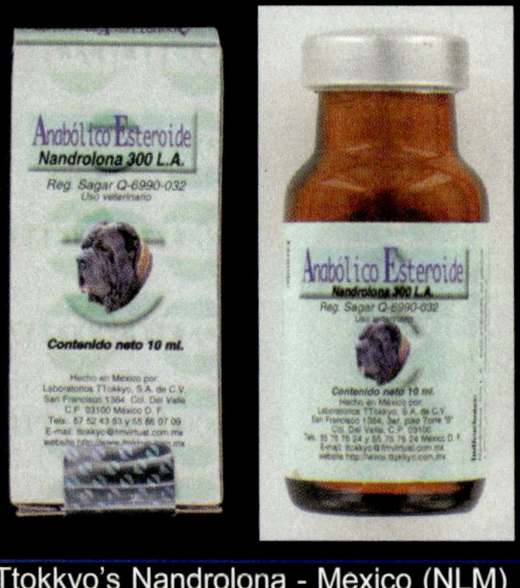

Ttokkyo's Nandrolona - Mexico (NLM)

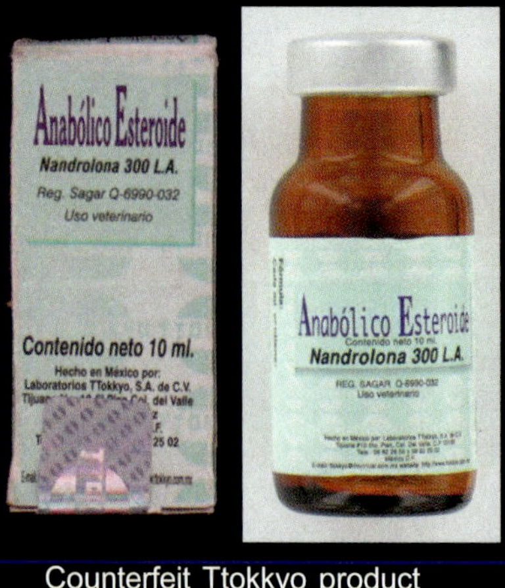

Counterfeit Ttokkyo product

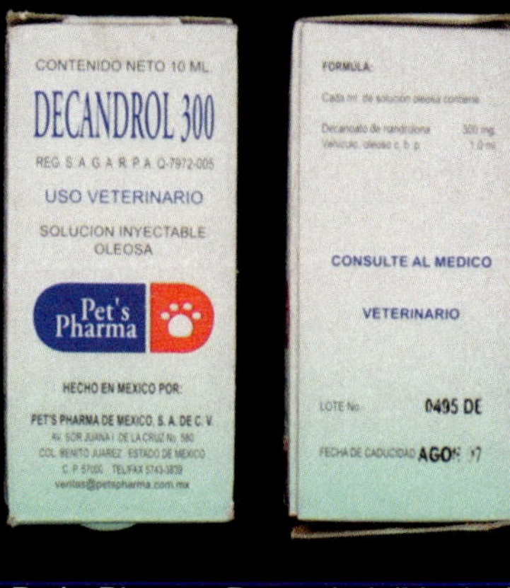

Pet's Pharma Decandrol (Mexico)

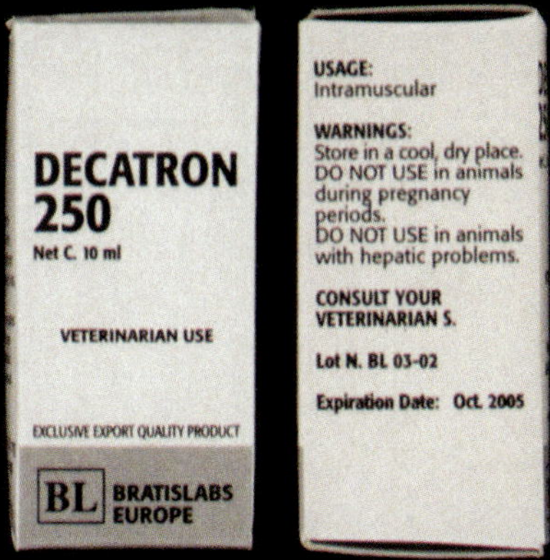

Bratis Decatron 250 (Mexico)

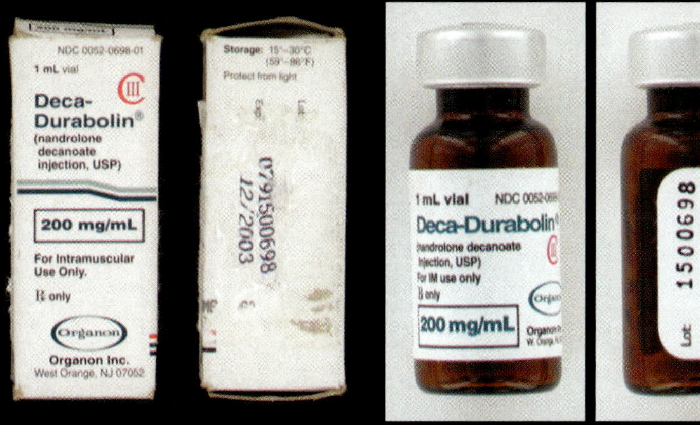

U.S. Deca-Durabolin® from Organon

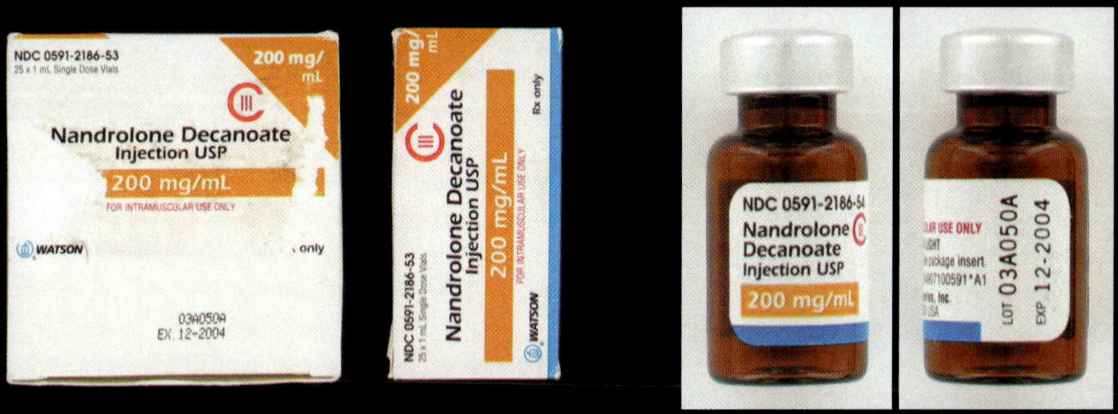

U.S. generic from Watson

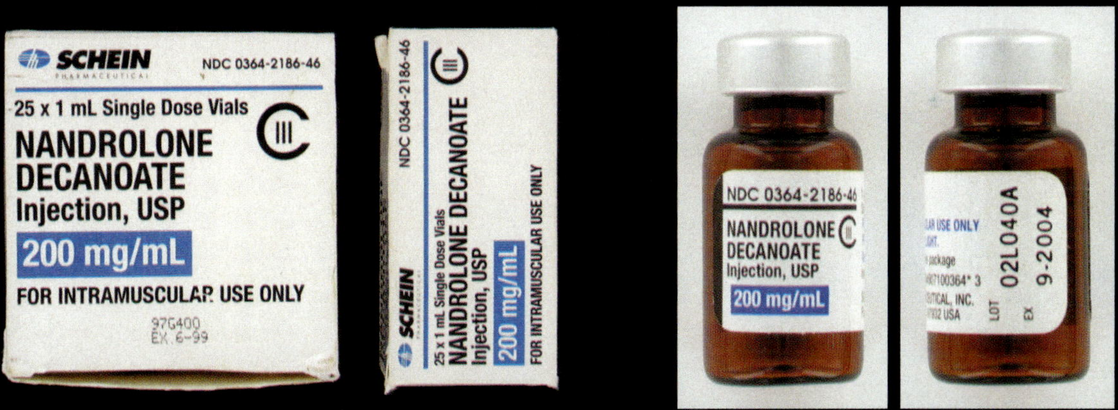

U.S. generic from Schein

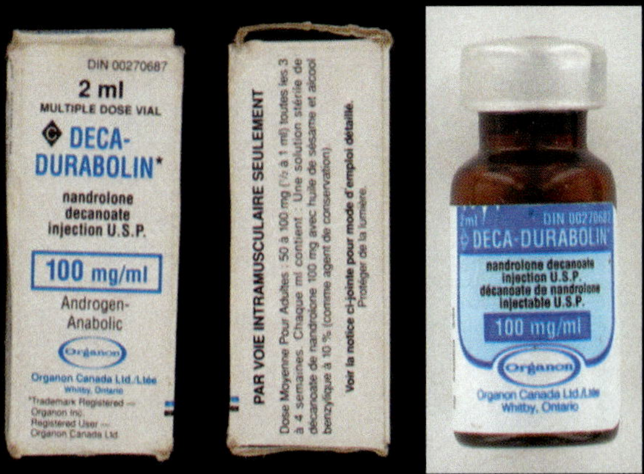

Canadian Deca-Durabolin®

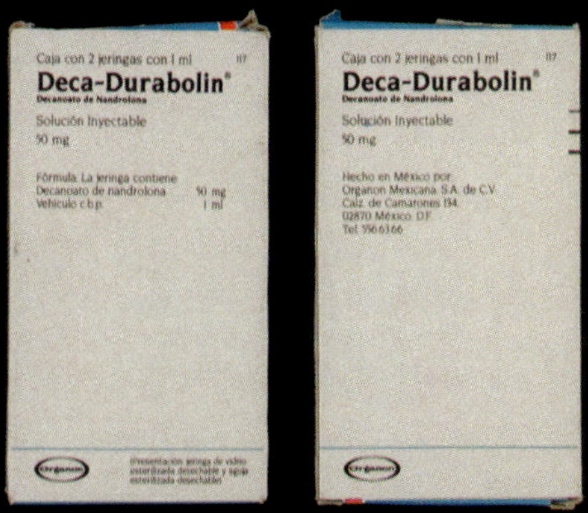

Deca-Durabolin® from Mexico

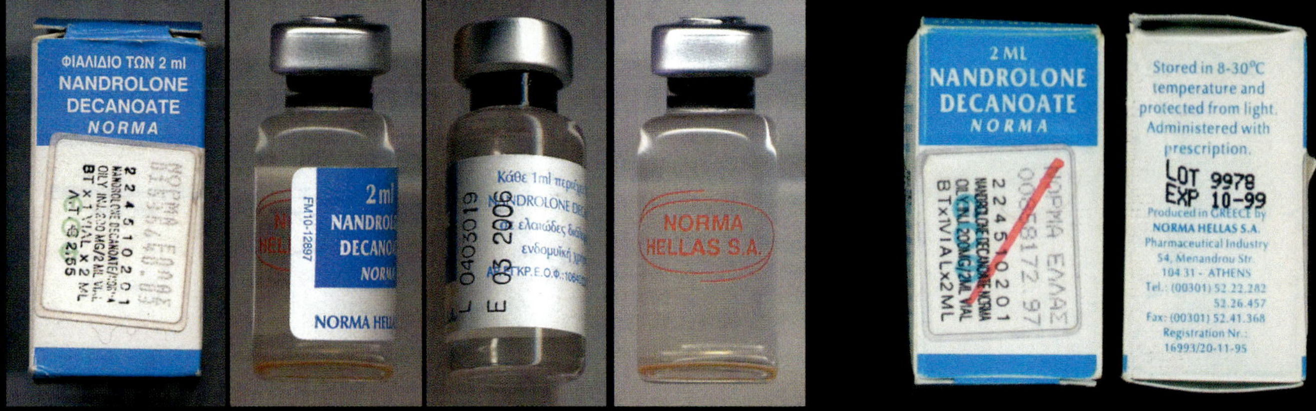

Norma Hellas Deca from Greece (newest version) — Old Box

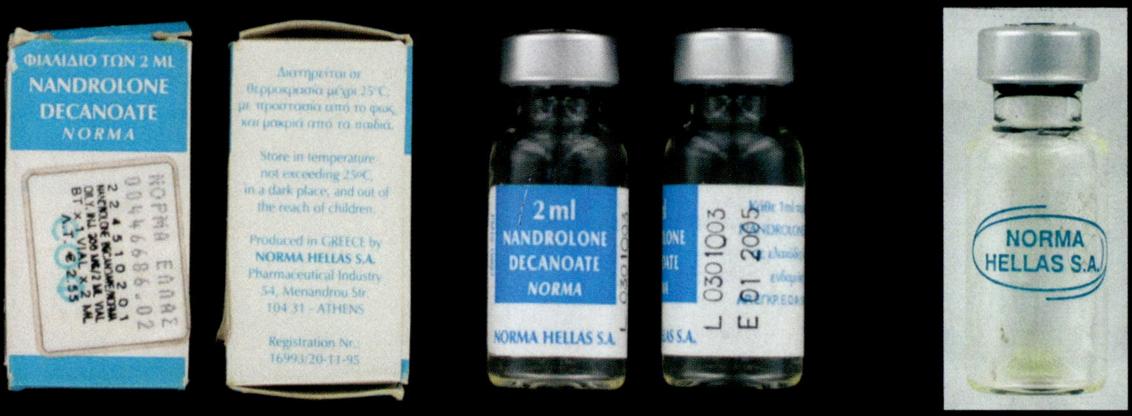

Norma Hellas Deca (2002) with blue etching under the label

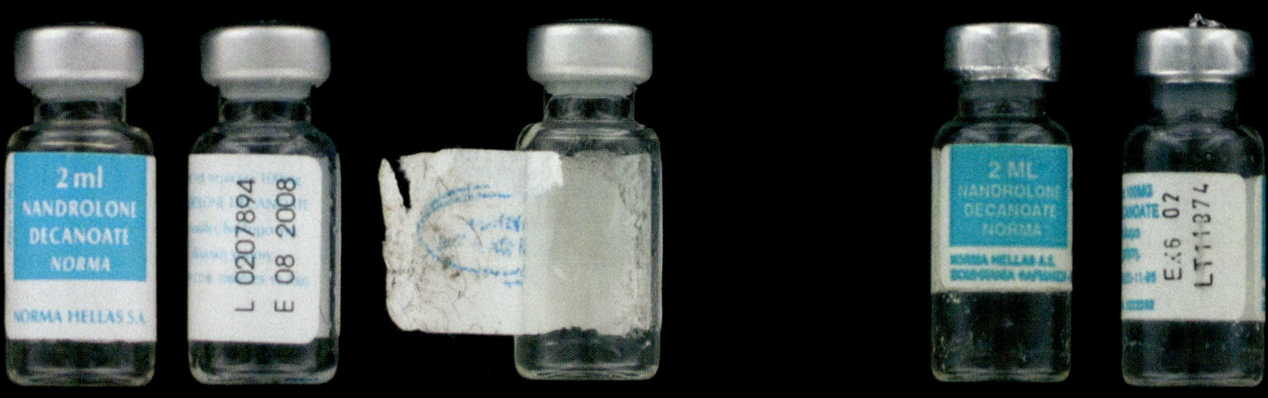

Counterfeit #1 - Norma Logo peels off with label — Counterfeit #2

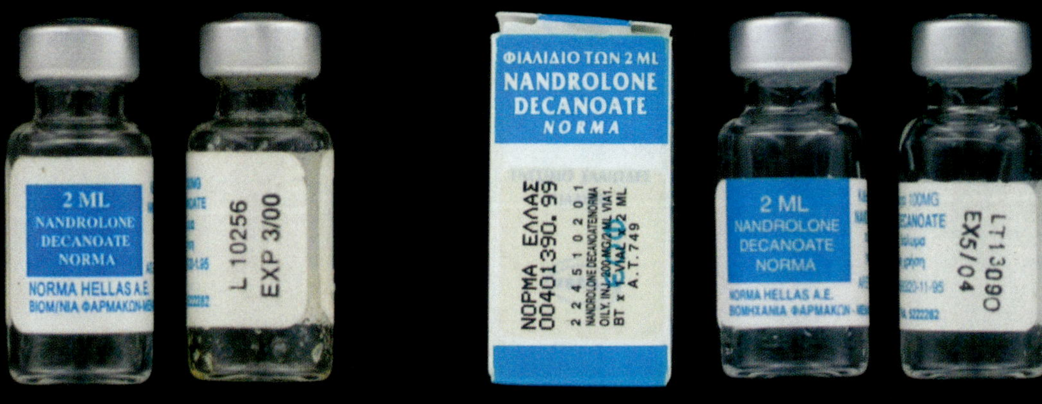

Counterfeit #3 — Counterfeit #4

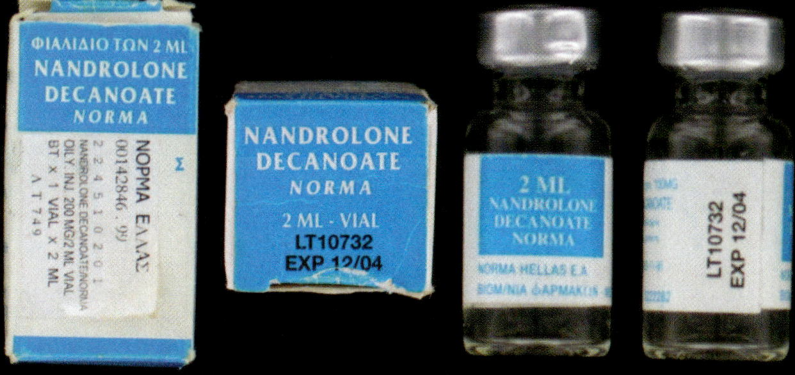

Counterfeit #5

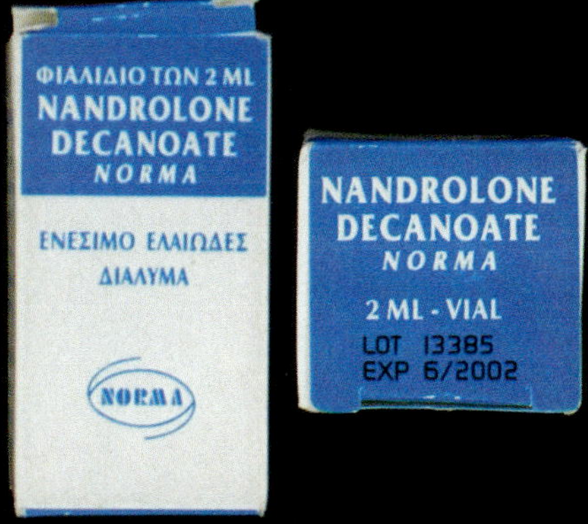

Counterfeit #6

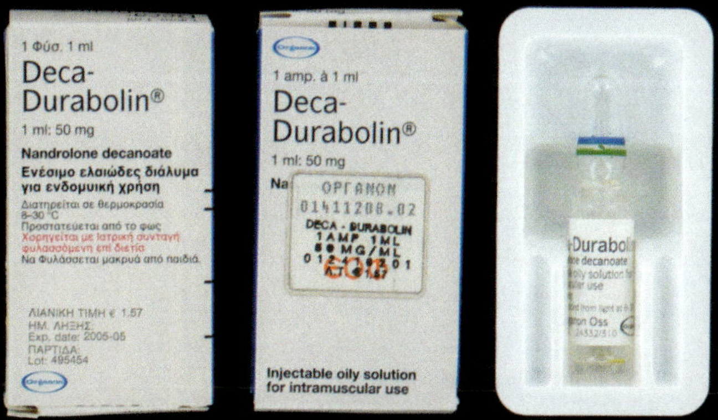

Deca-Durabolin® from Greece - 50mg ampule

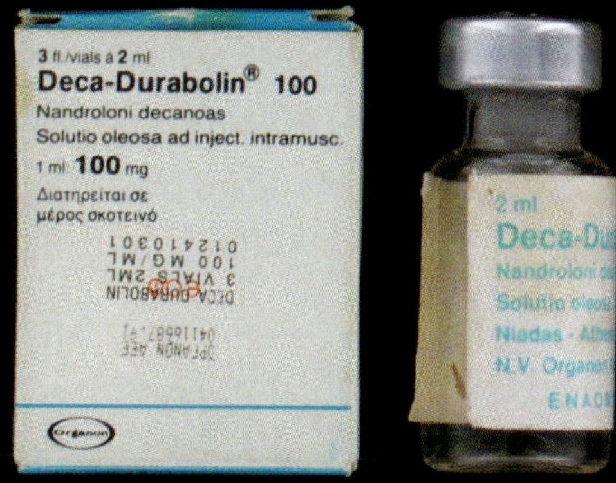

Old Deca 100mg/mL vial from Greece

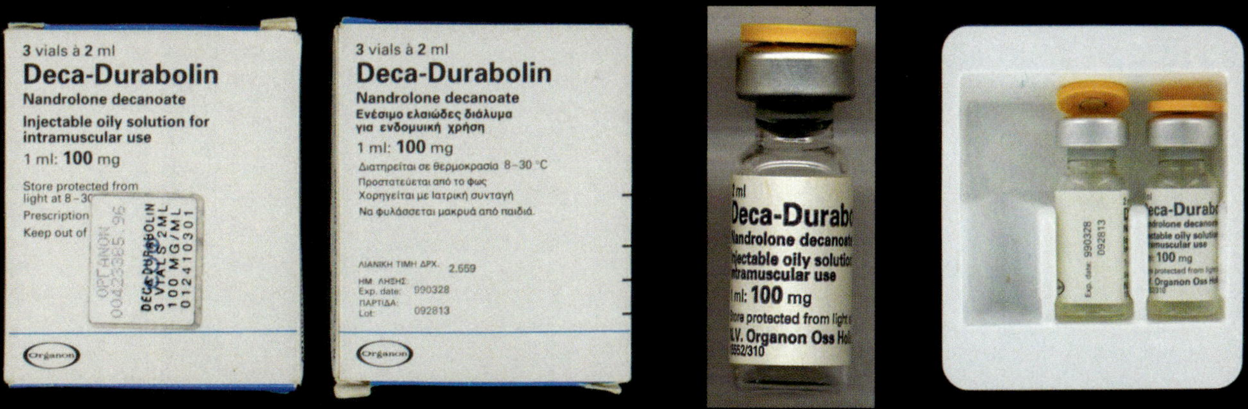

Older Style Greek "Yellow Top" Deca

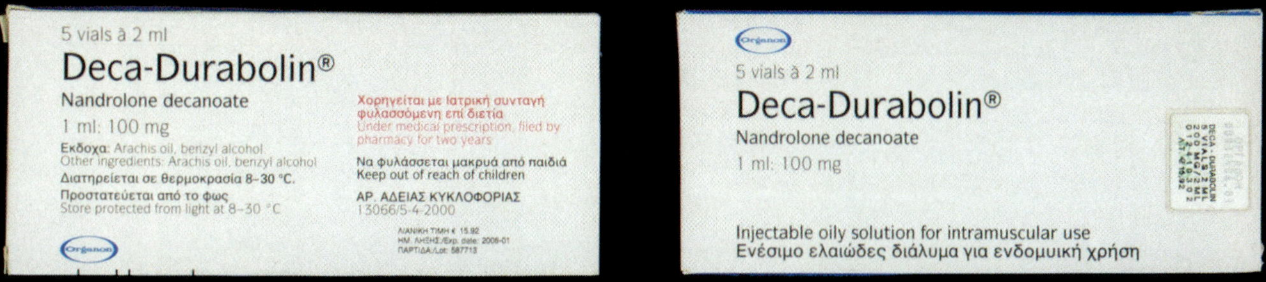

New style Deca-Durabolin® multi-dose vial product from Greece

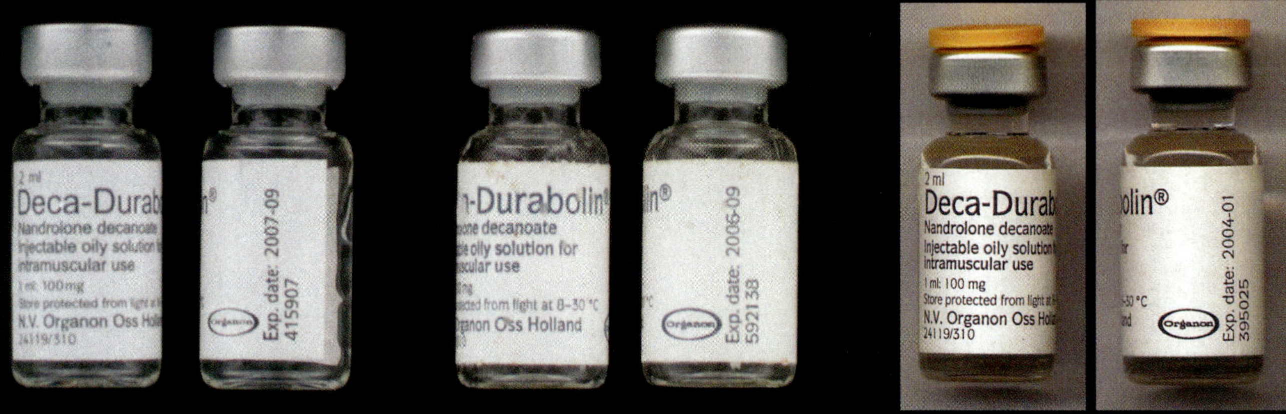

Real Greek vials of different dates of manufacture

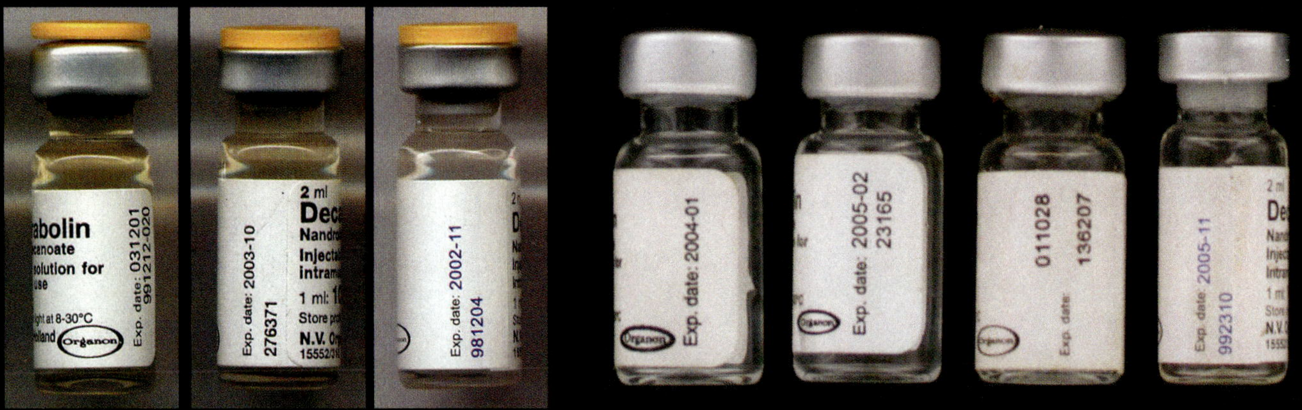

Seven different counterfeit Greek "Yellow Top" vials

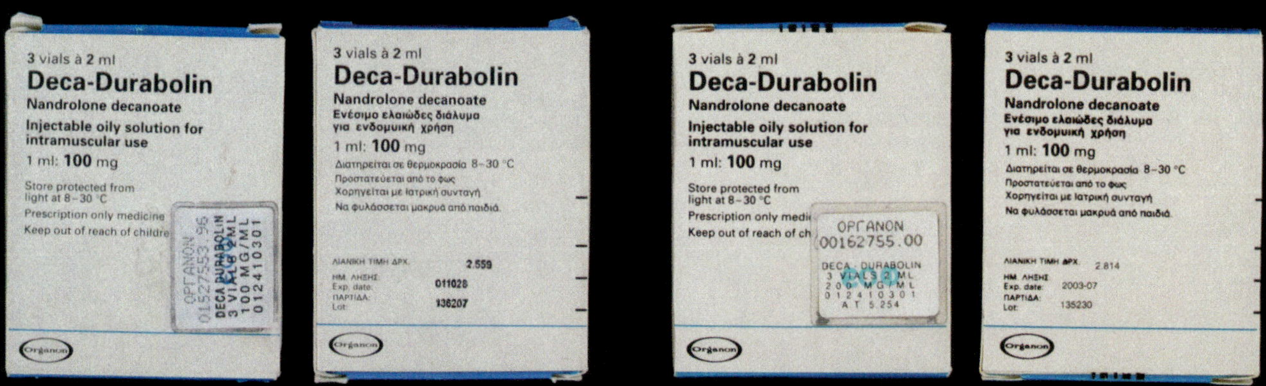

Two different sophisticated counterfeits, with fake Greek drug ID stickers

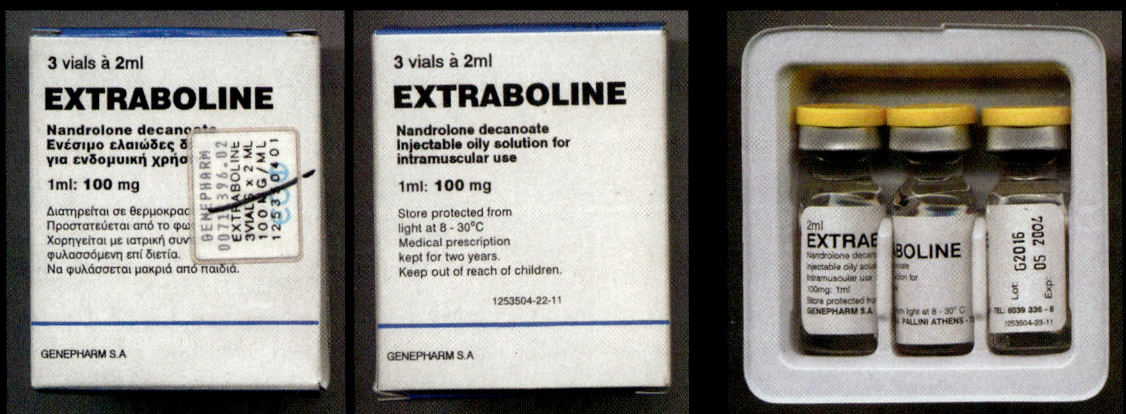

Greek Extraboline box and vials - new style

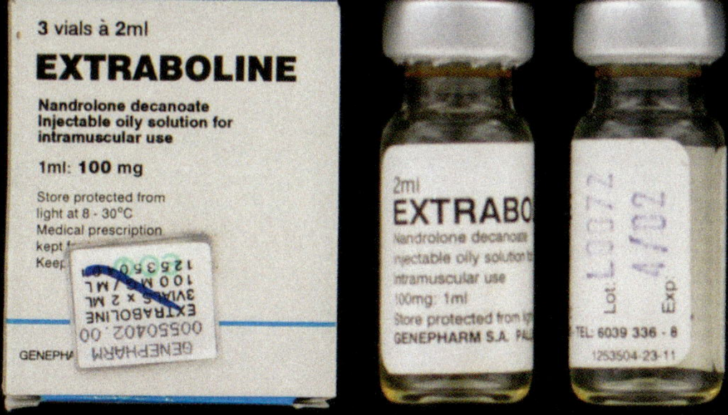

Old Greek Extraboline

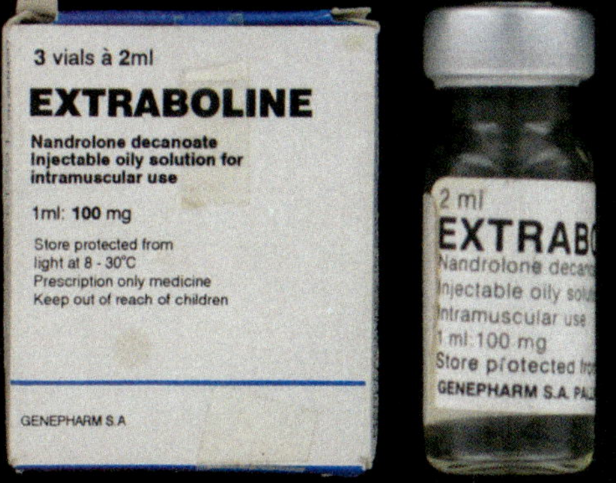

Counterfeit box and vial

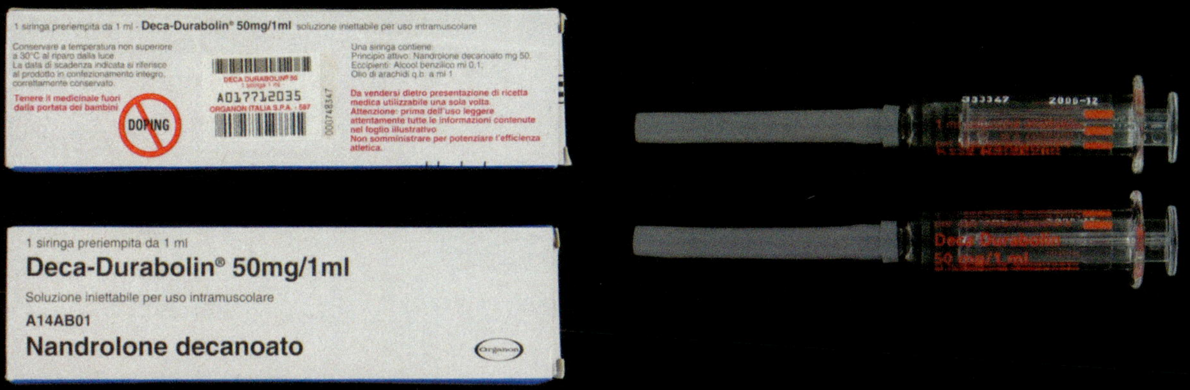

Deca-Durabolin® pre-loaded syringe from Italy

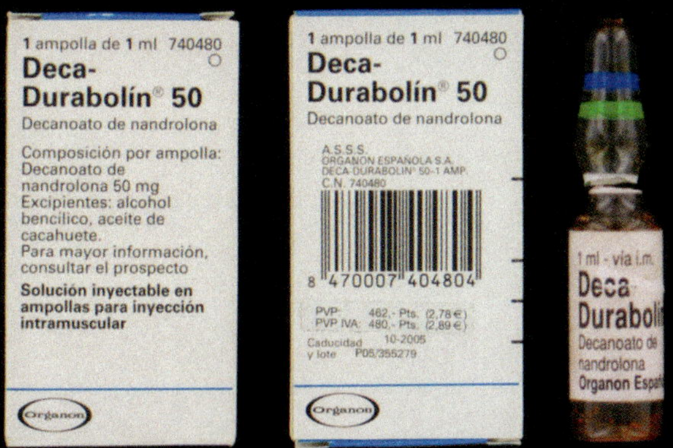

Spanish Deca, new style

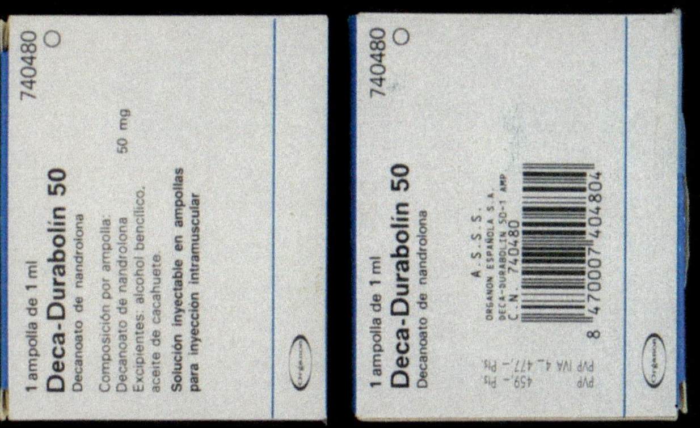

Old Spanish box

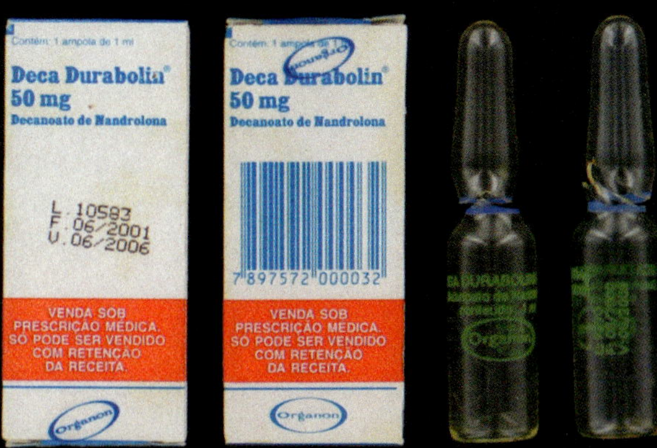

Deca-Durabolin® from Brazil

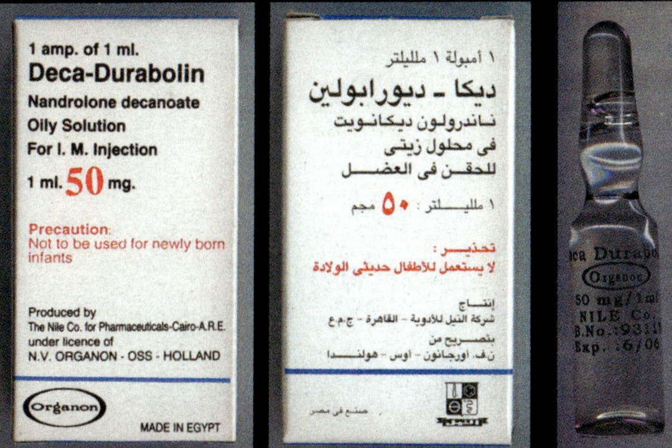

Deca from Egypt

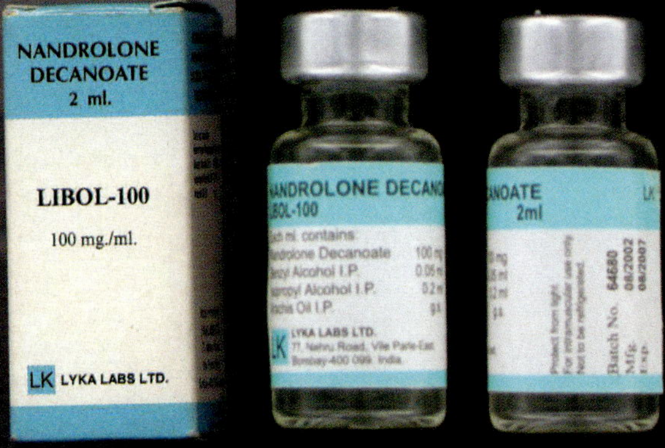

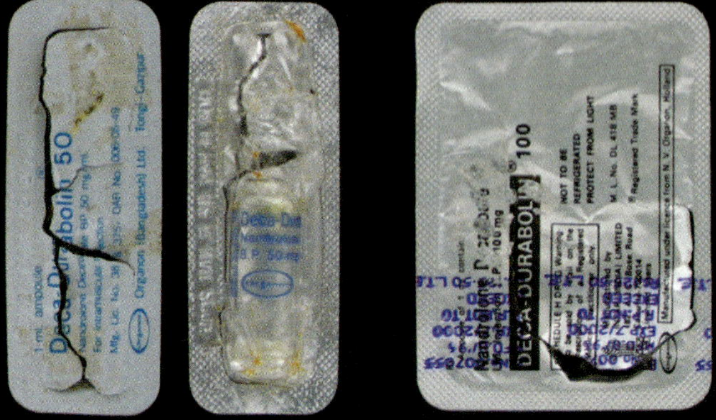

Libol from India

Deca-Durabolin® from Organon (left) and Infar (right) India

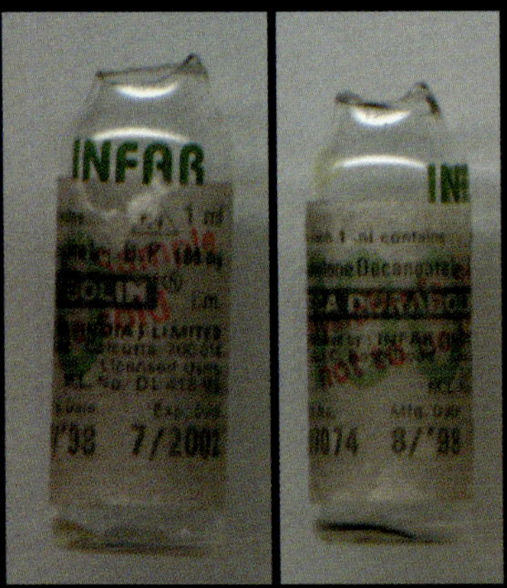

Infar ampule from India

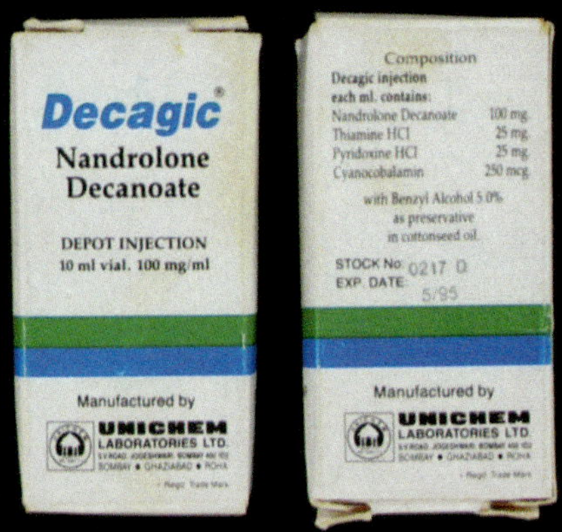

Decagic from India (NLM)

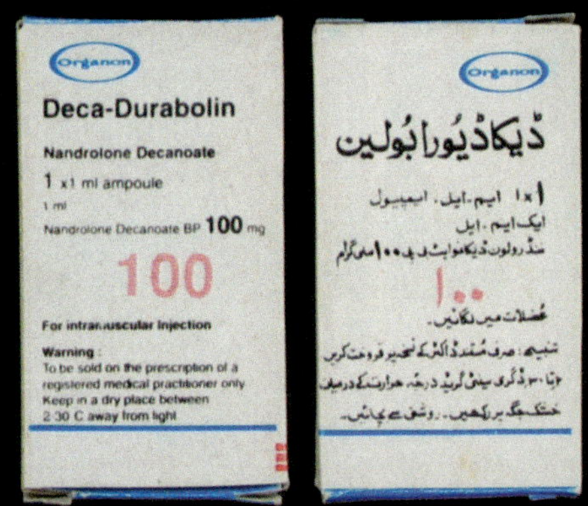

Deca from Pakistan (old style)

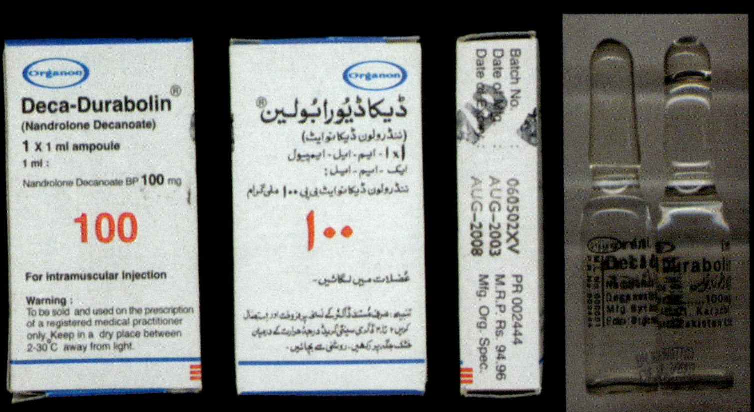

Deca-Durabolin® from Pakistan (new style)

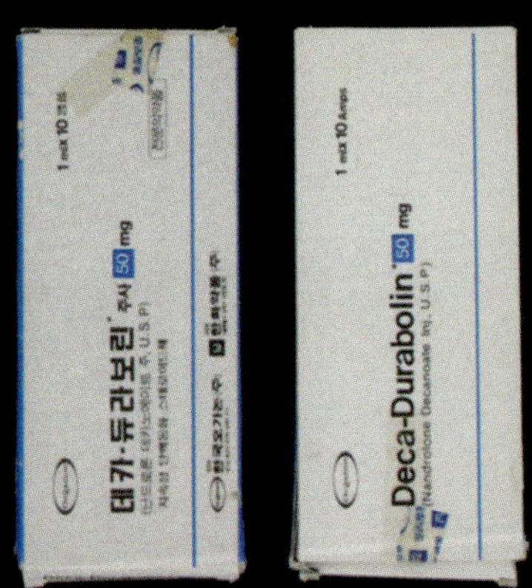

Deca from Korea

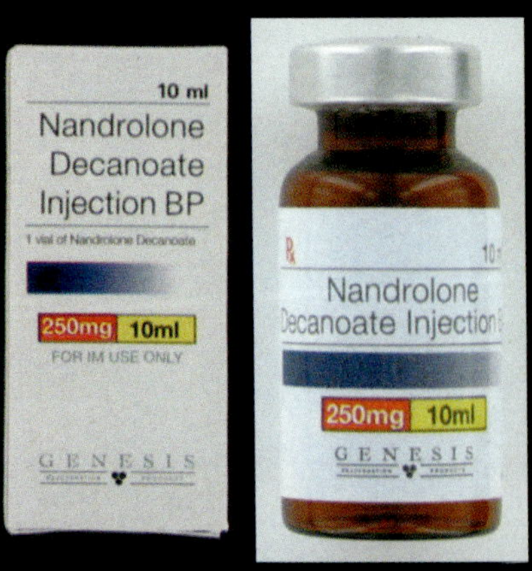

Generic from Genesis (Singapore)

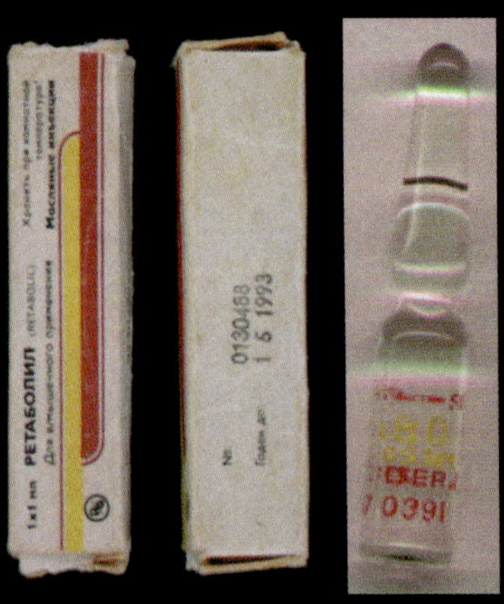

Retabolil (old) from Bulgaria

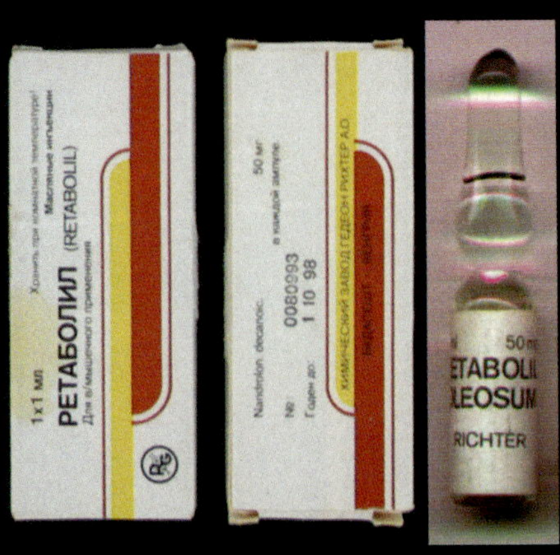

Newer style Retabolil box and ampule

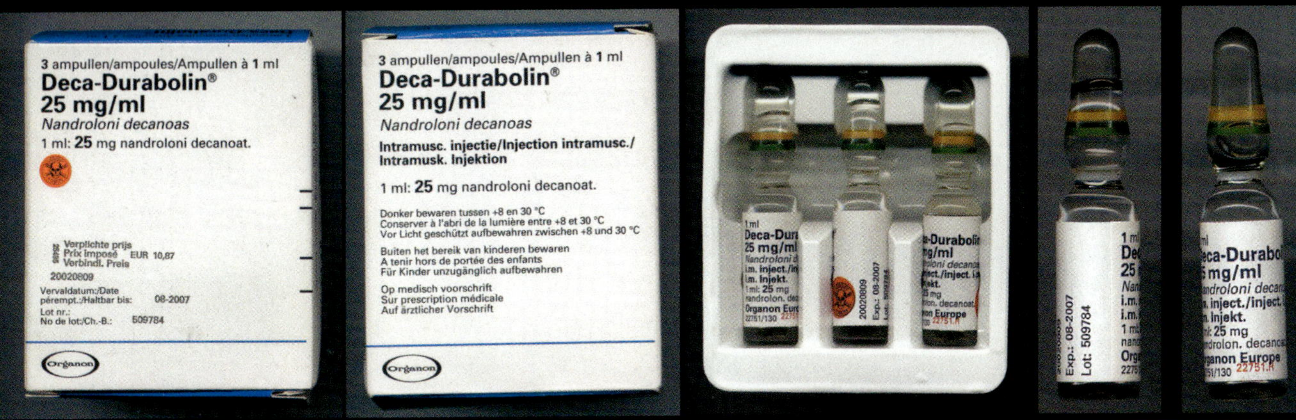

Deca-Durabolin® from Belgium

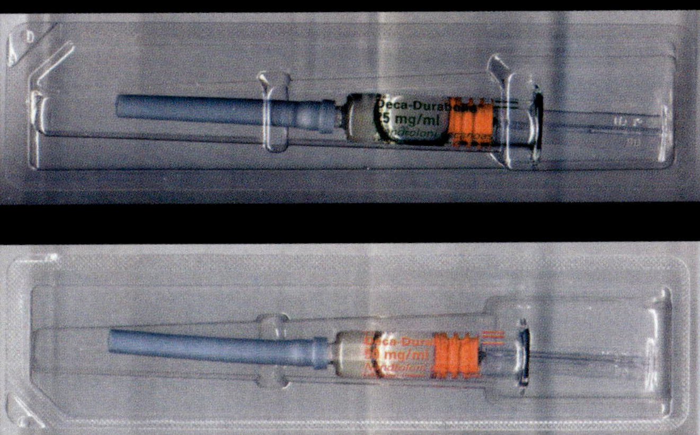
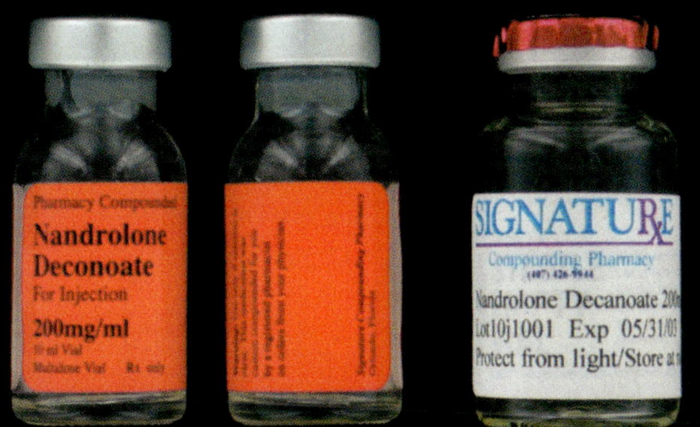

25mg/mL (top) and 50mg/mL (bottom) preload (Belgium)

Two U.S. private-label pharmacy generics

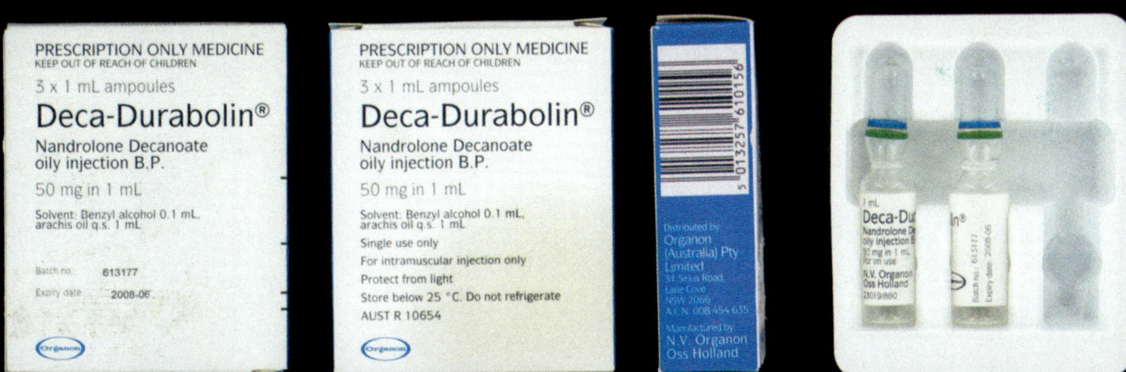

Deca-Durabolin® from Australia

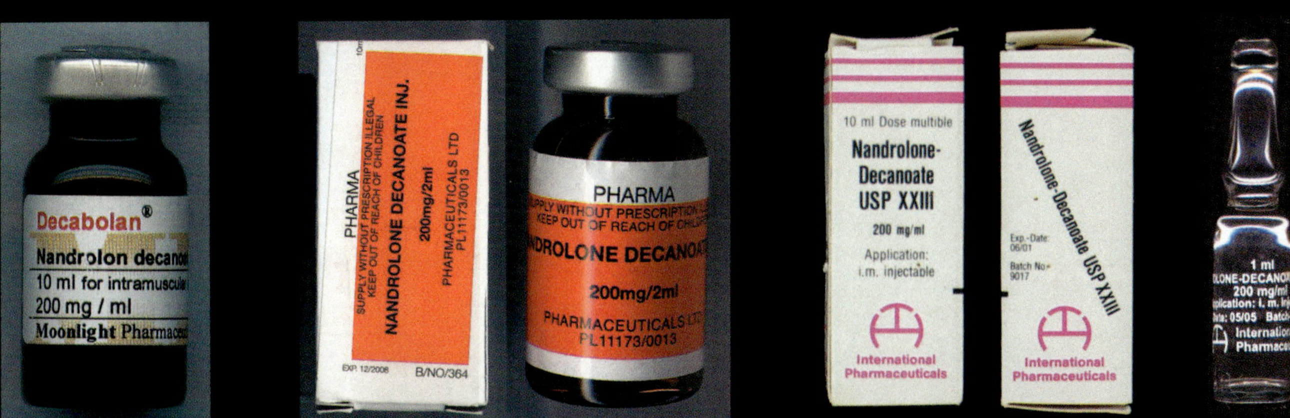

Four underground products, from Moonlight, Pharma, and International Pharmaceuticals (2)

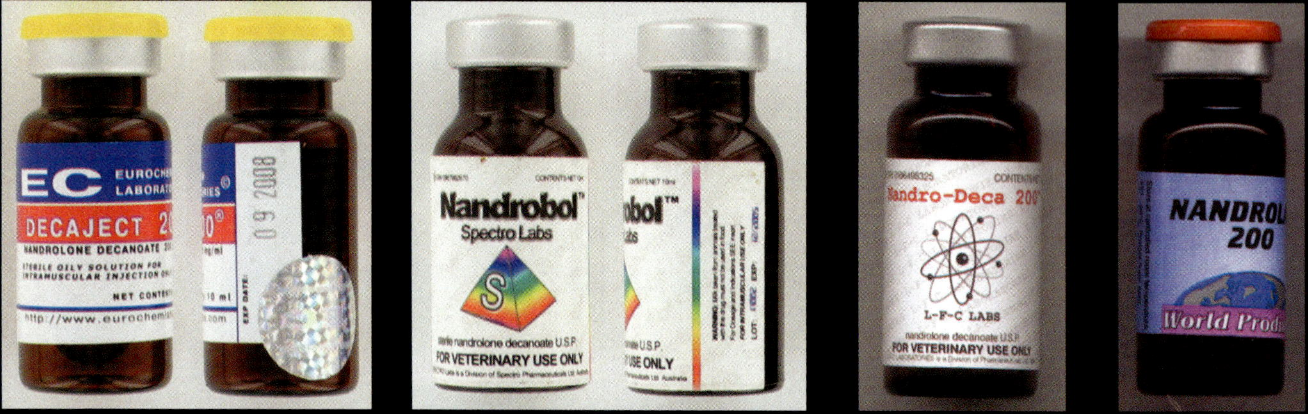

Four underground products, from Eurochem, Spectro (NLM), LFC and World

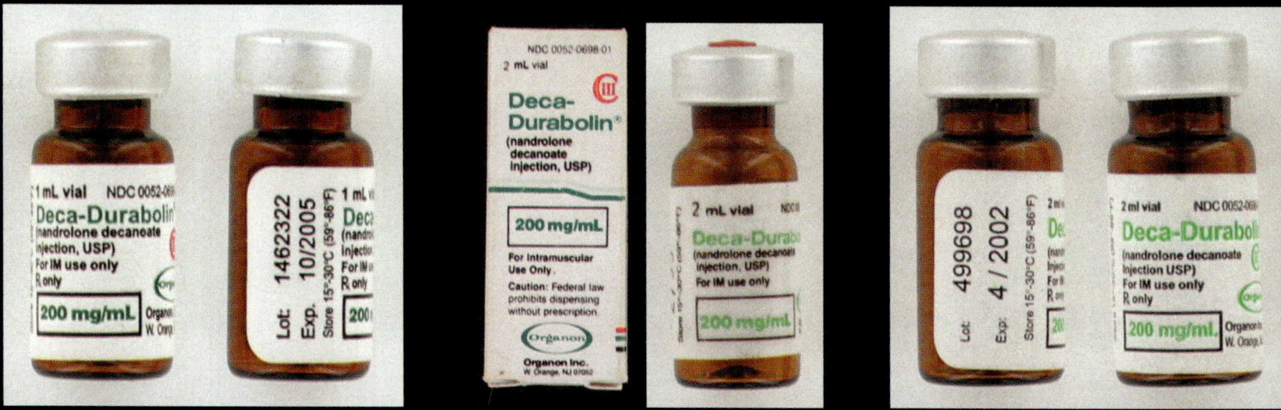

Three U.S. counterfeits

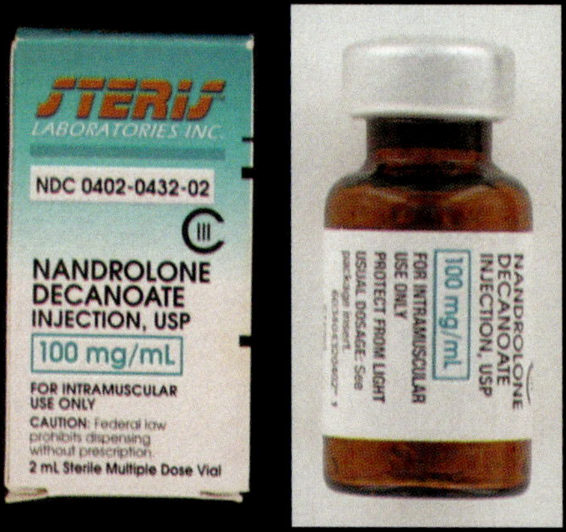

Counterfeit Steris 100mg/mL product

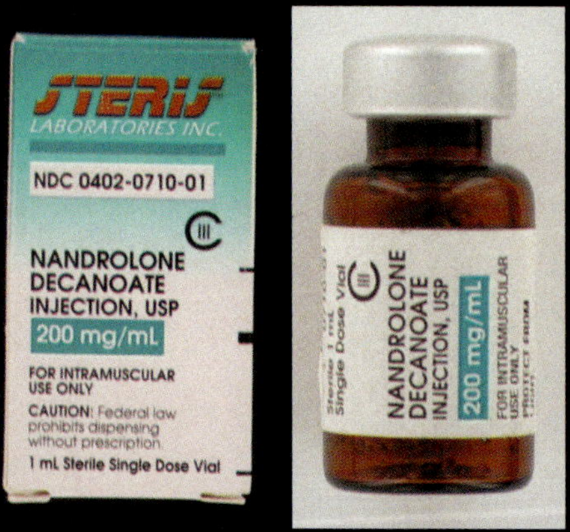

Counterfeit 200mg/mL

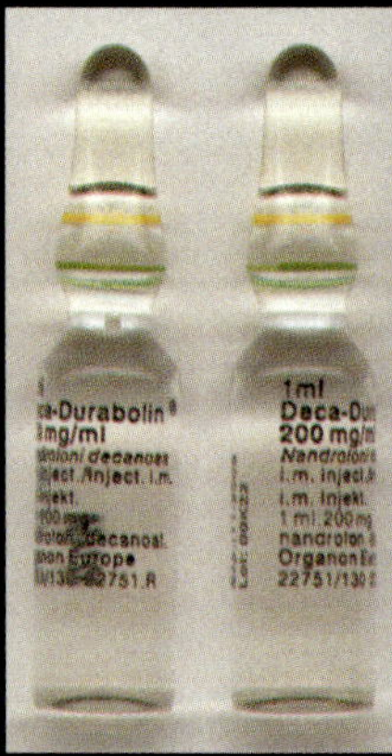

Fake "European" amp

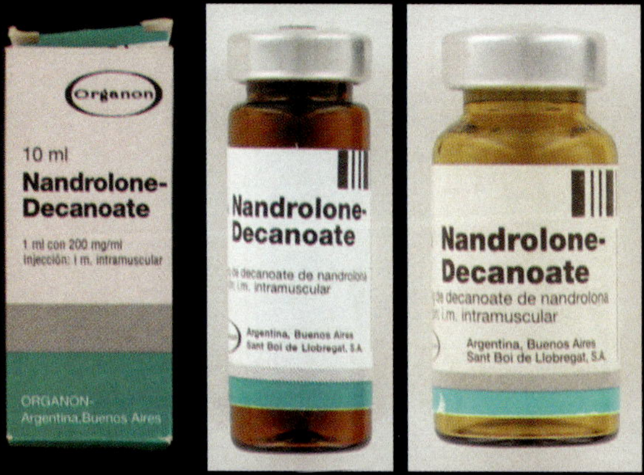

Fake Deca from Argentina - box and two vials

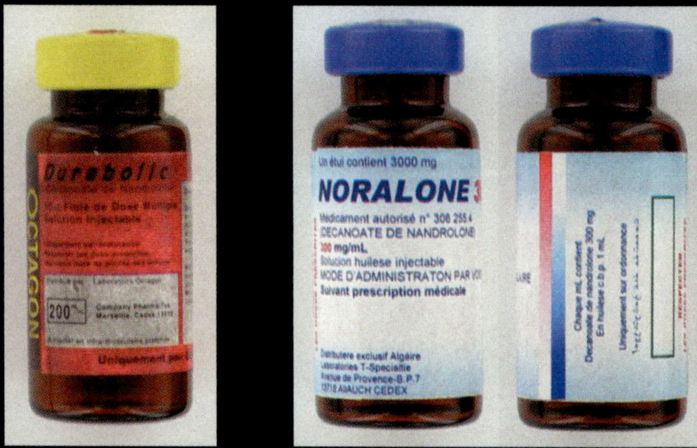

Two bogus French products

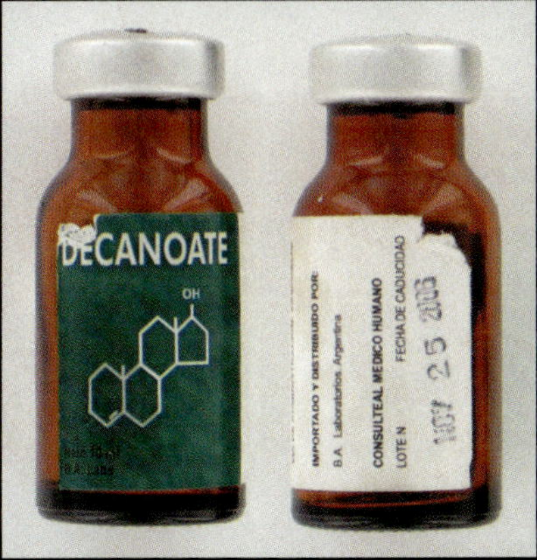

Bogus “Decanoate”

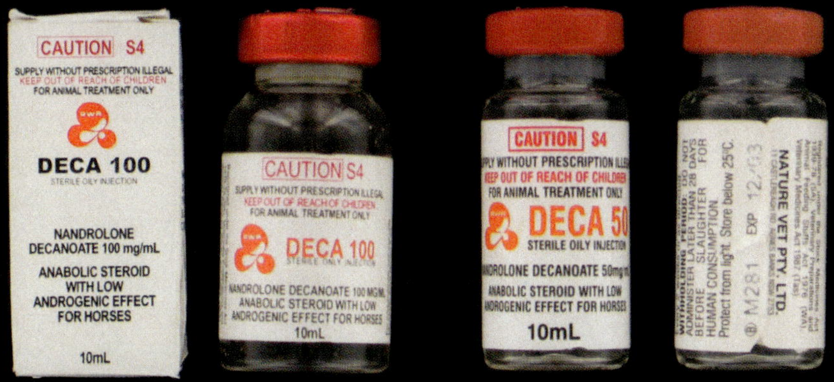

Counterfeit Australian RWR products - 100mg/mL and 50mg/mL

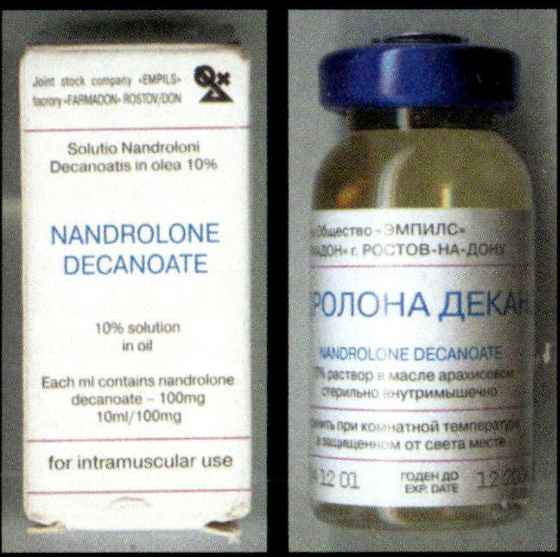

Counterfeit Farmadon generic

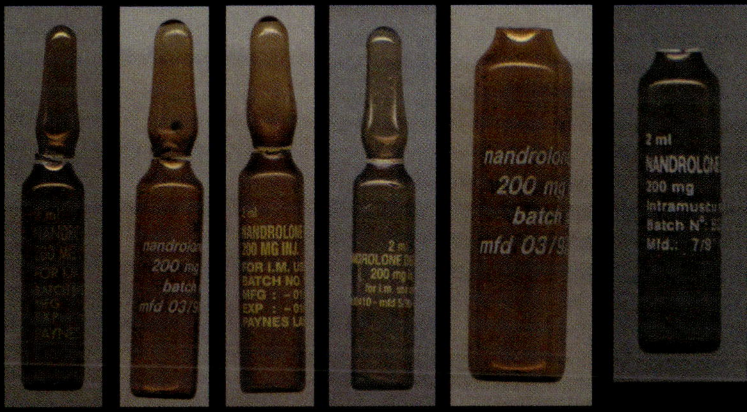

Various fake ampules

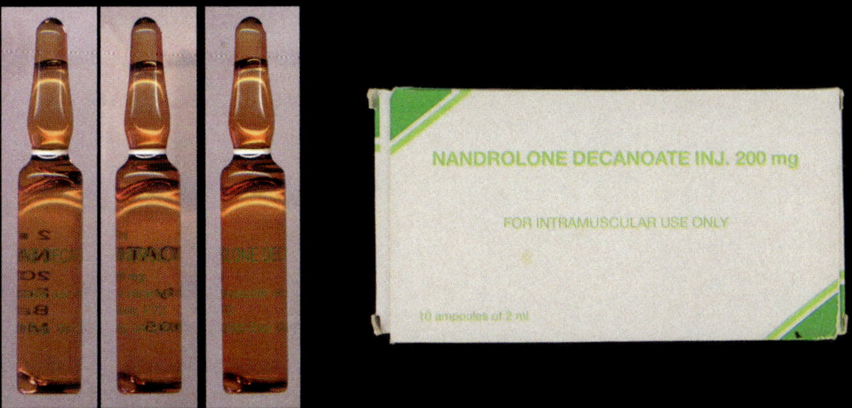

Counterfeit generic ampules and box with no name

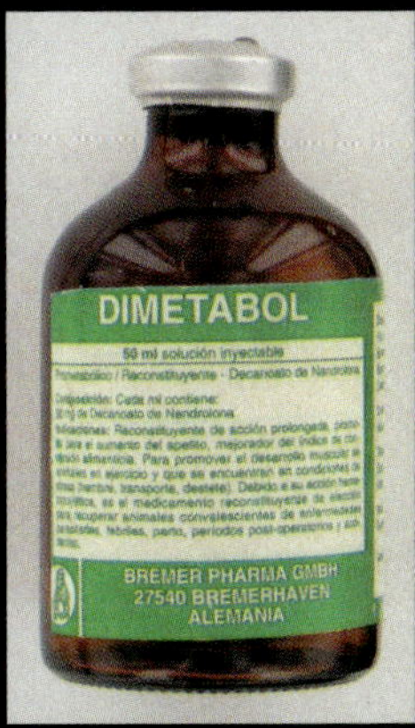

Counterfeit Dimetabol

Deposterona

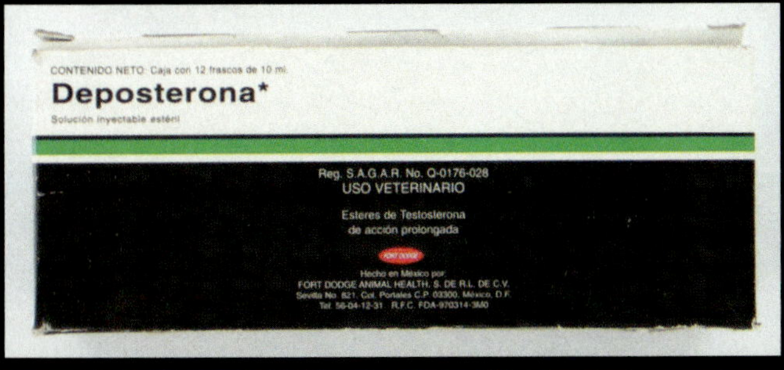

Fort Dodge Deposterona (Mexico)

Dianabol

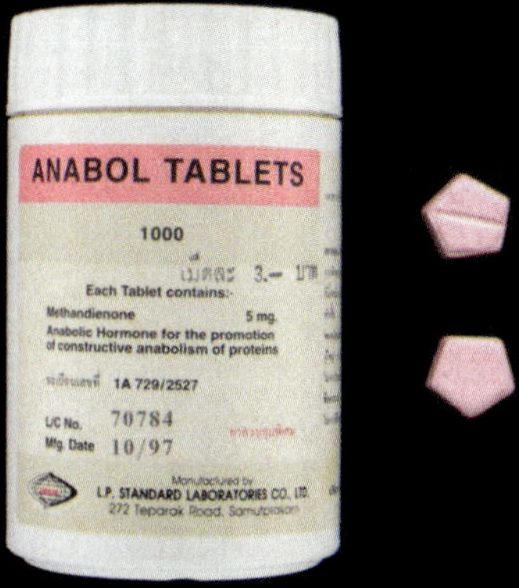

Anabol from LP Standard Thailand (NLM)

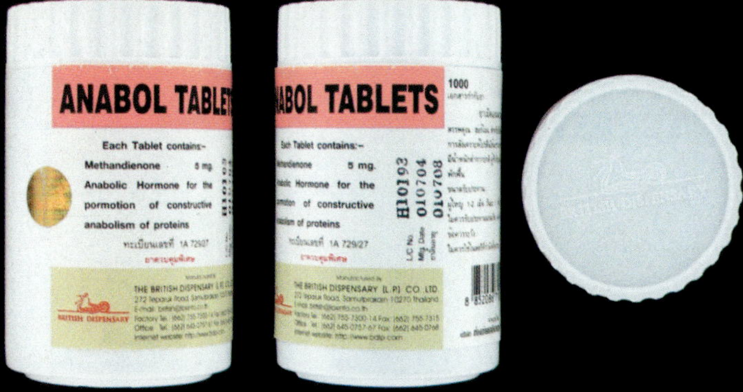

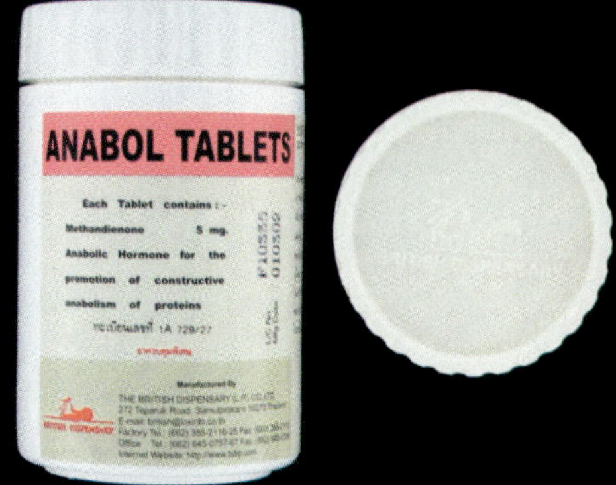

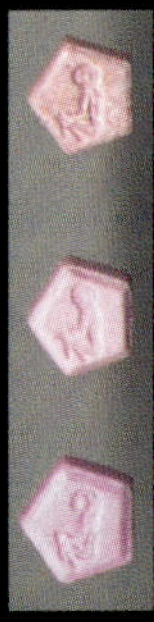

Anabol from British Dispensary (Thailand) Sophisticated fake bottle Real tab (middle)

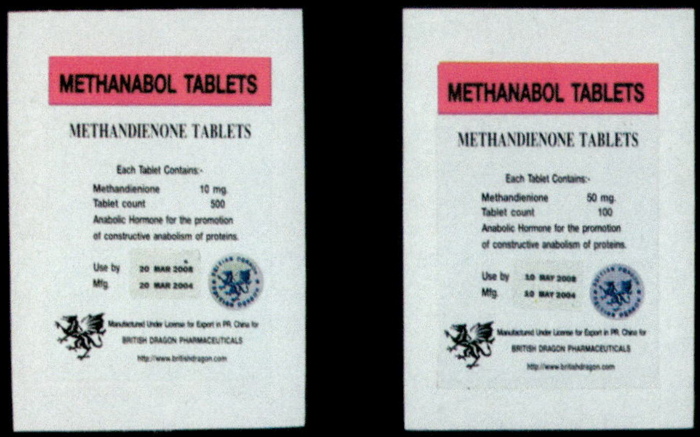

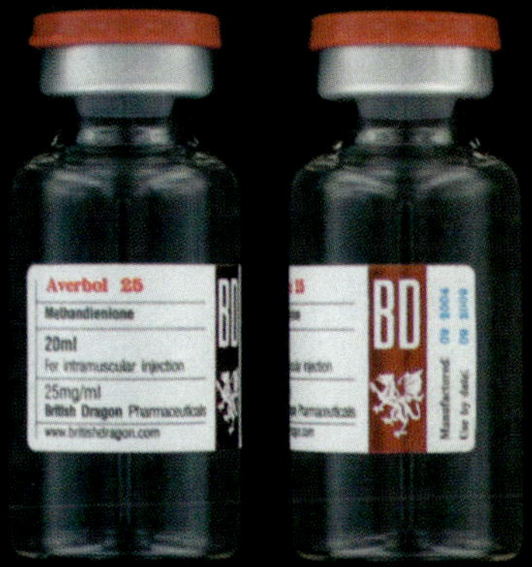

British Dragon 10mg and 50mg tablet products (Thailand) British Dragon injectable

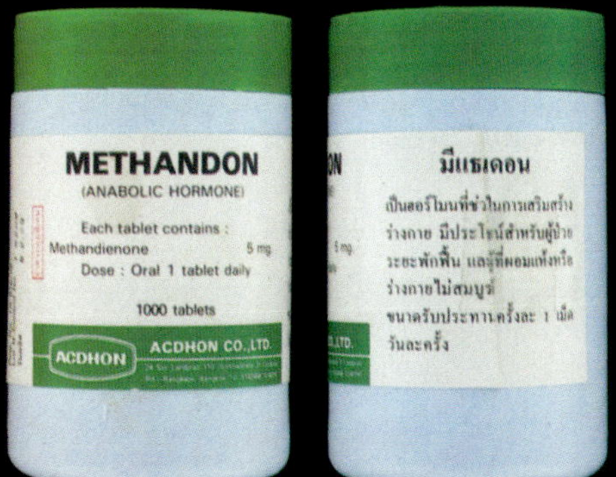

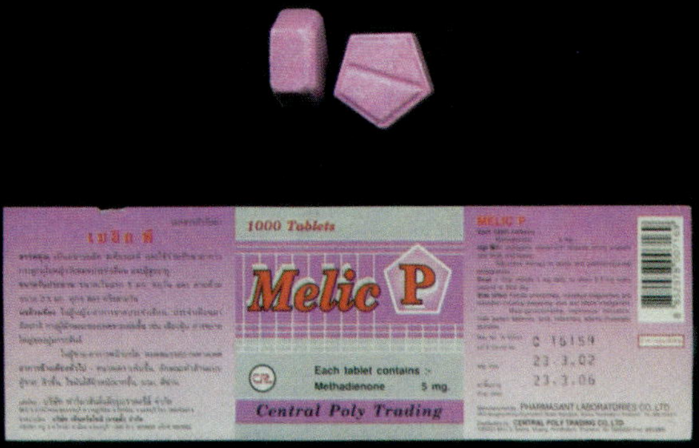

Thai Methandon Thai Melic (label and tablets)

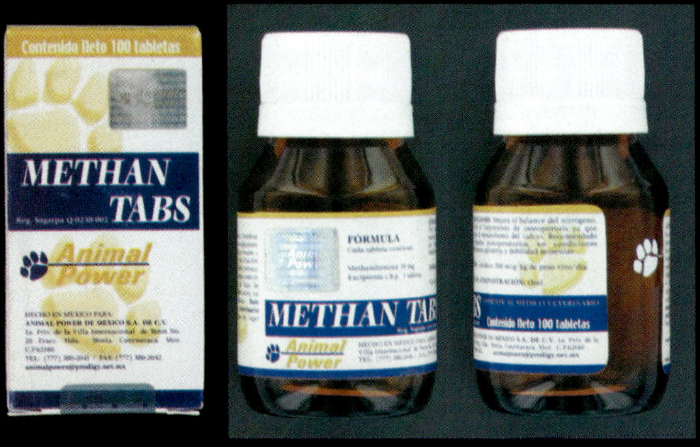

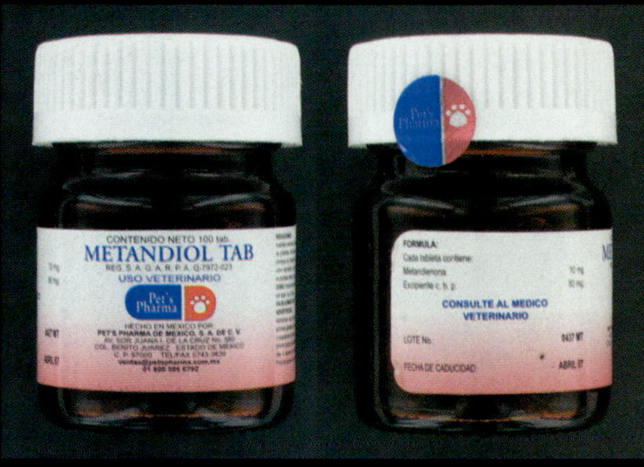

Methan tabs from Animal Power (Mexico) Metandiol Tab from Pet's Pharma (Mexico)

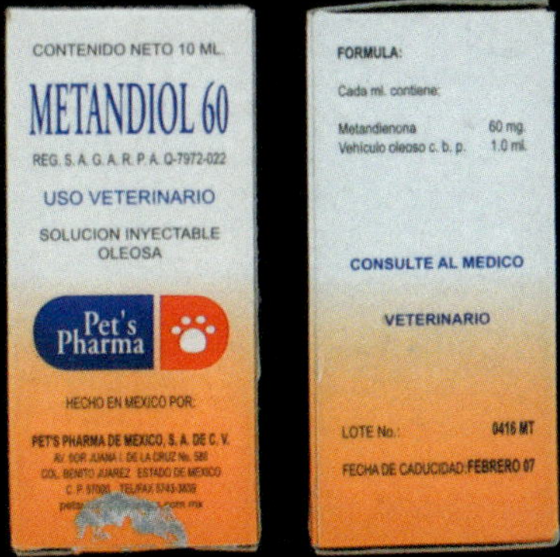

Pet's Pharma Injectable (Mexico)

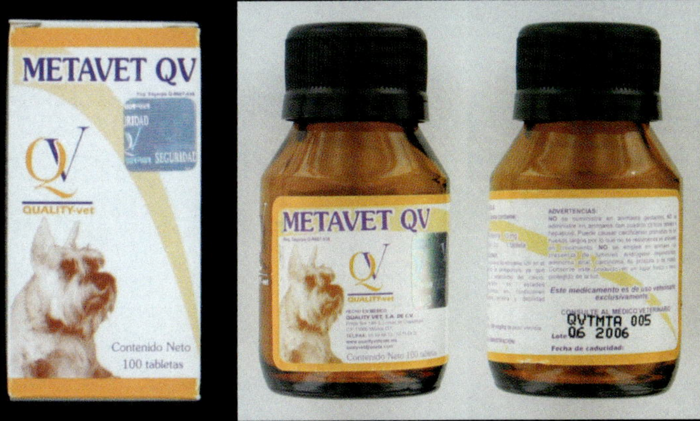

Metavet from Quality Vet (Mexico)

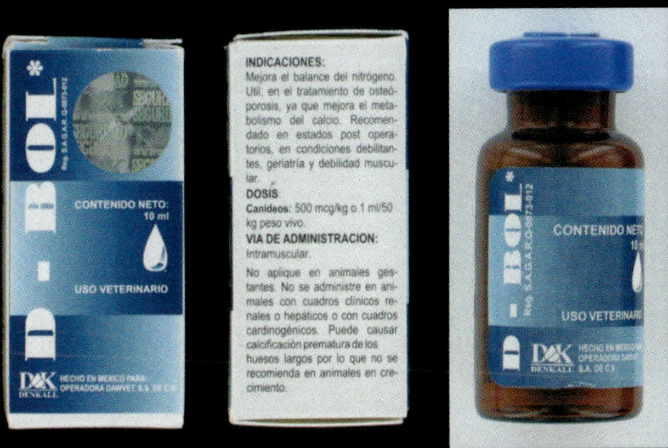

Denkall injectable (Mexico)

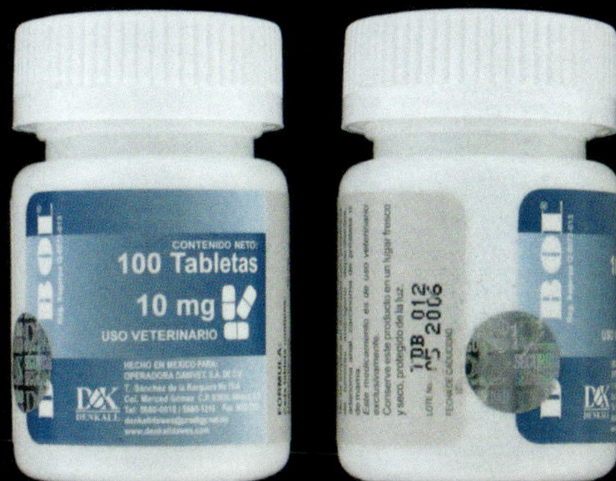

Denkall 100 tablet bottle

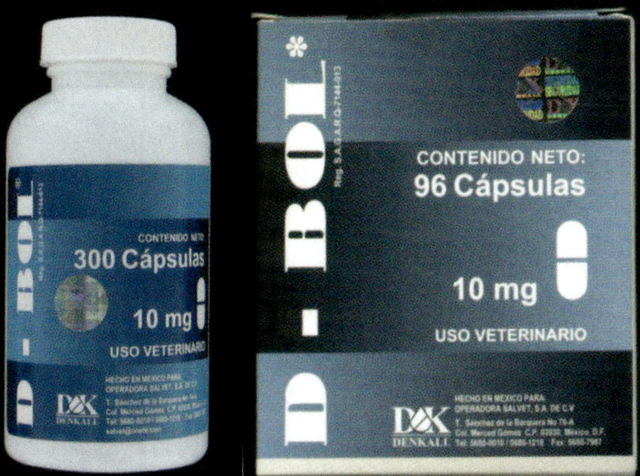

Denkall's D-Bol capsule products

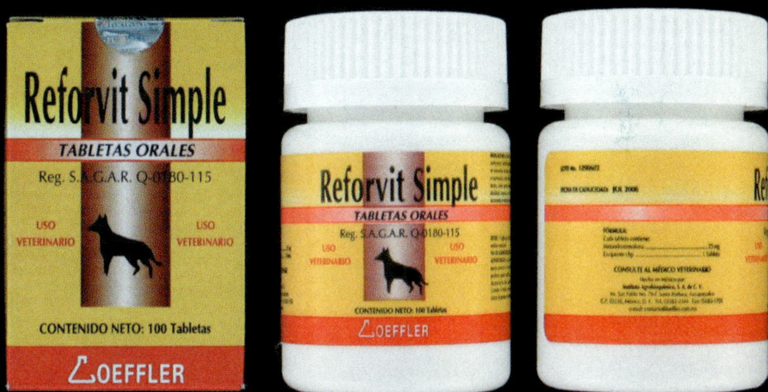

Loeffler Reforvit Simple (new style) from Mexico

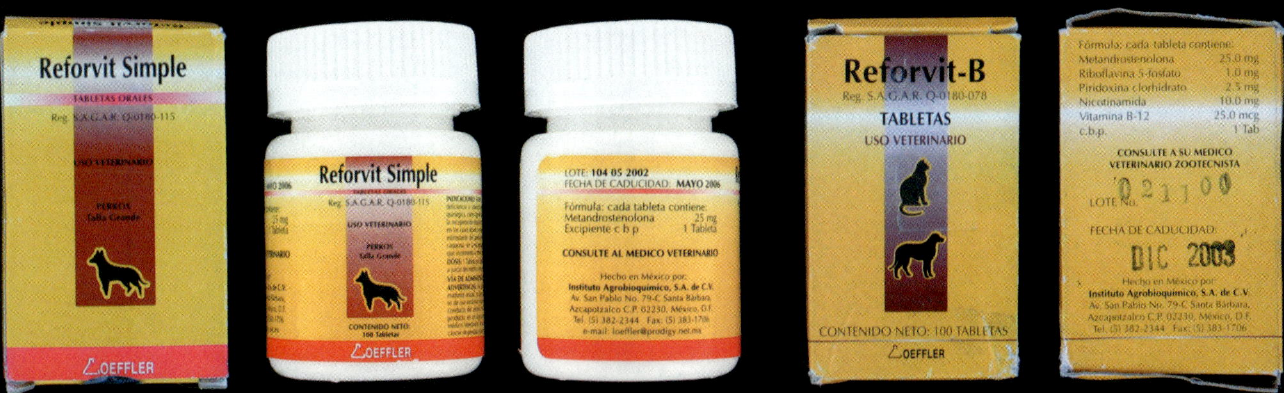

Two older style oral Reforvit products.

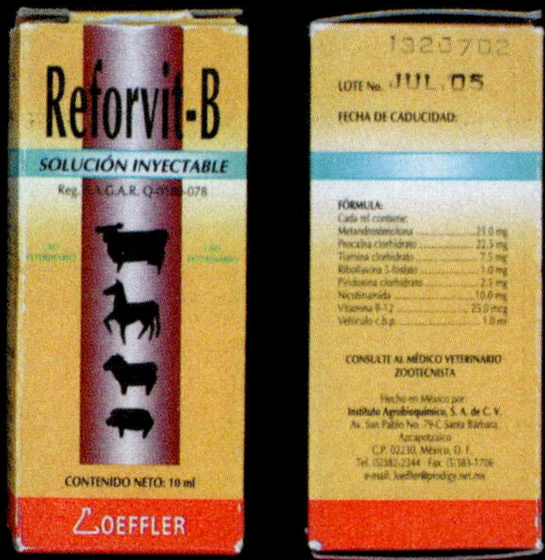

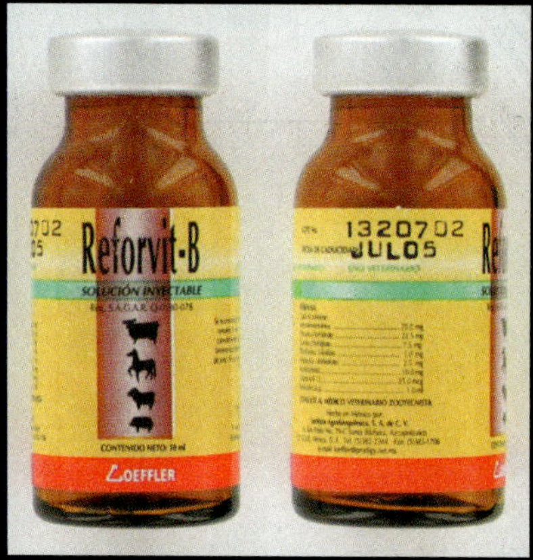

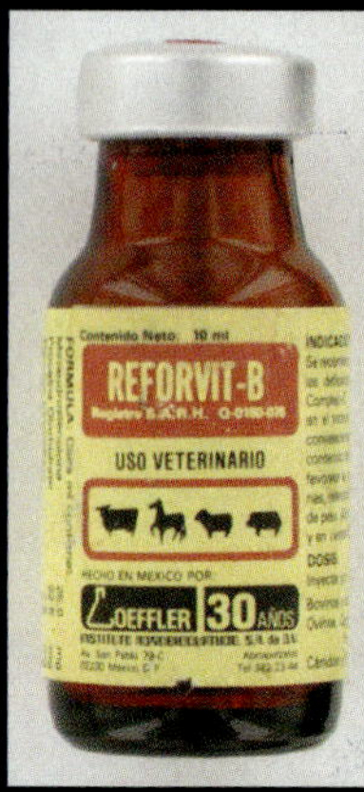

10ml injectable Reforvit from Loeffler (new style)

Old 10ml Reforvit vial

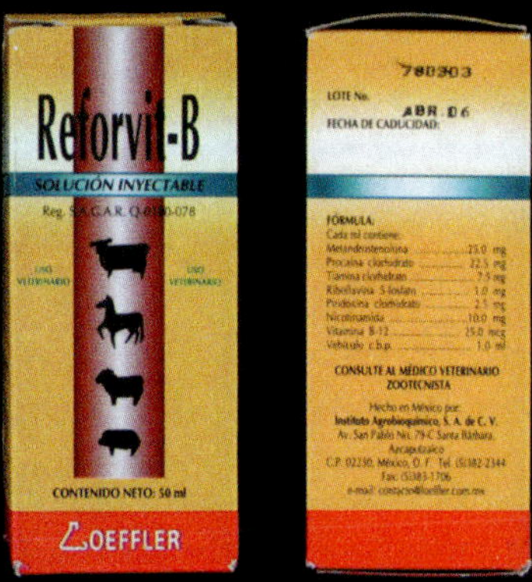

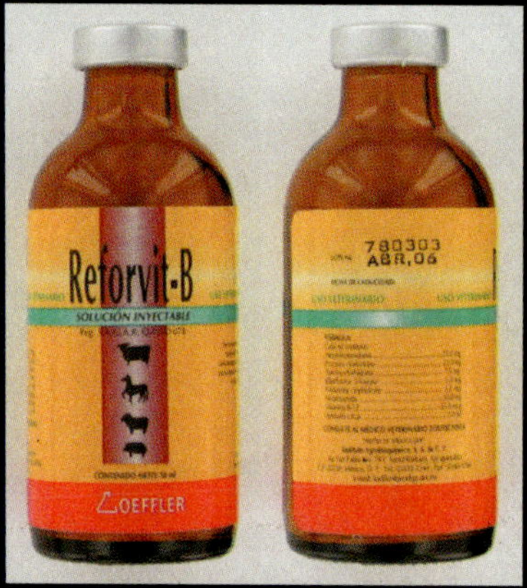

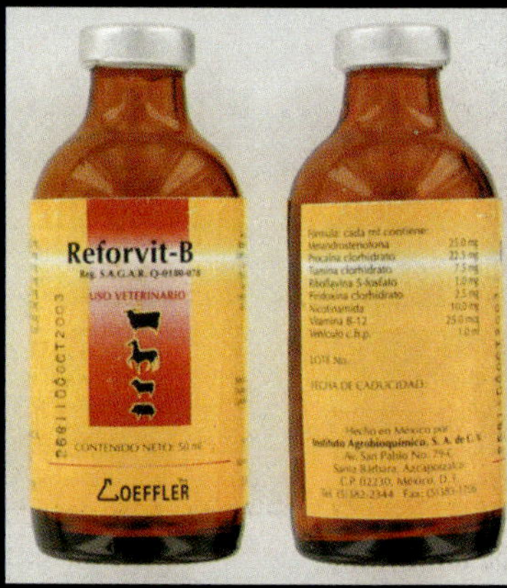

50ml Reforvit from Loeffler (new style)

Older Reforvit-B vial (50ml)

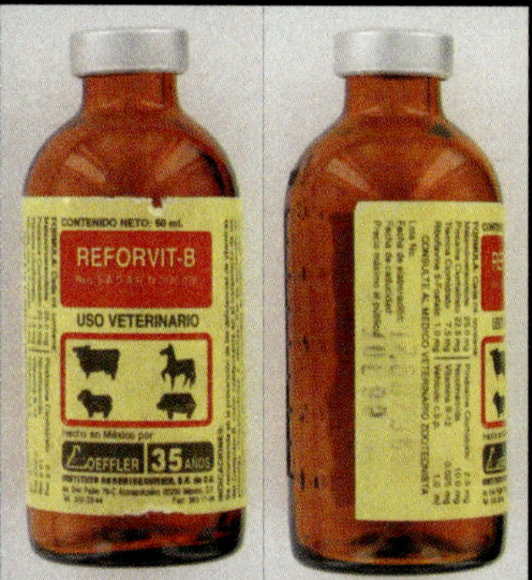

An even older 50ml Reforvit vial

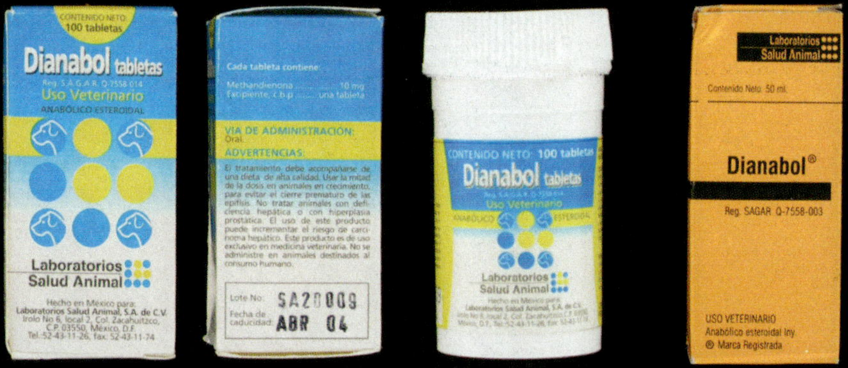

Dianabol tablets from Salud (Mexico), plus 50ml injectable box

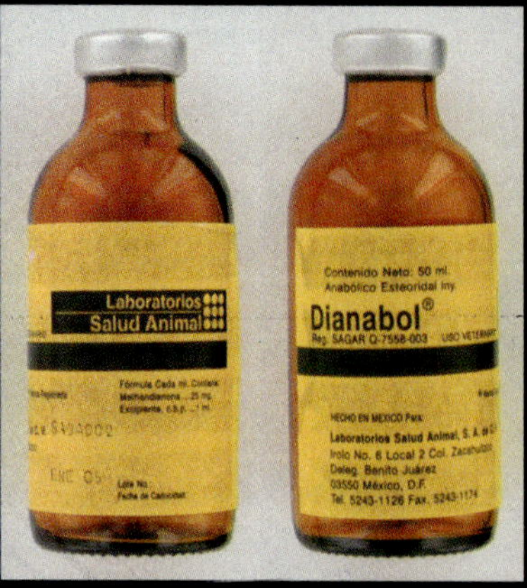

Salud 50ml vial

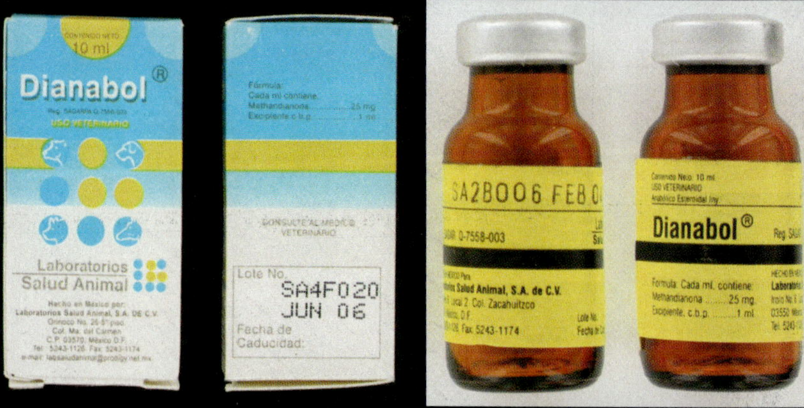

Salud 10ml box and vial

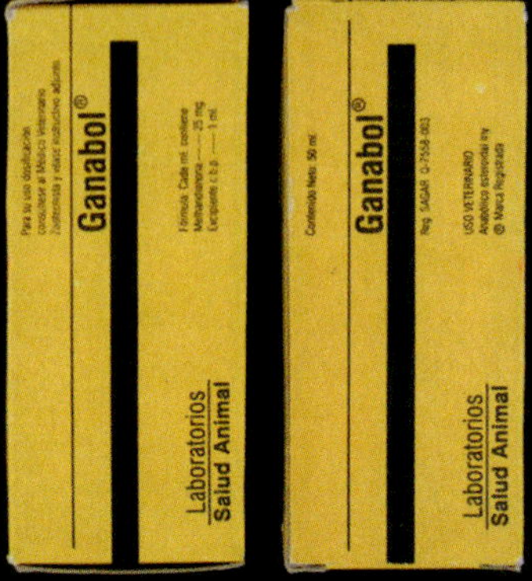

Salud's old Ganabol (NLM)

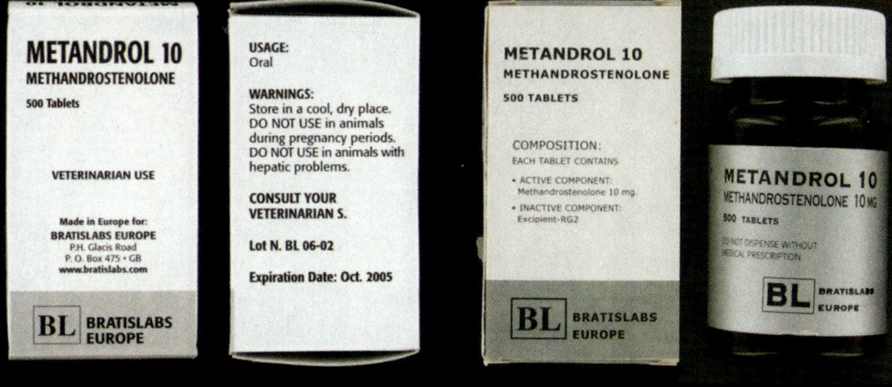

Bratis Metandrol 10, new (left) and old styles (Mexico)

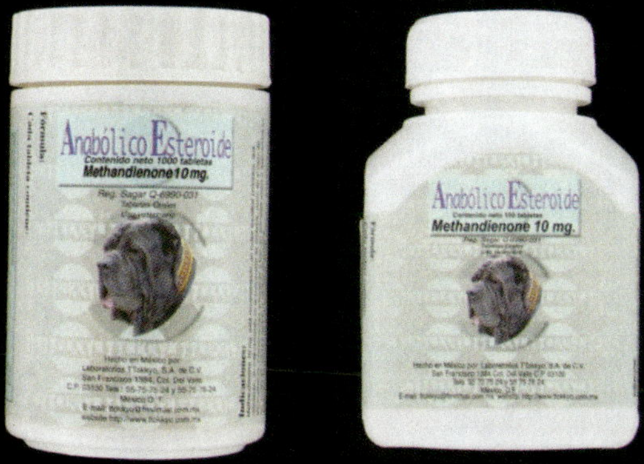

Ttokkyo 10mg (1000 and 100 tablets) from Mexico (NLM)

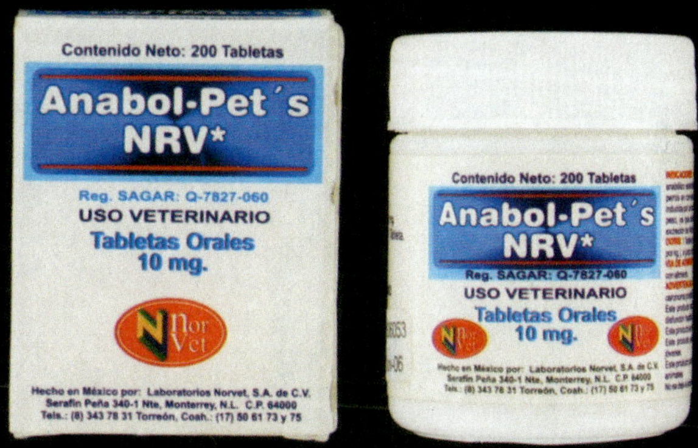

Anabol-Pet's from Norvet (Mexico)

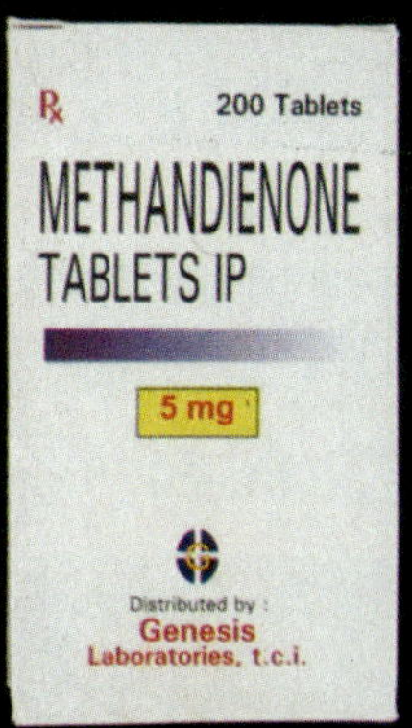

Genesis tabs (Singapore)

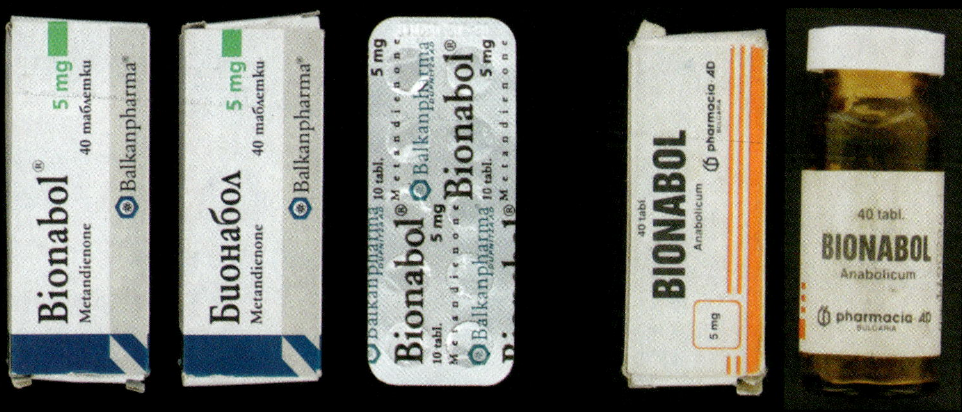

Bionabol from Bulgaria - New and old packaging

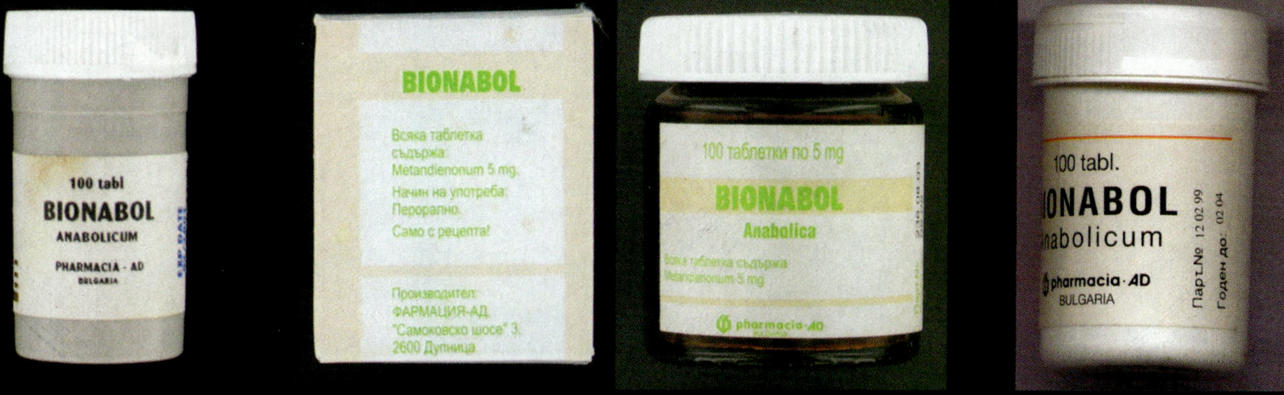

Three different counterfeits

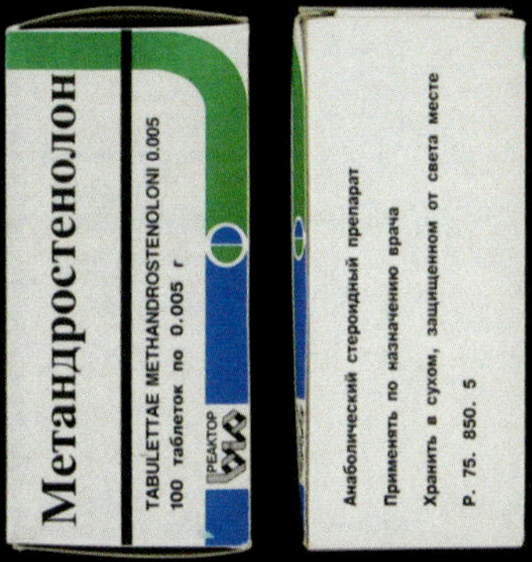

New Bioreaktor box from Russia

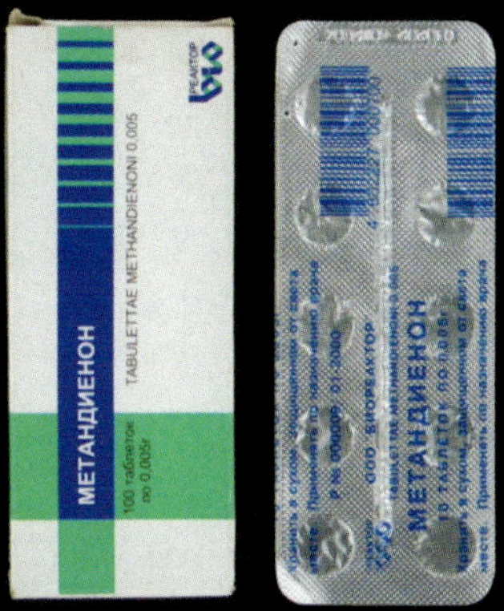

Previous box (2000-2004)

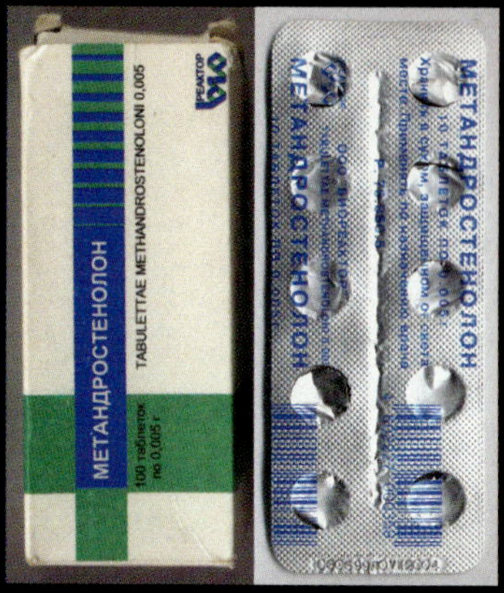

Pre-2000 box and strip

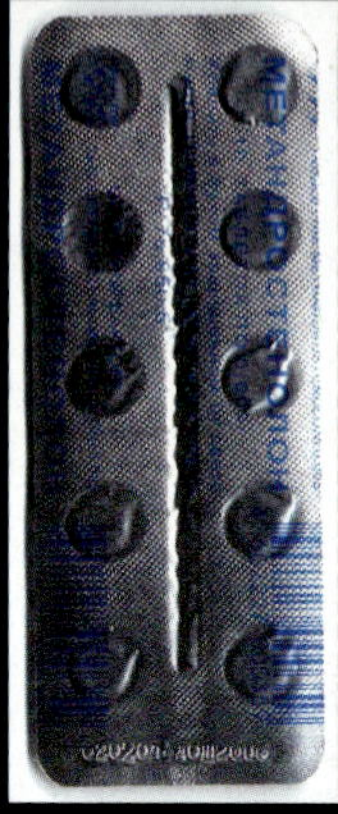

Counterfeit

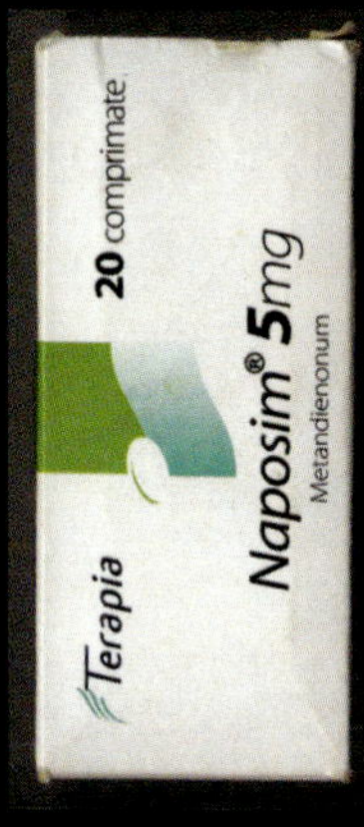

New Naposim box

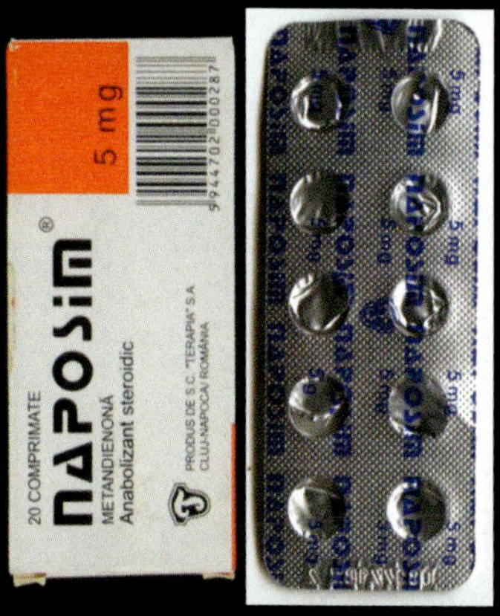

Previous Naposim (Rumania)

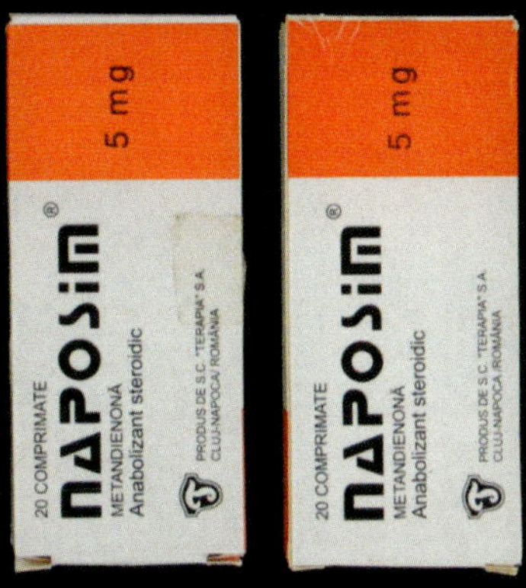

Older box, before barcoding

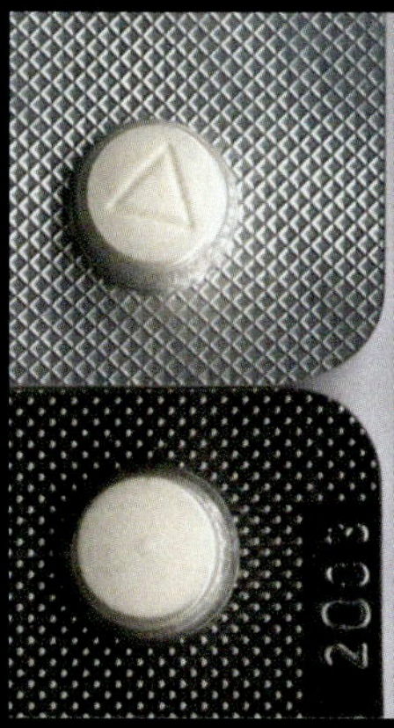

Fake on top

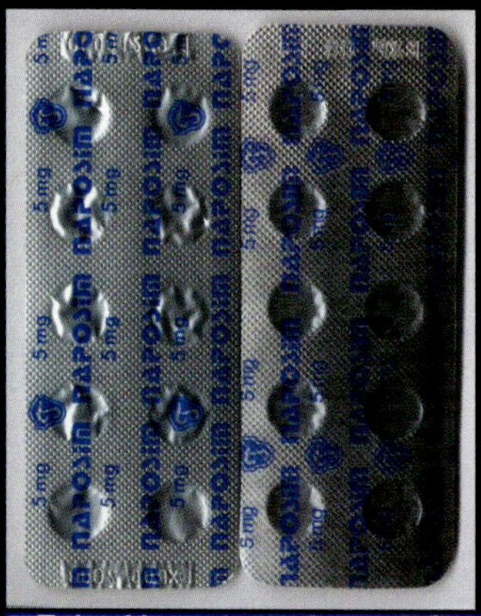

Fake Naposim strip on left

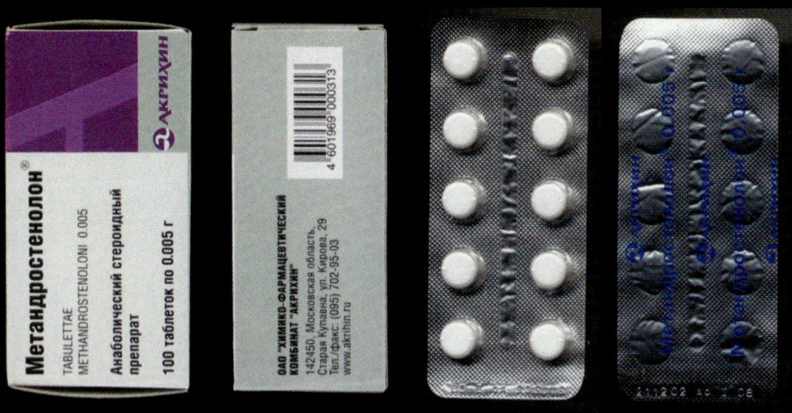

New look to Russian Dianabol

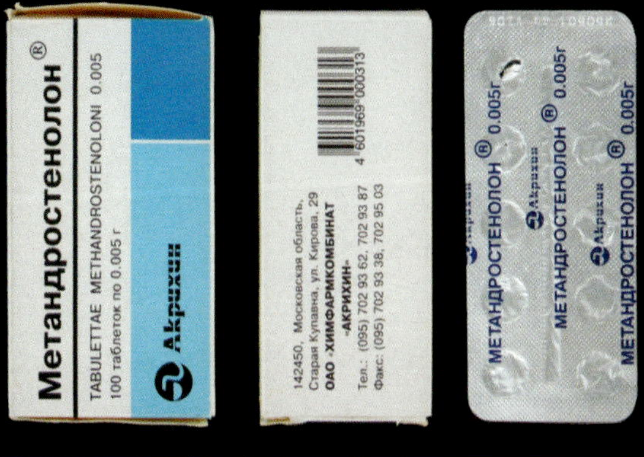

Previous packaging

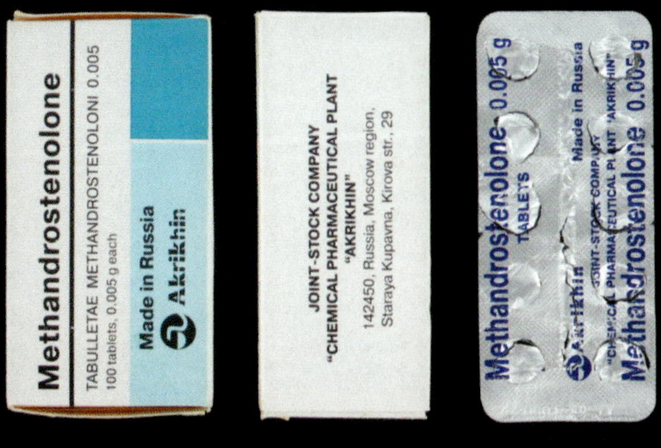

Counterfeit with English type

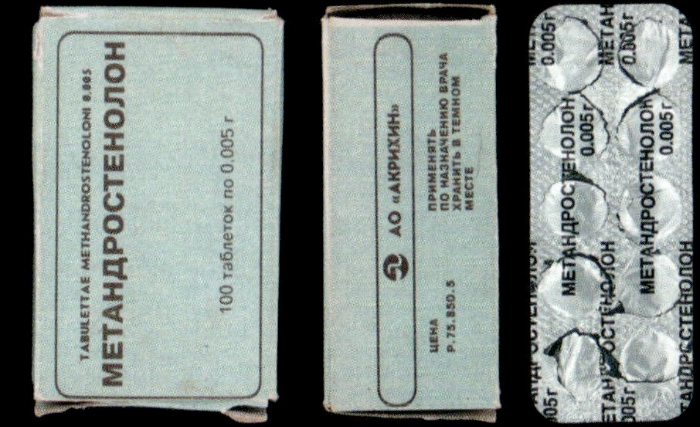

Old Russian Dianabol

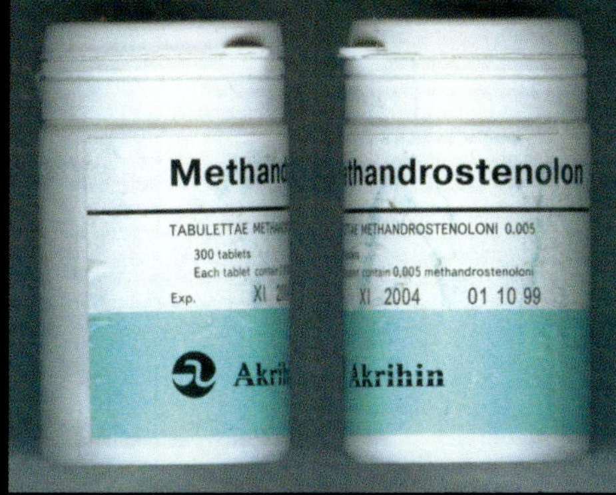

Counterfeit #2

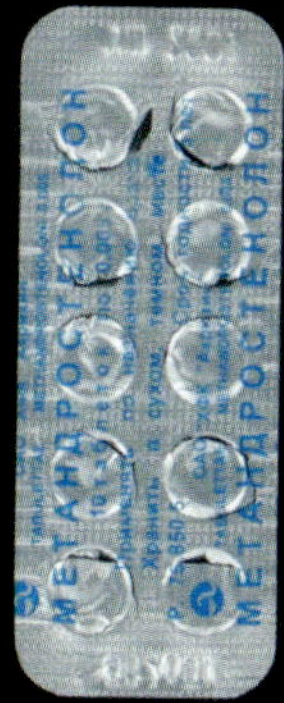

Counterfeit #3

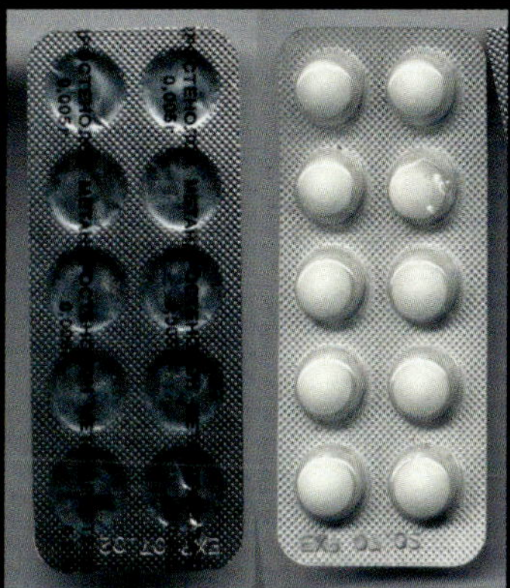

Counterfeit #4

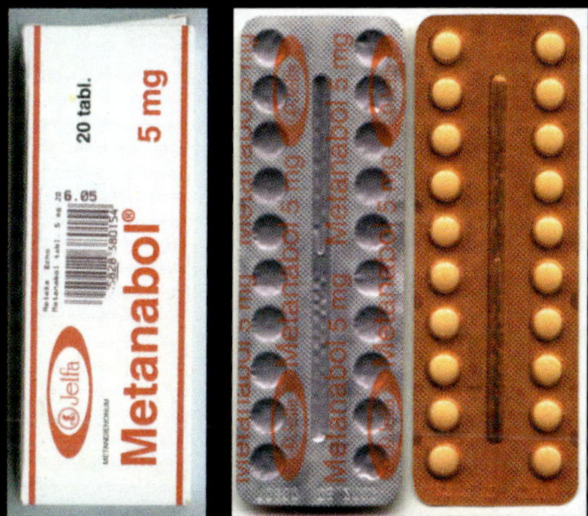

Metanabol from Poland

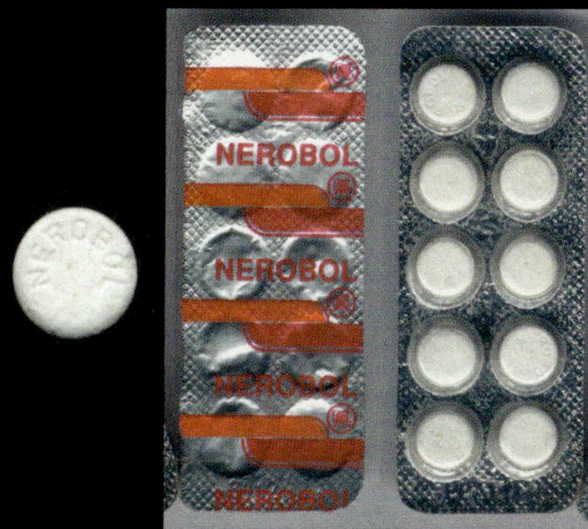

Nerobol from Hungary (NLM)

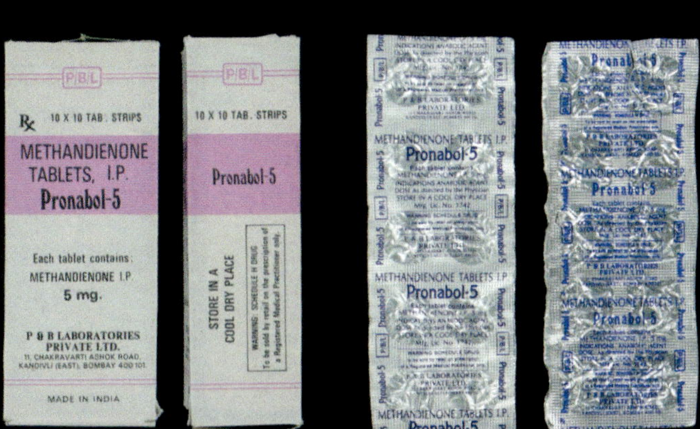

Pronabol from India (NLM)

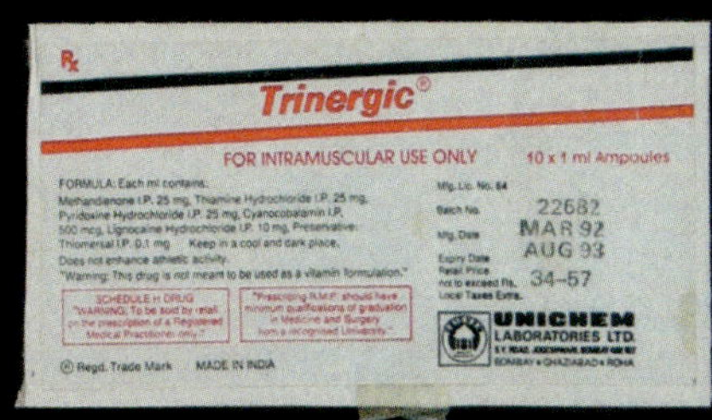

Trinergic from India (NLM)

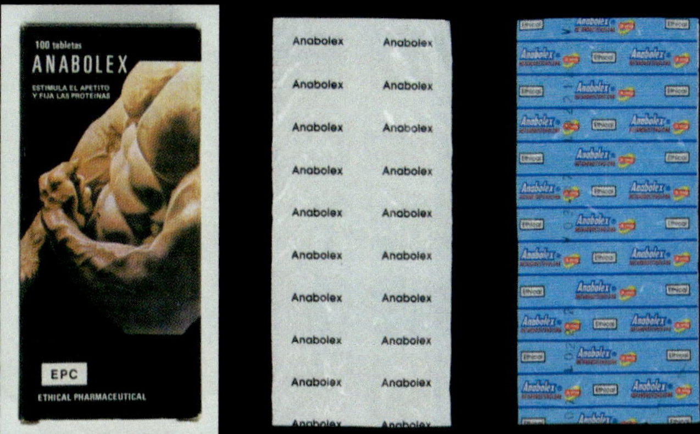

Anabolex from Dom. Rep. - New strip on right

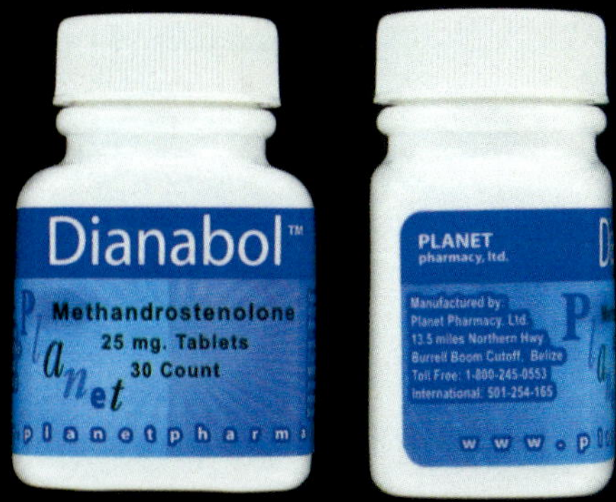

Dianabol from Planet Pharm (Belize)

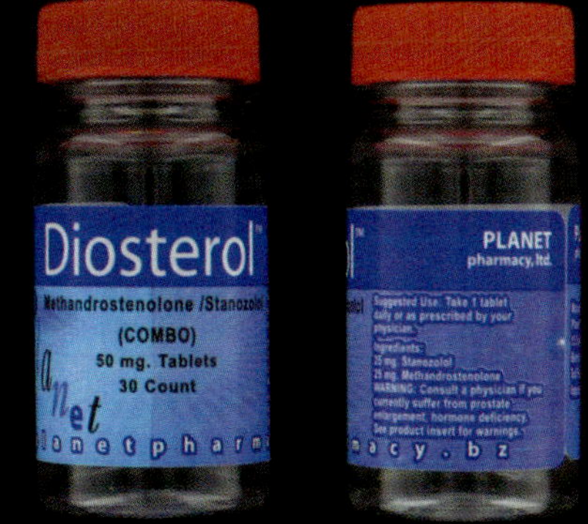

Diosterol (Dbol/Winny blend) - Belize

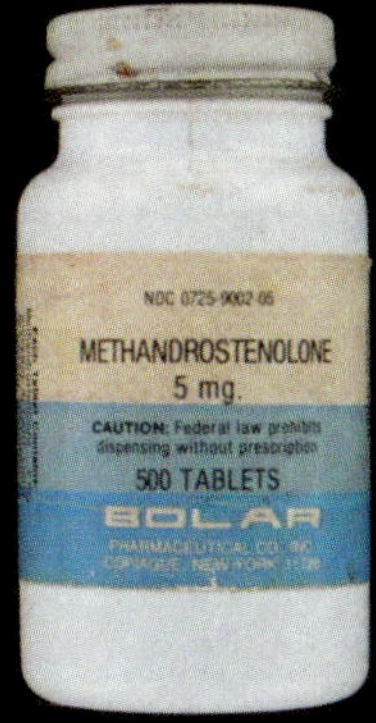

Old U.S. Generic (NLM)

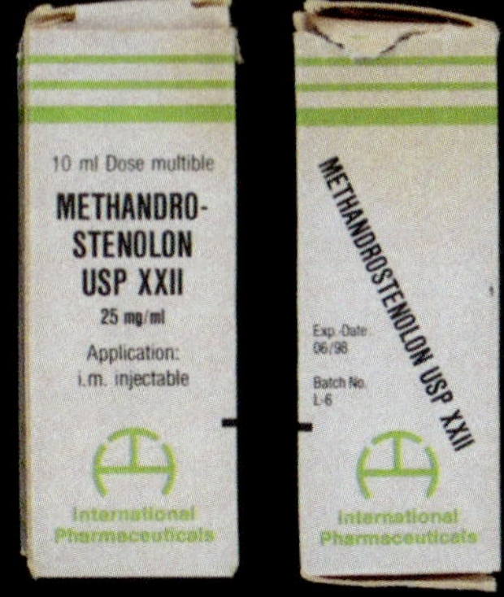

Underground IP box

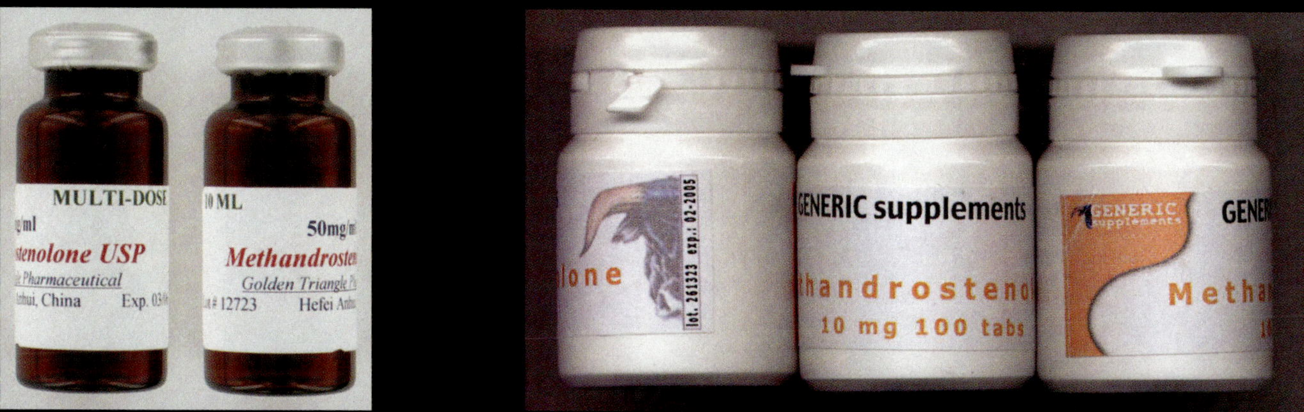

Underground products from Golden Triangle and Generic Supplements

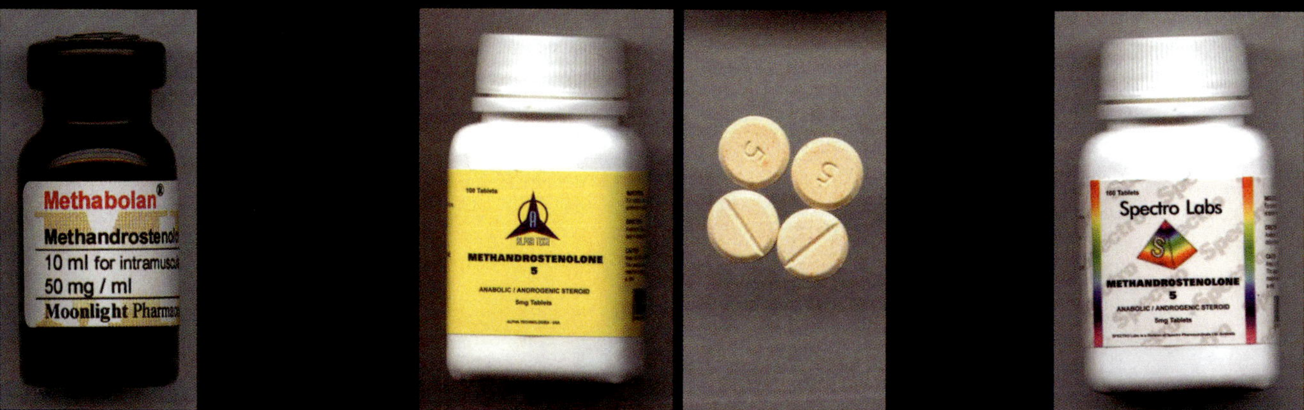

Underground products from Moonlight, Alpha Tech (NLM) and Spectro (NLM)

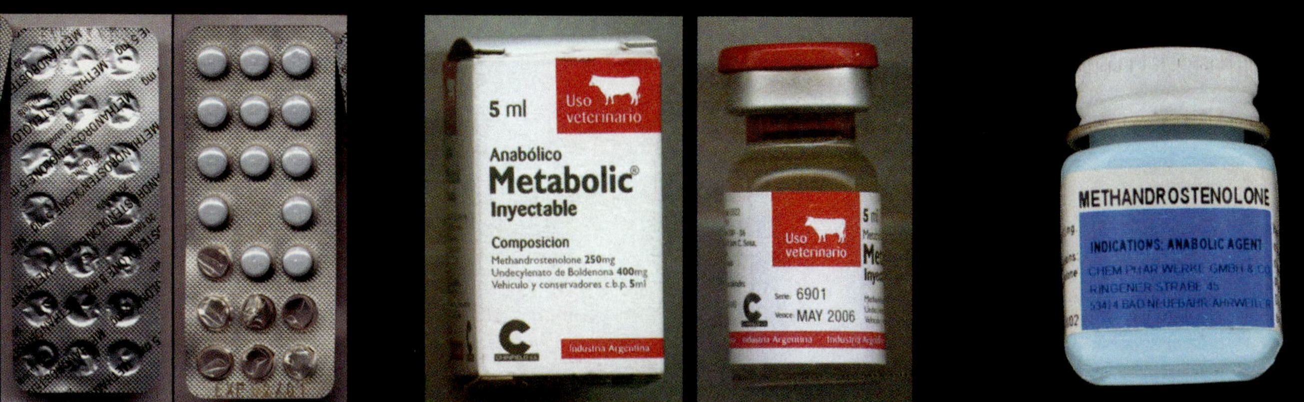

Three different counterfeit items

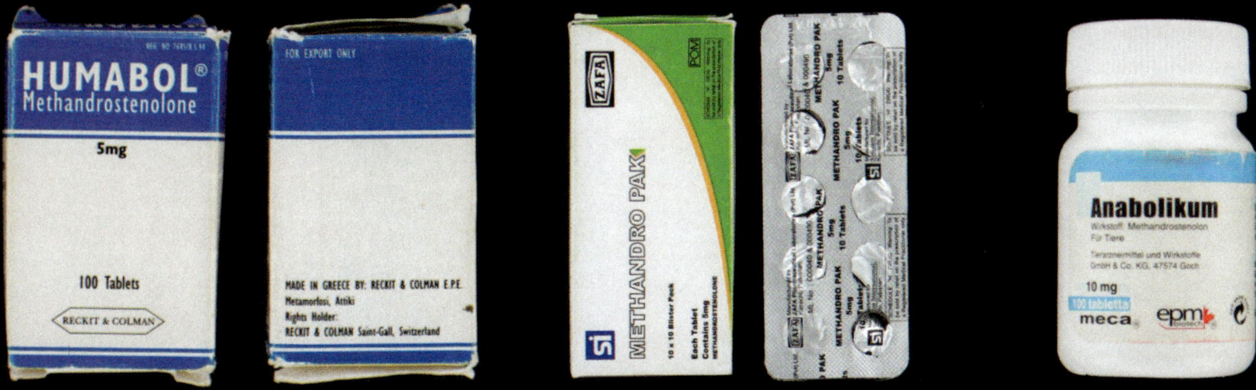

Three more counterfeits with fabricated brand names

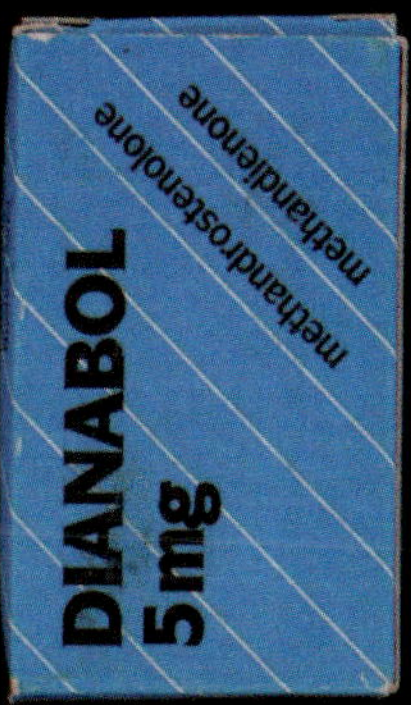

Old European fake

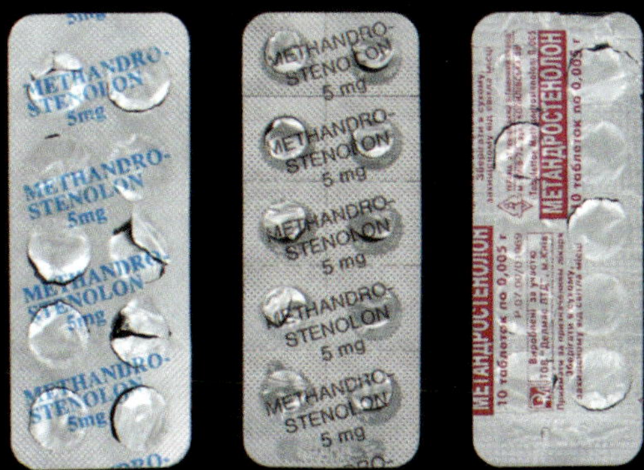

Three bogus tablet strips

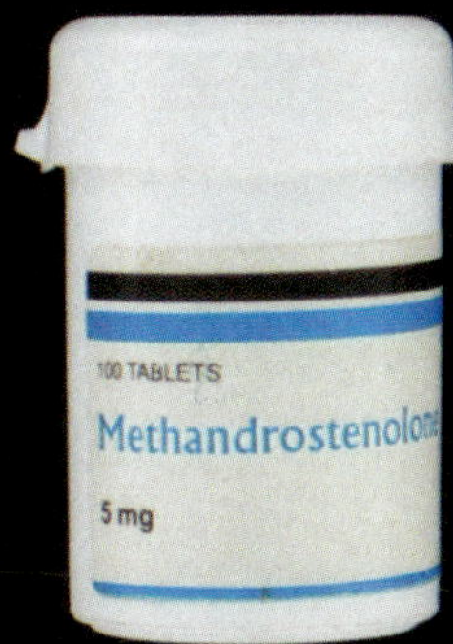

Fake bottle

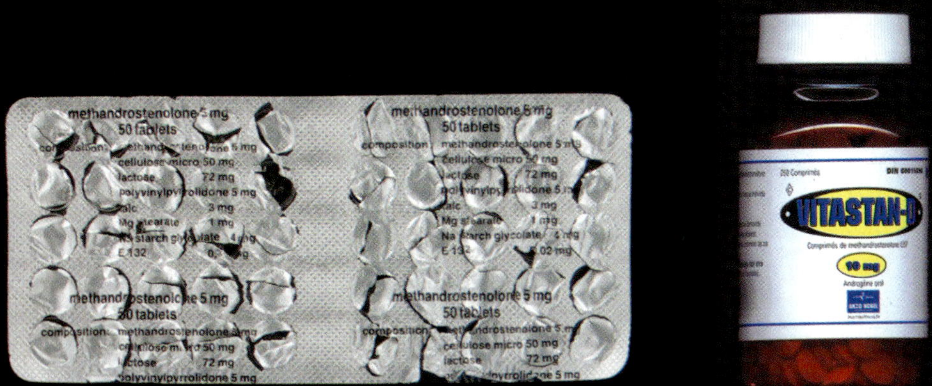

Counterfeit strip and “Vitastan” bottle (no such brand in made)

Dinandrol

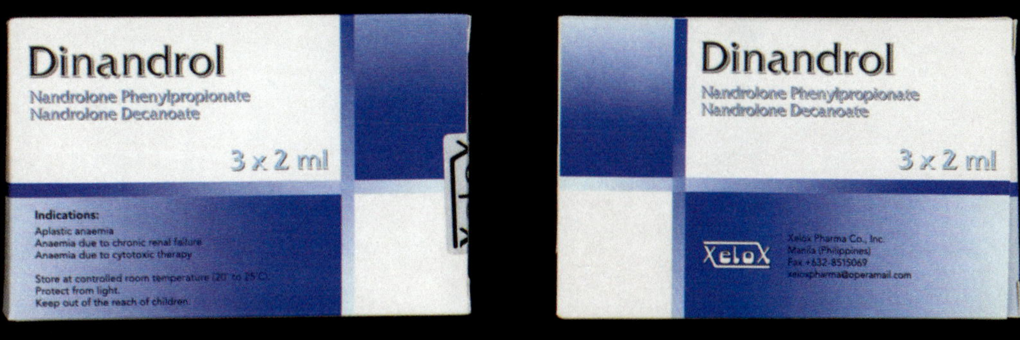

Dinandrol from Xelox Pharma (Philippines)

Drive

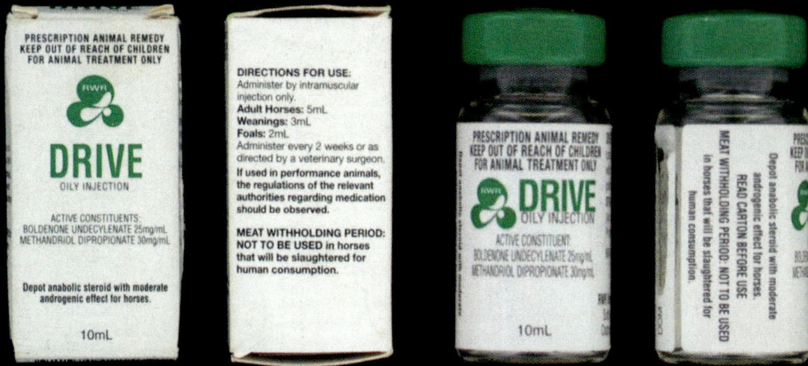

Drive from Australia

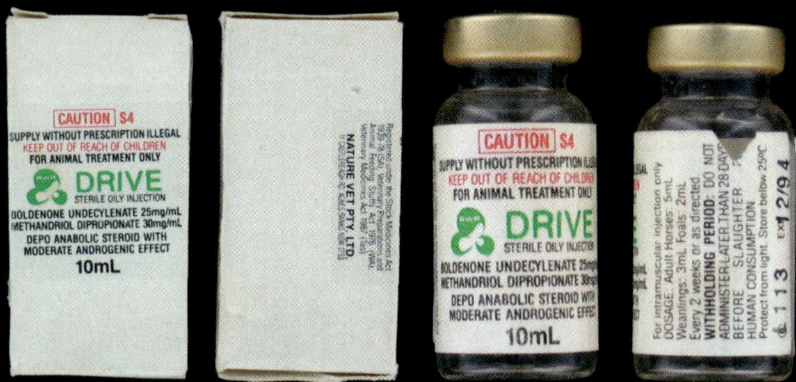

Counterfeit Drive box and vial

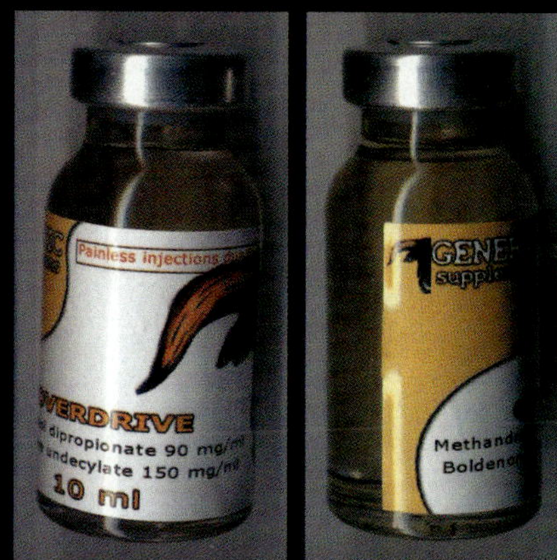

UG version from Generic Supplements

Durabolin

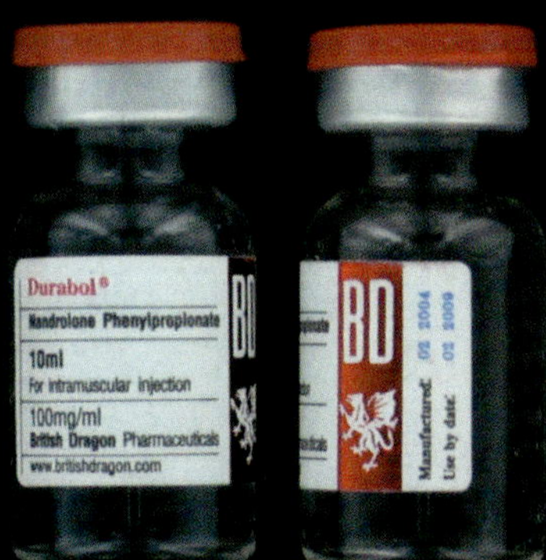

Durabol from British Dragon (Thailand)

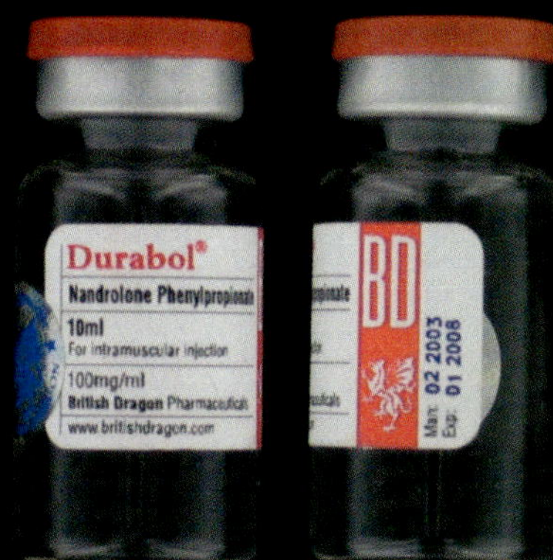

Older version BD vial

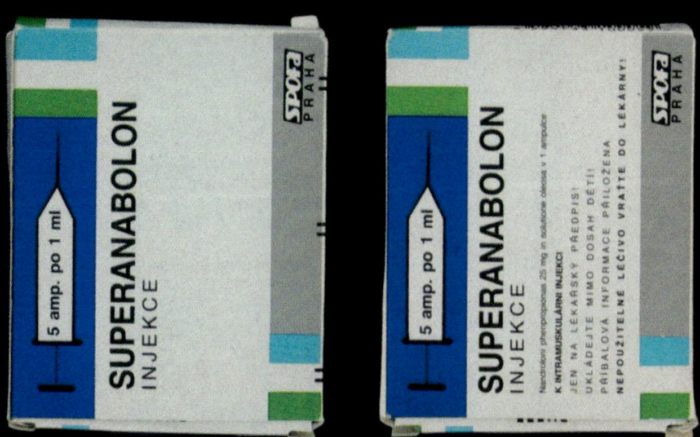

Superanabolon from the Czech Republic

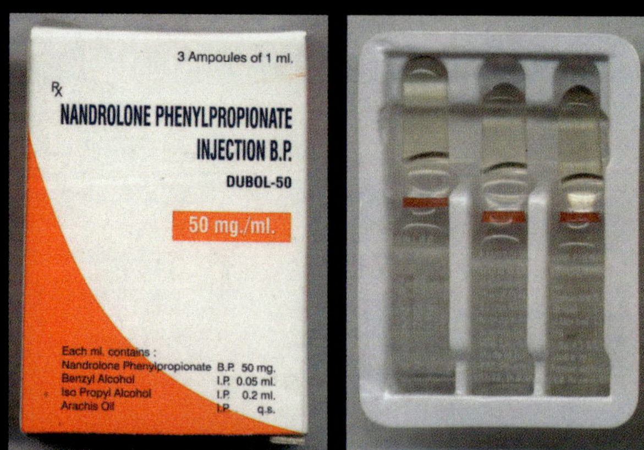

BM generic from India

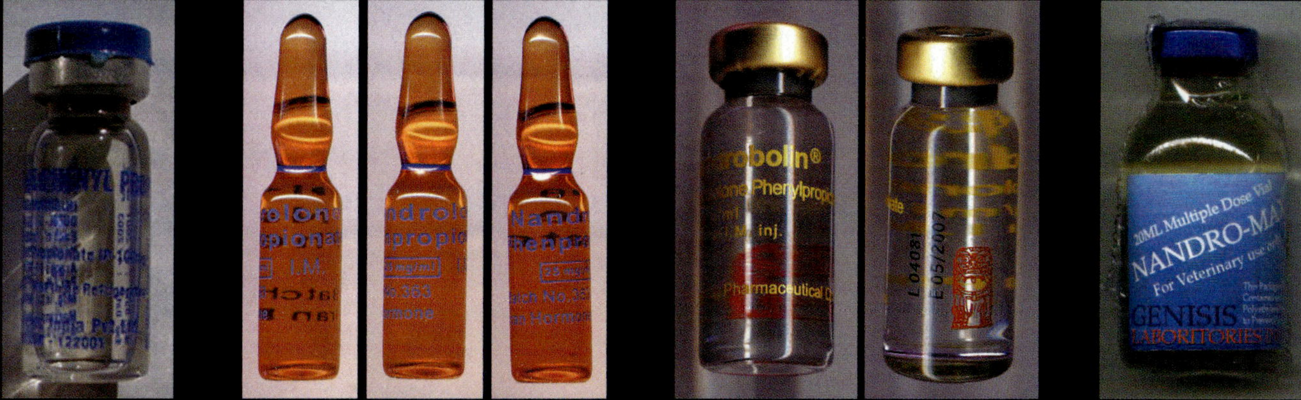

Hayrian vial India (NLM), ampules from Iran Hormone, vial Luoyang Pharm (China) and UG vial from Genisis

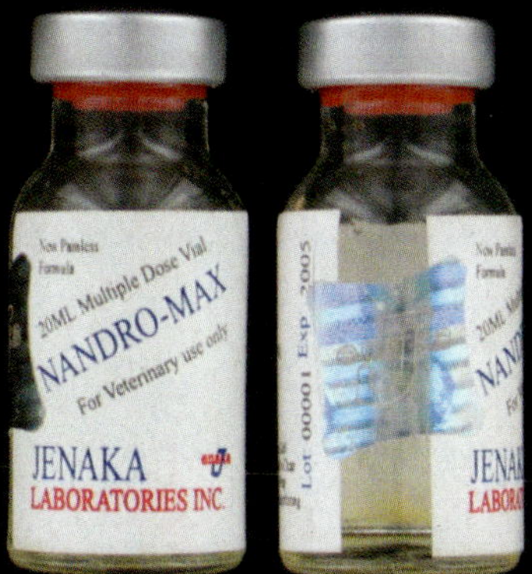

UG - Jenaka Nandro-Max (NLM)

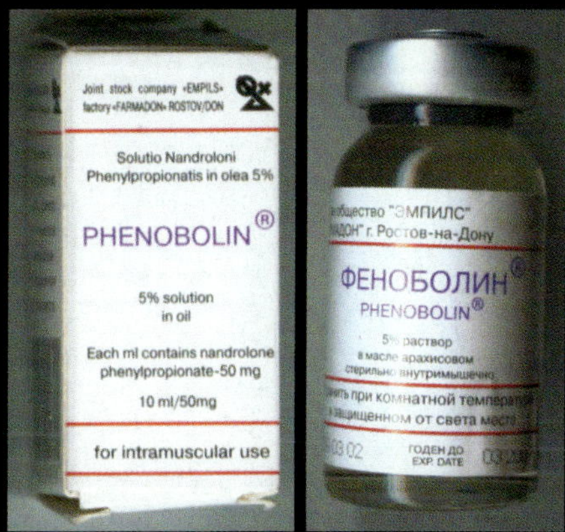

Counterfeit Farmadon product

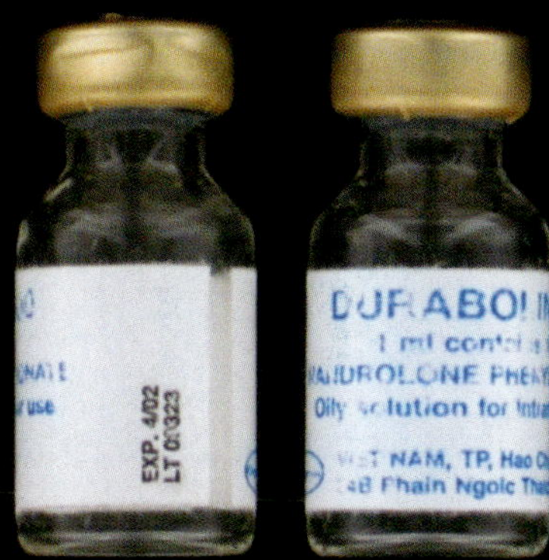

Fake Durabolin from Vietnam

Dynabolon

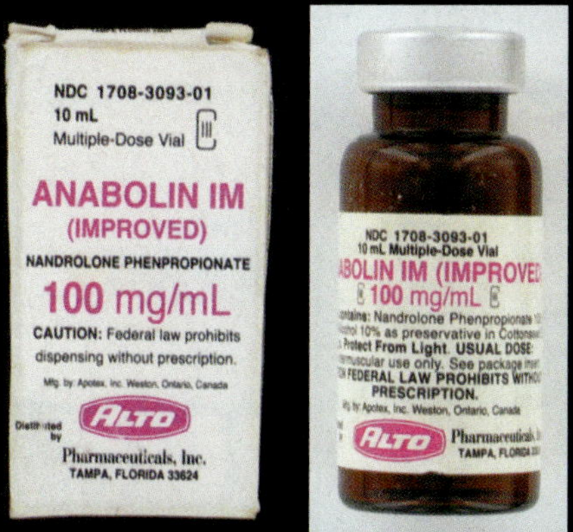

Counterfeit Anabolin

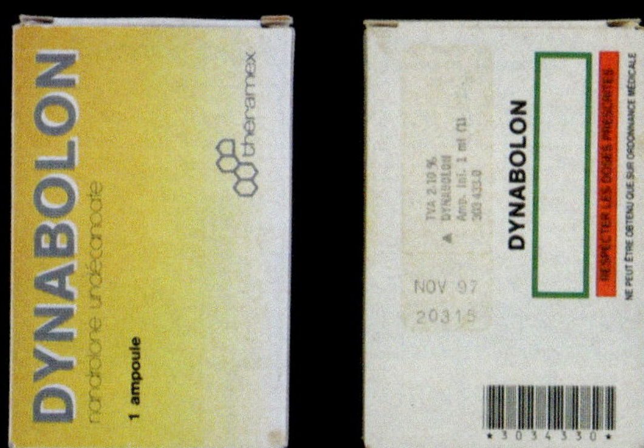

Dynabolon from France (NLM)

Equipoise

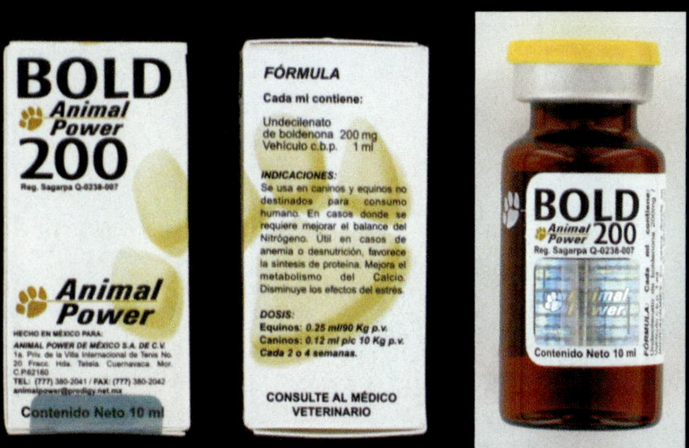

Bold 200 from Animal Power (Mexico)

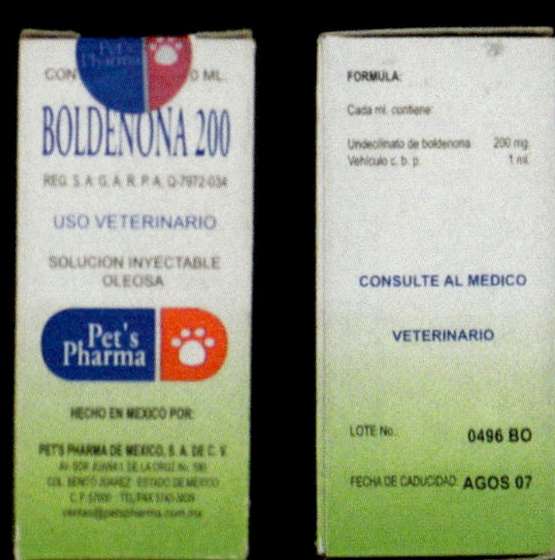

Generic from Pet's Pharma (Mexico)

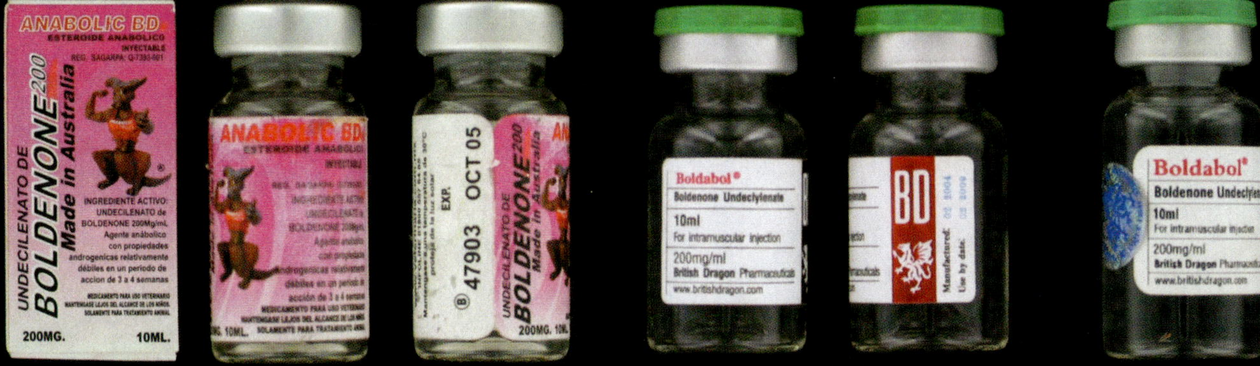

SYD Group Anabolic BD (Mexico) British Dragon Boldabol (Thailand) Old style BD vial

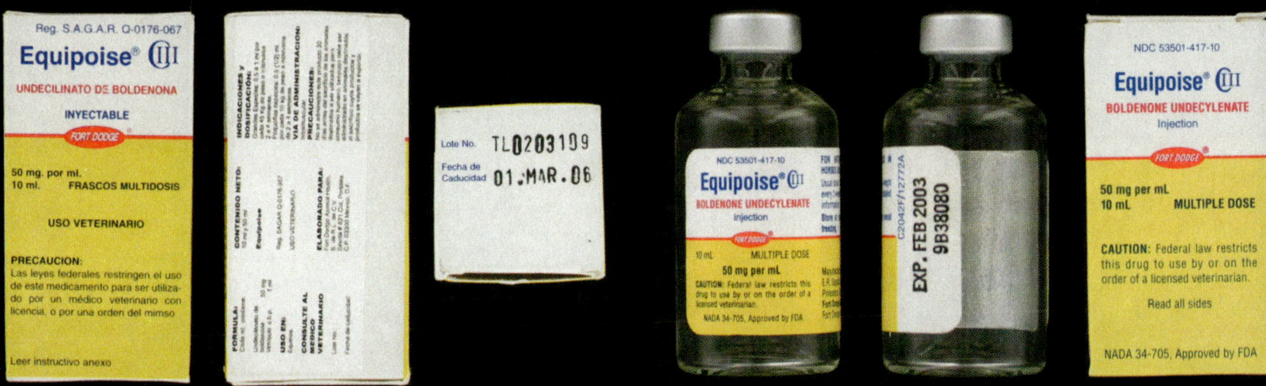

10ml U.S. Equipoise® from Fort Dodge (Mexican import) - New box on left

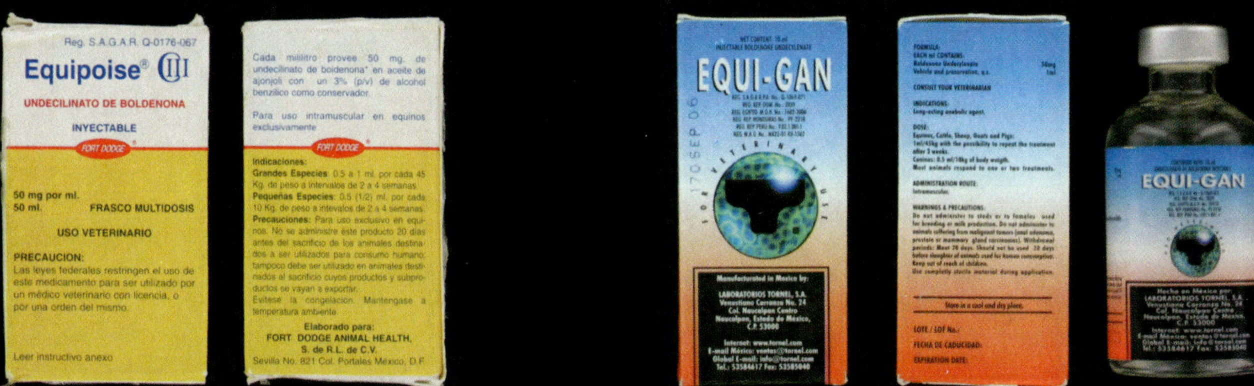

50ml Fort Dodge Equipoise® 10ml Equi-gan from Tornell (Mexico)

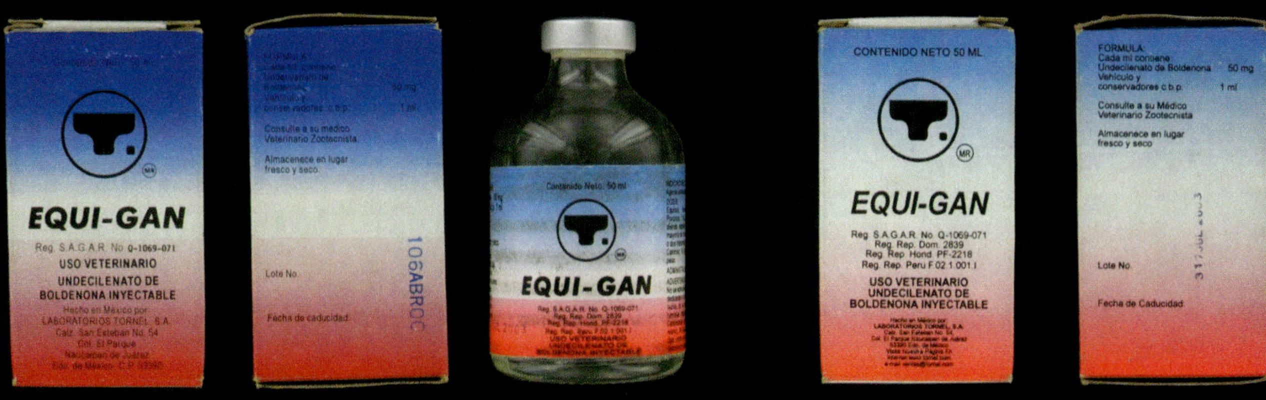

Older style 50ml box and vial Oldest style pictured

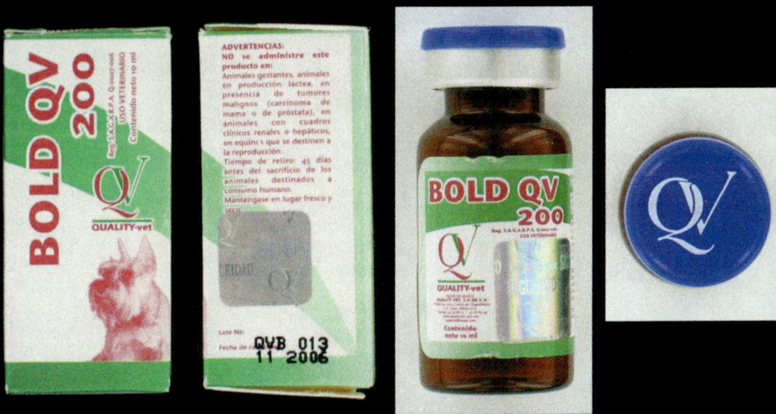

Bold QV from Quality Vet (Mexico)

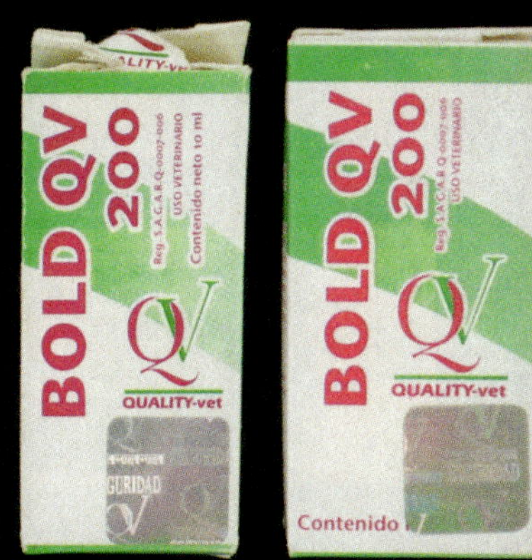

Two older QV boxes

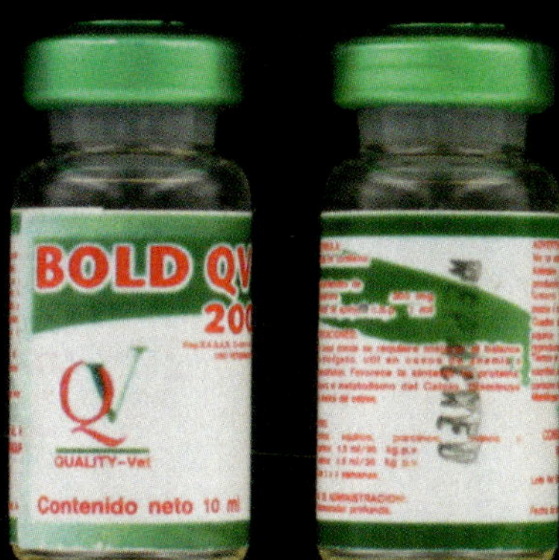

Counterfeit QV vial

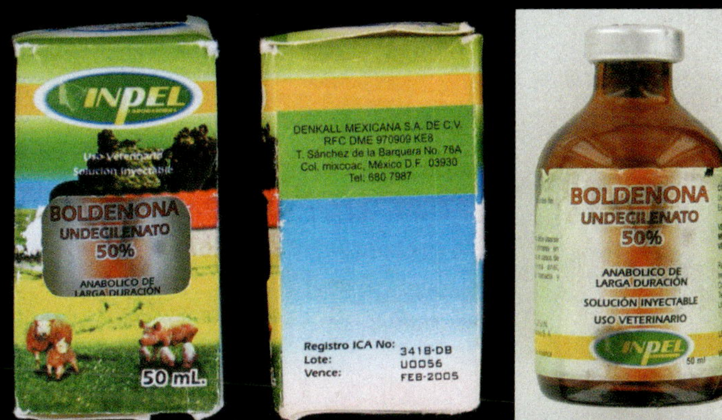

Inpel Maxigan from Mexico (NLM)

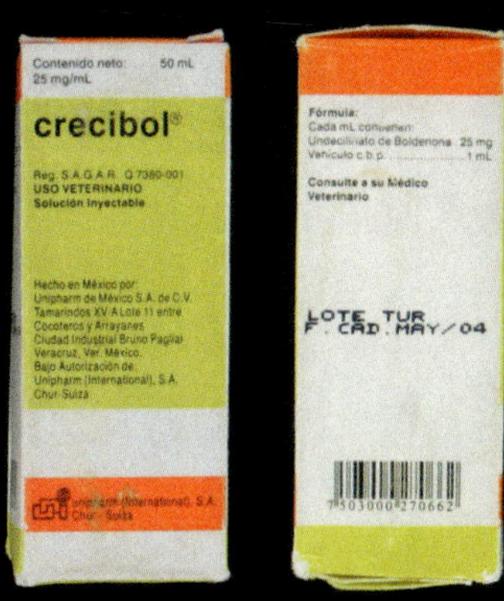

Mexican Crecibol

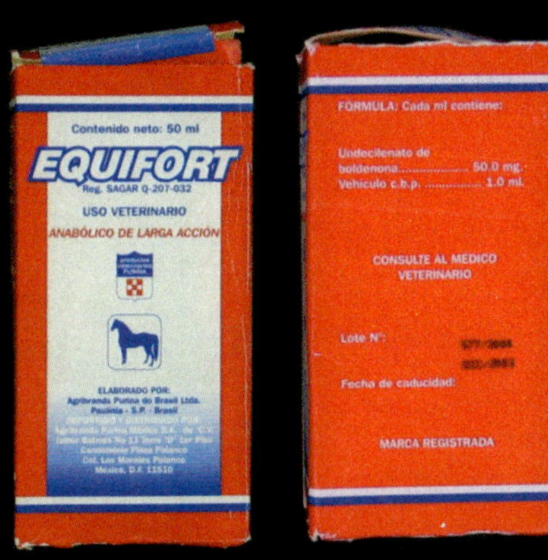

Equifort from Purina (Mexico)

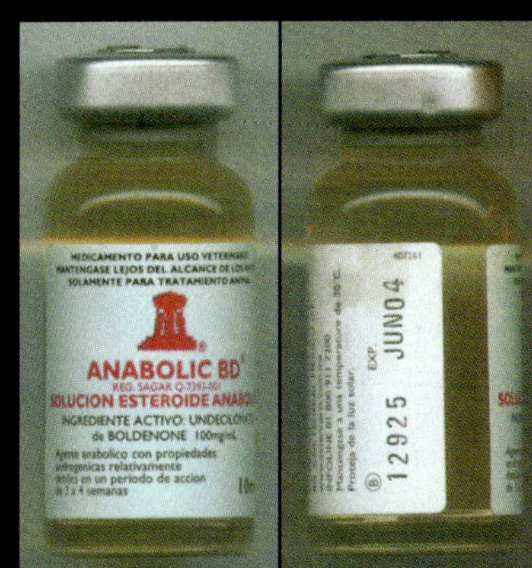

Anabolic BD - Grupo Mexico (NLM)

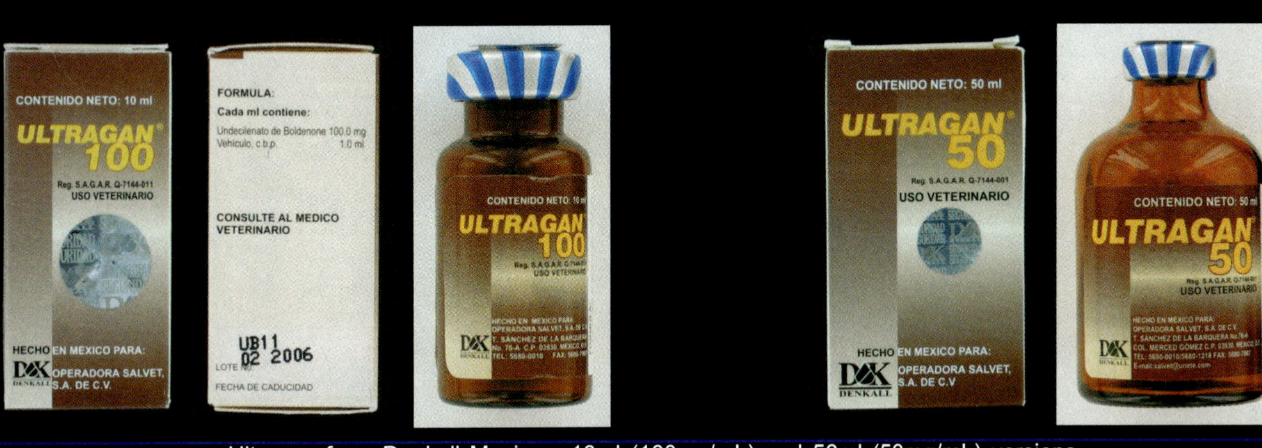

Ultragan from Denkall Mexico - 10ml (100mg/mL) and 50ml (50mg/mL) versions

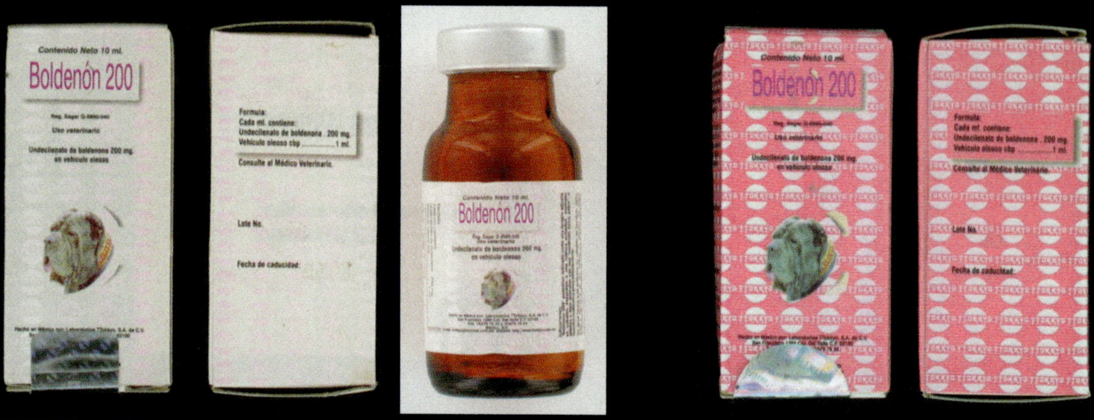

Boldenon 200 from Ttokkyo Mexico - New and older styles (both NLM)

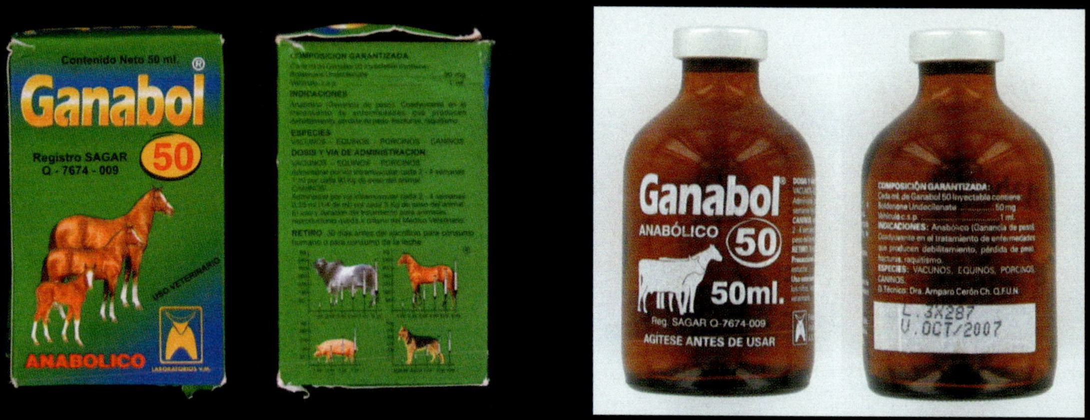

Ganabol from Colombia - New style packaging

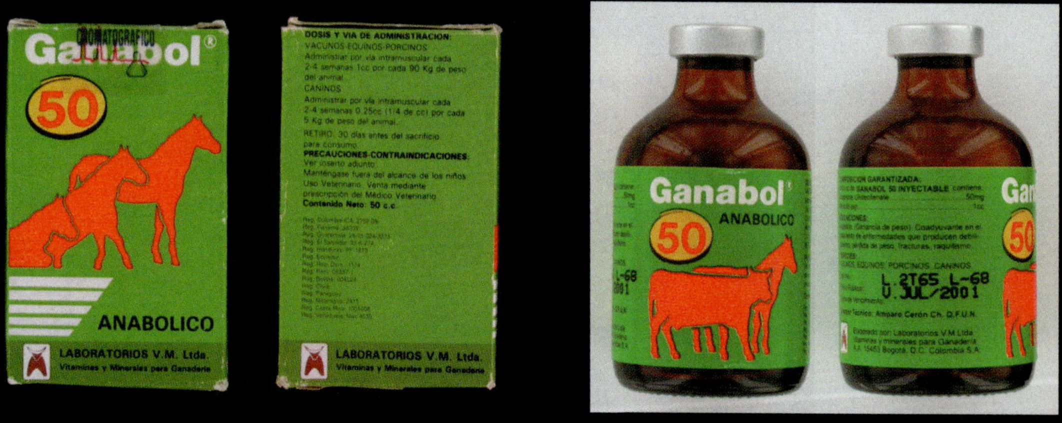

Older look to Ganabol

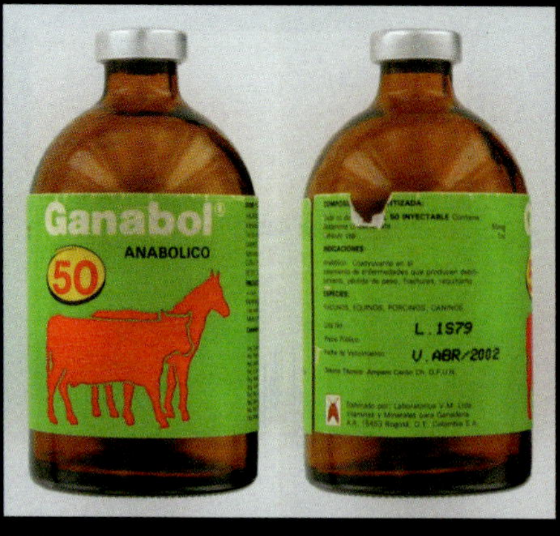

100mL vial

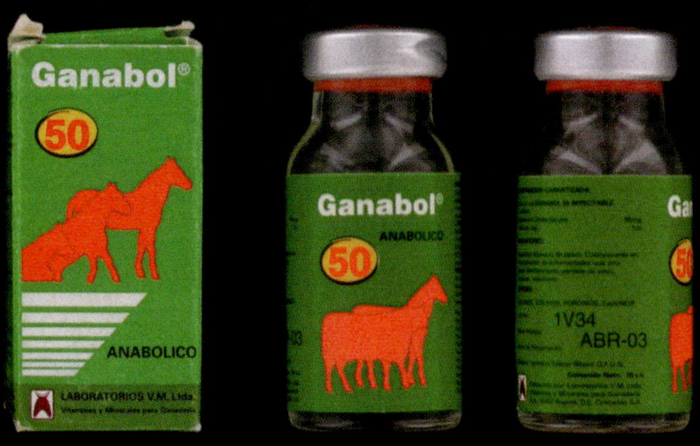

Counterfeit box and vial

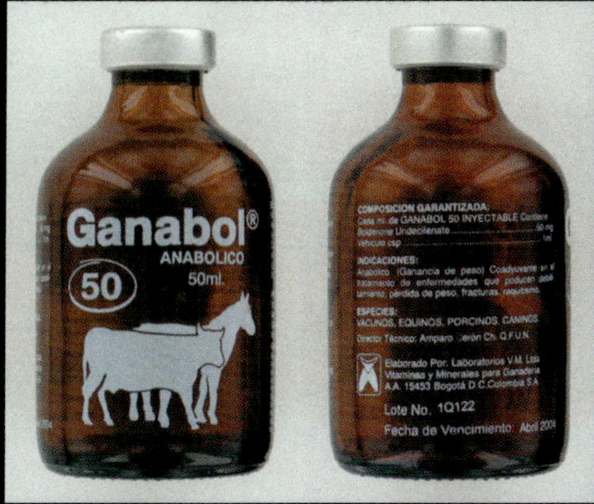

Counterfeit Ganabol vial

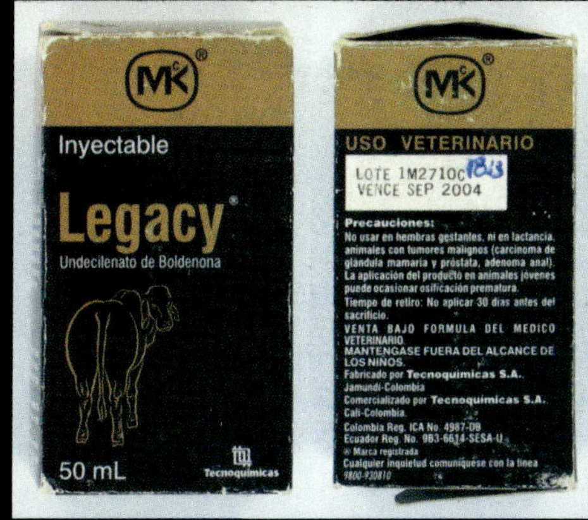

Legacy from Colombia

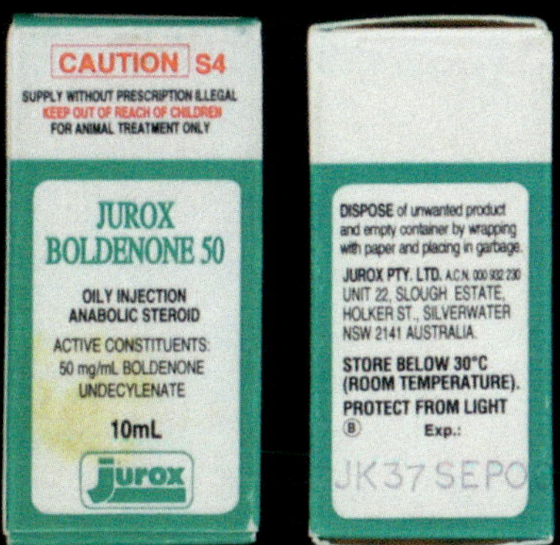

Jurox Boldenone - Australia (NLM)

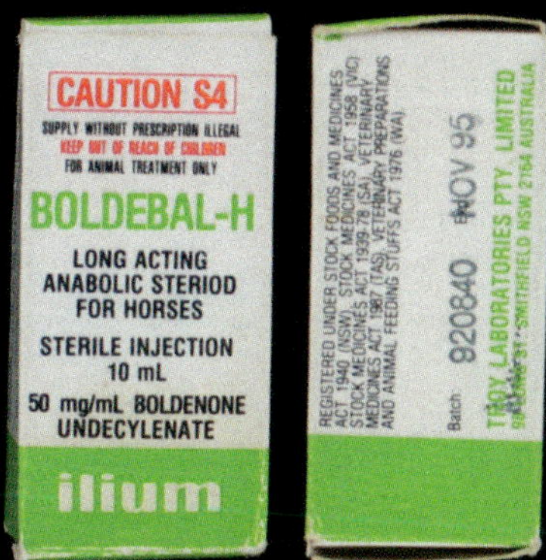

Ilium Boldebal-H (old style)

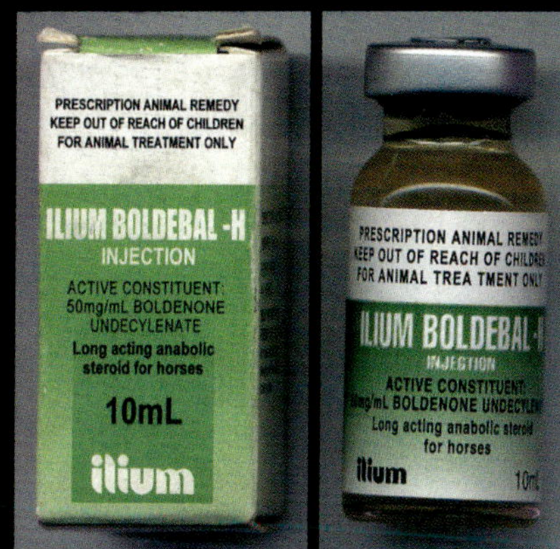

Counterfeit Ilium box and vial

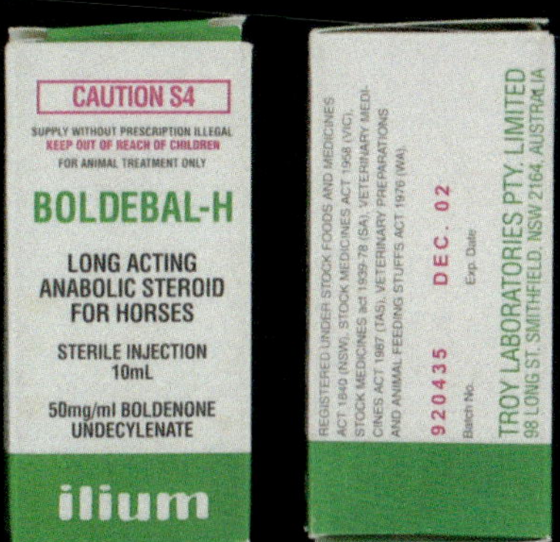

Counterfeit Boldebal-H

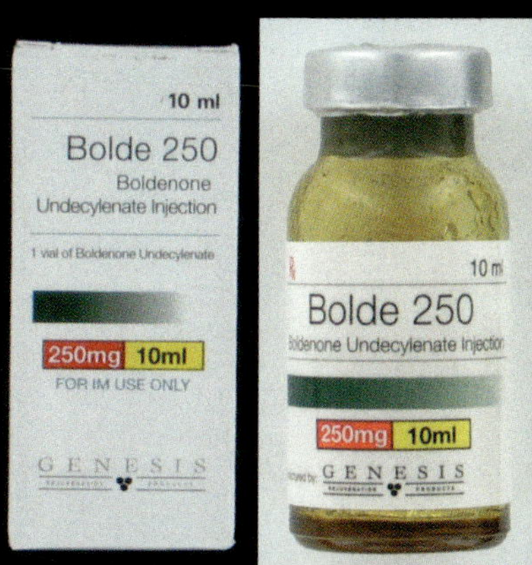

Bolde 250 (Singapore)

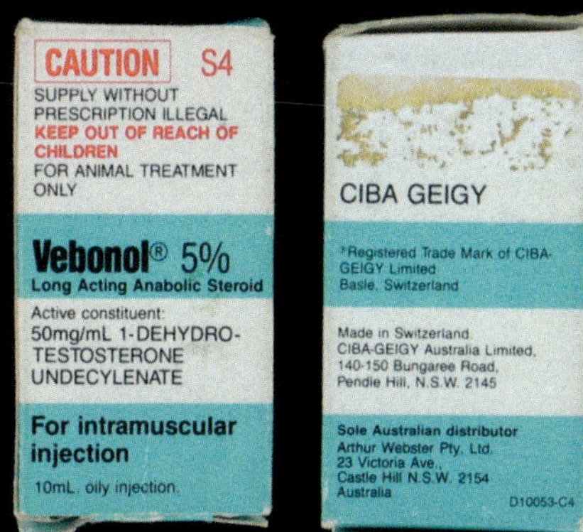

Australian Vebonol (NLM)

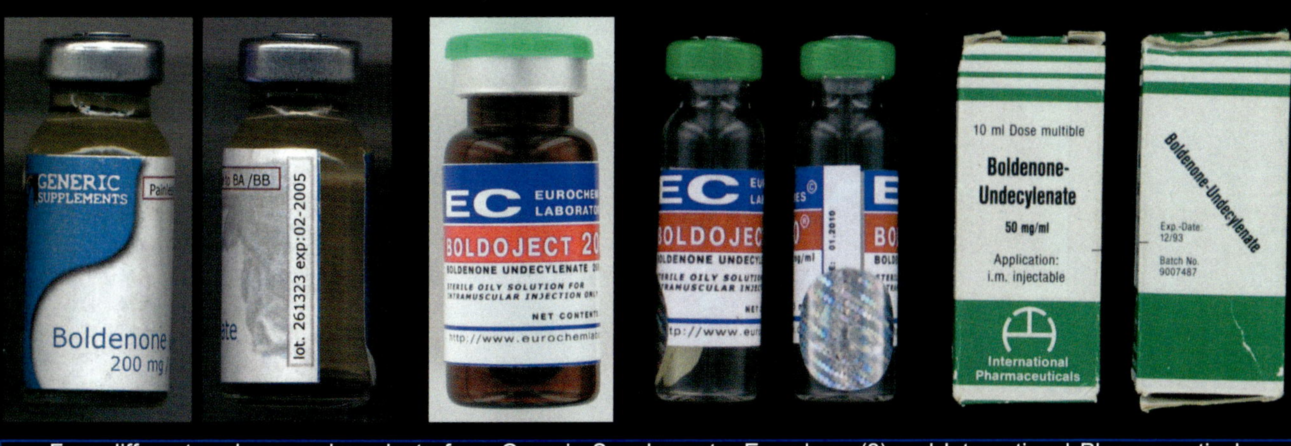

Four different underground products from Generic Supplements, Eurochem (2) and International Pharmaceuticals

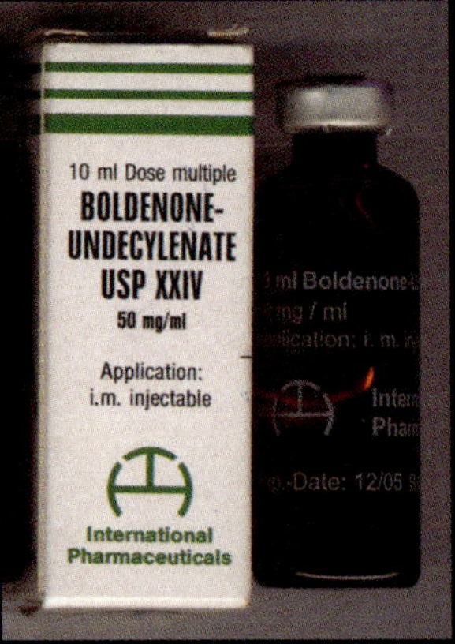

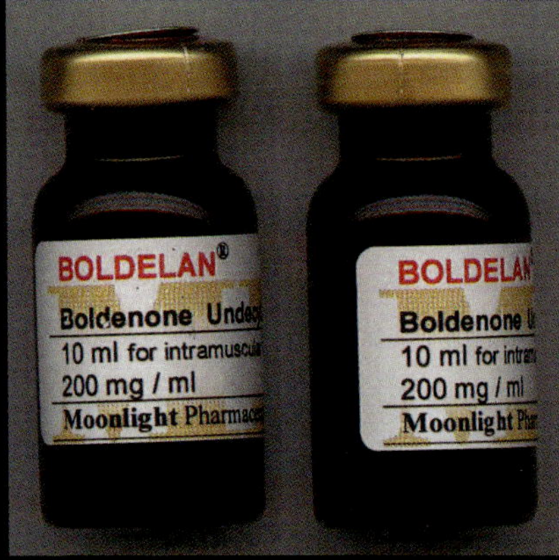

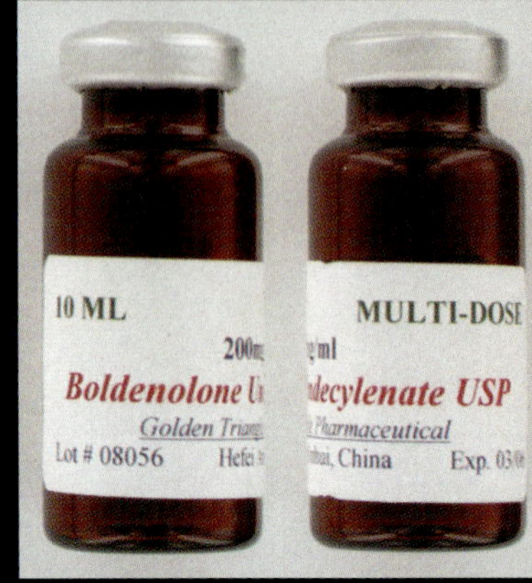

Newer IP box/vial

UG Moonlight product

UG Golden Triangle

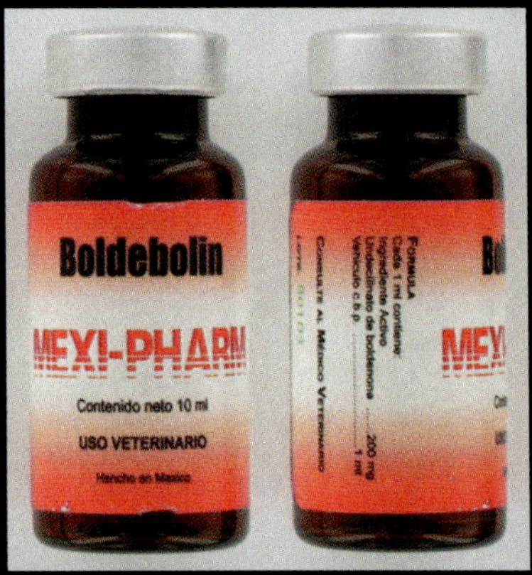

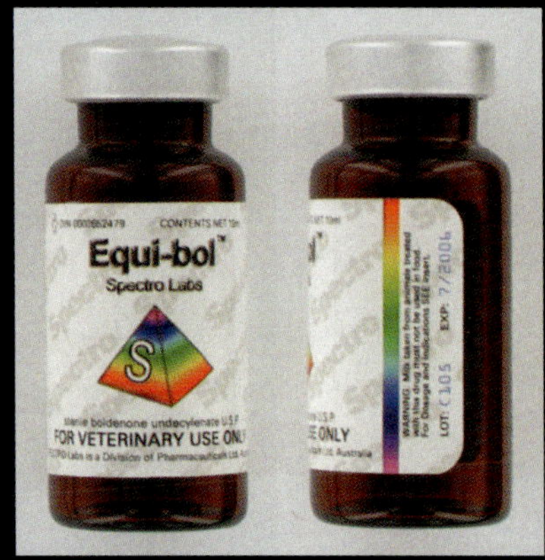

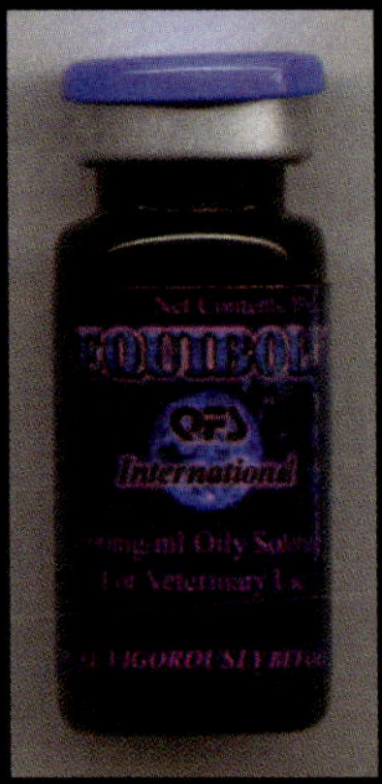

Underground products from Mexi-pharm, Spectro and QFS

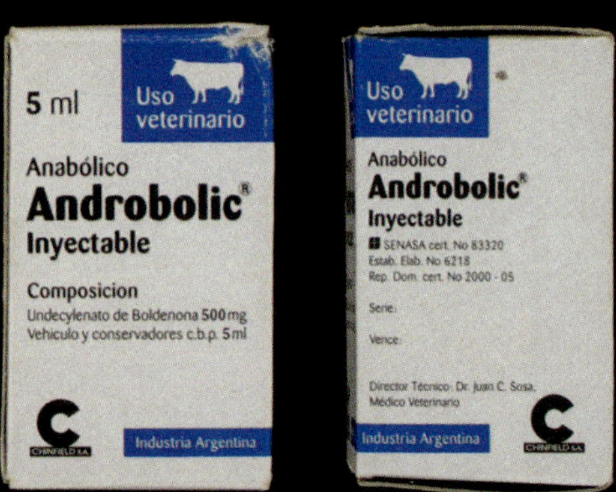

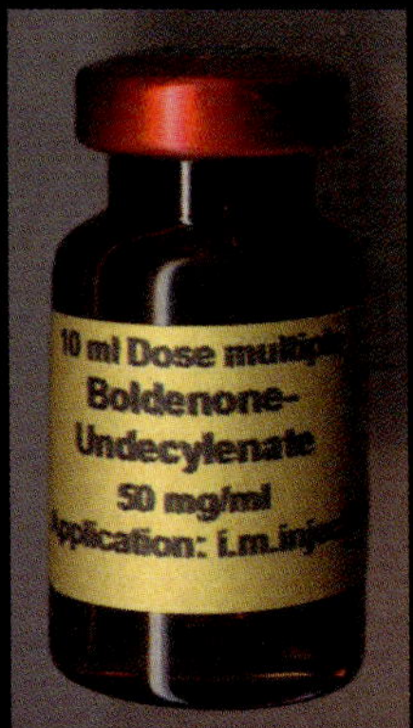

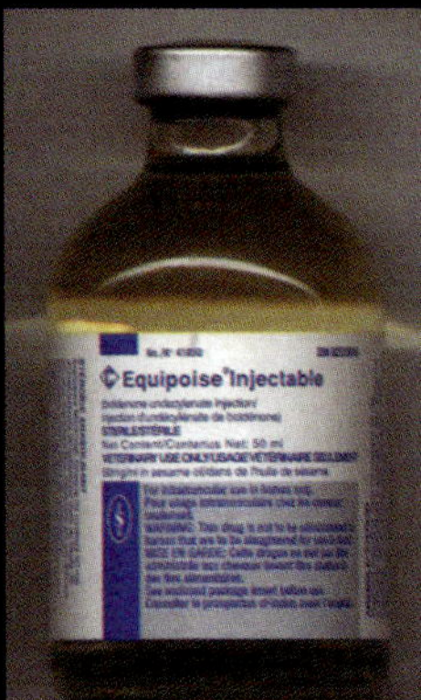

Bogus "Androbolic" from Argentina

Fake generic

Counterfeit Solvay EQ

Halotestin

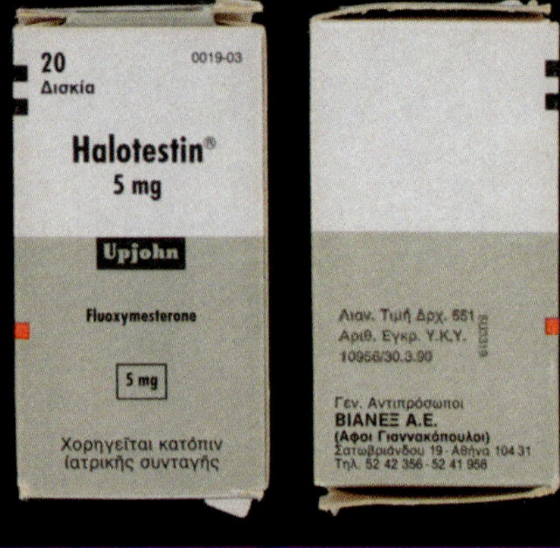

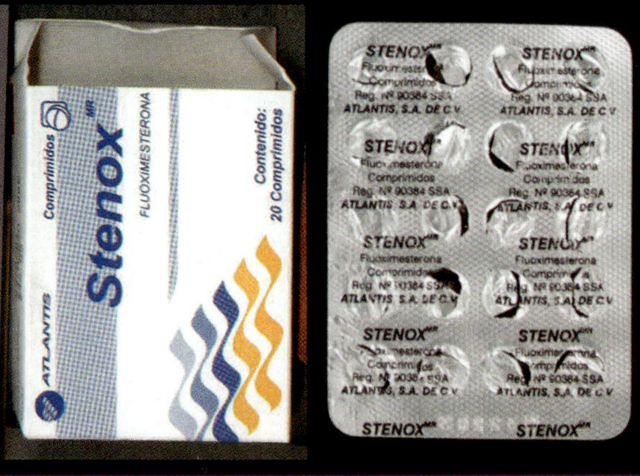

Greek Halotestin

Mexican Stenox

Laurabolin

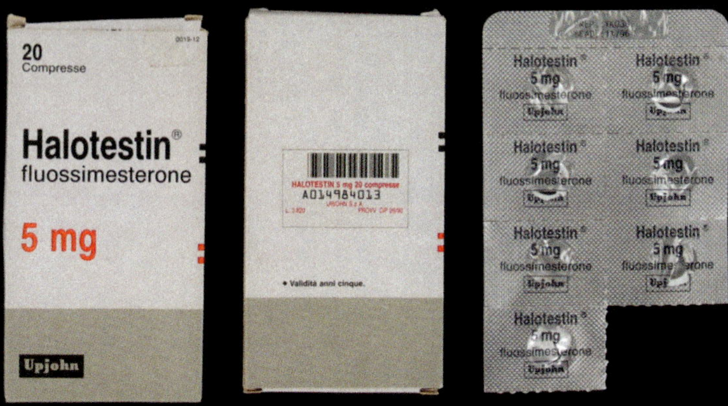

Halotestin from Italy

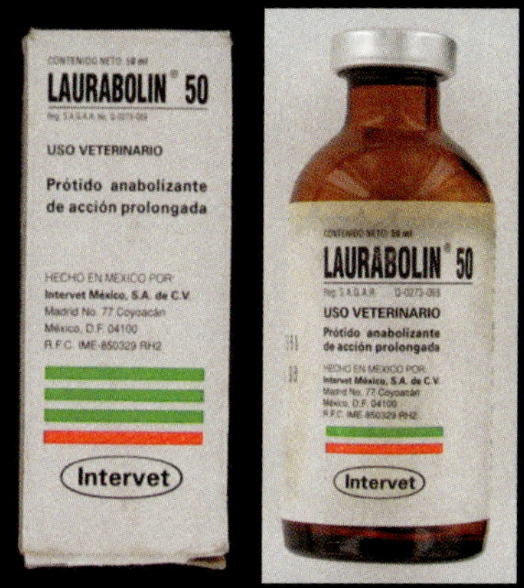

Old style Mexican Laurabolin

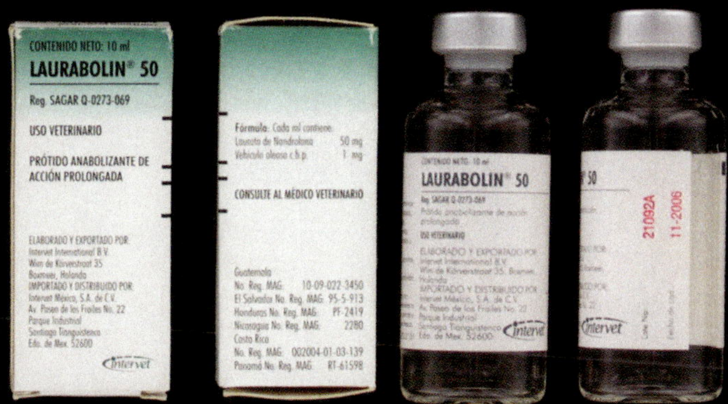

New Mexican Laurabolin from Intervet

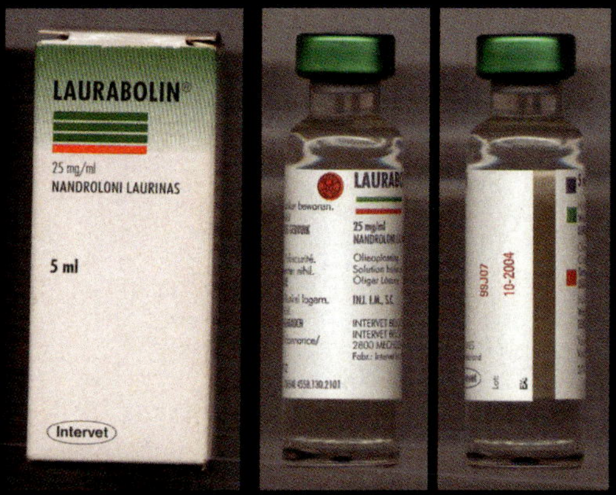

Laurabolin from Belgium (old style)

Libriol

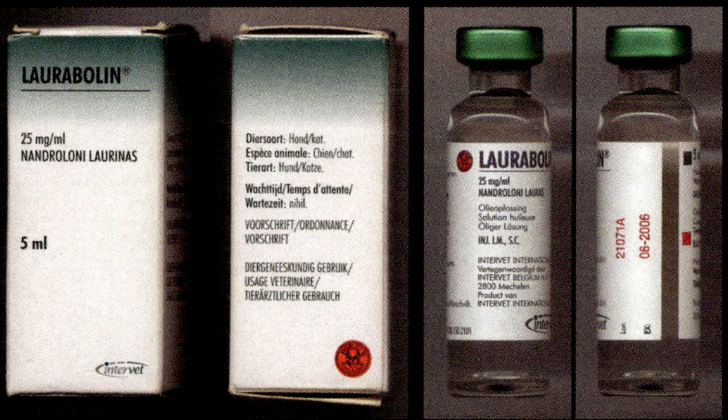

New look to Intervet Laurabolin (Belgium)

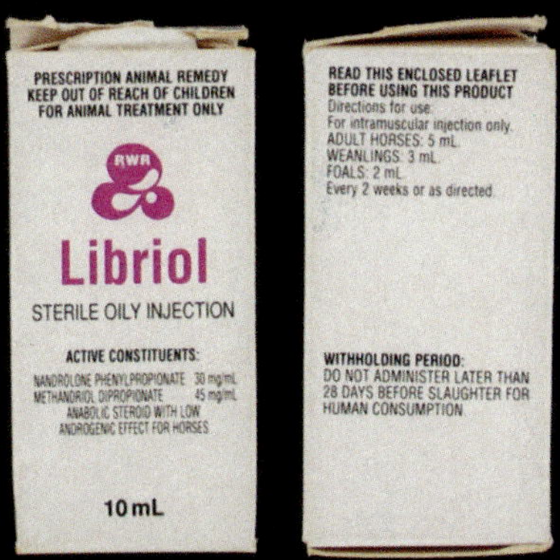

Libriol from RWR Australia

Masteron

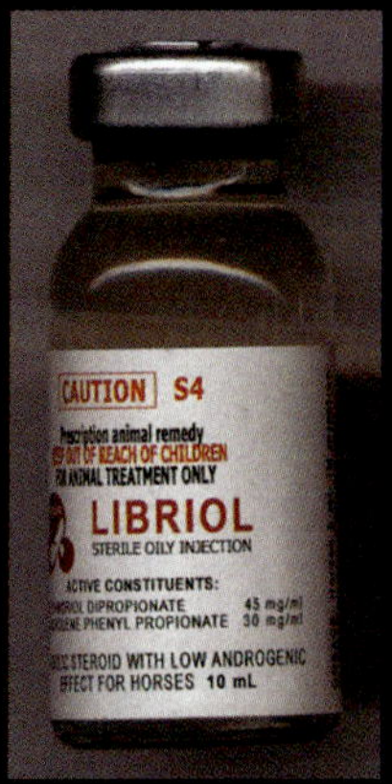

Counterfeit vial

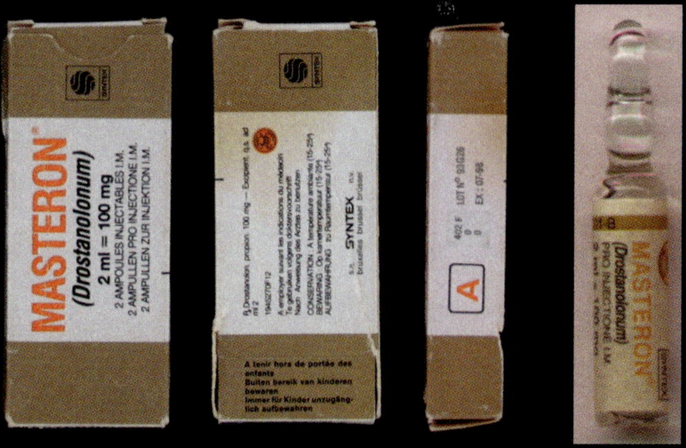

Masteron from Syntex Belgium (NLM)

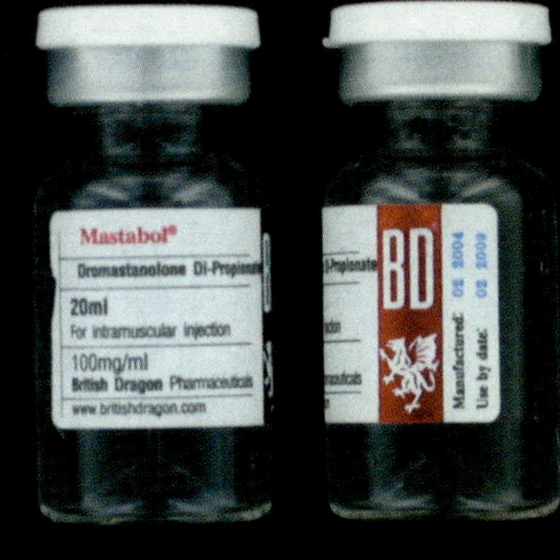

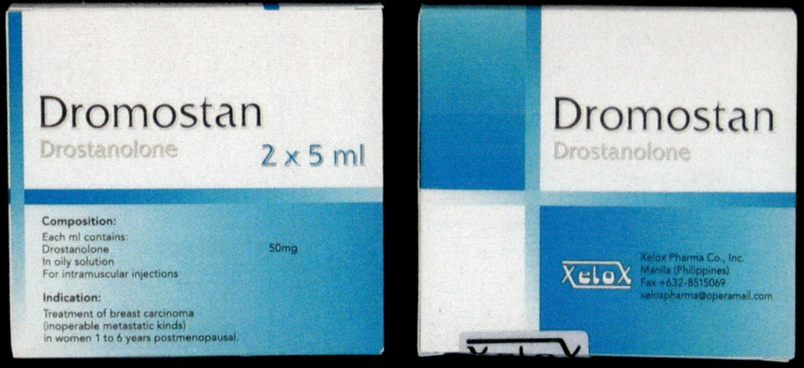

British Dragon Mastabol (Thailand) Dromostan (drostanolone base) from Xelox

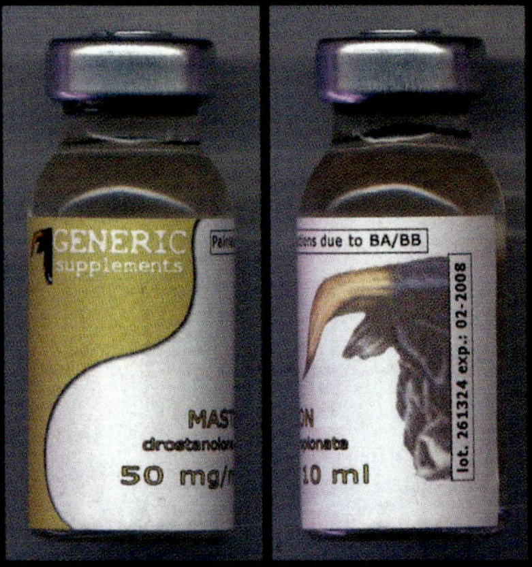

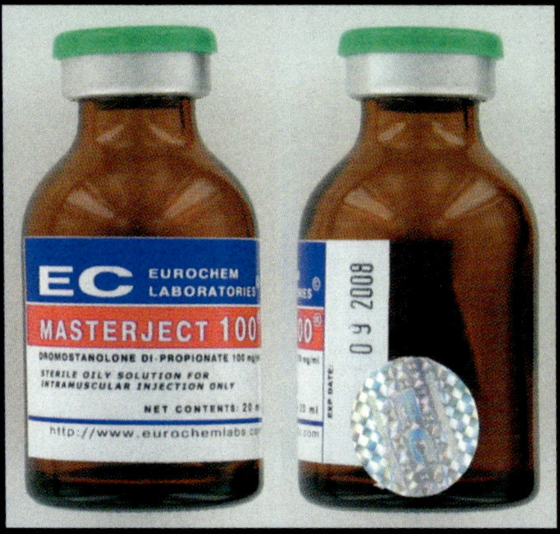

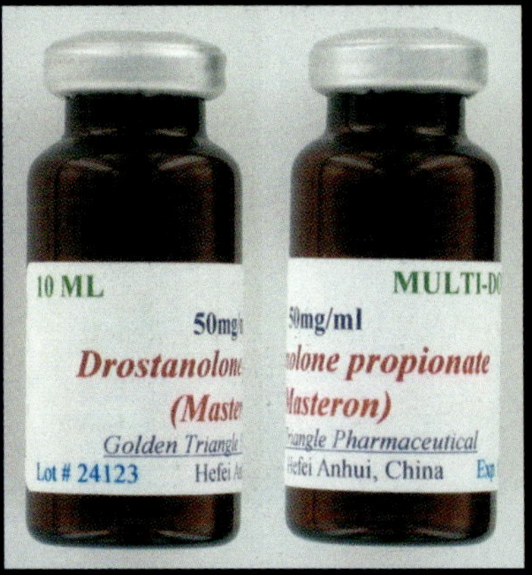

Generic Supplements (UG) Eurochem (UG product) UG vial from Golden Triangle

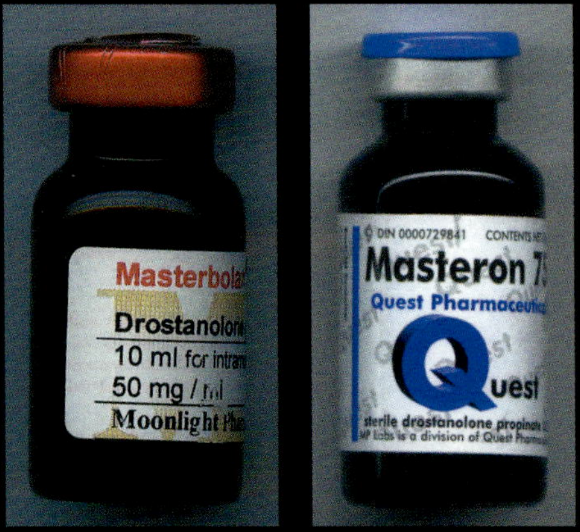

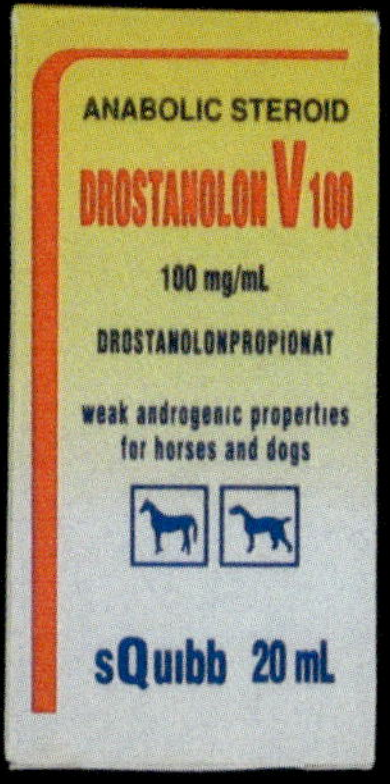

Methandriol

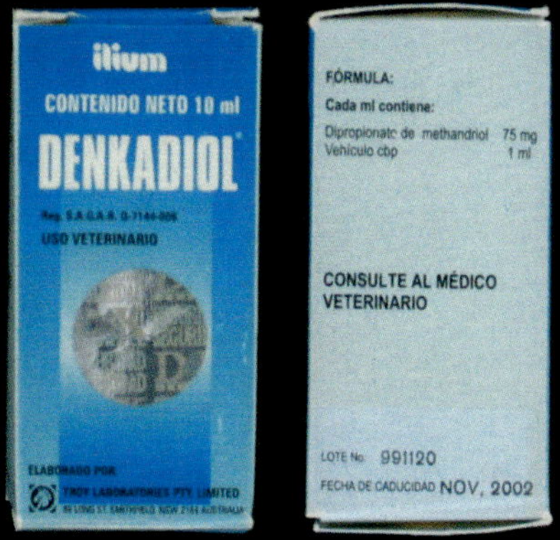

Two more underground products Bogus Canadian Squibb Denkadiol from Denkall Mexico

Methyltestosterone

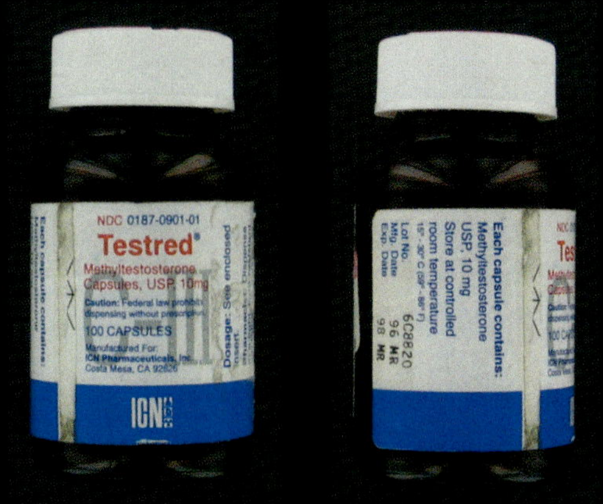

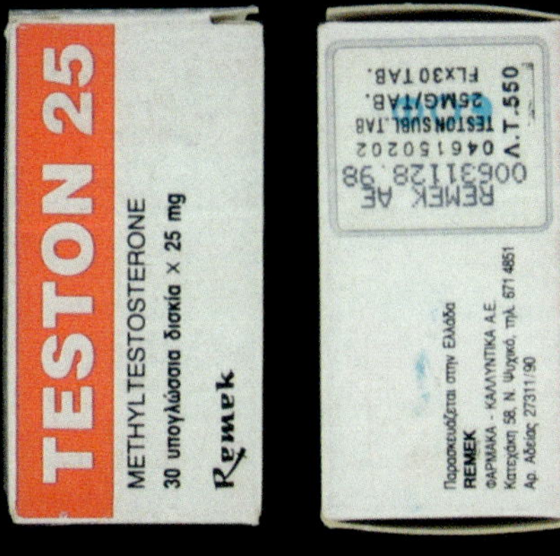

U.S. Testred bottle Teston 25 from Remek Greece

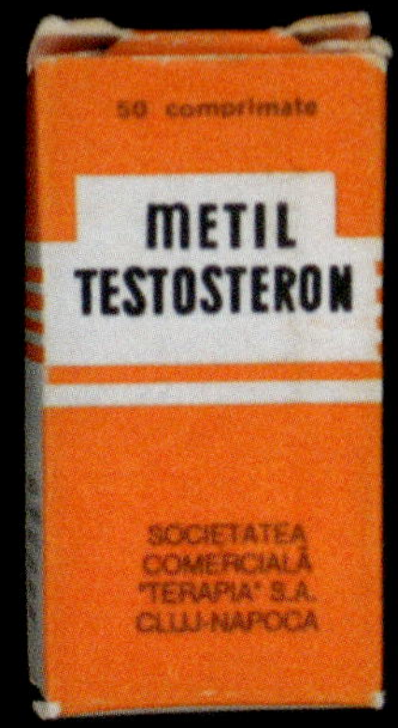

Generic from Rumania

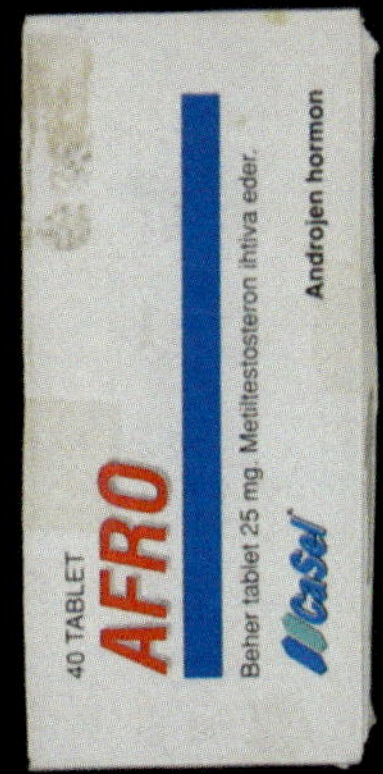

Afro (Turkey)

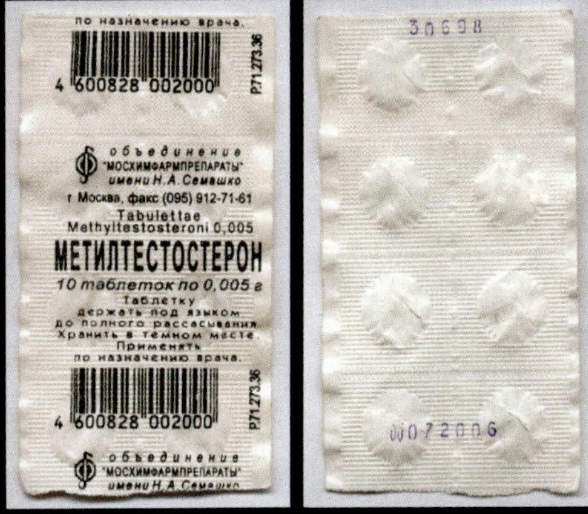

Russian generic

Nilevar

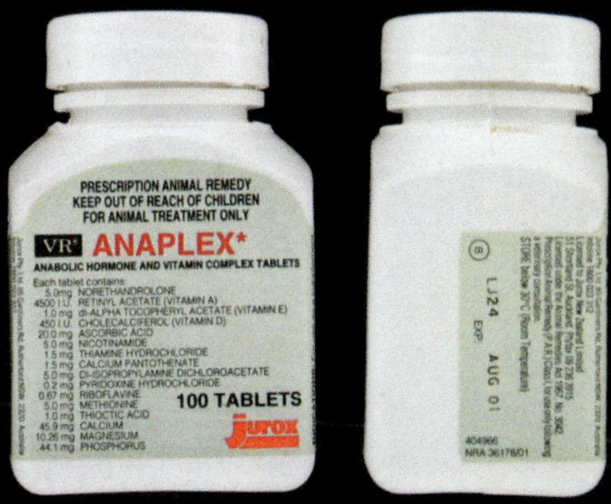

Anaplex from Jurox Australia

Omnadren

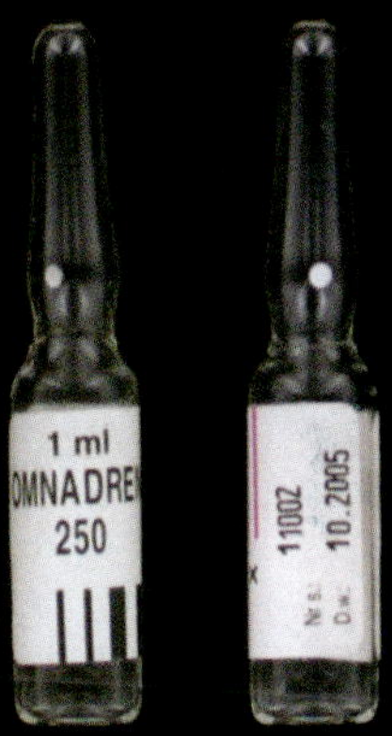

Omnadren Ampules

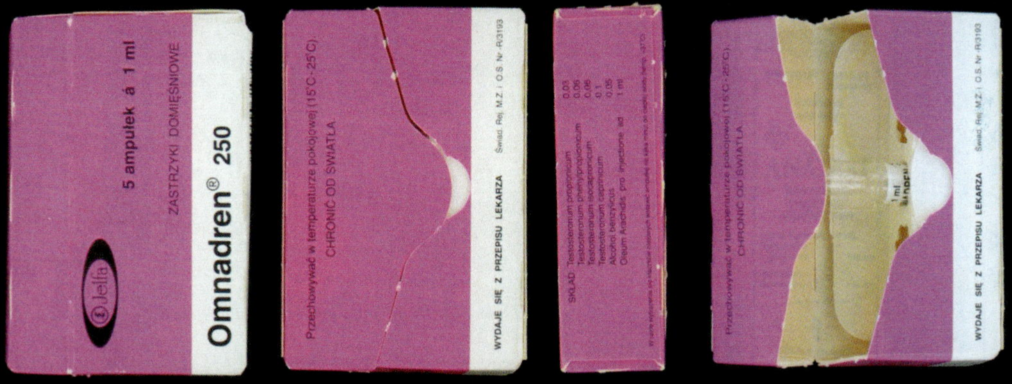

Current style Omnadren box and ampule

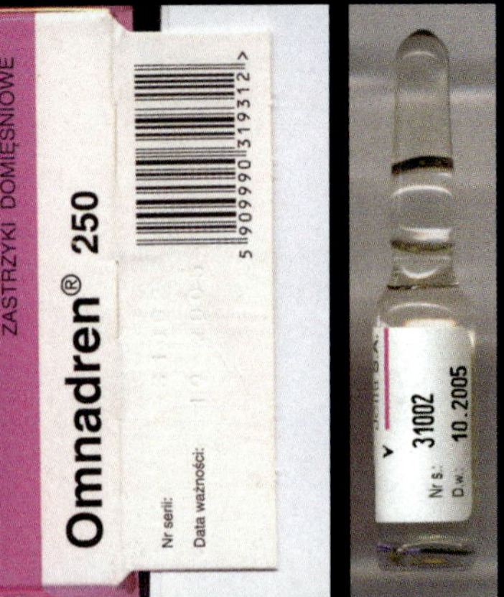

Real barcode and Ampule

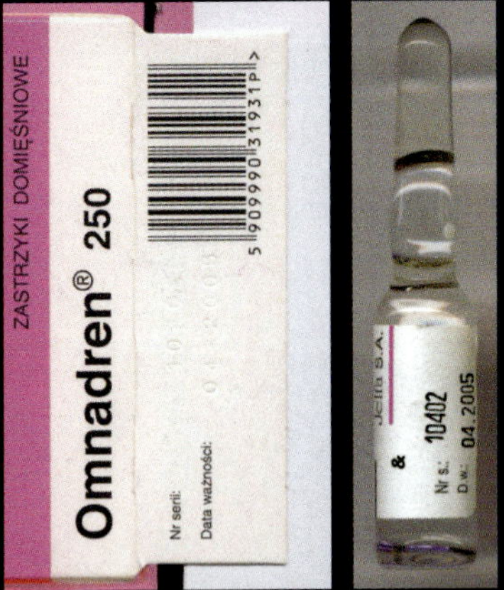

Counterfeit barcode and Ampule

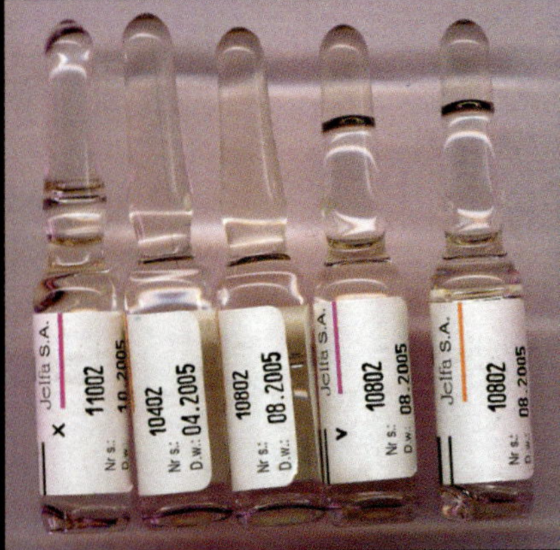

Various real ampules

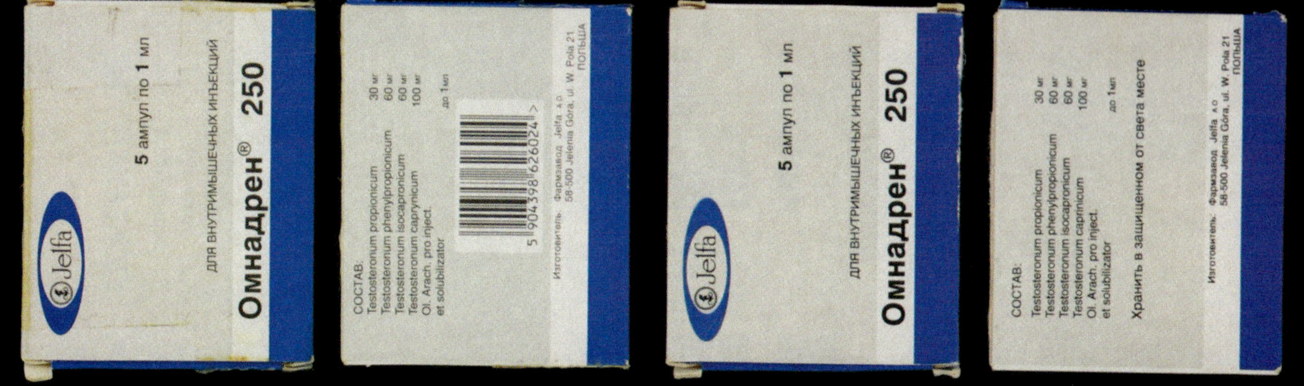

Two different out-of-date Omnadren boxes, made for Export to Russia

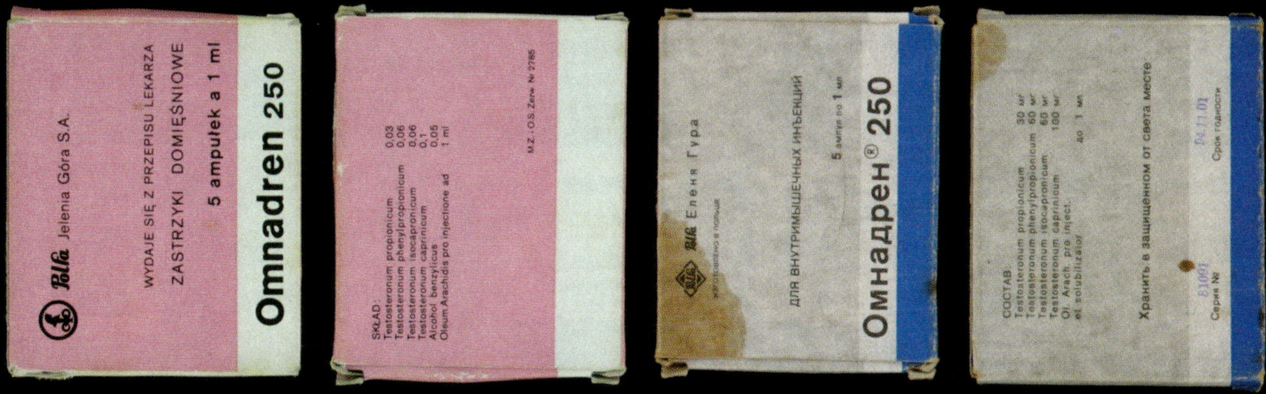

Old domestic (left) and export (right) products made under the State-owned Polfa company name

Orabolin

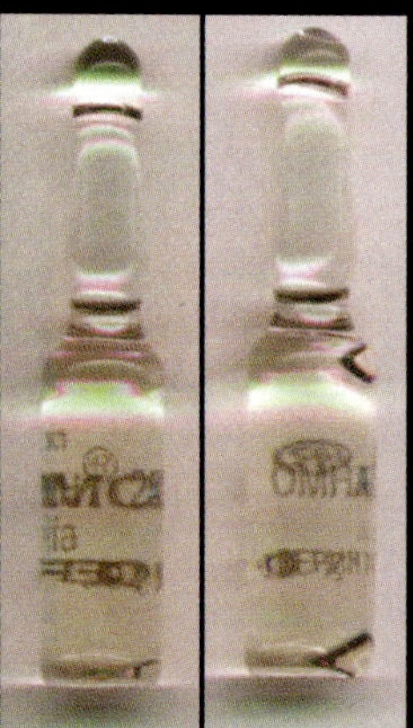

Older printed ampule

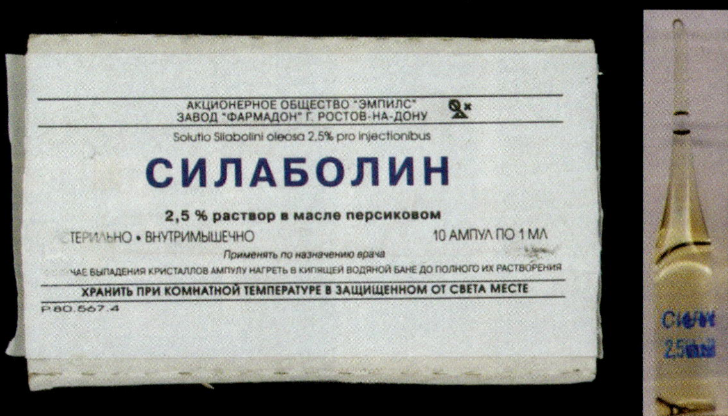

Russian Silabolin box and ampule

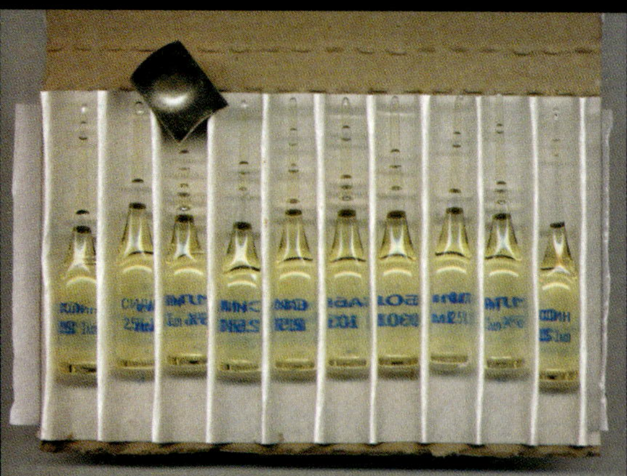

Open Silabolin box/ampules

Oral-Turinabol

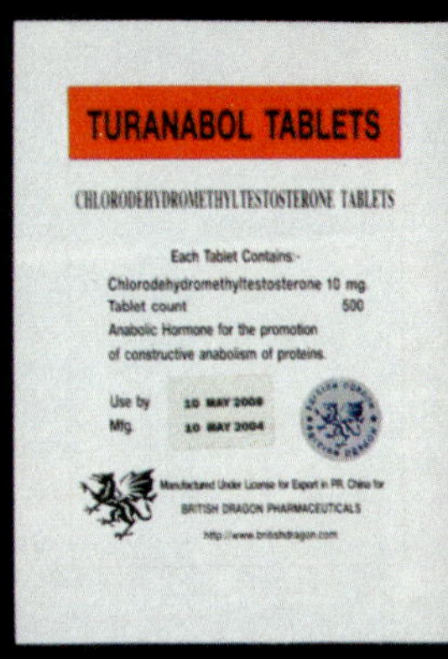

British Dragon Turanabol

Parabolan

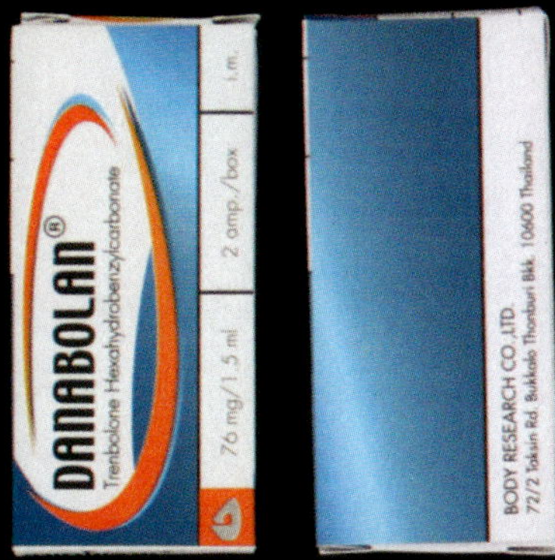

Danabolan from Thailand

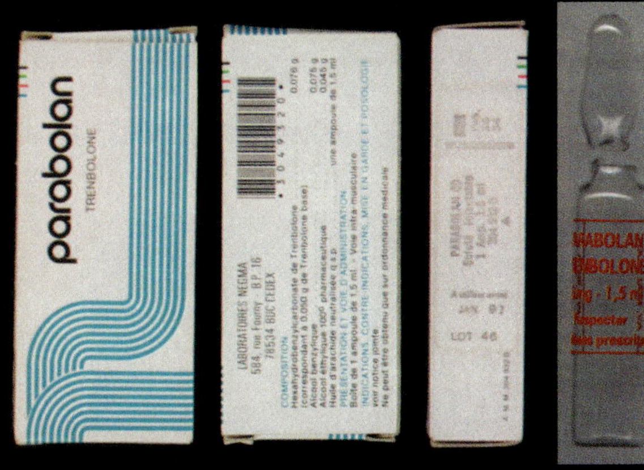

Real French Parabolan (NLM)

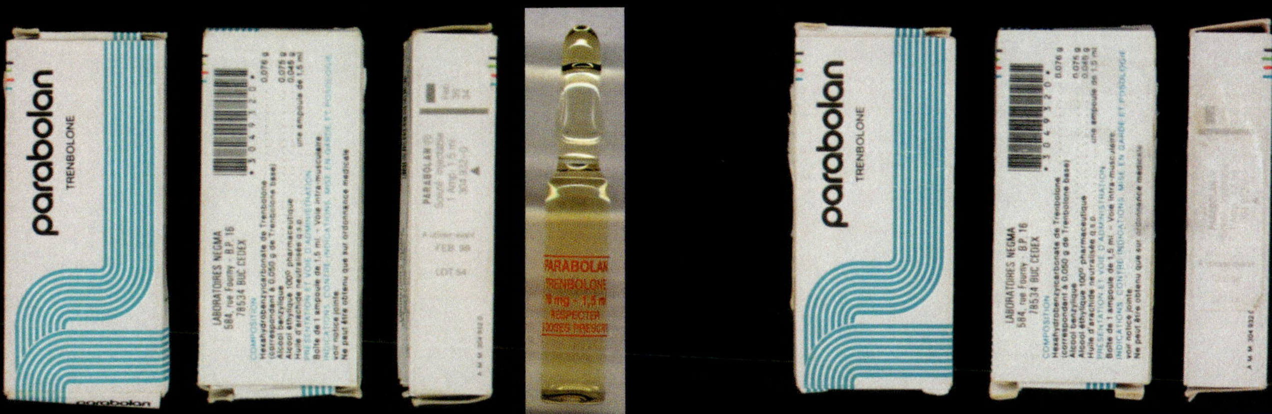

Two different counterfeits

Primobolan

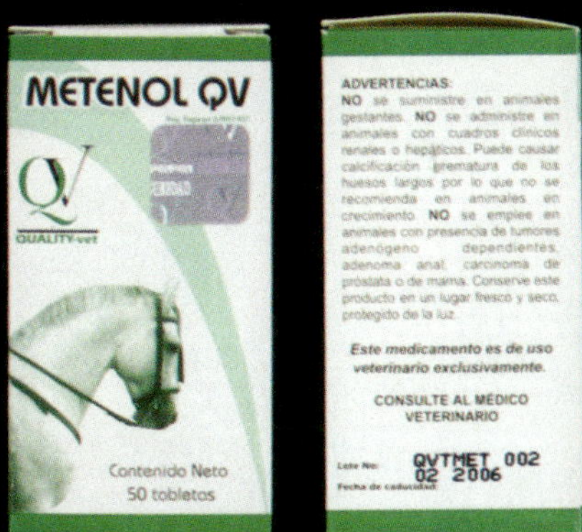

Metenol from Quality Vet (Mexico)

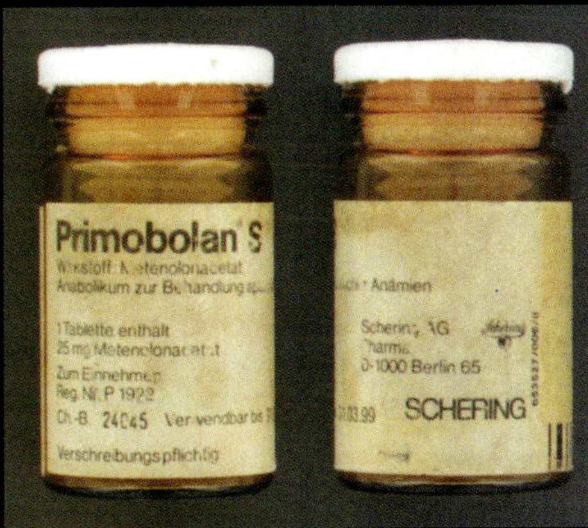

Old German bottle (NLM)

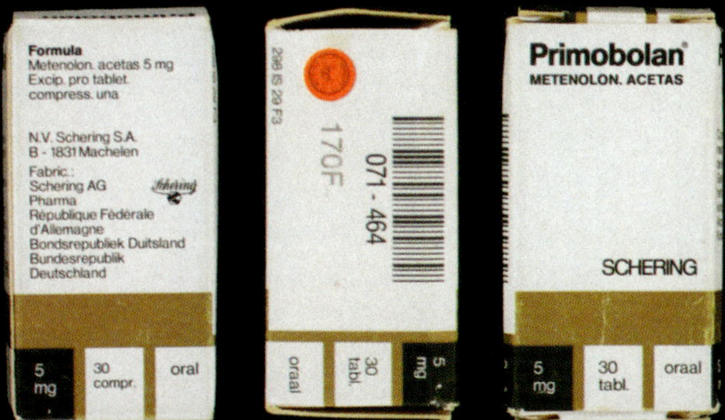

Belgian Primobolan tablets (NLM)

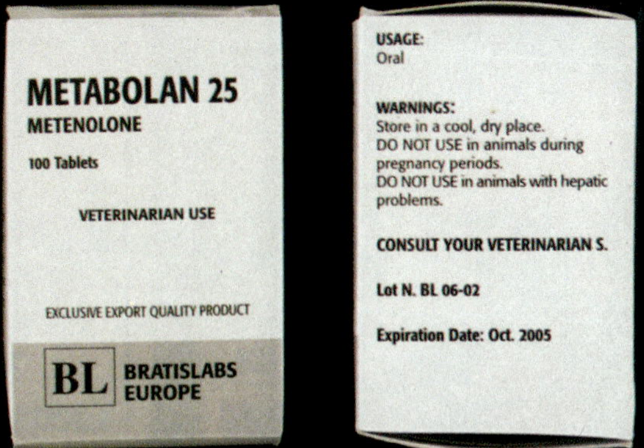

Bratis tablets from Mexico (newer packaging)

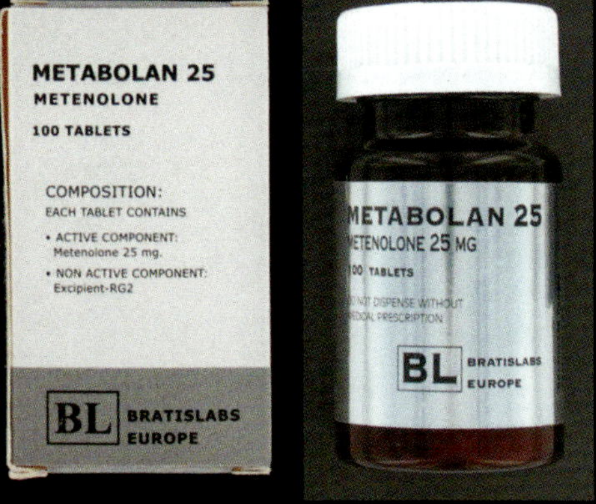

Old Bratis packaging (Mexico)

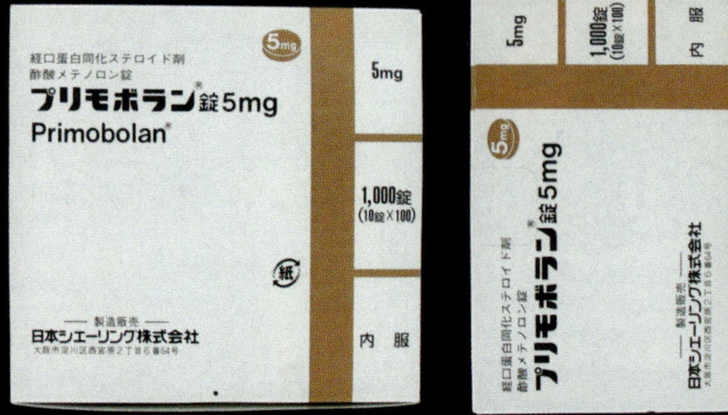

Primobolan from Japan (1000 tablet box)

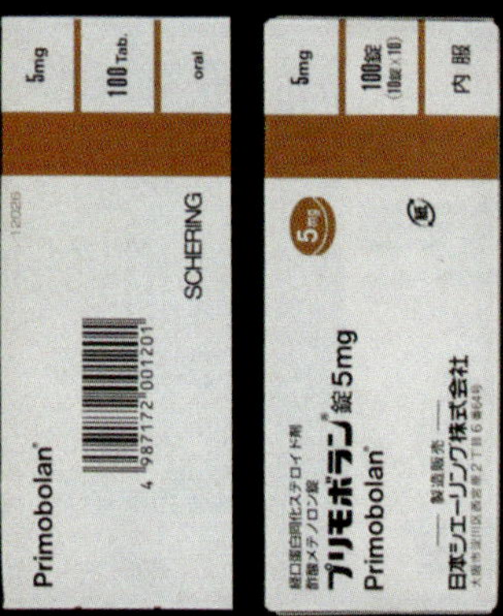

100 tablet box from Japan

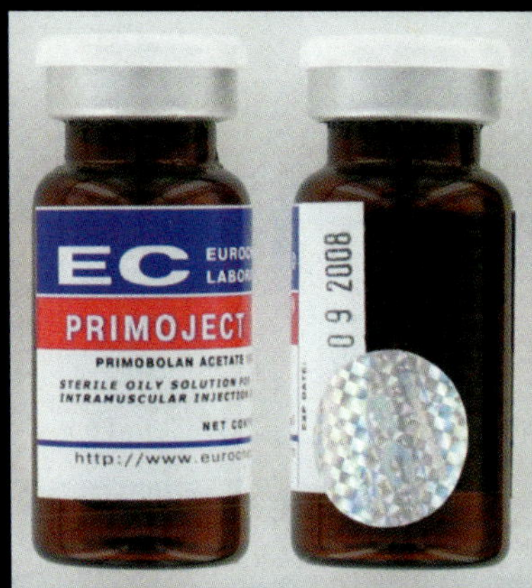

Underground Eurochem vial

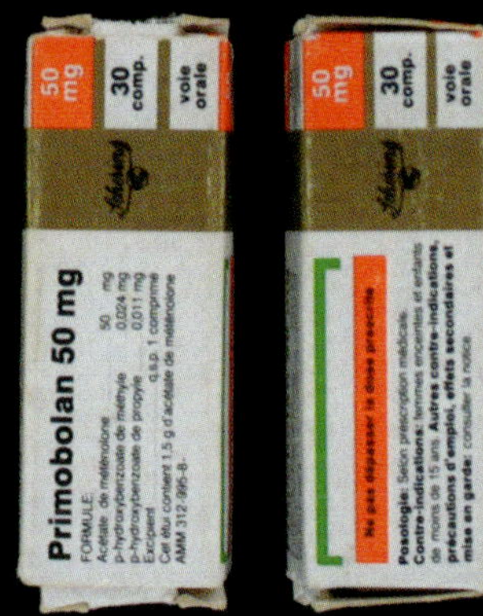

Counterfeit French tablets

Primobolan Depot

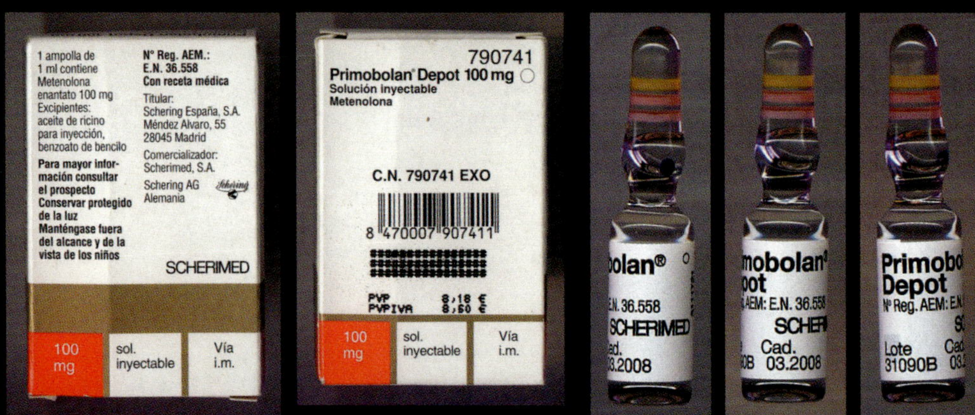

New Spanish "Scherimed" injectable box and ampules

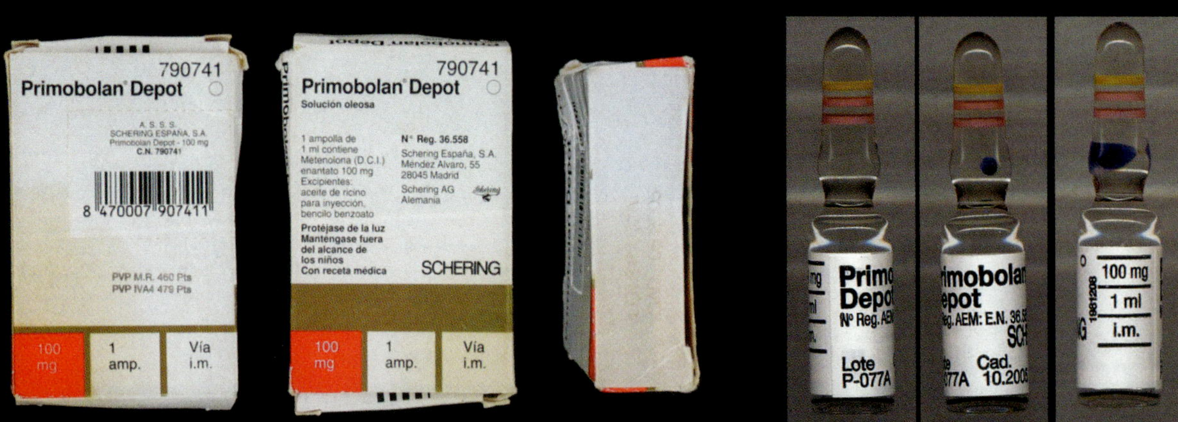

Older style packaging from Spain - box and ampules

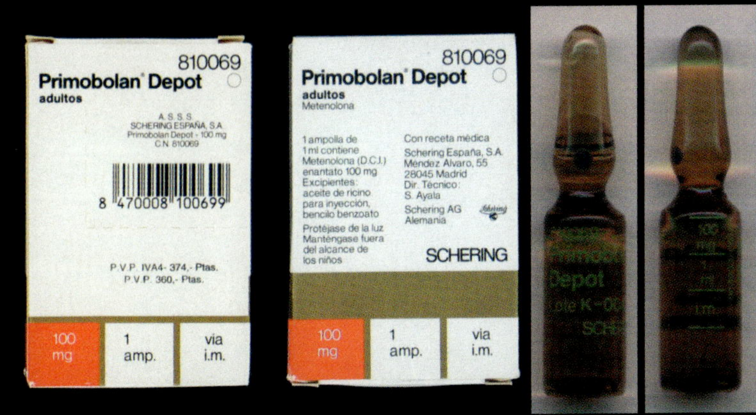

Another old version of Spanish Primobolan

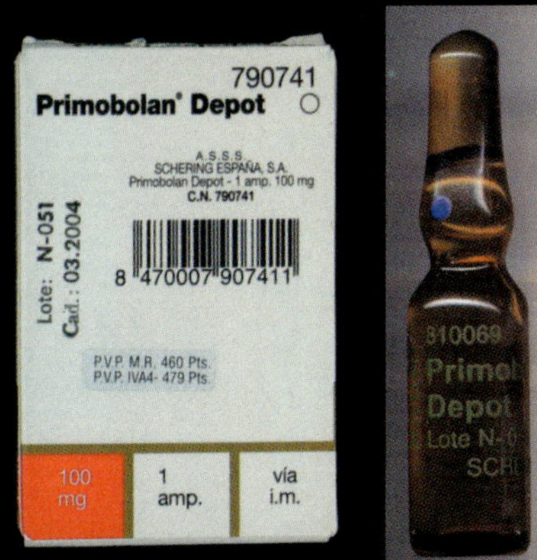

Counterfeit #1

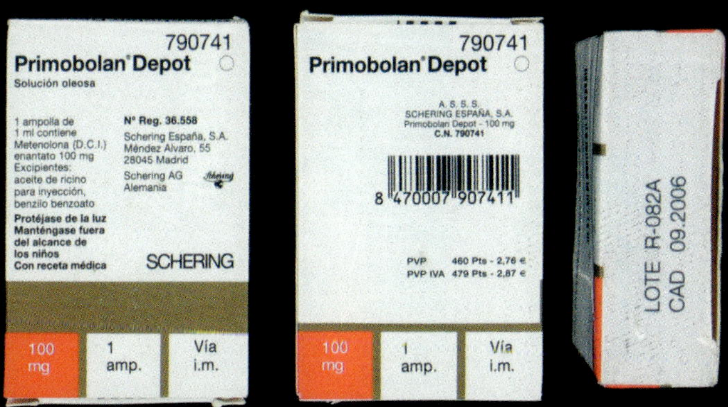

Counterfeit #2

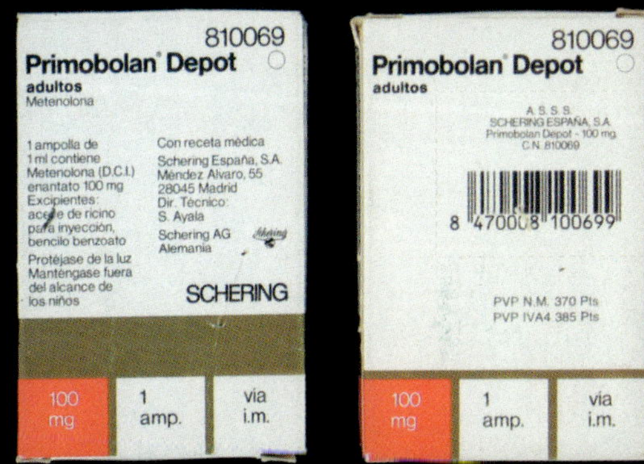

Counterfeit #3

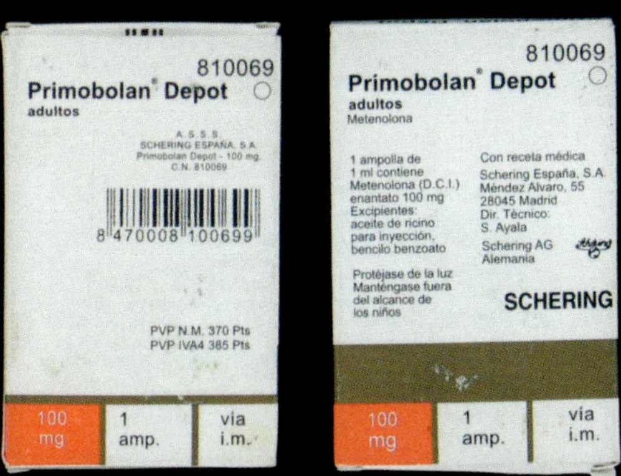

Counterfeit #4

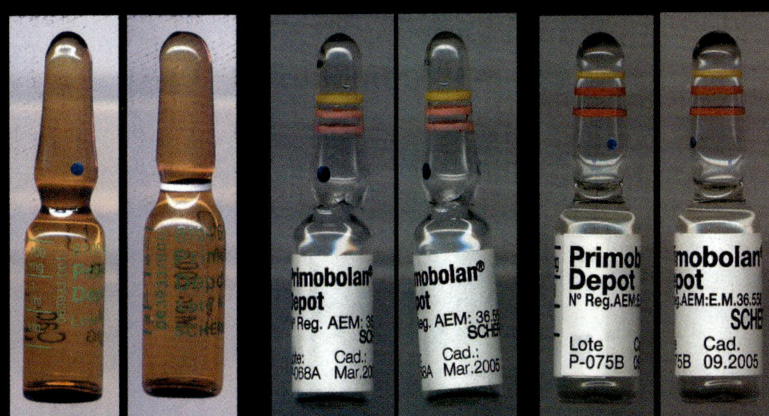

Three different countereit Spanish ampules

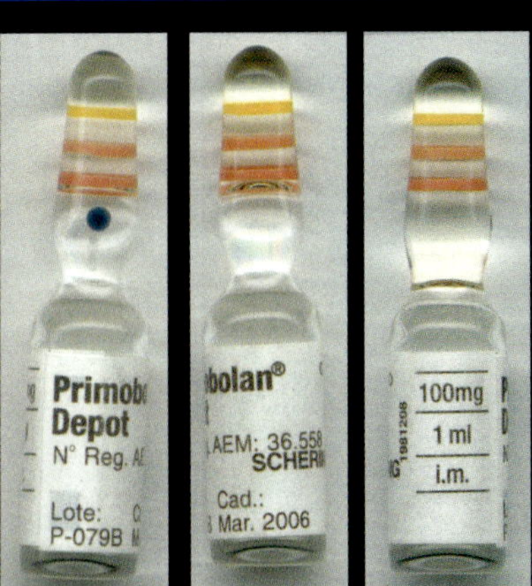

Counterfeit #8

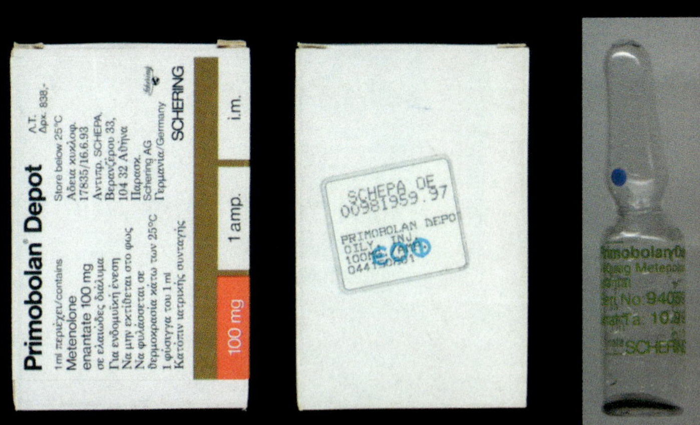

Greek Primobolan Depot (NLM)

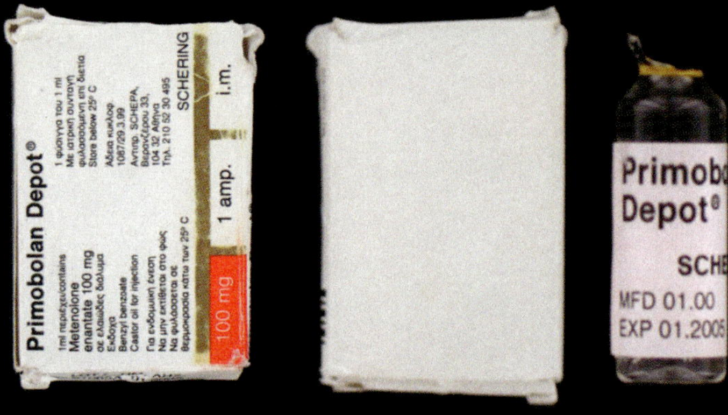

Counterfeit Greek Primobolan

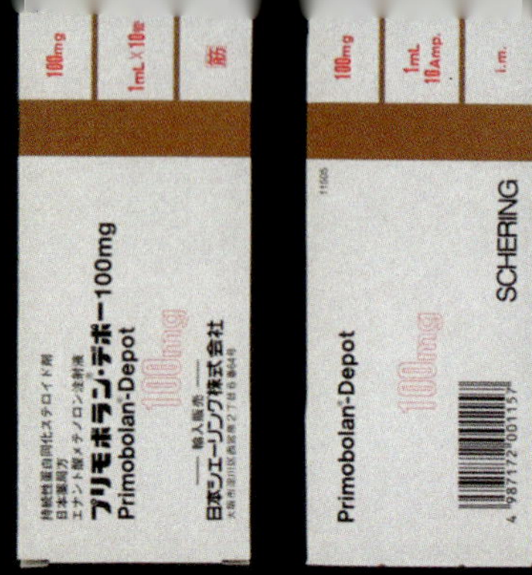

Primobolan from Japan

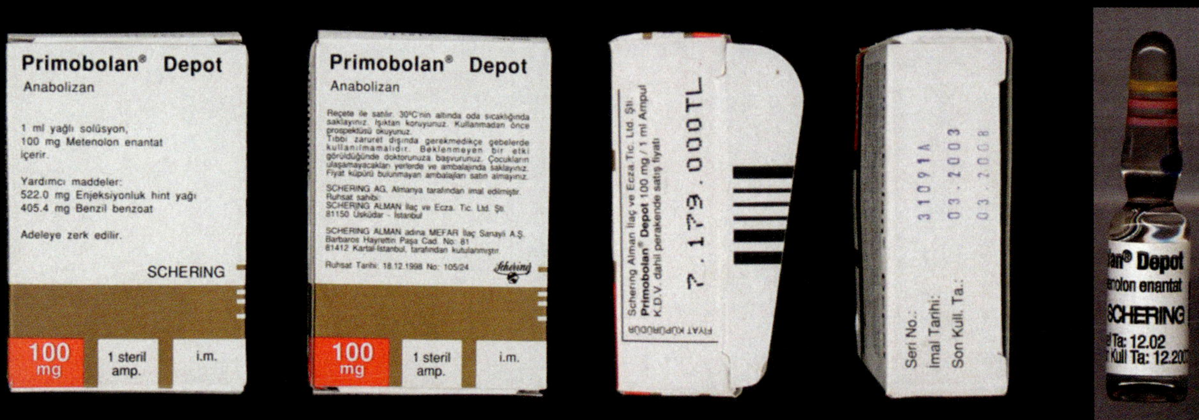

Primobolan from Turkey

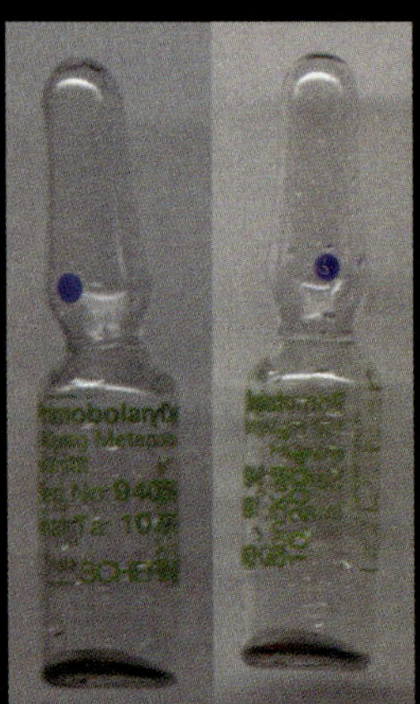

Old amp from Turkey

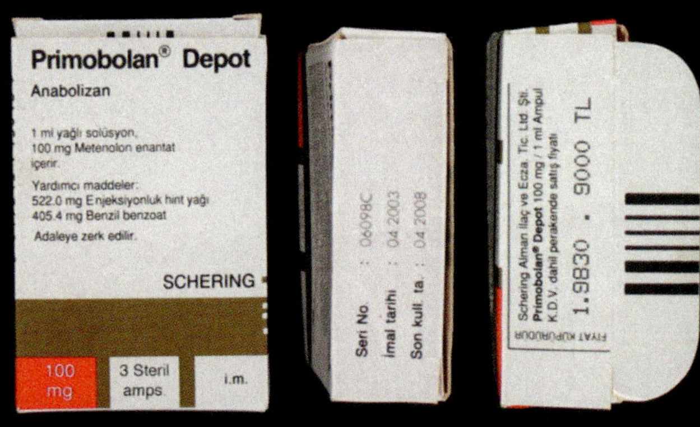

Counterfeit Primobolan from Turkey #1

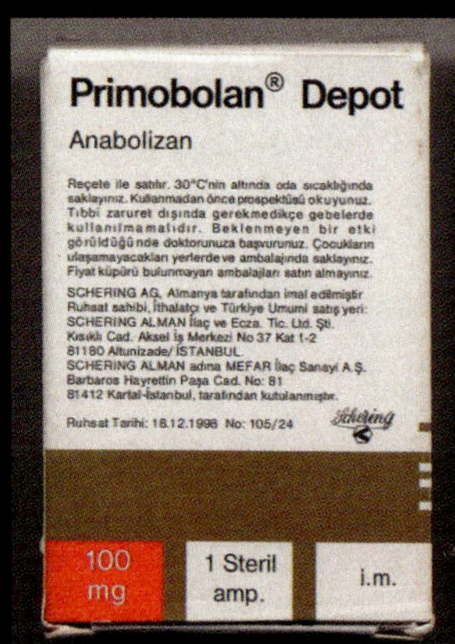

Counterfeit #2

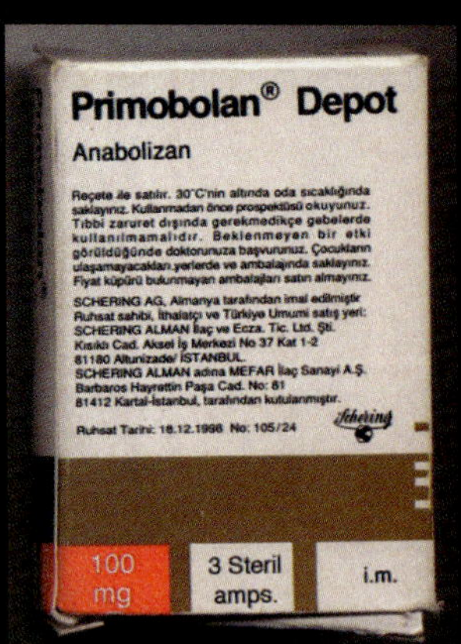

Counterfeit #3

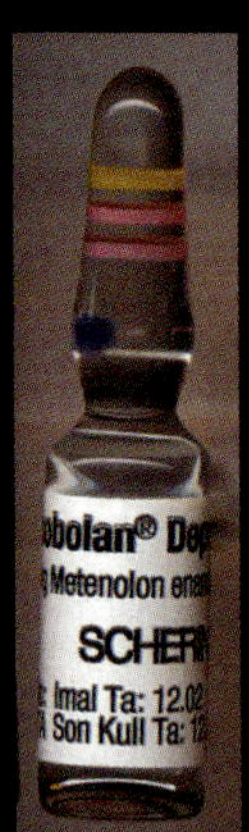

#4

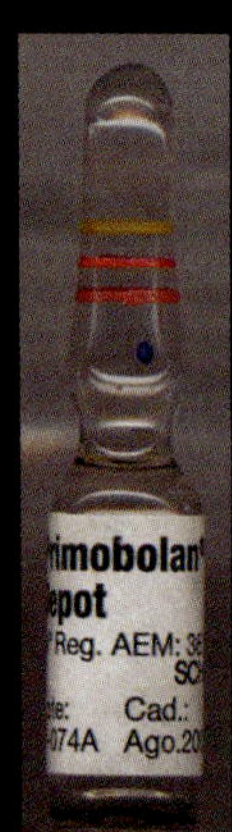

#5

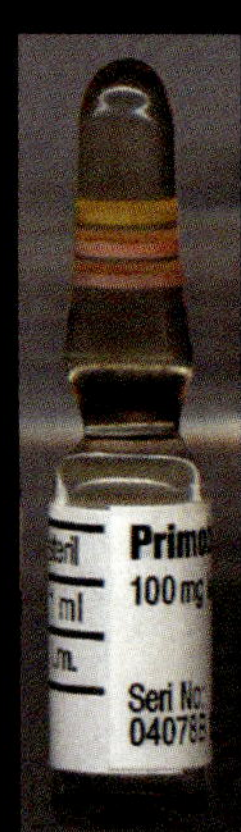

#6

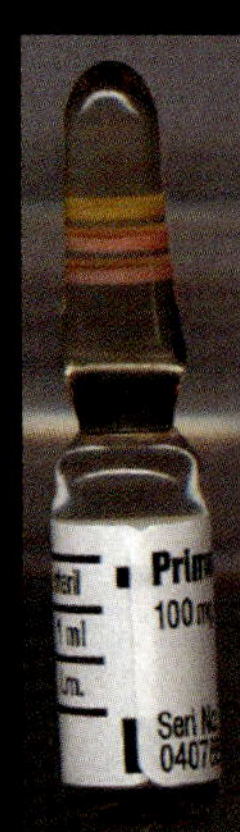

#7

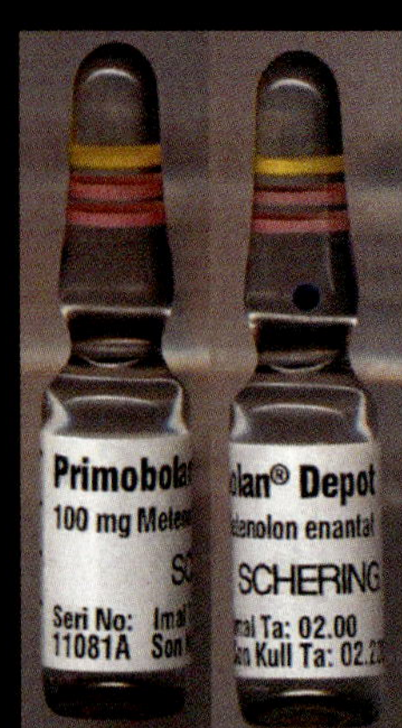

#8

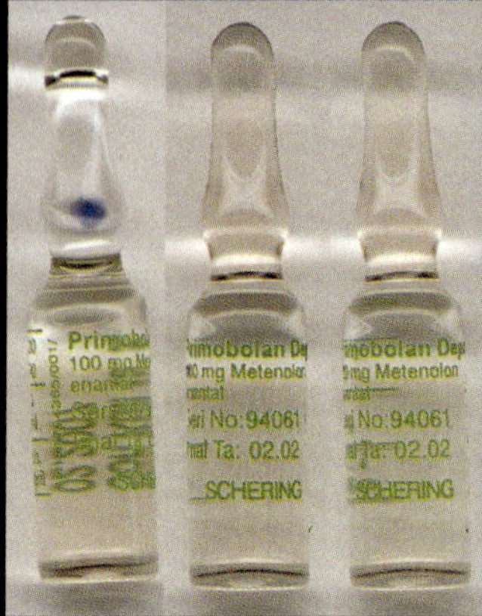

Turkish fake #9

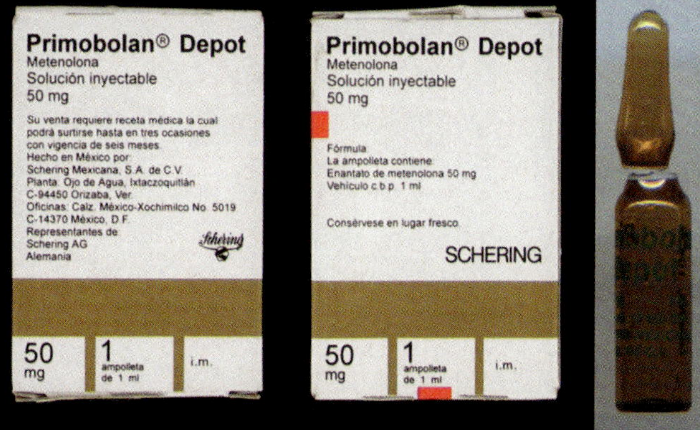

Primobolan Depot from Mexico

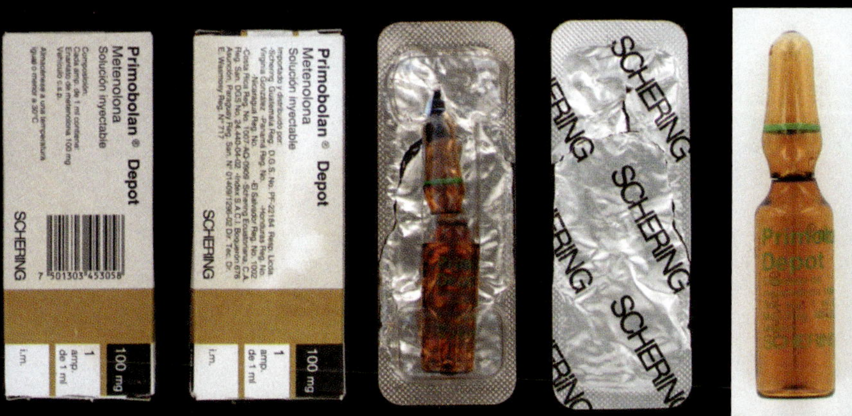

Primobolan Depot from Colombia

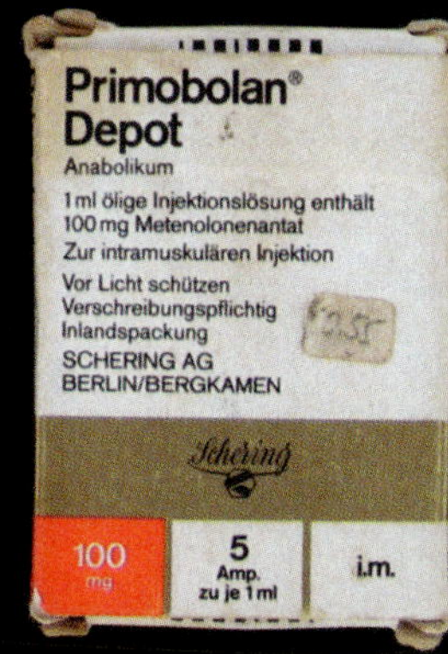

Old German Box (NLM)

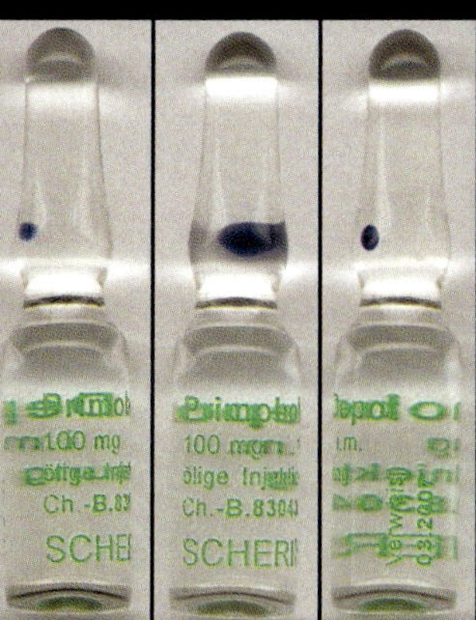

Counterfeit German Amps

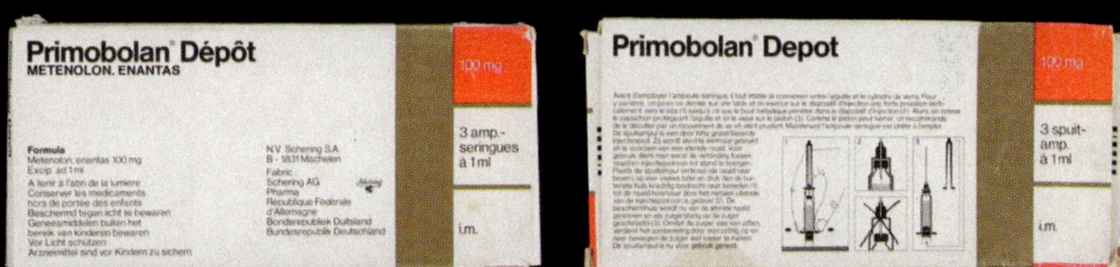

Preloaded syringe from Belgium

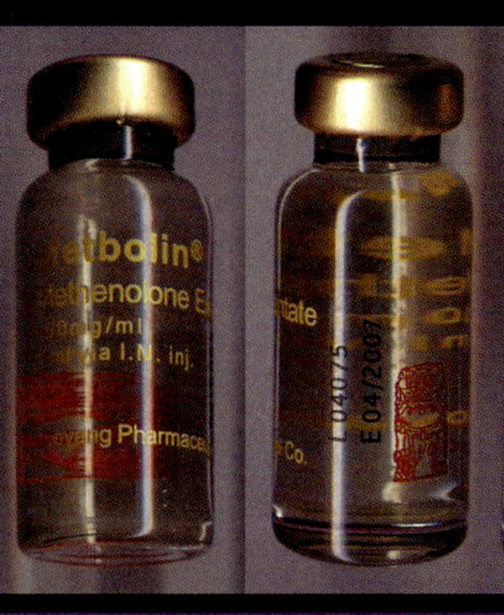

Metbolin from LP China

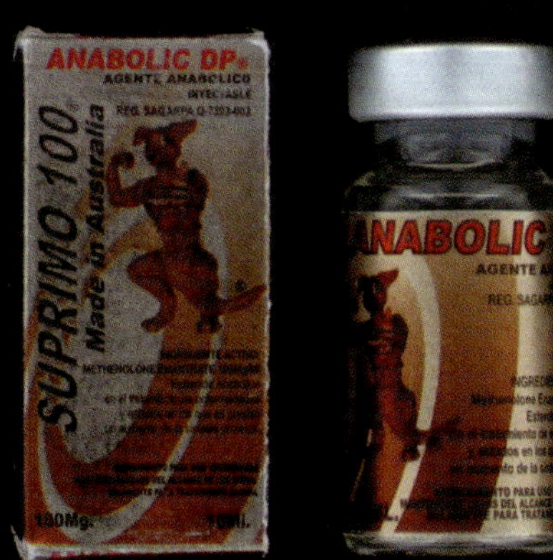

SYD Group Primo (Mexico)

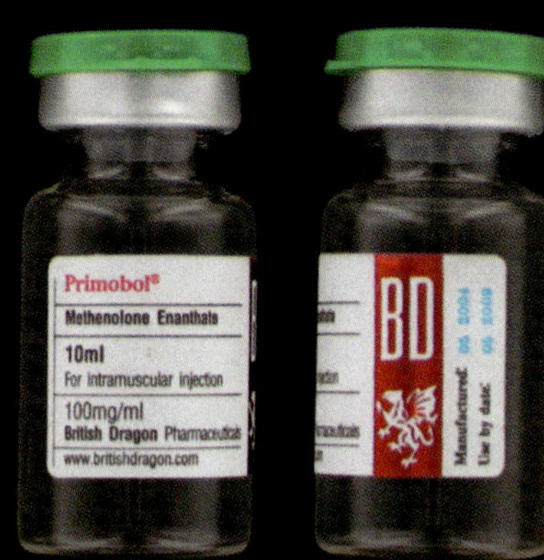

Primobol from British Dragon (Thailand)

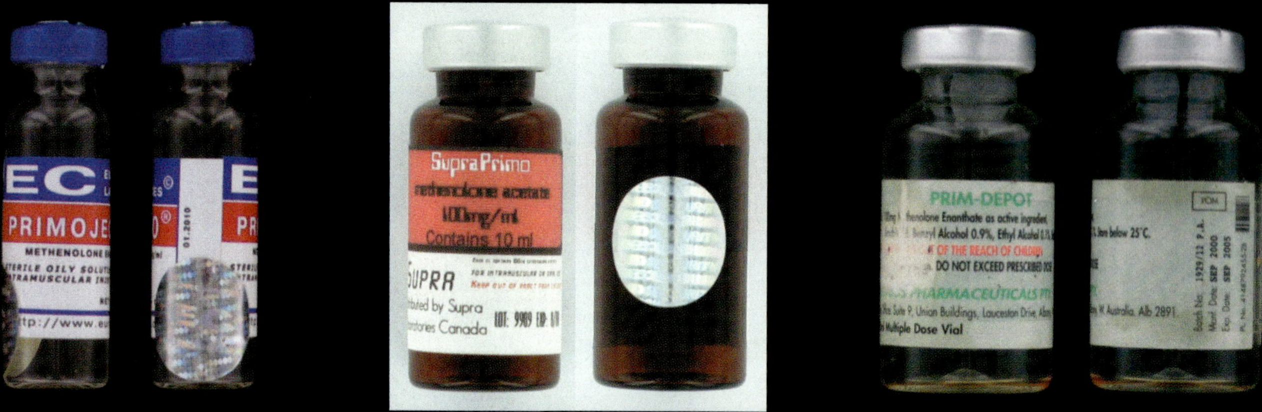

Underground products from Eurochem, Supra, and Pegasus

Proviron

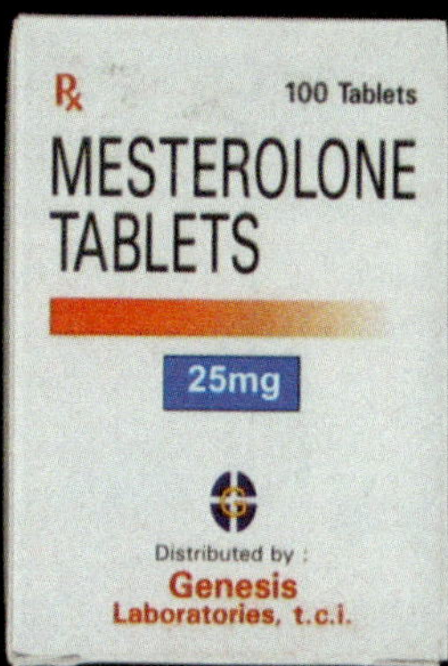

Generic from Singapore

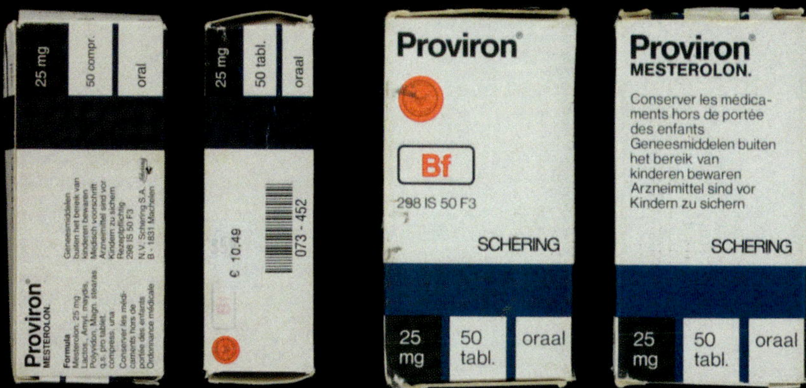

Proviron from Belgium - new (left) and old boxes

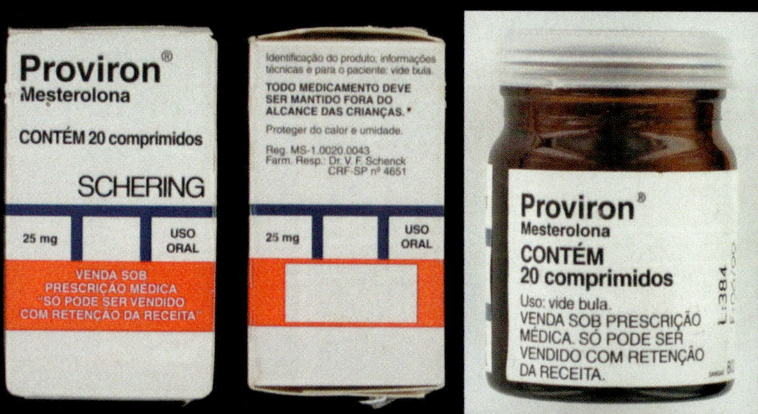

Proviron from Brazil

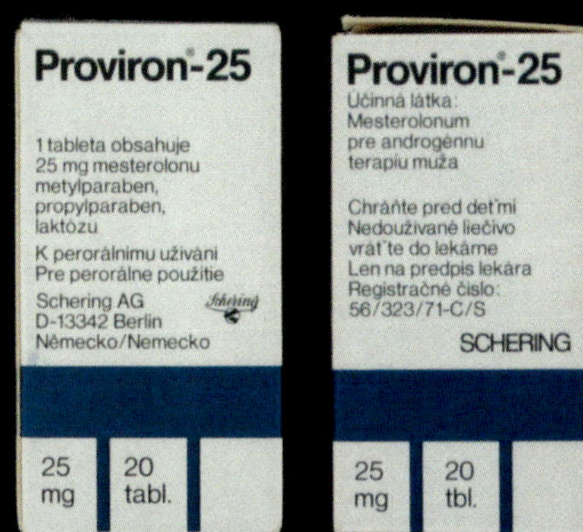

Box from Czech Republic

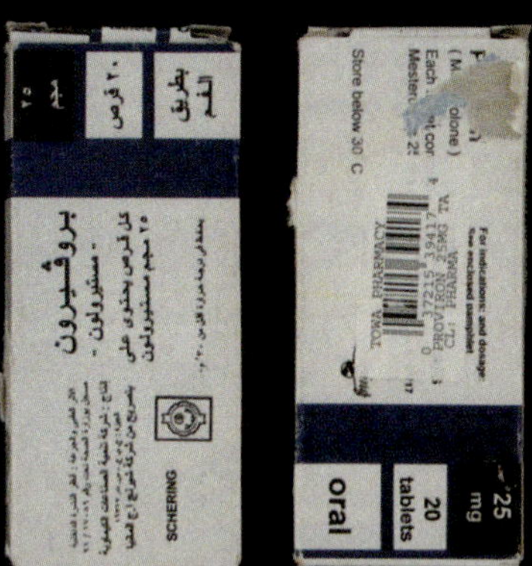

Proviron from Egypt

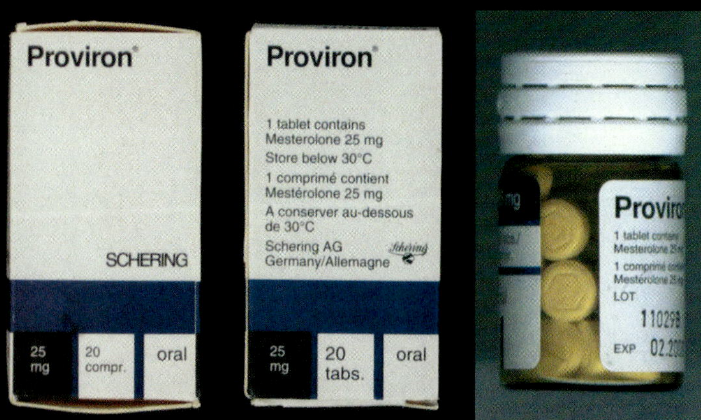

Older box and bottle from Egypt

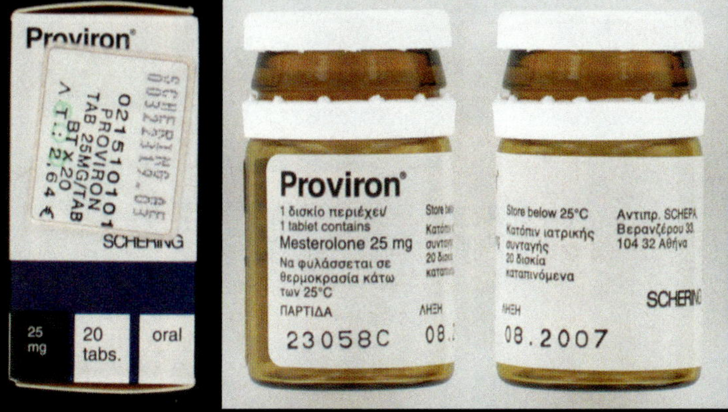

New style box and bottle from Greece

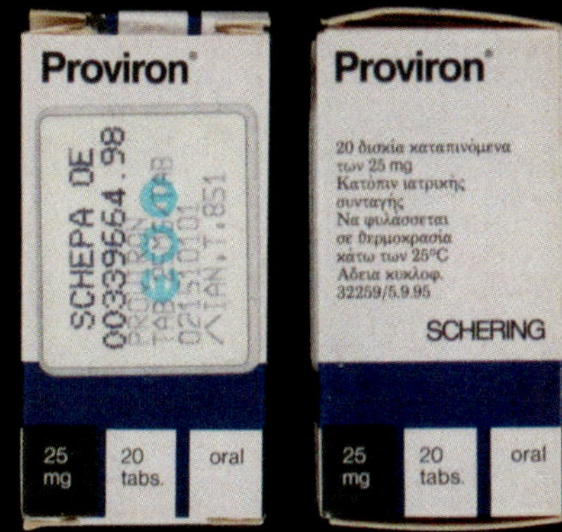

Older Greek box

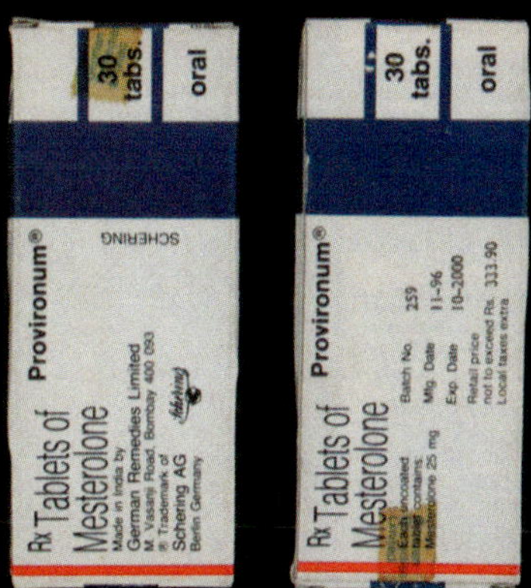

Provironum from India

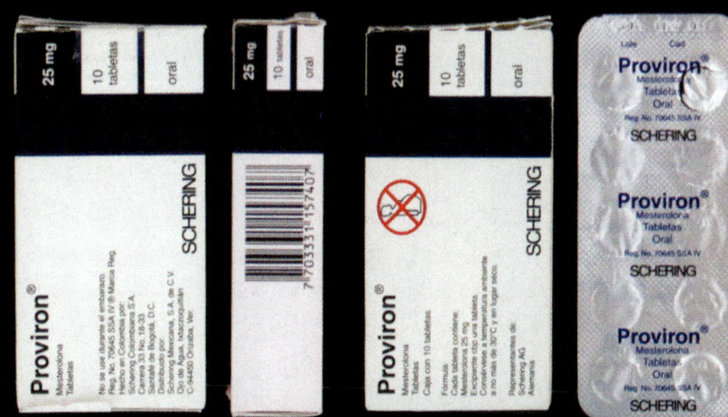

New style box and strip from Mexico

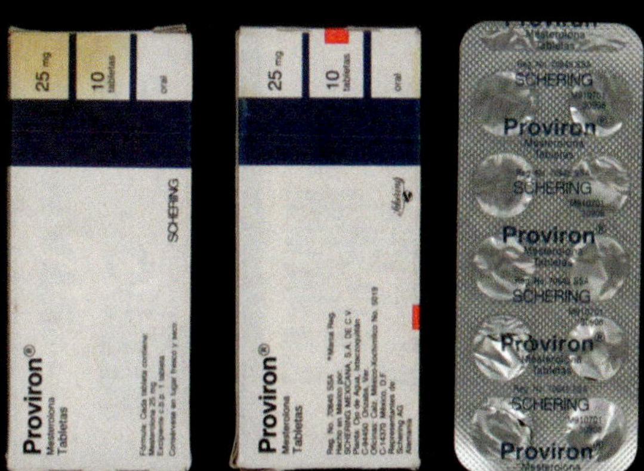

Older Mexican packaging

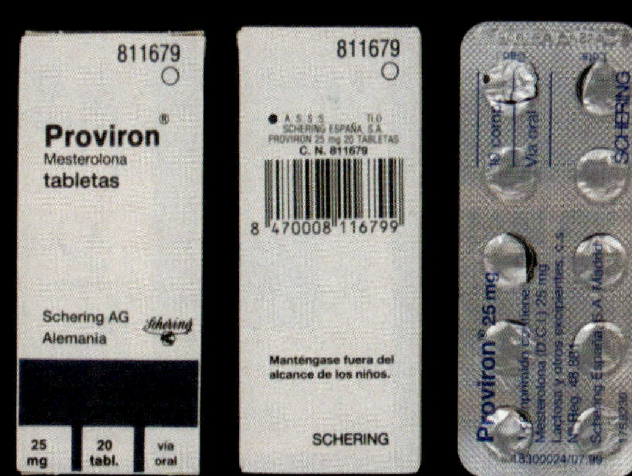

Old Spanish box and strip

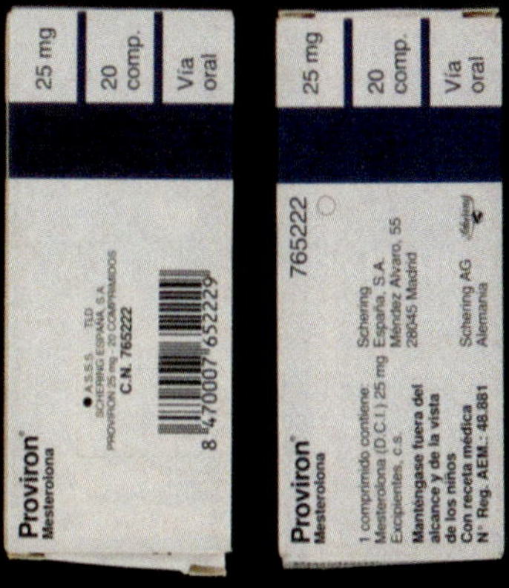

New Spanish box

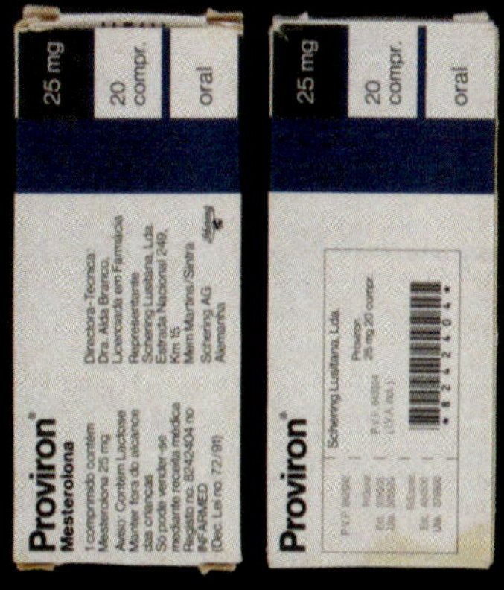

Box from Portugal

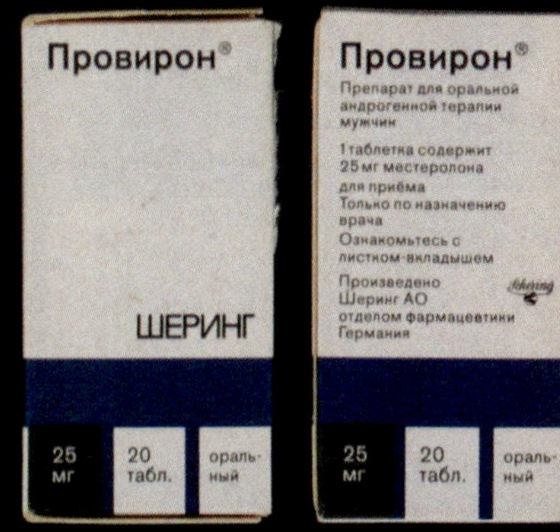

Russian Proviron

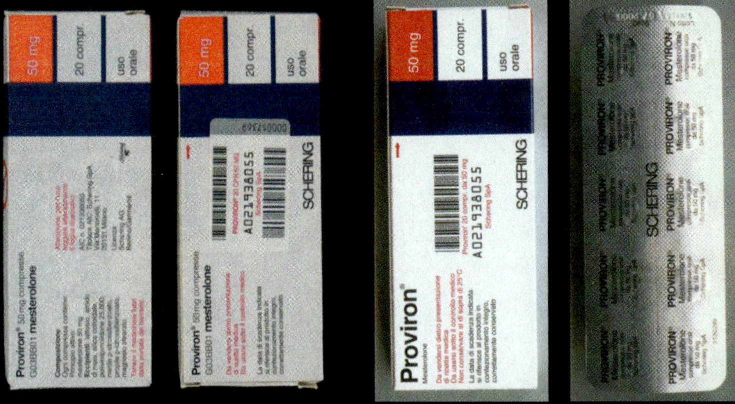

Spectriol

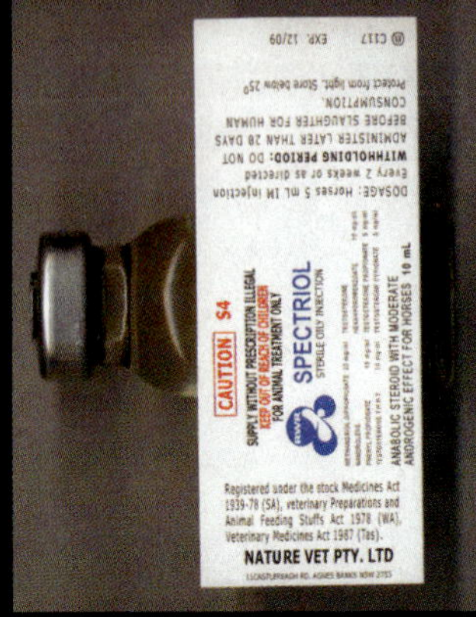

New and older style packaging from Italy

Counterfeit vial

Sten

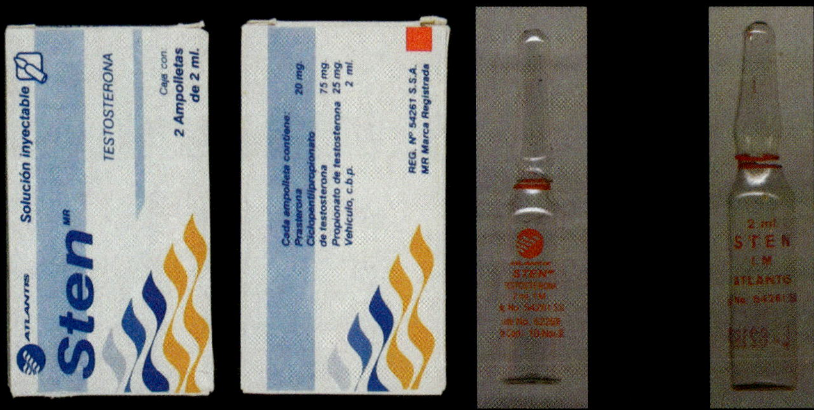

New style Sten (Mexico)

Old amp

Sustanon

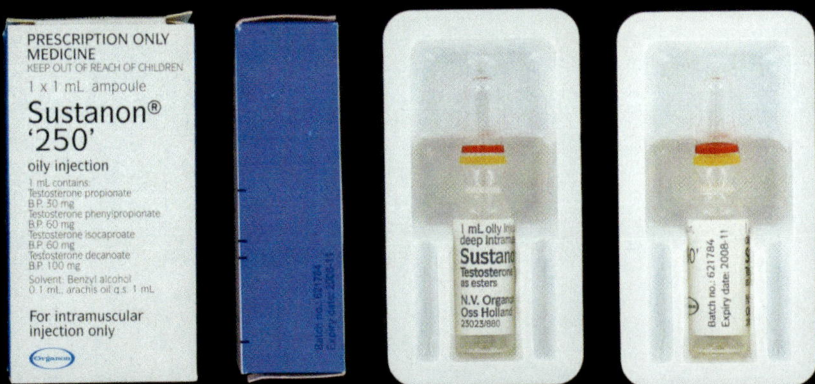

Sustanon from Australia

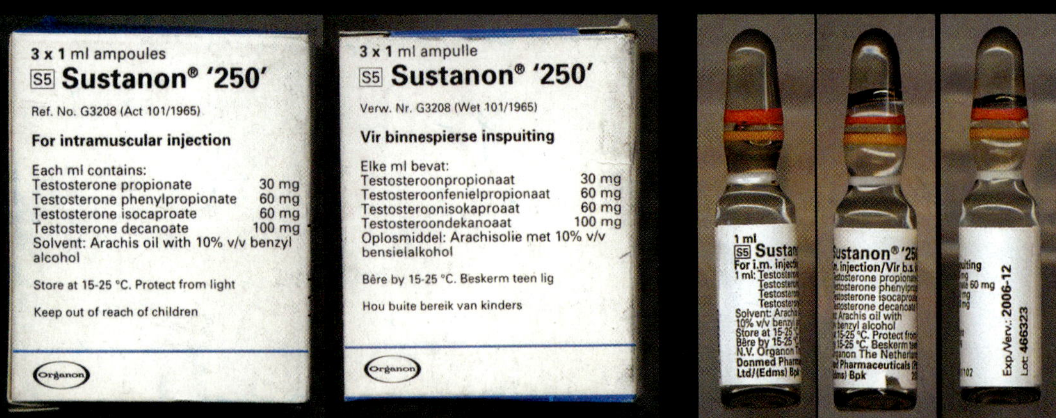

New style UK box and ampules

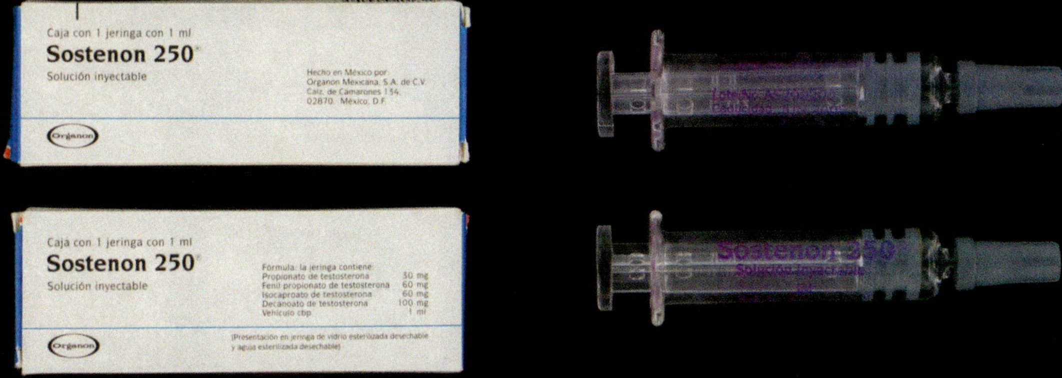

Pre-loaded syringe from Mexico - New style packaging

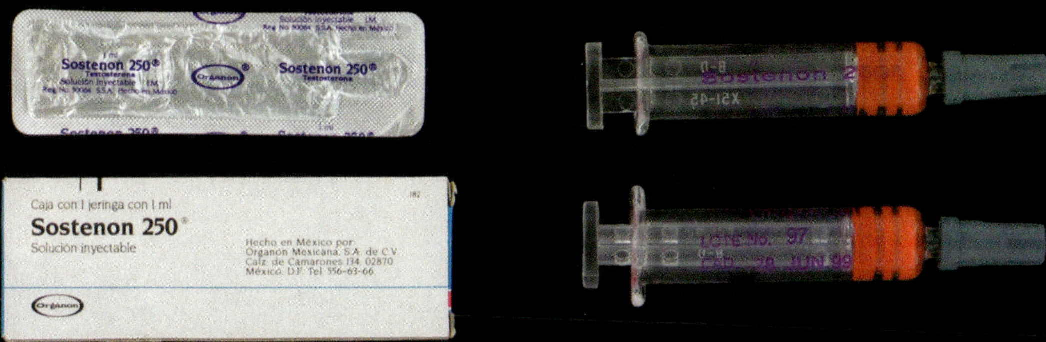

Older Mexican pre-load

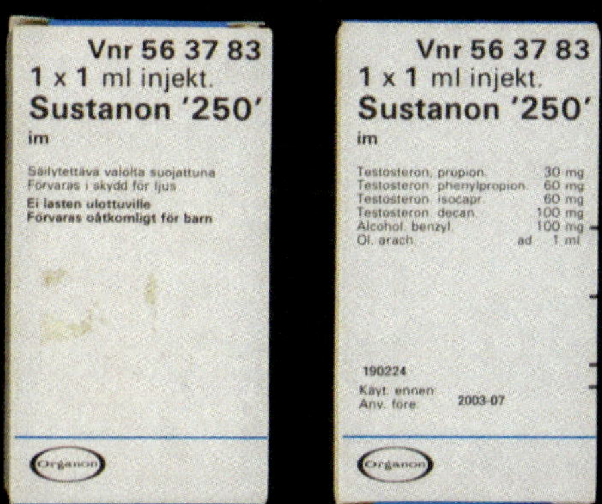

Sustanon '250' from Estonia

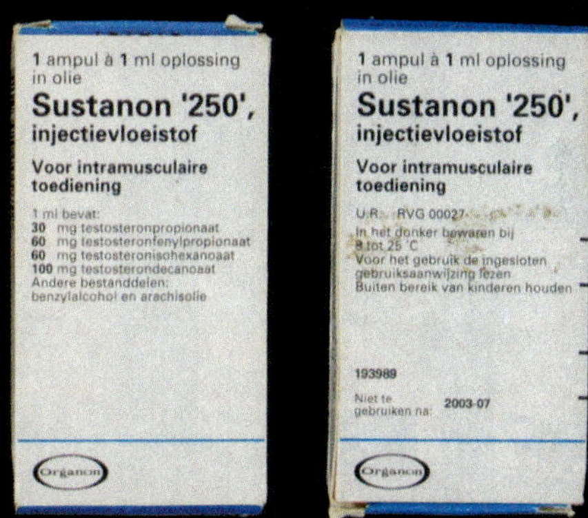

Sustanon '250' from Holland

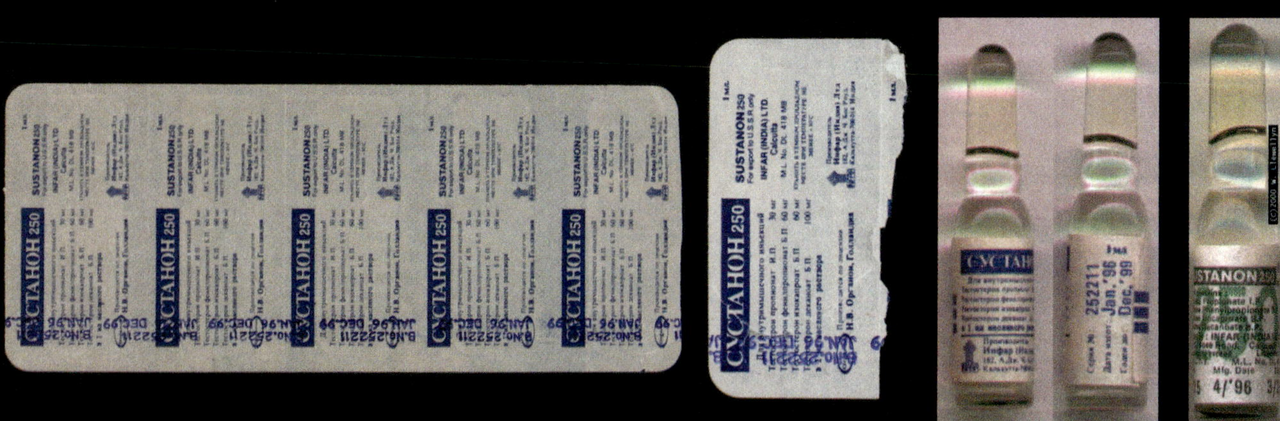

"Russian Sustanon" - Made in India by Infar, for export to Russia - New Green ampule on right

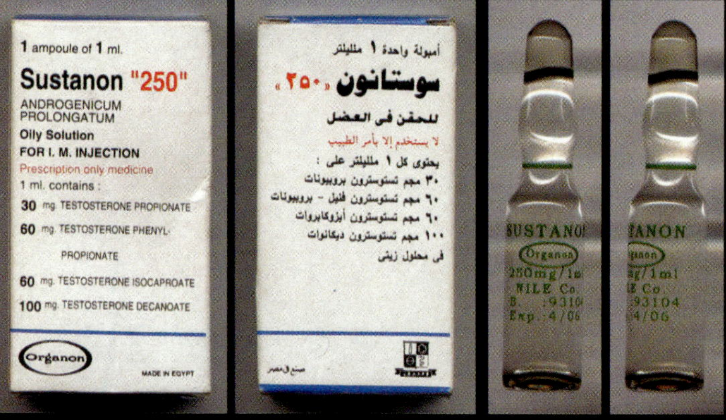

New Nile Sustanon from Egypt

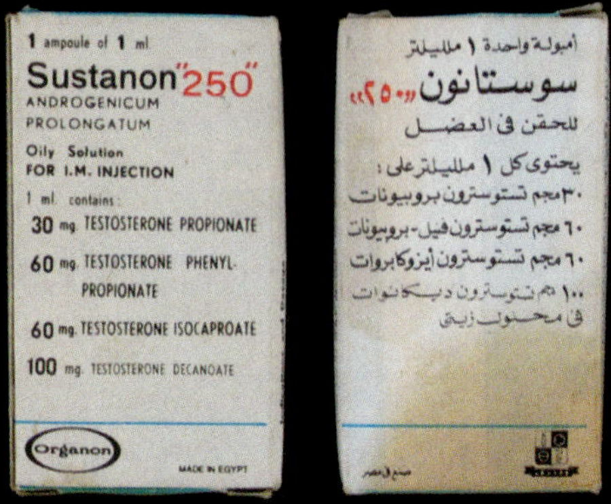

Older Nile packaging

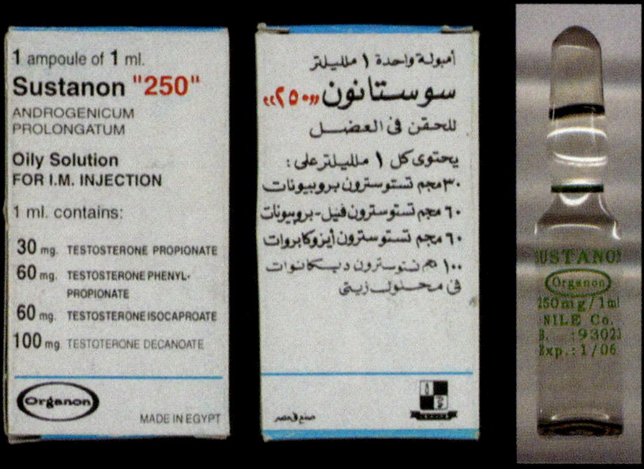

Excellent looking counterfeit Nile product

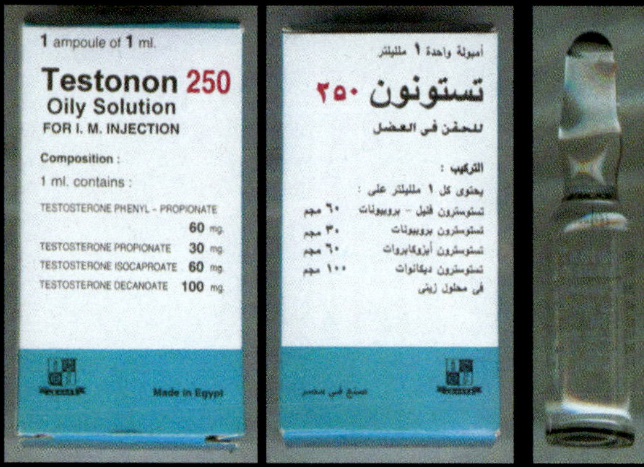

New Testonon from Nile Egypt

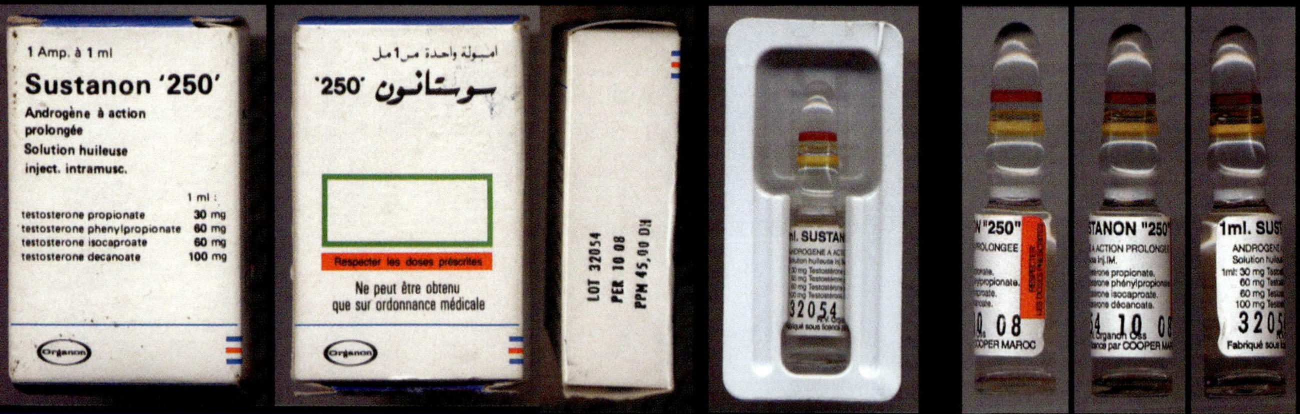

Sustanon '250' from Morocco

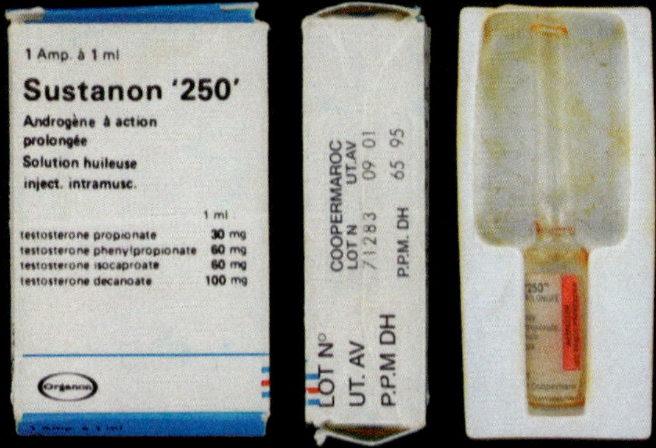

Counterfeit Sustanon from Morocco

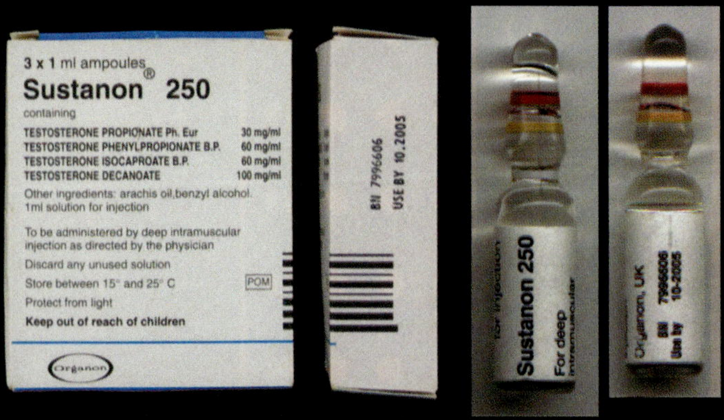

New style Sustanon 250 from the UK

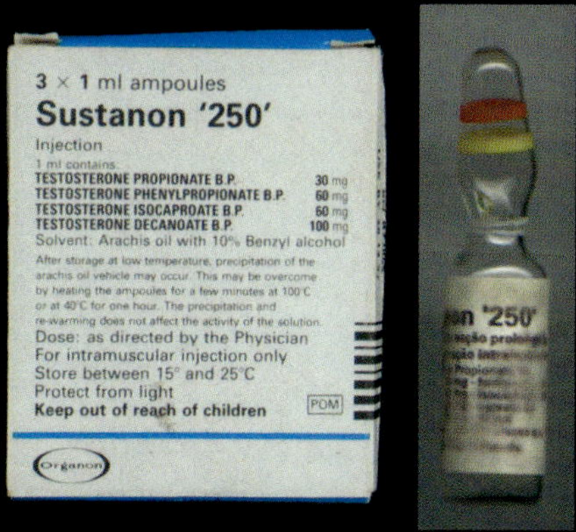

Old box and vial from the UK

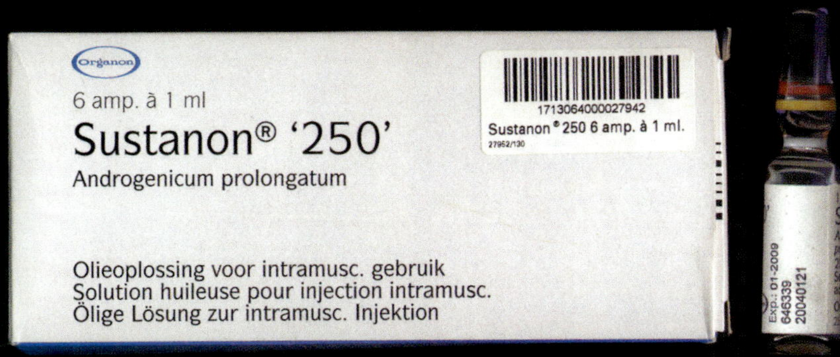

Sustanon '250' from Belgium - New style packaging

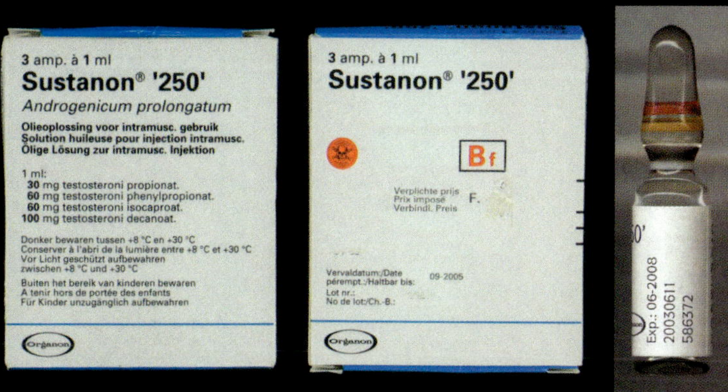

Older version from Belgium

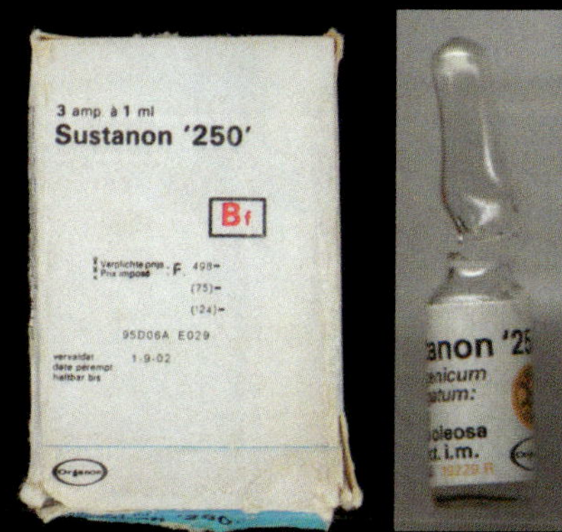

Belgian counterfeit

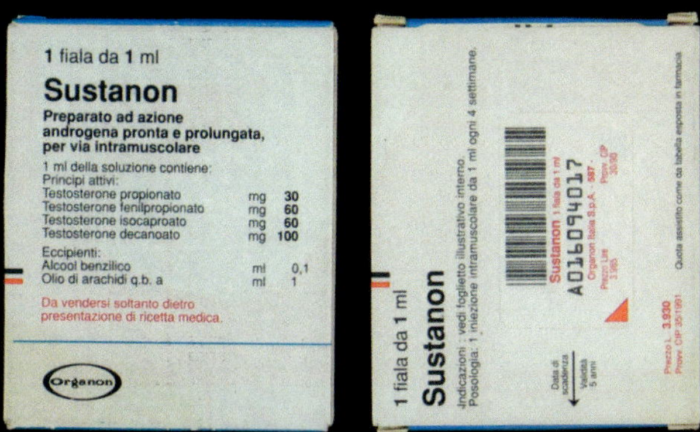

Sustanon from Italy - Older style packaging

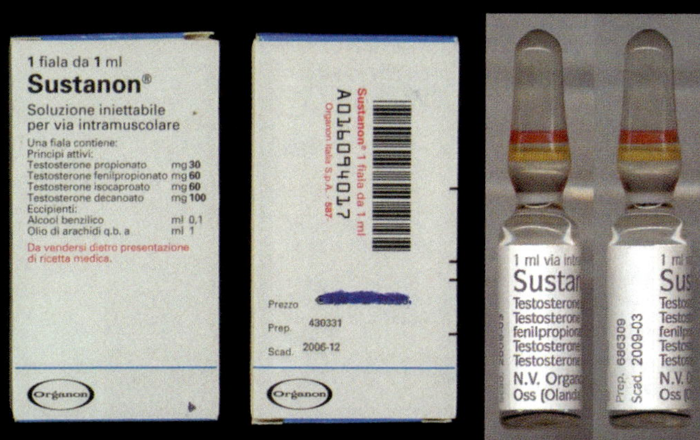

Newer Italian box and amp

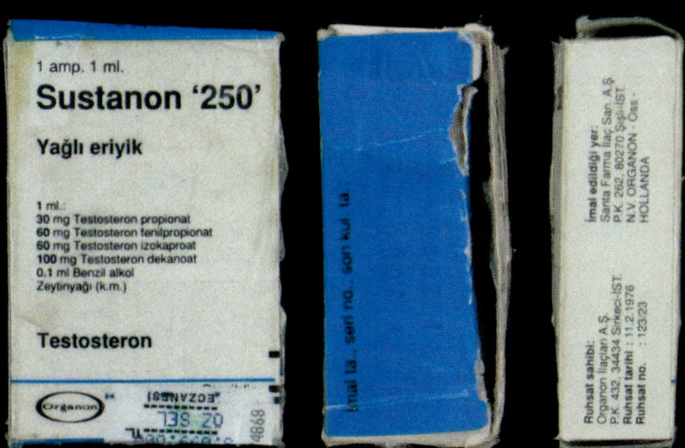

Sustanon '250' from Turkey

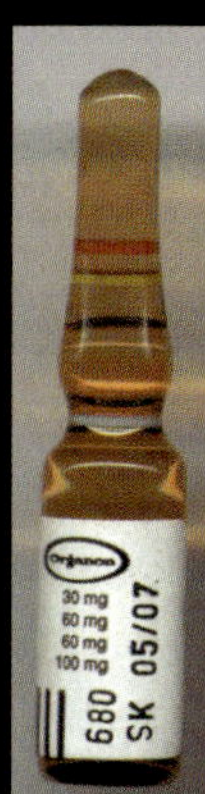

Real

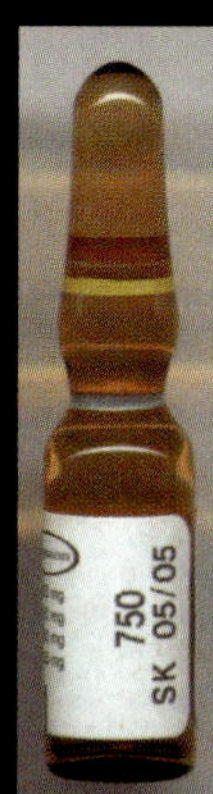

Fake

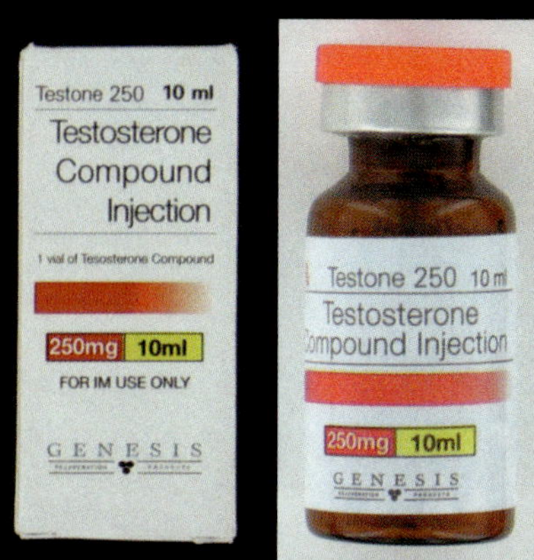

Genesis generic (Singapore)

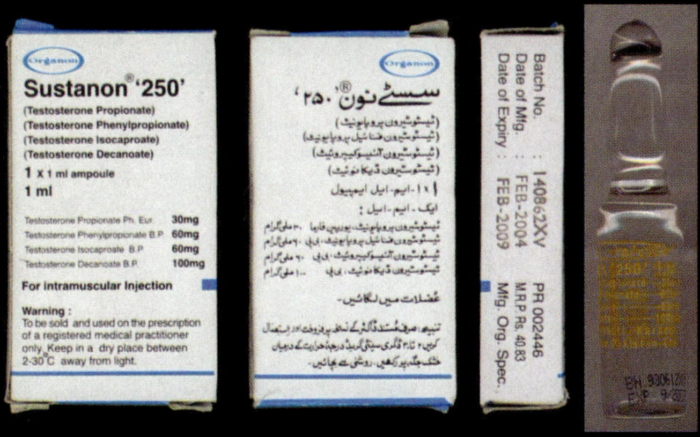

Sustanon from Pakistan

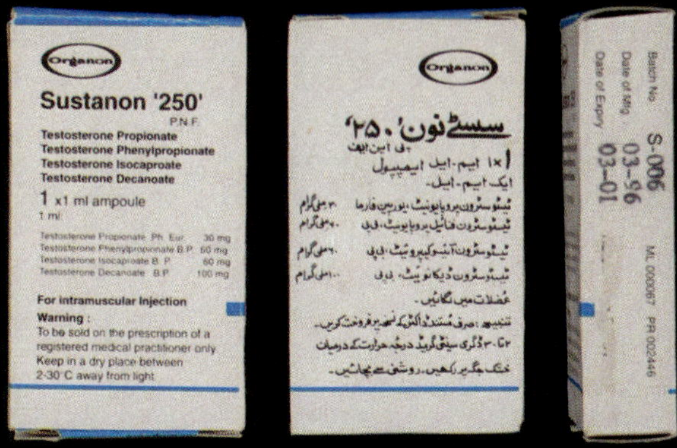

Older style box from Pakistan

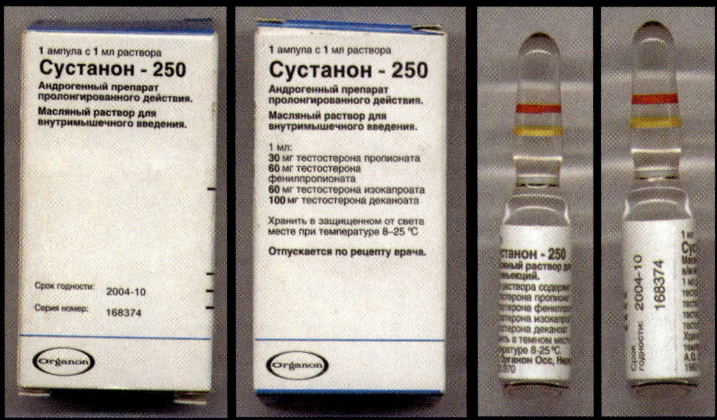

Organon Sustanon from Russia

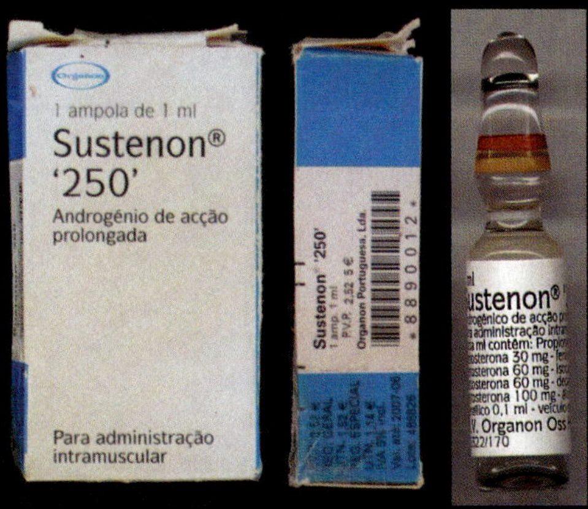

New packaging from Portugal

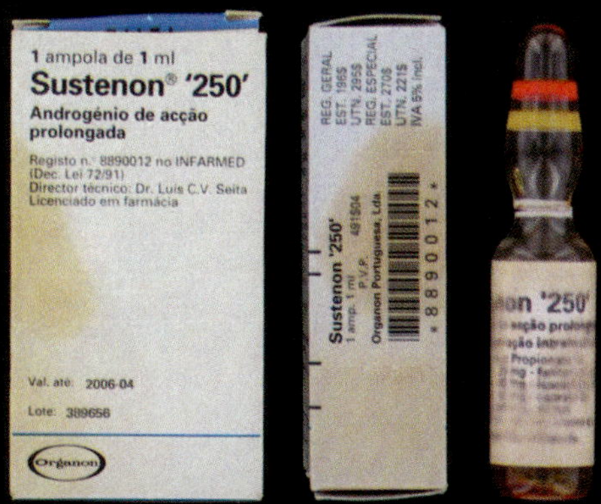

Older version from Portugal

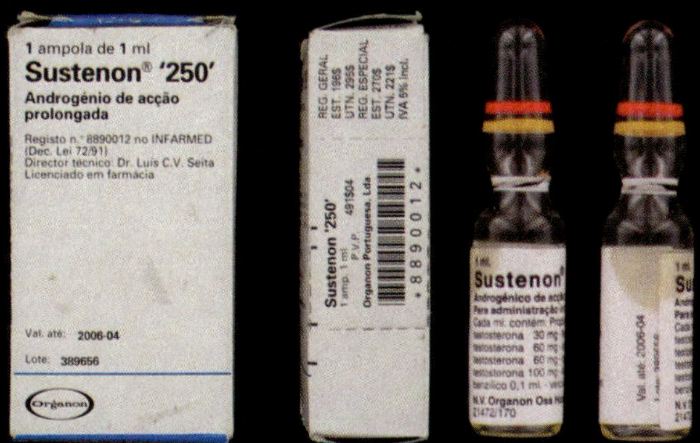

Counterfeit #1

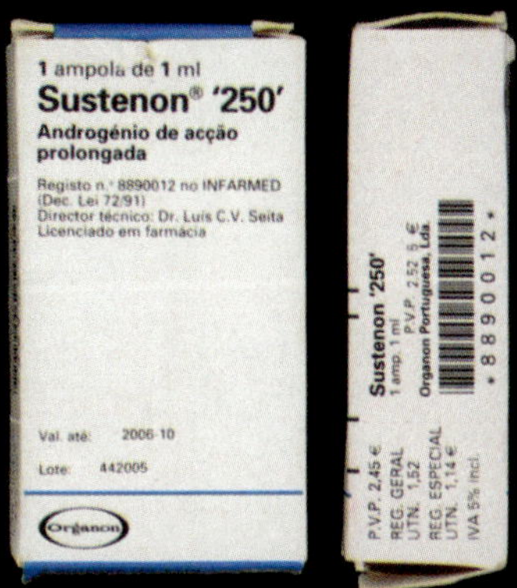

Counterfeit #2

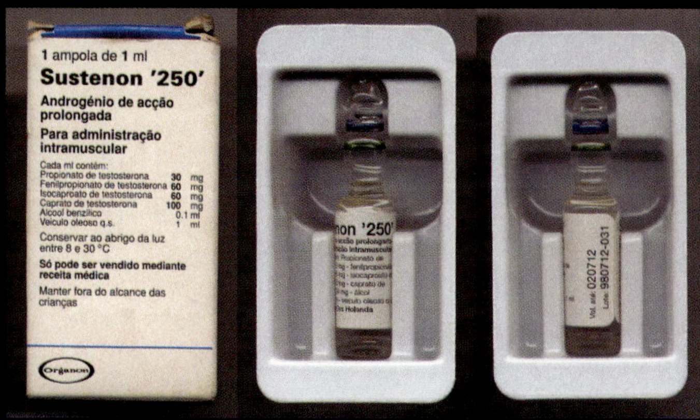

Counterfeit #3

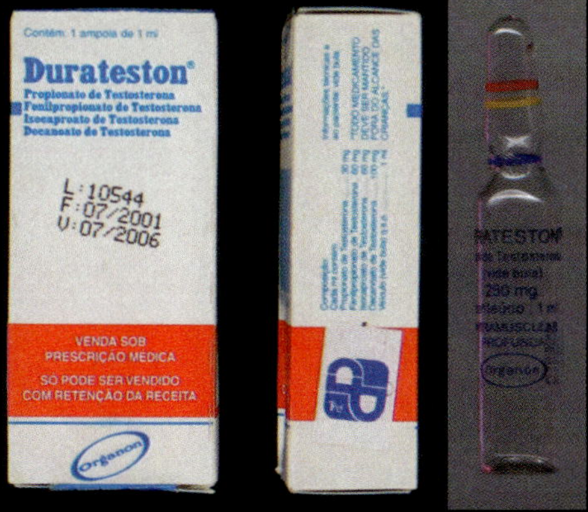

Durateston from Brazil

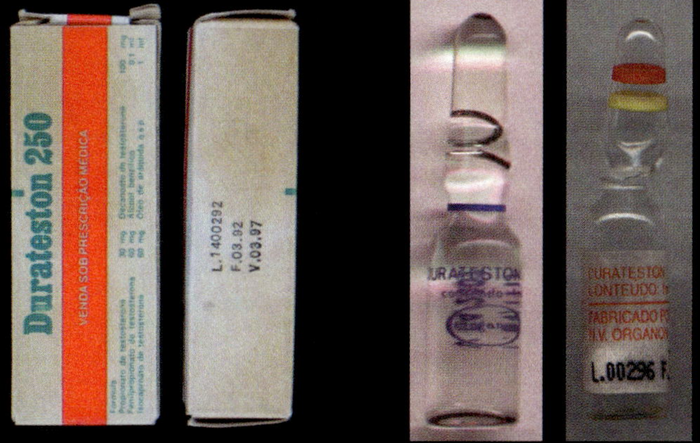

Older style box and ampules from Brazil

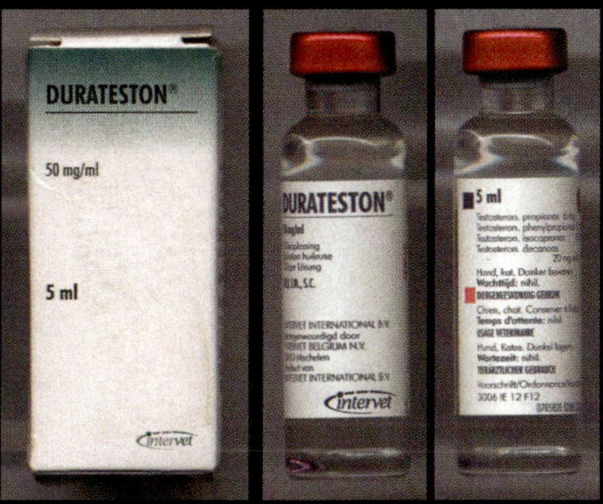

Durateston from Belgium

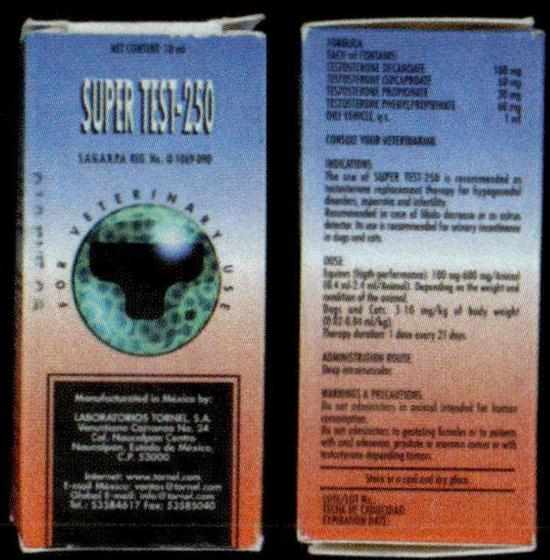

Supertest-250 from Tornel (Mexico)

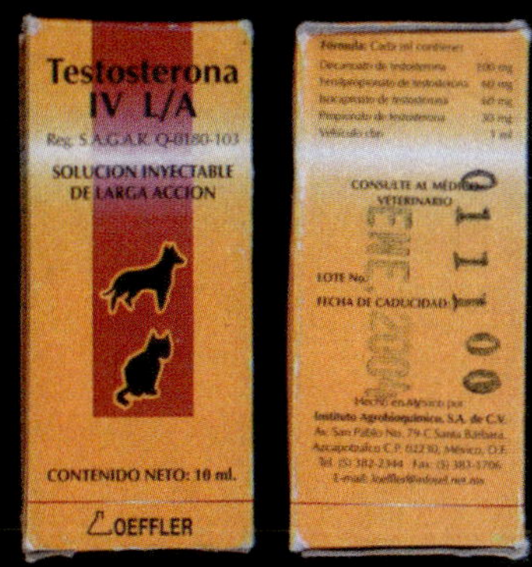

Loeffler Testosterona IV (Mexico)

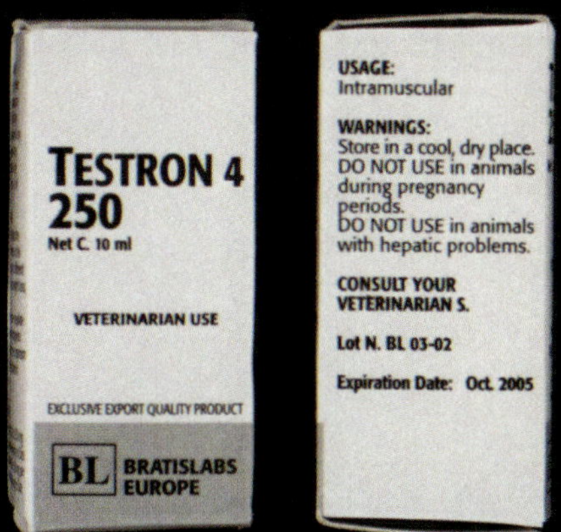

Testron from Bratis (Mexico)

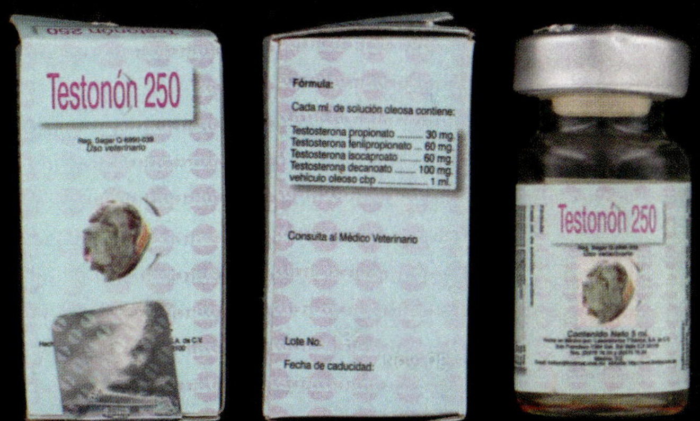

Testonon 250 from Ttokkyo Mexico (NLM)

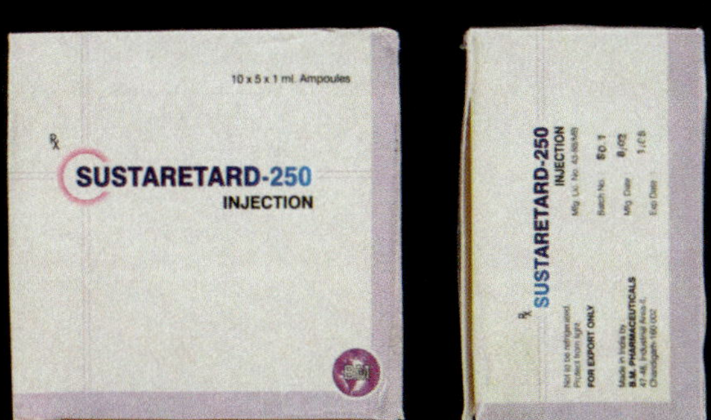

BM Sustaretard (India)

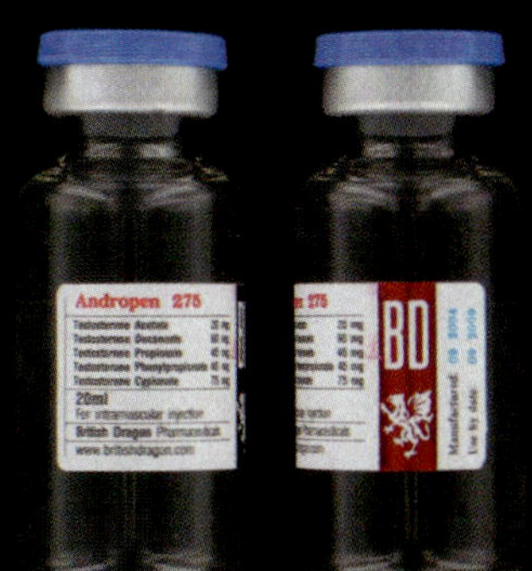

British Dragon vial (Thailand)

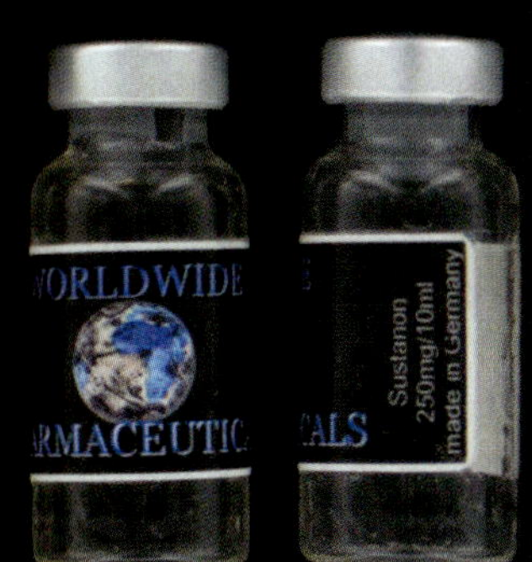

UG product from Worldwide

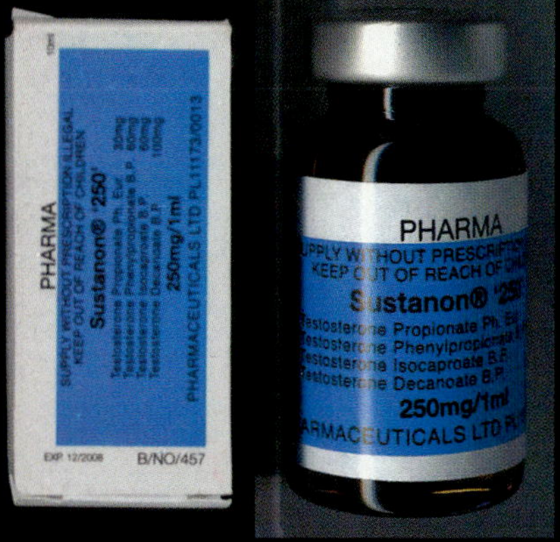

UG product from Pharma

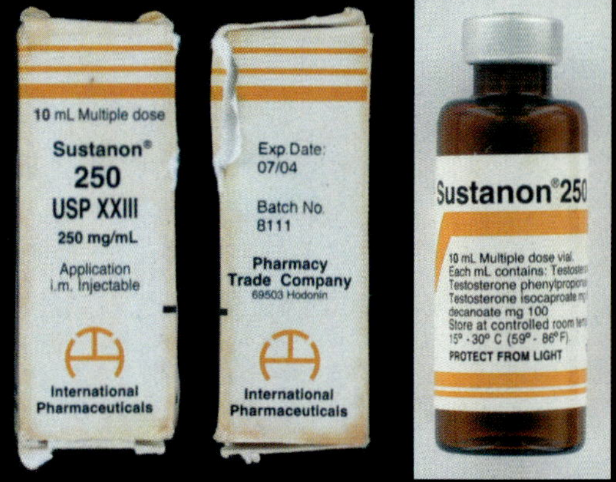

Counterfeit IP inectable

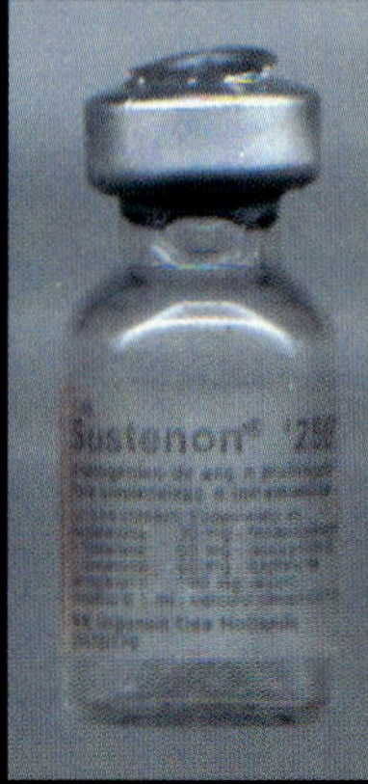

Fake vial

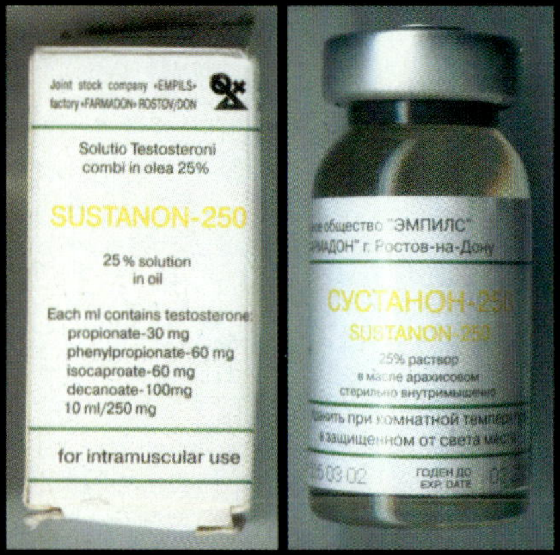

Fake Russian Farmadon product

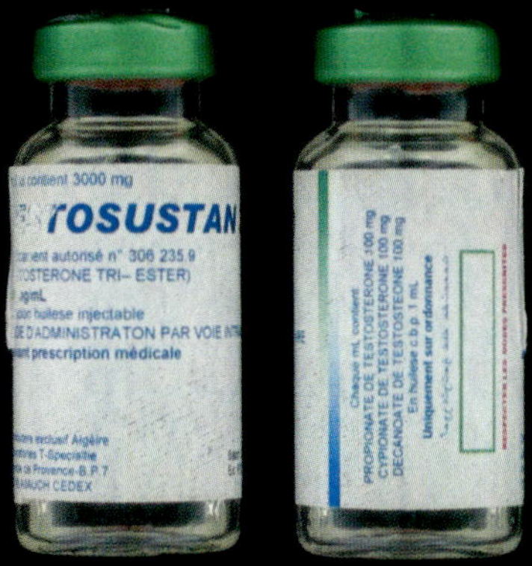

Counterfeit French “Testosustan”

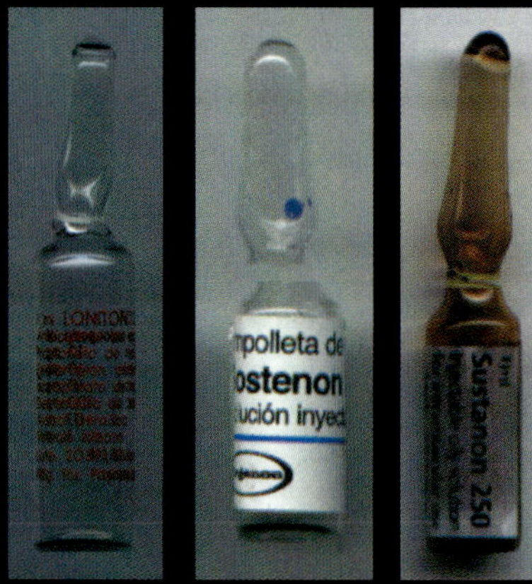

Three fake ampules

Synovex-H

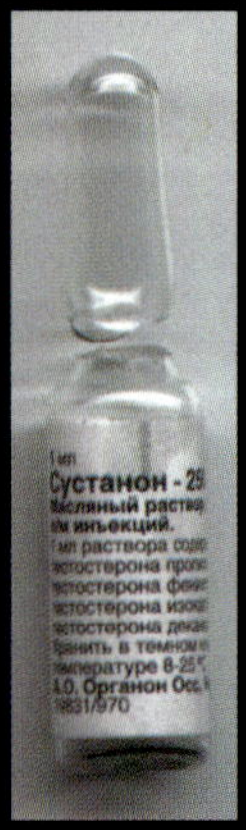

Russian Counterfeit

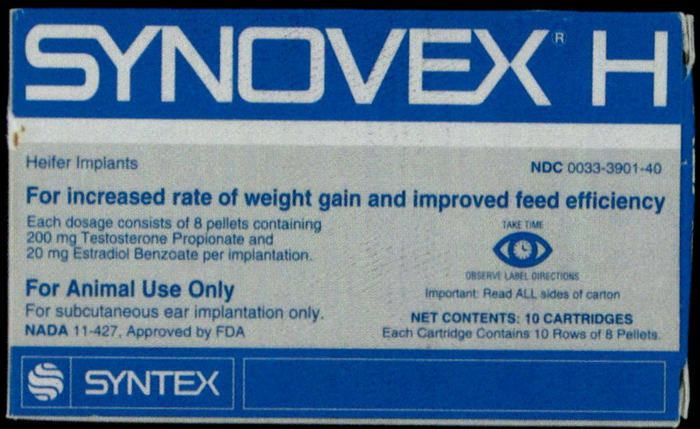

Synovex from Syntex U.S.

Test 400

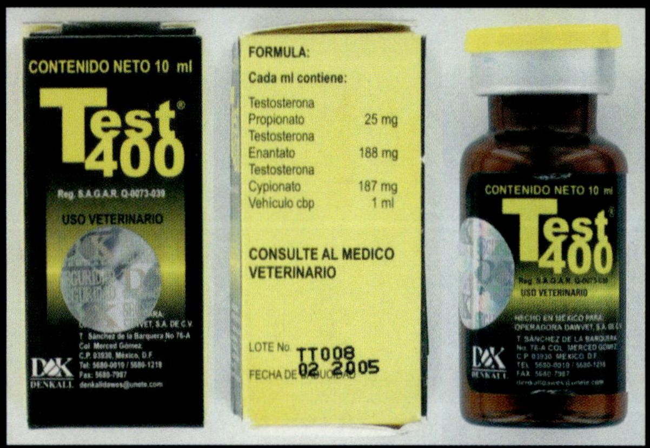

Test 400 from Denkall (Mexico)

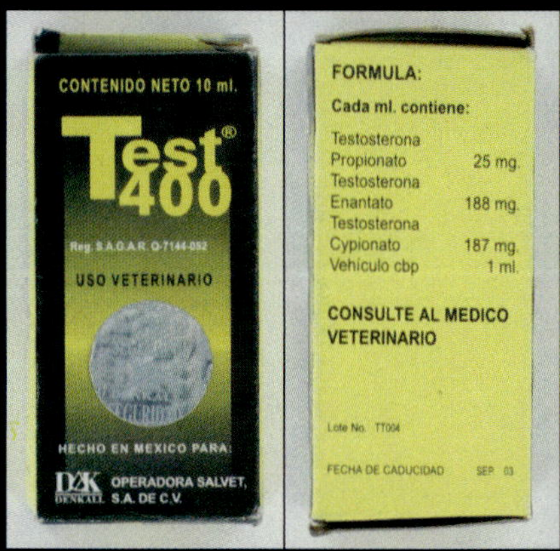

Counterfeit Test 400

Testolent

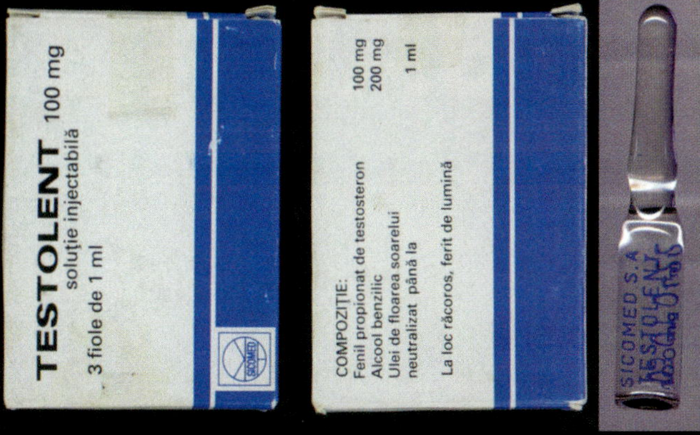

Testolent from Rumania (NLM)

T. Butyrate

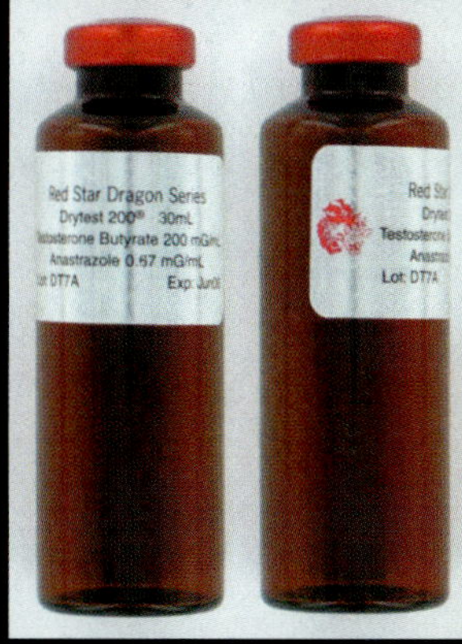

UG product from Red Star

T. Cypionate

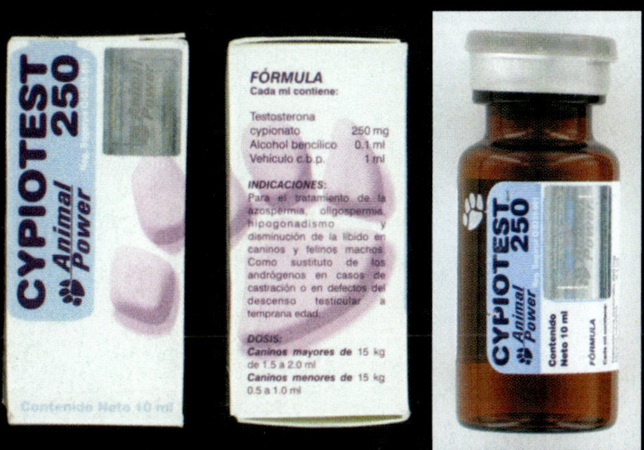

Animal Power Cypiotest 250 (Mexico)

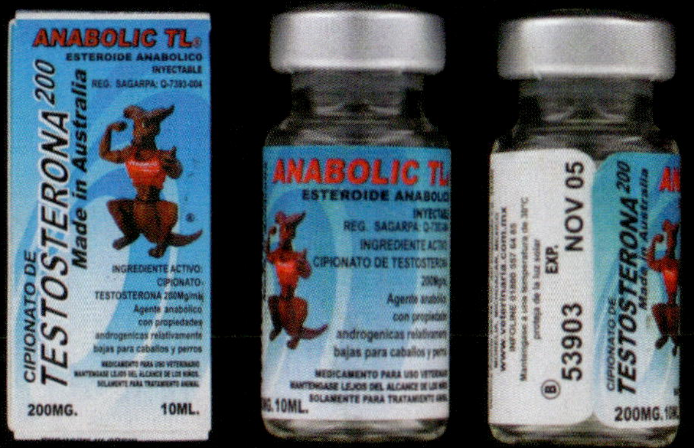

SYD Group Anabolic TL (Mexico)

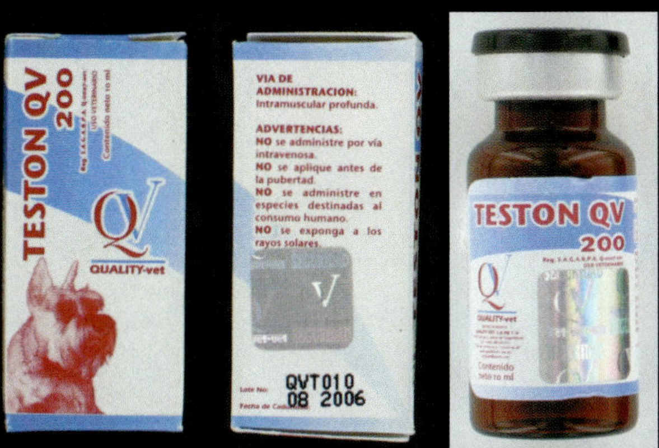

Teston from Quality Vet (Mexico)

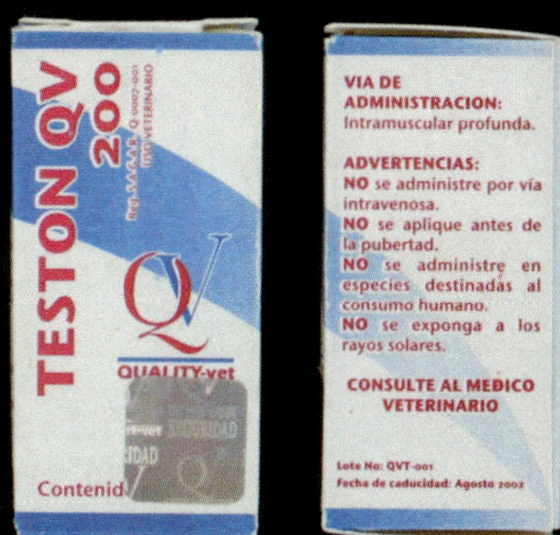

Older style QV box

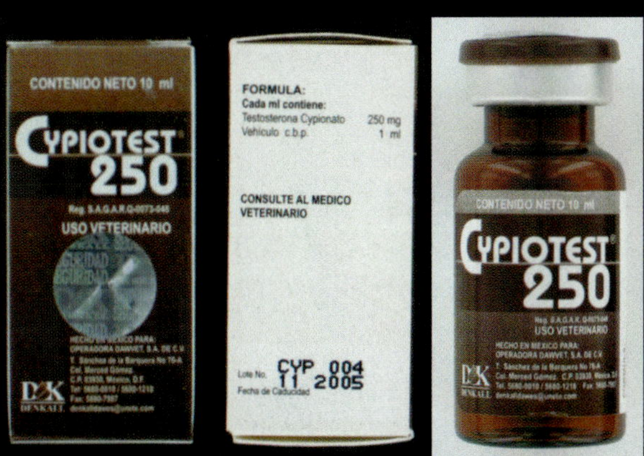

Cypiotest 250 from Denkall (Mexico)

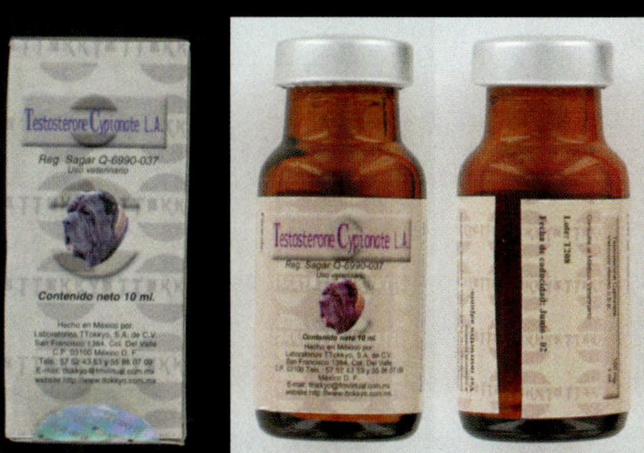

100mg/mL product from Ttokkyo Mexico (NLM)

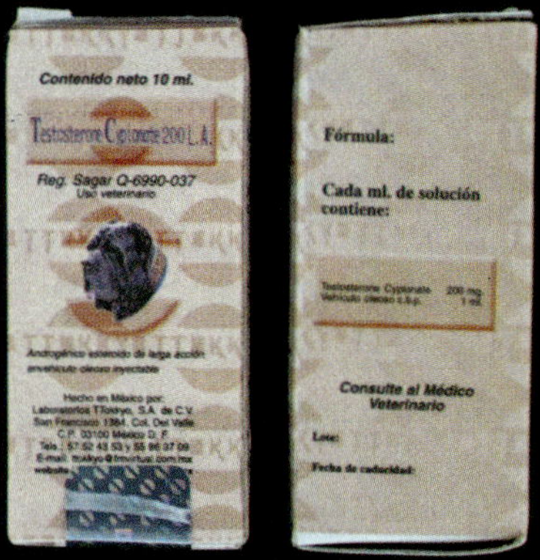

200mg/mL Ttokkyo box (NLM)

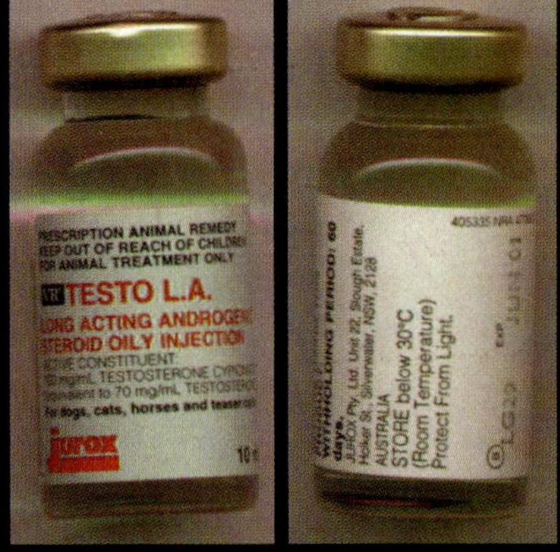

Testo L.A. from Jurox Australia(NLM)

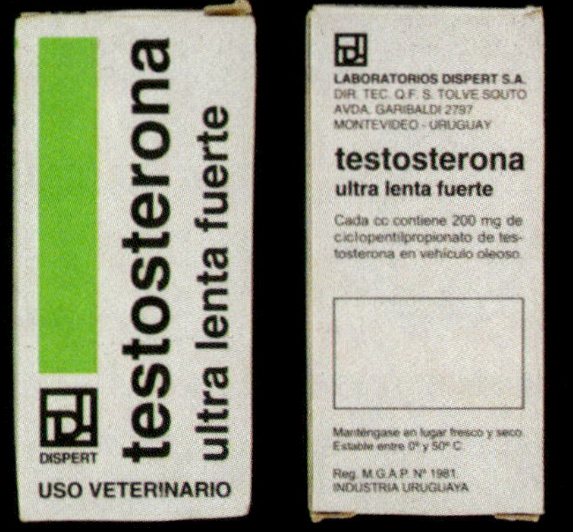

Testosterona Ultra 200mg (Uruguay)

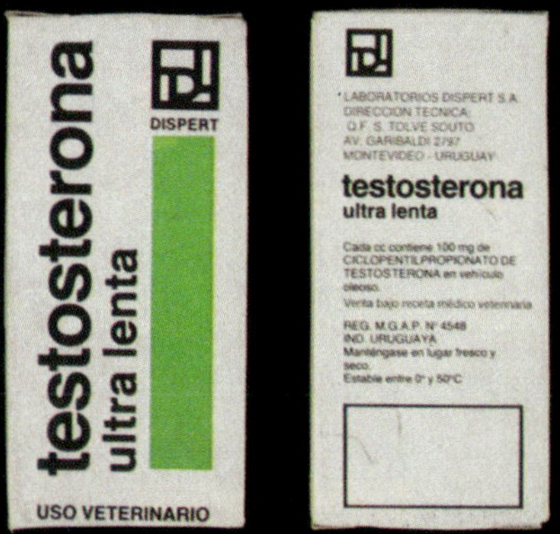

100mg/mL version

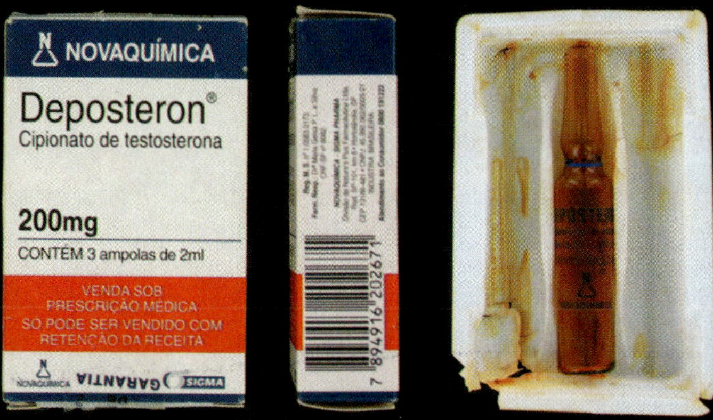

Deposteron from Brazil

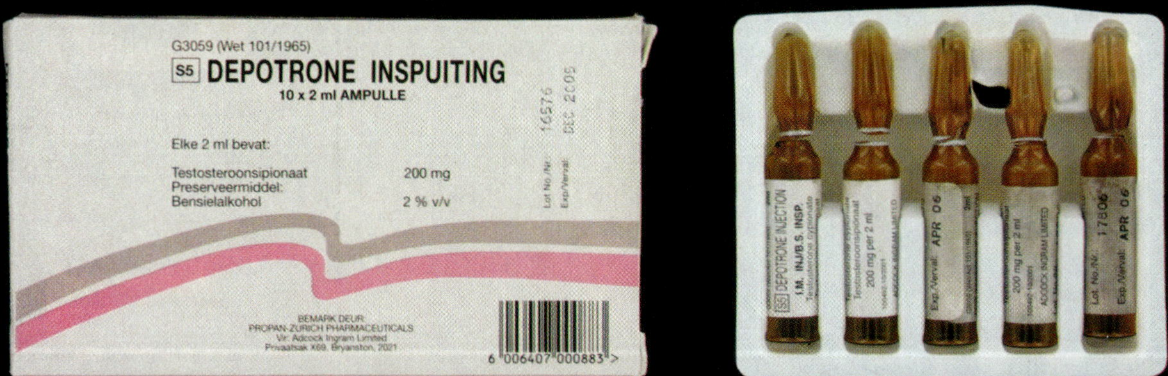

South African Depotrone

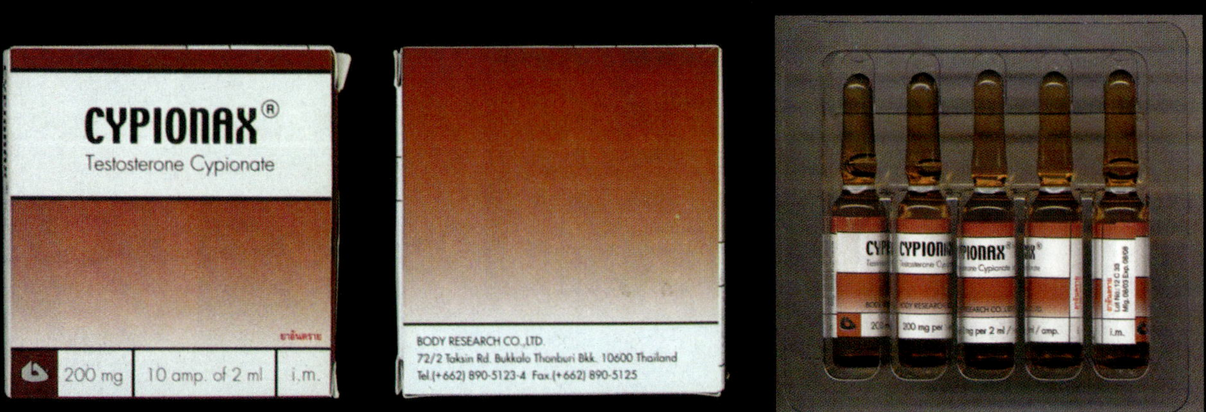

Cypionax from Body Research in Thailand

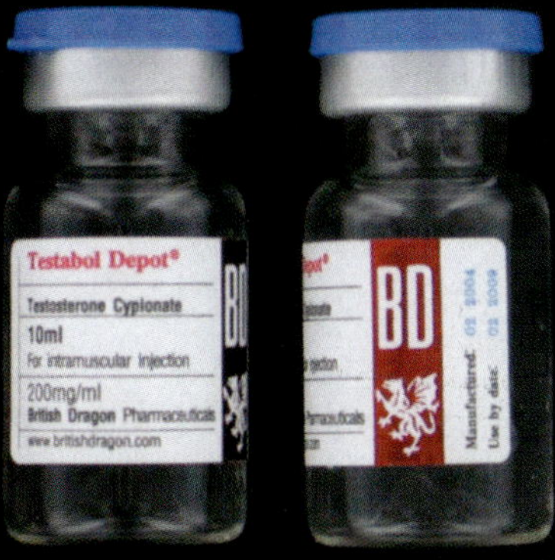

Testabol from British Dragon

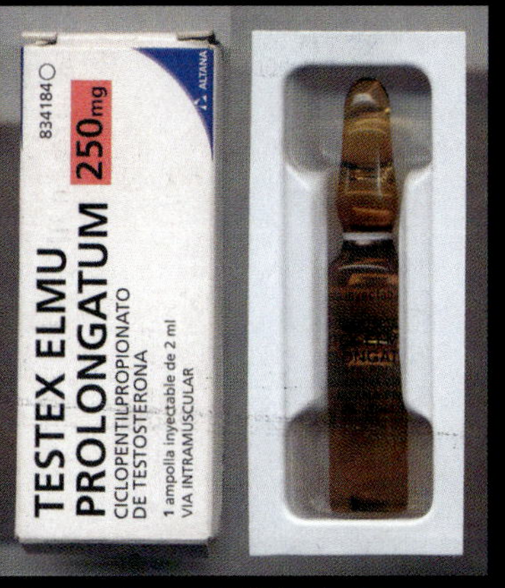

New Spanish Testex

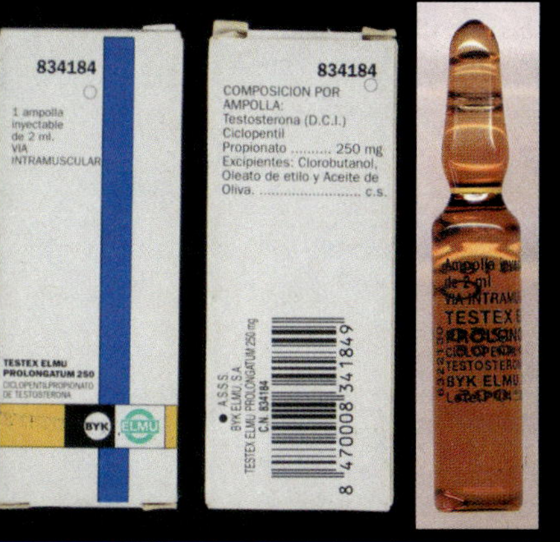

Older style Testex

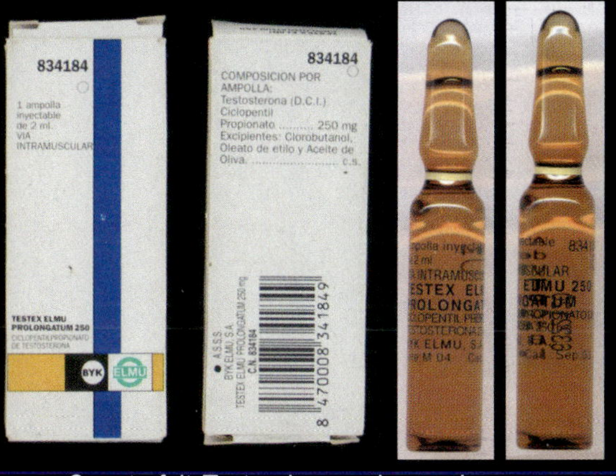

Counterfeit Testex box and ampules

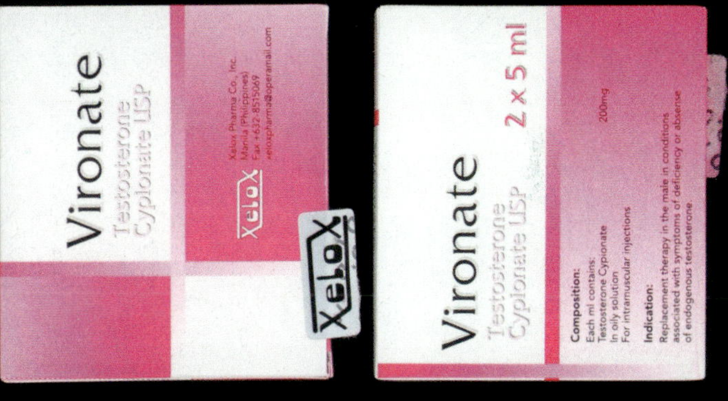

Vironate from Xelox (Philippines)

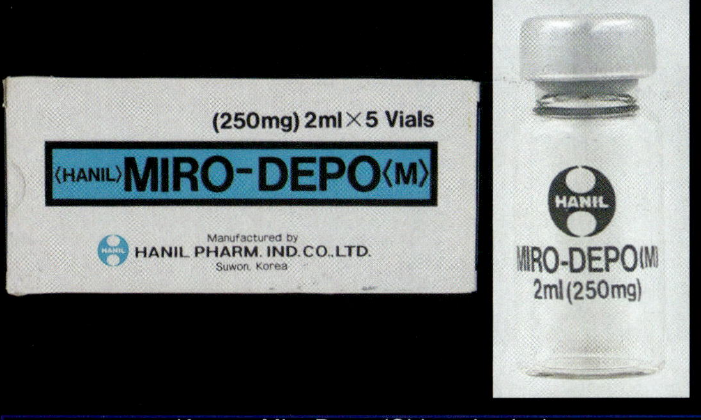

Korean Miro-Depo (Old packaging)

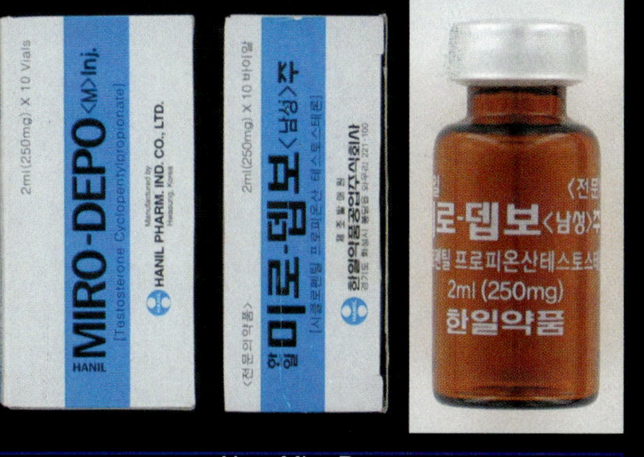

New Miro-Depo

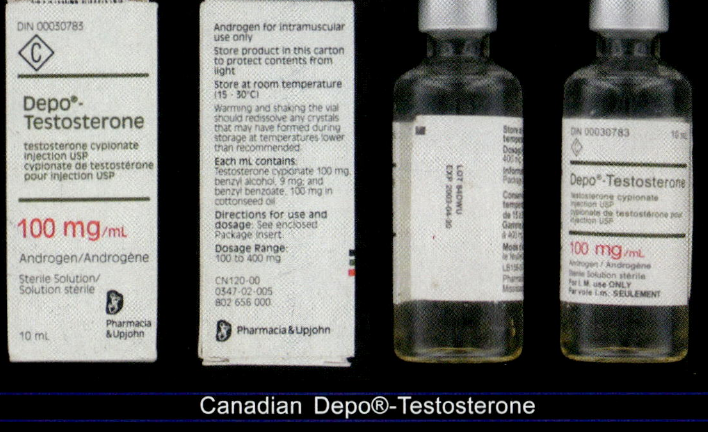

Canadian Depo®-Testosterone

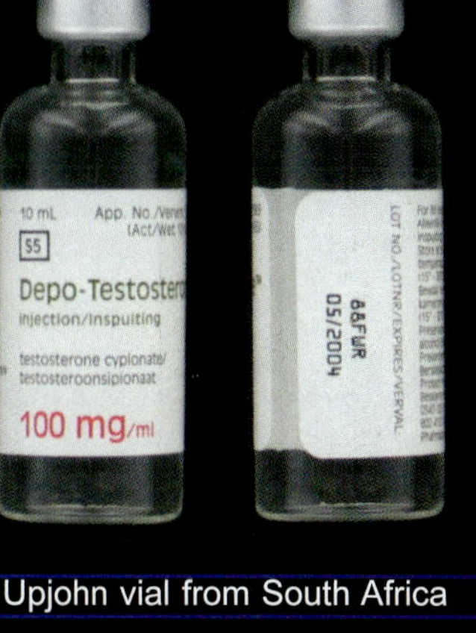

Upjohn vial from South Africa

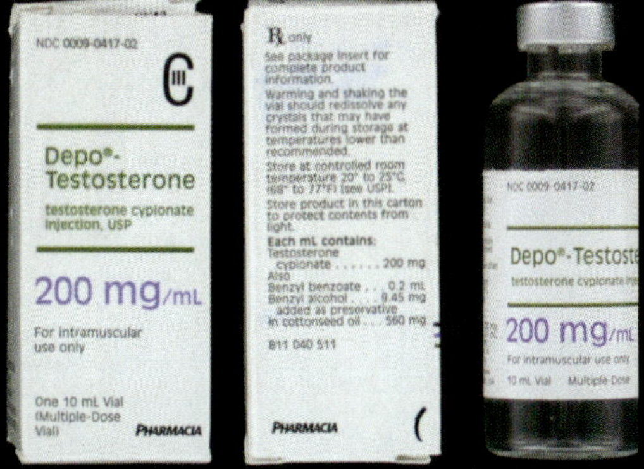

U.S. Depo®-Testosterone from Pharmacia

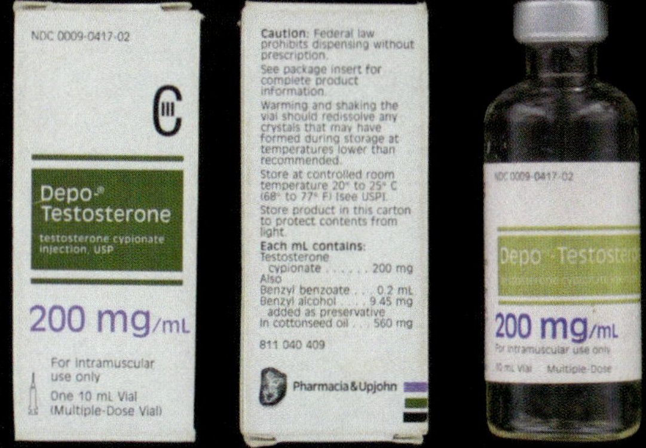

Older Style Box and vial

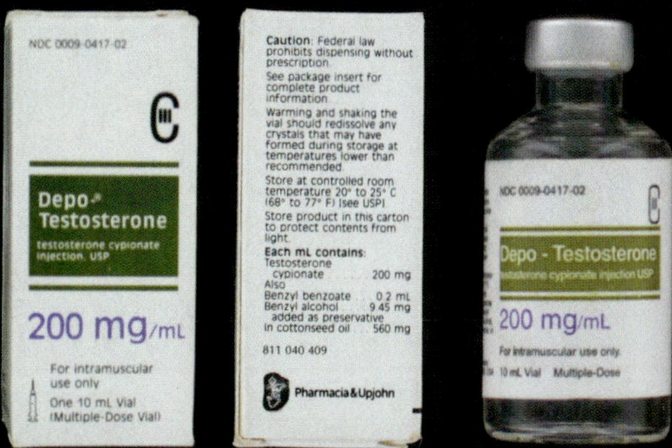

Counterfeit Depo-Test

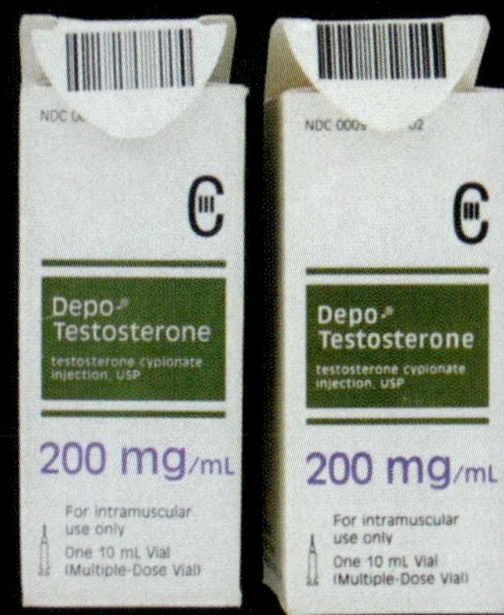

Real Fake

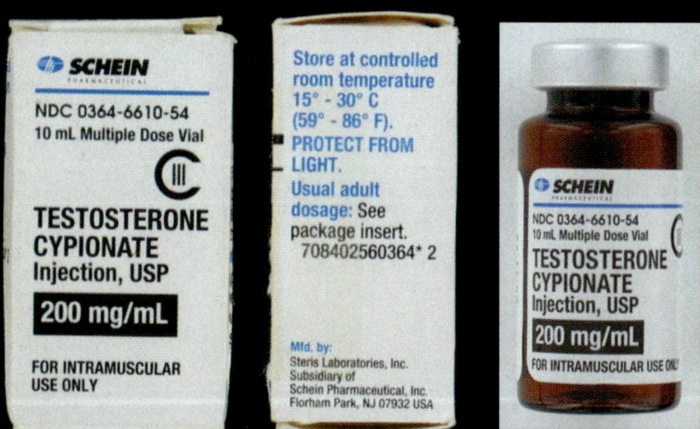

U.S. generic from Schein (NLM)

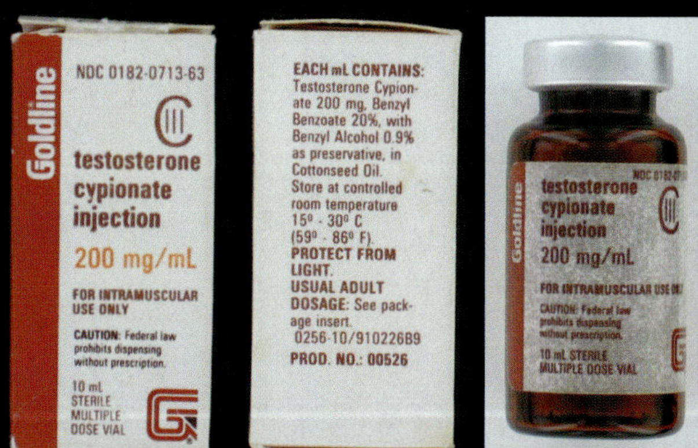

U.S. Goldline cyp (NLM)

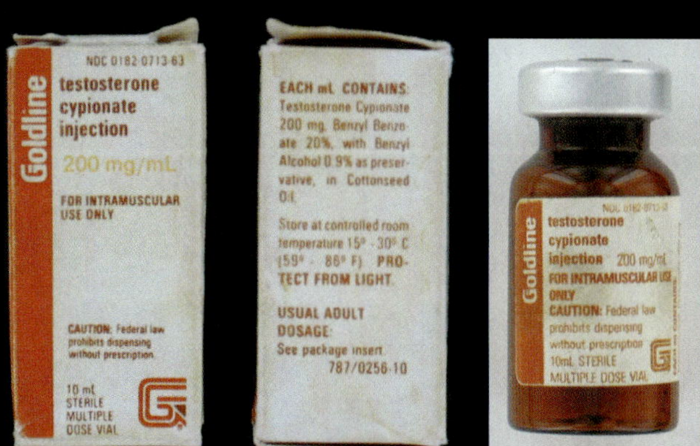

Counterfeit Goldline

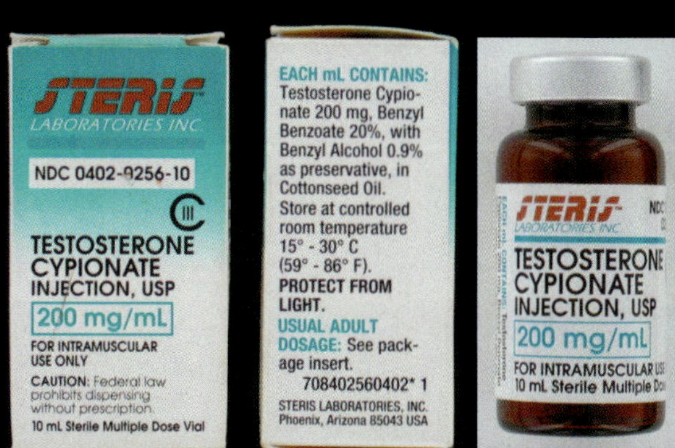

Counterfeit Steris

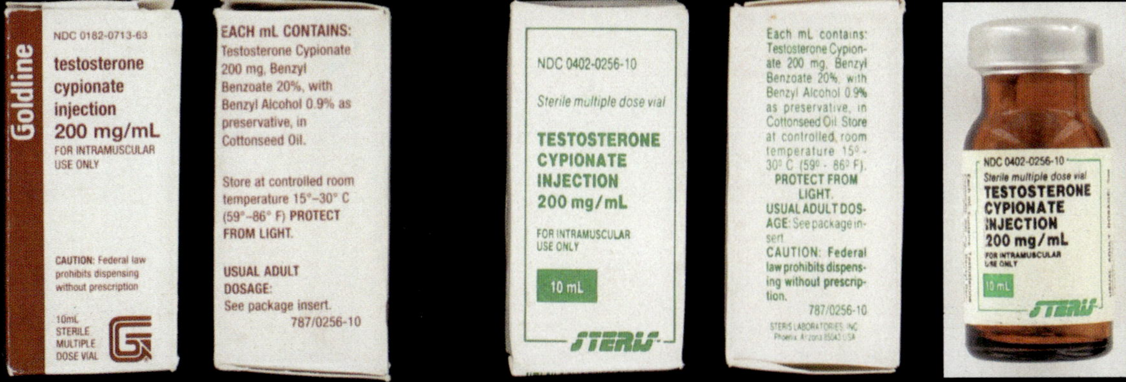

Two different counterfeit U.S. Steris products

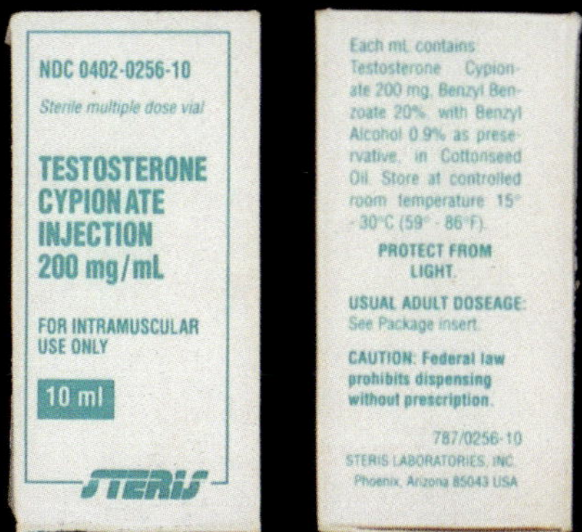

Another Steris fake

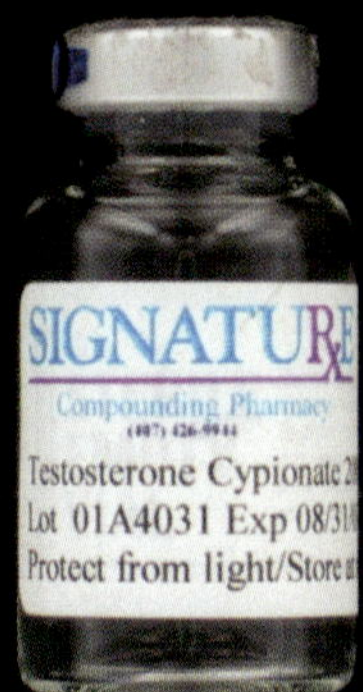

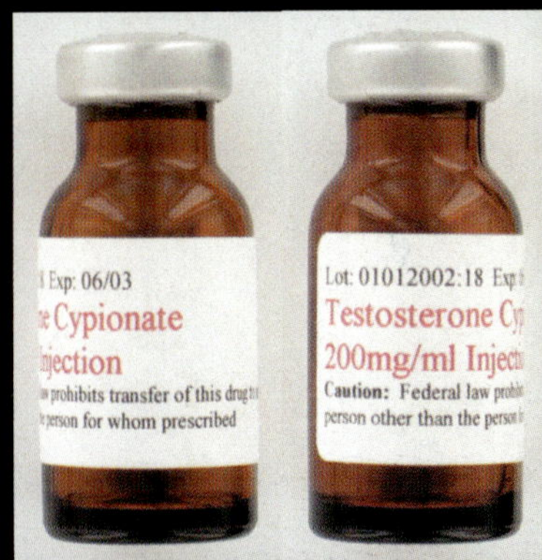

Two U.S. private-label products

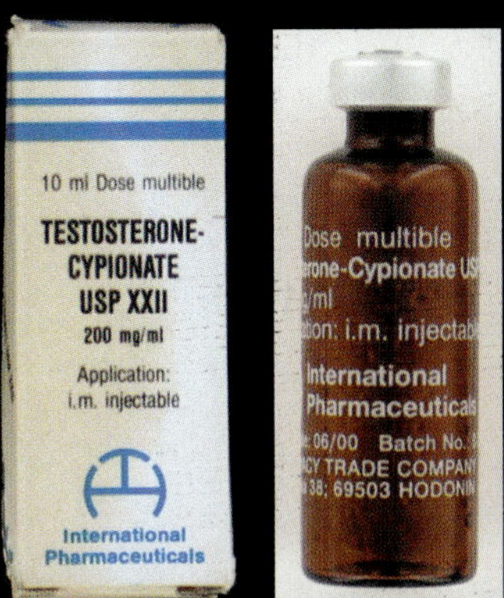

UG product from IP

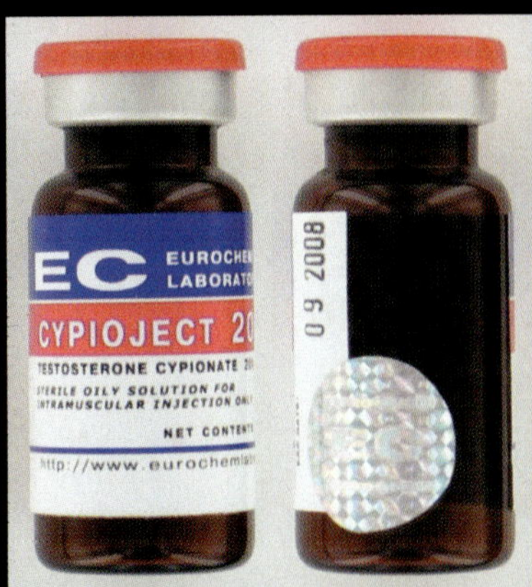

UG Eurochem vial

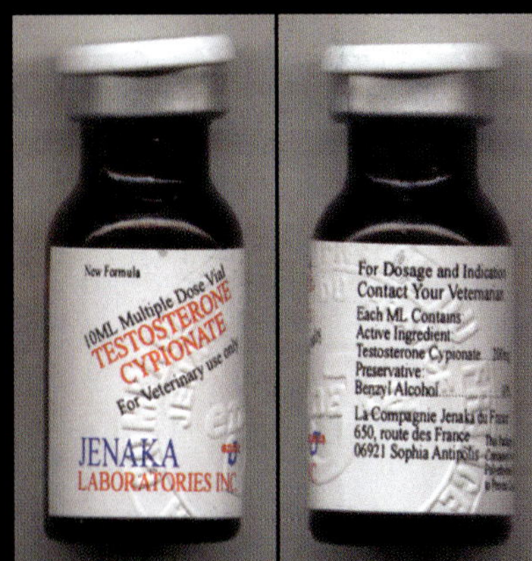

UG Jenaka vial (NLM)

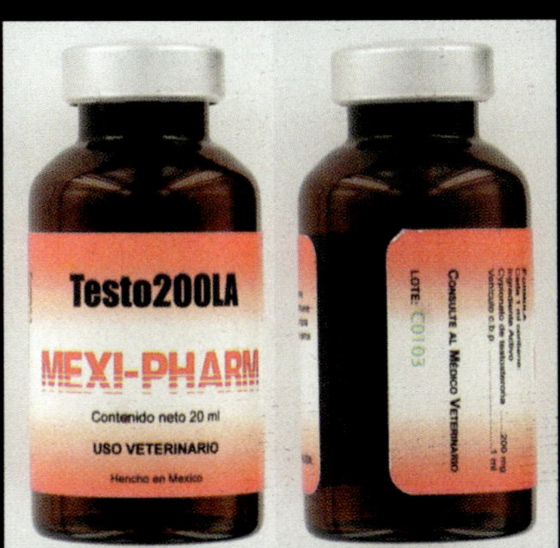

Mexi-pharm UG vial

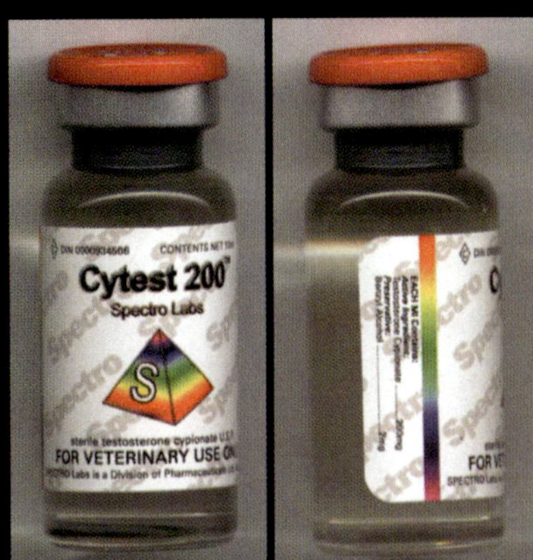

Cytest (UG) from Spectro (NLM)

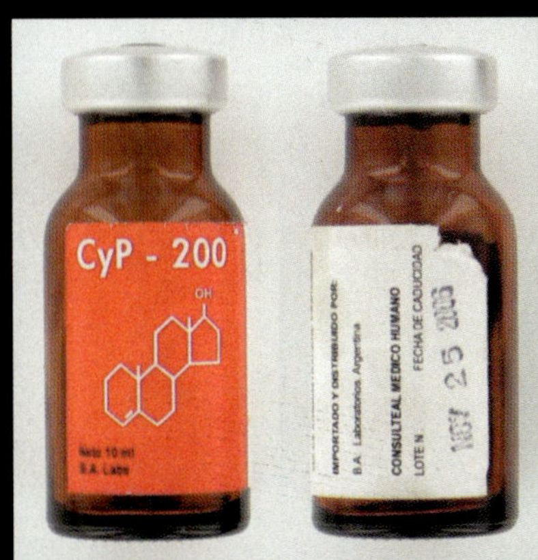

Bogus "Cyp-200"

T. Enanthate

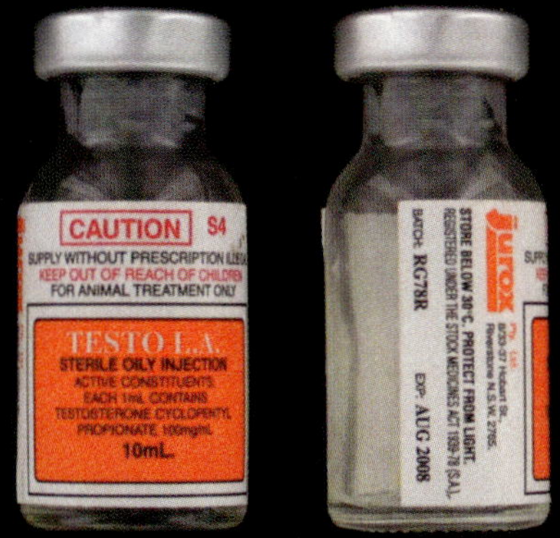

Jurox counterfeit

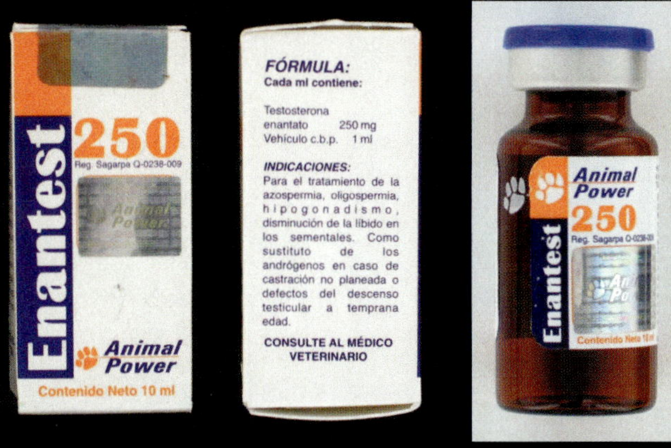

Enantest 250 from Animal Power (Mexico)

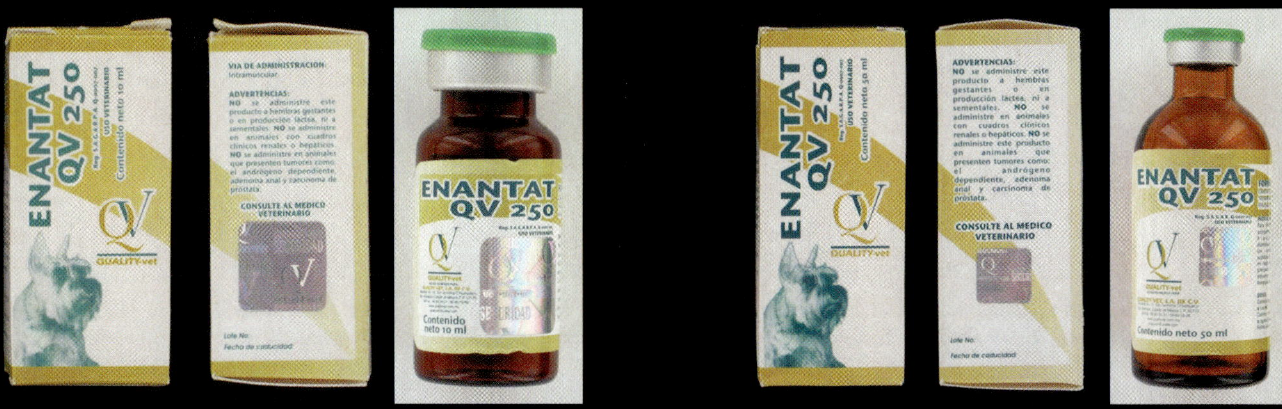

10ml and 50ml products from Quality Vet (Mexico)

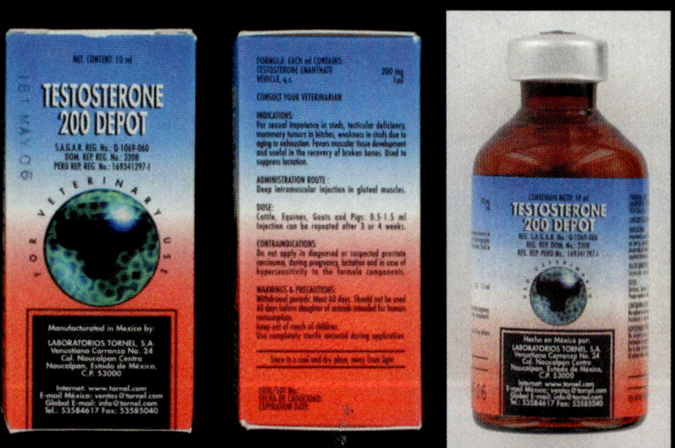

New version of Tornel generic (Mexico)

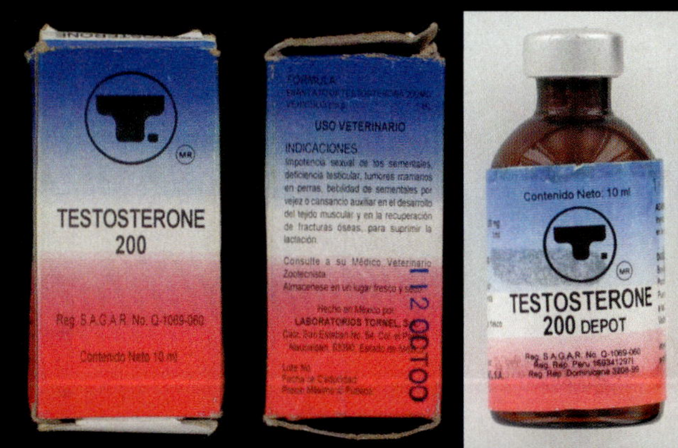

Older style packaging

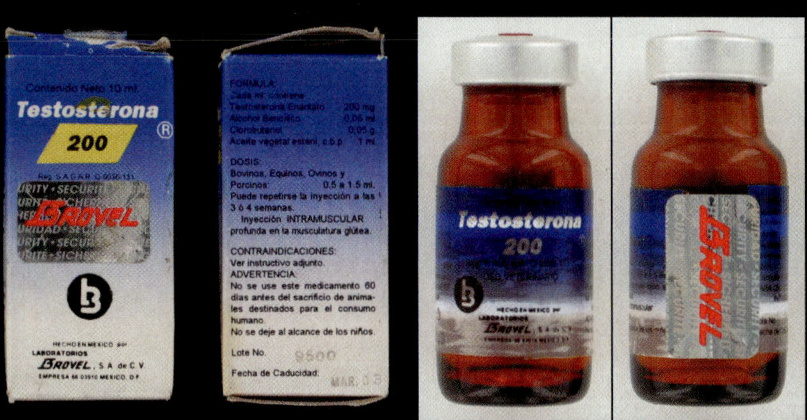

Brovel Testosterona 200 (Mexico)

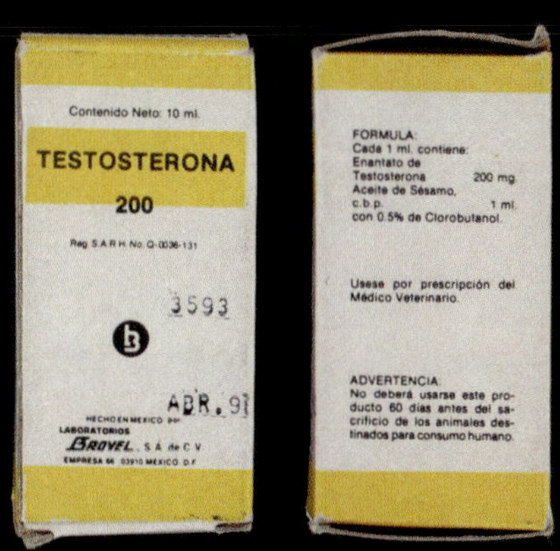

Very old packaging from Brovel

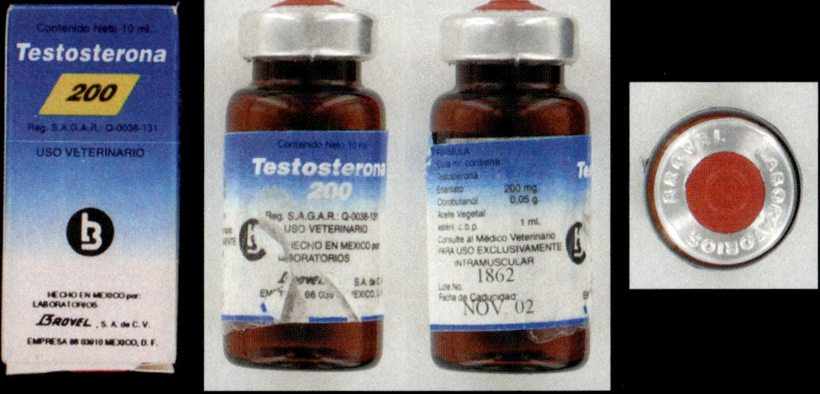

Brovel counterfeit #1

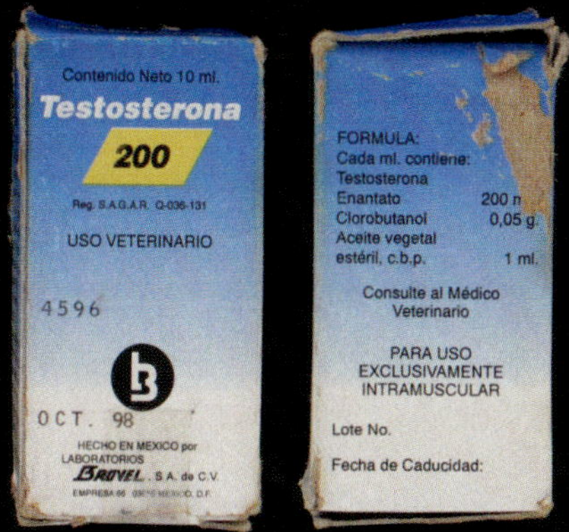

Counterfeit #2

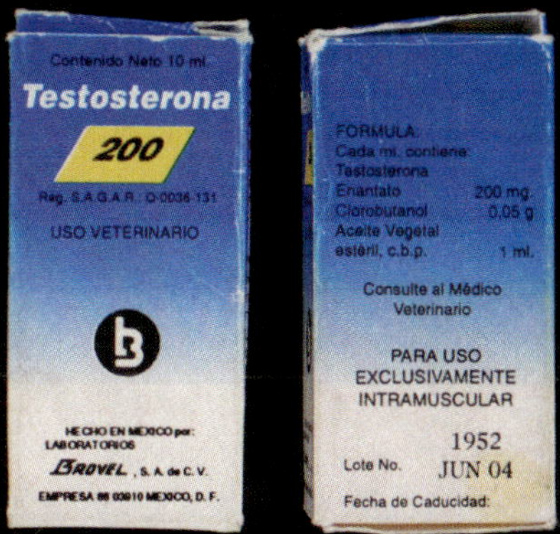

Counterfeit #3

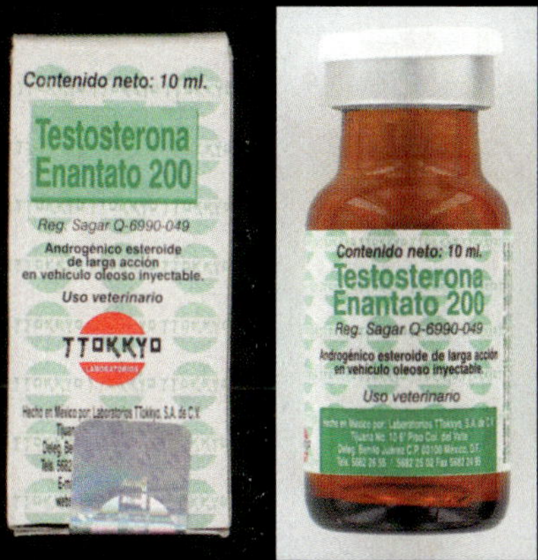

Enanthate from Ttokkyo Mexico (NLM)

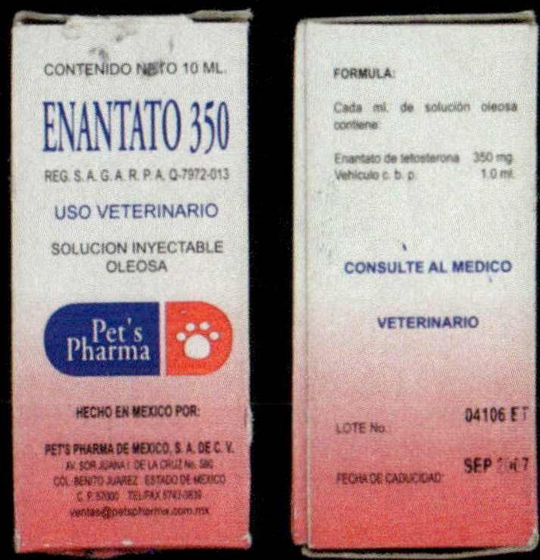

Pet's Pharma Enantato (Mexico)

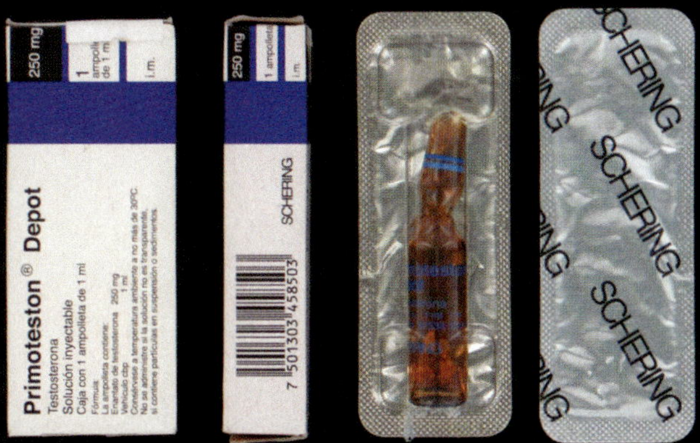

Primoteston Depot from Mexico

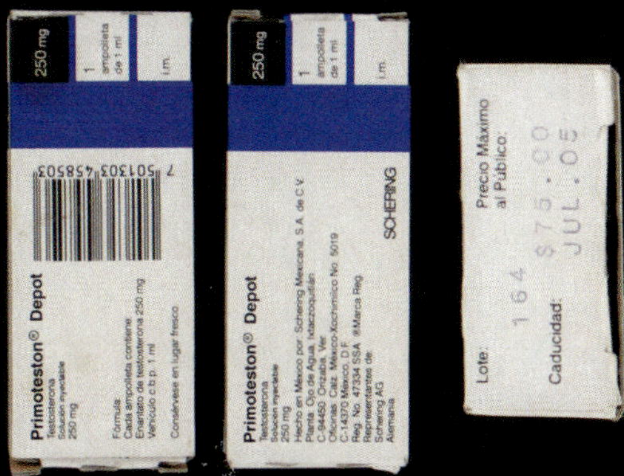

Older style Mexican box

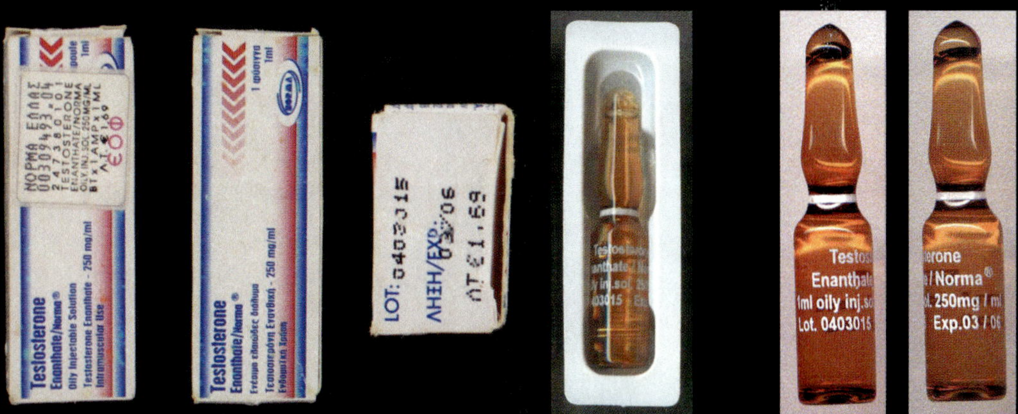

Enanthate from Norma Hellas Greece

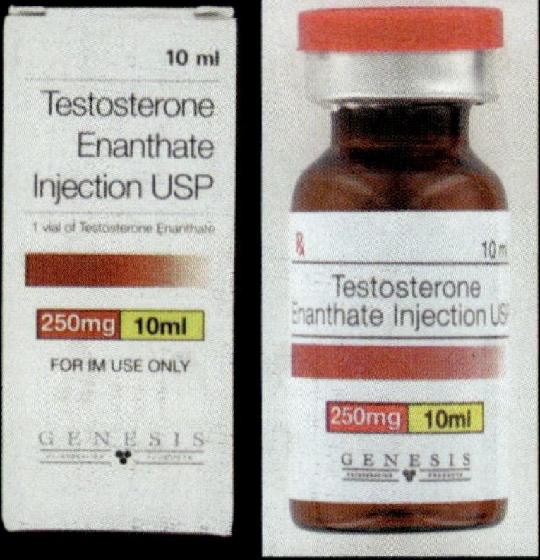

Generic from Singapore

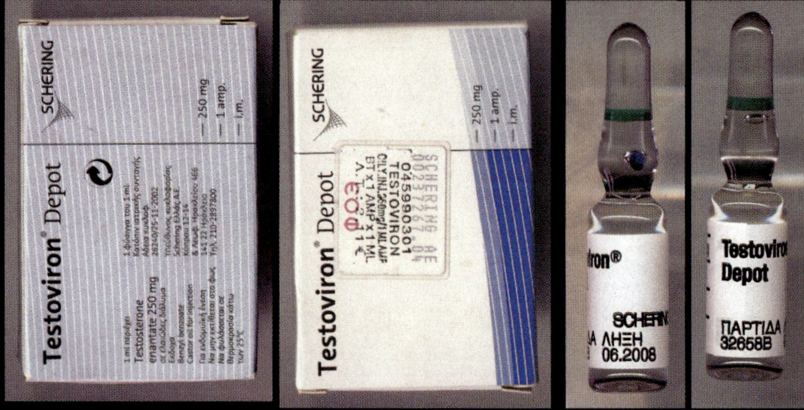

Greek Testoviron Depot

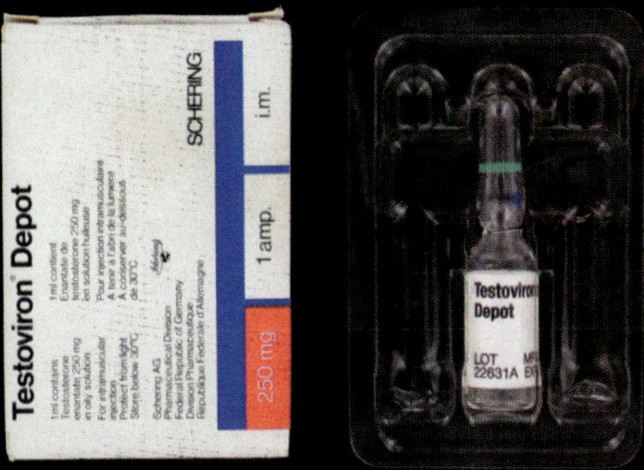

German Testoviron

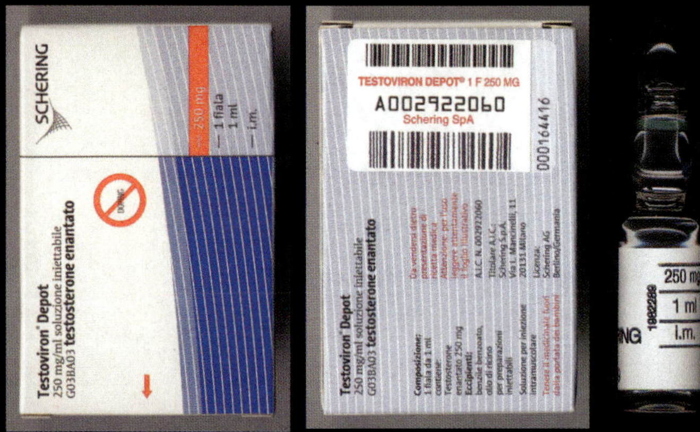

Italian box and ampule

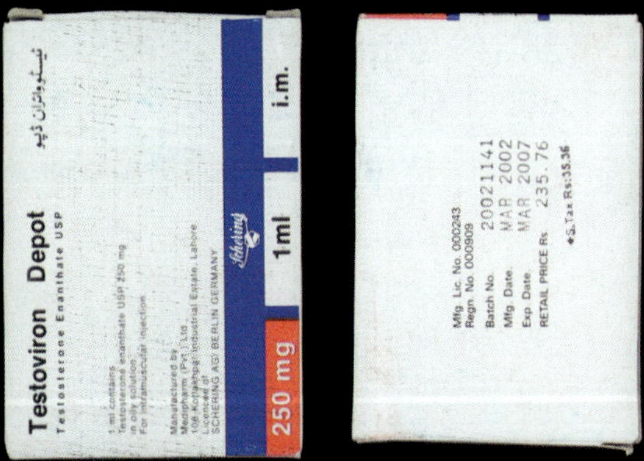

Testoviron from India

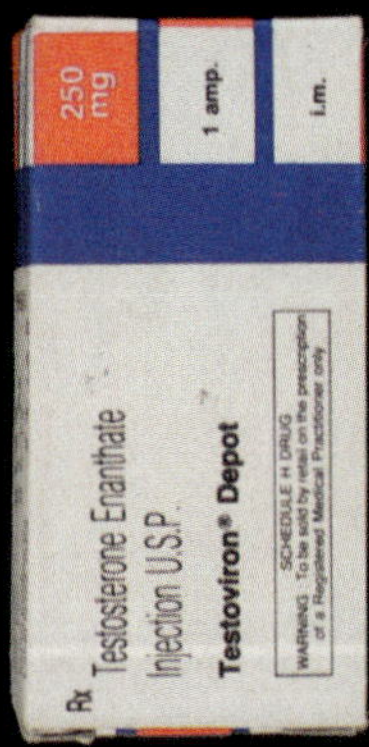

Older box from India

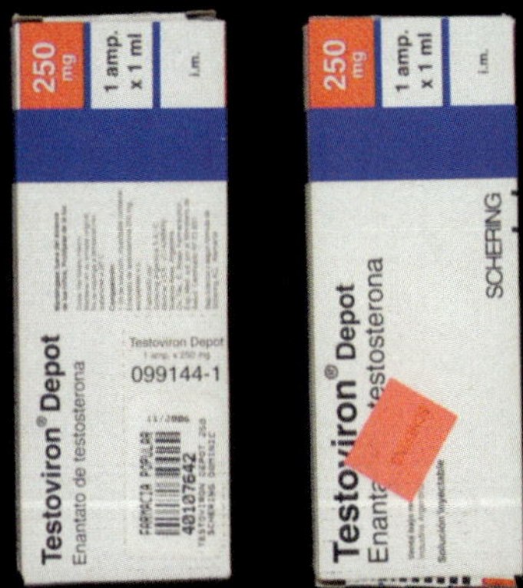

Testoviron from Argentina

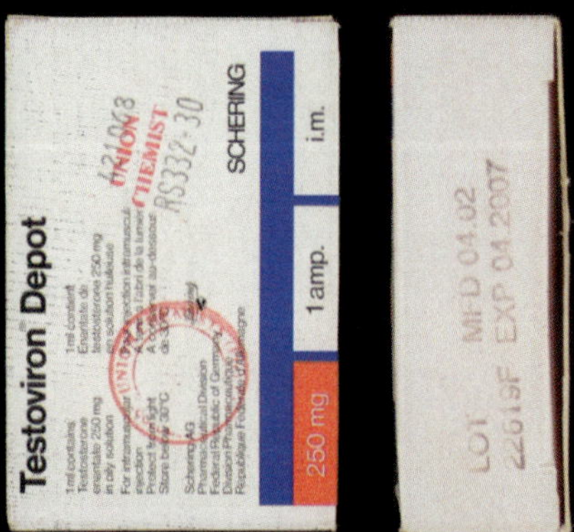

Box from Sri Lanka

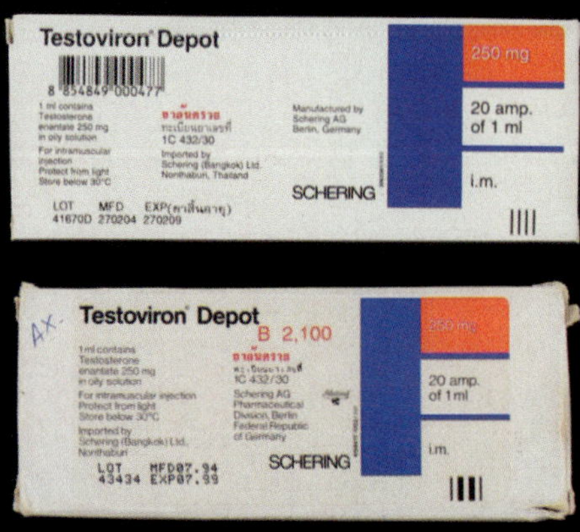

Thai packaging (new box on top)

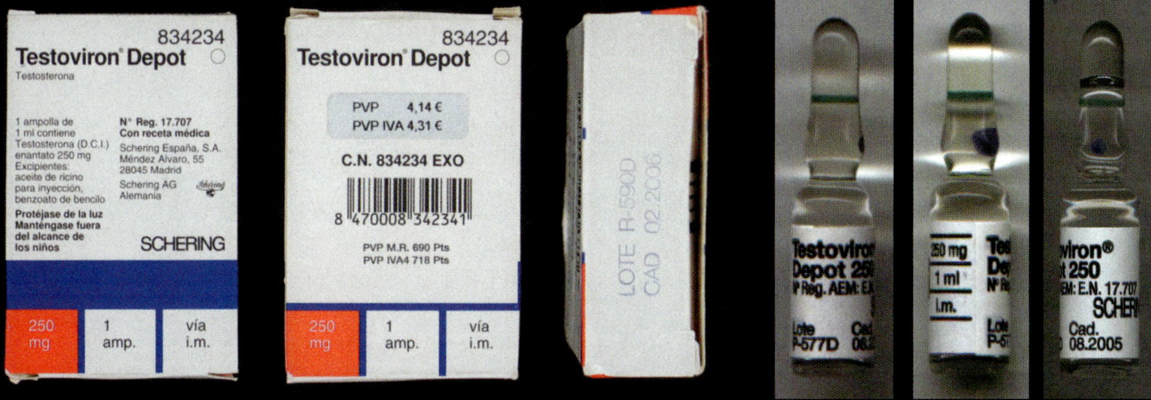

New look to Spanish Testoviron Depot (box and amp)

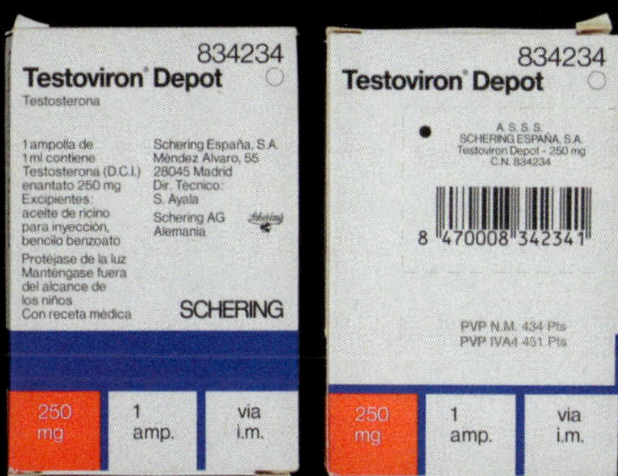

Older Spanish packaging

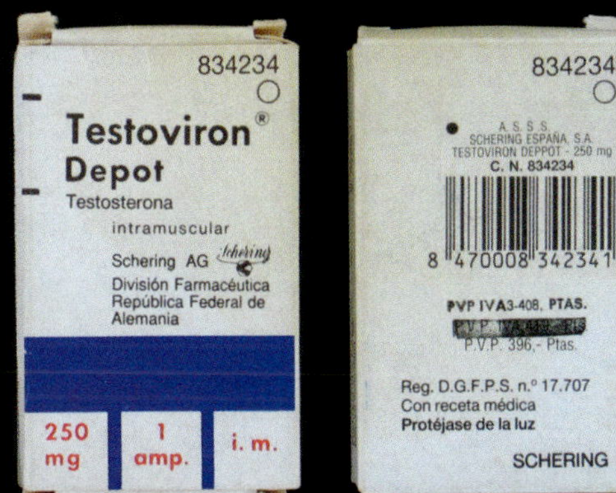

Very old Spanish box

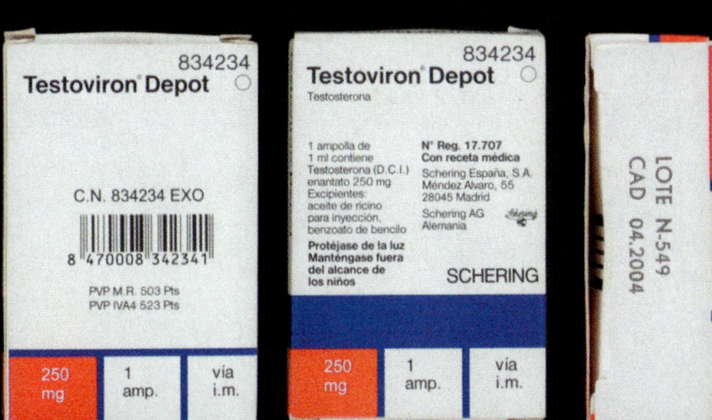

Counterfeit Spanish box

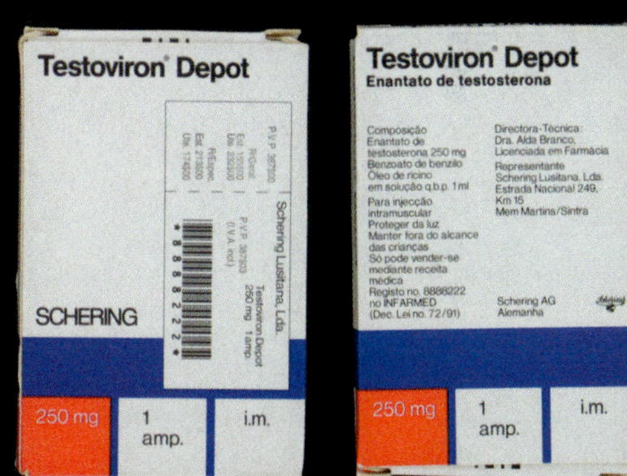

Testoviron from Portugal

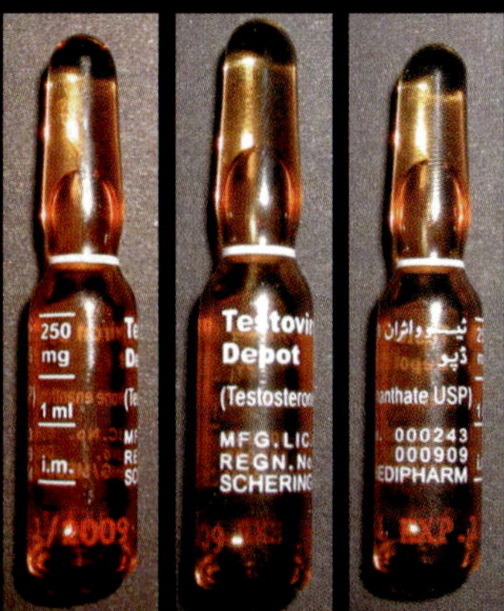

Ampules from Pakistan

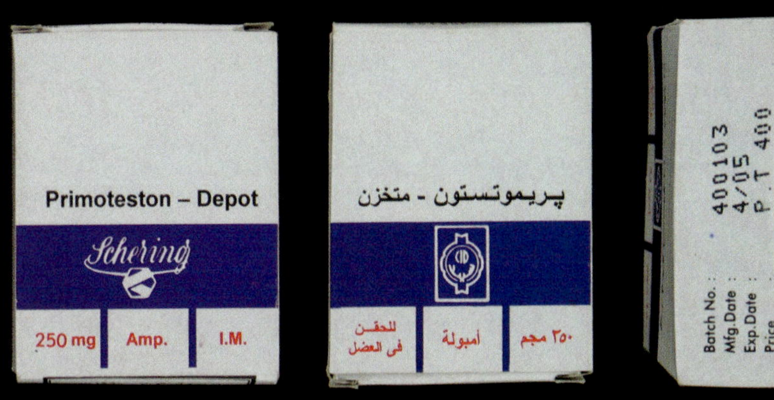

Primoteston-Depot from Schering/CID Egypt

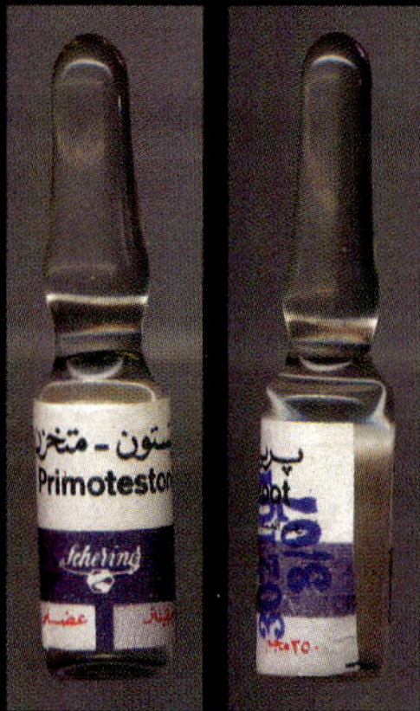

New Egyptian ampules

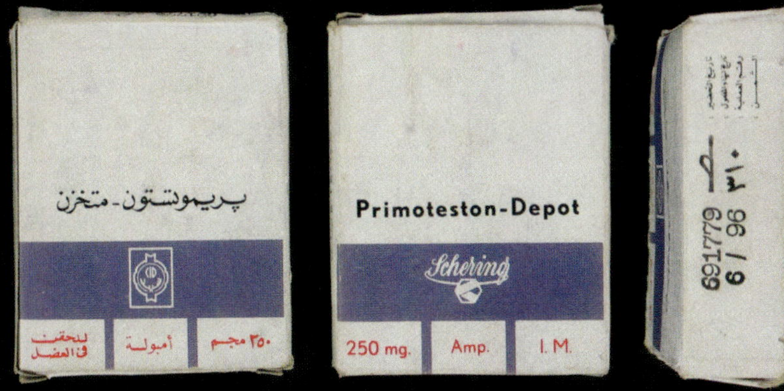

Older Egyptian box

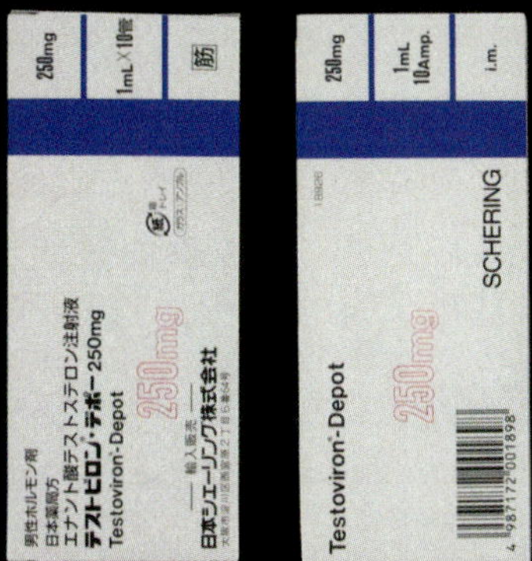

Testoviron from Japan

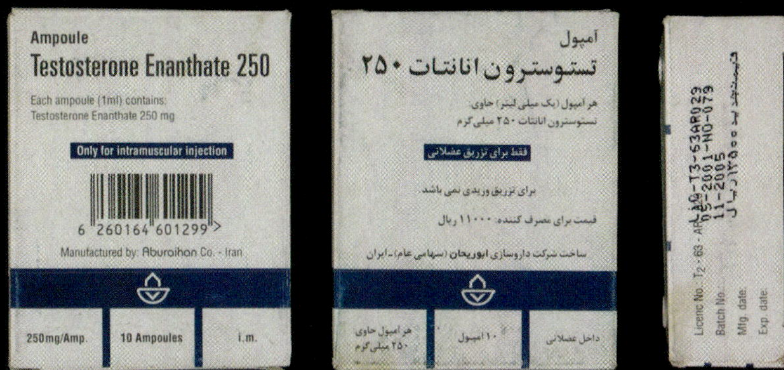

Enanthate from Iran

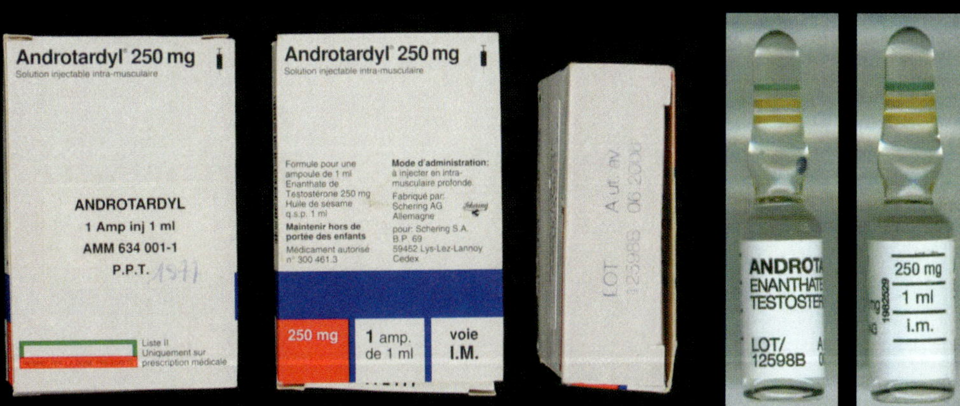

Androtardyl from France (box and ampule)

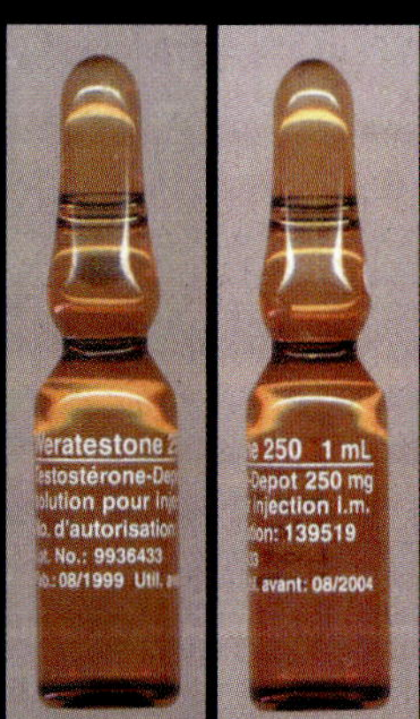

Weratestone (French export)

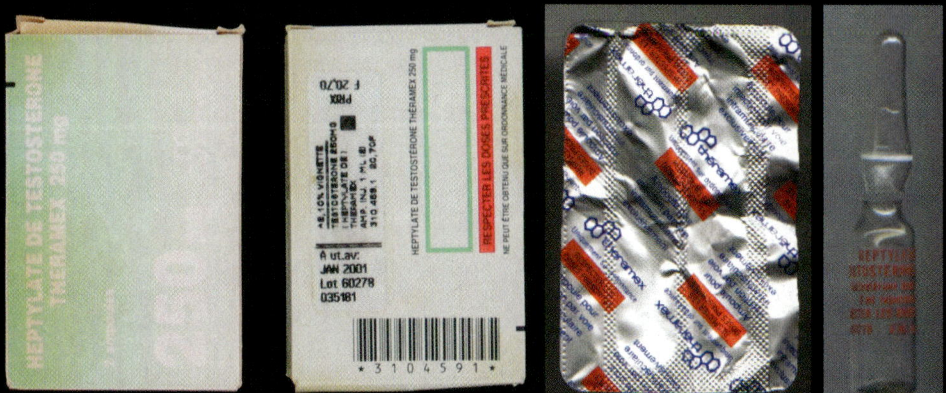

Testosterone Heptylate Theramex (enanthate from France)

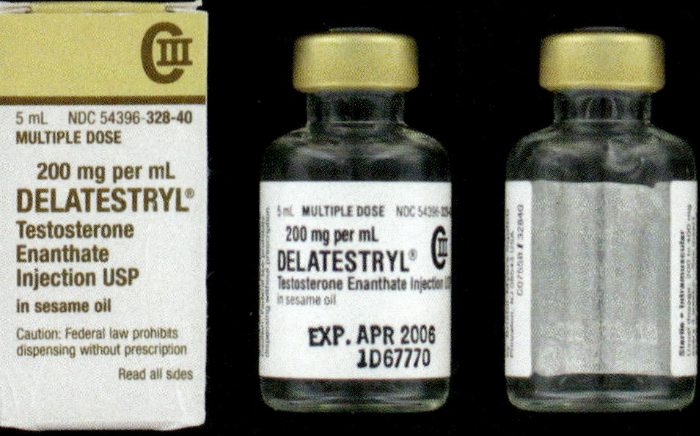

U.S. Delatestryl

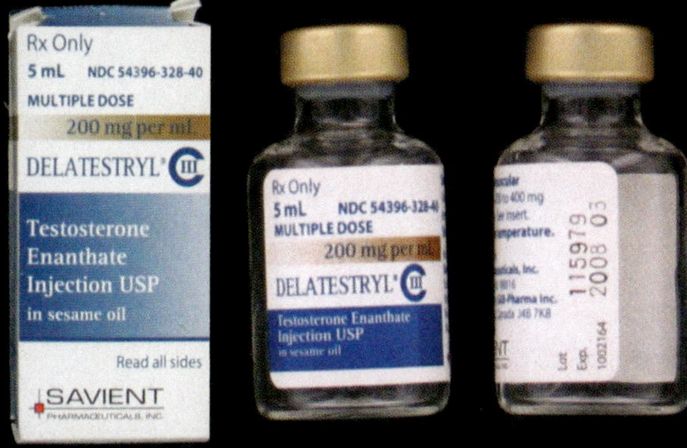

Delatestryl from Savient

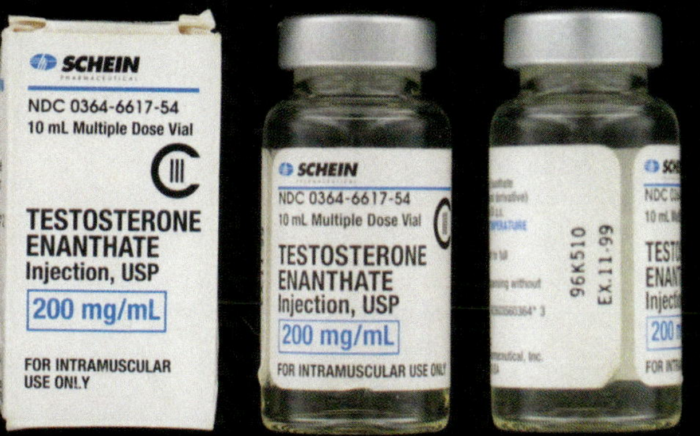

Generic from Schein (U.S.)

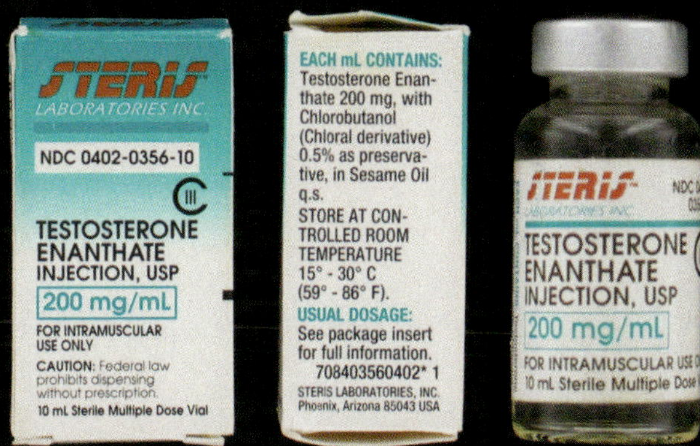

Counterfeit Steris box and vial

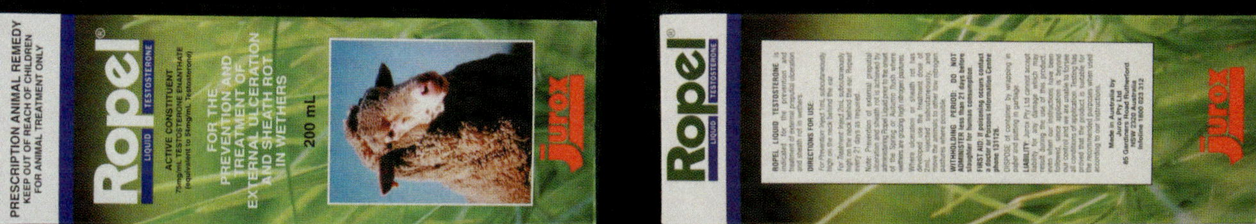

Ropel - Large-volume enanthate product from Jurox (Australia)

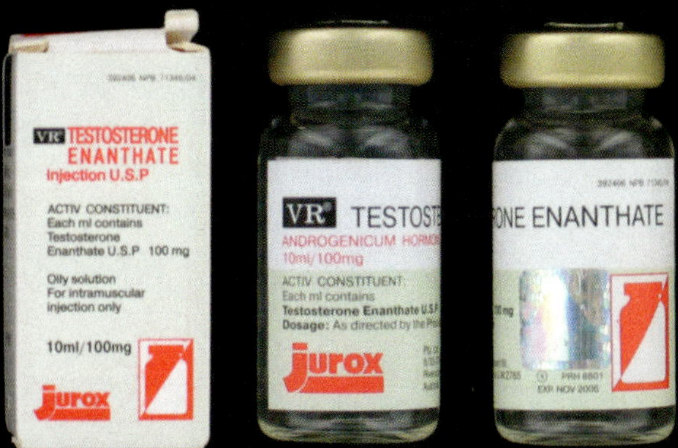

Jurox counterfeit - The real company has no hologram

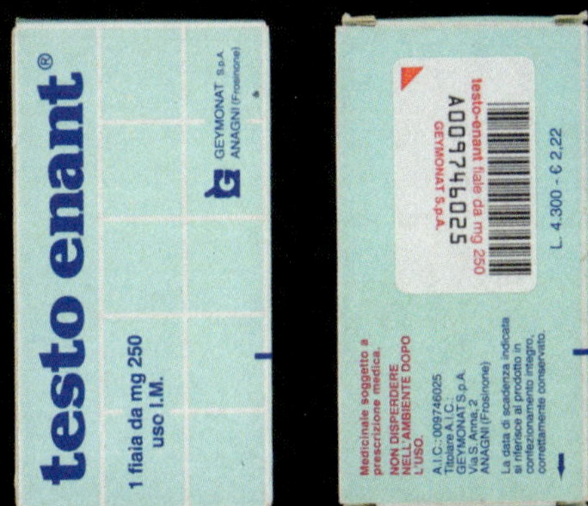

Testo Enant from Italy

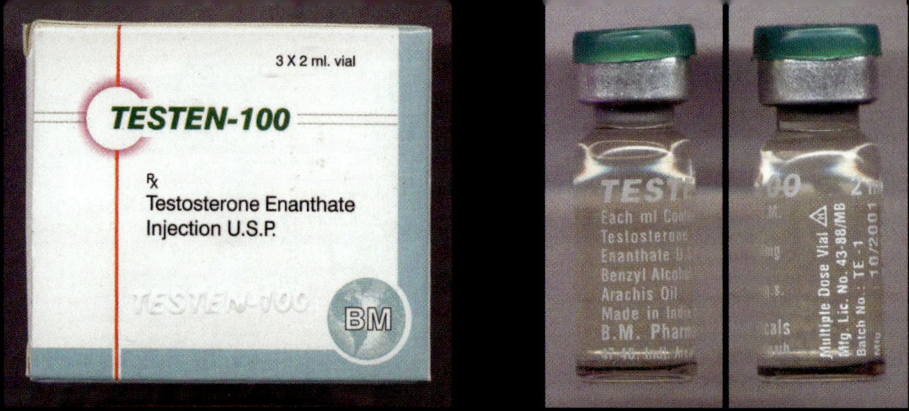

Testen-100 from BM Pharmaceuticals India

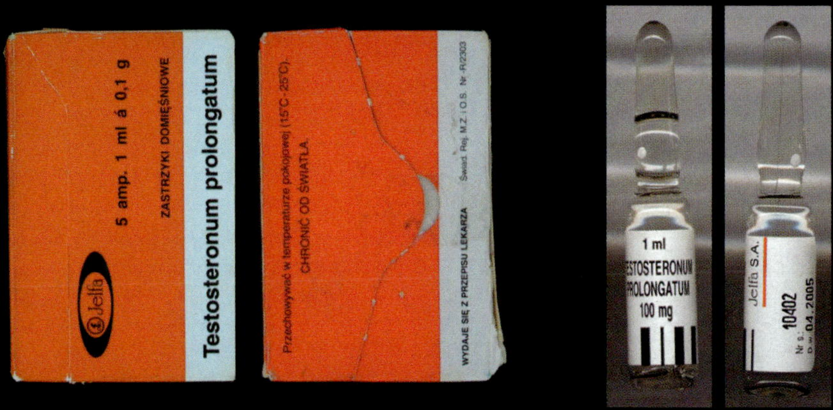

Testosteronum Prolongatum from Jelfa Poland

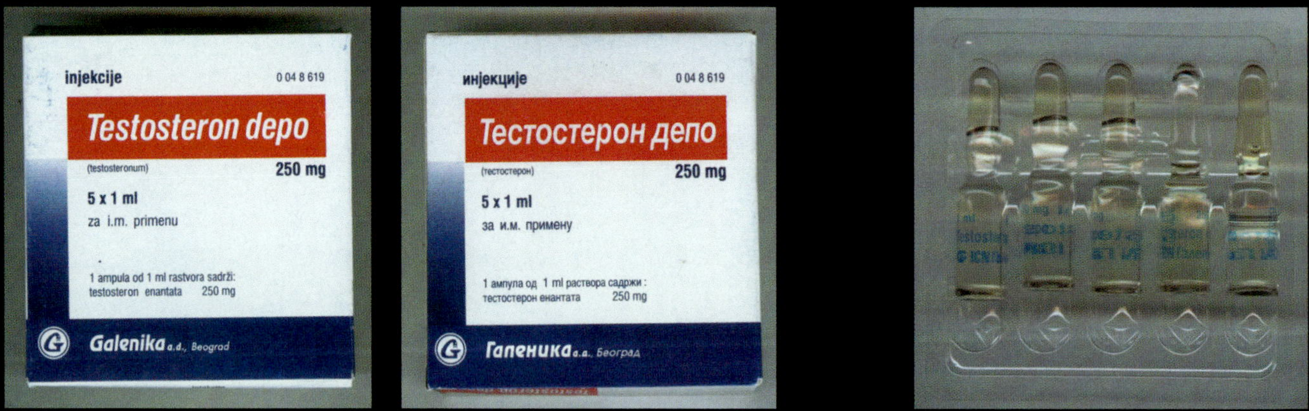

Testosteron Depo from Galenika Serbia (Former Yugoslavia)

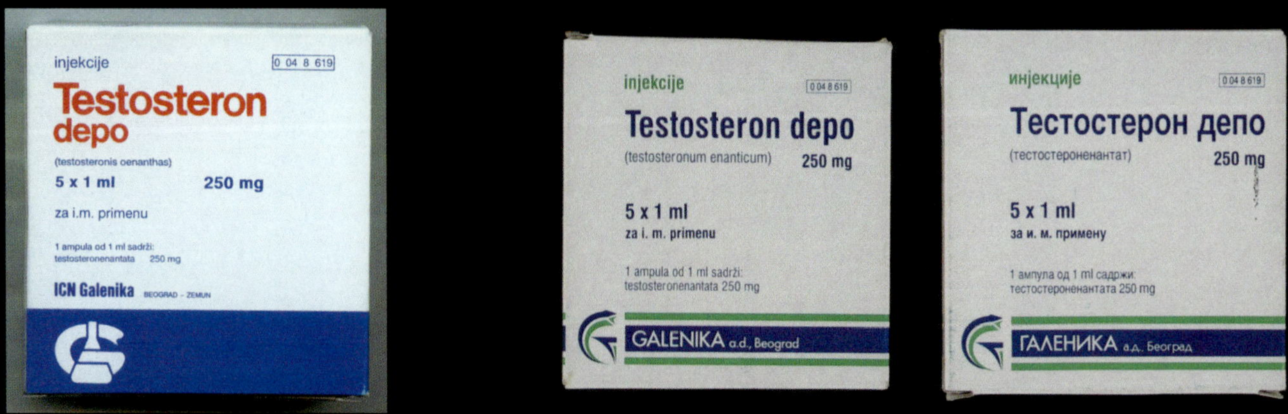

Two older style boxes from Galenika

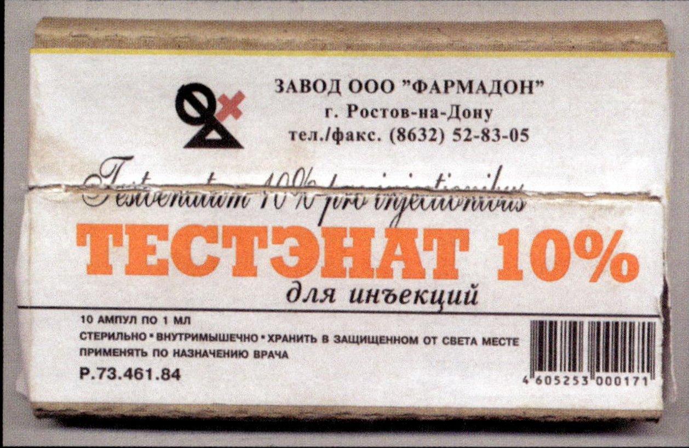

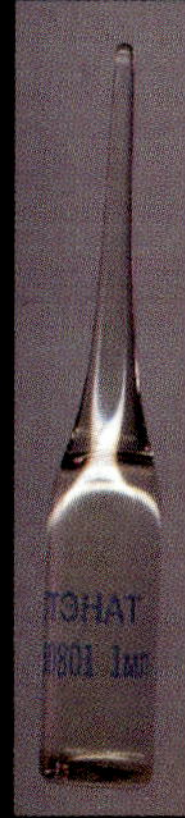

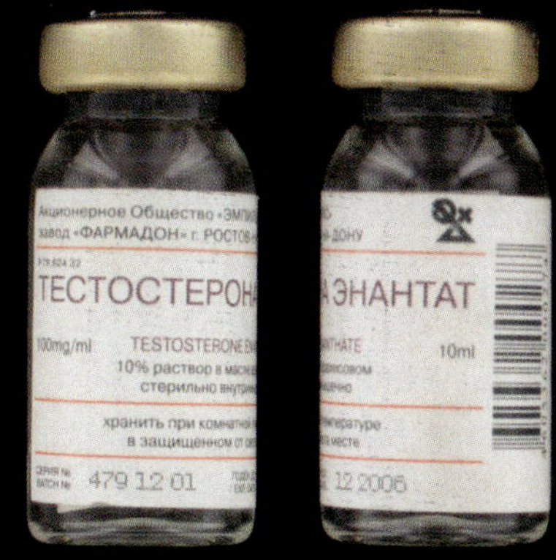

Testenat 10% by Farmadon (Russia)

Counterfeit Farmadon vial

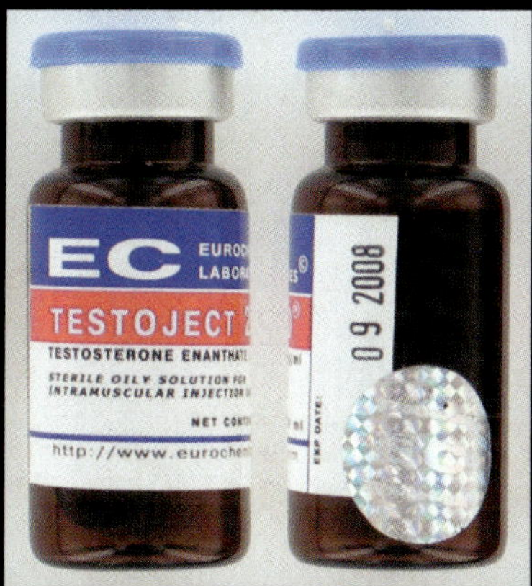

Eurochem vial (UG product)

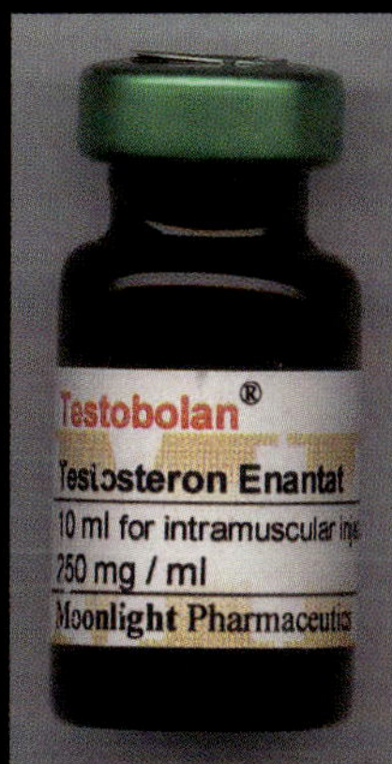

UG Moonlight vial

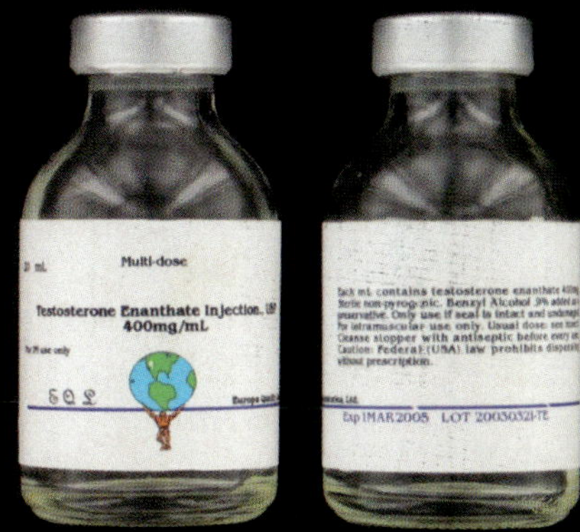

UG Europa enanthate

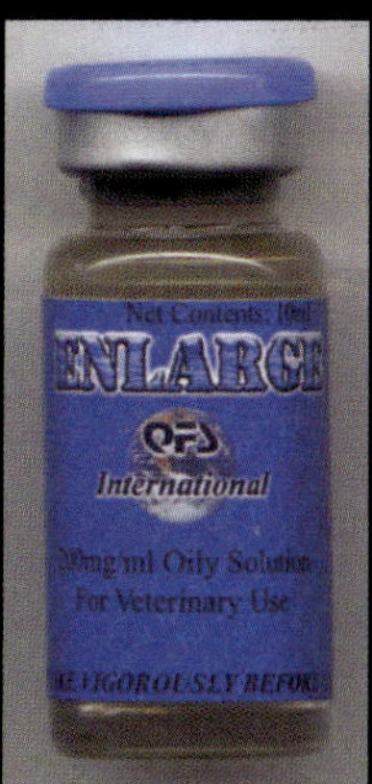

QFS UG product

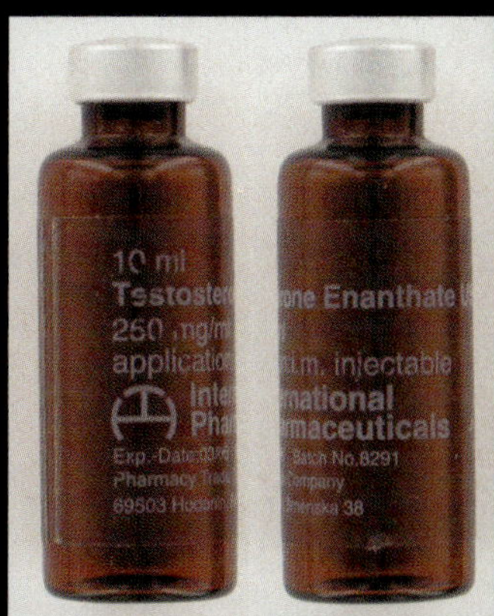

Counterfeit of the IP UG product

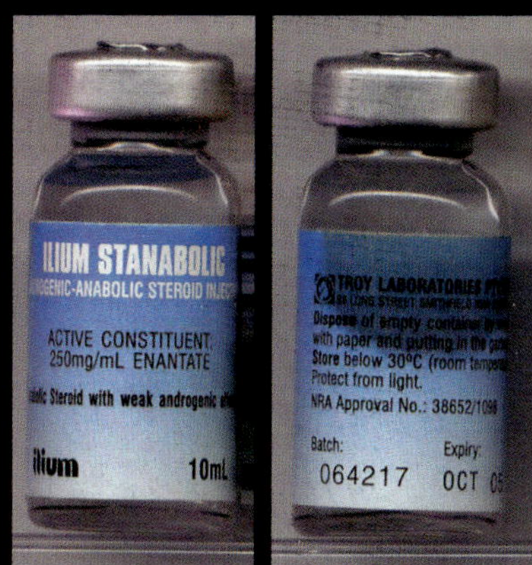

Counterfeit Stanabolic

T.Propionate

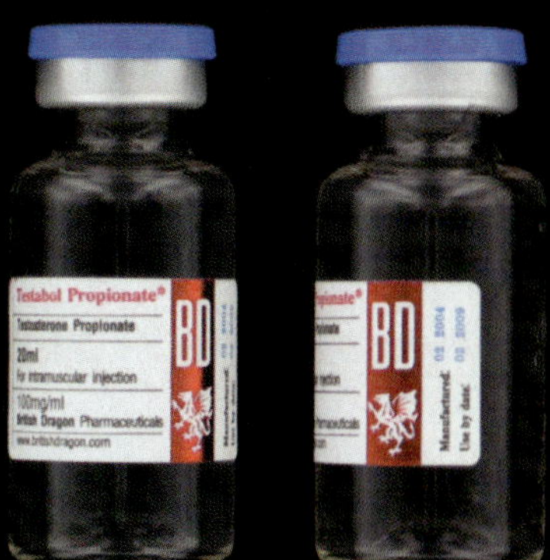

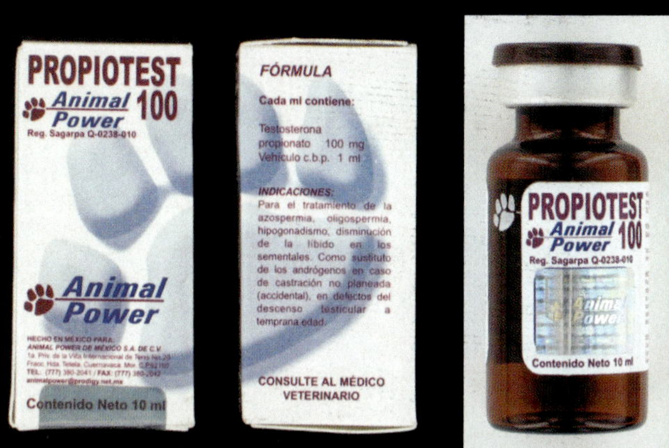

Propionate from British Dragon (Thailand)

Propiotest 100 from Animal Power (Mexico)

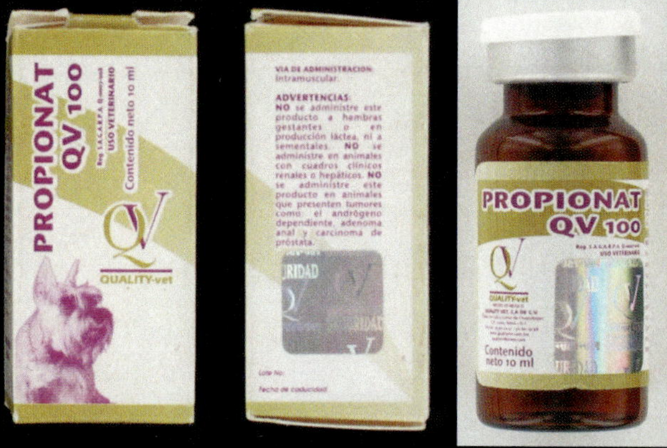

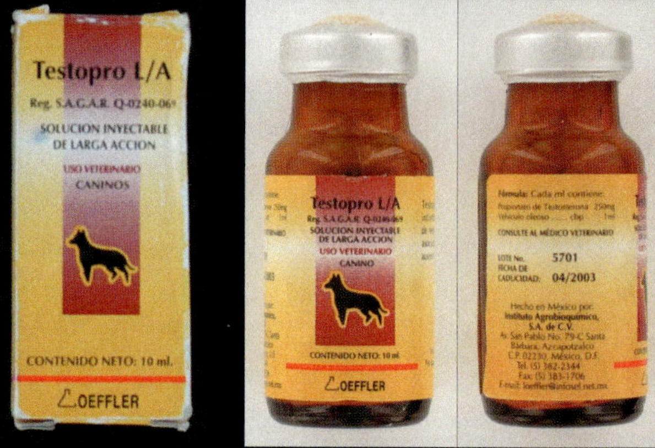

Propionat from Quality Vet (Mexico)

Testopro 250mg/mL product from Loeffler (Mexico)

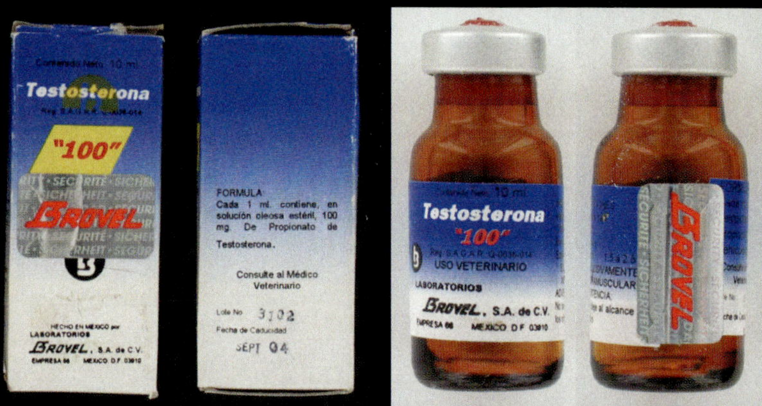

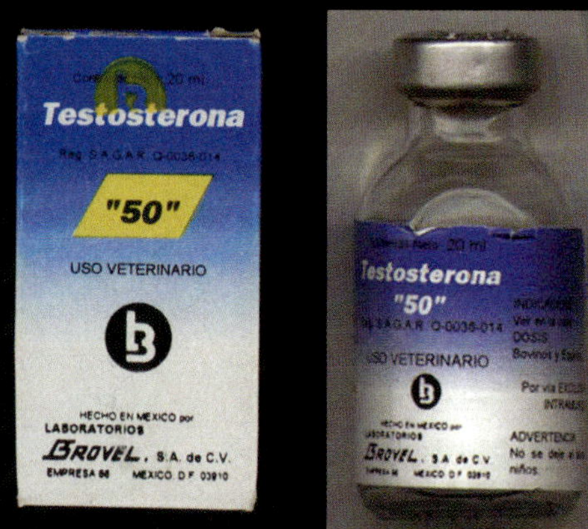

Testosterona “100” from Brovel (Mexico)

50mg/mL version from Brovel

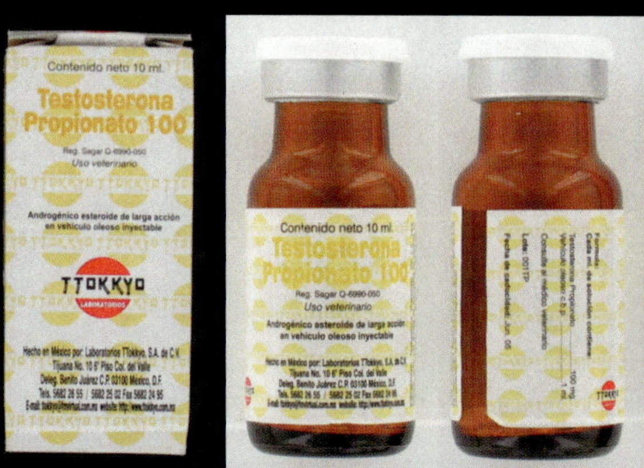

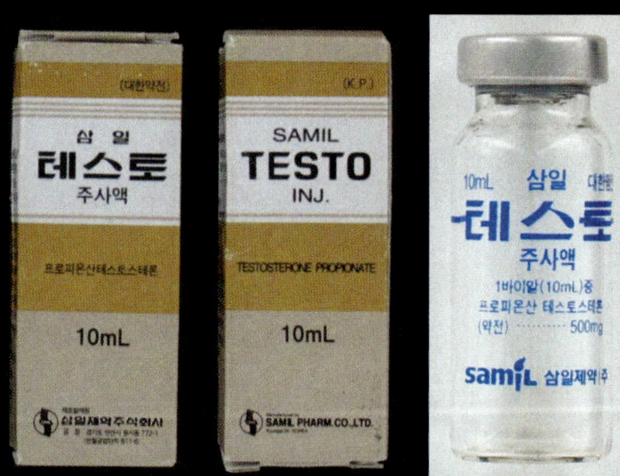

Mexican propionate from Ttokkyo (NLM)

Propionate from Samil Korea

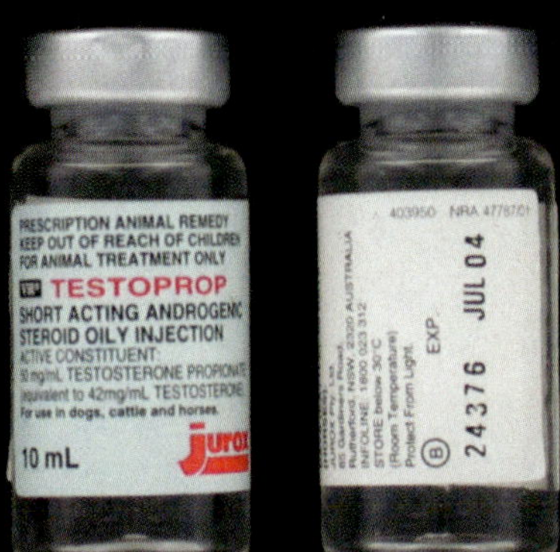

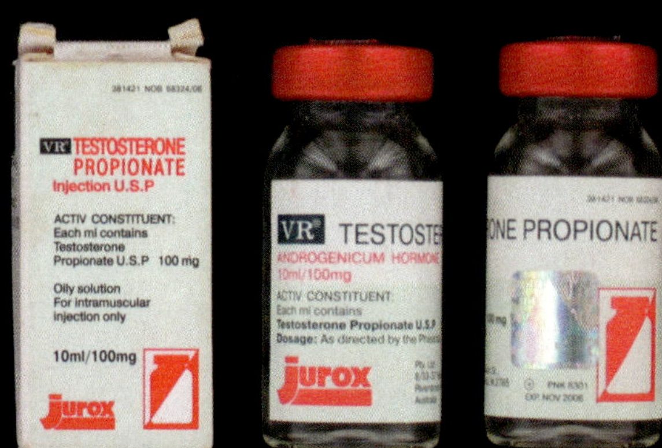

Jurox Testoprop

Counterfeit Jurox product with fabricated hologram

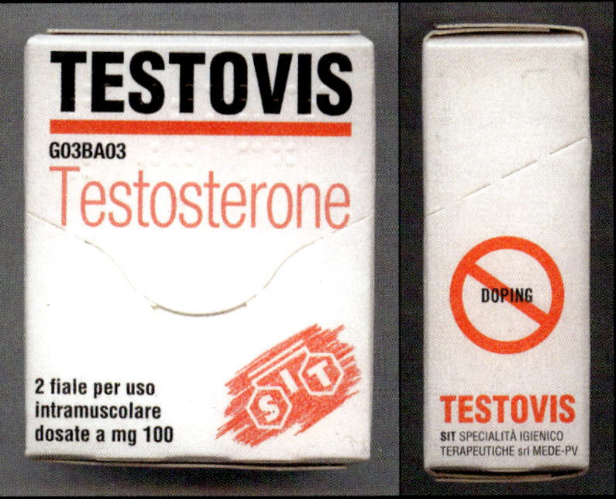

New Italian Testovis

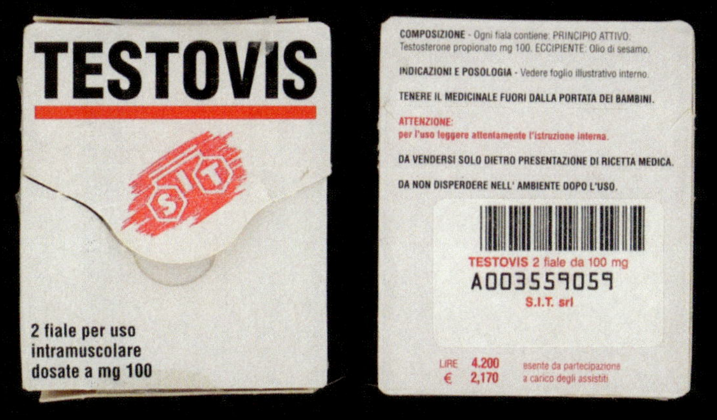

Previous box

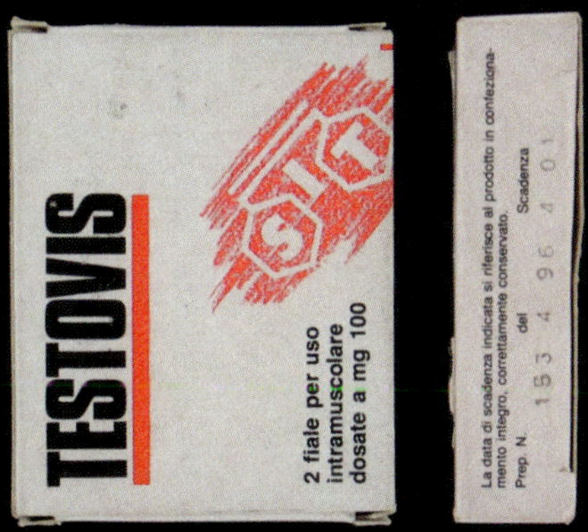

Very old Italian box

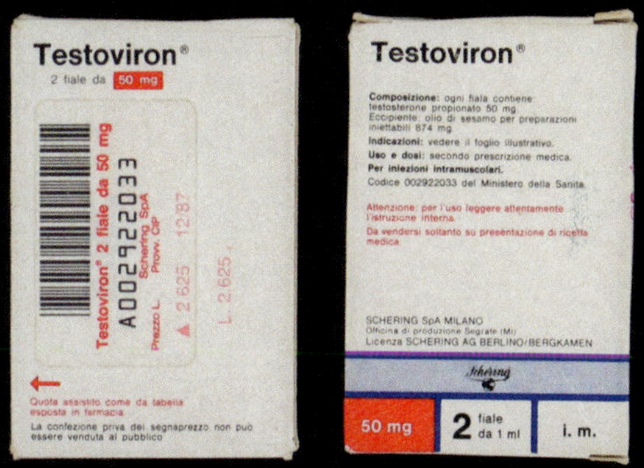

Italian Testoviron (NLM)

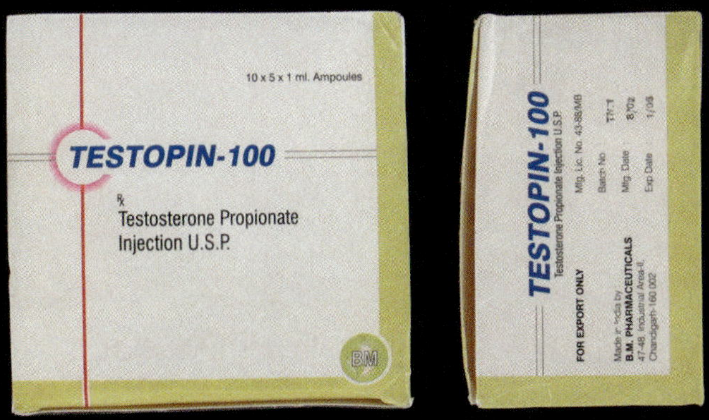

Testopin-100 from BM India - 50 amp box

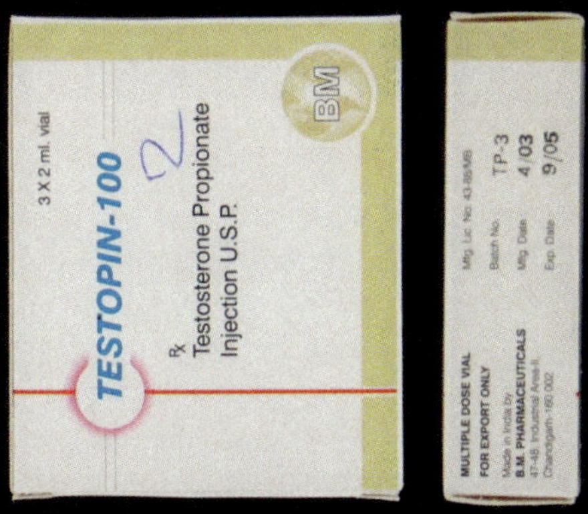

Testopin-100 version in 2ml vials

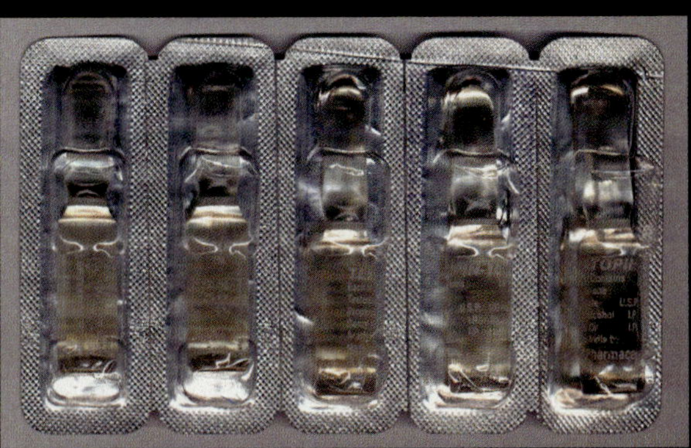

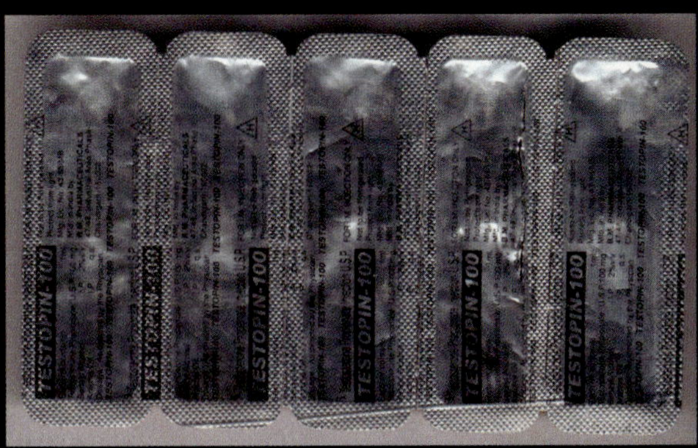

Testopin-100 ampules

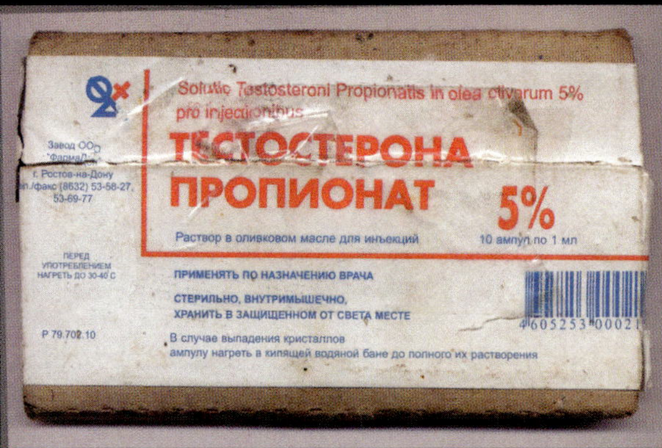

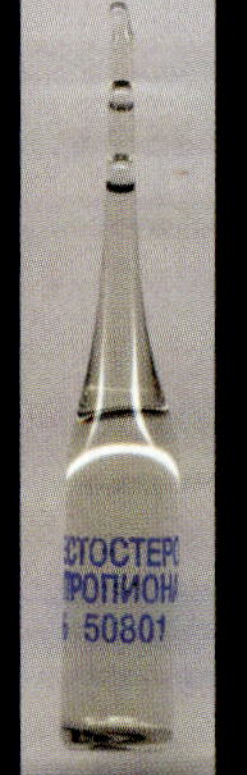

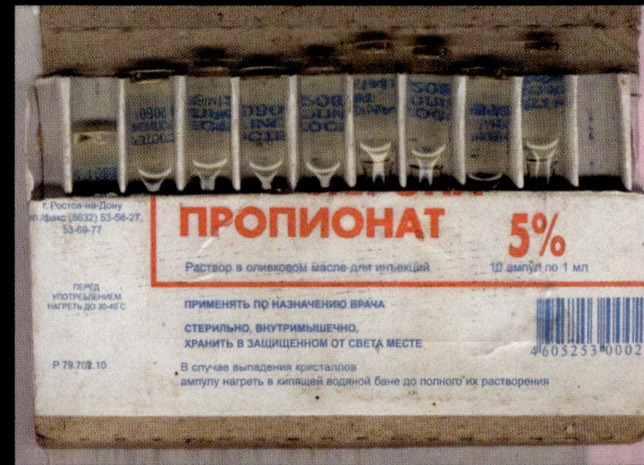

Russian propionate from Farmadon

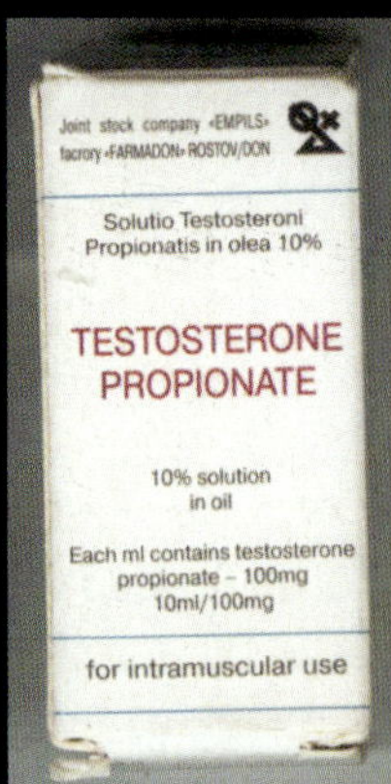

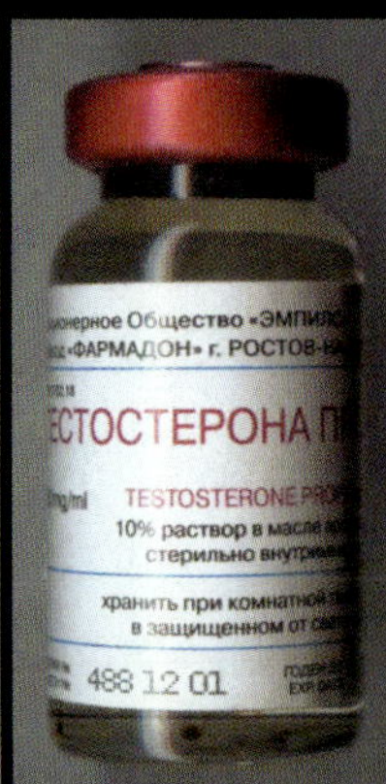

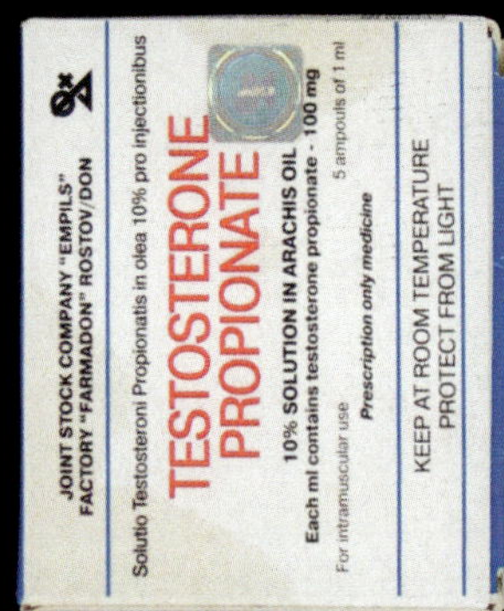

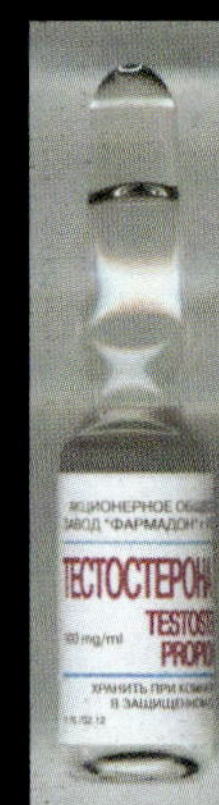

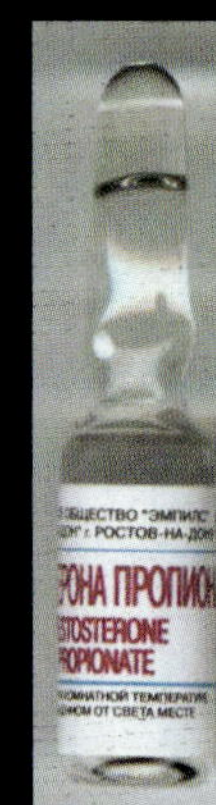

Two different counterfeits of Farmadon propionate

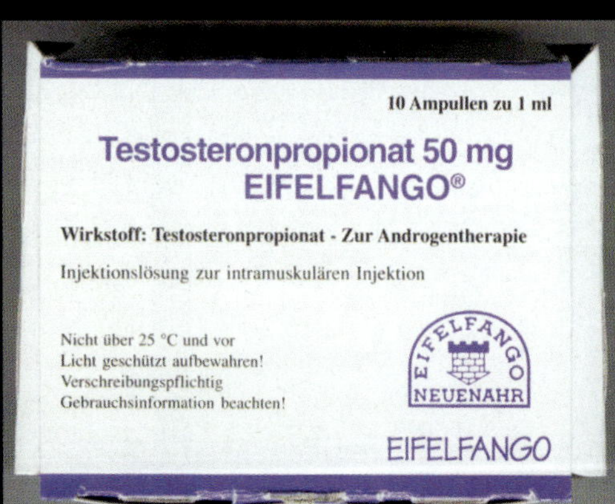

German Eifelfango box

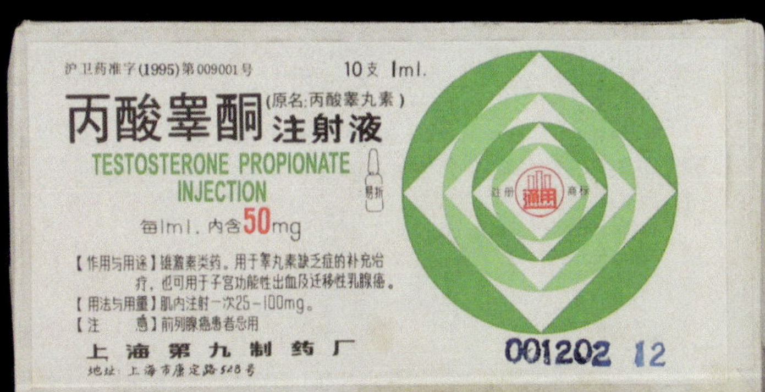

Generic from China

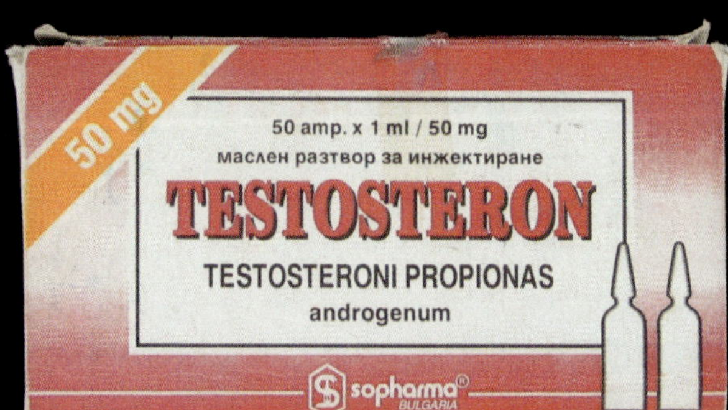

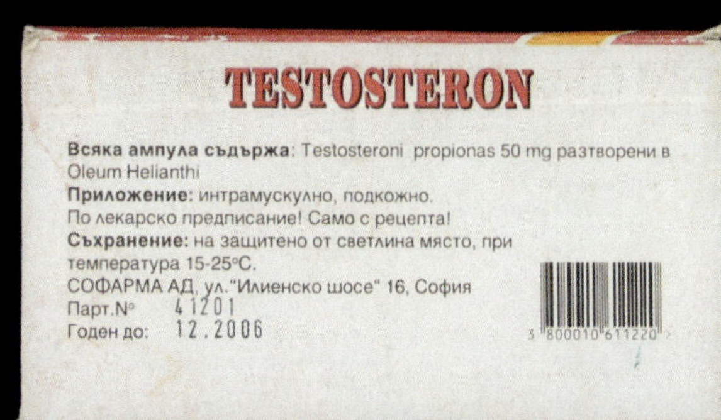

Testosteron 50mg/mL product from Bulgaria

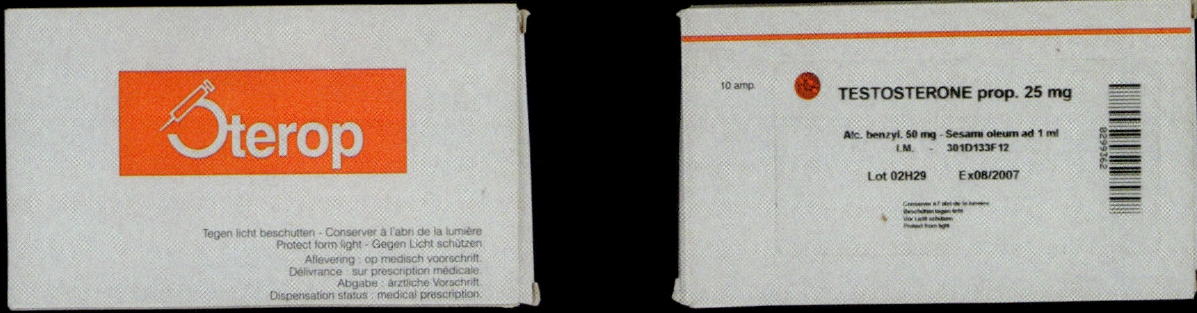

Sterop from Belgium

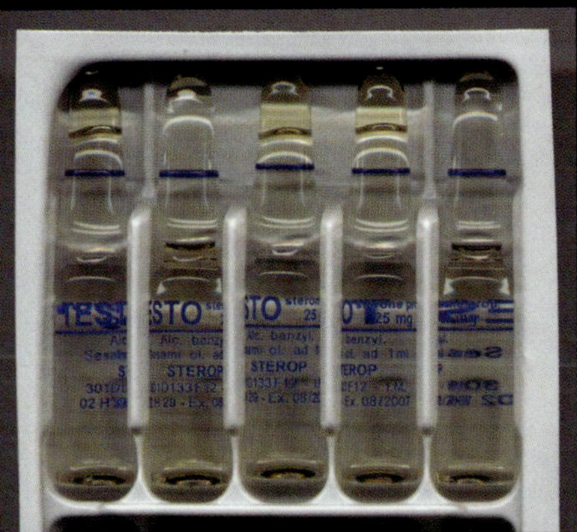

Sterop ampules

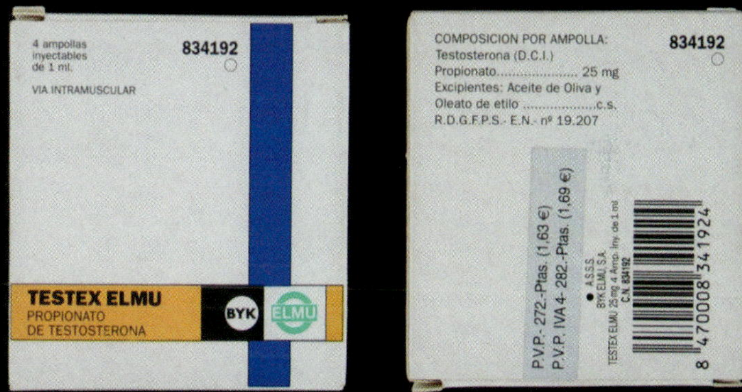

Testex from Spain

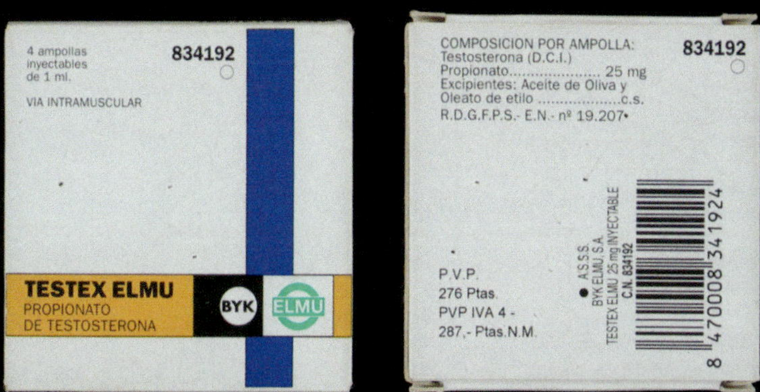

Older packaging - before the Euro pricing was added

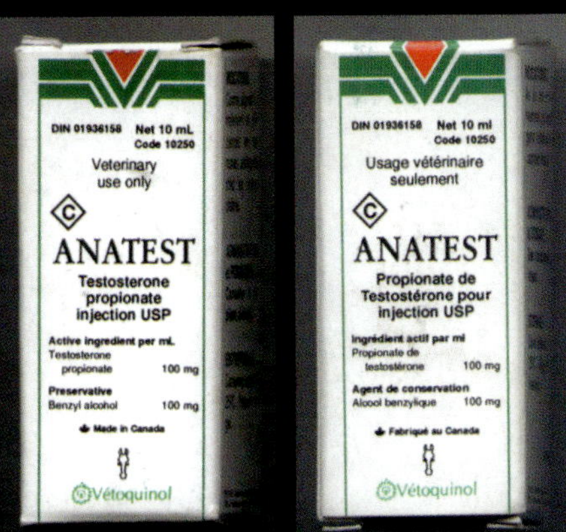

Anatest from Canada

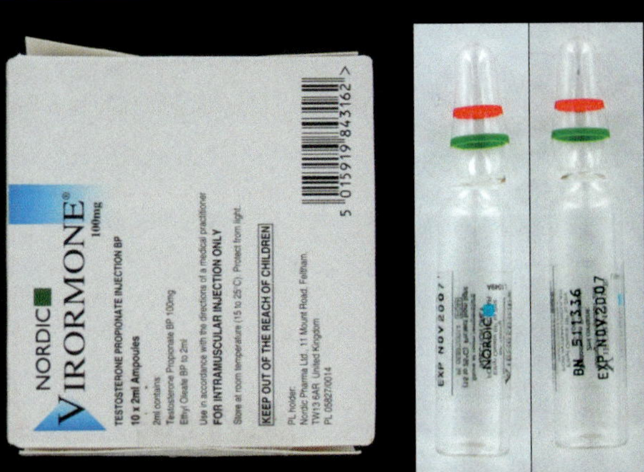

Virormone from Nordic (UK)

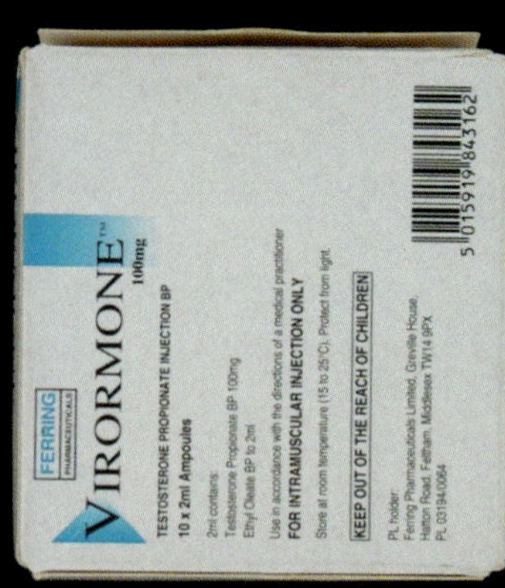

Old Ferring packaging

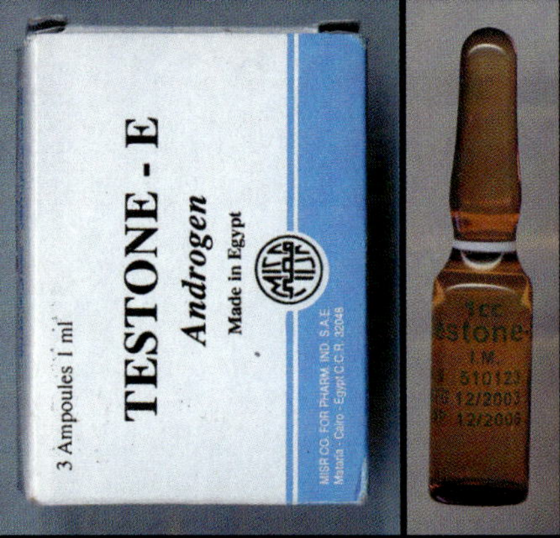

Testone-E box and amp from Egypt

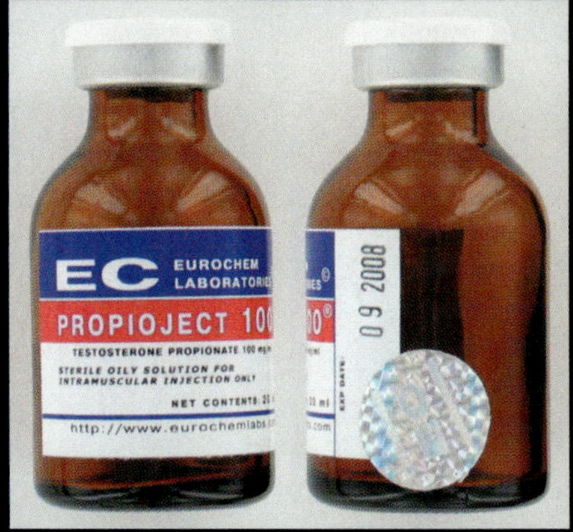

Eurochem - Underground product

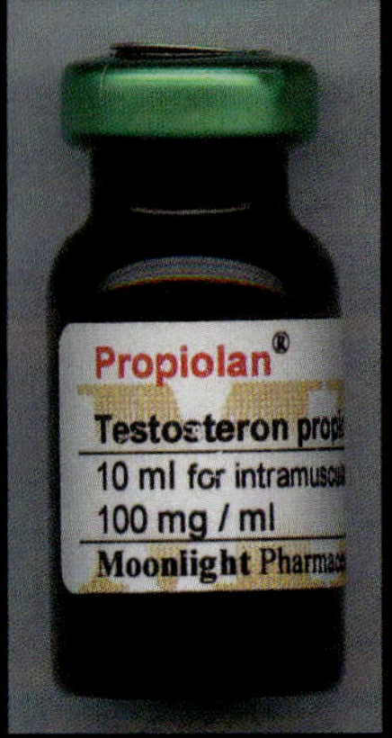

UG Moonlight vial

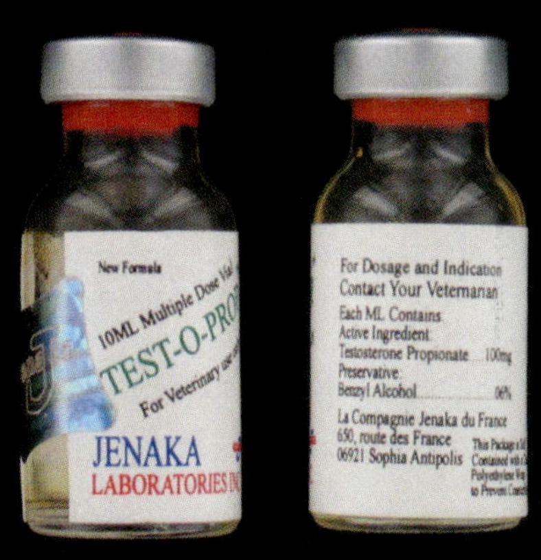

Jenaka UG vial (NLM)

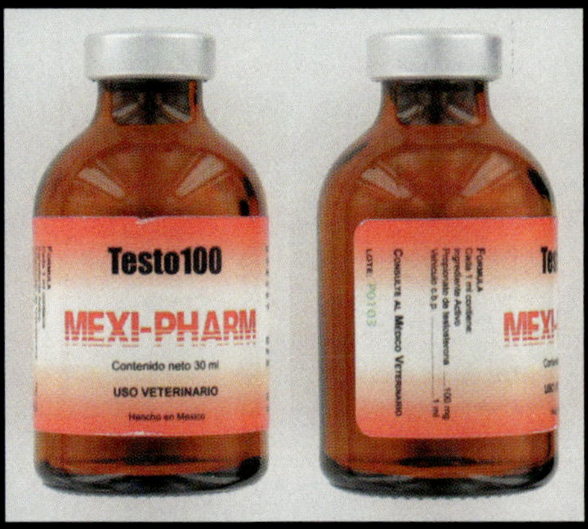

Mexi-pharm - Underground product

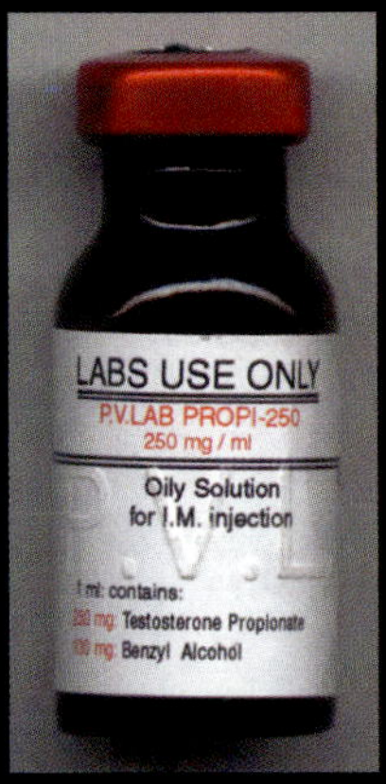

PVL - UG vial

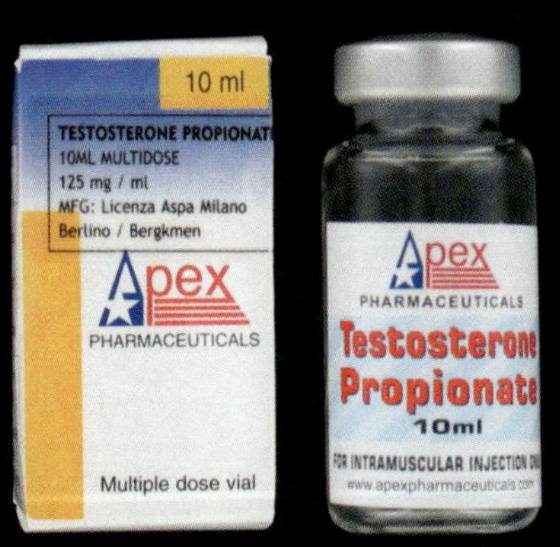

UG Apex box and vial

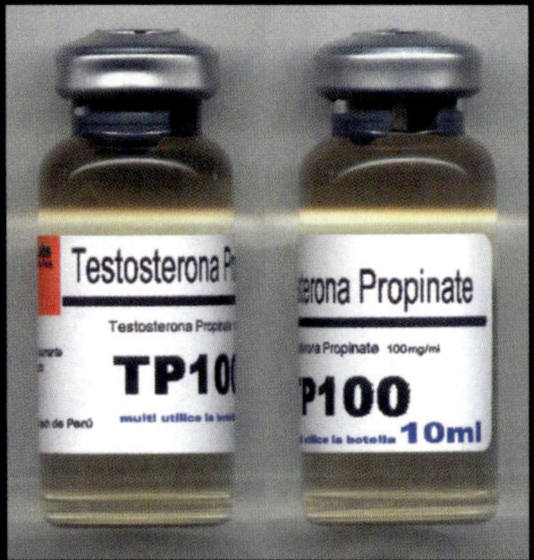

TP-100 from Peru - UG

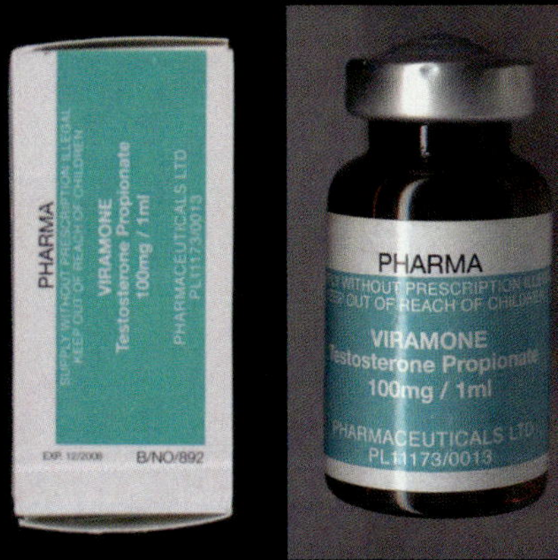

Pharma UG product

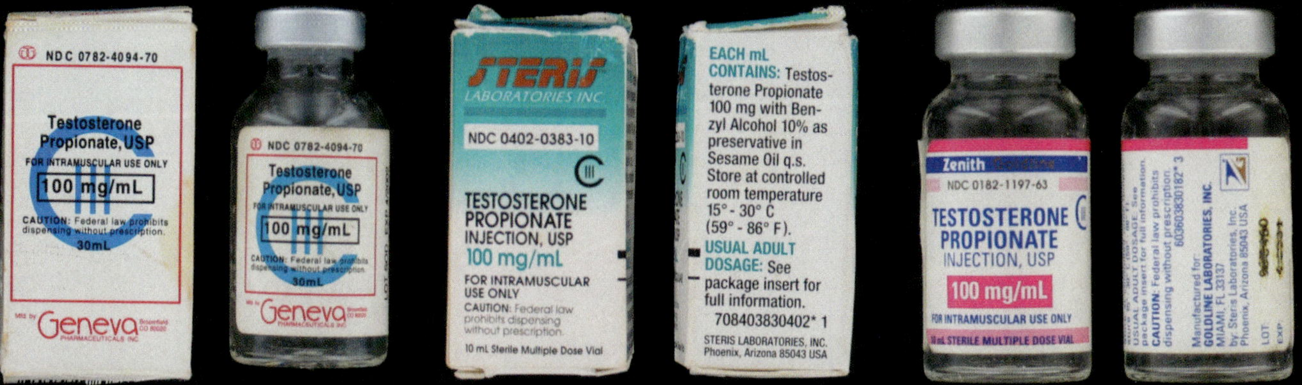

Three different counterfeit U.S. propionate products

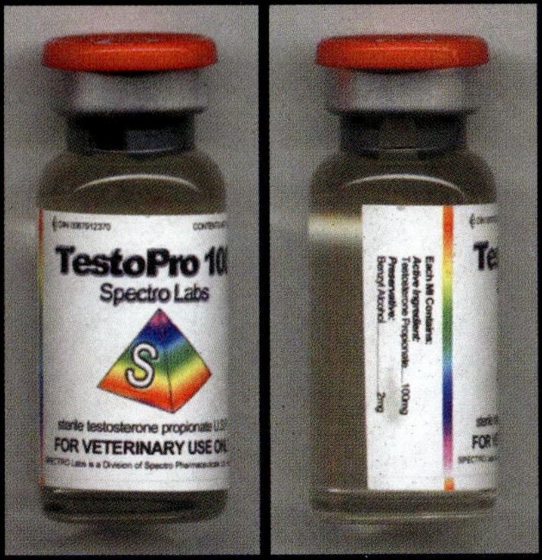

UG product from Spectro (NLM)

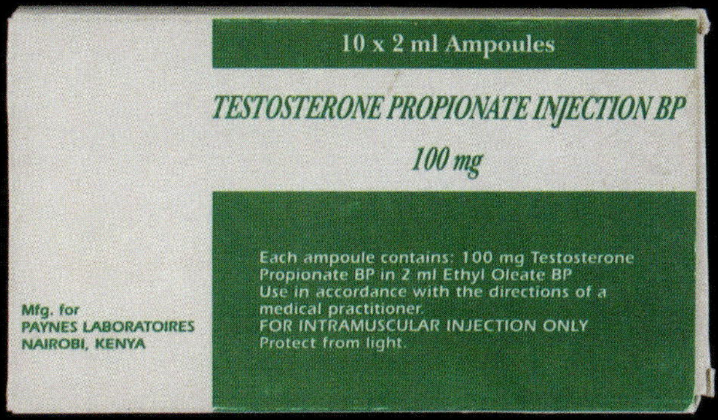

Counterfeit product from Paynes

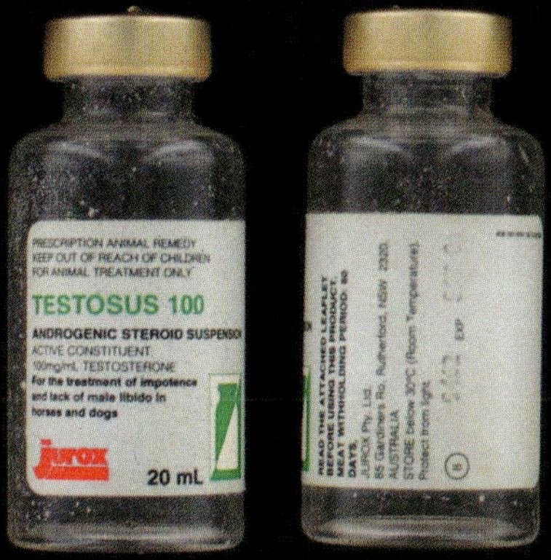

Testosus from Jurox Australia (NLM)

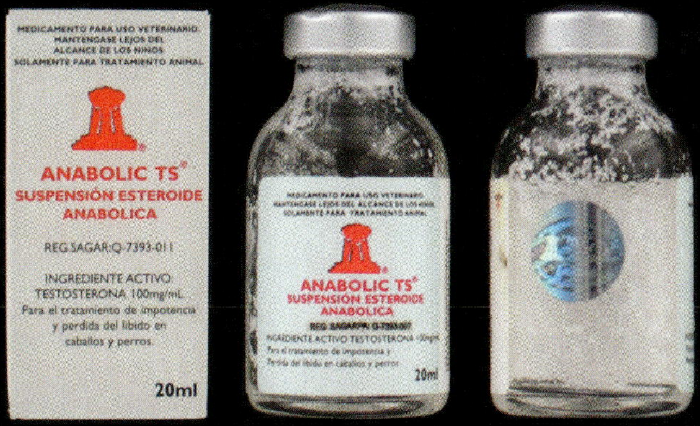

Anabolic TS - The old Grupo label (NLM)

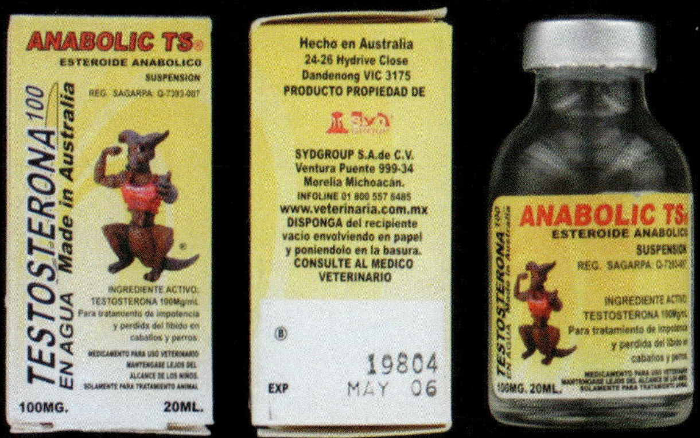

Anabolic TS from SYD Group (Mexico)

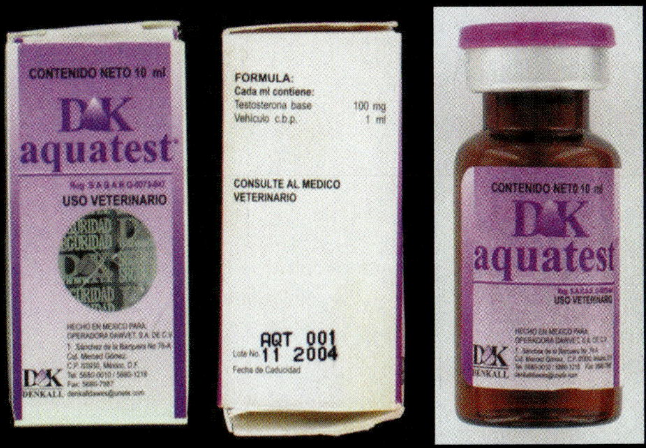

Denkall Aquatest (Mexico)

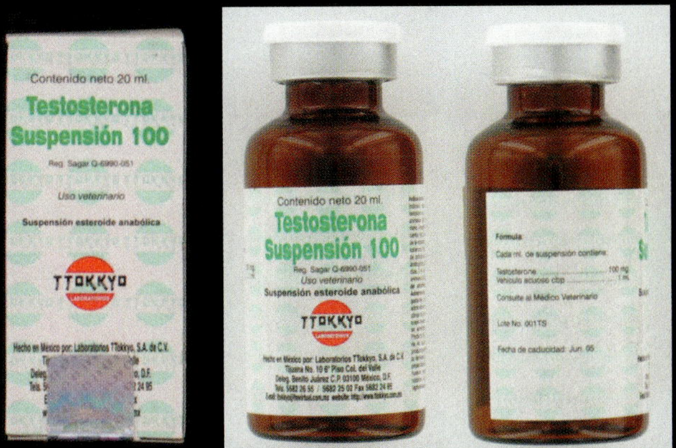

Ttokkyo suspension from Mexico (NLM)

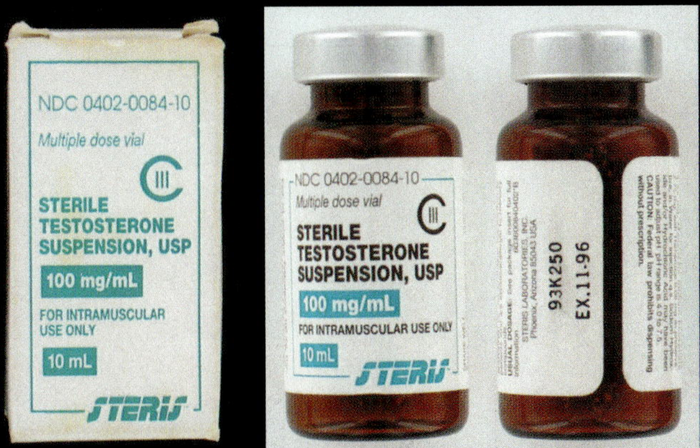

U.S. generic from Steris (NLM)

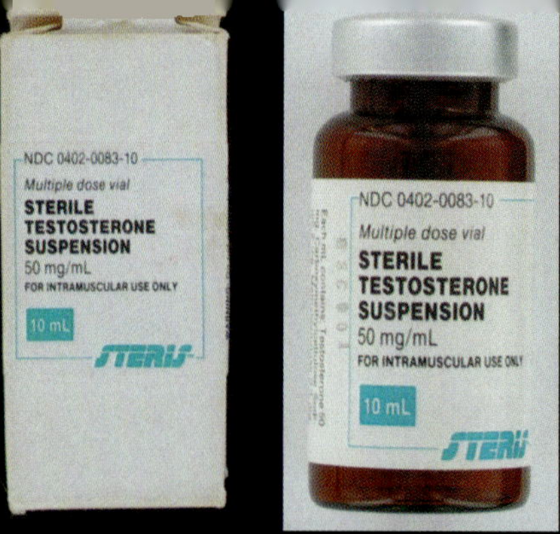

Steris counterfeit

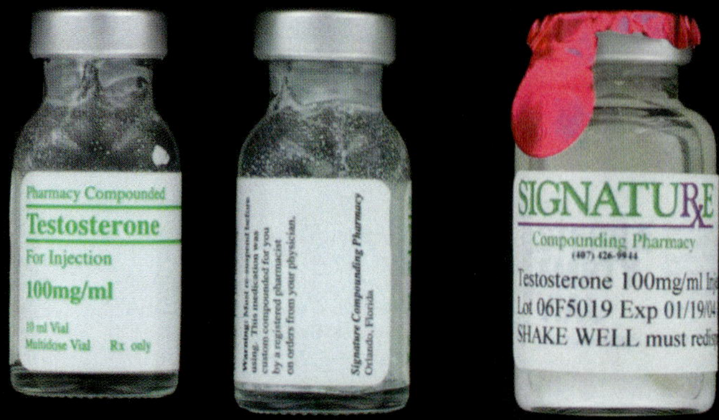

Two private-label generics - The only type of U.S. suspension now

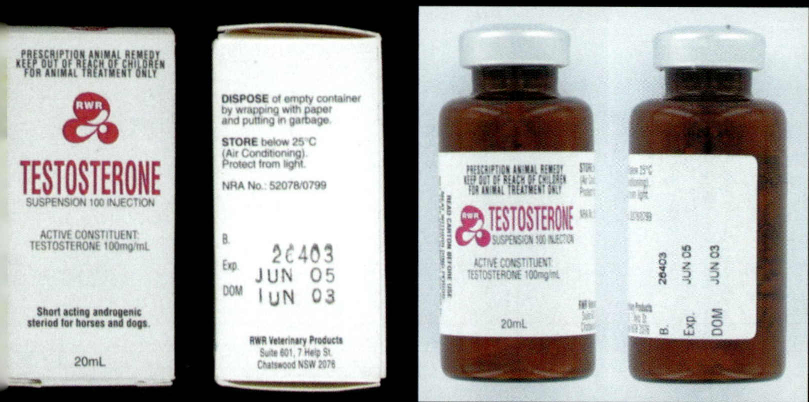

Suspension from RWR Australia

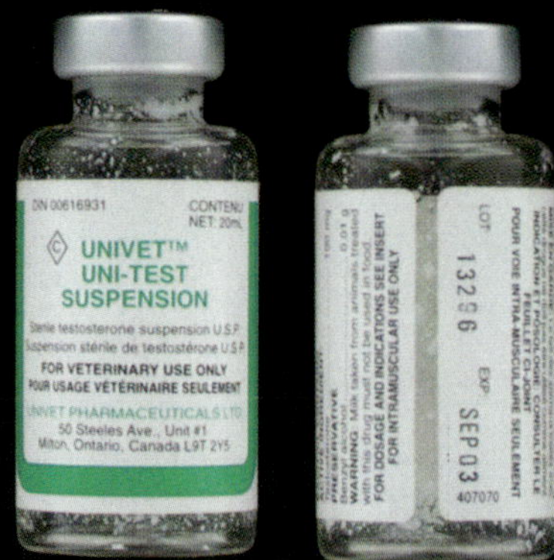

Canadian Univet Suspension

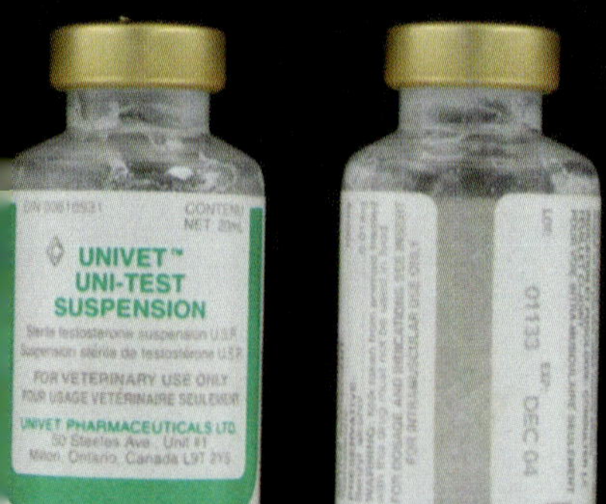

Counterfeit Canadian vial

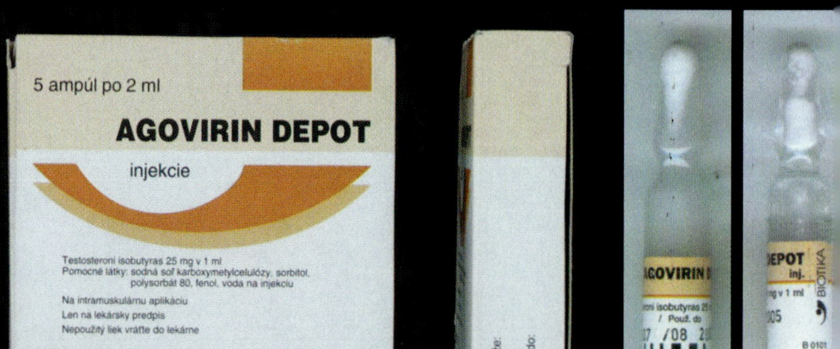

Agovirin Depot from Czech Rep.

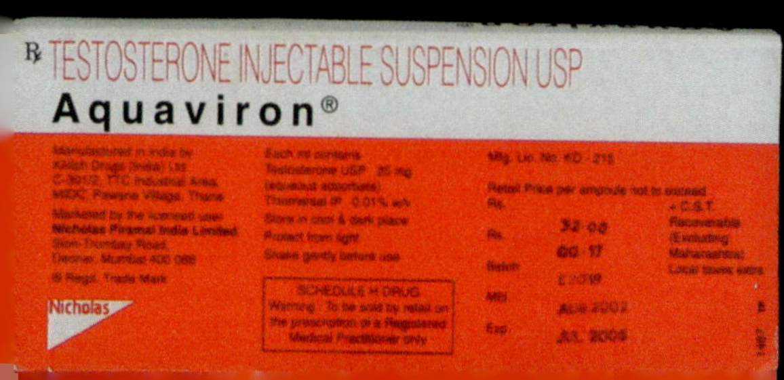

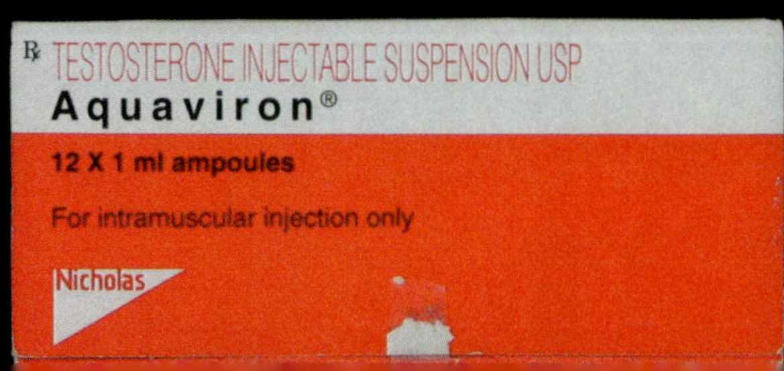

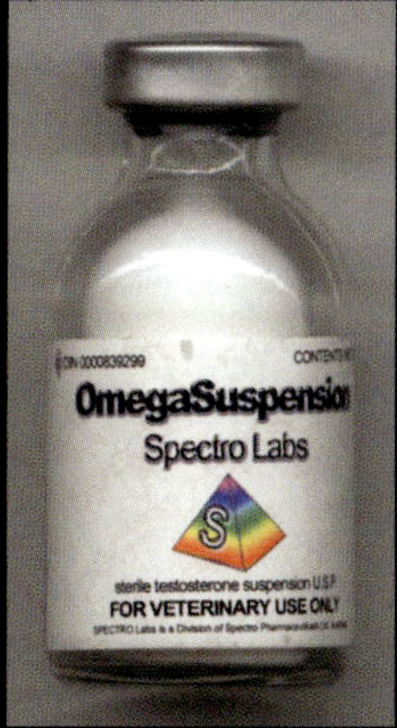

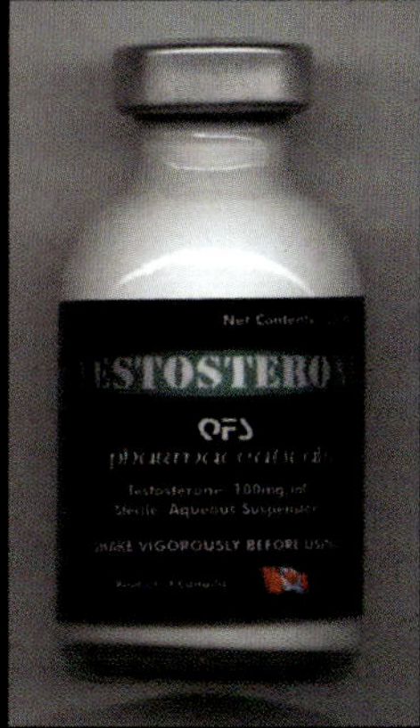

UG products from QFS and Spectro (NLM)

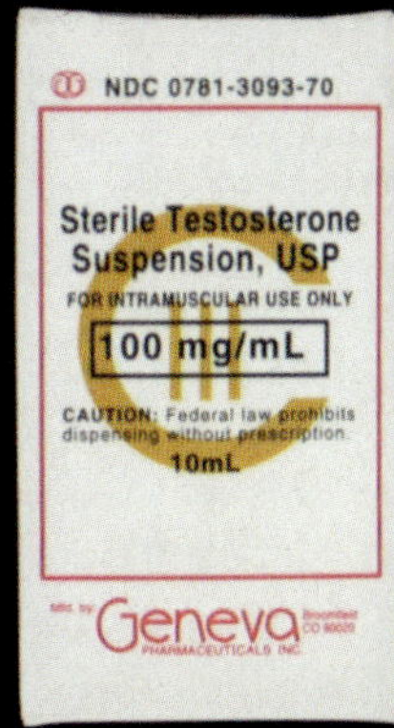

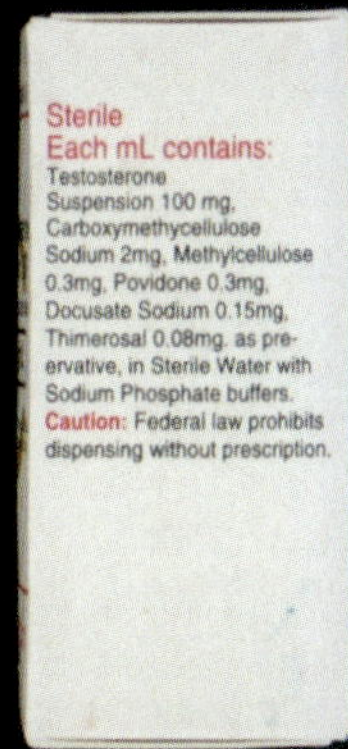

Counterfeit U.S. Geneva box

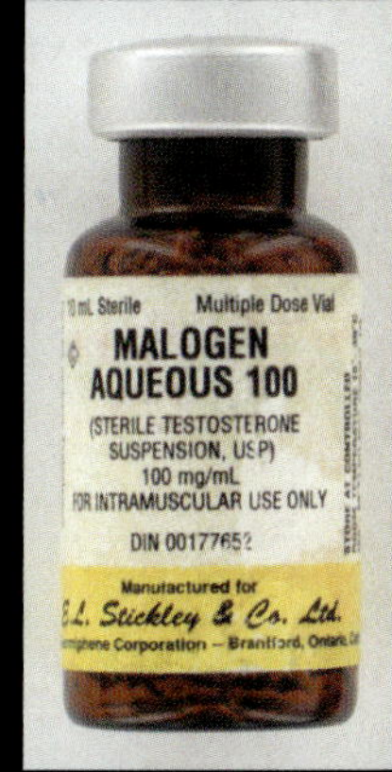

Fake Canadian Malogen

Testoviron

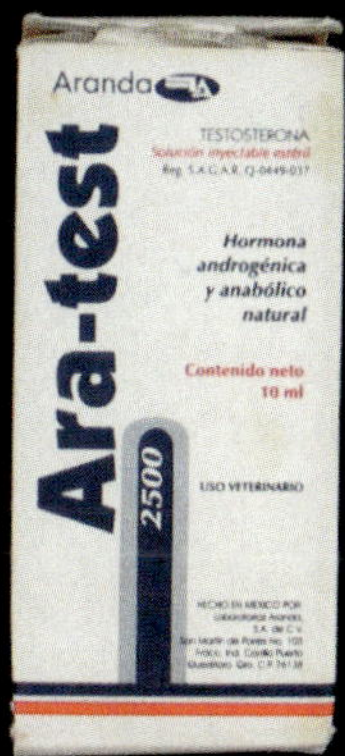

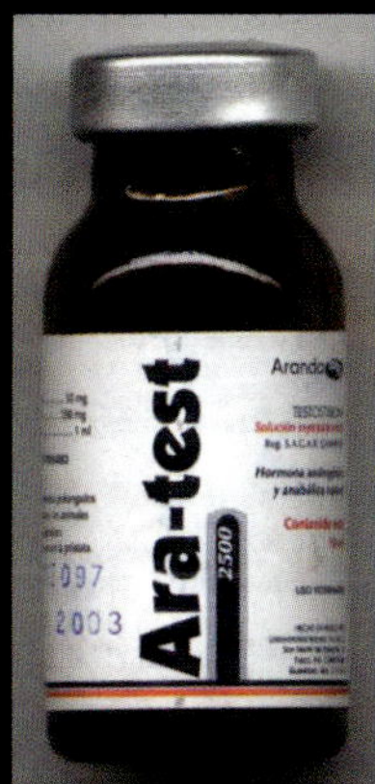

Ara-test from Mexico

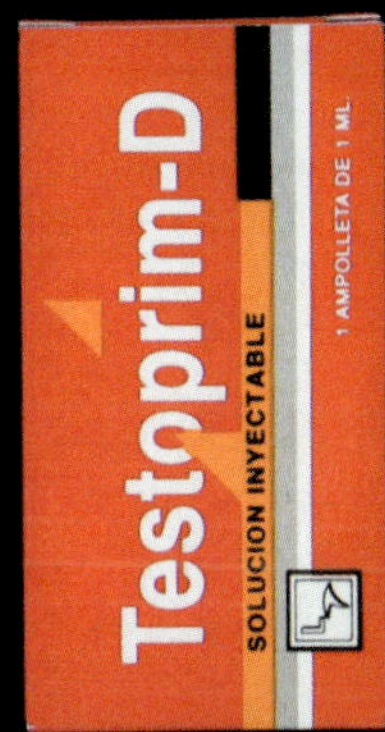

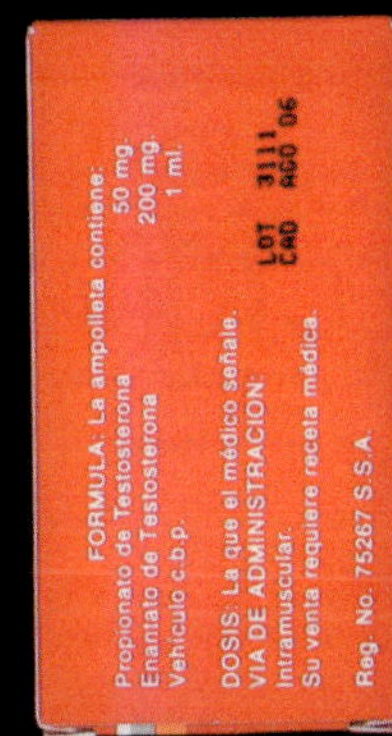

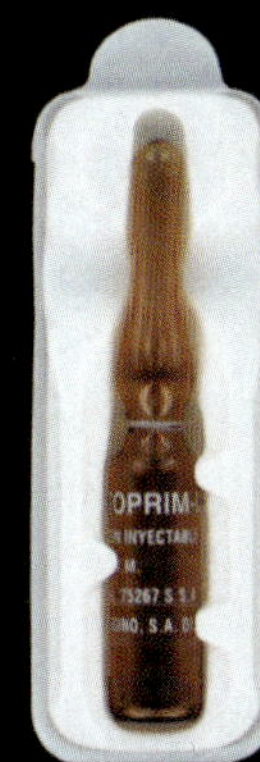

Testoprim-D from Mexico

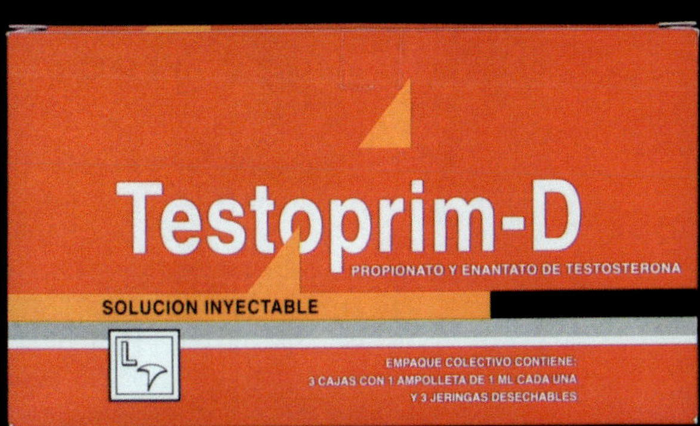

Large box with 3 ampules and syringes

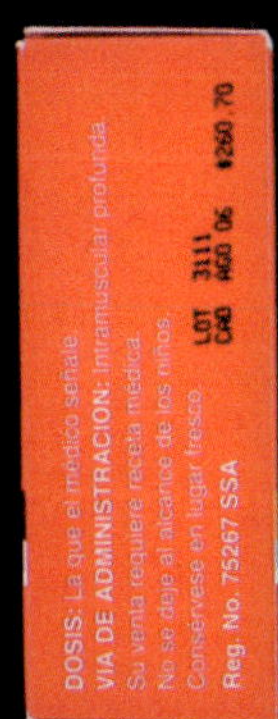

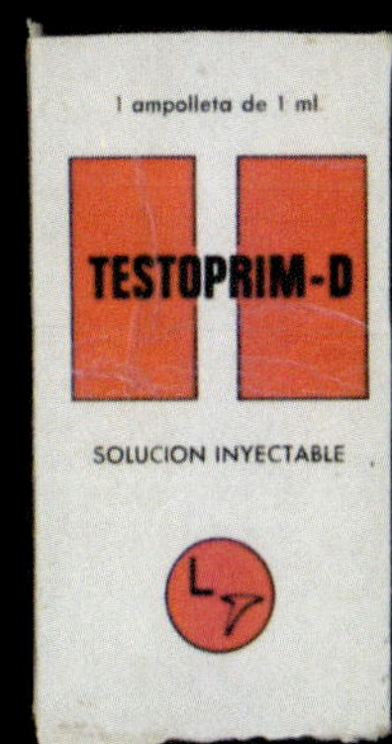

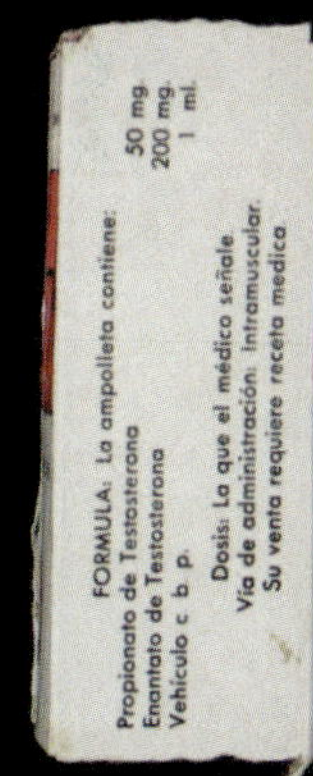

Old Testoprim packaging

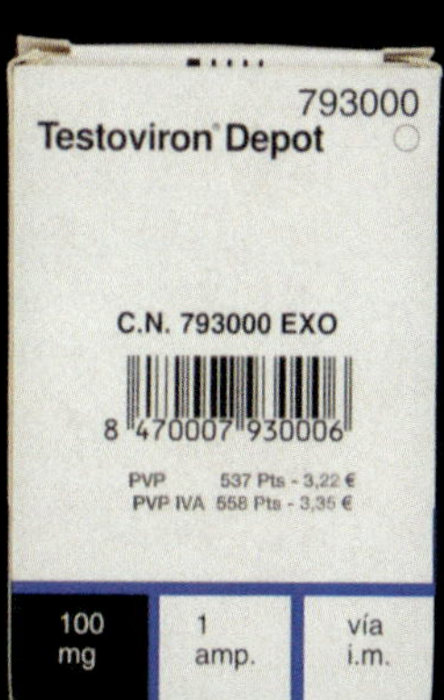

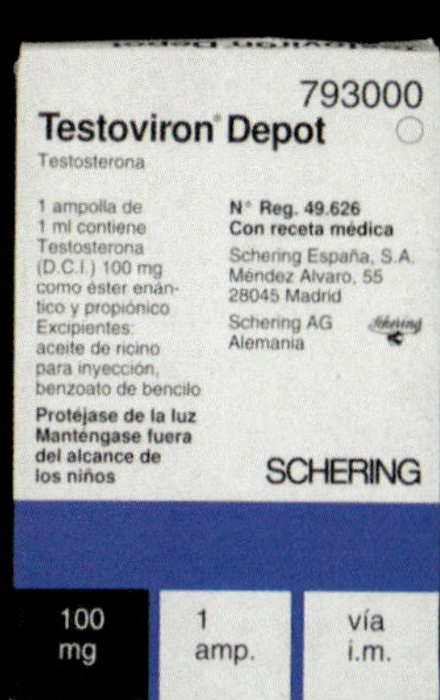

Spanish Testoviron (NLM)

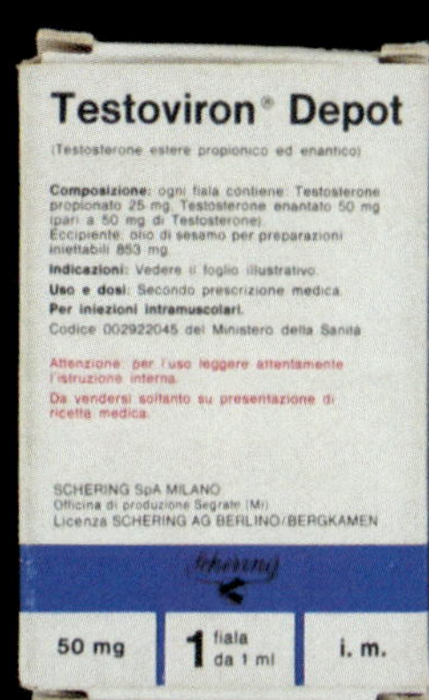

Italian Testoviron (NLM)

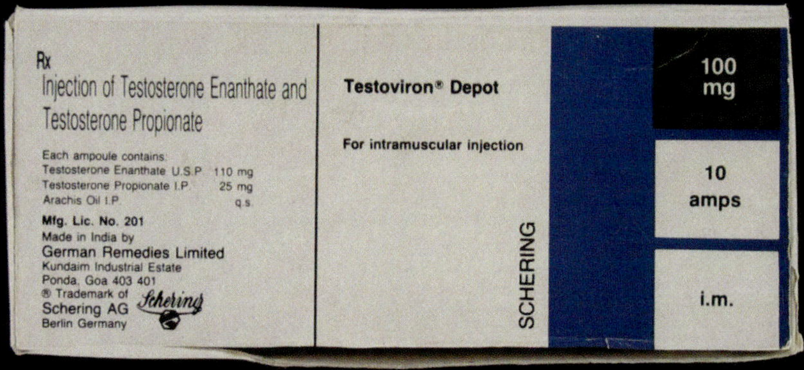

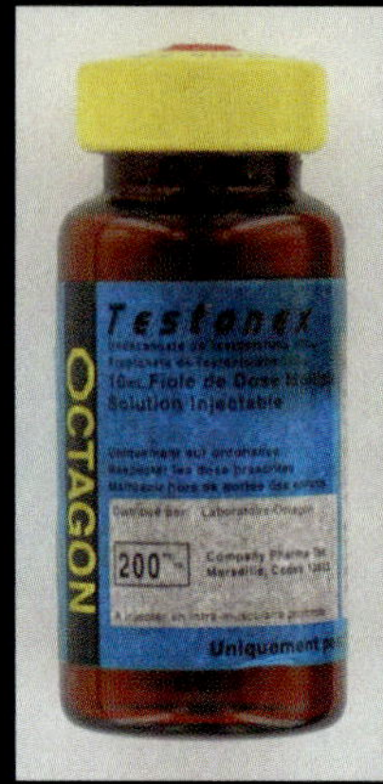

Testoviron from India (NLM) Bogus Octagon vial

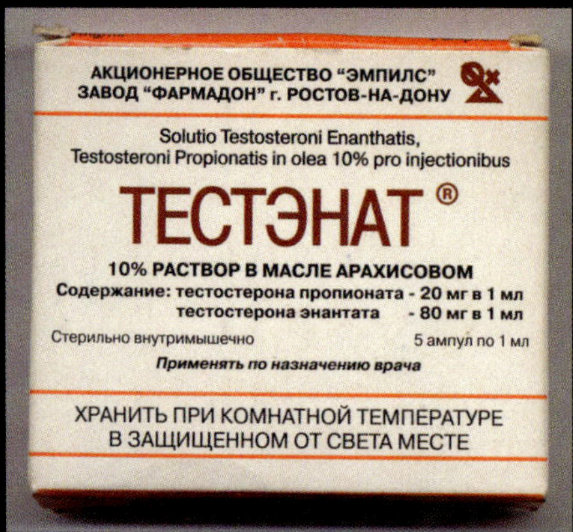

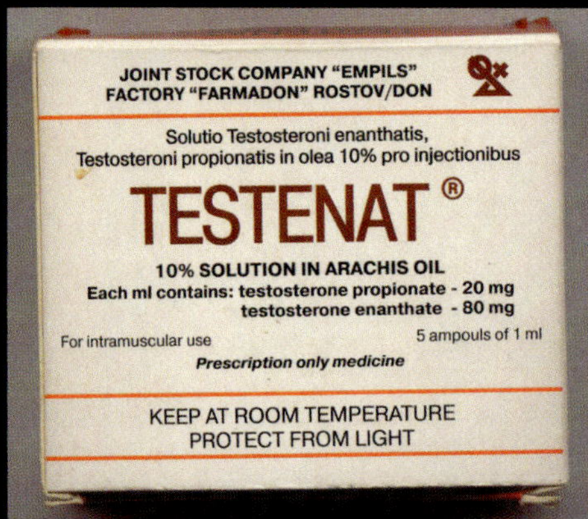

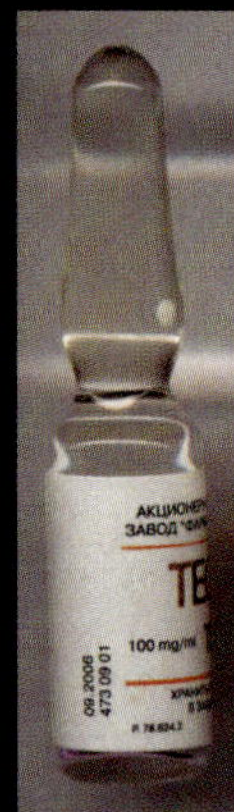

Fake Russian product from Farmadon

Trenbolone

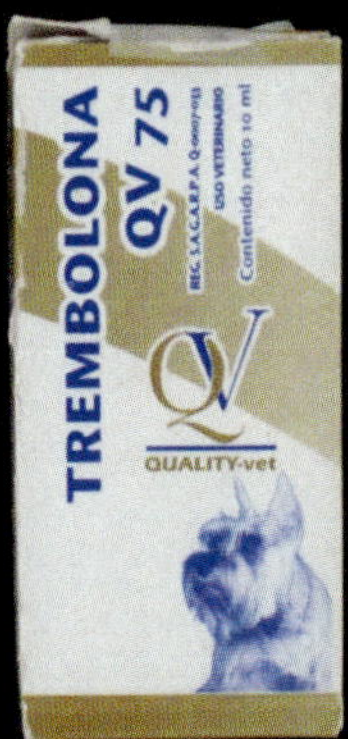

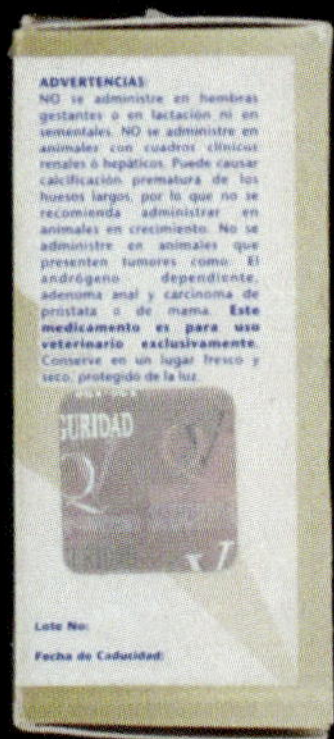

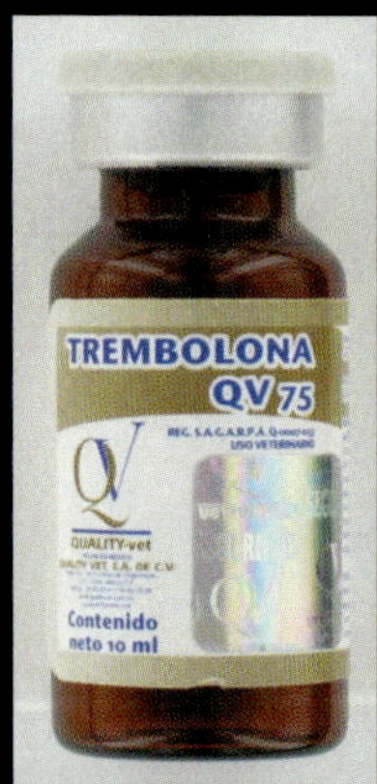

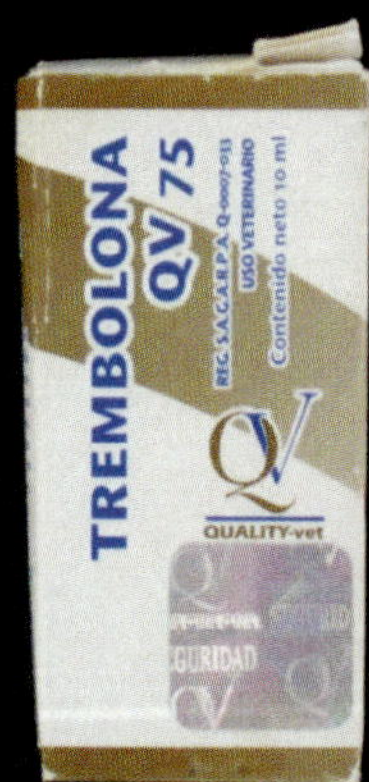

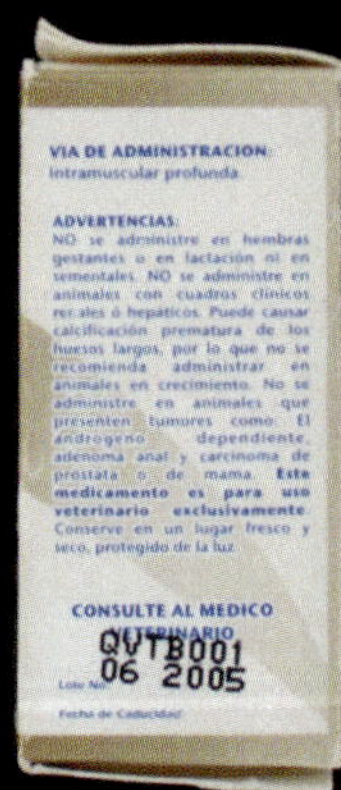

Quality Vet Trembolona (Mexico) Older style box

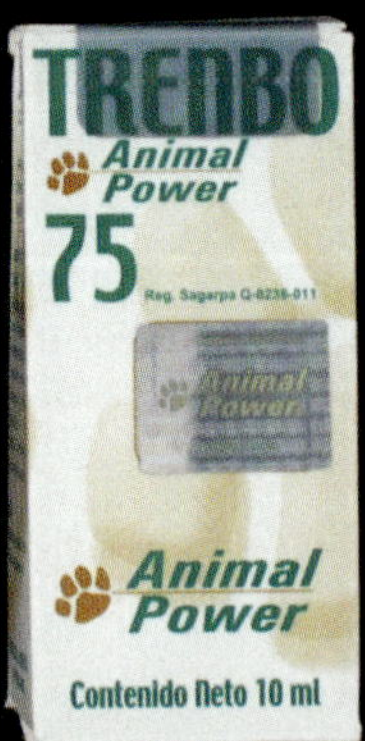

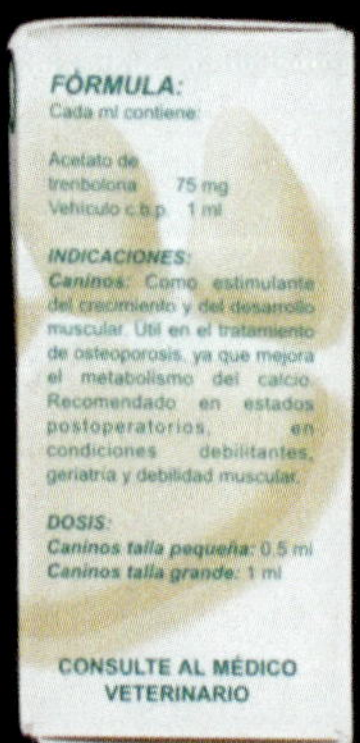

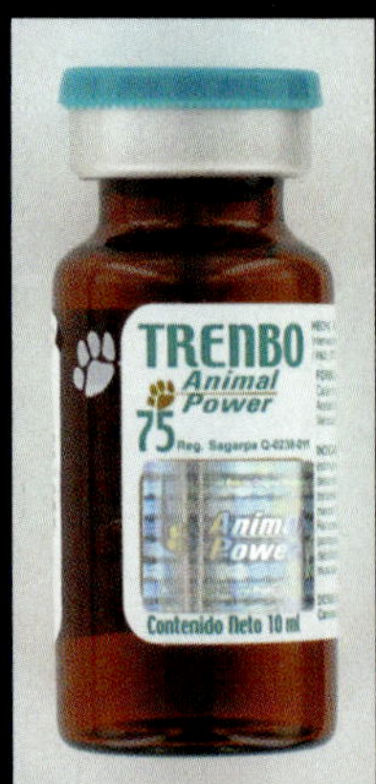

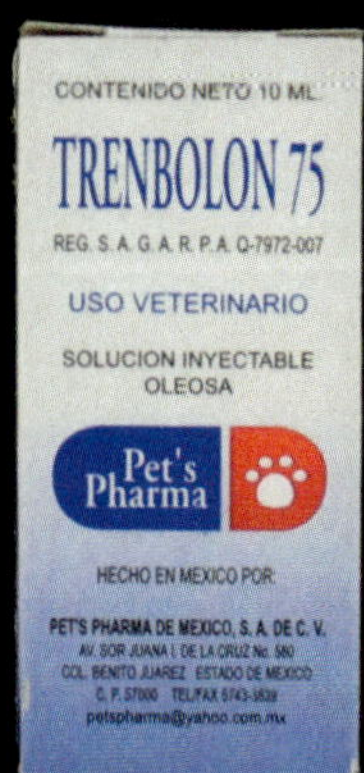

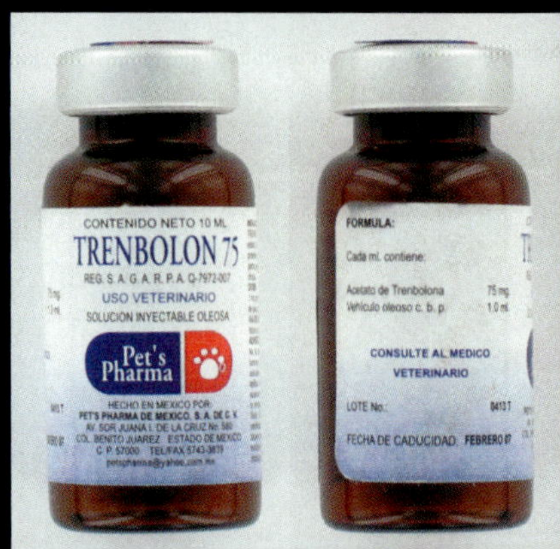

Trenbo 75 from Animal Power (Mexico) Trenbolon 75 - Pet's Pharma (Mexico)

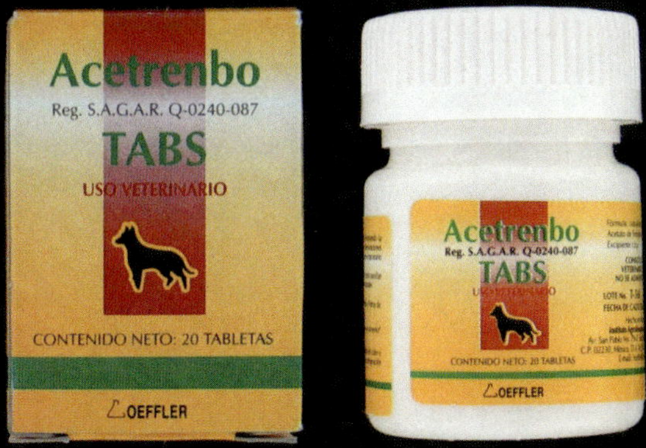

Loeffler Acetrenbo tabs (Mexico)

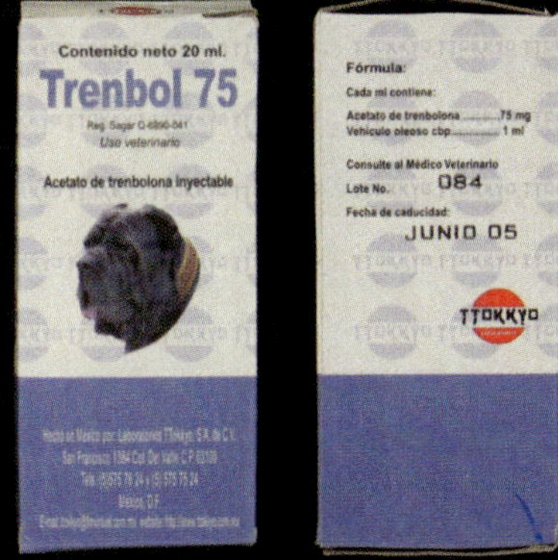

Ttokkyo Trenbol from Mexico (NLM)

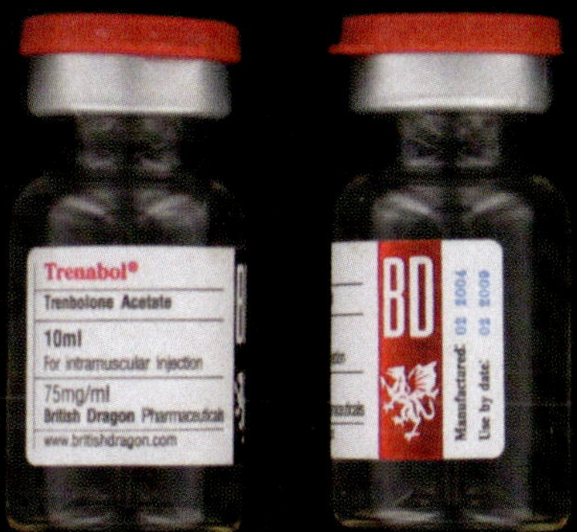

British Dragon Trenabol (Thailand)

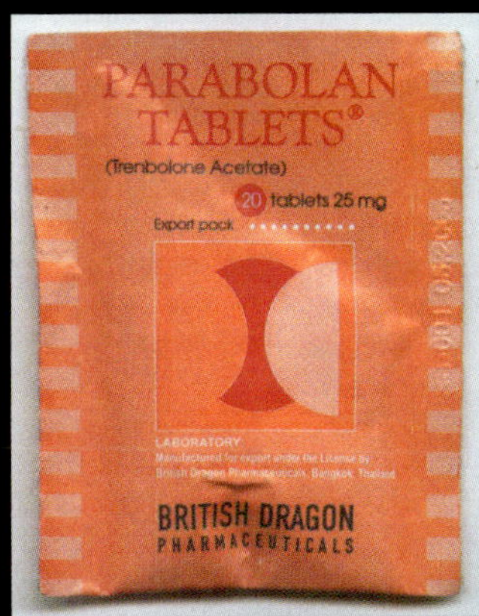

BD tablets (NLM)

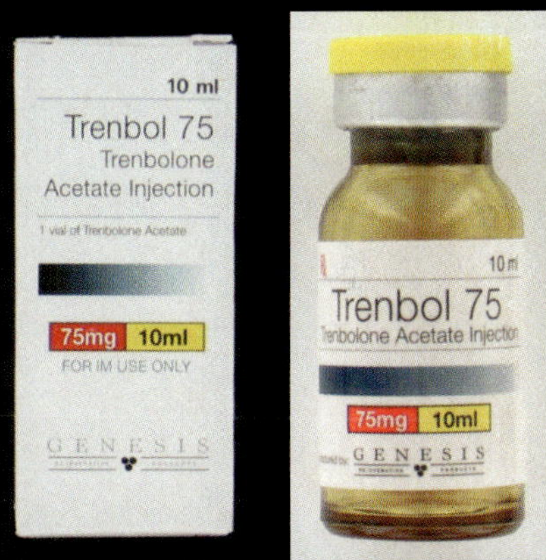

Trenbol 75 (Singapore)

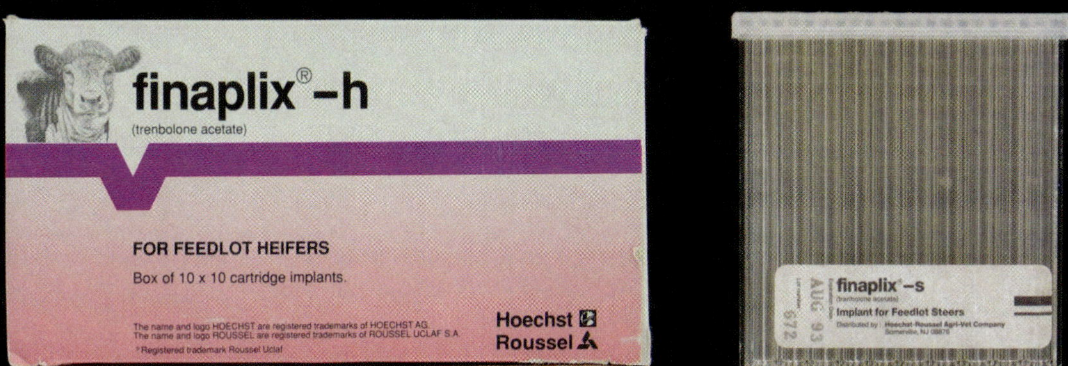

Older style Finaplix-H (U.S.)

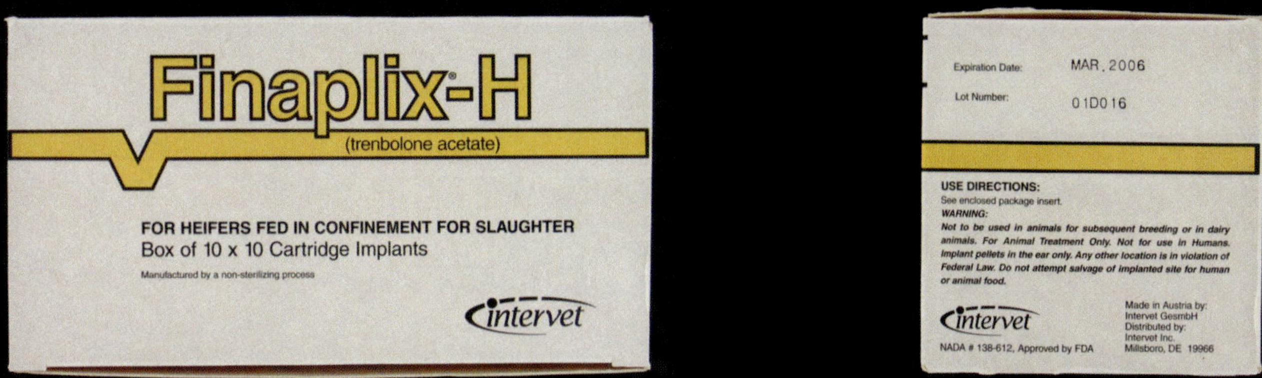

New Finaplix-H by Intervet (U.S.)

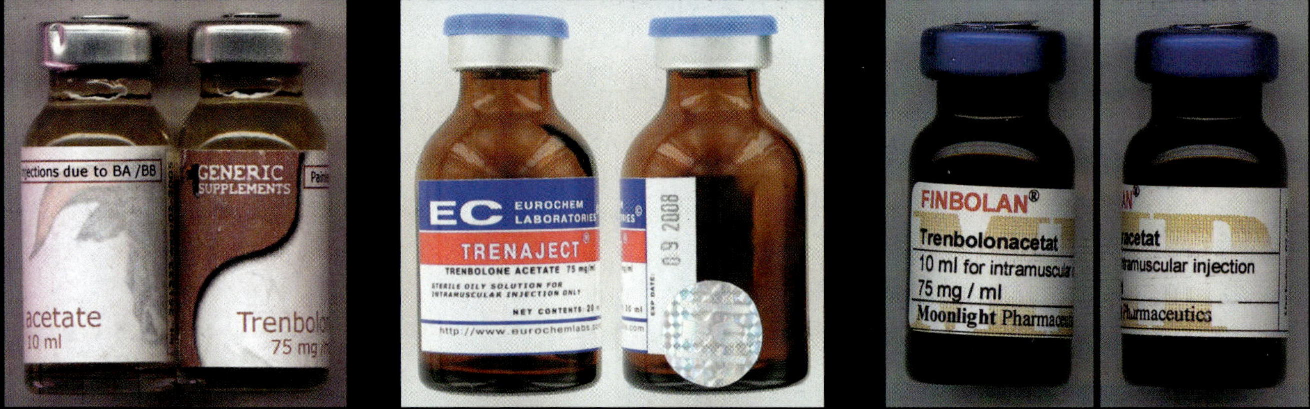

Three different underground products - Generic Supplements, Eurochem, and Moonlight

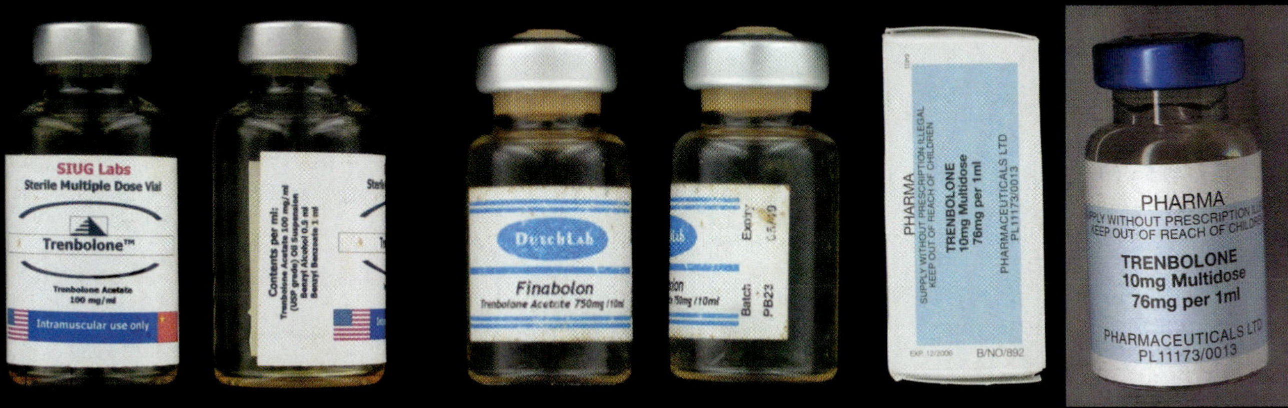

Three more underground products - SIUG, Dutch Labs, and Pharma

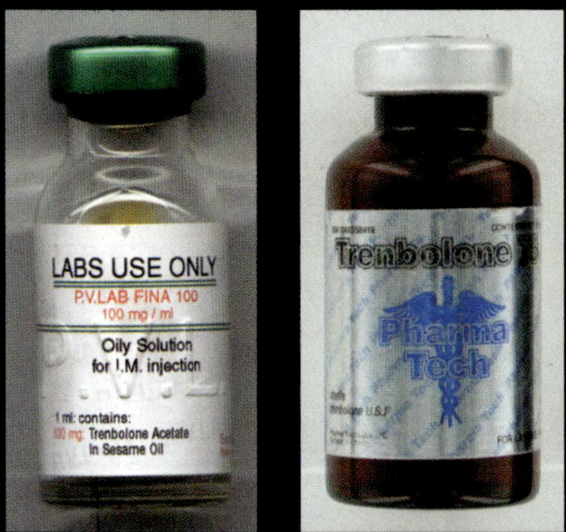

UG PVL and Pharma Tech

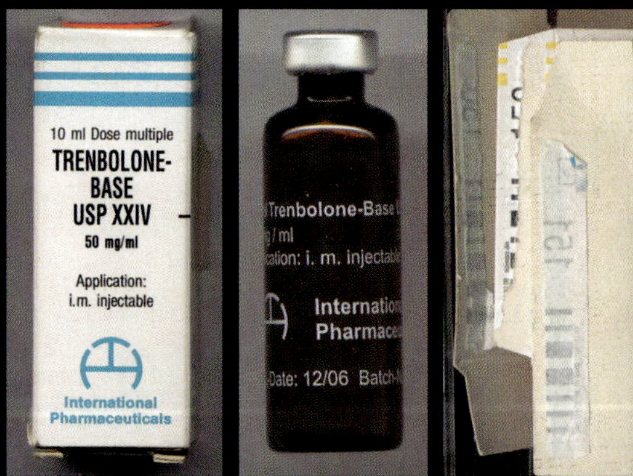

UG IP - Note the hidden numbers on the glue line

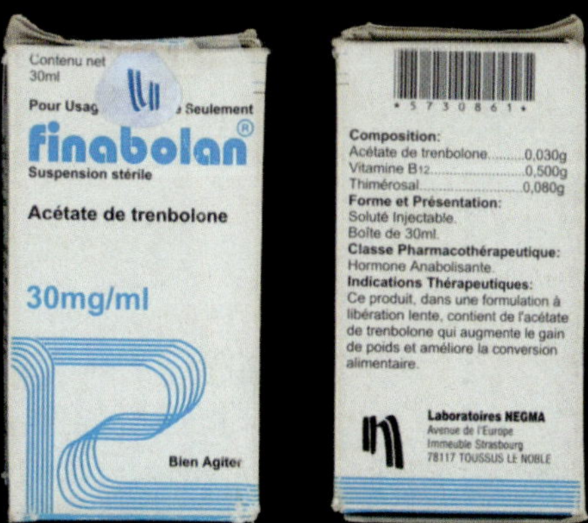

Counterfeit Finabolan

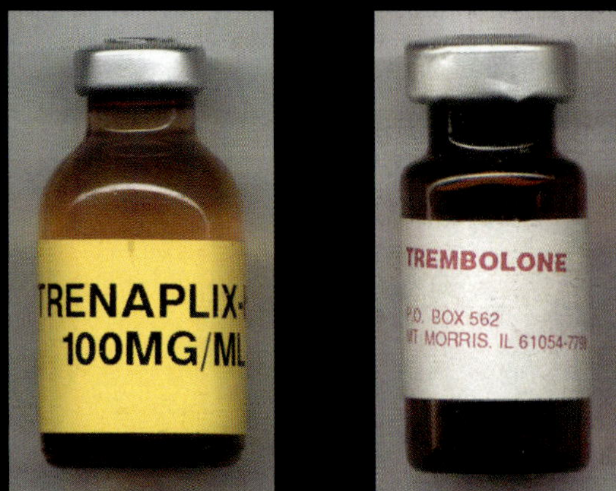

Two bogus vials

Tren. Enanthate

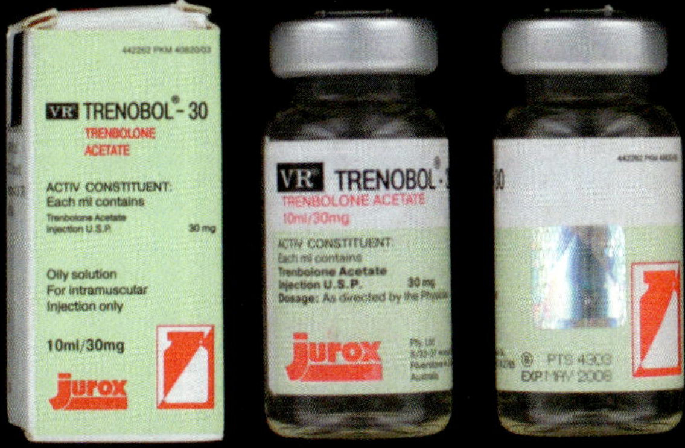

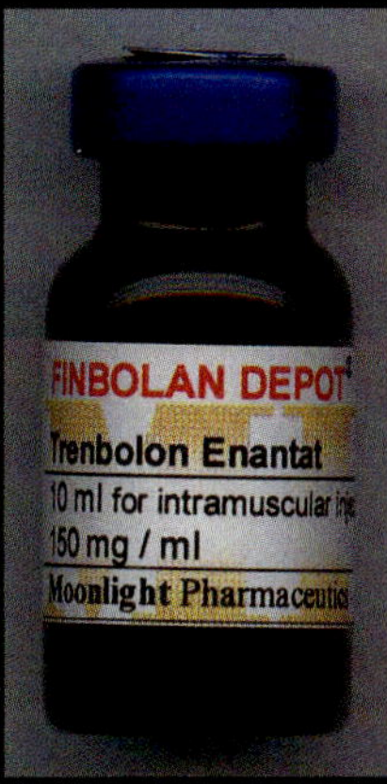

Counterfeit Jurox product (Jurox doesn't make trenbolone)

UG Moonlight vial

Trinabol

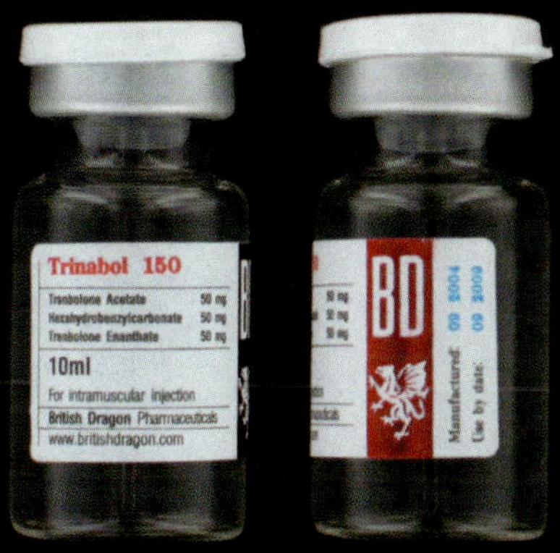

British Dragon Trinabol (Thailand)

Winstrol

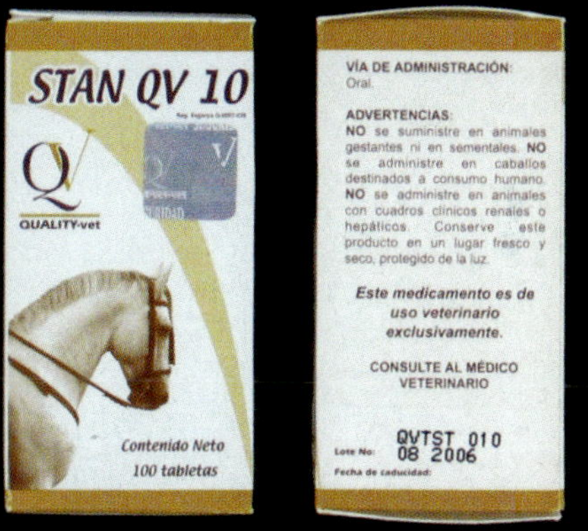

Quality Vet Stan QV tabs

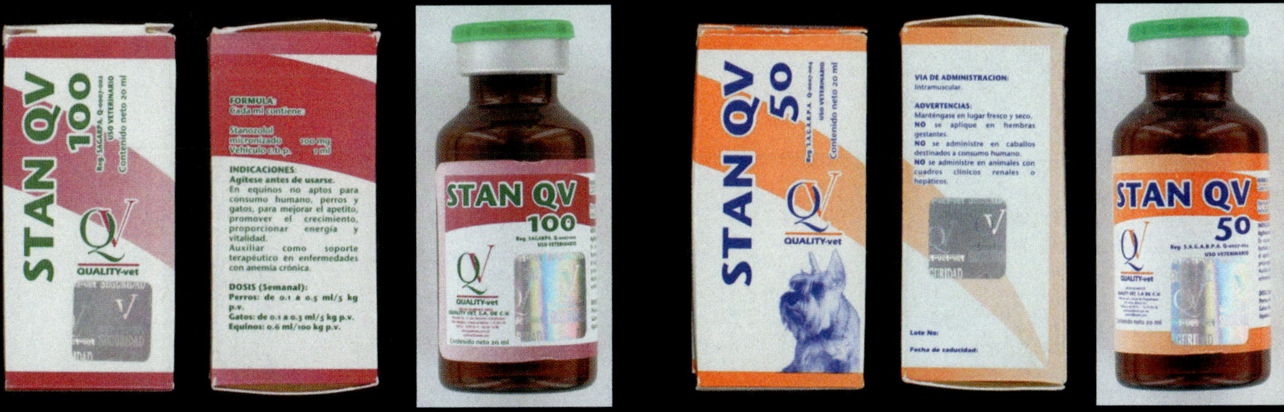

Quality Vet 100mg/mL and 50mg/mL injectable products (Mexico)

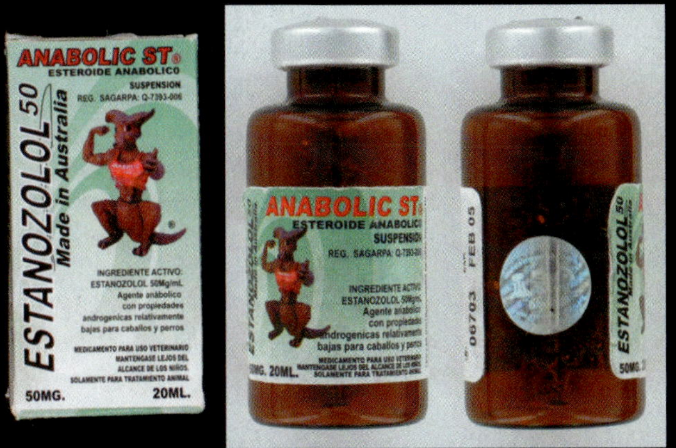

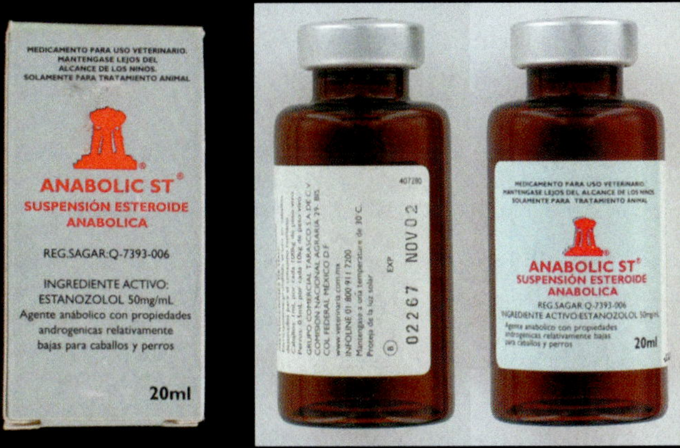

SYD Group product from Mexico

Anabolic ST under the old Mexican Grupo label (NLM)

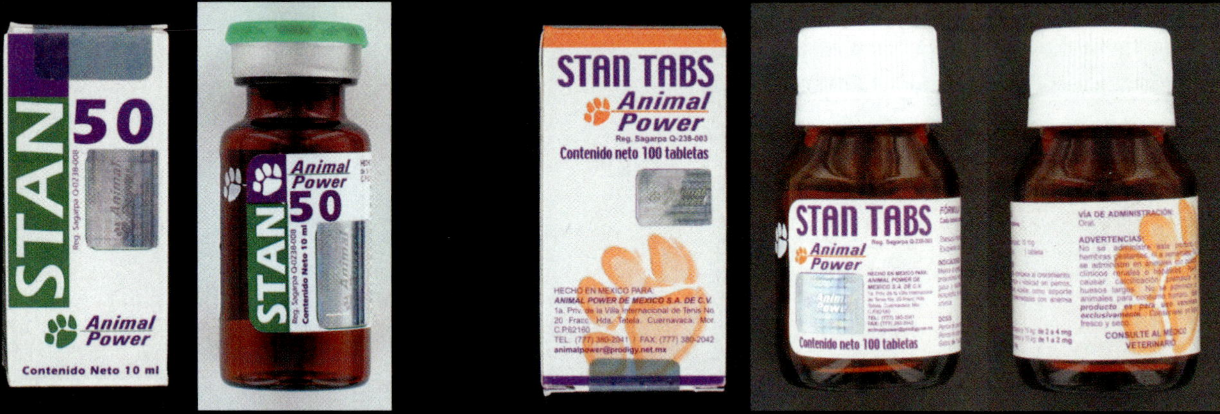

Injectable and oral products from Animal Power (Mexico)

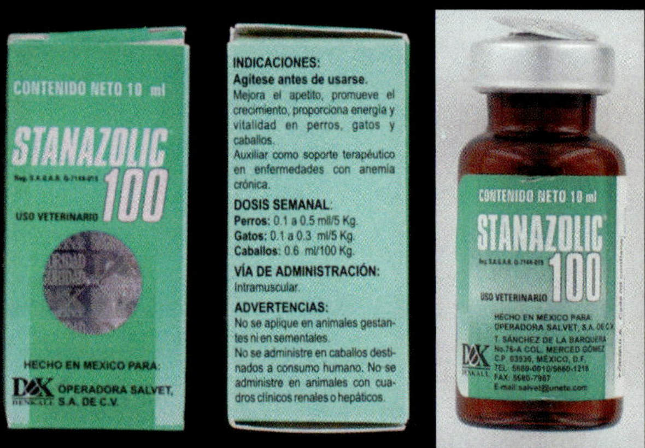

Stanazolic 100mg/mL from Denkall (Mexico)

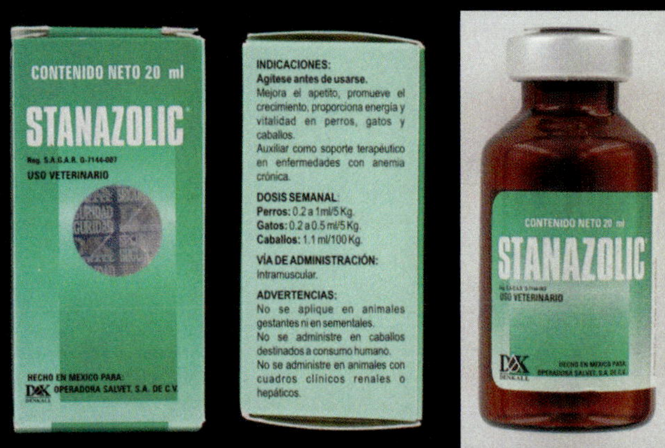

50mg/mL Stanazolic (Mexico)

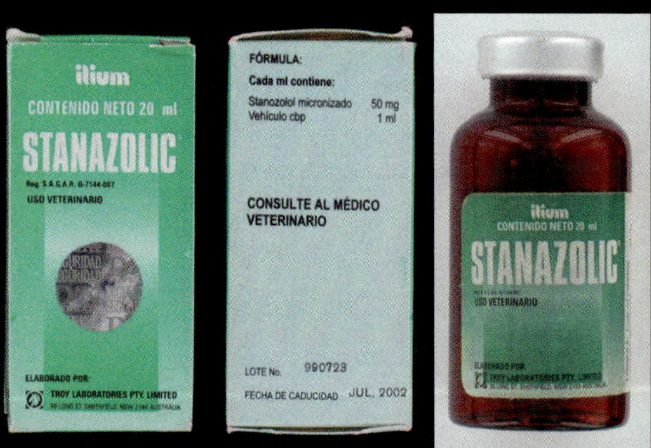

Stanazolic - Ilium export (Australia/Mexico)

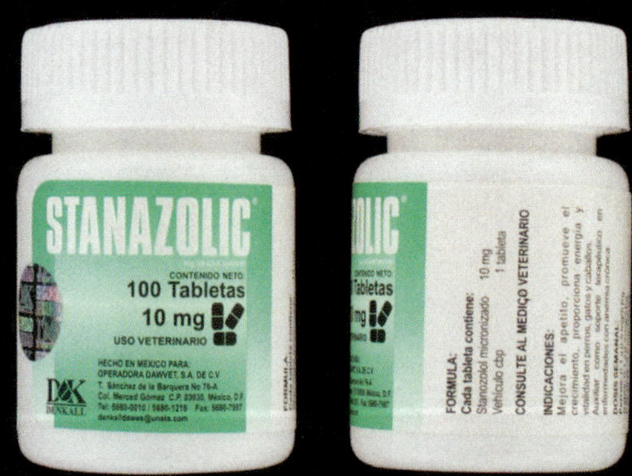

Denkall Stanazolic tabs

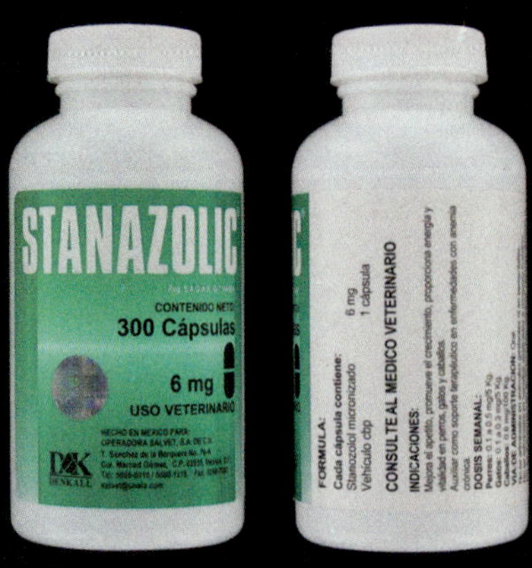

Stanazolic capsules

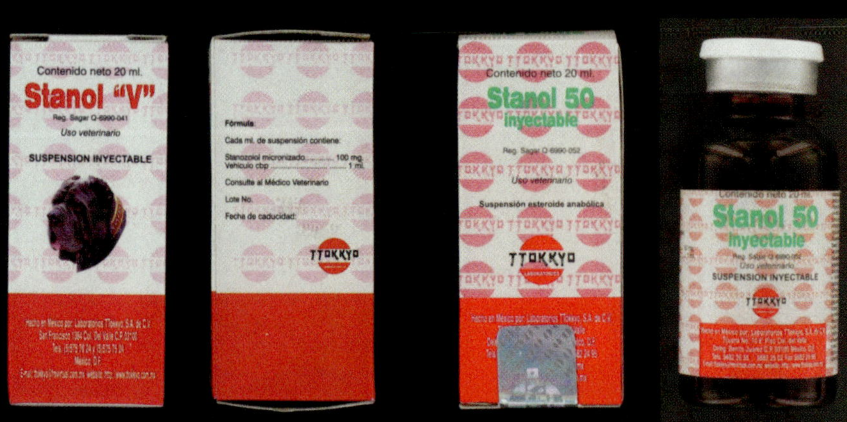

100mg/mL and 50mg/mL products from Ttokkyo Mexico (NLM)

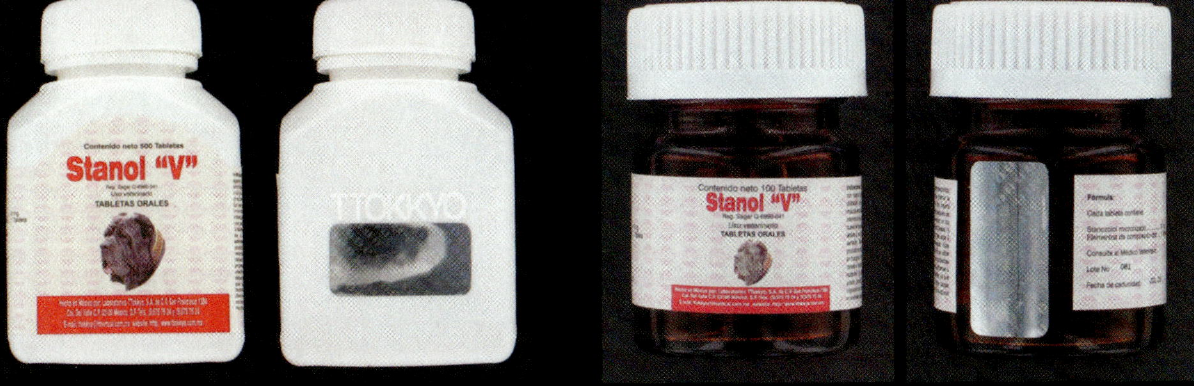

Stanol "V" tablets from Ttokkyo Mexico - 500 and 100 count bottles (NLM)

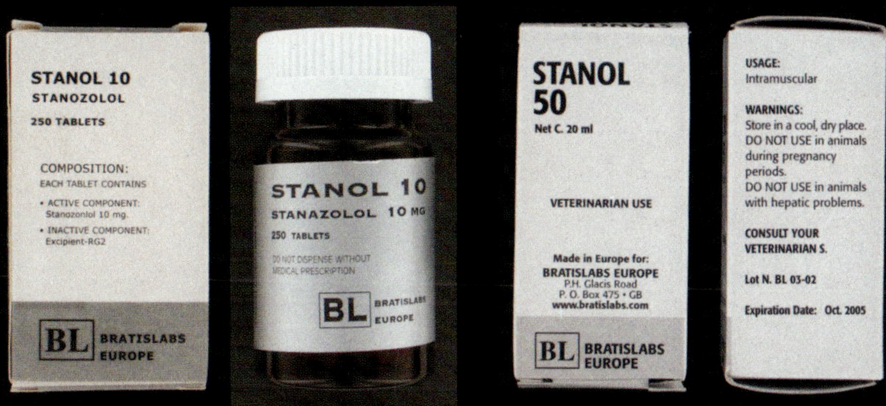

Stanol tablets and injectable from Bratis (Mexican "Import")

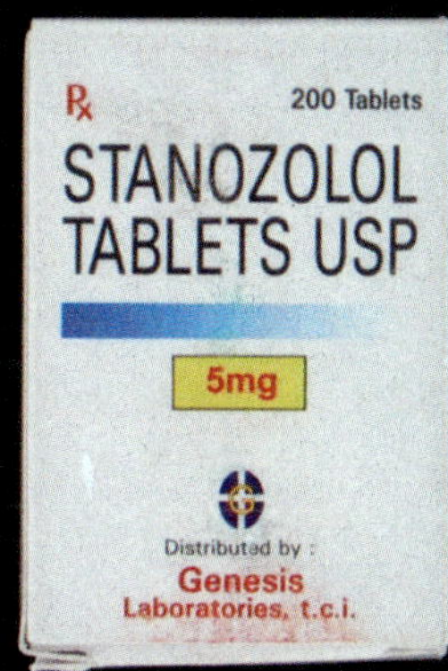

Genesis tabs (Singapore)

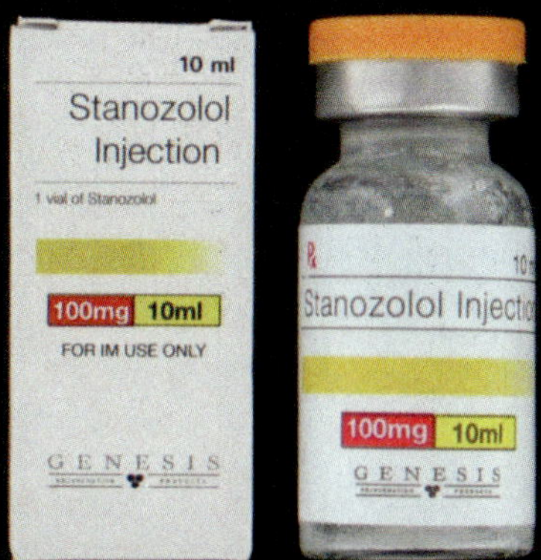

Genesis injectable

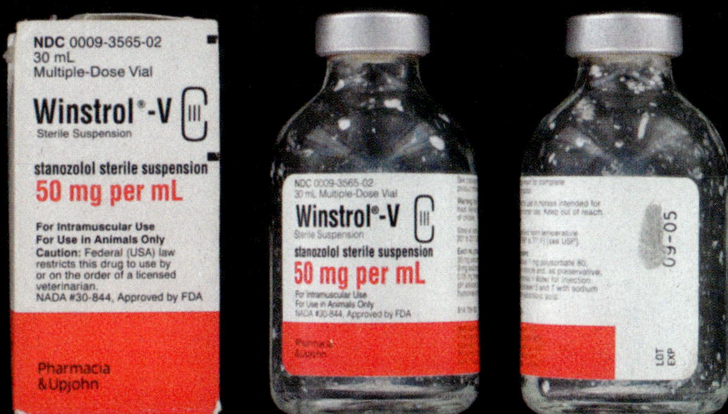

U.S. Winstrol®-V from Pharmacia & Upjohn

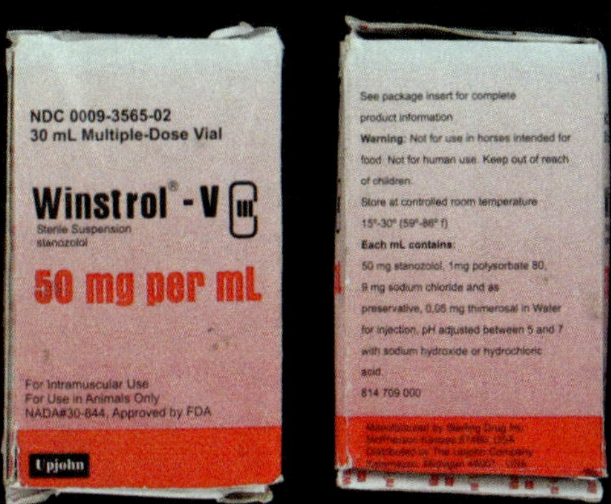

U.S. Upjohn counterfeit

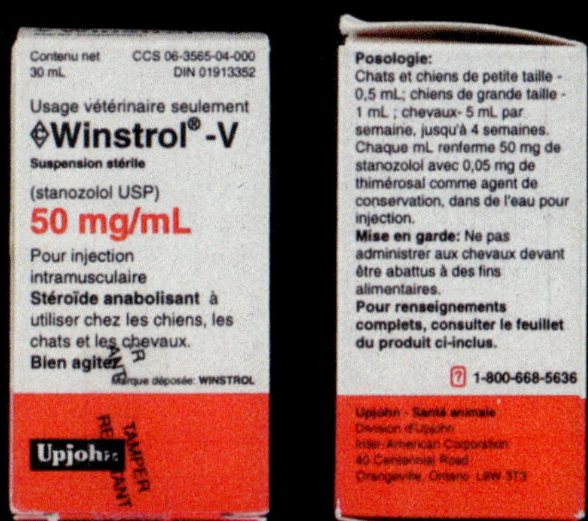

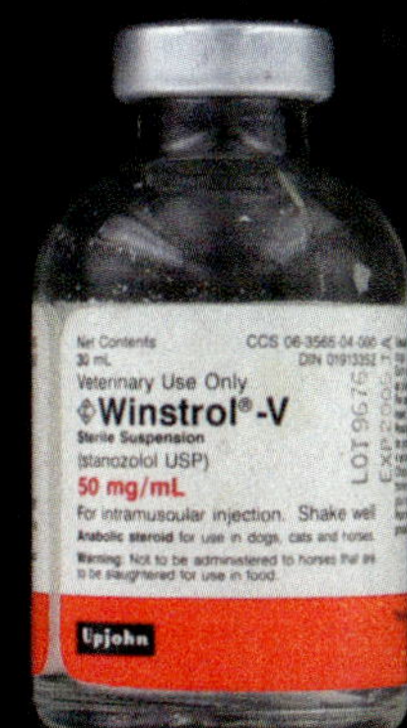

Canadian Winstrol®-V

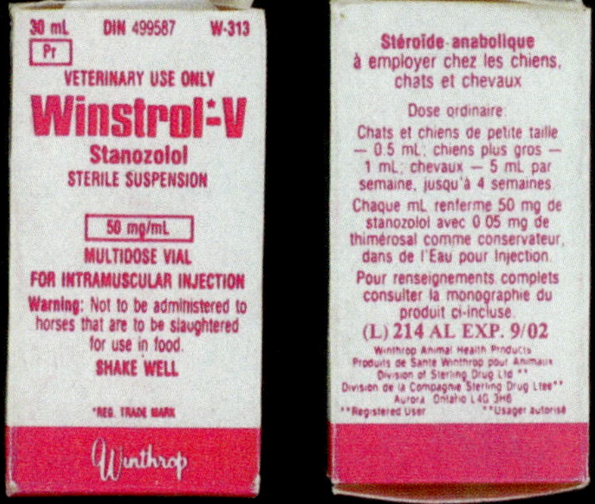

Canadian counterfeit

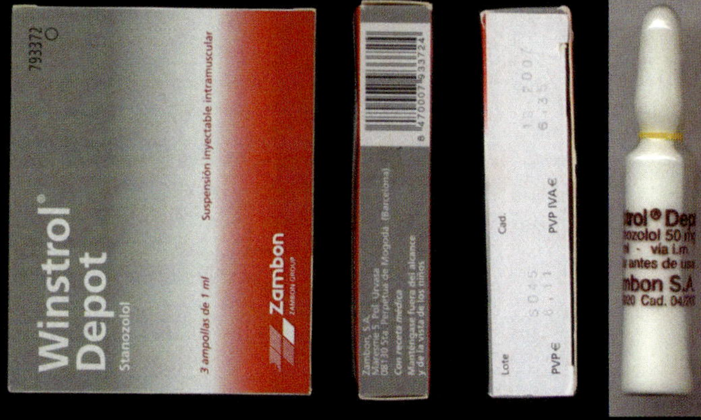

Winstrol Depot from Zambon (Spain)

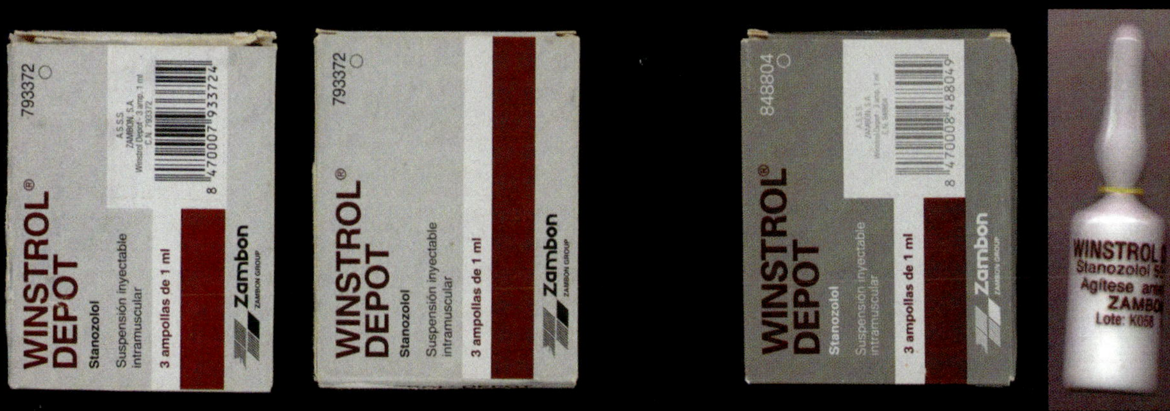

Two older versions of Spanish Winstrol Depot

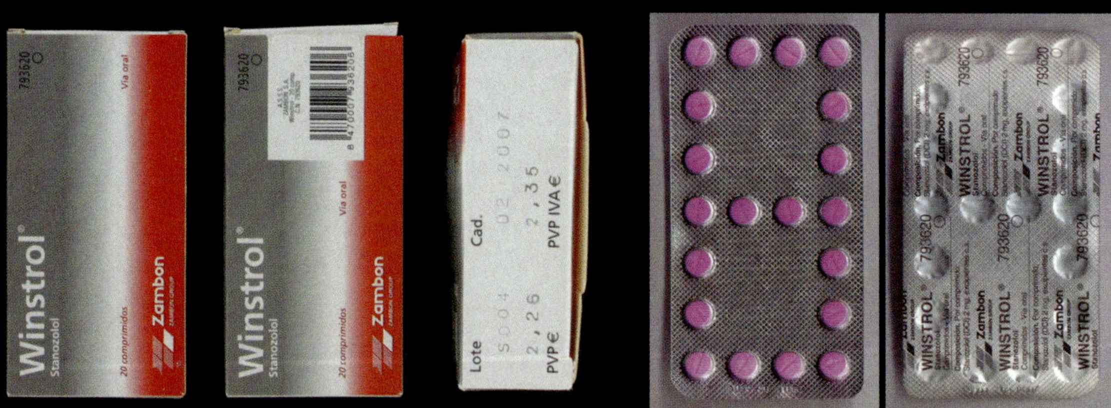

Winstrol tablets from Zambon (Spain)

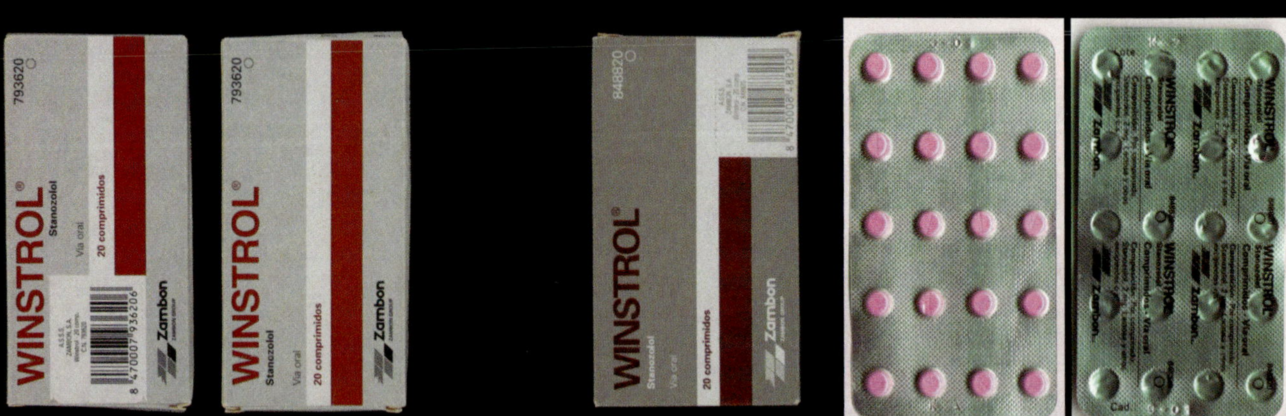

Two older versions of Spanish tablets

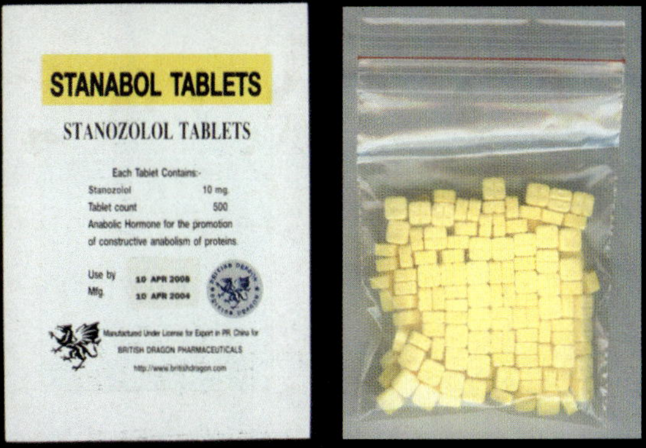

British Dragon 10mg Stanabol tablets

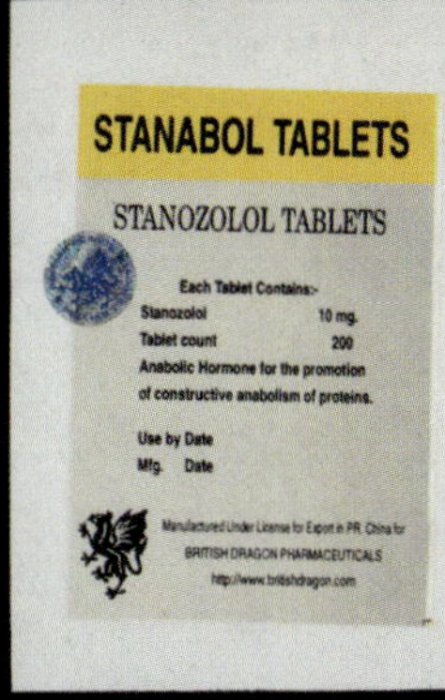

Older 10mg packaging

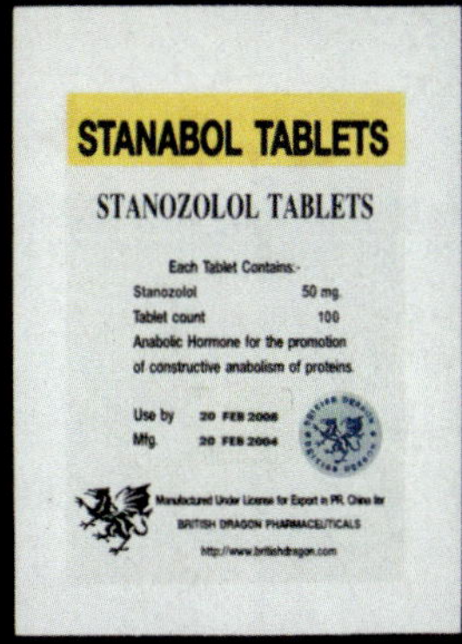

BD 50mg(!) tablets

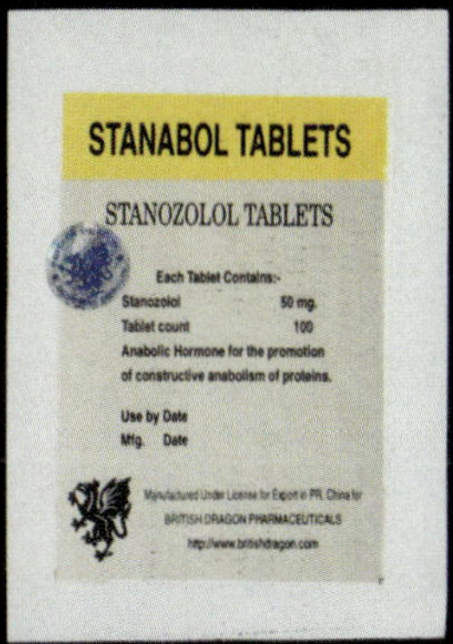

Older style 50's

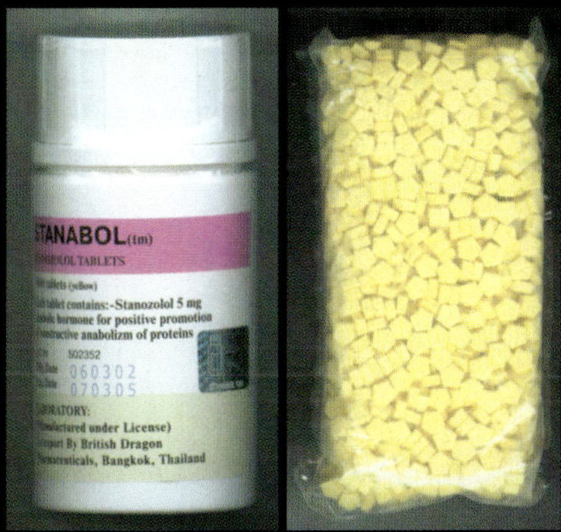

Old style BD 5mg

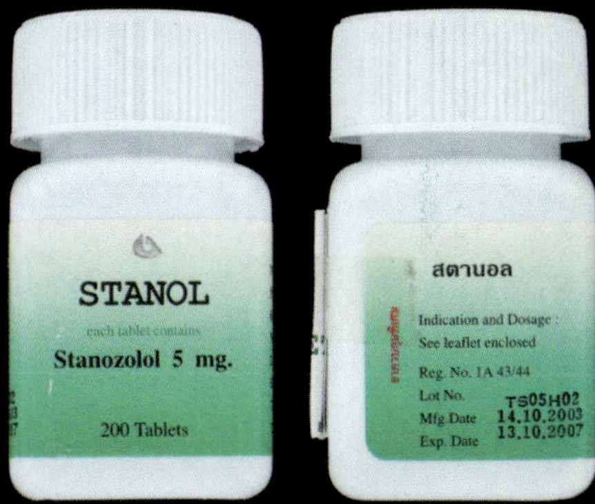

Stanol tablets from Thailand

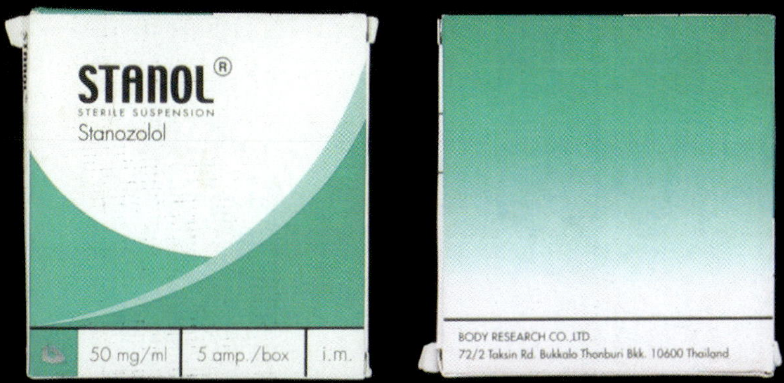

Stanol injectable (Thailand)

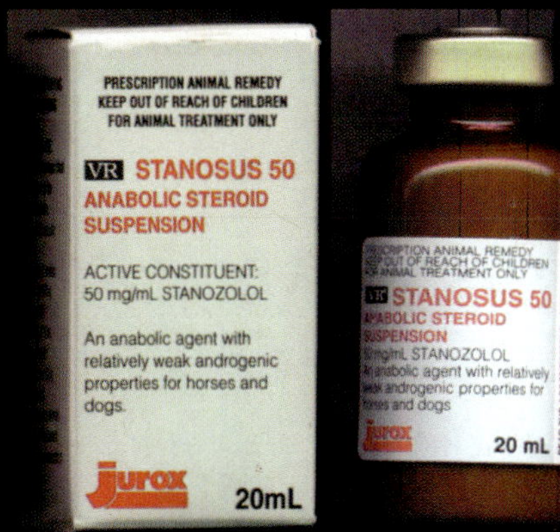

Jurox Stanosus from Australia (NLM)

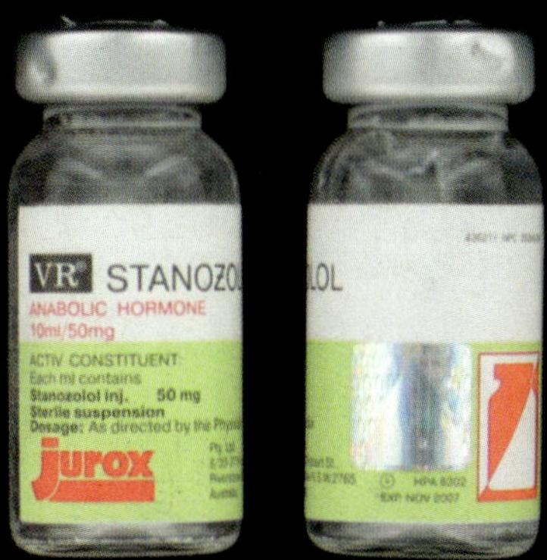

Counterfeit Jurox vial

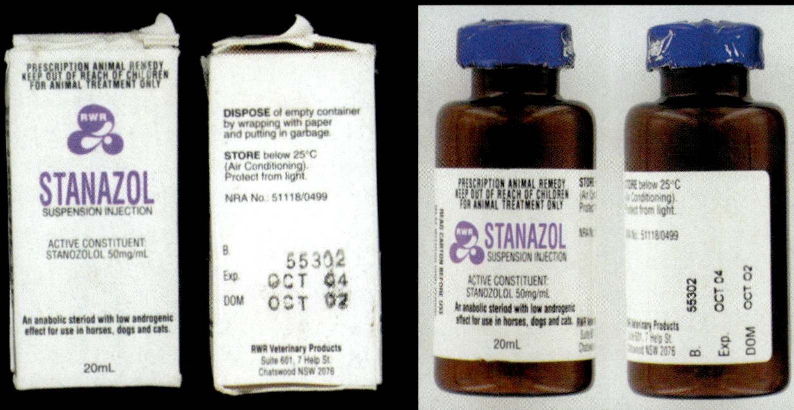

Stanazol from RWR (Australia)

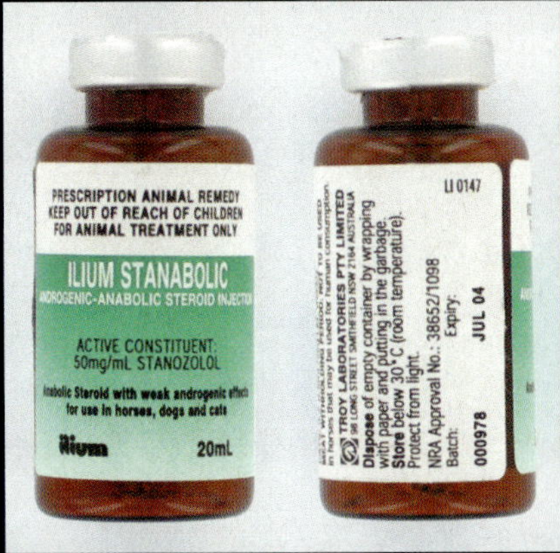

Ilium Stanabolic (Australia)

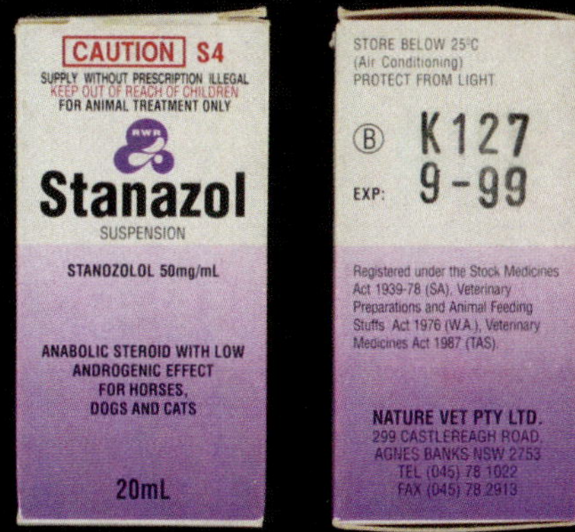

RWR Stanazol from Australia (NLM)

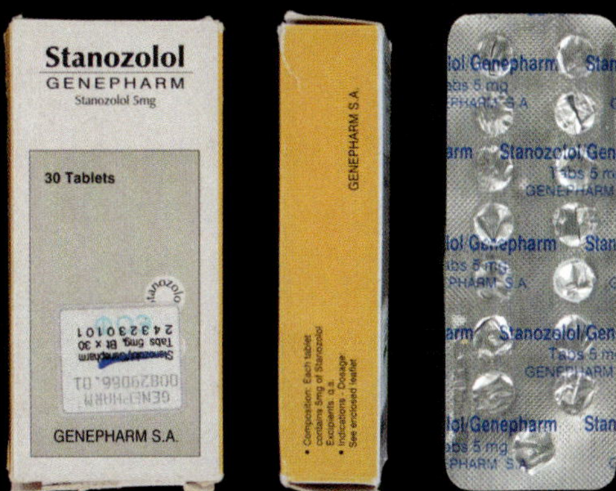

Stanozolol from Genepharm (Greece)

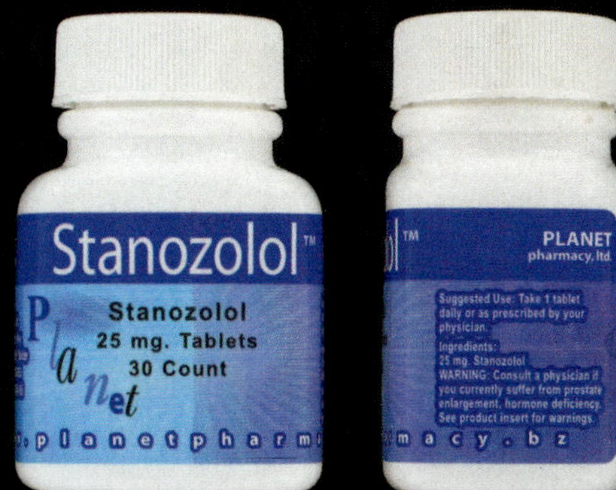

Generic from Planet Pharm (Belize)

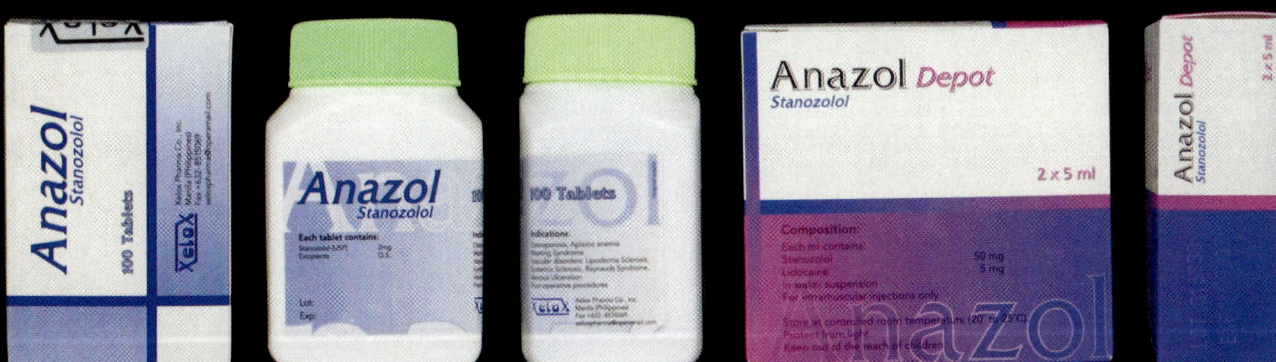

Anazol tablets and injectable from Xelox (Philippines)

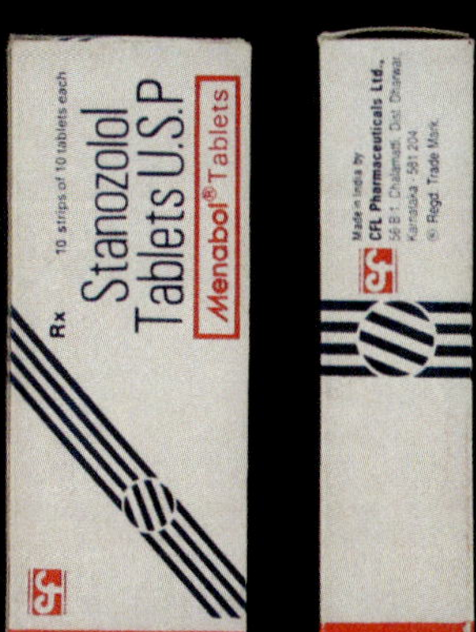

Menabol from India (NLM)

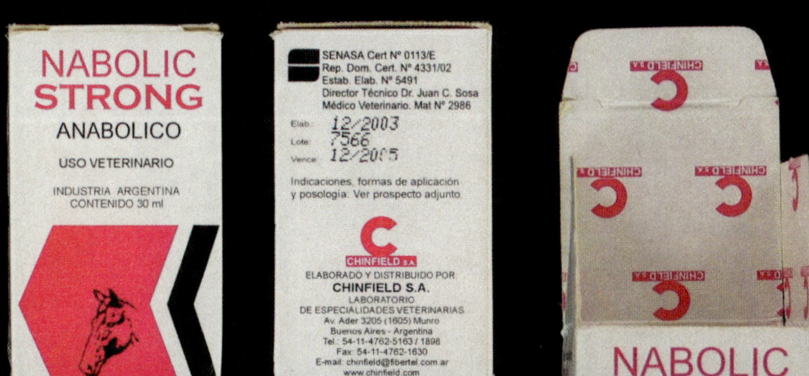

Nabolic Strong from Chinfield (Argentina)

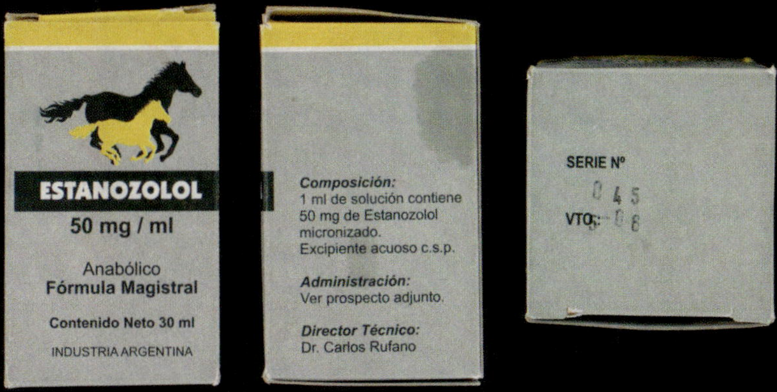

Injectable from Industria Argentina

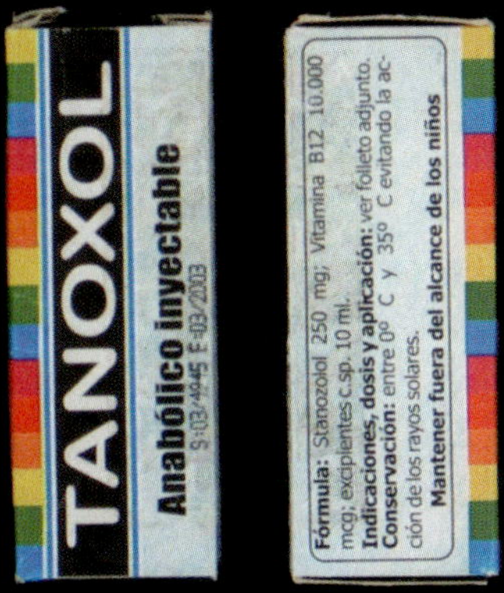

Tanoxol (Argentina)

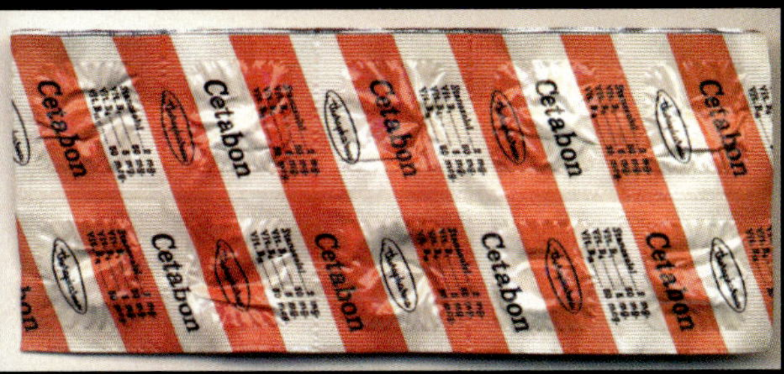

Thai Cetabon (NLM)

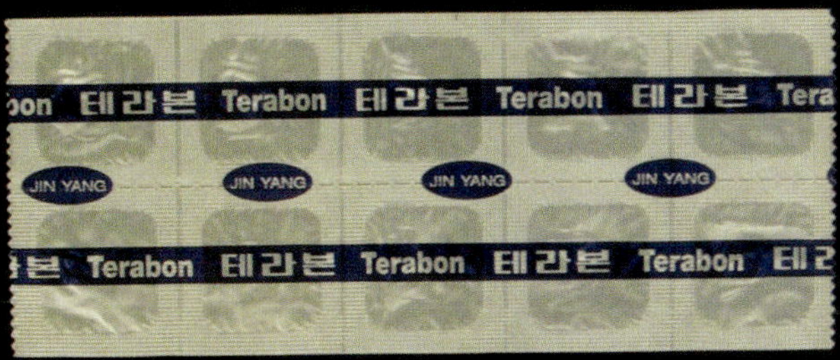

Terabon from Korea

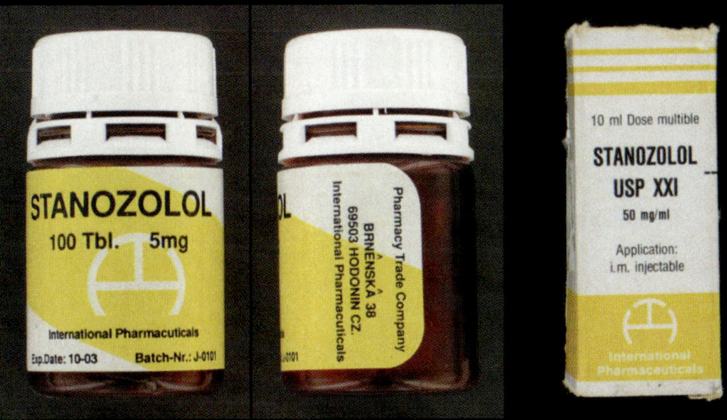

Underground tablets and injectable from IP

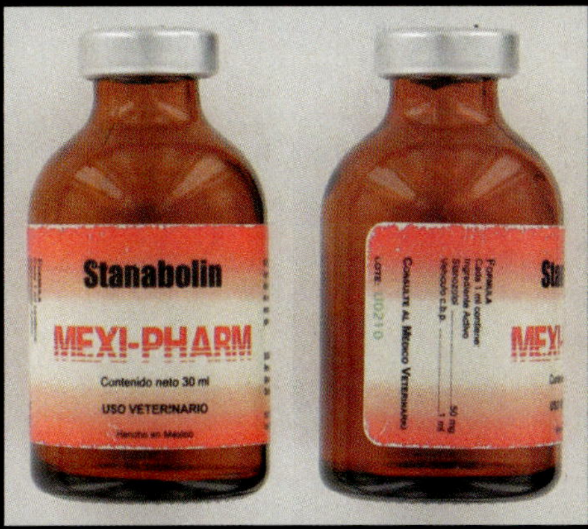

Mexi-pharm underground vial

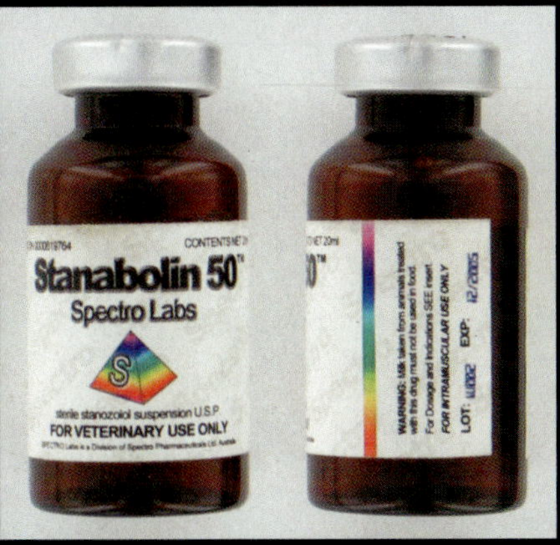

Spectro UG Stanabolin (NLM)

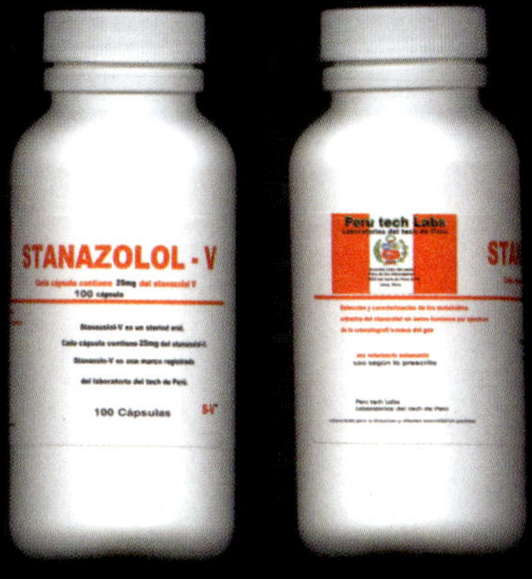

UG tablets from Peru Tech

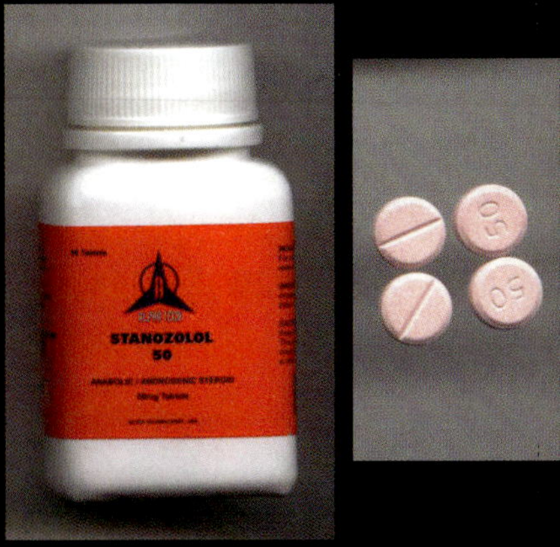

UG Alpha Tech (NLM)

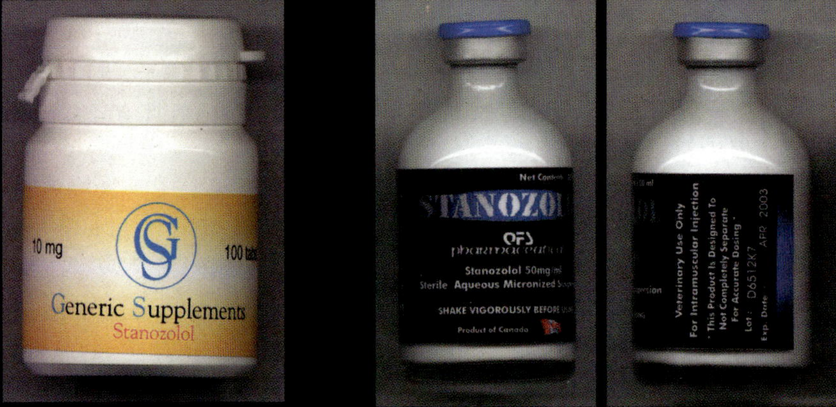

Underground products from Generic Supplements and QFS

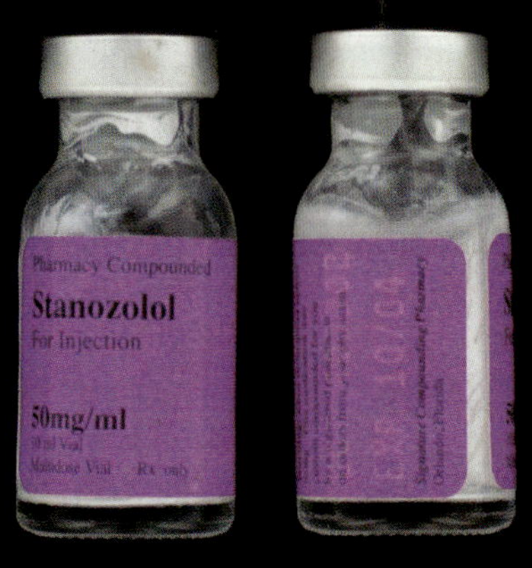

U.S. private -label generic

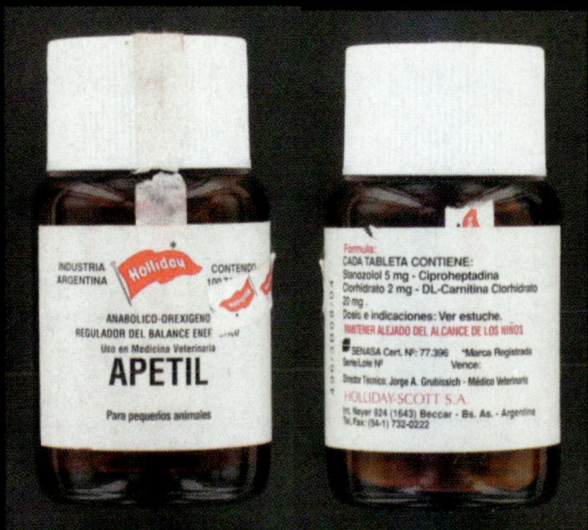

Counterfeit Apetil

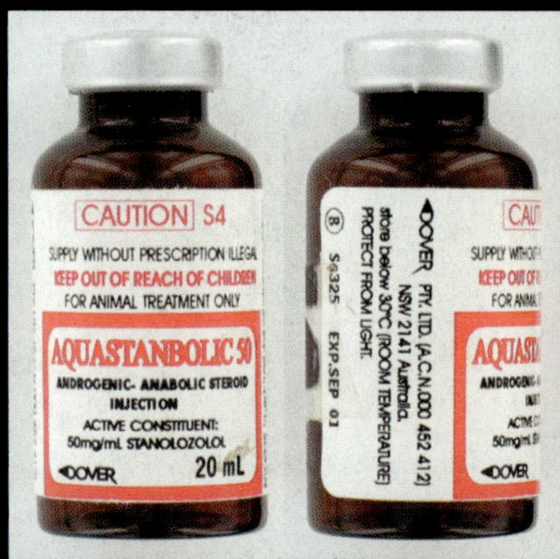

Bogus Aquastanbolic

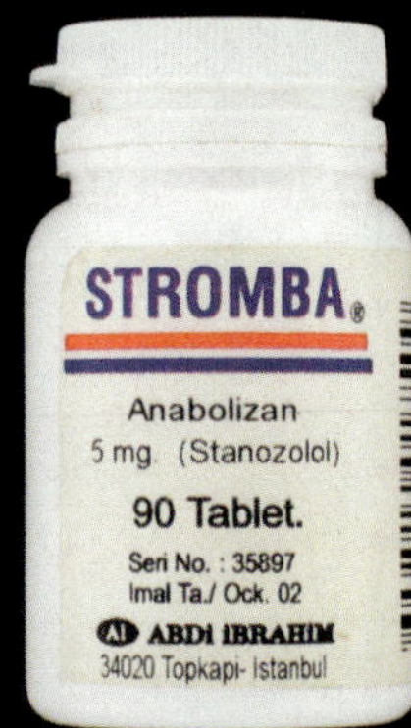

Fake Stromba

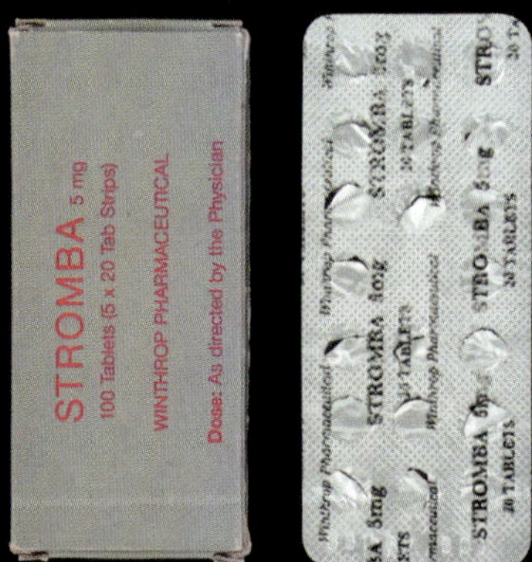

Fake Stromba Tablets

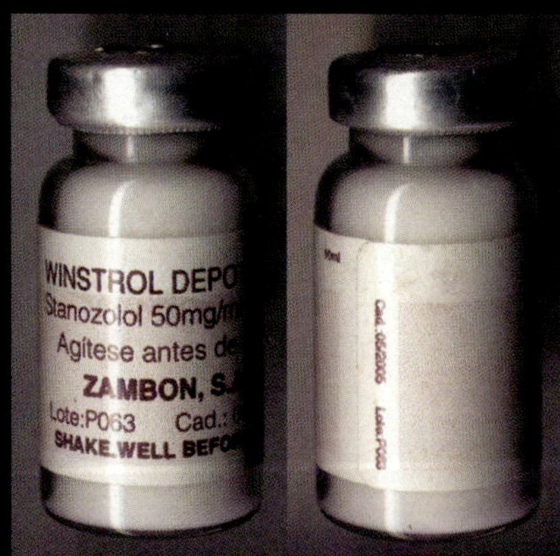

Counterfeit Italian Winstrol

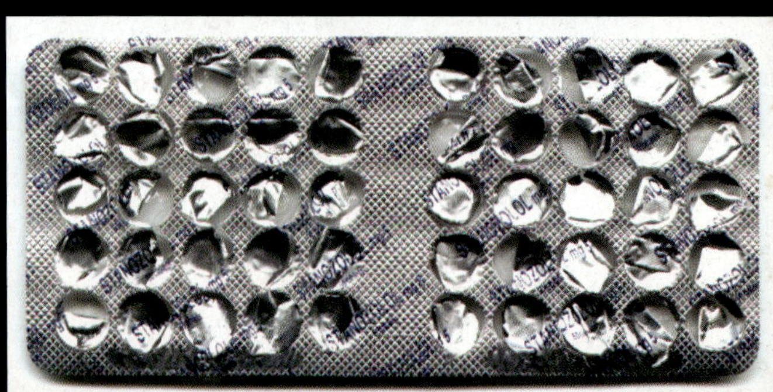

FREE ANABOLICS 2006!

Do you have an empty steroid box, vial, ampule, bottle, or tablet strip you don't see in ANABOLICS 2005? Send it to William Llewellyn at the address below. If he uses your sample, your copy of **ANABOLICS 2006** is **ABSOLUTELY FREE!**

ANABOLICS has become THE "standard-issue" global resource on performance-enhancing drugs because athletes know the information inside is the most recent and reliable! No other book of its type has ever been so comprehensive and up-to-date. The information in the latest update was aided in part by the efforts of readers all over the world, who share in William Llewellyn's thirst for knowledge. Bill receives thousands of letters every year containing empty steroid packaging samples for him to examine. This global web of supporters has helped make ANABOLICS the invaluable resource it is today. As a special thanks for the help, Llewellyn will send a free copy of the next book to anyone that submits an empty steroid packaging sample that he doesn't have. It helps other readers get the most current info, and helps you get your next copy **FIRST AND FREE**!

Send your CLEAN and EMPTY boxes, vials, or ampules to:

William Llewellyn
c/o Body of Science
5500 Military Trail
Ste. 22-318
Jupiter, FL 33458

Cleaning and Mailing Instructions:

Ampules/Vials: Empty contents completely. Flush with rubbing alcohol or water, if necessary, to remove residue. Mail all glass items in a box for protection.

Remember, EMPTY packaging samples only. Privacy protected.

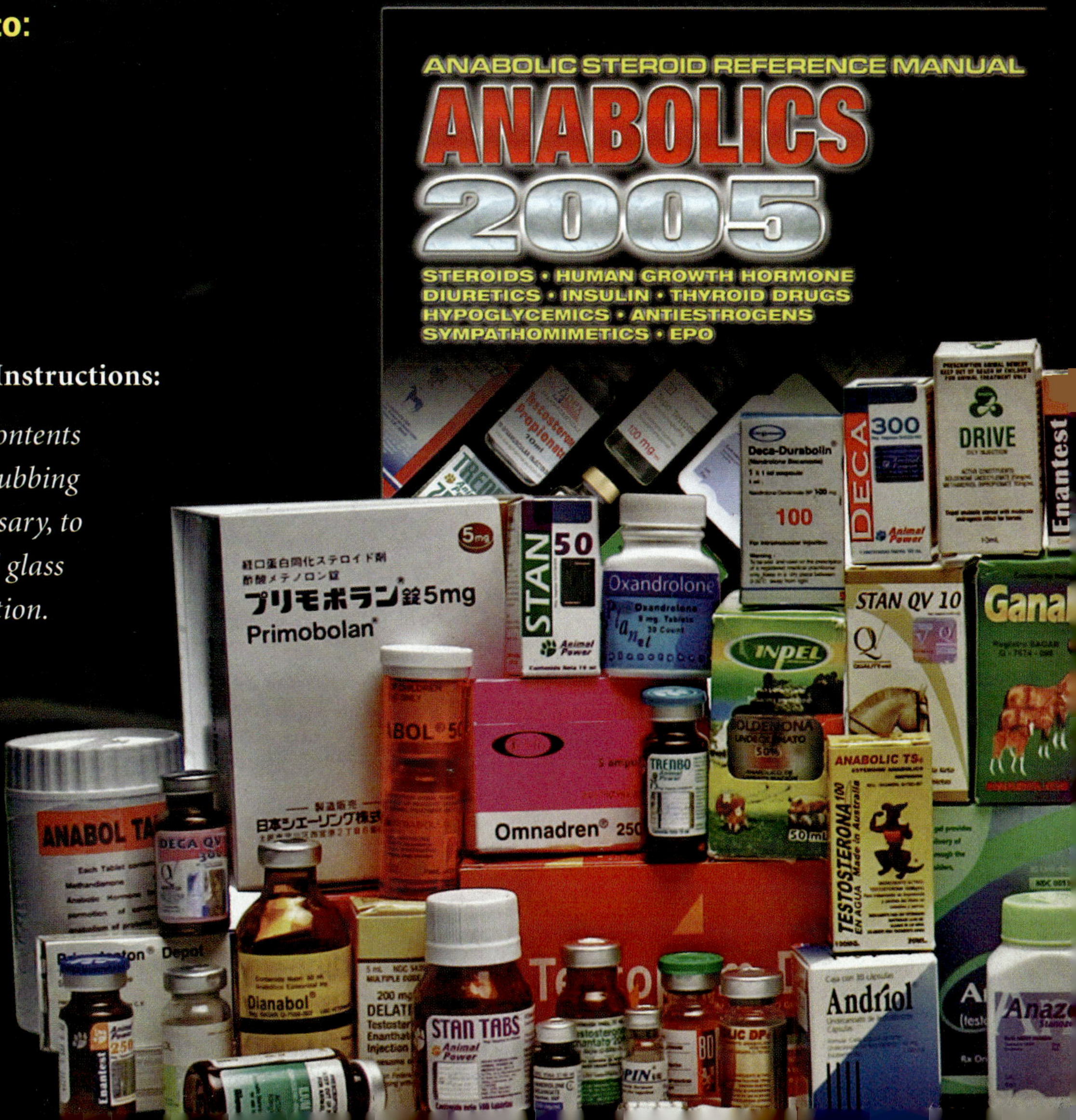

Drug Security Stickers

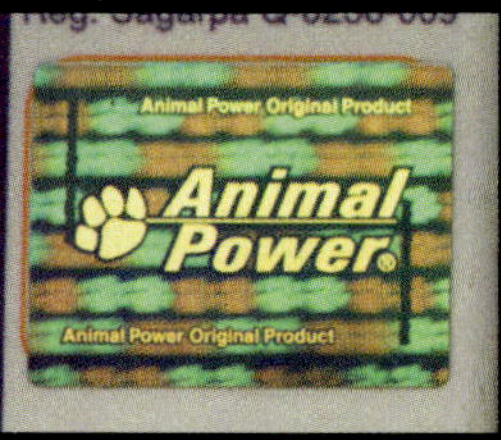

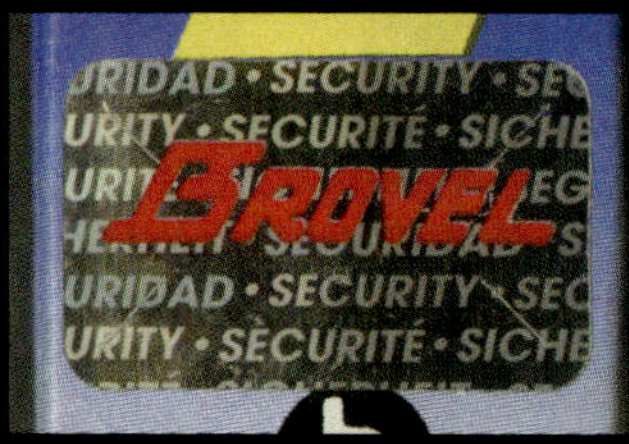

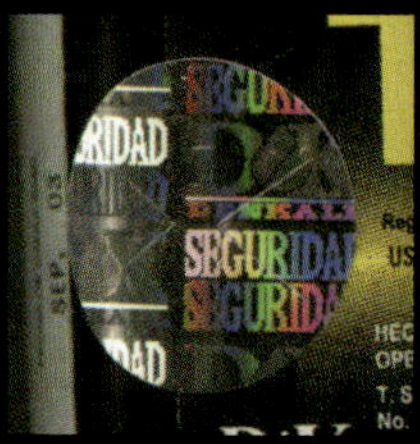

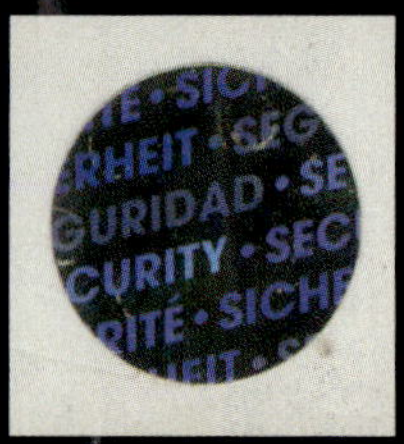

Animal Power (Mexico) Brovel (Mexico) Denkall (Mexico) Loeffler (Mexico)

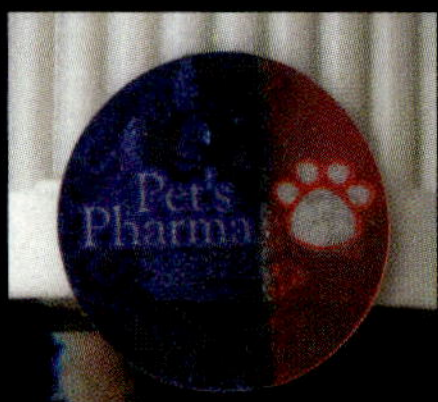

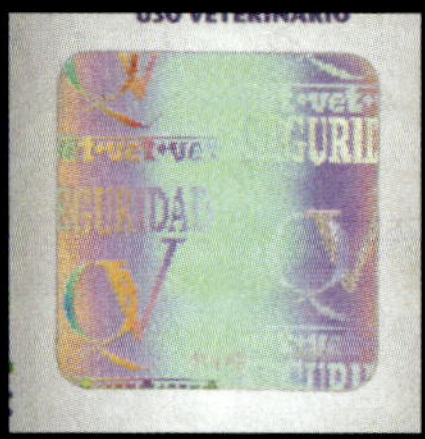

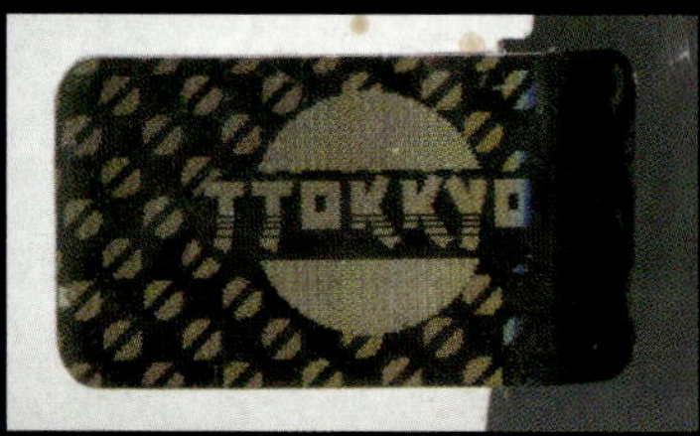

Pet's Pharma (Mexico) Quality Vet (Mexico) Ttokkyo (Mexico)

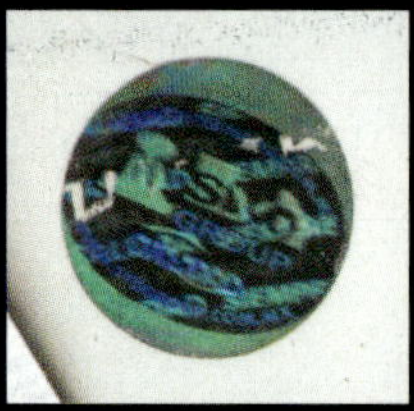

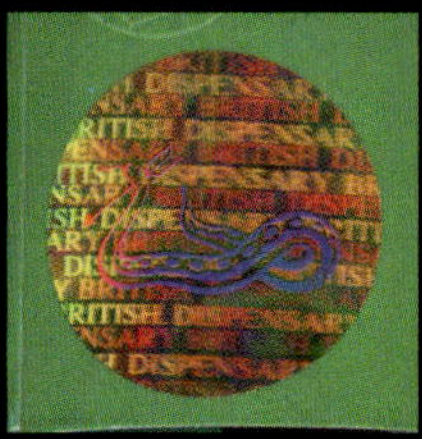

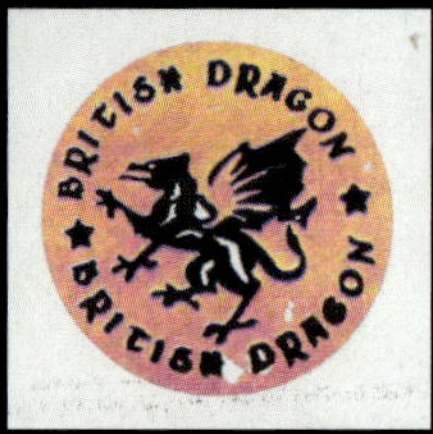

SYD Group (Mexico) British Dispensary (Thailand) British Dragon (Thailand)

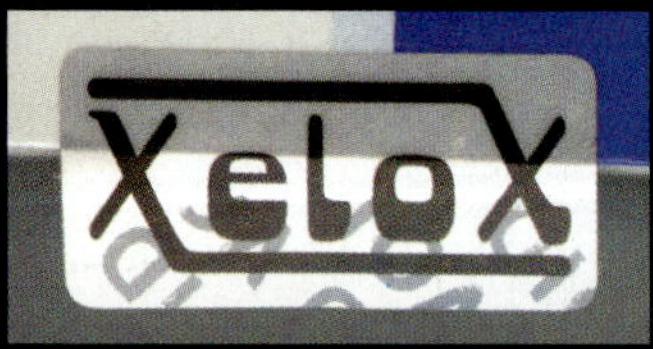

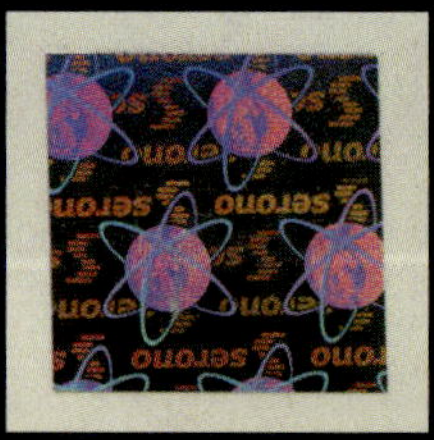

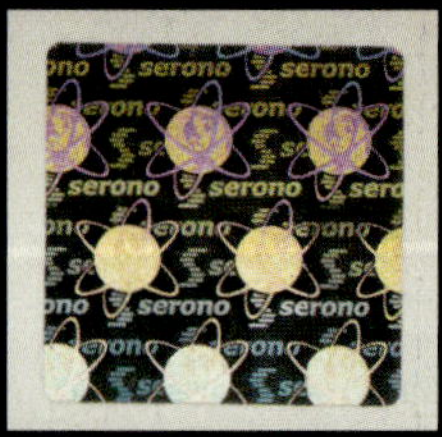

Xelox (Philippines) New Serono (U.S.) Old Serono (U.S.)

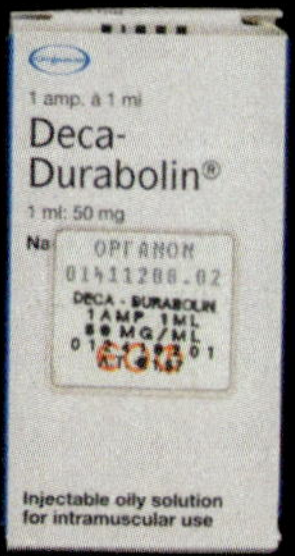

Under UV light:

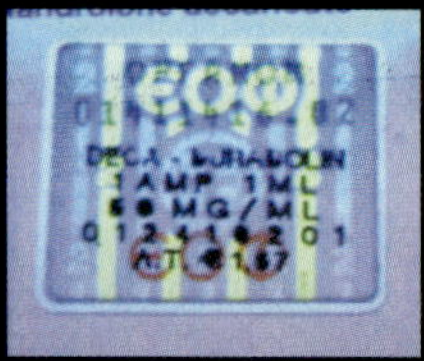

Greek Sticker (normal) (2001) (2002) (2003) (2004)